HIV AND AIDS – UPDATES ON BIOLOGY, IMMUNOLOGY, EPIDEMIOLOGY AND TREATMENT STRATEGIES

Edited by **Nancy Dumais**

HIV and AIDS – Updates on Biology, Immunology, Epidemiology and Treatment Strategies
Edited by Nancy Dumais

Published by InTech

Janeza Trdine 9, 51000 Rijeka, Croatia

Publishing Process Manager Alenka Urbancic

Technical Editor Teodora Smiljanic

Cover Designer InTech Design Team

Additional hard copies can be obtained from orders@intechopen.com

HIV and AIDS – Updates on Biology, Immunology,
Epidemiology and Treatment Strategies, Edited by Nancy Dumais
p. cm.
978-953-307-665-2

For EU product safety concerns:
IN TECH d.o.o., Prolaz Marije Krucifikse Kozulić 3, 51000 Rijeka, Croatia,
info@intechopen.com or visit our website at intechopen.com.

Meet the editor

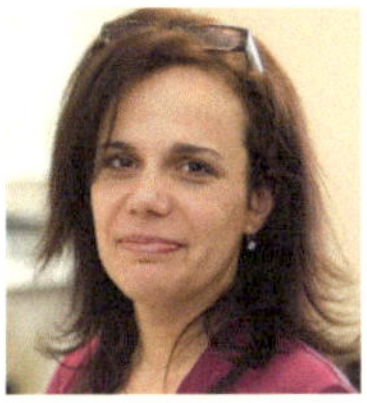

Dr. Nancy Dumais is a Professor of Virology at Université de Sherbrooke, Canada. She received her Diploma (M.Sc.) in Cellular and Molecular Biology and her Doctorate (Ph.D.) in Virology, in 1996 and 2001, respectively, both from Université Laval in Canada. Then, she was a Postdoctoral Researcher at McMaster University where she studied mucosal immunization against HIV. Her research interests include chemokines and chemokines receptors in HIV-1 pathogenesis. Her laboratory also investigates the roles of prostaglandins in HIV transcription and replication. In addition, she is interested in scientific and health education.

Contents

Preface

The ongoing research efforts that started even before our recognition of the HIV/AIDS syndrome and identification of HIV as the causative agent have made important inroads into our knowledge and understanding of this terrible disease. Nevertheless, the continuing AIDS pandemic and profound human and socio-economic impacts remind us that despite the unrelenting quest for knowledge since the early 1980s, we have much to learn about HIV and AIDS. Moreover, the copious amount of research performed on HIV and AIDS requires comprehensive overviews on this subject in order to provide clues and opportunities for future research. With this in mind, the purpose of this book is to aid clinicians, provide a source of inspiration for researchers, and serve as a guide for graduate and medical students in their continued search for an understanding and finally, a cure of HIV.

This volume has four sections grouped in two parts. The first part, "From the laboratory to the clinic," and the second part, "From the clinic to the patients," represent the unique but intertwined mission of this work: to provide basic and clinical knowledge on HIV/AIDS. The first two sections describe how basic research generates knowledge that impacts clinical practices. The first section details the multifaceted interactions that occur between HIV and host cells. Functions of the accessory protein Nef during the lentivirus replication cycle are reviewed in Chapter 1. Chapter 2 explains how HIV-1 proteins and therapeutic antiretroviral drugs cause oxidative stress-induced cardiovascular disease and neurological disorders. Chapter 3 is a comprehensive update on the prevalence of multiple HIV-1 subtypes, and how this influences pathogenesis, evasion on the immune system, and vaccine development. Insulin-like growth factor (IGF) levels are closely monitored in HIV/AIDS patients and help track the progression of the disease and Chapter 4 provides structural information on IGF and explains how understanding the IGF system may be useful for developing potent therapeutics. The information of Chapters 5 and 6 is presented to better understand the interactions between HIV and cellular proteins and the development of intrinsic immunity. These chapters discuss how host proteins are capable of inhibiting HIV-1 replication. These host proteins, termed cellular restriction factors, are a new and important research area that may provide new avenues for AIDS therapies.

The second section focuses on the relationship between HIV and the immune system. Continued study of the persistent HIV animal reservoir may provide insight into new vaccine strategies or therapeutic approaches for the treatment of HIV-infected humans. This very important area of HIV research is reviewed in Chapter 7. Chapters 8 and 9 approach some fundamental principles behind the design and development of effective vaccines and/or immunotherapies. These chapters are followed by a series of chapters (Chapter 10 to Chapter 13) that provide information on the role of cytokines, chemokines, and prostaglandins in HIV infection and pathogenesis.

The second part of this book is a compendium of chapters dedicated to AIDS and HIV epidemiology and clinical research. The third section entitled "HIV/AIDS and clinical manifestations" describes clinical manifestations of HIV/AIDS. Postmortem examinations provide important diagnostic and epidemiological data on the myriad diseases associated with HIV infection. Chapter 14 presents data from post-mortem surveillance from 1982 to 2011 showing differences in HIV epidemiology in Africa, Asia, the U.S., and Europe. Chapter 15 discusses the epidemiology, frequency, risk factors, clinical management, and treatment of HIV-infected lung cancer patients. Neuropsychiatric manifestations of HIV infection and AIDS are presented in Chapter 16. Chapter 17 presents information related to the treatment of HIV/AIDS patients in trauma units, an area of study that has been neglected. The aim of Chapter 18 is to highlight common cutaneous manifestations of HIV/AIDS in sub-Sahara Africa. Chapter 19 explores a number of the many possible HIV/AIDS associated disorders of the lymphoid system. Chapter 20 investigates the etiologic factors involved in the sexual dysfunctions of HIV/AIDS patients, proposes steps for assessment and diagnosis, and recommends therapeutic strategies for these patients. Chapter 21 explores consequences of condomization of women's sexuality on female diseases and dysfunctions. Several aspects of two devastating epidemics, breast cancer and AIDS, are discussed in this chapter.

The final set of chapters presented in the fourth section offers scientific data on epidemiology, transmission, diagnosis, and therapies for HIV. Lack of education increases the risk of HIV transmission and Chapter 22 gives strategies to better understand transmission of HIV through blood. Chapter 23 focuses on molecular epidemiology of HIV-1 infection in the Amazon region, while Chapter 24 presents data on HIV/AIDS in Nigeria. Methods for saliva testing for HIV screening are described in Chapter 25. In Chapter 26 examines paediatric HIV infection risk factors, causes of death, and the impact of HAART in HIV-1 infected children. The effect of nutritional status among persons with HIV and drug addictions is explored in Chapter 27. Chapter 28 reviews the influence of cannabinoids on the immune system and their potential use in supplementary therapy for HIV/AIDS, as well as the importance of food and nutrition security in the mitigation of HIV/AIDS in sub-Saharan Africa.

We are grateful to all the authors and researchers who contribute to the writing and content of this book on HIV/AIDS research. Their willingness to participate in this endeavour was fuelled by an unprecedented enthusiasm and I am privileged to be the editor of such a meaningful book. This book captures and describes in clear detail many aspects of basic and clinical research on HIV/AIDS, which is one of the most profound worldwide devastating diseases of our time.

Nancy Dumais
Département Biologie, Faculté des Sciences,
Université de Sherbrooke, Québec
Canada

Part 1

From the Laboratory to the Clinic: HIV and Cellular Interactions

1

Functions of the Lentiviral Accessory Protein Nef During the Distinct Steps of HIV and SIV Replication Cycle

Luciana J. Costa, Luiza M. Mendonça and Thatiane L. Sampaio
Departamento de Virologia, Instituto de Microbiologia Paulo de Góes, Universidade Federal do Rio de Janeiro
Brazil

1. Introduction

Human and Simian Immunodeficiency Viruses (HIV and SIV) are the etiological agents of the Acquired Immunodeficiency Syndrome (AIDS) in humans and the Simian AIDS (SAIDS) in macaques, respectively. HIVs and SIVs are members of the *Retroviridae* family, Lentivirus genera, and are considered complex retroviruses since its genome organization predicts the presence of at least 6 open reading frames (ORFs) in addition to the main Gag, Pol and Env ORFs present in the genomes of all retroviruses. These additional ORFs code for both regulatory (Tat and Rev) and accessory (Nef, Vif, Vpr, Vpu and Vpx) viral proteins and are all organized from the 5′ half of the genome in a way that overlap both with each other and with the Pol and Env ORFs and the non-coding 3′ Long Terminal Repeat (LTR) region (Figure 1). To ensure its expression and to achieve an optimal production of the viral progeny, complex mechanisms have evolved in these viruses that tightly control the expression of these ORFs during the viral replication cycle. The existence of such a number of viral proteins in addition to the viral structural (Gag and Env) and enzymatic (Pol) proteins allows the virus to explore new mechanisms to control the different steps of the replication cycle and to avoid the host cell defense. In this chapter we shall review the different steps of the HIV and SIV replication cycle with emphasis in the role taken by the viral accessory protein Nef, in both subverting the host cell machinery and influencing the function and activation of viral structural and enzymatic proteins in order to optimize viral progeny production as well as in evading the host cell defenses.

Lentiviral accessory proteins Vif, Vpr, Vpu and Nef were classically regarded as non-essential for virus production and/or infectivity since laboratory adapted HIV strains lacking the expression of these proteins could still replicate to several levels (Adachi et al., 1991). Since then, several studies demonstrated the crucial importance of these proteins to the efficient replication, infectivity and spread of both HIV and SIV (Kirchhoff, 2010).

Vif (Aguiar and Peterlin, 2008) and Vpu (Adachi et al., 1991) have now been acknowledged as crucial viral factors that counteract the host cell innate defense. Vif interacts and prompts the degradation of a family of cytidine deaminases DNA/RNA editing enzymes, known as Apoliprotein B mRNA-editing Enzymes (APOBECs), that otherwise would inhibit HIV and SIV replication by causing hypermutation of nascent retroviral genomes by deamination of cytidine residues (Aguiar and Peterlin, 2008). Vpu is a type-1 membrane associated protein that was first demonstrated to be involved in the downmodulation of the Cluster of Differentiation Antigen 4 (CD4) receptor from the infected cell surface by a mechanism of inducing the proteassomal degradation of the newly synthesized CD4 molecules in the Endoplasmic Reticulum (ER) (Schubert et al., 1998; Willey et al., 1992). Expression of Vpu is restricted to HIV-1 and a subset of SIV linages related to HIV-1. In HIV-2 and the related SIV*sooty mangabey* (SIVsm) linage, which lack the *vpu* gene, the cytoplasmic domain of the viral envelope protein gp41 mimicks this function of Vpu (Bour et al., 1996). For a long time it was considered to be the mechanism by which Vpu lead to an increase in HIV infectivity. Recently, however, it was demonstrated that Vpu in HIV-1 and related SIVs increases viral particle release from the infected cells by removing an Interferon-regulated protein (BST-2 or Theterin) from the surface of the infected cells, that otherwise would function as a host restriction factor inhibiting viral release (Neil et al., 2006; Neil et al., 2007; Neil et al., 2008).

Nef, the misnamed Negative Factor, is a myristoylated 27-35 kDa protein encoded at the far 3'end of the primate lentiviral genome (Figure 1). Nef is post-translationally modified by the addition of a myristic acid at glycine residue at amino acid position 2 (G2) on the N-terminal of the protein. This modification is required for the association of Nef to cellular membranes. Another post-translational modification in Nef is its cleavage by the virally encoded Protease (PR), which will be discussed further. The terciary structure of the Nef protein predicts an anchor domain encompassing the first 57 amino acids from the N-terminal, a highly structured central core domain encompassing amino acid residues 58-147, and a unstructures flexible C-terminal domain encompassing amino acid residues 148-180 which is commonly named C-terminal flexible-loop (Geyer et al., 2001)

Nef was first described as a negative regulator of the HIV-1 replication since in the absence of its expression levels of transcription from the viral LTR and viral replication were reported to be higher than in cells infected with the Nef positive virus counterpart (Ahmad and Venkatesan, 1988; Cheng-Mayer et al., 1989). Soon it was demonstrated that in fact the absence of Nef expression has a negative effect for virus spread in HIV-1-infected CD4 (+) cell cultures (Cheng-Mayer et al., 1989; Hammes et al., 1989; Kim et al., 1989; Lama et al., 1999; Ross et al., 1999). Moreover, evidences accumulated that the lack of Nef expression even in CD4 (-) cell cultures leads to reduction in the infectivity of the viral progeny (Chowers et al., 1995; Goldsmith et al., 1995). The effect of the Nef protein in virus infectivity is direct and specific since it can be rescued by providing Nef in *trans* to the virus producer cell (Miller et al., 1995; Pandori et al., 1996). The increase in virus infectivity by Nef is well-conserved amonsgst alleles from both HIVs and SIVs and can vary from 4-40-fold increase depending on the *nef* allele and the cell system being assayed. Nowdays, the increase in viral infectivity by Nef is the only consensus phenotype recognized for this primate lentiviral accessory protein.

The definitive proof of the crucial importance of Nef for HIV and SIV infections came from studies demonstrating that the disruption or the absence of the *nef* gene in both viruses was related to a slower or non-progression to AIDS in naturally infected humans and experimentally infected rhesus macaques, respectively (Daniel et al., 1992; Deacon et al., 1995; Kirchhoff et al., 1995). It was clearly demonstrated in these studies that in the absence of Nef expression infection with these viruses failed to mantain high levels of viremia and to progress to AIDS, defining Nef as a key factor for the pathogenesis of primate lentiviruses.

As soon as it was demonstrated that Nef has an important role for HIV and SIV infections several studies were conducted to ellucidate the mechanism by which this protein influences viral replication. The several functions described for Nef in the last two decades are reviewed in the sections bellow.

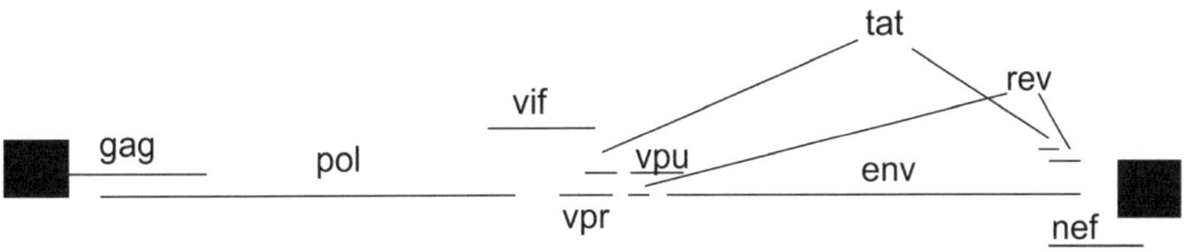

Fig. 1. Representative genomic organization of the provirus of the primate lentiviruses. The main (*gag, pol and env*); regulatory (*tat and rev*); and accessory (*vif, vpr, vpu and nef*) ORFs are represented by horizontal lines. The black squares represent the LTRs present at the 5′and 3′ extremities of the genome. The two exons of tat and rev are conected by angled lines. Note the extensive overlap of the structural, regulatory and accessory ORFs from the 3′half of the genome.

2. The classical functions of the HIV and SIV Nef proteins

2.1 Downmodulation of CD4 and MHC-I

The Nef protein from HIV and SIV have multiple functions and achieve its biochemical effects upon interactions with cellular components. Over thirty putative Nef targets have already been described. One of the first proteins that have been found associated with Nef is the human transmembrane CD4, which is downregulated from the cell surface by Nef (Garcia and Miller, 1991). Moreover, Nef also down-regulates other cell-surface proteins, as the major histocompatibility complex class I (MHC-I) molecules (Greenberg et al., 1998b; Swigut et al., 2000).

Observations from naturally HIV-1-infected individuals indicated that Nef functions on downmodulation of CD4 and MHC-I could be related to the pathogenesis of AIDS (Carl et al., 2001; Tobiume et al., 2002), however the real contribution of these functions still needs to be demonstrated (Crotti et al., 2006). The motifs in Nef that mediate CD4 downregulation were considered critical for SIVmac replication in rhesus macaques, however MHC-I downregulation by Nef is not sufficient for optimal virulence of SIVmac early in infection (Iafrate et al., 2000; Lang et al., 1997; Schindler et al., 2004). Moreover, the solely importance of the CD4 downmodulation for SIVmac pathogenesis in experimental models has been challenged (Jesus da Costa et al., 2009). The mechanisms by which Nef interferes with CD4 and MHC-I expression are described below.

CD4 is a type I integral membrane glycoprotein expressed primarily on T cells, thymocytes, and cells of the macrophage-monocyte lineage (Littman, 1987). CD4 is required for T-cell activation by the TCR signaling pathway and serves as the primary receptor for HIV and SIV. However, its continuous presence on the surface of HIV/SIV infected cell after viral entry is problematic for several reasons. First, because of their capacity to form complexes, co-expression of CD4 and the viral envelope protein gp120 disrupts the trafficking of both proteins (Lama et al., 1999; Ross et al., 1999). In addition, the presence of CD4 on the cell membrane reduces the ability of the newly formed particles to be properly released from the infected cell therefore reducing viral infectivity (Cortes et al., 2002; Lama et al., 1999). Finally, decreasing the number of viral receptors on the surface of an infected cell seems to prevent reinfection by HIV/SIV particles (the so-called superinfection) (Le Guern and Levy, 1992; Michel et al., 2005).

Nef reduces the steady-state levels of CD4 by several proposed models based on a premise: Nef binds to the cytoplasmatic tail and promotes the endocytosis of CD4 from the cell surface, which in turn results in CD4 degradation in lysosomes. Thus myristoylation of Nef, which is necessary for its membrane localization, is crucial for the downmodulation of CD4 (Bentham et al., 2003). For binding, a cluster of residues in the N-terminal half of HIV-1 Nef recognizes a dileucine motif within the cytoplasmatic tail of CD4 (Leu-413-414) exposed only when the serine residues in CD4 are phosphorylated (Aiken et al., 1994; Bentham et al., 2003; Pitcher et al., 1999). Subsequently, Nef acts as connector between mature CD4 and components of clathrin-dependent trafficking pathways at the cell surface (and to a lesser degree in the Golgi apparatus). For this purpose, Nef bridges the CD4 cytoplasmic tail with the adaptor protein complex of endosomal clathrin-coated pits (CCPs), thereby triggering the formation of CD4-specific endocytic vesicles, and the catalytic unit of the vacuolar proton pump v-ATPase (Bresnahan et al., 1998; Foti et al., 1997; Lu et al., 1998; Mandic et al., 2001; Mangasarian et al., 1997; Piguet et al., 1998). Furthermore, to target CD4 for lysosomal degradation Nef connects the receptor with the β subunit of the COP-I coatomer in endosomes, diverting Nef-bound CD4 molecules from a recycling to a degradation pathway (Piguet et al., 1999).

Another conserved function of Nef across HIV/SIV is the disruption of the transport of MHC-I to the cell surface in infected T cells to avoid immune recognition by cytotoxic T lymphocytes (CTLs) (Greenberg et al., 1998b; Swigut et al., 2000). The pathway is initiated by Nef binding to the phosphorin acidic cluster sorting protein-2 (PACS-2), which controls the endosome-to-Golgi trafficking of cytosolic sorting proteins, then targeting Nef and its cargo to the perinuclear region to bind and activate Scr family kinase (SFK). This Nef-SFK complex then phosphorylates ZAP-70 (Syk in monocytes and heterologous cells) on tyrosine, enabling ZAP-70-SFK complex to bind the SH2 domain of Phosphatidyl Inositol 3 Kinase (PI3K) (Swann et al., 2001). MHC-I is constitutively internalized and recycled via a GTPase ADP ribosylation factor 6 (ARF6) pathway. This multi-kinase complex triggers internalization of cell-surface MHC-I through a clathrin-independent, ARF6-dependent pathway, which connects vesicle trafficking with actin cytoskeletal rearrangement (Atkins et al., 2008; Blagoveshchenskaya et al., 2002; Hung et al., 2007).

Other authors showed evidence that Nef acts early in the secretory pathway to redirect MHC-I from the trans-Golgi network (TGN) to the endolysosomal pathway known as anteretrograde trafficking. Nef directs the MHC-I into the trans-Golgi compartment through association with clathrin adaptor protein complex (AP-1), thereby sorting these proteins into specific clathrin-coated transport vesicles addressed to the endolysosomal pathway (Greenberg et al., 1998b), moreover MHC-I molecules in the trans-Golgi are probably targeted for degradation. Consistent with this model, RNA interference (RNAi) against AP-1 blocks Nef-mediated disruption of MHC-1. AP-1 was also demonstrated to co-precipitate with MHC-I and Nef in HIV-infected primary T cells (Roeth et al., 2004). Therefore, Nef binds to the MHC-I and stabilizes the interaction of a tyrosine in the cytoplasmic tail of MHC-I with the natural tyrosine-binding pocket in AP-1 (Wonderlich et al., 2008). Nef targets early types of MHC-I molecules in the ER by preferentially binding hypophosphorylated cytoplasmic tails, thus preventing completion of the secretory pathway that would finally provide an antigen-presenting receptor on the cell surface to activate killing of the virus-infected cell (Kasper et al., 2005).

These models may not be mutually exclusive, a recent work shows that Nef simultaneously uses both antiretrograde and retrograde trafficking to down-regulate human leukocyte antigen class I (HLA-I) in the peripheral blood mononuclear cells and HeLa cells (Yi et al., 2010). Besides, another report used a small molecule to disrupt Nef-SFK binding and found that Nef orchestrates a highly regulated molecular program consisting of sequential use of signaling followed by stoichiometric modes to evade immune surveillance (Dikeakos et al., 2010).

Human MHC-I main function is to regulate the development of an immune response. HLA-I genes include HLA-A, B, and C (Tripathi and Agrawal, 2007) and its removal from the cell surface increases the potential susceptibility of infected cells to elimination by natural killer cells (NK). Nef downregulates highly polymorphic HLA-A and -B molecules as a mechanism of HIV-1 immune evasion, but not HLA-C or -E molecules which frequently serve as ligands to inhibit the activation of NK cells (Lanier, 2005). This selection is broadly conserved between SIV (smm/mac) and HIV-2 Nef alleles (DeGottardi et al., 2008). Moreover, differences in HLA downmodulation by Nef are based on amino acid modifications in HLA cytoplasmic domains, which implies that diverse properties of Nef are required to achieve the simultaneous evasion of the CTL and natural killer cell surveillance by HIV (DeGottardi et al., 2008; Lanier, 2005).

Nef is sufficiently adaptable to maintain downregulation of MHC-I and CD4 as a two independent functions and neither activity is optimized by the transmission event, despite the changing in immune pressure associated with sexual transmission (Noviello et al., 2007). In conclusion, the dramatic reduction of CD4 and MHCI expression in infected cells achieved by Nef seems to be in some degree important for the successful establishment of infection in a new host.

2.2 Downmodulation of MHC-II

In many ways Nef act in order to disrupt immune communication. Besides downmodulating MHC-I, CD80 and CD86, (Chaudhry et al., 2005; Greenberg et al., 1998a), Nef also interfere with MHC-II surface expression. However, for this surface marker, downmodulation is achieved by many mechanisms: i) Nef causes endocytosis of mature peptide-loaded MHC-II from the cell surface; ii) Nef can induce accumulation of immature MHC-II associated with the invariant chain (Ii) on the cell surface; iii) Nef reduces the rate of MHC-II delivery to the cell surface (Chaudhry et al., 2009; Stumptner-Cuvelette et al., 2001).

MHC-II depends extensively on the endocytic machinery in order to be properly mounted on the cell surface. After its translocation to the endoplasmatic reticulum a mechanism is needed in order to prevent association with its own peptides. This is achieved by MHC-II association with the Ii, which blocks the MHC-II peptide cleft, forming the immature MHC-II complex. This immature MHC-II complex exits the ER and move through the Golgi apparatus. Finally, vesicles containing immature MHC-II fuse to MIIC vesicles, a specialized MHC-II peptide-loading compartment containing all the components needed to Ii degradation and foreign peptide loading onto the MHC-II cleft. The mature MHC-II is then directed to the cell membrane where interaction with the TCR of a CD4+ cell can happen. A fraction of immature MHC-II travels to the plasma membrane and is subsequently internalized and directed to MIIC vesicles. A similar endocytosis mechanism was described to recycle mature MHC-II from the cell surface (Reid and Watts, 1992).

Nef selectively distinguishes between mature and immature MHC-II. While induces a two-fold reduction of peptide-loaded MHC-II from the cell surface, Nef induces a 15-fold more accumulation of immature MHC-II complexes composed of Ii, alpha and beta MHC-II chains. The motifs in Nef needed for one function or another are different. While for mature MHC-II endocytosis, the acidic motif EEEE65 is important, for upregulation of immature MHC-II WL57,58 motif is required. For both of them the poliproline (PxxP) and dileucine (LL164) motifs in Nef are required. The amount of Nef needed also vary depending on the phenomena. It was observed in transient expression experiments that even small quantities of Nef were enough for Ii upregulation, while for MHC-II downmodulation high expression of Nef was required. Of note, those high levels of Nef expression were considered physiologically relevant, as experiments using HIV infected cells showed quantities of Nef similar to that seen on super expression experiments (Stumptner-Cuvelette et al., 2001).

Nef also acts slowing the delivery rate of newly synthesized MHC-II molecules to the plasma membrane, however this molecular mechanism is less explored (Chaudhry et al., 2009).

Loss of cell surface MHC-II induced by Nef is observed during HIV-1 host cell infection. In the presence of Nef, mature MHC-II are found at high levels in intracellular lysossomal compartments, marked with Lamp-1, while delivery of immature MHC-II to the endolysossomal compartment is impaired. MHC-II Nef-mediated endocytosis was described as dependent on Rab5, Lyst, cholesterol and Phosphatidyl Inositol Kinases, and dispenses Dynamin 2 (Dyn2) (Chaudhry et al., 2009).

This downmodulation of mature and upregulation of immature MHC-II is a function conserved in many *nef* alleles from HIV-1/2 and SIVs. Contrary to what is seen in MHCI downmodulation, Nef activity on MHC-II and Ii do not change significantly during the stages of infection. Of note, the strong Ii upregulation observed in the presence of wild type Nef is lost in some *nef* alleles derived from Long-term infected HIV-1 patients which do not progress to AIDS, suggesting that this feature of Nef may contribute to immune evasion (Schindler et al., 2003).

Although Nef has been described to directly bind to the citoplasmatic tail of many receptors that it modulates (Chaudhry et al., 2005), there is still no evidence that it can bind MHC-II, suggesting that Nef might interact with proteins involved in the physiological turnover pathways of this surface marker, disrupting the natural balance of MHC-II surface expression. The model postulates that recycling MHC-II enters sorting endossomes for a decision on whether they will be recycled back to surface or not, which is where Nef intervene and reroute them to the Golgi apparatus. This model takes advantage of the observation that mature MHC-II is short-lived on the cell surface and thus, Nef subversive action on the endocytic program responsible for the removal of MHC-II is plausible (Chaudhry et al., 2009).

Another model has been proposed for Ii upregulation. In this simpler model, Nef would increase Ii surface expression by competing for the endocytic machinery. More specifically, the dileucine motif in Nef would tritate AP-2, the adaptor protein responsible for Ii endocytosis (Mitchell et al., 2008). Although elegant, this model encounters some conflicting data, showing that a small amount of Nef is able to induce strong accumulation of Ii. Also, other receptors that depend on AP-2 for its endocytosis, such as the Transferrin receptor, are not upregulated by Nef (Schindler et al., 2003). Nevertheless, this could be another mechanism used for Ii upregulation and still cannot be discarded.

2.3 Cellular activation by Nef

It is now clear that Nef is capable of mimicking transcriptional programs in order to manipulate the cell activation status in a way that favors HIV pathogenesis in a myriad of ways. The Nef protein can deliver antiapoptotic signals to the infected cells in order to sustain a prolonged infection, create a viral reservoir, or increase the number of permissive cells for viral infection (Mahlknecht et al., 2000). In a contrary fashion, it can stimulate apoptosis in bystander CD8+ T lymphocytes to evade immune response (Xu et al., 1999). In any case, the cell reprogramming induced by Nef is not only limited to manipulation of apoptosis. It also includes the activation or suppression of cell signaling pathways (Mahlknecht et al., 2000; Mangino et al., 2007; Percario et al., 2003; Varin et al., 2003).

Although the effects of Nef sometimes seem contradictory it must be stressed out that its functions are the product of many protein-protein interactions that can take place during different steps of the viral replication cycle in the infected cell and are subjected to Nef cellular trafficking and conformational status. As a myristoylated protein, Nef is addressed to cellular membranes. However, it has been shown that less than 50% of the protein locates at this site, and that the majority of Nef is cytossolic (Fackler et al., 1997; Kaminchik et al., 1994; Niederman et al., 1993; Welker et al., 1998). After membrane targeting, Nef is rapidly internalized though interaction of its C-terminal flexible loop and cell proteins involved in the endocytic pathways. It has been shown that while Nef is in its membrane-bound form it appears more compactly folded, suggesting that membrane-bound and cytossolic Nef shown distinct accessible interaction domains (Breuer et al., 2006), which could explain the distinct phenotypes of Nef. Nef's ability to dimerize or even oligomerize can also function as a mechanism of regulating Nef's effects (Breuer et al., 2006; Dennis et al., 2005).

Exogenous Nef have been shown to enter monocytes/macrophages, B cells and Dendritic Cells (DC) by adsorptive endocytosis. Nef also binds to the surface of T cells, but is not internalized by this cell type. No specific receptor to this protein has yet been identified (Alessandrini et al., 2000). The finding that Nef is found in sera of HIV+ positive subjects in a concentration of 10ng/ml show that this protein is somehow secreted and that this event should have a role in pathogenesis. It is assumed that this concentration could be even higher in lymphnodes or other sites where virus-producing and target cells are tightly packaged (Fujii et al., 1996). Until now no mechanism by which Nef is secreted from cells have been identified. However, since it is involved in cellular trafficking and the biogenesis of the Multi-Vesicular Bodies (MVBs), it is possible that Nef is packaged in some of these vesicles that are later exocyted from the cell. Uninfected cells could internalize Nef by endocytosis, pinocytosis or other unknown mechanisms. Exogenous Nef recapitulates in part the effects described for endogenous produced Nef (Quaranta et al., 2006; Varin et al., 2003). Still, some divergences appear, as some evidences showing that Nef can have distinct effects on an infected or uninfected cell (as the stimulation of apoptotic or non apoptotic status). Thus, Nef's delivering route is also a determining factor of the phenotype modulated by Nef. Therefore, Nef fits the Trojan horse hypothesis, which suggests that the virus take advantage of the deliberate secretion of highly immunogenic virions proteins, not packaged into viral particles, capable of modulating phenotypes on nearby cells, favoring HIV infection (Gould et al., 2003).

Nef activates many cells types to, ultimately, activate CD4+ T cells (and also activates the CD4+ T cell itself). The effect of Nef on cellular activation has been described in DCs, B cells, and macrophages, all cell types known to activate CD4+ T cells (Mahlknecht et al., 2000;

Quaranta et al., 2006; Xu et al., 2009). By activating CD4+ T cells, Nef favours infection spread, as well as increases the pool of permissive cells and transcription from the virus promoter on cells already infected.

Nef interacts with a number of serine and tyrosine protein kinases usually by its PxxP domain, known to bind proteins with SH3 domains (Saksela et al., 1995). Binding of Nef to these proteins lead to their activation, and activation of the pathway in which they are included. Some of these kinases include Hck, PAK1, Lyn, c-Raf, and p53, but many more have been described (Arold et al., 1998; Baur et al., 1997; Cheng et al., 1999; Greenway et al., 2002; Hodge et al., 1998; Lu et al., 1996; Saksela et al., 1995). Nef recruits several molecules involved in TCR signaling, as Lck and Vav (Baur et al., 1997; Djordjevic et al., 2004; Fackler et al., 1999), to glycolipid-enriched domains, leading the T-cell to a preactivation state (Simmons et al., 2001). Furthermore, Nef can activate T cells independently of TCR, stimulating calcium-dependent signaling by interaction with inositol triphosfate receptor on these cells (Manninen and Saksela, 2002).

Interestinglly, some effects of Nef on signaling can be seen even in the absence of the PxxP domain, as STAT3 phosphorilation. For STAT3 phosphorilation the domains necessary for interaction with the endocytic machinery, as the diacid domains EE155 and DD174 and the dileucine domain LL164 were needed, showing that interaction with SH3 domain containing proteins is not the only event related to manipulation of signaling pathways by Nef (Percario et al., 2003).

Activation of the signaling pathways by Nef leads, for instance, to the induction NFkB nuclear translocation by inducing phosphorilation of IKK alpha and beta and their subsequent degradation (Mangino et al., 2007; Varin et al., 2003). This activation leads to the secretion of pro-inflammatory mediators, as IL-1beta, IL-6 and TNFalpha, and chemokines as MIP1alpha and beta. Other pathways activated by Nef include AP-1, c-Jun, and MAPK ERK1/2, JNK and p38 (Mangino et al., 2007). This effect can take place in many cell types as promonocytic cells, Monocyte-Derived Macrophages (MDMs), and DCs (Olivetta et al., 2003; Quaranta et al., 2006; Varin et al., 2003). The soluble mediators synthesized as the result of the activation of these pathways, as IL-6 and MIP-1alpha, activate JAK, leading to dimmerization of STAT1 and 3 (Mangino et al., 2007; Percario et al., 2003). Also, as Nef activates IRF3, leading to the synthesis of IFNbeta, it also leads to STAT2 activation (Mangino et al., 2007). NFkB activation also contributes to synthesis of viral proteins, since NFkB is one of the main regulators of the viral promoter (Nabel and Baltimore, 1987).

Signaling through NFkB and STAT3 are responsible for regulation of antiapoptotic genes on infected cells, preventing their death, prolonging viral production and spread (Quaranta et al., 2006). Along with TNF, Nef stimulation of NFkB may act blocking caspase 8 activation (Wang et al., 1998).

It has been described that treatment of cells with exogenous Nef are similar to the treatment with TNFalpha, and lead to the same outcomes (Mahlknecht et al., 2000; Varin et al., 2003), as NFkB, AP-1 and JNK activation. It is thus believed that Nef might engage interactions with some actor of the TNFalpha signaling pathway, but such protein have not yet been identified (Varin et al., 2003).

Nef was found in the germinal centers of infected lymphoid follicules, and its presence has been observed in IgD+ B cells, although these cells showed no signs of infection, as they lack any other viral protein or RNA. On B cells, Nef inhibits CD40-dependent activation and IgG2 and IgA class-switch. Interestingly, Nef can reach these cells by inducing conduit formation on infected nearby macrophages, and trafficking through them in vesicles that are delivered to B cells (Xu et al., 2009).

AIDS is by many authors considered as the outcome of many immunological disorders. The solely expression of Nef in SCID human/mouse model recapitulates many of the AIDS symptoms (Hanna et al., 1998; Lindemann et al., 1994; Skowronski et al., 1993). Nef completely transfigures signaling of DCs, T cells, monocytes/macrophages, B cells and probably many others cell types. These attributes make this protein probably the major pathogenicity factor of HIV.

2.4 Downmodulation of TCR/CD3

HIV-1 infection in humans and SIVmac infection in rhesus macaques induces overall levels of immune activation associated with accelerated T cell turnover rates and increased susceptibility to apoptotic cell death that culminates in progression to AIDS in the absence of an effective anti-HIV therapy. Moreover, the accessory protein Nef from both HIV and SIV has been implicated in immune activation and disease progression as discussed previously. HIV-1 Nef has also been reported to directly enhance the responsiveness of T cells to activation (Fenard et al., 2005; Fortin et al., 2004; Wang et al., 2000). Nonetheless, non-human primates naturally infected with their species-specific SIVs (e.g., sooty mangabeys (SMs) and African green monkeys (AGMs)) generally do not show signs of progression to SAIDS (Silvestri et al., 2007; VandeWoude and Apetrei, 2006). The mechanism underlying the remarkable difference in the outcome of infection between these primate hosts include T cell activation as a strong predictor of progression to AIDS (Giorgi et al., 1999; Sousa et al., 2002).

The signaling cascade which leads to T-cell activation and differentiation depends on the immunoreceptor tyrosine activation motifs (ITAMs) of the TCR/CD3 complex localized in cell surface for initiation of signaling cascades, thereby resulting in recruitment and activation of multiple protein tyrosine kinases, signaling intermediates, and adapter molecules (Guy and Vignali, 2009). TCR/CD3 complexes are composed of the clonotypic αβ heterodimer, the CD3 δε and γε heterodimers, the ζ homodimer and contain a total of 10 ITAMs (Alcover and Alarcon, 2000). TCR/CD3 complexes are relatively stable but are constantly internalized and recycled back to the cell surface by the endocytosis and intracellular trafficking pathway of membrane receptors. Besides the host TCR/CD3 complexes equilibrium, SIV and HIV-2 Nef bypasses the mechanisms that normally mediate the recruitment of TCR/CD3 complexes to the endocytic machinery, therefore, SIV and HIV-2 Nef target the CD3-ζ subunit and accelerate its endocytosis rate (Howe et al., 1998; Swigut et al., 2003). The proposed mechanisms for TCR-CD3 endocytosis induced by SIVmac and HIV-2 Nef proteins are based on the interaction of Nef with the CD3-ζ subunit via the AP-2 clathrin adaptor pathway (Bell et al., 1998; Howe et al., 1998; Swigut et al., 2003).

Although HIV-1 Nef fails to downregulate CD3 (Foster and Garcia, 2008) essentially all SIV Nefs, except for a small subset, downmodulate TCR/CD3 complexes to suppress T cell activation and programmed cell death (Kirchhoff et al., 2008). The exceptions include the chimpanzee precursor of HIV-1, SIVcpz, as well as SIVgsn, SIVmus, SIVmon, SIVgor and SIVolc. In contrast, the majority of *nef* alleles, including those of SIVsmm, SIVmac, and HIV-2 but also those of SIVrcm, SIVdeb, SIVsyk, SIVblu, SIVsun, SIVtan, SIVsab, SIVden, SIVwrc, SIVgri, SIVlho, and SIVasc downmodulated TCR/CD3 efficiently (Schindler et al., 2006; Schmokel et al., 2011).

In a previous report, an association between Nef proteins of all *vpu*-containing viruses and the loss of ability to down-modulate the TCR/CD3 was demonstrated, hence only *vpu*-containing viruses were predicted to be unable to down-modulate the TCR/CD3 complexes, e.g. HIV-1, SIVcpz, SIVgor, SIVgsn, SIVmus, SIVmon (Schindler et al., 2006). Exceptions to this association has been demonstrated since in SIVden strain, in which Nef retains the ability to downmodulate TCR/CD3, the *vpu* gene is present, whereas in SIVolc, which does not contain Vpu, Nef protein is unable to perform this function (Schmokel et al., 2011).

Besides the role of Nef in TCR/CD3 downmodulation a question remains to be understood: does CD3 downregulation contribute to the nonpathogenic phenotype of natural SIV infections? The reports suggest that a protective role of Nef-mediated TCR/CD3 downmodulation is needed to reduce the stimulation of virally infected CD4+ helper T cells by antigen-presenting cells and might contribute to the nonpathogenic phenotype of natural SIV infections. Inefficient CD4+ helper T cell activation would weaken the antiviral immune response and might allow the virus to persist at high levels. Indeed, reduced T cell activation, proliferation and apoptosis might also allow the host to maintain a functional immune system (Kirchhoff et al., 2008). However, two models of experimental SIV infection appear to be contradictory to this hypothesis. First, SIVmac, a virus inadvertently transmitted from naturally infected SMs to macaques in captivity (Daniel et al., 1985), causes immunodeficiency and SAIDS in macaques despite the fact that its Nef protein efficiently downmodulates TCR/CD3. Second, SIVmac viruses harboring the HIV-1 *nef* gene (the so-called Nef-SHIVs) do not induce greater pathogenicity than wild-type SIVmac in experimentally infected macaques (Alexander et al., 1999). Taken together, further analyses are required to clarify the biological significance of CD3 downregulation to the pathogenicity of SIV, HIV-1, and HIV-2 for their hosts.

Although compeling evidences that the functions of Nef described above can be related to primate lentiviral pathogenesis, each one of them individually can be excluded as the mechanism by which this protein increases viral infectivity by a number of other evidences. Nef is a multifunctional protein and besides interacting with a multitude of host cellular factors and to contribute to virus pathogenesis it seems to play a key role during the primate lentiviral replication cycle to make viral particles optimally infectious. The participation of Nef during the different steps of the primate lentiviral replication cycle will be reviwed in the next sections.

2.5 Interference with cell cytoskeleton

It has been demonstrated that HIV-1 takes advantage of the cytoskeleton dynamics in order to ensure viral entry and transport within and egress from target cells, as well as to interfere with other cellular processes (Fackler and Krausslich, 2006). The specific interference of Nef with cell cytoskeleton for virus entry will be discussed on section 4.1.

Nef's interference on the actin dynamics is also an important mechanism for Nef-induced alterations of T-cell receptor (TCR) signaling (Haller et al., 2006; Rudolph et al., 2009). TCR engagement triggers actin rearrangements that control receptor clustering for signal initiation and dynamic organization of signaling protein complexes to form an immunological synapse. Nef inhibits immunological synapse formation by a dynamic process involving rapid actin modifications (Thoulouze et al., 2006). TCR signaling events at the immunological synapse, including F-actin remodeling and re-localization of Lck, are evolutionary conserved activities of highly divergent lentiviral Nef proteins (Rudolph et al.,

2009). Indeed, alteration of the endocytic and signaling pathways at the immunological synapse likely impacts the function and destiny of HIV-1-infected cells. T-cell chemotaxis constitutes an essential function of the immune response, since active secretion of chemokines controls homing and recruitment of leukocytes into tissues. A number of studies have reported that Nef affects T-cell chemotaxis through the modulation of Rho-GTPase-regulated signaling pathways (Janardhan et al., 2004; Lee et al., 2008; Swingler et al., 1999).

HIV-1 infection of primary human macrophages induces the formation of tunneling nanotubes (TNT) by Nef (Lamers et al., 2010). TNT is a novel communication system observed in immune cells, including B, T and NK cells, neutrophils and monocytes, as well as in neurons and glial cells, which can be utilized by HIV to spread viral particles by an intercellular route (Gerdes et al., 2007).

The effect of Nef is dependent on its myristoylation and SH3 domains. While Nef myristoylation is required for its membrane association, the proline-rich SH3-binding domain is involved in Nef association with Vav, DOCK2-ELMO1, Rac and the cellular kinase Pak2 (Roeth and Collins, 2006). First, Vav is activated by the interaction between its C-terminal SH3 domain and PxxP motif in Nef leading to Vav's downstream effectors activation, resulting in morphological changes, cytoskeleton rearrangements and the activation of the c-Jun N-terminal kinase (JNK)/stress-activated protein kinase (SAPK) cascade (Fackler et al., 1999). Then, Nef activates Rac by binding the DOCK2-ELMO1 complex, a key activator of Rac in antigen- and chemokine-initiated signaling pathways, and this interaction is linked to the abilities of Nef to inhibit chemotaxis and promote T cell activation (Janardhan et al., 2004). Finally, Nef association with Pak2 prevents actin remodeling to impair host cell motility by disregulation of cofilin, which is an actin-depolymerizing factor that promotes actin turnover and subsequent cell motility (Stolp et al., 2010).

The cytoskeleton reorganization induced by Nef is associated with an impairment of cell movements combined with induction of long filopodium-like structures in T lymphocytes (Stolp et al., 2010). In summary, Nef displays a variety of complex effects on the motility and cellular morphology of HIV-1-infectected T lymphocyte, thus resulting in a strategy to improve immune evasion and viral spread in the infected host.

3. SIV Nef to counteract a cellular restriction factor?

3.1 Tetherin and Nef

The cellular protein Tetherin (also known as BST-2, CD317, or HM1.24) is a membrane protein with a number of distinct characteristics indicating that it plays a straight role in suppressing the release of virions from infected cells. Tetherin was discovered in 2008 when groups of Bieniasz and Guatelli were investigating the HIV-1 Vpu anti-Tetherin activity during the virus life cycle (Neil et al., 2008; Van Damme et al., 2008). The N-terminal of this protein is localized in the cytoplasm, followed by a transmembrane domain and a coiled-coil extracellular domain. The extracellular domain contains two N-linked glycosylation sites that are modified by a glycosyl phosphatidyl inositol (GPI) membrane anchor at the C-terminus (Kupzig et al., 2003; Rollason et al., 2007).

Tetherin functions as a broadly acting antiviral factor because besides lentiviruses, Tetherin restricts the release of different retroviruses, including alpha-, beta-, delta-, spumaviruses, and other viruses as arena- (Lassa), filo- (Marbuburg, Ebola), and herpesviruses (KSHV) (Mansouri et al., 2009). Tetherin belongs to the three main classes of restriction factors in addition to

APOBEC3G, which induces hypermutation in the retroviral genome, and the Tripartide Motif Protein 5α (TRIM 5α), which acts as new incoming retroviral capsid restriction factor (Neil et al., 2008). HIV-1 overcomes these restrictions factors by the action of accessory proteins as Vif and Vpu that act against cellular substrates APOBEC3G and Tetherin, respectively, to ensure viral persistence, replication, dissemination, and transmission (Malim and Emerman, 2008).

Tetherin is antagonized by the HIV-1 protein Vpu (Neil et al., 2008; Van Damme et al., 2008). Vpu interact directly with the transmembrane domain of Tetherin with a high specificity (Gupta et al., 2009; McNatt et al., 2009). The mechanism by which Vpu remove Tetherin from the cell surface was proposed as Vpu recruits β-TrCP, a substrate adaptor for an SCF E3 ubiquitin ligase complex, to remove Tetherin via post-endocytic membrane trafficking events (Douglas et al., 2009; Mitchell et al., 2009). As a consequence, Vpu leads to moderately reduced levels of Tetherin at the host cell surface and a modest decrease in total cellular Tetherin (Douglas et al., 2009; Mitchell et al., 2009; Van Damme et al., 2008).

Anti-Tetherin factors are also found in other viruses. Kaposi's sarcoma-associated herpesvirus (KSHV) uses K5/MIR2 protein to ubiquitinate and target Tetherin for degradation (Mansouri et al., 2009). Ebola virus glycoprotein antagonizes Tetherin-mediated restriction (Kaletsky et al., 2009; Lopez et al., 2010). Vpu functions as an anti-Tetherin factor in lentiviruses as SIV from Skye's monkeys (Lopez et al., 2010). Since lentiviruses of the SIVsmm/mac/HIV-2 lineage do not have a *vpu* gene to impair Tetherin aactivity, this role was taken by other viral proteins. Some primate lentiviruses (e.g., SIVsmm, SIVmac, and SIVagm) use the Nef protein to antagonize Tetherin (Jia et al., 2009). SIVcpz from chimpanzees and SIVgor from gorillas, which contain the *vpu* gene and are the ancestors of HIV-1, also use Nef to antagonize Tetherin (Yang et al., 2010). HIV-2 on the other hand, uses its envelope glycoprotein Env (and not Nef) to downmodulate Tetherin (Bour et al., 1996; Le Tortorec and Neil, 2009; Ritter et al., 1996). SIVtan from Tantalus monkeys uses both Env and Nef to antagonize Tetherin (Gupta et al., 2009; Zhang et al., 2009).

Analyses of the interactions between Tetherins from different primate species and the antagonist proteins used by viruses that infect those hosts have revealed a high degree of species-specificity. For example, the HIV-1 Vpu protein antagonizes human but not monkey Tetherin (Gupta et al., 2009; McNatt et al., 2009). These antiviral factors have sequence divergences that may constitute barriers to zoonotic viral transmission from animal reservoirs. For instance, the specificity of SIV Nef for rhesus Tetherin mapped to a four amino acid sequence in the cytoplasmatic domain that is missing from the human protein, whereas the specificity of HIV-1 Vpu for human Tetherin mapped to amino acid differences in the transmembrane domain (Jia et al., 2009).

Tetherin is usually only expressed efficiently in plasmacytoid dendritic cells, some cancer cells, terminally differentiated B cells, and bone marrow stromal cells (Blasius et al., 2006; Goto et al., 1994; Ishikawa et al., 1995) and its expression is strongly induced by type I Interferons (Neil et al., 2007). Tetherin is constitutively expressed on the surface of HeLa, Hep-2 and Jurkat cells lines but is not detected in other cell lines, such as 293T, HOS and Cos-7 cells (Van Damme et al., 2008). The absence of Tetherin expression in some cell lines suggest that the anti-Tetherin function of Vpu or Nef may not be obligatory for efficient viral replication *in vitro* and disease progression *in vivo*. It also remains to be determined whether Tetherin will promote or block cell-to-cell transmission (Gummuluru et al., 2000; Neil et al., 2006; Neil et al., 2008; Vendrame et al., 2009). Thus, further studies on the effect of Tetherin for primate lentiviral replication are necessary.

4. Nef and the basic steps of the HIV and SIV replication cycle

4.1 Nef and virus entry and uncoating

HIV and SIV enter target cells by fusion of the viral envelope with the cell membrane followed by the delivery of the virion core inside the cell cytoplasm. The host cell cytoskeleton imposes the first physical barrier to viral invasion upon entry and Retroviruses have evolved mechanisms to interfere with cytoskeleton arrangement. More specifically, it has been proposed that Nef could reorganize actin to ensure initial viral core movement. Association of Nef with viral cores (Kotov et al., 1999) and cellular proteins involved in actin cytoskeleton dynamics such as Vav and PAK (a member of the p21-activated kinase family) could account to the early movement of the viral cores through cortical actin and into microtubules (Roeth and Collins, 2006). Therefore, it has been proposed that this function of Nef could account to the increase in virus infectivity (Campbell et al., 2004).

Lentiviruses infect non-dividing cells implying that the recently formed viral DNA enters the nucleus through the nuclear pore. In fact, the so-called Pre-Integration Complex (PIC), formed by the double strand viral DNA associated with the viral Integrase (IN) and other viral and cellular proteins gains access to the nucleus by being actively transported through the nuclear pore. This phenomena imposes the necessity of an uncoating step because the diameter of the viral core (60 nm wide) exceeds that of the nuclear pore (30 nm) (Arhel, 2010). Uncoating is the process of core disassembly that takes place after virus entry into the host cell. Three distinct models of lentivirus uncoating have been proposed: i) in the first model it is predicted that disassembly occurs spontaneously and immediately after the viral core has entered the cell cytoplasm; ii) in the second model disassembly occurs in a time frame when the reverse transcription of the viral RNA has already started; iii) in the third model core disassembly occurs later on when the synthesis of the viral DNA is already completed and the Reverse Transcription Complex (RTC) is in close proximity of the nuclear membrane. Recent evidences favor the third model.

Disassembly of the viral cores has to occur in an optimal rate to ensure that reverse transcription is successfully completed. This was evident from studies demonstrating that mutations in Gag affecting core stability reduced reverse transcription in cells (Brun et al., 2008; Forshey et al., 2002). Since Nef-deleted viruses have a defect in reverse transcription unrelated to a direct role of Nef in the Reverse Transcriptase (RT) activity (which will be discussed in section 4.2), it was proposed that the absence of Nef in the incoming viruses would affect core stability, compromising uncoating and therefore reverse transcription. However, studies failed to show this effect of Nef ruling out a role for Nef during viral uncoating (Cavrois et al., 2004; Forshey and Aiken, 2003).

Interestingly, the route of viral entry seems to dictate the Nef requirement for optimal infectivity. Whereas wild type HIV-1 or amphotropic murine leukemia glycoprotein-pseudotyped HIV-1 virions that promote membrane fusion and cell entry through the plasma membrane are dependent on Nef to be fully infectious, HIV-1 virions pseudotyped with the glycoproteins for which fusion and entry take place after endocytosis and upon endosome acidification (e.g. Vesicular Stomatitis Virus glycoprotein - VSV-G) do not require Nef to increase infectivity (Aiken, 1997; Chazal et al., 2001; Luo et al., 1998). As pointed out previously, the treatment of target cells with drugs that disrupt the cortical actin cytoskeleton complements the infectivity defect of Nef-deleted virus (Campbell et al., 2004). Therefore, taken together, and discarding the role of Nef in facilitating viral uncoating (Cavrois et al., 2004; Forshey and Aiken, 2003), these findings have been interpreted as evidence for a role of Nef in facilitating the penetration of the viral cores through the cortical acting barrier, a function that would become dispensable if entry occurs through endocytosis. However, it was recently demonstrated that the presence of Nef itself in viral particles by means of its incorporation through Vpr (Nef.Vpr fusion protein) was not sufficient to increase viral infectivity (Laguette et al., 2009). Moreover, it has been shown that in some cases the requirement for Nef to achieve optimal viral infectivity is not circumvent by directing viral entry through endocytocis followed by exposure to low pH. In an elegant study it was shown that pseudotyping HIV-1 cores with the Rous Sarcoma Virus A (RSV-A) receptor, the Tva molecule, and using this pseudotypes to infect cells harboring the RSV-A glycoprotein Nef was still necessary for optimal infectivity (Pizzato et al., 2008). Therefore it remains to be fully established that the importance of Nef to the increase of viral infectivity is solely related to its effect on the actin rearrangement upon viral entry and whether other components of the viral core also contribute in the process.

4.2 Nef and reverse transcription

Upon entry to the target cell the reverse transcription step of the Retroviral replication cycle is initiated. Reverse transcription is defined as the synthesis of the viral double strand DNA (dsDNA) from the viral single strand RNA genome (ssRNA), which is catalyzed by the two sub unities of the viral Reverse Transcriptase (RT), p66 (polymerase and RNase H) and p51 (polymerase). A pre-requisite to reverse transcription is the formation of a pre-initiation RTC during viral maturation within the producer cell. Minimally, the pre-initiation RTC is composed by two copies of the viral ssRNA genome, the tRNA primer and the viral enzymes RT and IN. Other viral proteins including nucleocapsid (NC) and the accessory proteins Vpr and Nef are also part of the pre-initiation RTC (Warrilow et al., 2009). An important characteristic of the pre-initiation RTC for most of the retroviruses is that, in virions, it undergoes minimal reverse transcription and this event is trigged in the target cell by factors that are still not completely understood. One of the major events triggering reverse transcription seems to be the exposure of the RTC to the non-limiting concentration of deoxyribonucleotides within the target cells. Once the reverse transcription is initiated structural changes occur releasing most of the protein content of the pre-initiation RTC, turning it into a mature RTC. For instance, most of the RT and the Nef content is shed at this time. It is being now recognized that cellular proteins such as helicases and other cellular factors are also present at the RTC and must play important roles during reverse transcription (Warrilow et al., 2010). The RTC migrates towards the nuclear pore through association with the cell cytoskeleton and once reverse transcription is completed the RTC is fully maturated in the PIC to enter the nucleus for the next step of viral dsDNA integration (Warrilow et al., 2009). One of the models of uncoating discussed previously predicts that only at the stage of fully maturation of the RTC into PIC is that most of the CA protein content is shed. Therefore, uncoating occurs later after reverse transcription and implies that an optimal core microenvironment is maintained in order to avoid dilution of the crucial RTC contents and the attack of deleterious cellular factors (Arhel, 2010).

Reverse transcription occur in two distinct phases; the early phase encompasses the formation of the negative strand DNA (cDNA) from the genomic RNA, while in the late phase the positive strand DNA is synthesized from the cDNA generating the dsDNA. RT is the sole enzyme that catalyses the DNA synthesis and the degradation of the viral RNA template. However, IN has a crucial role during the initiation of the reverse transcription by physically interacting and increasing the processivity of the RT (Dobard et al., 2007; Wu et al., 1999). Therefore, not only the high stoichiometry of the RT must be maintained during reverse transcription but also that of the IN. Other viral proteins have been implicated in facilitating or participating in reverse transcription. For instance, NC and Vpr physically interact with RT as well as with IN and may play an important role during the initiation of reverse transcription (Warrilow et al., 2009).

The presence of Nef in the RTC is well documented (Forshey and Aiken, 2003; Kotov et al., 1999), as well as its function in stimulating the synthesis of the viral dsDNA during reverse transcription in the target cell (Aiken and Trono, 1995; Schwartz et al., 1995). However, Nef does not influence RT activity *per se* since the *in vitro* activity of RT from Nef-deleted viruses is not altered and the treatment of these viruses with deoxyribonucleotides previous to infection of the target cells restores viral infectivity (Aiken and Trono, 1995; Khan et al., 2001). These observations prompt to the conclusion that Nef would function in an early step during the viral replication cycle before reverse transcription. Studies have failed to demonstrate any influence of Nef in virus entry, delivery of the viral cores to the cell cytoplasm or core disassembly (Cavrois et al., 2004; Forshey and Aiken, 2003; Miller et al., 1995). Other study had shown however that this early effect of Nef can be attributed to a post-entry event like facilitating the movement of the viral core through cortical actin located beneath the plasma membrane (Campbell et al., 2004), however this has recently being disputed since two different studies demonstrated that the effect of Nef in increasing viral infectivity derives not from its presence in the viral particles but from some effect on the virus producer cell (Laguette et al., 2009; Pizzato et al., 2008).

4.3 Nef and virus assembly

The viral genomic RNA is transported to the cytoplasm were it leads to the synthesis of the Gag and GagPol polyprotein precursors. These precursors oligomerize and traffic to the plasma membrane by still not completely understood pathway(s). Concomitantly, the Env glycoproteins are translated in the ER and are transported to the plasma membrane via the secretory pathway. Membrane-targeted Gag and GagPol polyproteins recruit the viral genomic RNAs and assemble at the plasma membrane, leading to the induction of membrane curvature at the site of assembly, while the Env glycoproteins are incorporated into the budding particles during the assembly process. Experimental evidences suggest an important role for lipids and especialized cell membrane microdomains for the optimal assembly of HIV-1.

Also, HIV and SIV and many other viruses infect their target cells by interacting with the surface membrane microdomains enriched with cholesterol, sphingolipids and other saturated lipids, as well as specific types of proteins, referred as lipid rafts or detergent-resistance membranes (DRMs) (Nayak and Hui, 2004). Lipid rafts form a liquid-ordered state through lipid-lipid interactions and are central for attachment of proteins when membranes are moved around inside the cell and during signaling transduction (Verkade and Simons, 1997). Glycosylphosphatidylinositol (GPI)-anchored proteins, transmembrane proteins and doubly acylated tyrosine kinases of the Src family all associate and are incorporated into DRMs.

Moreover, Nef has been proposed to have a role during the assembly step of the viral replication cycle. Several studies reported that HIV-1 Nef expression alters the lipid composition of virions by increasing cholesterol biosynthesis and its incorporation into

DRMs, therefore Nef increases the concentration of Gag and colocalizes with viral structural components in the DRMs. These features were linked to the increase in viral infectivity and the facilitation of virus spread (Wang JK, 2000; Zheng et al., 2003). Also, it seems that infectivity enhancement by Nef requires its association with components of the assembling HIV/SIV particles. Gag from HIV/SIV associates with DRMs and disruption of Gag-raft interactions impairs virus particle production (Chukkapalli et al., 2010). It has been demonstrated that fusion of the host protein cyclophilin A (CypA) to Nef allowed controlled incorporation of Nef into HIV-1 particles via association with Gag during viral particle assembly for enhancement of HIV-1 infectivity (Qi and Aiken, 2008).

Besides the effect of Nef association with DRMs to viral infectivity, Nef also associates with these membrane microdomains together with several proteins involved in the initiation and propagation of T cell signaling and could therefore affect the later steps of the replication cycle. Nef was shown to interact with Pak-2 in lipid rafts (Krautkramer et al., 2004), which may result in increased frequency of cells expressing transcriptionally active forms of NF-κB and NFAT and increased T cell activation (Fenard et al., 2005). The interaction of Nef with PAK2 is conserved for many Nef proteins derived from HIV-1, HIV-2, and SIV strains (Sawai et al., 1995), and was demonstrated to be mediated by Cdc42 and Rac, which are PAK 2 activators, and being dependent on raft integrity (Krautkramer et al., 2004). While delivers activation stimulus to CD4 T cells Nef also mediates exclusion of molecules such as Lck, Vav, and TCRζ E2 known as ubiquitin-conjugating enzyme (UbcH7) from rafts in lipid rafts to avoid the negative regulation of T cell signaling (Simmons et al., 2005).

Rafts were also initially proposed to act as platforms for virus entry, facilitating interactions between CD4 receptors and the incoming virions (Chukkapalli et al., 2010). This role has been, however, questioned, because CD4 molecules unable to associate with rafts still allow virus entry (Percherancier et al., 2003; Popik and Alce, 2004). Moreover, Sol-Foulon and co-workers proposed that the effects of Nef on CD4 downregulation and the increase in viral infectivity were independent of lipid rafts (Sol-Foulon et al., 2004). Discrepancies in methodological approaches from these authors with the reports described before could account for the observed differences on this effect of Nef. Therefore, more detailed studies are needed in order to establish a connection between the localization and the effects of Nef in DRMs and its importance for virus replication and infectivity.

Endocytosis may be classified into two categories, clathrin dependent and independent. The role of Nef in inducing clathrin-dependent endocytosis of some surface receptors, as CD4 (Aiken et al., 1994; Chaudhuri et al., 2007; Garcia and Miller, 1991; Mariani and Skowronski, 1993), triggering the *de novo* formation of clathrin coated pits and acting as a connector between receptor cargo and the endocytic machinery (Foti et al., 1997) has been addressed here. Dyn2 was identified as a Nef binding partner through immunopreciptation assays, and is intrinsically related to clathrin-dependent endocytosis (Pizzato et al., 2007). It is a ubiquitously expressed member of large GTPases that is thought to aid the fission step that separates clathrin-coated vesicles from the plasma membrane (Hinshaw, 2000). Nef distinguishes between the three isoforms of Dyn, binding specifically to Dyn2, and this interaction is conserved among different *nef* alleles. The interaction is dependent of the Middle and GTPase Effector domains of Dyn2 and surface-exposed core domain residues in Nef, as L112, F121 and D123. Loss of Dyn2 interaction leads to loss of infectivity, however, Nef mutants that are able to bind Dyn2, as LL164,165AA, also show infectivity impairment, showing that Dyn2 interaction is not sufficient for Nef induced infectivity enhancement

(Pizzato et al., 2007). Interestingly, this was the same domain considered crucial for sorting of Nef on clathrin coated vesicles, showing that Nef may have multiple mechanisms in order to gain access to clathrin-dependent endocytosis (Greenberg et al., 1998a).
Furthermore, the increase in viral infectivity by Nef through binding to Dyn2 is dependent on clathrin and the proposed mechanism predicts that by binding to Dyn2 Nef would gain access and selectively modify specific membrane domains in the infected cell from which viral assembly occurs (Pizzato et al., 2007). On the other hand, clathrin by its turn may also have another direct role during HIV infection. At least for HIV-2 and SIVmac, the p6 peptide within Gag is thought to directly engage clathrin, by a motif that resembles the classic clathrin box, LLpL(-), where p is a polar residue and (-) a negatively charged one (Kirchhausen, 2000; Popov et al., 2011). It was also shown that although HIV-1 lacks such sequence in Gag or GagPol, it may also engage clathrin through GagPol, in a mechanism dependent of the IN region of this polyprotein (Popov et al., 2011). This might be explained by the enhanced GagPol dimerization rate that a GagPol precursor deleted in the IN domain possess, which could occlude a putative clathrin interaction surface (Bukovsky and Gottlinger, 1996). Since Nef interacts with GagPol and PR, it may also decrease GagPol dimerization, resulting in a better-exposed clathrin interacting surface (Costa et al., 2004; Miller et al., 1997; Pandori et al., 1998).

4.4 Nef and virus budding

The endo-lysosomal sorting machinery was first described in yeasts, but is well conserved in mammals. In yeasts it is called VPS pathway (for Vacuolar protein sorting), and the proteins of this pathway are denominated class E proteins, as their inactivation leads to the formation of an enlarged and abnormal membrane compartment. Class E proteins can present themselves as isolated proteins or as hetero-oligomeric complexes of high molecular weight known as ESCRT (Endosomal Sorting Complex Requires for Transport) (von Schwedler et al., 2003).
In mammals, this machinery is involved in the sorting of proteins to many cellular compartments, as endosomes, lysosomes, Golgi complex and endoplasmatic reticullum. The pathway initiates with the ESCRT-I recruitment to the already ubiquitinated (ESCRT tagging) cytoplasmatic portion of the protein to be sorted. This first recruitment is made by the cellular proteins STAM and HRS (referred by some authors as ESCRT-0). From this point, two pathways might be taken: ESCRT-I activates a second complex named ESCRT-II, or it recruits Alix/AIP-1, a central protein of the ESCRT pathway, but that is not a stable part of any of the three complexes. In both cases, the ESCRT-III is recruited, whose factors bind directly to intracellular membranes and promote its invagination, usually to an endosome. Due to its morphology, endosomal compartments that contain vesicles in its interior are called Multivesicular Bodies (MVBs). This structure might have two fates, lysosomes fusion, delivering its content to degradation, or fusion with the plasmatic membrane, liberating its vesicles as exosomes (Strack et al., 2003).
The topology of viral budding is analogous to the MVBs formation, and to the membrane fission event that happens on mitosis. Therefore it is reasonable that the same cytoplasmatic machinery used for the MVBs biogenesis is co-opted by viral specific motifs in viral proteins named late domains in order to perform viral budding (Fujii et al., 2007).
Three types of late domains have been characterized in a variety of viral proteins: P(T/S)AP, responsible for the interaction with the ESCRT-I component, Tsg101; PPxY, that engage

interactions with the Nedd4 ubiquitin ligase family; and YPxL, that interact with Alix/AIP-1 (Freed and Mouland, 2006). The fact that these late domains maintain its functionality even when translocated to other regions of viral proteins or swapped between distinct viruses suggest that they serve as anchoring sites to cellular factors, rather than structural elements (Garrus et al., 2001).

On HIV-1 and SIV, the budding process initiates concomitantly with the end of the viral particle assembly, which is orchestrated by the different Gag domains. The PTAP motif contained in p6 peptide within Gag is considered the main late domain of HIV. However, the HIV genome holds two more late domains, the YPxL also located in p6 and the YPLT domain in Nef, both capable of interacting with Alix/AIP-1. Nef physical and direct interaction with Alix/AIP-1 has been demonstrated both *in vivo* and *in vitro* (Costa et al., 2006). Nef can substitute for the L domain of a p6-deleted Gag polyprotein when fused to its C-terminal, restoring viral budding. Also, a Vpr.Nef chimera was able to restore viral budding when the PTAP domain in p6 was disrupted (Costa et al., 2006).

In CEM and SupT1 cell lines, Nef was shown to increase biogenesis of MVBs, a feature that can be useful for budding (Costa et al., 2006; Stumptner-Cuvelette et al., 2001). HIV budding toward MVB was seen in many cell lines, and can be especially decisive in macrophages, a lineage known to have well-developed endosomal machinery. Accumulation of late endosomes was dependent of the YPLT domain in Nef, and requires Nef interaction with Alix/AIP-1.

4.5 Nef and virus maturation

The retrovirus enzymatic and structural proteins are produced by the translation of a polycistronic RNA and originate the polyprotein precursors Gag and GagPol (Frankel and Young, 1998). The viral PR (Navia et al., 1989) catalyses the hydrolysis of the peptide bonds of the polyproteins' cleavage sites originating the mature proteins capable of generating an infectious particle (Louis et al., 2000).

The lentiviral PR is composed of 99 amino acids, and is synthesized as part of the GagPol precursor polyprotein. As it contains an aspartic acid in the center of the catalytic domain, the HIV and SIV PR are classified as members of the aspartyl PR family (Navia et al., 1989). Some features separate cellular aspartyl PRs from primate lentiviral PR. Unlike cellular aspartyl PRs, which are monomeric, viral aspartyl PRs are dimeric and must dimerize in order to gain catalytic activity. Therefore, the first step of PR activation is the dimerization of two GagPol molecules (Pettit et al., 2005; Weber, 1990). Other feature is that the cleavage sites recognized by HIV and SIV PR do not share amino acid identity on the cleavage sequence, or on its flanking regions (Hellen et al., 1989; Krausslich et al., 1988). Finally, the last characteristic that separate HIV and SIV PR from its cellular relatives is that, as for cellular PRs the whole catalytic machinery is pre-formed, and its activation lies mostly on the cleavage of a zymogen (Tang and Wong, 1987), for HIV and SIV PR the activation is extremely controlled by mechanisms involving protein folding, zymogen cleavage, PR context, interactions and pH (Gatlin et al., 1998; Partin et al., 1991; Pettit et al., 2004). These abundant regulatory mechanisms point out that the correct PR activation is essential for the formation of infectious particles, and that a premature activation must be avoided. Such activation could lead to complete viral processing before the completion of budding, resulting in the diffusion of viral constituents on the cytosol and altering the protein ratio in the budding particle (Pettit et al., 2004).

After dimerization, the first cleavages events occur in *cis*. The first cleavage site is located between sp1 and NC, and the second is inside the p6* region of the GagPol precursor polyprotein, divinding p6* in an octapeptide (sometimes referred as Transframe Peptide, TFP) and a 48 amino acids region that is immediately upstream the PR. These two cleavages generate the processing intermediates MA-CA-sp1 (42KDa), NC-TFP (7,4KDa) from Gag and p6*-PR-RT-IN (113KDa) from Pol (Pettit et al., 2004). It is thought that at this point p6* acts as a zymogen, lying on the catalityc center and blocking further cleavages (Partin et al., 1991). In order to continue processing an event capable of dislodging p6* from the catalic site is needed. Many events have been alleged as capable of so. The pH decay that occurs during the budding is the fit theory. However, it is not excluded that some cellular or viral protein may participate in this process. For instance, it has been demonstrated that the viral accessory protein Nef binds specifically to the p6* region of the GagPol precursor (Costa et al., 2004; Jesus da Costa et al., 2009).

It is well established that the Nef protein from both HIV-1 (Chen et al., 1998; Freund et al., 1994; Miller et al., 1997; Pandori et al., 1998) and -2 (Schorr et al., 1996) is cleaved by the viral PR. Initially, the cleavage site within Nef was demonstrated to localize to the N-terminal region generating a 9kDa membrane anchor domain and a 20kDa Nef core domain (30kDa core domain in the case of HIV-2). These cleavage forms of Nef are recognized only inside the viral particles, implying that cleavage takes place during the viral maturation step that culminates with the formation of mature infectious viruses. Although the HIV-2 PR cleaves Nef from HIV-1 (Schorr et al., 1996), there is no amino acid sequence conservation of the cleavage sites between Nef from HIV-1 and HIV-2. While in the HIV-1 Nef the well established cleavage site localizes between the Tryptophan 57 and Leucine 58, in the amino acid sequence context 54DCAW*LEAQ61, in HIV-2 Nef the cleavage site is localized between the Tyrosine 39 and Serine 40 in the amino acid sequence context 36GGEY*SQFQ43. Another cleavage site within HIV-1 Nef must exist since two independent groups reported a C-terminal cleavage form of Nef with an apparent molecular weight of 13kDa (Laguette et al., 2009; Miller et al., 1997). Recent data from our group demonstrated that the SIVcpz PR also cleaves Nef from SIVcpz during the virus replication cycle probably at the same residues as in HIV-1 Nef. Moreover, we have also observed that the SIVcpz PR has the capacity of cleaving Nef from HIV-1 generating a Nef core domain with the same apparent molecular weight when cleaved by the HIV-1 PR (Sampaio, manuscript in preparation). Since there is a great degree of conservation between the *nef* genes from HIV-2 and SIVmac it is likely that the Nef protein from SIVmac is also cleaved by the viral PR.

The fact that Nef is cleaved by the viral PR implicates that these proteins interact during the viral replication cycle, however the consequences of this cleavage for viral infectivity is still a matter of controversy. Mutations introduced at the main cleavage site on Nef, which prevent PR cleavage, does not necessarily correlates with a loss of infectivity. For instance, in one study the deletion of the cleavage site of Nef (ΔDCAWL 54-58) prevented its cleavage and reduced viral infectivity by 80% (Miller et al., 1997), while in another study a similar deletion, which again prevented Nef cleavage, reduced viral infectivity by only 20% (Pandori et al., 1998) (Table 1). On the other hand, mutations at the same cleavage site that did not disrupt cleavage, like W57A, had a great impact on viral infectivity (Chen et al., 1998; Miller et al., 1997). A summary of mutations and deletions introduced at the cleavage site of Nef and its impact on viral infectivity are listed on Table

1. From this data we can observe that most of the mutations that prevented cleavage correlated with a reduction in viral infectivity, however some mutations that still allow cleavage to happen also had an impact on viral infectivity. Based on these observations authors excluded that processing of Nef by the viral PR could be related to the capacity of the former to increase viral infectivity.

Nevertheless, one can draw some conclusions from these data. First, some of the mutations considered not disrupting cleavage of Nef did in fact altered the normal rate of cleavage, as for mutations W57A and WL57AA there was much less cleavage observed (Chen et al., 1998; Miller et al., 1997), while for mutation CAW55LLL it could be observed a higher cleavage rate of the Nef protein (Miller et al., 1997). Therefore, alteration of the cleavage rate could interfere with the properties of Nef to increase viral infectivity without disrupting cleavage entirely. Second, a complicating issue is that the cleavage site of Nef is also involved with downmodulation of CD4 therefore, disruption of this domain could have consequences for viral infectivity that could be related to this well established function of Nef. But it must be pointed out that the viral infectivity data described here was obtained from CD4 negative cells ruling out the effect that these mutations would have on CD4 downmodulation. Lastly, as pointed out previously 55CAWL58 is the main viral PR cleavage site but other sites exist within Nef (Laguette et al., 2009; Miller et al., 1997). This could explain that however impairing the cleavage at the major site viral infectivity increase by Nef would not be greatly affected.

It is not the presence of Nef in the viral particles *per se* that increases viral infectivity. This was proven by a study by Laguette and co-workers (Laguette et al., 2009) where it was demonstrated that increasing the amounts of Nef being incorporated within HIV-1 particles by means of a Nef-Vpr fusion protein was not sufficient to make viral particles more infectious. In any case, this Nef-Vpr fusion was normally processed by the viral PR and retained classical Nef functions such as downmodulation of CD4 from the surface of virus producer cells. This data therefore indicates that the role of Nef related to the increase in viral infectivity occurs during the late stages of the replication cycle in the virus producer cells, probably by optimally regulating/modifying the structural and/or enzymatic viral components. Some aspects related to this possible function of Nef will be discussed further.

Interestingly, besides connecting viral PR since being recognized as a specific substrate, Nef can also connect the structural/enzymatic polyprotein precursor GagPol through different domains either in Nef and in GagPol (Costa et al., 2004; Jesus da Costa et al., 2009). These studies demonstrated that the Nef protein from both HIV-1 (Costa et al., 2004) and SIVmac (Jesus da Costa et al., 2009) can interact with the GagPol precursor through the flexible-loop domain in Nef and the p6* regulatory region of GagPol. Although the specific amino acid residues involved in this interaction in both Nef and p6* were not yet demonstrated, its specificity and the biological relevance were. Interaction of GagPol and Nef occurs in cells during the HIV-1 replication cycle and was sufficient to explain the dominant negative phenotype of an laboratory adapted allele of HIV-1 *nef* (Nef F12) which localizes to the ER and inhibits the release of Gag and its processing by the viral PR (Fackler et al., 2001; Olivetta et al., 2000). The F12 phenotype was recapitulated by a Nef with an ER retention signal, meaning that by interacting with GagPol Nef retained this polyprotein precursor inside the producer cell avoiding both release and maturation of viral particles (Costa et al., 2004). Furthermore, the relevance of this interaction was confirmed by an experiment demonstrating that release of a late-domain defective HIV-1 from producer cells was rescued by a Nef-Tsg101 fusion protein, indicating that, besides interacting early during the expression of GagPol, Nef and the viral structural/enzymatic precursors are present concomitantly at the sites of virus budding. While investigating what influence the binding of Nef and GagPol would have for HIV-1 infectivity we have also established that Nef from HIV binds the cellular Alix protein and correlated these findings with optimal viral replication in cells (Costa et al., 2006). We demonstrated that this interaction correlated with the property of Nef to stimulate the synthesis of MVBs in cells and the optimal infection of MDMs. Taken together, the fact that Nef binds both the viral precursor GagPol and to the cellular Alix protein, which is involved in virus budding, suggest that Nef actively participates in a late step of viral replication. We further extended these observations to SIVmac, demonstrating that the binding of Nef to both GagPol and Alix is conserved in Nef from this virus (Jesus da Costa et al., 2009). The functional relevance of these bindings was clearly demonstrated in rhesus macaques. First, informative mutations were introduced into the *nef* gene of infectious SIVmac and this mutant virus used to infect four rhesus macaques. Whereas rhesus macaques infected with the WT virus developed high viral loads and progressed rapidly to SAIDS, only two of four monkeys inoculated with the mutant virus displayed a similar picture, albeit with much delayed kinetics. Importantly, in both cases, we observed reversions in SIVNef that restored its binding to SIVGagPol and Alix. In two other rhesus macaques, mutant Nef sequences persisted and they developed neither high viral loads nor SAIDS. Further studies in cells provided additional support for these findings. Taken together these studies suggest that interactions between Nef, GagPol and Alix are important for optimal viral replication and progression to disease in the monkey model of AIDS and possibly also pertinent to the human disease since these interactions are preserved in both HIV-1 and SIVmac.

Still, what would be the mechanism by which interacting with GagPol and Alix, Nef would stimulate viral infectivity? Recent work from our group demonstrated that Nef that from SIVcpz also binds to GagPol from both SIVcpz and HIV-1. Furthermore, our results showed that Nef exerts a direct influence upon the viral PR activity: i) first by characterizing a SIVcpz provirus that expresses a N-terminal truncated peptide of Nef that is a potent inhibitor of viral processing and consequently viral infectivity and exerts a dominant negative activity both against PR from SIVcpz and HIV-1 (Sampaio et al. - manuscript in preparation); second by demonstrating that in the absence of Nef expression during the replication cycle of HIV-1 the processing kinetics of the Gag and GagPol precursors are accelerated, resulting in slightly lower concentration of the structural (p24-Capsid protein) and 2-fold lower concentration of the enzymatic (IN) components within viral particles (Mendonça et al. - manuscript in preparation). Moreover, the accelerated activity of the viral PR in the absence of Nef expression in the producer cells was also demonstrated by the fact that higher concentrations of PR inhibitors (e.g. Lopinavir) are required to inhibit virus replication at the same levels as of the wild type viruses. Based on this preliminary results a working model was drawn (Figure 2), in which the role of Nef for virus infectivity is explained by the following: upon binding of the p6* and PR regions, within the GagPol precursor, Nef would function as a fine regulator of PR activation, holding it to an optimal timing when budding of the viral particles is almost complete.

Therefore, the right content of the viral constituents is achieved. In the absence of Nef, PR activation would occur earlier on before the completion of budding, consequently some of the protein content is lost during the formation of the viral particles, especially the IN, since it is one of the first enzymes to be processed out from the GagPol precursor. How would this explain the decreased infectivity of the Nef-deficient viruses? Since IN is important not only for the integration step of the viral DNA to the host genome but also participates during the Reverse Transcription of the viral RNA, lower concentrations of the IN would affect reverse transcription of the incoming virus impacting on viral infectivity. Our results conciliates previous data demonstrating an impairment in the HIV-1 ability to reverse transcribe the viral RNA genome in Nef-deficient viruses, which could not be explained by a role of Nef in facilitating an early step of the replication cycle as enhancement of viral capsid delivery to the cytosol of the target cell (Cavrois et al., 2004; Miller et al., 1995; Tobiume et al., 2001), trafficking of the viral cores through the cortical actin network since (Campbell EM, 2004; Pizzato et al., 2008), or capsid uncoating (Cavrois et al., 2004; Kotov et al., 1999).

Mutation	Nef cleavage	Infectivity reduction (%)	Literature
W57A	Yes *	70 50	(Miller et al., 1997) (Chen et al., 1998)
L58A	Yes	50	(Chen et al., 1998)
WL57GG	No	75	(Miller et al., 1997)
WL57AA	No Yes *	50 75	(Chen et al., 1998) (Miller et al., 1997)
CAW (55-57) LLL	Yes **	70	(Miller et al., 1997)
ΔCAW (55-57)	No	75	(Miller et al., 1997) (Fackler et al., 2006)
ΔDCAWL (54-57)	No	20	(Pandori et al., 1998)
ΔLEAQ (58-61)	Yes	50	(Pandori et al., 1998)
ΔAWLEA (56-60)	No	80	(Pandori et al., 1998)
ΔDCAWL (54-61)-ATIM***	Yes**	30	(Pandori et al., 1998)

Table 1. Mutations within the cleavage site of Nef and its effect on viral infectivity* Less cleavage of the Nef protein was observed (Miller et al., 1997). ** A higher cleavage rate of the Nef protein was observed (Miller et al., 1997). *** A cleavage site (ATIM) from the viral Nucleocapsid protein was introduced at amino acid position 55 in Nef, accelerated cleavage of Nef was observed (Pandori et al., 1998).

5. Conclusion

Nef is a multifunctional accessory protein only present in the primate lentiviruses. Its influence on viral infectivity and pathogenesis is undisputable. However, the mechanism by which Nef contributes to the optimal infectivity of these viruses is still a matter of controversy. The classical functions described for Nef are the downmodulation of the CD4 and MHC-I molecules from the cell surface and the activation of signaling cascades in Nef-expressing or HIV/SIV-infected cells. While the downmodulation of immune system molecules from the surface of cells, as described here, could all contribute to the effect of Nef on pathogenesis and disease progression, these functions failed to be correlated with the contribution of Nef to the optimal infectivity of HIV/SIV. Some experimental evidences prompt to the conclusion that Nef participates in an early step of the replication cycle post-entry and before reverse transcription to increase infectivity. However it is becoming more evident that the requirement for Nef occurs in the producer cell, possibly by modifying or regulating the last steps of the viral replication cycle (assembly, budding and/or maturation) Nef would promote the formation of optimally infectious virus progeny.

In our model, the specific interaction of Nef with the precursor polyprotein GagPol and its influence on the kinetics of processing of the viral precursor proteins, predicts that in the absence of Nef viral PR will be activated earlier on during budding resulting in the incorporation of lower amounts of the viral enzymes into viral cores, especially IN. Since IN is crucial to the initiation of reverse transcription and that Nef-deleted viruses have a defect in viral DNA synthesis, our model conciliates these findings to explain the optimal infectivity of the viral particles in the presence of Nef.

If that is the case, very important implications for this function of Nef in the current anti-retroviral therapy can be predicted. First, Nef could become a target to anti-retroviral drugs that would act in synergism with PR inhibitors currently in use to achieve a more efficient inhibition of virus replication. Second, we should predict a co-evolution of both Nef and PR during the therapy with PR inhibitors, which will have a direct impact on the selection of resistance mutations that is still not appreciated.

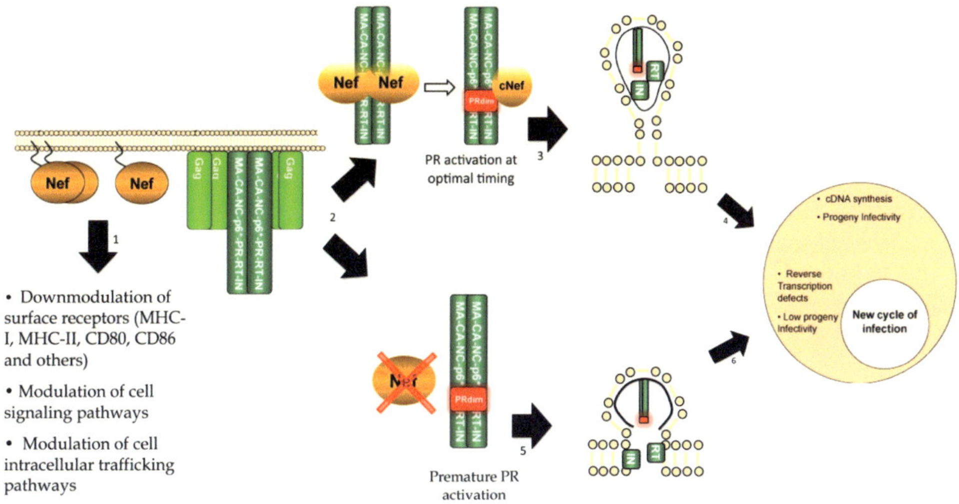

Fig. 2. Schematic representation of the working model for the functions of Nef during the last steps of the primate Lentiviral replication cycle. Nef associates with cellular membranes and classically exerts several functions that do not necessarily correlate with its role in increasing viral infectivity and promote disease progression (arrow 1). Nef from both HIV-1 and SIVmac binds to the p6*PR within the GagPol precursor (Costa et al., 2004; Jesus da Costa et al., 2009) (arrow 2). In the presence of Nef the viral PR is activated at an optimal time during the budding step, assuring the correct amount of the viral IN and RT inside the viral core (arrow 3). IN influences the activity of RT during the initiation of reverse transcription, therefore the normal amounst of IN in viral particles will promote optimal cDNA synthesis and viral infectivity of the incoming viruses (arrow 4). On the other hand, in the absence of Nef viral PR is prematurely activated, consequently the processing of the GagPol precursor would occur before the formation of the viral cores leading to a lesser incorporation of IN (arrow 5), what would impact reverse transcription and viral infectivity (arrow 6).

6. References

Adachi, A., Ono, N., Sakai, H., Ogawa, K., Shibata, R., Kiyomasu, T., Masuike, H., Ueda, S., 1991. Generation and characterization of the human immunodeficiency virus type 1 mutants. Arch Virol 117, 45-58.

Aguiar, R.S., Peterlin, B.M., 2008. APOBEC3 proteins and reverse transcription. Virus research 134, 74-85.

Ahmad, N., Venkatesan, S., 1988. Nef protein of HIV-1 is a transcriptional repressor of HIV-1 LTR. Science 241, 1481-1485.

Aiken, C., 1997. Pseudotyping human immunodeficiency virus type 1 (HIV-1) by the glycoprotein of vesicular stomatitis virus targets HIV-1 entry to an endocytic pathway and suppresses both the requirement for Nef and the sensitivity to cyclosporin A. J Virol 71, 5871-5877.

Aiken, C., Konner, J., Landau, N.R., Lenburg, M.E., Trono, D., 1994. Nef induces CD4 endocytosis: requirement for a critical dileucine motif in the membrane-proximal CD4 cytoplasmic domain. Cell 76, 853-864.

Aiken, C., Trono, D., 1995. Nef stimulates human immunodeficiency virus type 1 proviral DNA synthesis. J Virol 69, 5048-5056.

Alcover, A., Alarcon, B., 2000. Internalization and intracellular fate of TCR-CD3 complexes. Crit Rev Immunol 20, 325-346.

Alessandrini, L., Santarcangelo, A.C., Olivetta, E., Ferrantelli, F., d'Aloja, P., Pugliese, K., Pelosi, E., Chelucci, C., Mattia, G., Peschle, C., Verani, P., Federico, M., 2000. T-tropic human immunodeficiency virus (HIV) type 1 Nef protein enters human monocyte-macrophages and induces resistance to HIV replication: a possible mechanism of HIV T-tropic emergence in AIDS. J Gen Virol 81, 2905-2917.

Alexander, L., Du, Z., Howe, A.Y., Czajak, S., Desrosiers, R.C., 1999. Induction of AIDS in rhesus monkeys by a recombinant simian immunodeficiency virus expressing nef of human immunodeficiency virus type 1. J Virol 73, 5814-5825.

Arhel, N., 2010. Revisiting HIV-1 uncoating. Retrovirology 7, 96.

Arold, S., O'Brien, R., Franken, P., Strub, M.P., Hoh, F., Dumas, C., Ladbury, J.E., 1998. RT loop flexibility enhances the specificity of Src family SH3 domains for HIV-1 Nef. Biochemistry 37, 14683-14691.

Atkins, K.M., Thomas, L., Youker, R.T., Harriff, M.J., Pissani, F., You, H., Thomas, G., 2008. HIV-1 Nef binds PACS-2 to assemble a multikinase cascade that triggers major histocompatibility complex class I (MHC-I) down-regulation: analysis using short interfering RNA and knock-out mice. J Biol Chem 283, 11772-11784.

Baur, A.S., Sass, G., Laffert, B., Willbold, D., Cheng-Mayer, C., Peterlin, B.M., 1997. The N-terminus of Nef from HIV-1/SIV associates with a protein complex containing Lck and a serine kinase. Immunity 6, 283-291.

Bell, I., Ashman, C., Maughan, J., Hooker, E., Cook, F., Reinhart, T.A., 1998. Association of simian immunodeficiency virus Nef with the T-cell receptor (TCR) zeta chain leads to TCR down-modulation. J Gen Virol 79 (Pt 11), 2717-2727.

Bentham, M., Mazaleyrat, S., Harris, M., 2003. The di-leucine motif in the cytoplasmic tail of CD4 is not required for binding to human immunodeficiency virus type 1 Nef, but is critical for CD4 down-modulation. J Gen Virol 84, 2705-2713.

Blagoveshchenskaya, A.D., Thomas, L., Feliciangeli, S.F., Hung, C.H., Thomas, G., 2002. HIV-1 Nef downregulates MHC-I by a PACS-1- and PI3K-regulated ARF6 endocytic pathway. Cell 111, 853-866.

Blasius, A.L., Giurisato, E., Cella, M., Schreiber, R.D., Shaw, A.S., Colonna, M., 2006. Bone marrow stromal cell antigen 2 is a specific marker of type I IFN-producing cells in the naive mouse, but a promiscuous cell surface antigen following IFN stimulation. J Immunol 177, 3260-3265.

Bour, S., Schubert, U., Peden, K., Strebel, K., 1996. The envelope glycoprotein of human immunodeficiency virus type 2 enhances viral particle release: a Vpu-like factor? J Virol 70, 820-829.

Bresnahan, P.A., Yonemoto, W., Ferrell, S., Williams-Herman, D., Geleziunas, R., Greene, W.C., 1998. A dileucine motif in HIV-1 Nef acts as an internalization signal for CD4 downregulation and binds the AP-1 clathrin adaptor. Curr Biol 8, 1235-1238.

Breuer, S., Gerlach, H., Kolaric, B., Urbanke, C., Opitz, N., Geyer, M., 2006. Biochemical indication for myristoylation-dependent conformational changes in HIV-1 Nef. Biochemistry 45, 2339-2349.

Brun, S., Solignat, M., Gay, B., Bernard, E., Chaloin, L., Fenard, D., Devaux, C., Chazal, N., Briant, L., 2008. VSV-G pseudotyping rescues HIV-1 CA mutations that impair core assembly or stability. Retrovirology 5, 57.

Bukovsky, A., G˄ttlinger, H., 1996. Lack of integrase can markedly affect human immunodeficiency virus type 1 particle production in the presence of an active viral protease. J Virol 70, 6820-6825.

Campbell EM, N.R., Hope TJ, 2004. Disruption of the actin cytoskeleton can complement the ability of Nef to enhance human immunodeficiency virus type 1 infectivity. J Virol 78, 5745-5755.

Campbell, E.M., Nunez, R., Hope, T.J., 2004. Disruption of the actin cytoskeleton can complement the ability of Nef to enhance human immunodeficiency virus type 1 infectivity. J Virol 78, 5745-5755.

Carl, S., Greenough, T.C., Krumbiegel, M., Greenberg, M., Skowronski, J., Sullivan, J.L., Kirchhoff, F., 2001. Modulation of different human immunodeficiency virus type 1 Nef functions during progression to AIDS. J Virol 75, 3657-3665.

Cavrois, M., Neidleman, J., Yonemoto, W., Fenard, D., Greene, W.C., 2004. HIV-1 virion fusion assay: uncoating not required and no effect of Nef on fusion. Virology 328, 36-44.

Chaudhry, A., Das, S.R., Hussain, A., Mayor, S., George, A., Bal, V., Jameel, S., Rath, S., 2005. The Nef protein of HIV-1 induces loss of cell surface costimulatory molecules CD80 and CD86 in APCs. J Immunol 175, 4566-4574.

Chaudhry, A., Verghese, D.A., Das, S.R., Jameel, S., George, A., Bal, V., Mayor, S., Rath, S., 2009. HIV-1 Nef promotes endocytosis of cell surface MHC class II molecules via a constitutive pathway. J Immunol 183, 2415-2424.

Chaudhuri, R., Lindwasser, O.W., Smith, W.J., Hurley, J.H., Bonifacino, J.S., 2007. Downregulation of CD4 by human immunodeficiency virus type 1 Nef is dependent on clathrin and involves direct interaction of Nef with the AP2 clathrin adaptor. J Virol 81, 3877-3890.

Chazal, N., Singer, G., Aiken, C., Hammarskjold, M.L., Rekosh, D., 2001. Human immunodeficiency virus type 1 particles pseudotyped with envelope proteins that fuse at low pH no longer require Nef for optimal infectivity. J Virol 75, 4014-4018.
Chen, Y.L., Trono, D., Camaur, D., 1998. The proteolytic cleavage of human immunodeficiency virus type 1 Nef does not correlate with its ability to stimulate virion infectivity. J Virol 72, 3178-3184.
Cheng, H., Hoxie, J.P., Parks, W.P., 1999. The conserved core of human immunodeficiency virus type 1 Nef is essential for association with Lck and for enhanced viral replication in T-lymphocytes. Virology 264, 5-15.
Cheng-Mayer, C., Iannello, P., Shaw, K., Luciw, P.A., Levy, J.A., 1989. Differential effects of nef on HIV replication: implications for viral pathogenesis in the host. Science 246, 1629-1632.
Chowers, M.Y., Pandori, M.W., Spina, C.A., Richman, D.D., Guatelli, J.C., 1995. The growth advantage conferred by HIV-1 nef is determined at the level of viral DNA formation and is independent of CD4 downregulation. Virology 212, 451-457.
Chukkapalli, V., Oh, S.J., Ono, A., 2010. Opposing mechanisms involving RNA and lipids regulate HIV-1 Gag membrane binding through the highly basic region of the matrix domain. Proc Natl Acad Sci U S A 107, 1600-1605.
Cortes, M.J., Wong-Staal, F., Lama, J., 2002. Cell surface CD4 interferes with the infectivity of HIV-1 particles released from T cells. J Biol Chem 277, 1770-1779.
Costa, L.J., Chen, N., Lopes, A., Aguiar, R.S., Tanuri, A., Plemenitas, A., Peterlin, B.M., 2006. Interactions between Nef and AIP1 proliferate multivesicular bodies and facilitate egress of HIV-1. Retrovirology 3, 33.
Costa, L.J., Zheng, Y.H., Sabotic, J., Mak, J., Fackler, O.T., Peterlin, B.M., 2004. Nef binds p6* in GagPol during replication of human immunodeficiency virus type 1. J Virol 78, 5311-5323.
Crotti, A., Neri, F., Corti, D., Ghezzi, S., Heltai, S., Baur, A., Poli, G., Santagostino, E., Vicenzi, E., 2006. Nef alleles from human immunodeficiency virus type 1-infected long-term-nonprogressor hemophiliacs with or without late disease progression are defective in enhancing virus replication and CD4 down-regulation. J Virol 80, 10663-10674.
Daniel, M.D., Kirchhoff, F., Czajak, S.C., Sehgal, P.K., Desrosiers, R.C., 1992. Protective effects of a live attenuated SIV vaccine with a deletion in the nef gene. Science 258, 1938-1941.
Daniel, M.D., Letvin, N.L., King, N.W., Kannagi, M., Sehgal, P.K., Hunt, R.D., Kanki, P.J., Essex, M., Desrosiers, R.C., 1985. Isolation of T-cell tropic HTLV-III-like retrovirus from macaques. Science 228, 1201-1204.
Deacon, N.J., Tsykin, A., Solomon, A., Smith, K., Ludford-Menting, M., Hooker, D.J., McPhee, D.A., Greenway, A.L., Ellett, A., Chatfield, C., Lawson, V.A., Crowe, S., Maerz, A., Sonza, S., Learmont, J., Sullivan, J.S., Cunningham, A., Dwyer, D., Dowton, D., Mills, J., 1995. Genomic structure of an attenuated quasi species of HIV-1 from a blood transfusion donor and recipients. Science 270, 988-991.
DeGottardi, M.Q., Specht, A., Metcalf, B., Kaur, A., Kirchhoff, F., Evans, D.T., 2008. Selective downregulation of rhesus macaque and sooty mangabey major histocompatibility complex class I molecules by Nef alleles of simian immunodeficiency virus and human immunodeficiency virus type 2. J Virol 82, 3139-3146.

Dennis, C.A., Baron, A., Grossmann, J.G., Mazaleyrat, S., Harris, M., Jaeger, J., 2005. Co-translational myristoylation alters the quaternary structure of HIV-1 Nef in solution. Proteins 60, 658-669.

Dikeakos, J.D., Atkins, K.M., Thomas, L., Emert-Sedlak, L., Byeon, I.J., Jung, J., Ahn, J., Wortman, M.D., Kukull, B., Saito, M., Koizumi, H., Williamson, D.M., Hiyoshi, M., Barklis, E., Takiguchi, M., Suzu, S., Gronenborn, A.M., Smithgall, T.E., Thomas, G., 2010. Small molecule inhibition of HIV-1-induced MHC-I down-regulation identifies a temporally regulated switch in Nef action. Mol Biol Cell 21, 3279-3292.

Djordjevic, J.T., Schibeci, S.D., Stewart, G.J., Williamson, P., 2004. HIV type 1 Nef increases the association of T cell receptor (TCR)-signaling molecules with T cell rafts and promotes activation-induced raft fusion. AIDS Res Hum Retroviruses 20, 547-555.

Dobard, C.W., Briones, M.S., Chow, S.A., 2007. Molecular mechanisms by which human immunodeficiency virus type 1 integrase stimulates the early steps of reverse transcription. J Virol 81, 10037-10046.

Douglas, J.L., Viswanathan, K., McCarroll, M.N., Gustin, J.K., Fruh, K., Moses, A.V., 2009. Vpu directs the degradation of the human immunodeficiency virus restriction factor BST-2/Tetherin via a {beta}TrCP-dependent mechanism. J Virol 83, 7931-7947.

Fackler, O.T., d'Aloja, P., Baur, A.S., Federico, M., Peterlin, B.M., 2001. Nef from human immunodeficiency virus type 1(F12) inhibits viral production and infectivity. J Virol 75, 6601-6608.

Fackler, O.T., Kienzle, N., Kremmer, E., Boese, A., Schramm, B., Klimkait, T., K¸cherer, C., Mueller-Lantzsch, N., 1997. Association of human immunodeficiency virus Nef protein with actin is myristoylation dependent and influences its subcellular localization. Eur J Biochem 247, 843-851.

Fackler, O.T., Krausslich, H.G., 2006. Interactions of human retroviruses with the host cell cytoskeleton. Curr Opin Microbiol 9, 409-415.

Fackler, O.T., Luo, W., Geyer, M., Alberts, A.S., Peterlin, B.M., 1999. Activation of Vav by Nef induces cytoskeletal rearrangements and downstream effector functions. Mol Cell 3, 729-739.

Fackler, O.T., Moris, A., Tibroni, N., Giese, S.I., Glass, B., Schwartz, O., Krausslich, H.G., 2006. Functional characterization of HIV-1 Nef mutants in the context of viral infection. Virology 351, 322-339.

Fenard, D., Yonemoto, W., de Noronha, C., Cavrois, M., Williams, S.A., Greene, W.C., 2005. Nef is physically recruited into the immunological synapse and potentiates T cell activation early after TCR engagement. J Immunol 175, 6050-6057.

Forshey, B.M., Aiken, C., 2003. Disassembly of human immunodeficiency virus type 1 cores in vitro reveals association of Nef with the subviral ribonucleoprotein complex. J Virol 77, 4409-4414.

Forshey, B.M., von Schwedler, U., Sundquist, W.I., Aiken, C., 2002. Formation of a human immunodeficiency virus type 1 core of optimal stability is crucial for viral replication. J Virol 76, 5667-5677.

Fortin, J.F., Barat, C., Beausejour, Y., Barbeau, B., Tremblay, M.J., 2004. Hyper-responsiveness to stimulation of human immunodeficiency virus-infected CD4+ T cells requires Nef and Tat virus gene products and results from higher NFAT, NF-kappaB, and AP-1 induction. J Biol Chem 279, 39520-39531.

Foster, J.L., Garcia, J.V., 2008. HIV-1 Nef: at the crossroads. Retrovirology 5, 84.
Foti, M., Mangasarian, A., Piguet, V., Lew, D.P., Krause, K.H., Trono, D., Carpentier, J.L., 1997. Nef-mediated clathrin-coated pit formation. J Cell Biol 139, 37-47.
Frankel, A.D., Young, J.A., 1998. HIV-1: fifteen proteins and an RNA. Annu Rev Biochem 67, 1-25.
Freed, E.O., Mouland, A.J., 2006. The cell biology of HIV-1 and other retroviruses. Retrovirology 3, 77.
Freund, J., Kellner, R., Houthaeve, T., Kalbitzer, H.R., 1994. Stability and proteolytic domains of Nef protein from human immunodeficiency virus (HIV) type 1. Eur J Biochem 221, 811-819.
Fujii, K., Hurley, J.H., Freed, E.O., 2007. Beyond Tsg101: the role of Alix in 'ESCRTing' HIV-1. Nat Rev Microbiol 5, 912-916.
Fujii, Y., Otake, K., Tashiro, M., Adachi, A., 1996. Soluble Nef antigen of HIV-1 is cytotoxic for human CD4+ T cells. FEBS Lett 393, 93-96.
Garcia, J.V., Miller, A.D., 1991. Serine phosphorylation-independent downregulation of cell-surface CD4 by nef. Nature 350, 508-511.
Garrus, J.E., von Schwedler, U.K., Pornillos, O.W., Morham, S.G., Zavitz, K.H., Wang, H.E., Wettstein, D.A., Stray, K.M., CÙtÈ, M., Rich, R.L., Myszka, D.G., Sundquist, W.I., 2001. Tsg101 and the vacuolar protein sorting pathway are essential for HIV-1 budding. Cell 107, 55-65.
Gatlin, J., Arrigo, S.J., Schmidt, M.G., 1998. HIV-1 protease regulation: the role of the major homology region and adjacent C-terminal capsid sequences. J Biomed Sci 5, 305-308.
Gerdes, H.H., Bukoreshtliev, N.V., Barroso, J.F., 2007. Tunneling nanotubes: a new route for the exchange of components between animal cells. FEBS Lett 581, 2194-2201.
Geyer, M., Fackler, O.T., Peterlin, B.M., 2001. Structure--function relationships in HIV-1 Nef. EMBO Rep 2, 580-585.
Giorgi, J.V., Hausner, M.A., Hultin, L.E., 1999. Detailed immunophenotype of CD8+ memory cytotoxic T-lymphocytes (CTL) against HIV-1 with respect to expression of CD45RA/RO, CD62L and CD28 antigens. Immunol Lett 66, 105-110.
Goldsmith, M.A., Warmerdam, M.T., Atchison, R.E., Miller, M.D., Greene, W.C., 1995. Dissociation of the CD4 downregulation and viral infectivity enhancement functions of human immunodeficiency virus type 1 Nef. J Virol 69, 4112-4121.
Goto, T., Kennel, S.J., Abe, M., Takishita, M., Kosaka, M., Solomon, A., Saito, S., 1994. A novel membrane antigen selectively expressed on terminally differentiated human B cells. Blood 84, 1922-1930.
Gould, S.J., Booth, A.M., Hildreth, J.E., 2003. The Trojan exosome hypothesis. Proc Natl Acad Sci U S A 100, 10592-10597.
Greenberg, M., DeTulleo, L., Rapoport, I., Skowronski, J., Kirchhausen, T., 1998a. A dileucine motif in HIV-1 Nef is essential for sorting into clathrin-coated pits and for downregulation of CD4. Curr Biol 8, 1239-1242.
Greenberg, M.E., Iafrate, A.J., Skowronski, J., 1998b. The SH3 domain-binding surface and an acidic motif in HIV-1 Nef regulate trafficking of class I MHC complexes. Embo J 17, 2777-2789.
Greenway, A.L., McPhee, D.A., Allen, K., Johnstone, R., Holloway, G., Mills, J., Azad, A., Sankovich, S., Lambert, P., 2002. Human immunodeficiency virus type 1 Nef binds

to tumor suppressor p53 and protects cells against p53-mediated apoptosis. J Virol 76, 2692-2702.

Gummuluru, S., Kinsey, C.M., Emerman, M., 2000. An in vitro rapid-turnover assay for human immunodeficiency virus type 1 replication selects for cell-to-cell spread of virus. J Virol 74, 10882-10891.

Gupta, R.K., Mlcochova, P., Pelchen-Matthews, A., Petit, S.J., Mattiuzzo, G., Pillay, D., Takeuchi, Y., Marsh, M., Towers, G.J., 2009. Simian immunodeficiency virus envelope glycoprotein counteracts tetherin/BST-2/CD317 by intracellular sequestration. Proc Natl Acad Sci U S A 106, 20889-20894.

Guy, C.S., Vignali, D.A., 2009. Organization of proximal signal initiation at the TCR:CD3 complex. Immunol Rev 232, 7-21.

Haller, C., Rauch, S., Michel, N., Hannemann, S., Lehmann, M.J., Keppler, O.T., Fackler, O.T., 2006. The HIV-1 pathogenicity factor Nef interferes with maturation of stimulatory T-lymphocyte contacts by modulation of N-Wasp activity. J Biol Chem 281, 19618-19630.

Hammes, S.R., Dixon, E.P., Malim, M.H., Cullen, B.R., Greene, W.C., 1989. Nef protein of human immunodeficiency virus type 1: evidence against its role as a transcriptional inhibitor. Proc Natl Acad Sci U S A 86, 9549-9553.

Hanna, Z., Kay, D.G., Rebai, N., Guimond, A., Jothy, S., Jolicoeur, P., 1998. Nef harbors a major determinant of pathogenicity for an AIDS-like disease induced by HIV-1 in transgenic mice. Cell 95, 163-175.

Hellen, C.U., de Crombrugghe, M., Wimmer, E., Seeger, M.A., Kaufman, T.C., 1989. Amalgamated sequences. Nature 340, 682.

Hinshaw, J.E., 2000. Dynamin and its role in membrane fission. Annu Rev Cell Dev Biol 16, 483-519.

Hodge, D.R., Dunn, K.J., Pei, G.K., Chakrabarty, M.K., Heidecker, G., Lautenberger, J.A., Samuel, K.P., 1998. Binding of c-Raf1 kinase to a conserved acidic sequence within the carboxyl-terminal region of the HIV-1 Nef protein. J Biol Chem 273, 15727-15733.

Howe, A.Y., Jung, J.U., Desrosiers, R.C., 1998. Zeta chain of the T-cell receptor interacts with nef of simian immunodeficiency virus and human immunodeficiency virus type 2. J Virol 72, 9827-9834.

Hung, C.H., Thomas, L., Ruby, C.E., Atkins, K.M., Morris, N.P., Knight, Z.A., Scholz, I., Barklis, E., Weinberg, A.D., Shokat, K.M., Thomas, G., 2007. HIV-1 Nef assembles a Src family kinase-ZAP-70/Syk-PI3K cascade to downregulate cell-surface MHC-I. Cell Host Microbe 1, 121-133.

Iafrate, A.J., Carl, S., Bronson, S., Stahl-Hennig, C., Swigut, T., Skowronski, J., Kirchhoff, F., 2000. Disrupting surfaces of nef required for downregulation of CD4 and for enhancement of virion infectivity attenuates simian immunodeficiency virus replication in vivo. J Virol 74, 9836-9844.

Ishikawa, J., Kaisho, T., Tomizawa, H., Lee, B.O., Kobune, Y., Inazawa, J., Oritani, K., Itoh, M., Ochi, T., Ishihara, K., et al., 1995. Molecular cloning and chromosomal mapping of a bone marrow stromal cell surface gene, BST2, that may be involved in pre-B-cell growth. Genomics 26, 527-534.

Janardhan, A., Swigut, T., Hill, B., Myers, M.P., Skowronski, J., 2004. HIV-1 Nef binds the DOCK2-ELMO1 complex to activate rac and inhibit lymphocyte chemotaxis. PLoS Biol 2, E6.

Jesus da Costa, L., Lopes Dos Santos, A., Mandic, R., Shaw, K., Santana de Aguiar, R., Tanuri, A., Luciw, P.A., Peterlin, B.M., 2009. Interactions between SIVNef, SIVGagPol and Alix correlate with viral replication and progression to AIDS in rhesus macaques. Virology 394, 47-56.

Jia, B., Serra-Moreno, R., Neidermyer, W., Rahmberg, A., Mackey, J., Fofana, I.B., Johnson, W.E., Westmoreland, S., Evans, D.T., 2009. Species-specific activity of SIV Nef and HIV-1 Vpu in overcoming restriction by tetherin/BST2. PLoS Pathog 5, e1000429.

Kaletsky, R.L., Francica, J.R., Agrawal-Gamse, C., Bates, P., 2009. Tetherin-mediated restriction of filovirus budding is antagonized by the Ebola glycoprotein. Proc Natl Acad Sci U S A 106, 2886-2891.

Kaminchik, J., Margalit, R., Yaish, S., Drummer, H., Amit, B., Sarver, N., Gorecki, M., Panet, A., 1994. Cellular distribution of HIV type 1 Nef protein: identification of domains in Nef required for association with membrane and detergent-insoluble cellular matrix. AIDS Res Hum Retroviruses 10, 1003-1010.

Kasper, M.R., Roeth, J.F., Williams, M., Filzen, T.M., Fleis, R.I., Collins, K.L., 2005. HIV-1 Nef disrupts antigen presentation early in the secretory pathway. J Biol Chem 280, 12840-12848.

Khan, M., Garcia-Barrio, M., Powell, M.D., 2001. Restoration of wild-type infectivity to human immunodeficiency virus type 1 strains lacking nef by intravirion reverse transcription. J Virol 75, 12081-12087.

Kim, S., Ikeuchi, K., Byrn, R., Groopman, J., Baltimore, D., 1989. Lack of a negative influence on viral growth by the nef gene of human immunodeficiency virus type 1. Proc Natl Acad Sci U S A 86, 9544-9548.

Kirchhausen, T., 2000. Clathrin. Annu Rev Biochem 69, 699-727.

Kirchhoff, F., 2010. Immune evasion and counteraction of restriction factors by HIV-1 and other primate lentiviruses. Cell Host Microbe 8, 55-67.

Kirchhoff, F., Greenough, T.C., Brettler, D.B., Sullivan, J.L., Desrosiers, R.C., 1995. Brief report: absence of intact nef sequences in a long-term survivor with nonprogressive HIV-1 infection. N Engl J Med 332, 228-232.

Kirchhoff, F., Schindler, M., Specht, A., Arhel, N., Munch, J., 2008. Role of Nef in primate lentiviral immunopathogenesis. Cell Mol Life Sci 65, 2621-2636.

Kotov, A., Zhou, J., Flicker, P., Aiken, C., 1999. Association of Nef with the human immunodeficiency virus type 1 core. J Virol 73, 8824-8830.

Krausslich, H.G., Schneider, H., Zybarth, G., Carter, C.A., Wimmer, E., 1988. Processing of in vitro-synthesized gag precursor proteins of human immunodeficiency virus (HIV) type 1 by HIV proteinase generated in Escherichia coli. J Virol 62, 4393-4397.

Krautkramer, E., Giese, S.I., Gasteier, J.E., Muranyi, W., Fackler, O.T., 2004. Human immunodeficiency virus type 1 Nef activates p21-activated kinase via recruitment into lipid rafts. J Virol 78, 4085-4097.

Kupzig, S., Korolchuk, V., Rollason, R., Sugden, A., Wilde, A., Banting, G., 2003. Bst-2/HM1.24 is a raft-associated apical membrane protein with an unusual topology. Traffic 4, 694-709.

Laguette, N., Benichou, S., Basmaciogullari, S., 2009. Human immunodeficiency virus type 1 Nef incorporation into virions does not increase infectivity. J Virol 83, 1093-1104.

Lama, J., Mangasarian, A., Trono, D., 1999. Cell-surface expression of CD4 reduces HIV-1 infectivity by blocking Env incorporation in a Nef- and Vpu-inhibitable manner. Curr Biol 9, 622-631.

Lamers, S.L., Fogel, G.B., Huysentruyt, L.C., McGrath, M.S., 2010. HIV-1 nef protein visits B-cells via macrophage nanotubes: a mechanism for AIDS-related lymphoma pathogenesis? Curr HIV Res 8, 638-640.

Lang, S.M., Iafrate, A.J., Stahl-Hennig, C., Kuhn, E.M., Nisslein, T., Kaup, F.J., Haupt, M., Hunsmann, G., Skowronski, J., Kirchhoff, F., 1997. Association of simian immunodeficiency virus Nef with cellular serine/threonine kinases is dispensable for the development of AIDS in rhesus macaques. Nat Med 3, 860-865.

Lanier, L.L., 2005. Missing self, NK cells, and The White Album. J Immunol 174, 6565.

Le Guern, M., Levy, J.A., 1992. Human immunodeficiency virus (HIV) type 1 can superinfect HIV-2-infected cells: pseudotype virions produced with expanded cellular host range. Proc Natl Acad Sci U S A 89, 363-367.

Le Tortorec, A., Neil, S.J., 2009. Antagonism to and intracellular sequestration of human tetherin by the human immunodeficiency virus type 2 envelope glycoprotein. J Virol 83, 11966-11978.

Lee, C.M., Gala, S., Stewart, G.J., Williamson, P., 2008. The proline-rich region of HIV-1 Nef affects CXCR4-mediated chemotaxis in Jurkat T cells. Viral Immunol 21, 347-354.

Lindemann, D., Wilhelm, R., Renard, P., Althage, A., Zinkernagel, R., Mous, J., 1994. Severe immunodeficiency associated with a human immunodeficiency virus 1 NEF/3'-long terminal repeat transgene. J Exp Med 179, 797-807.

Littman, D.R., 1987. The structure of the CD4 and CD8 genes. Annu Rev Immunol 5, 561-584.

Lopez, L.A., Yang, S.J., Hauser, H., Exline, C.M., Haworth, K.G., Oldenburg, J., Cannon, P.M., 2010. Ebola virus glycoprotein counteracts BST-2/Tetherin restriction in a sequence-independent manner that does not require tetherin surface removal. J Virol 84, 7243-7255.

Louis, J.M., Weber, I.T., T^zsÈr, J., Clore, G.M., Gronenborn, A.M., 2000. HIV-1 protease: maturation, enzyme specificity, and drug resistance. Adv Pharmacol 49, 111-146.

Lu, X., Wu, X., Plemenitas, A., Yu, H., Sawai, E.T., Abo, A., Peterlin, B.M., 1996. CDC42 and Rac1 are implicated in the activation of the Nef-associated kinase and replication of HIV-1. Curr Biol 6, 1677-1684.

Lu, X., Yu, H., Liu, S.H., Brodsky, F.M., Peterlin, B.M., 1998. Interactions between HIV1 Nef and vacuolar ATPase facilitate the internalization of CD4. Immunity 8, 647-656.

Luo, T., Douglas, J.L., Livingston, R.L., Garcia, J.V., 1998. Infectivity enhancement by HIV-1 Nef is dependent on the pathway of virus entry: implications for HIV-based gene transfer systems. Virology 241, 224-233.

Mahlknecht, U., Deng, C., Lu, M.C., Greenough, T.C., Sullivan, J.L., O'Brien, W.A., Herbein, G., 2000. Resistance to apoptosis in HIV-infected CD4+ T lymphocytes is mediated by macrophages: role for Nef and immune activation in viral persistence. J Immunol 165, 6437-6446.

Malim, M.H., Emerman, M., 2008. HIV-1 accessory proteins--ensuring viral survival in a hostile environment. Cell Host Microbe 3, 388-398.

Mandic, R., Fackler, O.T., Geyer, M., Linnemann, T., Zheng, Y.H., Peterlin, B.M., 2001. Negative factor from SIV binds to the catalytic subunit of the V-ATPase to internalize CD4 and to increase viral infectivity. Mol Biol Cell 12, 463-473.

Mangasarian, A., Foti, M., Aiken, C., Chin, D., Carpentier, J.L., Trono, D., 1997. The HIV-1 Nef protein acts as a connector with sorting pathways in the Golgi and at the plasma membrane. Immunity 6, 67-77.

Mangino, G., Percario, Z.A., Fiorucci, G., Vaccari, G., Manrique, S., Romeo, G., Federico, M., Geyer, M., Affabris, E., 2007. In vitro treatment of human monocytes/macrophages with myristoylated recombinant Nef of human immunodeficiency virus type 1 leads to the activation of mitogen-activated protein kinases, IkappaB kinases, and interferon regulatory factor 3 and to the release of beta interferon. J Virol 81, 2777-2791.

Manninen, A., Saksela, K., 2002. HIV-1 Nef interacts with inositol trisphosphate receptor to activate calcium signaling in T cells. J Exp Med 195, 1023-1032.

Mansouri, M., Viswanathan, K., Douglas, J.L., Hines, J., Gustin, J., Moses, A.V., Fruh, K., 2009. Molecular mechanism of BST2/tetherin downregulation by K5/MIR2 of Kaposi's sarcoma-associated herpesvirus. J Virol 83, 9672-9681.

Mariani, R., Skowronski, J., 1993. CD4 down-regulation by nef alleles isolated from human immunodeficiency virus type 1-infected individuals. Proc Natl Acad Sci U S A 90, 5549-5553.

McNatt, M.W., Zang, T., Hatziioannou, T., Bartlett, M., Fofana, I.B., Johnson, W.E., Neil, S.J., Bieniasz, P.D., 2009. Species-specific activity of HIV-1 Vpu and positive selection of tetherin transmembrane domain variants. PLoS Pathog 5, e1000300.

Michel, N., Allespach, I., Venzke, S., Fackler, O.T., Keppler, O.T., 2005. The Nef protein of human immunodeficiency virus establishes superinfection immunity by a dual strategy to downregulate cell-surface CCR5 and CD4. Curr Biol 15, 714-723.

Miller, M.D., Warmerdam, M.T., Ferrell, S.S., Benitez, R., Greene, W.C., 1997. Intravirion generation of the C-terminal core domain of HIV-1 Nef by the HIV-1 protease is insufficient to enhance viral infectivity. Virology 234, 215-225.

Miller, M.D., Warmerdam, M.T., Page, K.A., Feinberg, M.B., Greene, W.C., 1995. Expression of the human immunodeficiency virus type 1 (HIV-1) nef gene during HIV-1 production increases progeny particle infectivity independently of gp160 or viral entry. J Virol 69, 579-584.

Mitchell, R.S., Chaudhuri, R., Lindwasser, O.W., Tanaka, K.A., Lau, D., Murillo, R., Bonifacino, J.S., Guatelli, J.C., 2008. Competition model for upregulation of the major histocompatibility complex class II-associated invariant chain by human immunodeficiency virus type 1 Nef. J Virol 82, 7758-7767.

Mitchell, R.S., Katsura, C., Skasko, M.A., Fitzpatrick, K., Lau, D., Ruiz, A., Stephens, E.B., Margottin-Goguet, F., Benarous, R., Guatelli, J.C., 2009. Vpu antagonizes BST-2-mediated restriction of HIV-1 release via beta-TrCP and endo-lysosomal trafficking. PLoS Pathog 5, e1000450.

Nabel, G., Baltimore, D., 1987. An inducible transcription factor activates expression of human immunodeficiency virus in T cells. Nature 326, 711-713.

Navia, M.A., Fitzgerald, P.M., McKeever, B.M., Leu, C.T., Heimbach, J.C., Herber, W.K., Sigal, I.S., Darke, P.L., Springer, J.P., 1989. Three-dimensional structure of aspartyl protease from human immunodeficiency virus HIV-1. Nature 337, 615-620.

Nayak, D.P., Hui, E.K., 2004. The role of lipid microdomains in virus biology. Subcell Biochem 37, 443-491.

Neil, S.J., Eastman, S.W., Jouvenet, N., Bieniasz, P.D., 2006. HIV-1 Vpu promotes release and prevents endocytosis of nascent retrovirus particles from the plasma membrane. PLoS Pathog 2, e39.

Neil, S.J., Sandrin, V., Sundquist, W.I., Bieniasz, P.D., 2007. An interferon-alpha-induced tethering mechanism inhibits HIV-1 and Ebola virus particle release but is counteracted by the HIV-1 Vpu protein. Cell Host Microbe 2, 193-203.

Neil, S.J., Zang, T., Bieniasz, P.D., 2008. Tetherin inhibits retrovirus release and is antagonized by HIV-1 Vpu. Nature 451, 425-430.

Niederman, T.M., Hastings, W.R., Ratner, L., 1993. Myristoylation-enhanced binding of the HIV-1 Nef protein to T cell skeletal matrix. Virology 197, 420-425.

Noviello, C.M., Pond, S.L., Lewis, M.J., Richman, D.D., Pillai, S.K., Yang, O.O., Little, S.J., Smith, D.M., Guatelli, J.C., 2007. Maintenance of Nef-mediated modulation of major histocompatibility complex class I and CD4 after sexual transmission of human immunodeficiency virus type 1. J Virol 81, 4776-4786.

Olivetta, E., Percario, Z., Fiorucci, G., Mattia, G., Schiavoni, I., Dennis, C., J‰ger, J., Harris, M., Romeo, G., Affabris, E., Federico, M., 2003. HIV-1 Nef induces the release of inflammatory factors from human monocyte/macrophages: involvement of Nef endocytotic signals and NF-kappa B activation. J Immunol 170, 1716-1727.

Olivetta, E., Pugliese, K., Bona, R., D'Aloja, P., Ferrantelli, F., Santarcangelo, A.C., Mattia, G., Verani, P., Federico, M., 2000. cis expression of the F12 human immunodeficiency virus (HIV) Nef allele transforms the highly productive NL4-3 HIV type 1 to a replication-defective strain: involvement of both Env gp41 and CD4 intracytoplasmic tails. J Virol 74, 483-492.

Pandori, M., Craig, H., Moutouh, L., Corbeil, J., Guatelli, J., 1998. Virological importance of the protease-cleavage site in human immunodeficiency virus type 1 Nef is independent of both intravirion processing and CD4 down-regulation. Virology 251, 302-316.

Pandori, M.W., Fitch, N.J., Craig, H.M., Richman, D.D., Spina, C.A., Guatelli, J.C., 1996. Producer-cell modification of human immunodeficiency virus type 1: Nef is a virion protein. J Virol 70, 4283-4290.

Partin, K., Zybarth, G., Ehrlich, L., DeCrombrugghe, M., Wimmer, E., Carter, C., 1991. Deletion of sequences upstream of the proteinase improves the proteolytic processing of human immunodeficiency virus type 1. Proc Natl Acad Sci U S A 88, 4776-4780.

Percario, Z., Olivetta, E., Fiorucci, G., Mangino, G., Peretti, S., Romeo, G., Affabris, E., Federico, M., 2003. Human immunodeficiency virus type 1 (HIV-1) Nef activates STAT3 in primary human monocyte/macrophages through the release of soluble factors: involvement of Nef domains interacting with the cell endocytotic machinery. J Leukoc Biol 74, 821-832.

Percherancier, Y., Lagane, B., Planchenault, T., Staropoli, I., Altmeyer, R., Virelizier, J.L., Arenzana-Seisdedos, F., Hoessli, D.C., Bachelerie, F., 2003. HIV-1 entry into T-cells is not dependent on CD4 and CCR5 localization to sphingolipid-enriched, detergent-resistant, raft membrane domains. J Biol Chem 278, 3153-3161.

Pettit, S.C., Clemente, J.C., Jeung, J.A., Dunn, B.M., Kaplan, A.H., 2005. Ordered processing of the human immunodeficiency virus type 1 GagPol precursor is influenced by the context of the embedded viral protease. J Virol 79, 10601-10607.

Pettit, S.C., Everitt, L.E., Choudhury, S., Dunn, B.M., Kaplan, A.H., 2004. Initial cleavage of the human immunodeficiency virus type 1 GagPol precursor by its activated protease occurs by an intramolecular mechanism. J Virol 78, 8477-8485.

Piguet, V., Chen, Y.L., Mangasarian, A., Foti, M., Carpentier, J.L., Trono, D., 1998. Mechanism of Nef-induced CD4 endocytosis: Nef connects CD4 with the mu chain of adaptor complexes. Embo J 17, 2472-2481.

Piguet, V., Gu, F., Foti, M., Demaurex, N., Gruenberg, J., Carpentier, J.L., Trono, D., 1999. Nef-induced CD4 degradation: a diacidic-based motif in Nef functions as a lysosomal targeting signal through the binding of beta-COP in endosomes. Cell 97, 63-73.

Pitcher, C., Honing, S., Fingerhut, A., Bowers, K., Marsh, M., 1999. Cluster of differentiation antigen 4 (CD4) endocytosis and adaptor complex binding require activation of the CD4 endocytosis signal by serine phosphorylation. Mol Biol Cell 10, 677-691.

Pizzato, M., Helander, A., Popova, E., Calistri, A., Zamborlini, A., Pal˘, G., Gˆttlinger, H.G., 2007. Dynamin 2 is required for the enhancement of HIV-1 infectivity by Nef. Proc Natl Acad Sci U S A 104, 6812-6817.

Pizzato, M., Popova, E., Gottlinger, H.G., 2008. Nef can enhance the infectivity of receptor-pseudotyped human immunodeficiency virus type 1 particles. J Virol 82, 10811-10819.

Popik, W., Alce, T.M., 2004. CD4 receptor localized to non-raft membrane microdomains supports HIV-1 entry. Identification of a novel raft localization marker in CD4. J Biol Chem 279, 704-712.

Popov, S., Strack, B., Sanchez-Merino, V., Popova, E., Rosin, H., Gˆttlinger, H.G., 2011. Human Immunodeficiency Virus Type 1 and Related Primate Lentiviruses Engage Clathrin through Gag-Pol or Gag. J Virol 85, 3792-3801.

Qi, M., Aiken, C., 2008. Nef enhances HIV-1 infectivity via association with the virus assembly complex. Virology 373, 287-297.

Quaranta, M.G., Mattioli, B., Giordani, L., Viora, M., 2006. The immunoregulatory effects of HIV-1 Nef on dendritic cells and the pathogenesis of AIDS. FASEB J 20, 2198-2208.

Reid, P.A., Watts, C., 1992. Constitutive endocytosis and recycling of major histocompatibility complex class II glycoproteins in human B-lymphoblastoid cells. Immunology 77, 539-542.

Ritter, G.D., Jr., Yamshchikov, G., Cohen, S.J., Mulligan, M.J., 1996. Human immunodeficiency virus type 2 glycoprotein enhancement of particle budding: role of the cytoplasmic domain. J Virol 70, 2669-2673.

Roeth, J.F., Collins, K.L., 2006. Human immunodeficiency virus type 1 Nef: adapting to intracellular trafficking pathways. Microbiol Mol Biol Rev 70, 548-563.

Roeth, J.F., Williams, M., Kasper, M.R., Filzen, T.M., Collins, K.L., 2004. HIV-1 Nef disrupts MHC-I trafficking by recruiting AP-1 to the MHC-I cytoplasmic tail. J Cell Biol 167, 903-913.

Rollason, R., Korolchuk, V., Hamilton, C., Schu, P., Banting, G., 2007. Clathrin-mediated endocytosis of a lipid-raft-associated protein is mediated through a dual tyrosine motif. J Cell Sci 120, 3850-3858.

Ross, T.M., Oran, A.E., Cullen, B.R., 1999. Inhibition of HIV-1 progeny virion release by cell-surface CD4 is relieved by expression of the viral Nef protein. Curr Biol 9, 613-621.

Rudolph, J.M., Eickel, N., Haller, C., Schindler, M., Fackler, O.T., 2009. Inhibition of T-cell receptor-induced actin remodeling and relocalization of Lck are evolutionarily conserved activities of lentiviral Nef proteins. J Virol 83, 11528-11539.

Saksela, K., Cheng, G., Baltimore, D., 1995. Proline-rich (PxxP) motifs in HIV-1 Nef bind to SH3 domains of a subset of Src kinases and are required for the enhanced growth of Nef+ viruses but not for down-regulation of CD4. Embo J 14, 484-491.

Sawai, E.T., Baur, A.S., Peterlin, B.M., Levy, J.A., Cheng-Mayer, C., 1995. A conserved domain and membrane targeting of Nef from HIV and SIV are required for association with a cellular serine kinase activity. J Biol Chem 270, 15307-15314.

Schindler, M., Munch, J., Brenner, M., Stahl-Hennig, C., Skowronski, J., Kirchhoff, F., 2004. Comprehensive analysis of nef functions selected in simian immunodeficiency virus-infected macaques. J Virol 78, 10588-10597.

Schindler, M., Munch, J., Kutsch, O., Li, H., Santiago, M.L., Bibollet-Ruche, F., Muller-Trutwin, M.C., Novembre, F.J., Peeters, M., Courgnaud, V., Bailes, E., Roques, P., Sodora, D.L., Silvestri, G., Sharp, P.M., Hahn, B.H., Kirchhoff, F., 2006. Nef-mediated suppression of T cell activation was lost in a lentiviral lineage that gave rise to HIV-1. Cell 125, 1055-1067.

Schindler, M., W¸rfl, S., Benaroch, P., Greenough, T.C., Daniels, R., Easterbrook, P., Brenner, M., M¸nch, J., Kirchhoff, F., 2003. Down-modulation of mature major histocompatibility complex class II and up-regulation of invariant chain cell surface expression are well-conserved functions of human and simian immunodeficiency virus nef alleles. J Virol 77, 10548-10556.

Schmokel, J., Sauter, D., Schindler, M., Leendertz, F.H., Bailes, E., Dazza, M.C., Saragosti, S., Bibollet-Ruche, F., Peeters, M., Hahn, B.H., Kirchhoff, F., 2011. The presence of a vpu gene and the lack of Nef-mediated downmodulation of T cell receptor-CD3 are not always linked in primate lentiviruses. J Virol 85, 742-752.

Schorr, J., Kellner, R., Fackler, O., Freund, J., Konvalinka, J., Kienzle, N., Krausslich, H.G., Mueller-Lantzsch, N., Kalbitzer, H.R., 1996. Specific cleavage sites of Nef proteins from human immunodeficiency virus types 1 and 2 for the viral proteases. J Virol 70, 9051-9054.

Schubert, U., Anton, L.C., Bacik, I., Cox, J.H., Bour, S., Bennink, J.R., Orlowski, M., Strebel, K., Yewdell, J.W., 1998. CD4 glycoprotein degradation induced by human immunodeficiency virus type 1 Vpu protein requires the function of proteasomes and the ubiquitin-conjugating pathway. J Virol 72, 2280-2288.

Schwartz, O., Marechal, V., Danos, O., Heard, J.M., 1995. Human immunodeficiency virus type 1 Nef increases the efficiency of reverse transcription in the infected cell. J Virol 69, 4053-4059.

Silvestri, G., Paiardini, M., Pandrea, I., Lederman, M.M., Sodora, D.L., 2007. Understanding the benign nature of SIV infection in natural hosts. J Clin Invest 117, 3148-3154.

Simmons, A., Aluvihare, V., McMichael, A., 2001. Nef triggers a transcriptional program in T cells imitating single-signal T cell activation and inducing HIV virulence mediators. Immunity 14, 763-777.

Simmons, A., Gangadharan, B., Hodges, A., Sharrocks, K., Prabhakar, S., Garcia, A., Dwek, R., Zitzmann, N., McMichael, A., 2005. Nef-mediated lipid raft exclusion of UbcH7 inhibits Cbl activity in T cells to positively regulate signaling. Immunity 23, 621-634.

Skowronski, J., Parks, D., Mariani, R., 1993. Altered T cell activation and development in transgenic mice expressing the HIV-1 nef gene. Embo J 12, 703-713.

Sol-Foulon, N., Esnault, C., Percherancier, Y., Porrot, F., Metais-Cunha, P., Bachelerie, F., Schwartz, O., 2004. The effects of HIV-1 Nef on CD4 surface expression and viral infectivity in lymphoid cells are independent of rafts. J Biol Chem 279, 31398-31408.

Sousa, A.E., Carneiro, J., Meier-Schellersheim, M., Grossman, Z., Victorino, R.M., 2002. CD4 T cell depletion is linked directly to immune activation in the pathogenesis of HIV-1 and HIV-2 but only indirectly to the viral load. J Immunol 169, 3400-3406.

Stolp, B., Abraham, L., Rudolph, J.M., Fackler, O.T., 2010. Lentiviral Nef proteins utilize PAK2-mediated deregulation of cofilin as a general strategy to interfere with actin remodeling. J Virol 84, 3935-3948.

Strack, B., Calistri, A., Craig, S., Popova, E., G^ttlinger, H.G., 2003. AIP1/ALIX is a binding partner for HIV-1 p6 and EIAV p9 functioning in virus budding. Cell 114, 689-699.

Stumptner-Cuvelette, P., Morchoisne, S., Dugast, M., Le Gall, S., Raposo, G., Schwartz, O., Benaroch, P., 2001. HIV-1 Nef impairs MHC class II antigen presentation and surface expression. Proc Natl Acad Sci U S A 98, 12144-12149.

Swann, S.A., Williams, M., Story, C.M., Bobbitt, K.R., Fleis, R., Collins, K.L., 2001. HIV-1 Nef blocks transport of MHC class I molecules to the cell surface via a PI 3-kinase-dependent pathway. Virology 282, 267-277.

Swigut, T., Greenberg, M., Skowronski, J., 2003. Cooperative interactions of simian immunodeficiency virus Nef, AP-2, and CD3-zeta mediate the selective induction of T-cell receptor-CD3 endocytosis. J Virol 77, 8116-8126.

Swigut, T., Iafrate, A.J., Muench, J., Kirchhoff, F., Skowronski, J., 2000. Simian and human immunodeficiency virus Nef proteins use different surfaces to downregulate class I major histocompatibility complex antigen expression. J Virol 74, 5691-5701.

Swingler, S., Mann, A., Jacque, J., Brichacek, B., Sasseville, V.G., Williams, K., Lackner, A.A., Janoff, E.N., Wang, R., Fisher, D., Stevenson, M., 1999. HIV-1 Nef mediates lymphocyte chemotaxis and activation by infected macrophages. Nat Med 5, 997-103.

Tang, J., Wong, R.N., 1987. Evolution in the structure and function of aspartic proteases. J Cell Biochem 33, 53-63.

Thoulouze, M.I., Sol-Foulon, N., Blanchet, F., Dautry-Varsat, A., Schwartz, O., Alcover, A., 2006. Human immunodeficiency virus type-1 infection impairs the formation of the immunological synâpse. Immunity 24, 547-561.

Tobiume, M., Takahoko, M., Yamada, T., Tatsumi, M., Iwamoto, A., Matsuda, M., 2002. Inefficient enhancement of viral infectivity and CD4 downregulation by human immunodeficiency virus type 1 Nef from Japanese long-term nonprogressors. J Virol 76, 5959-5965.

Tobiume, M., Tokunaga, K., Kiyokawa, E., Takahoko, M., Mochizuki, N., Tatsumi, M., Matsuda, M., 2001. Requirement of nef for HIV-1 infectivity is biased by the expression levels of Env in the virus-producing cells and CD4 in the target cells. Arch Virol 146, 1739-1751.

Tripathi, P., Agrawal, S., 2007. The role of human leukocyte antigen E and G in HIV infection. Aids 21, 1395-1404.

Van Damme, N., Goff, D., Katsura, C., Jorgenson, R.L., Mitchell, R., Johnson, M.C., Stephens, E.B., Guatelli, J., 2008. The interferon-induced protein BST-2 restricts HIV-1 release and is downregulated from the cell surface by the viral Vpu protein. Cell Host Microbe 3, 245-252.

VandeWoude, S., Apetrei, C., 2006. Going wild: lessons from naturally occurring T-lymphotropic lentiviruses. Clin Microbiol Rev 19, 728-762.

Varin, A., Manna, S.K., Quivy, V., Decrion, A.Z., Van Lint, C., Herbein, G., Aggarwal, B.B., 2003. Exogenous Nef protein activates NF-kappa B, AP-1, and c-Jun N-terminal kinase and stimulates HIV transcription in promonocytic cells. Role in AIDS pathogenesis. J Biol Chem 278, 2219-2227.

Vendrame, D., Sourisseau, M., Perrin, V., Schwartz, O., Mammano, F., 2009. Partial inhibition of human immunodeficiency virus replication by type I interferons: impact of cell-to-cell viral transfer. J Virol 83, 10527-10537.

Verkade, P., Simons, K., 1997. Robert Feulgen Lecture 1997. Lipid microdomains and membrane trafficking in mammalian cells. Histochem Cell Biol 108, 211-220.

von Schwedler, U.K., Stuchell, M., M¸ller, B., Ward, D.M., Chung, H.Y., Morita, E., Wang, H.E., Davis, T., He, G.P., Cimbora, D.M., Scott, A., Kr‰usslich, H.G., Kaplan, J., Morham, S.G., Sundquist, W.I., 2003. The protein network of HIV budding. Cell 114, 701-713.

Wang, C.Y., Mayo, M.W., Korneluk, R.G., Goeddel, D.V., Baldwin, A.S., 1998. NF-kappaB antiapoptosis: induction of TRAF1 and TRAF2 and c-IAP1 and c-IAP2 to suppress caspase-8 activation. Science 281, 1680-1683.

Wang JK, K.E., Verdin E, Trono D., 2000. The Nef protein of HIV-1 associates with rafts and primes T cells for activation. Proc Natl Acad Sci U S A 97, 394-399.

Wang, J.K., Kiyokawa, E., Verdin, E., Trono, D., 2000. The Nef protein of HIV-1 associates with rafts and primes T cells for activation. Proc Natl Acad Sci U S A 97, 394-399.

Warrilow, D., Tachedjian, G., Harrich, D., 2009. Maturation of the HIV reverse transcription complex: putting the jigsaw together. Rev Med Virol 19, 324-337.

Warrilow, D., Warren, K., Harrich, D., 2010. Strand transfer and elongation of HIV-1 reverse transcription is facilitated by cell factors in vitro. PLoS One 5, e13229.

Weber, I.T., 1990. Comparison of the crystal structures and intersubunit interactions of human immunodeficiency and Rous sarcoma virus proteases. J Biol Chem 265, 10492-10496.

Welker, R., Harris, M., Cardel, B., Kr‰usslich, H.G., 1998. Virion incorporation of human immunodeficiency virus type 1 Nef is mediated by a bipartite membrane-targeting signal: analysis of its role in enhancement of viral infectivity. J Virol 72, 8833-8840.

Willey, R.L., Maldarelli, F., Martin, M.A., Strebel, K., 1992. Human immunodeficiency virus type 1 Vpu protein induces rapid degradation of CD4. J Virol 66, 7193-7200.

Wonderlich, E.R., Williams, M., Collins, K.L., 2008. The tyrosine binding pocket in the adaptor protein 1 (AP-1) mu1 subunit is necessary for Nef to recruit AP-1 to the major histocompatibility complex class I cytoplasmic tail. J Biol Chem 283, 3011-3022.

Wu, X., Liu, H., Xiao, H., Conway, J.A., Hehl, E., Kalpana, G.V., Prasad, V., Kappes, J.C., 1999. Human immunodeficiency virus type 1 integrase protein promotes reverse transcription through specific interactions with the nucleoprotein reverse transcription complex. J Virol 73, 2126-2135.

Xu, W., Santini, P.A., Sullivan, J.S., He, B., Shan, M., Ball, S.C., Dyer, W.B., Ketas, T.J., Chadburn, A., Cohen-Gould, L., Knowles, D.M., Chiu, A., Sanders, R.W., Chen, K., Cerutti, A., 2009. HIV-1 evades virus-specific IgG2 and IgA responses by targeting systemic and intestinal B cells via long-range intercellular conduits. Nat Immunol 10, 1008-1017.

Xu, X.N., Laffert, B., Screaton, G.R., Kraft, M., Wolf, D., Kolanus, W., Mongkolsapay, J., McMichael, A.J., Baur, A.S., 1999. Induction of Fas ligand expression by HIV involves the interaction of Nef with the T cell receptor zeta chain. J Exp Med 189, 1489-1496.

Yang, S.J., Lopez, L.A., Hauser, H., Exline, C.M., Haworth, K.G., Cannon, P.M., 2010. Anti-tetherin activities in Vpu-expressing primate lentiviruses. Retrovirology 7, 13.

Yi, L., Rosales, T., Rose, J.J., Chowdhury, B., Knutson, J.R., Venkatesan, S., 2010. HIV-1 Nef binds a subpopulation of MHC-I throughout its trafficking itinerary and down-regulates MHC-I by perturbing both anterograde and retrograde trafficking. J Biol Chem 285, 30884-30905.

Zhang, F., Wilson, S.J., Landford, W.C., Virgen, B., Gregory, D., Johnson, M.C., Munch, J., Kirchhoff, F., Bieniasz, P.D., Hatziioannou, T., 2009. Nef proteins from simian immunodeficiency viruses are tetherin antagonists. Cell Host Microbe 6, 54-67.

Zheng, Y.H., Plemenitas, A., Fielding, C.J., Peterlin, B.M., 2003. Nef increases the synthesis of and transports cholesterol to lipid rafts and HIV-1 progeny virions. Proc Natl Acad Sci U S A 100, 8460-8465.

2

The Role of Human Immunodeficiency Virus Type 1 (HIV-1) Proteins and Antiretroviral Drug Therapy in HIV-1-Induced Oxidative Stress

Edna Maria Vissoci Reiche and Andréa Name Colado Simão
Clinical Immunology and Molecular Diagnosis Laboratories, University Hospital of Londrina, State University of Londrina, Brazil

1. Introduction

Over 33 million people worldwide are infected with human immunodeficiency virus type 1 (HIV-1). In addition, over 2.7 million new cases are diagnosed each year with half of these infections occurring in individuals younger than 25 years (UNAIDS, 2008). Fortunately, since the emergence of highly active antiretroviral therapy (HAART) in 1996, morbidity and mortality associated with HIV-1 infection have been markedly decreased. HIV-1 infected patients have demonstrated dramatic decreases in viral burden and opportunistic infections, and an overall increase in life expectancy. Despite the positive HAART-associations outcomes, including the improvement of the clinical course, prognosis, and survival of patients infected with HIV-1, it has become increasingly clear that HIV-1 infected patients have an enhanced risk for developing noninfectious consequences of HIV-1 infection over time. In the last few years, lipodystrophy, characterized by redistribution of body fat, and insulin resistance, have been reported in many HIV-1 infected patients, and their relationship with antiretroviral drugs and HIV-1 infection *per se* have become a subject of debate and researches worldwide. Evidence suggests that HIV-1 infected patients are under chronic oxidative stress that may be involved in the development and progression of the disease. Oxidative stress is enhanced by the chronic inflammation that is associated with activation of lymphocytes and phagocytes, and is accompanied by the direct or indirect effects of several opportunistic pathogens. In addition, HIV-1 proteins and various components of current HAART regimes contribute to oxidative stress-induced disturbances such as cardiovascular disease (including metabolic syndrome and endothelial dysfunction), neurological disorders (HIV-1 dementia), and ocular complications (retinopathy). Cardiovascular complications are been recognized with increasing frequency and are associated with the greatest risk of death in HIV-1 patients. Studies demonstrated that not only do various components of HAART contribute to endothelial cell damage and vascular dysfunction in patients, but also the viral proteins themselves increase cardiovascular risk. HIV-1-associated cardiovascular disease progression is thus most likely a multifactorial process, resulting from a combination of distinct HIV-1 proteins as well as various components of current multidrug antiretroviral therapy (Kline et al., 2008).

It is estimated that one-third of adults infected with HIV-1 develop dementia (Janssen et al., 1992). It was reported that oxidative stress has been demonstrated in the brain and cerebrospinal fluid (CSF) from HIV-1 infected individuals, showing important implications for therapeutic approaches for HIV-1-induced dementia (HIVD).
The aim of this chapter is to review the roles of both HIV-1 proteins and antiretroviral drugs in the development of oxidative stress-induced disturbances such as cardiovascular disease and neurological disorders. For this purpose, studies, *in vitro* and *in vivo*, were identified by a systematic search through PubMed for English-language literature, included original and review articles published up to 2011.

2. Oxidative stress and biomarkers

Oxidative stress is defined as an imbalance between the antioxidant and pro-oxidant systems with the shift towards the pro-oxidant system. Oxidative stress is also defined as the modification and accumulation of biological molecules altered by various kinds of reactive oxygen species (ROS) and reactive nitrogen species (RNS). ROS and RNS affect gene transcription and cell growth/proliferation, and they have been considered intercellular signal molecules.
ROS and RNS are highly reactive, toxic oxygen or nitrogen moieties, respectively, such hydroxyl radical, peroxyl radical, superoxide anion, hydrogen peroxide, nitric oxid (NO), and peroxynitrite. The half-life of ROS species varies from nanoseconds for the hydroxyl radical to seconds for NO and peroxyl radicals. Because of the differences in half-lives, the ROS reactivity differs from the aqueous environment in which they were formed to reacting deep within the membrane (Pocernich et al., 2005).
In biological systems, the cellular membrane constitutes in a main target of the ROS and RNS. In addition to the cellular membrane, other intracellular membranes are important target of the oxidative stress such as mitochondrial, nuclear and endoplasmic reticulum membranes that can suffer the lesive action of the ROS and RNS by changing their form and function. Not only enzymes but also receptors and transport proteins can be important early targets of oxidative damage. While most ROS do not diffuse more than a few femtometres (fm), the lipid peroxides that are resulted from the ROS-induced peroxidation of membrane phospholipids, such as malondialdehyde (MDA), can transverse the circulation and cell membranes, with resultant dysfunction of vital cellular processes including membrane transport and mitochondrial respiration (Haliwell, 1987).
ROS can attack double bonds in polyunsaturated fatty acids (PUFAs), inducing lipid peroxidation (LPO), which may result in more oxidative cellular damage. LPO has been defined as the oxidative deterioration of polyunsaturated lipids and its measurement is a laboratorial approach for determining oxidative stress. Peroxides and aldehydes generated are not only passive biomarkers of oxidative stress, but also cytotoxic products (Zwart et al., 1999).
MDA is a three carbon, low molecular weight aldehyde that can be produced from free radicals that attack on PUFAs of biological membranes. The determination of MDA is used for monitoring LPO in biological samples. LPO has been the focus of attention in recent researches because it was commonly thought that the thiobarbituric acid (TBA) test, the commonest assay of LPO *in vitro*, measures free MDA. It arises largely from peroxidation of PUFAs with more than two double bonds, such as linolenic, arachidonic and docosahexaenoic acids. MDA can also be formed enzimatically during eicosanoid

metabolism. Under physiological conditions, proteins are more readily attacked by MDA than are free amino acids, resulting in modification of several residues, especially lysine, as well as intra- and intermolecular protein cross-links.

One particular class of toxic products of LPO is the isoprostanes, a series of prostaglandin-like compounds formed during peroxidation of arachidonic acid. Because they are structurally similar to prostaglandin F2α, isoprostanes are collectively referred as F2-isoprostane. F2-isoprostane is useful marker of LPO and can be measured in human plasma and urine (Halliwell & Gutteridge, 1999).

Collectively, ROS can lead to oxidation of proteins, and DNA, peroxidation of lipids, and ultimately cell death (Butterfield et al., 2001). These protein carbonyl moieties result from a direct oxidation of many amino acids such as lysine, arginine, histidine, proline and threonine, β-scission of the peptide backbone, or from binding of the LPO product 4-hydroxy-2-nonenal (HNE) to proteins. Alterations in proteins can lead to aggregation, changes in secondary and tertiary structure, susceptibility to proteolysis, fragmentation, and loss-of function. LPO produces large amounts of aldehydes, such as HNE, MDA, and acrolein, and leads to isoprostanes formation (Butterfield et. al, 2002). HNE and acrolein contribute to membrane damage and cell death induced by various oxidative insults, and through alterations of protein structure, these molecules are capable of inhibiting DNA, RNA, and protein synthesis, glycolysis, and degradation of enzymes (Pocernick et al., 2005).

ROS produce a multiplicity of change in proteins, including oxidation of -SH groups, hydroxylation of thyrosine and phenylalanine, conversion of methionine to its sulphoxide and generation of protein peroxides. Several assays for damage to specific amino acid residues in proteins have been developed and can be used to assess steady-state levels of oxidative protein damage *in vivo*. The carbonyl assay is a general approach for evaluating oxidation protein damage. It is based on the fact that several ROS attack amino acid residues in proteins that results products with carbonyl groups, which can be measured after reaction with 2,4-dinitrophenylhydrazine (Halliwell & Gutteridge, 1999). Oxidative stress also increases the levels of protein oxidation measured by the Advanced Oxidation Protein Products (AOPPs). AOPPs are novel biomarkers of oxidative damage and are considered as reliable markers to estimate de degree of oxidant-mediated protein damage. AOPPs resulted from the interaction between oxidants and plasma proteins with the oxidation of amino acid residues such as tyrosine, leading to the formation of dityrosine-containing protein cross-linking products detected by spectrophotometry (Witko-Sarsat et al., 1998). Neutrophils that constitute the most important source of chlorined oxidants due to their high content in myeloperoxidase might be involved in plasma AOPPs formation. *In vivo* plasma levels of AOPPs closely correlate with level of dityrosine, a hallmark of oxidized proteins, and with pentosidine, a marker of protein glycation closely related with oxidative stress (Witko-Sarsat et al., 1998).

2.1 NO and HIV-1 infection

NO is a free-radical gas, a diffusible messenger that displays a variety of physiological functions, including vasorelaxation, bronchodilatation, inhibition of platelet aggregation, and neurotransmission (Radi, 2004). Additionally, it appears to be involved in the macrophage-dependent killing of intracellular parasites and functions as a tumoricidal and antimicrobial molecule *in vitro* and *in vivo* (Torre et al., 2002). NO represents an important component of the host immune response against DNA and RNA viral infections, including HIV-1 infection (Mannick et al., 1995).

NO is synthesized by the family of enzymes called nitric oxide synthase (NOS). Various isoenzymes of NOS, such as endothelial nitric oxide synthase (eNOS), inducible NOS (iNOS), and neuronal NOS (nNOS) are localized in endothelium, macrophages, and the brain, respectively. In normal endothelial cells, the amino acid L-arginine is constitutively converted to L-citrulline and NO by eNOS.

The iNOS expression is increased by oxidative stress or pro-inflammatory cytokines (Nathan, 1997). However, interleukin 1 beta (IL-1β), interleukin 6 (IL-6), interferon alfa-2b (IFN-α2b), interferon gamma (IFN-γ), and interleukin 17 (IL-17) induce iNOS, whereas transforming growth factor beta (TGF-β), interleukin 4 (IL-4), interleukin 10 (IL-10), interleukin 11 (IL-11), and interleukin 13 (IL-13) suppress the induction of NO released from macrophages (Torre et al., 2002). In addition, HIV-1 also stimulates NO production by human macrophages, inasmuch as concentration of recombinant gp120 HIV-1 envelope glycoprotein *in vitro* increases production of NO by human monocyte-derived macrophages (Pietraforte et al., 1994).

The excessive production of NO by iNOS may contribute to tissue damage in several inflammatory and infectious diseases and this damage may be the price to pay for equipping so many host cells with the ability to deploy this compound against infections. Although NO production can be increased by the iNOS, the biodisponibility of NO can be impaired because NO is consumed in a reaction with superoxide anion yielding a strong oxidant species, the peroxynitrite ($ONOO^{-}$), which in turn accelerates the LPO reaction (Li et al., 2007; Tao et al., 2007). Peroxynitrite production is also supported by the elevated levels of nitrotyrosine, a marker of endogenous peroxynitrite generation found in both human and animal models (Yamaguchi et al., 2006).

Since NO is a very labile free radical with a half-life of only a few seconds and is rapidly oxidized by tissue oxygen to the stable end products, nitrite (NO_2^-) and nitrate (NO_3^-), it is difficult to measure NO levels in the tissue directly with real time. NO can be evaluated by several methods, including the assessment of NO metabolite (NOx) levels. Commonly, serum NO levels are assessed on the basis of nitrite and nitrate concentration according to the Griess reaction supplemented by the enzymatic reduction of nitrate to nitrite with cadmium (Guevara et al., 1998; Navarro-Gonzales et al., 1998). Following up the changes in nitrite/nitrate levels in the human tissues and plasma samples can be an important tool in understanding NO involvement.

Although NO is an important mediator of the immune response against microorganisms, NO that is produced during the infectious diseases may be also deleterious, particularly in HIV-1 infection where may contribute to AIDS pathogenesis by enhancing viral replication in lymphocytes (Jimenez et al., 2001) and monocytes (Blond et al., 2000), increasing lymphocyte apoptosis (Mossalayi et al., 1999), and participating in the pathogenesis of AIDS-related dementia complex (Adamson et al., 1996). A study demonstrated impaired iNOS mRNA expression and NO levels in peripheral blood mononuclear cells from HIV-1 infected patients, either *in vivo* or *in vitro* HIV-1 infection of normal cells (Cairoli et al., 2008). Low levels of NO have been implicated in lymphocyte activation and proliferation (Barbul et al., 1990). NO donors such as sodium nitroprusside and to a lesser degree gaseous NO, increase lymphocyte uptake of glucose (an early event during lymphocyte activation), stimulate TNF-α production and the transcriptional nuclear factor kappa beta (NF-kB) binding activity, and enhance activity of tyrosine kinase, p56, which is implicated in lymphocyte signaling events (Lander et al., 1993). Paradoxically, high concentrations of NO, which occur following macrophage activation, suppress antigen presenting cell activity and T cell proliferation (Holt et al., 1991).

In addition, vascular dysfunction and damage have been shown to be associated with impaired endothelial NO metabolism and function. Therefore, iNOS-derived NO mediates the inflammatory response and has been shown to cause vascular dysfunction in a number of experimental models (Gunnett et al., 2003).

The data of NO levels obtained in HIV-1 infected individual samples are controversial. Groeneveld et al. (1996) have shown that serum nitrate concentrations are higher in asymptomatic HIV-1 infected patients than in healthy individuals. In addition, increased production of NO was correlated with RNA-HIV-1 viral load and activation of mononuclear phagocytes in HIV-1 infected patients. Torre et al. (1996a, 1996b) have shown that NO production is increased in AIDS patients with opportunistic infection, whereas nitrite concentrations were normal in asymptomatic patients. These authors have also confirmed increased production of NO and IL-1β, TNF-α, and IFN-γ in the sera of children with HIV-1 infection and they postulated that the increase in the concentration of these cytokines may represent a substantial stimulation of NO production. Zangerle et al. (1995) noted high nitrite and nitrate concentrations in 39 patients with AIDS without opportunistic infections, especially in those with lower $CD4^+$ T cell counts, whereas in asymptomatic patients no such increase was seen. However, a previous study showed no altered endogenous nitrate formation in eight patients with AIDS, most of whom had opportunistic infections (Evans et al., 1994).

However, some aspects must be taken in to account when these apparent controversial results are discussed including the fact that the oxidative stress was evaluated in HIV-1 infected individuals that differed in the clinical course of the disease and in the presence or absence of opportunistic infections. Increases in the NO production may not be observed due the consume resources by the oxidative stress. Anyway, further studies may be necessary to confirm these previous results.

2.2 Antioxidants

To neutralize the damaging oxidative stress, natural antioxidant systems have evolved, including enzymes like glutathione (GSH) peroxidase, glutathione reductase, glutathione transferase, superoxide dismutase (SOD), S-methyl transferase, and catalase. Protection against free radicals can also come from small non-protein, cellular antioxidants, nonenzymatic, such as vitamin C, vitamin E, carotenoids, flavonoids, thioredoxin, and uric acid (Butterfield, et al., 1997).

GSH is a tripeptide (γ glutamate-cysteine-glycine) present in high concentrations in all mammalian cells that has many critical protective and metabolic functions. GSH detoxifies electrophilic metabolites of xenobiotics and protects cells from the toxic effects of free radicals and ROS (Bleuter, 1989). It is also important in the immune response against infections and plays an important role in lymphocyte proliferation, antibody-dependent and cell-mediated cytotoxicity, and protection of lymphocytes against superoxides that are produced to destroy invading pathogens (Droge et al., 1991; Smyth, 1991). N-acetyl-L-cysteine (NAC) acts as an indirect precursor of GSH by raising levels of cysteine, a precursor of GSH. Whey proteins have been shown to increase GSH levels in human, most likely by supplying the amino acid cysteine necessary for the synthesis of GSH (Pocernich et al., 2005).

Vitamin C represents the major water-soluble antioxidant in the human body. Ascorbate protects cell components from free radical damage by quenching water soluble radicals, scavenging lipid-peroxidation-derived radicals, or reducing tocopherol radical to tocopherol (Stehbens, 2004).

SOD is an endogenous antioxidant that catalyses de dismutation of the superoxide anion radical (Stambullian et al., 2007).

Vitamin E, a potent chain breaking lipid soluble antioxidant, reacts with lipid peroxyl radical eventually by terminating the peroxidation chain reaction and thereby by reducing oxidative damage. Vitamin E acts as an antioxidant on biomembranes and it is the principal lipid soluble chain-breaking antioxidant in mitochondria, microsomes, and lipoproteins.

Selenium is an essential nonmetal trace element that is necessary for normal immune function. Selenium also increases the GSH peroxidase activity and its deficiency diminishes cell-mediated immunity and depresses B-cell function (Stehbens, 2004).

3. Evidences of oxidative stress in individuals infected with HIV-1

The hallmark of HIV-1 infection is the cellular $CD4^+$ T cell immunodeficiency; however, the real cause of the loss of these cells is unknown. The most widely accepted hypothesis is that HIV-1 primes the cell to apoptotic death. Different agents appear to trigger apoptosis in $CD4^+$ T cells, including viral protein, inappropriate secretion of inflammatory cytokines by activated macrophages and toxins produced by opportunistic microorganisms. Since oxidative stress can also induce apoptosis, it can be hypothesized that it could participate in $CD4^+$ T cell apoptosis observed in AIDS (Reppeto et al., 1996).

Evidence suggested that HIV-1 infected patients are under chronic oxidative stress. This effect is subsequent to depletion of endogenous antioxidant moieties and to an increased production of ROS. Observation of the multiple pathogenic interactions between ROS and the HIV-1 has drawn attention to the possibility that these types of the interaction may play a role in the pathogenesis of many other viruses as well. ROS has been suggested to be involved in many aspects of HIV-1 disease pathogenesis, including increase viral replication, inflammatory response, decrease of immune cell proliferation, loss of immune function, chronic weight loss, and increase sensitivity to drug toxicity. In addition, antiretroviral combination therapy increases protein oxidation as well as the level of oxidative stress already present in HIV-1 infection (Ngondi et al., 2006).

One aspect of the role of ROS in HIV-1 pathogenesis is the positive modulatory effect on the immune activation, important both in eradication of viral infection but also in immune-induced cellular injury (Schwarz, 1996). HIV-1 infections causes a chronic inflammation as shown by high plasma levels of pro and inflammatory cytokines, chemokines and ROS in seropositive individuals (Israel & Gougerot-Pocidalo, 1997). Increased production of ROS such as superoxide anion, hydroxyl radical, and hydrogen peroxide may be related to an increased activation of polymorphonuclear leukocytes during HIV-1 infection or influenced by the pro-oxidant effect of pro-inflammatory cytokines produced by activated macrophages during the course of HIV-1 infection (Das et al., 1990)

In HIV-1 infected patients, the increased oxidative stress has been implicated in increased HIV-1 transcription through the activation of NF-kB. NF-kB is bound to kinase inhibitor nuclear factor-kB (IkB) in the cytoplasm in its active form, but various factors, such as TNF-

α and ROS, can cause the release of NF-kB from factor IkB, and NF-kB translocates to the nucleus and binds to DNA. In this way, the NF-kB is available to bind in the nuclear DNA and to induce HIV-1 gene transcription (Schereck et al., 1991). Thus, oxidative stress may potentially be involved in the pathogenesis of HIV-1 infection through direct effects of cells and through interactions with NF-kB and activation of HIV-1 replication (Greenspan & Aruoma, 1994; Israel & Gougerot-Pocidalo, 1997).

The activation of phagocytes induced by HIV-1 is associated with oxidative stress, not only because ROS are released but also the fact that activated phagocytes may release pro-oxidant cytokines, such as TNF-α and IL-1, which promote iron uptake by the monocyte macrophage system. TNF-α is synthesized in infected host cells, produces pro-oxidant effects in mitochondria, and inhibits mitochondrial respiration at Site II, the site of superoxide production (Schulze-Osthoff et al., 1992). Other cytokine that is involved in the oxidative stress is the IL-1. Activated monocytes produce IL-1 that stimulates neutrophils to release lysosomal proteins, including lactoferrin. This protein rapidly binds iron and this complex accumulates in the monocyte macrophage system. If the accumulated iron exceeds cellular iron-binding capacity, unbound pro-oxidant iron could interact with the superoxide via Fenton's reaction and produces hydroxyl radicals (Halliwell, 1987).

Oxidative stress biomarkers (pro-oxidants and antioxidants) have been investigated in HIV-1 patients serum samples; however, previous studies show inconsistent findings regarding MDA levels in these patients. One study showed significantly elevated serum MDA concentration in HIV-1 infected patients, where HIV-1 symptomatic presented higher levels than asymptomatic patients, suggesting that the infection results in oxidative stress of the host lipids (Sönnerborg et al., 1988; Jordão Júnior et al. 1998; Suresh et al., 2009). The oxidative stress was evaluated by the LPO and GSH plasma levels in 150 HIV-1 infected individuals and in 30 healthy controls, and the results showed that the mean LPO plasma levels were significantly higher in HIV-1 infected individuals as compared to healthy controls, and the mean GSH level in HIV-1 infected individuals was significantly lower compared to healthy controls. In addition, there was a significant positive correlation between absolute $CD4^+$ T cells and GSH levels. However, there was no significant difference in the levels of LPO and GSH among HIV-1 infected individuals receiving antiretroviral therapy (ART) and those without ART (Wanchu et al., 2009).

Jordão Júnior et al. (1998) evaluated 28 serologically positive HIV-1 patients, 16 patients with AIDS (with < $200/mm^3$ $CD4^+$T lymphocytes) and 12 HIV-1 infected and asymptomatic patients (with $200\text{-}500/mm^3$ $CD4^+$ T lymphocytes). The control group consisted of 11 healthy individuals. All individuals showed normal plasma vitamin A levels. However, urinary excretion of vitamin A and MDA was higher in AIDS patients than in HIV-1 asymptomatic patients and considerably higher than in the control subjects. Therefore, the severe oxidative stress that occurs in the HIV-1 seropositive patients in comparison with seronegative individuals can exert a role in the progression of disease (Suresh et al., 2009)

4. Oxidative stress and cardiovascular diseases associated with HIV-1 infection

Endothelium dysfunction is an initial step in the development of cardiovascular diseases, especially atherosclerosis, and is associated with an increase in oxidative stress. HIV-1 infection is associated with increased ROS production and chronic oxidative stress, suggesting a role of ROS in HV-1-induced endothelial cells dysfunction. Evidence from experimental, observational, and clinical studies suggests that HIV-1 infection itself and the associated pro-inflammatory response can increase the risk of cardiovascular disease.

Multiple mechanisms, both specific and overlapping ways, are proposed to explain how HIV-1 proteins damage the endothelium, considering that viral genome contains nine main genes (*gag, pol, env, tat, rev, vpu, vpr, vif,* and *nef*) and encodes for approximately 15 mature HIV-1 proteins that may interact with any number of unique targets. Proteolytic cleavage of the Gag-Pol precursor protein yields the major structural components of the viral core including matrix p17, capsid p24, nucleocapsides p9 and p6, reverse transcriptase (RT), protease and integrase. Proteolytic cleavage of Env produces the important envelope glycoprotein (gp) gp120 and gp41. The remaining genes encode for the regulatory proteins Tat and Rev, and the accessory proteins Vpu, Vpr, Vif, and Nef (Greene, 1991).

The gp120, Tat, Vpu, and Nef proteins exert some important effects on endothelial cell homeostasis (reviewed by Kline & Sutliff, 2008). HIV-1 proteins can activate several inflammatory pathways in the vascular wall with cytokines release and expression of endothelial molecules, such as vascular cell adhesion molecule-1 (VCAM-1), intracellular adhesion molecule-1 (ICAM-1), and E-selectin (Seigneur et al., 1997; Greenwood et al., 1998; Wolf et al. 2002). The gp120 increases the expression of ICAM-1, but not VCAM-1 or E-selectin, in human coronary artery, lung, brain, umbilical vein, and dermal microvascular endothelial cells. The gp120 also induces the apoptosis in human coronary endothelial cells, the adhesion of monocytes and lymphocytes to the endothelium; gp120 increases the endothelium permeability through cytoskeletal rearrangement, downregulation of tight junction proteins, and increases ROS production. The gp120 negatively affects endothelium function through the production of potent vasoconstrictors. The nonstructural Tat protein contains 86-101 amino acids that are formed from two exons. The first exon contributes to the first 72 amino acids and acts as a transacting nuclear regulatory protein actively secreted by infected cells that is essential for viral replication.

Similar to gp120, Tat protein can promote the apoptosis, monocyte chemoattraction and adhesion, endothelium permeability, proliferation, angiogenesis, and an increase in the expression of matrix metalloproteinases and ROS. It has been demonstrated that viral Tat protein liberated by HIV-1 infected cells interferes with calcium homeostasis, activates caspases and induces mitochondrial generation and accumulation of ROS, all being important events in the apoptotic cascade of several cell types. When activated, peripheral blood T lymphocytes are induced to express Fas/APO-1/CD95 receptor that mediates apoptosis when binding to Fas ligand. $CD4^+$ T cell subset depletion in HIV-1/AIDS patients is the most dramatic effect of apoptosis mediated by redox abnormalities and induction of Fas/APO-1/CD95 receptor expression (Westendorp et al., 1995; Kruman et al., 1998; Jaworowski & Crowe, 1999).

In patients with uncontrolled HIV-1 infection, vasculitis are also observed in small blood vessels, aneurysms in medium and large arteries, significantly decreased levels of high-density lipoprotein (HDL) cholesterol, and elevated plasma levels of von Willebrand factor, plasminogen activator inhibitor-1 (PAI-1) antigen, and tissue-type plasminogen activator (tPA). Although HIV-1 is likely not vasculotropic, the virus affects endothelium homeostasis and function in important ways (Kline & Sutliff, 2008).

The vascular endothelium is exposed continually to a number of viral stimuli in the bloodstream. These stimuli include: a) HIV-1 infected $CD4^+$ T cells, monocytes, and macrophages; b) freely circulating HIV-1 viruses; c) HIV-1 proteins released upon host cell lysis; d) actively secreted proteins (Tat and gp120); and e) viral-induced pro-inflammatory cytokines. HIV-1-induced cytokines may also activate the endothelium, leading to enhanced production of ROS, and the release of chemoattractant at localized areas of vascular inflammation. HIV-1-infected individuals have higher plasma levels of hydroperoxides and MDA compared with uninfected individuals, indicating enhanced ROS-mediated LPO. HIV-1-induced ROS likely contribute to endothelium dysfunction through direct effects on the endothelium and/or indirectly through monocytes and macrophages contacting the vessel wall.

Elevated ROS in HIV-1 infection could play a role in various signaling pathways, among which are the mitogen-activated protein kinases (MAPKs). MAPKs are serine and threonine protein kinases, which have three major classes, including extracellular signal-regulated kinase 1 and 2 (ERK1/2) and BMK1, c-Jun N-terminal protein kinases (JNKs) and p38. ROS may mediate activation of MAPKs in a variety of cells, leading to changes in gene expression (Blenis, 1993), downregulation of eNOS, and alteration of other gene expression involved in the endothelium dysfunction. Taken together, these data indicate that oxidative stress activating MAPKs, may be one of the major mechanisms in HIV-1-induced endothelium dysfunction.

HIV-1 infected patients have low circulating levels of the antioxidant vitamin C, cysteine, and GSH, a situation that can lead to increased oxidative stress. Serum GSH levels and GSH peroxidase activity are decreased in HIV-1 patients, while the LPO product MDA, DNA fragmentation in lymphocytes, and total hydroperoxides are increased. These observations have important implications for therapeutic approaches. Clinical studies showed that selenium, and β carotene supplementation increased serum GSH levels. Dual vitamin C and E supplementation reduced plasma LPO and oxidative stress in HIV-1 patients. Supplementation with α-tocopherol or selenium also decreased plasma viral load and improved T-cell numbers and viability (Suresh et al, 2009; Stehbens, 2004).

These clinical findings suggest that vascular endothelial cells are exposed to ROS in the form of LPO products, pro-inflammatory cytokines, activated monocytes and phagocytes of the immune system.

5. Oxidative stress associated with antiretroviral therapy

Nearly 25 antiretroviral drugs have been licensed for the treatment of HIV-1 infected individuals and are divided mechanistically into five classes (reviewed by Estrada & Portilla, 2011): (1) nucleoside reverse transcriptase inhibitor (NRTI), including abacavir (ABC), didanosine (ddI), stavudine (d4T), lamivudine (3TC), tenofovir (TDF), zidovudine (AZT), and emtricitabine (FTC); (2) non-nucleoside reverse transcriptase inhibitor (NNRTI), including nevirapine (NVP), efavirenz (EFV), and etravirine (ETR); (3) protease inhibitor (PI) including atazanavir (ATV), indinavir (IDV), lopinavir (LPV), nelfinavir (NFV), ritonavir (RTV), saquinavir (SQV), darunavir (DRV), fosamprenavir (FPV), and amprenavir (APV); (4) fusion inhibitor, entry inhibitor (chemokine receptor CCR5 inhibitor) including enfuvirtide and maraviroc (MVC); and (5) integrase inhibitor, including raltegravir (RAL).

The HAART for management of HIV-1 infection that includes an association of the two NRTIs plus NNRTI and/or PI has been effective to suppress HIV-1 replication.

In addition to HIV-1 proteins, the HAART has been related with endothelium dysfunction. Experimental evidence shows that NRTIs are associated with endothelial cell toxicity. NRTIs induce oxidative stress, particularly mitochondrial ROS and seem to play an important role in cell culture and animal models of endothelial cell toxicity. However, clinical evidence for NRTIs-induced vascular/endothelium toxicity is indirect and difficult to define because NRTIs are not prescribed as monotherapy, and cardiovascular effects are often attributed to other components of HAART, such as PIs.

NNRTIs show, in general, the best lipid profile of all anti –HIV-1 drugs because they are associated with an increase in HDL cholesterol and a significant reduction in cholesterol total/HDL ratio. NNRTIs have been associated with a lower risk of myocardial infarction (Worm et al., 2010) that could hypothetically be associated with this good lipid profile. As regard NVP, the mechanism of HDL elevation may be an increase in the production of apolipoprotein-A1 (Franssen et al., 2009).

Among the PIs, lopinavir/ritonavir (LVP/r), DRV/r and ATV alone or with RTV (ATV/r) are the most extensively used PIs at present. PIs-associated dyslipidemia is a frequent class-related event and can limit their use especially in patients with preexisting increase cardiovascular risk. A meta-analysis of major clinical trials performed in 2009 (Hill et al., 2009) showed that patients randomized to LPV/r or FPV/r presented greater elevations of total cholesterol and triglycerides than those assigned to SQV/r, ATV/r, or DRV/r, without differences in low density lipoprotein cholesterol (LDL) or HDL.

The integrase inhibitor RAL is the first drug in this class and shows a remarkable lack of relevant adverse effects (Emery et al., 2010) and patients treated with RAL presented a significantly low frequency of dyslipidemia (Martinez et al., 2010).

Trials with HIV-1 patients treated with chemokine receptor-5 antagonist MVC have shown that it has a very favorable safety profile. MCV was associated with non-significant changes in total cholesterol, LDL, HDL and triglycerides (Cooper et al., 2010).

The LDL receptor (LDLR) plays a critical role in the regulation of plasma LDL levels (Brown & Goldstein, 1986). By controlling LDL catabolism, the number of hepatic LDLR directly governs the plasma LDL concentrations. The expression of LDLR is under metabolic, hormonal, and genetic control. Growth hormone (GH), insulin, estrogen, and dehydroepiandrosterone (DHEA) may stimulate LDLR expression and reduce plasma LDL cholesterol levels (Wade et al., 1989; Pascale et al., 1995; Rudling et al., 1996). As important hormonal modifications occur in HIV-1 infected patients with lipodystrophy, particularly insulin and DHEA changes, the LDLR expression was evaluated in HIV-1 infected patients with or without lipodystrophy. The results revealed that HIV-1-lipodystrophy is associated with a low expression of LDLR and this decreased expression seems independent of DHEA or insulin secretion (Petit et al., 2002). These authors suggested that the decreased expression of the LDLR may be explained by a direct effect of the PIs (Rayes et al., 1996). Other hypothesis is that PIs lead to dyslipidemia by inhibition of LDLR-related protein (LRP), which has homology to the catalytic site of HIV-1 protease, to which all PIs bind (Carr et al., 1998).

The HIV-1 infected patients with lipodystrophy have also an impaired metabolism of DHEA and insulin, all known to regulate LDLR (Meyer et al., 1998; Walli et al., 1998; Christeff et al., 1999; Behrens et al., 1999;). In addition, HIV-1 PIs also can modulate the function of certain LDLR family members. Tran et al., (2003) demonstrated that among six different HIV-1 PIs evaluated, NFV, specifically, decreased mRNA and protein levels of the LDLR and LRP, which, in turn, decreased the functional activity of these two receptors. One study showed that exposure of IDV or NFV, combined with AZT and EFV, increased ICAM-1 gene expression and that concomitant exposure to TNF-α further increased ICAM-1 gene expression, VCAM-1, and endothelial-leukocyte adhesion molecule cell surface protein levels (Mondal et al., 2004).

The Figure 1 shows the production of NO induced by HIV-1 and its viral proteins (mainly gp120 and Tat proteins), and by PIs in promoting beneficial and deleterious effects in the host cells. The NO is synthesized via MAPK signaling pathway when the macrophage is activated by pro-inflammatory and inflammatory cytokines as result of the HIV-1 infection. Despite the protective effect of NO in the host defense against this pathogen, NO has been associated with a harmful effect in many systems.

The Figure 2 summarizes some of the effects of ROS and RNS that are induced by HIV-1 proteins and PIs.

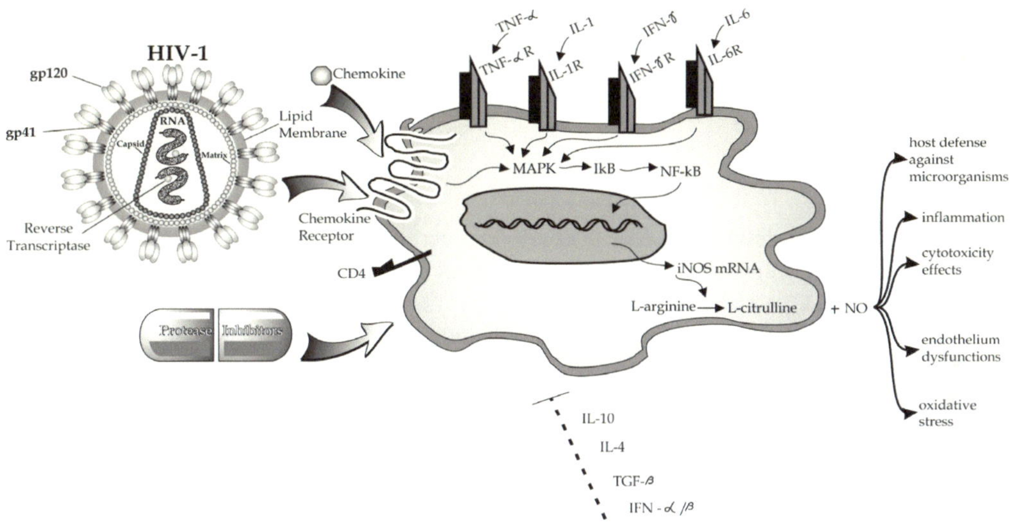

Fig. 1. Mechanisms of nitric oxide (NO) production induced by human immunodeficiency virus type 1 (HIV-1) and the viral proteins (mainly gp120 and Tat proteins), and by protease inhibitors (PIs) in promoting beneficial and deleterious effects in the host cells. TNF-α: tumor necrosis factor alpha;

TNF-αR: tumor necrosis factor alpha receptor; IL-1: interleukin 1; IL-1R: interleukin 1 receptor; IFN-γ: interferon gamma; IFN-γR: interferon gamma receptor; IL-6: interleukin 6; IL-6R: interleukin 6 receptor; IL-10: interleukin 10; IL-4: interleukin 4; TGF-β: transforming growth factor beta; IFN-α/β: interferon alpha and interferon beta; MAPK: mitogen-activated protein kinase; IkB: kinase inhibitor nuclear factor-kB; transcriptional nuclear factor kappa beta (NF-kB); iNOS: inducible nitric oxide synthase; mRNA: messenger RNA; NO: nitric oxide.

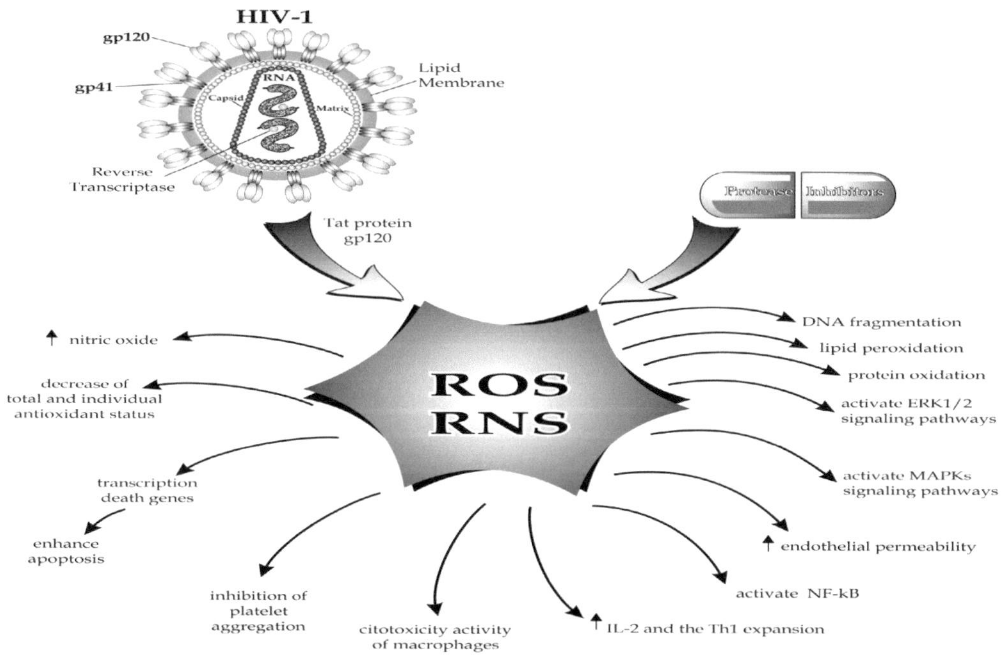

Fig. 2. Beneficial and deleterious effects of the endogenous reactive oxygen species (ROS) and reactive nitrogen species (RNS) that are induced by both human immunodeficiency virus type 1 (HIV-1) proteins and the antiretroviral therapy with protease inhibitors (PIs). ROS and RNS that are accumulated by the imbalance of oxidants and antioxidants molecules exert effects on DNA, lipids, proteins, signaling pathways, immune system cells, neuronal tissue, and endothelial functions. ERK1/2: extracellular signal-regulated kinase 1 and 2; MAPKs: mitogen-activated protein kinases; transcriptional nuclear factor kappa beta (NF-kB).

6. Molecular mechanisms of HIV-1 PI-induced endothelium dysfunction

It is well-known that the endothelium acts as the first-line defense mechanism against the development of vascular injury. It exerts is protective action through modulation of vascular tone, vascular structure, and the interaction of blood components. Endothelial dysfunction may contribute to the systemic manifestations of many diseases, including atherosclerosis. Several reviews have been focused on metabolic disorders such as systemic insulin resistance, dyslipidemia, and peripheral lipodystrophy associated with endothelial dysfunction (Shankar & Dube, 2003; Koutkin & Grinspoon, 2004).

The molecular mechanisms of PIs toxicity in endothelial cells have been described in greatly detail. The effect of PIs on endothelium-depending vasorelaxation was first suggested by the significant reduction of flow-mediated vasodilatation of the brachial artery in HIV-1 infected patients receiving PIs as compared with the patients without PIs treatment (Stein et al., 2001). Other study showed that RTV, APV, or SQV individually caused a significant reduction in endothelium-dependent vasorelaxation of porcine coronary arteries (Conklin et al., 2004). The expression of eNOS was significantly decreased in porcine coronary arteries treated by RTV, SQV, and APV. In parallel, RTV also caused a significant reduction of eNOS messenger RNA (mRNA) and protein levels in cultured human coronary artery endothelial cells (Fu et al., 2005).

PIs produces serious mitochondrial disturbances as evidenced by reduced cellular respiration and ATP production, decrease mitochondrial membrane potential, increase mitochondrial production of ROS, and enhanced mitochondrial DNA (mtDNA) damage. PIs also increase endothelial cell permeability and leukocyte adhesion in cell culture models. PIs contribute to cardiovascular risk by dysregulating fat cell homeostasis that may explain the high incidence of lipodystrophy and hyperlipidemia in HIV-1 patients. PIs prevent the differentiation of preadipocytes by decreasing matrix metalloproteinase expression, inhibiting adiponectin secretion, and inhibiting triglyceride and very low-density lipoprotein (VLDL) cholesterol clearance and catabolism (Wang et al., 2007). Evidences point to adipocytes as a complex and active endocrine tissue whose secretory products, including adiponectin, play an important role in the regulation of human metabolic alterations and vascular biology (Hamdy, 2005). Adiponectin accounts for approximately 0.01% of total plasma protein and has been shown to be related to lipodystrophy, metabolic alterations, and HIV-1 PIs use. Unlike other adipocyte products, adiponectin correlates with decreased free fatty acid blood concentrations and reduced body mass index. Adiponectin provides protection from vascular diseases by inhibiting local inflammatory signals, preventing preatherogenic plaque formation, and impeding arterial wall thickening (Schondorf et al., 2005). However, HIV-1 PIs such as RTV selectively decreased expression of adiponectin (Kim et al., 2006) suggesting that hypoadiponectinemia is partially responsible for the metabolic disorders induced by HIV-1 PIs, and adiponectin or its agonists might be used for the treatment of these disorders (Xu et al., 2004) .

HIV-1 PIs may also activate different types of MAPKs in different cell types or different culture conditions (Wang et al., 2007), leading to changes in gene expression in the same manner of the HIV-1 induced ROS.

Some studies have showed high oxidative stress among the effects of HAART. Mandas et al. (2009) assessed serum oxidant and antioxidant levels in HIV-1 infected population treated with HAART and compared them with those untreated HIV-1 seropositive and HIV-1 seronegative individuals. Serum oxidant levels were significantly higher in the HIV-1 treated group as compared to untreated and control groups. In addition, a decrease of serum total antioxidant status was observed in HIV-1 treated individuals. An important result obtained is that patients who rigorously followed antiretroviral therapy have significantly higher oxidative status than those who have poor HAART adherence. These results indicate that HAART may affect oxidative stress in HIV-1 infected patients and also suggested that antiretroviral therapy may exert a synergic effect with HIV-1 in the oxidative stress induction.

Another study (Gil et al., 2010) evaluated the effect of two HAART combinations on redox indicators and on progression markers of disease. A cohort of 84 healthy and 84 HIV-1 seropositive subjects was followed for six months. Fifty-six HIV-1 seropositive subjects were distributed in group I (AZT, 3TC, IND) and group II (d4T, 3TC, NEV) according to drug combination. Biomarkers of oxidative stress were evaluated including peroxidation potential (PP), MDA, total hydroperoxides (HPO), AOPP and, percent of DNA fragmentation (% FDNA). There were also evaluated biomarkers of antioxidant status, including catalase, SOD and GSH at baseline and six months after HAART started. In this study, the concentration of antioxidants was low at baseline, and LPO index and DNA fragmentation were increased. After HAART had been started, catalase values for both groups receiving treatment showed no significant difference. For group II, all other parameters of oxidative stress were significantly higher than those for group I and the HIV-1 positive not treated, except for GSH values in group II which was lower than group I values. These data suggest poor prognostic for group II. The findings suggest that increased oxidative stress occurs additionally to persistent redox imbalance associated to HIV-1 infection during apparently successfully HAART.

HAART may increase chemically reactive species in circulation, possibly by producing more oxidized metabolites derived from the interaction between ROS and infected-cell biomolecules. This is supported by several biochemical mechanisms, such as mitochondrial interference, following treatment with HAART-NRTI and activation of the P450 hepatic system by HAART, when comprising PIs (La Asuncion et al., 1998; Kumar et al., 1999; Hulgan et al., 2003; Lewis, 2003; Cossarizza & Moyle, 2004; Day & Lewis, 2004).

7. Oxidative stress in HIV-1 infection associated with neurological disorders

The mechanisms by which HIV-1 first enters in the central nervous system (CNS) remain obscure. However, loss of blood-brain-barrier (BBB) integrity may be an important part of some of the tissue damage that accompanies HIV-1 infection of the brain, and may facilitate viral entry into the CNS. The active replication of HIV-1 into macrophages and microglia represents a reservoir for the virus and an important step for the neuropathogenesis of HIV-1 infection. This process leading to the production of inflammatory products and, in turn, to the production of an excess formation of free radical species, is involved in the subsequent increased permeability of the BBB and has been suggested to play a key role in the neuropathogenesis of HIV-1 infection. The combination of BBB damage and elevated plasma viral load is associated with neurocognitive impairment and an increased risk for development of HIV-1-induced dementia (HIVD). In addition, oxidative stress has been demonstrated in the brain and cerebrospinal fluid (CSF) from HIV-1-infected individuals and it is proposed to be a key event in the pathophysiology of HIVD.

One of the neurotoxins that is suggested to be involved in neuronal damage is NO. NO is a nitrogen free radical generates in many tissues, including the CNS, via bioconversion of L-arginine into L-citrulline by nNOS (Lamas et al., 1998). It can be released constitutively by neurons in response to many neurochemical stimuli, including excitatory neurotransmission and changes of Ca^{2+} influx (Moncada et al., 1991). NO release has been induced *in vitro* from glial cells following the addition of inflammatory cytokines and soluble antigens such as the HIV-1 coating gp120 glycoprotein (Dawson et al., 1993; Mollace & Nistico, 1995). Pro-inflammatory cytokines including IL-1, TNF-α, and IFN-γ which are released in HIV-1 infected brain tissue have been shown to upregulate the iNOS. To modulate this response, the NO formation is downregulated by the cytokines tissue grown factor beta (TGF-β), and IFN alpha/beta (IFN-α/β), according to Hua et al., (1998).

Evidences show that although the direct neurotoxic effects of NO are modest, they are greatly enhanced by reacting with superoxide anion to form peroxynitrite. Superoxide anion is produced by myeloid-monocytic cell lines following HIV-1 infection and the production of this molecule results in subsequent changes in the antioxidant status of these cells because SOD, a superoxide anion scavenger, is generated. Neurofilament, a protein that provides structural stability to neurons, is one of the target proteins of peroxynitrite and the resulting nitration results in disrupted neurofilament assembly and thus neuronal damage (Coyle & Puttfarcken, 1993).

Neurotoxic levels of ROS and RNS are especially produced by the macrophages recruited to the CNS as well as by astrocytes and glial cells activated following different stimuli such as cytokine, endotoxin, and soluble antigens in the CSN.

In vitro studies show that gp120 and Tat HIV-1 proteins can be directly toxic to human endothelial cells, compromises BBB integrity by reducing tight junction (occludin) protein expression and enhances monocytes migration across BBB. Protein oxidation was increased in the CSF of HIV-1 patients with mild and severe dementia compared to non-dement HIV-1 patients. Nitrated tyrosine residues, evidence of peroxynitrite reaction with proteins, are increased in brain of HIVD patients. Activation of cytokine receptors and oxidative stress can induce the production of ceramide from membrane sphingomyelin, and recent findings suggest that ceramide is an important mediator of apoptosis. The HIV-1 Tat protein can also induce increase of ceramide and sphingomyelin in culture neurons. Tat can be transported efficiently across the intact BBB. In HIV-1 infected astrocytes, the regulatory gene *tat* is overexpressed, and mRNA levels for Tat protein are elevated in brain extracts from individuals with HIVD. The Tat sequences from brains of patients with HAD are mutated with glutamate substitutions in the second exon, which may decrease its ability to be taken up by cells, thus increasing its extracellular concentrations and possibly neurotoxicity effects in the cell. Brain regions particularly susceptible to Tat toxicity are striatum, hippocampal dentate gyrus, and the CA3 region of the hippocampus.

Tat has been hypothesized by many studies as a potential contributor to HIVD by many mechanisms (reviewed by Pocernich et al., 2005). Tat protein released by astrocytes produces trimming of neuritis, mitochondrial dysfunction, and cell death in neurons. Tat-induced neurotoxicity is though to be mediated through excitotoxic mechanisms involving calcium. Tat can also induce markers of oxidative stress such as protein and LPO in synaptosomal membranes and neuronal cell cultures. To neutralize the oxidative stress, the GSH protects neurons against ROS directly and indirectly, and binds LPO products. GSH is the major cellular thiol participating in the maintenance of cellular redox status of the neuron and neuronal mitochondria. The biosynthesis of GSH may be compromised by Tat protein. It was hypothesized that the chronic inflammation of CSN by HIV-1, the activation of microglia, and increased lipid and protein oxidation, all observed in HIV-1 infected patients, can lead to the decrease of GSH serum levels and potentially HIVD. Low serum level of GSH is associated with poor survival in HIV-1-infected patients, while administration of GSH to HV-1-infected patients decreases mortality.

The production of superoxide anions by HIV-1 infected cells is counteracted by SOD, which, in turn, generates hydrogen peroxide (H_2O_2). Under basal conditions this is scavenged by catalase. To date, clear evidence exists that catalase activity is modified in brain tissue of AIDS patients. However, it has recently been reported that catalase is diminished in $CD8^+$ T lymphocytes from HIV-1 positive individuals, suggesting the H_2O_2 scavenger activity might be decreased during HIV-1 infection (Yano et al., 1998).

8. Antioxidant status in HIV-1 infection

Although the concentration of plasma antioxidant components can be measured individually, these measurements may be time- and cost-consuming and labor intensive. In addition, it may not accurately reflect the total antioxidant status (Wayner et al., 1987). Total antioxidant capacity considers the cumulative effect of all oxidants present in blood and any fluids (Nagy et al., 2006) and it could be evaluated by several assays including total peroxyl radical trapping antioxidant parameter (TRAP), total antioxidant capacity (TAC), ferric reducing ability (FRAP), and their variations.

It has been previously shown that the HIV-1 infected individuals are oxidative stressed and have significantly lower antioxidant concentrations than HIV-1 seronegative individuals.

There is experimental evidence that different metabolic events that occur as consequence of HIV-1 infection directly influence the consumption of antioxidant components thus contributing to the increase of oxidative stress. Studies have found impaired antioxidant defense in HIV-1 infected patients and the antioxidant depletion indicates a decrease in immune function. Cells of immune system generally require a higher antioxidant concentration than other cells to retain redox balance, and preserve integrity and function (De La Fuente et al., 2002).

There are numerous studies reporting GSH deficiency in HIV-1 infection. The concentration of GSH is low in plasma, lung epithelial lining fluid, and peripheral blood mononuclear cells of HIV-1 infected individuals (Buhl et al., 1989; Roederer et al., 1993). Studies *in vitro* have shown that low GSH levels impair T cell function and also promote HIV-1 expression, suggesting a link between GSH deficiency and progression of HIV-1 disease (Kalebic et al., 1991; Roederer et al., 1993). Poor survival rates of HIV-1 seropositive individuals with low GSH levels and improved survival when GSH was replenished were also reported (Herzenberg et al., 1997). Taken together, these data can proposed that a persistent oxidative stress leads an accelerated rate of consumption of GSH that is not matched by an equal in the rate of synthesis of the tripeptide.

Gil et al. (2003) showed both a reduction of GSH levels and an increased in MDA and total hydroperoxides levels were detected in the plasma of HIV-1 seropositive individuals. These patients also showed an increase of DNA fragmentation in lymphocytes, reduction of glutathione peroxidase, and an increase in SOD activity in erythrocytes. There are several studies of disturbed GSH metabolism in HIV-1 infected patients. Arkrust et al. (2003) showed that, during HAART, the decrease in virus load and the increase in $CD4^+$ T cell count are accompanied by both an improvement in the abnormal GSH-redox status and an increase in the subnormal levels of antioxidant vitamins. They have shown that HIV-1 infected patients are characterized by a decrease in both reduced GSH and vitamin C, the two most important hydrophilic antioxidants.

HIV-1 infection results in considerably reduced α-tocopherol concentrations and very low plasma zinc and selenium levels. Zinc and copper ions inhibit intracellular HIV-1 replication (Sprietsma, 1997). The precise mechanism by which the antioxidant effects of zinc is accomplished stems from its involvement in SOD and other enzymatic process. In humans, marked zinc deficiency strongly compromises the immune function and often enhances vulnerability to fatal opportunistic infections. It decreases $CD4^+$ T helper cell function, $CD8^+$ T cell cytotoxic activity, serum thymulin activity, and the interleukin-2 (IL-2) production by peripheral blood mononuclear cells. It also reduces the natural killer cells lytic activity, DNA repair, the antibodies formation, and macrophage and neuthrophil function. In experimental and human models, the zinc deficiency caused an imbalance between Th1 and Th2 functions resulting in decreased production of IFN-γ. These specific effects on T cell proliferation and function are not duplicated by other micronutrients (Stehbens, 2004).

Selenium deficiency diminishes cell-mediated immunity and depresses B-cell function, and it is associated with the occurrence, virulence, and disease progression to overt AIDS (Stehbens, 2004). Apoptosis of the cells is fundamental to progression of the disease that correlates with the decrease in plasma zinc, selenium, and vitamin E (Farvier et al., 1994).

Many antioxidants have been tried for AIDS therapy including selenium, vitamin C, vitamin E, lipoic acid, β carotene, whey proteins, and the epigallocatechin gallate (EGCG), the major component of green tee.

However, there are conflicting reports in the values of antioxidant vitamin E and vitamin C and SOD enzyme activity among HIV-1 infected patients in various stages in the literature (Allard et al., 1998; Stambullian et al., 2007). Suresh et al. (2009) showed that vitamin E, vitamin C, SOD, and TAC levels are decreased in HIV-1 patients, and the depletion was pronounced in HIV-1 symptomatic compared to HIV-1 asymptomatic individuals, in contrast to previous studies where were no significant differences in antioxidant vitamins in both groups (Allard et al., 1998).

McDermid et al. (2002) investigated the relation between dietary antioxidant intake and oxidative stress in clinically stable HIV-1 positive and HIV-1 negative adults. The results suggested dietary selenium intake was strongly and inversely associated with plasma MDA, but dietary antioxidant intakes were not related to peripheral blood mononuclear cell GSH concentration.

Total antioxidant status has been reduced in HIV-1 infected patients, probably due depletion of antioxidant molecules when they are consumed in the process of protecting cells against ROS induced oxidative damage in a magnitude that is related to advancement of the disease to AIDS (Ogunro et al., 2005).

Endothelial dysfunction induced by HIV-1 PIs may possible be reversed by antioxidants, including ginsenosides, selenium, curcumin (Chai et al., 2005a; Chai et al., 2005b), and resveratrol (Touzet & Philips, 2010). Therefore, it has been proposed by some researches that the oxidative stress and antioxidant status of HIV-1 seropositive patients could be monitored periodically during the disease progression. The possibility of counteracting oxidative stress by a pool of proper antioxidant plus an appropriate diet, mainly in patients whose blood antioxidant deficiencies can be easily rebalanced may have real health benefit and represent a promising way of inhibiting the progression of disease.

A new class of non-peptidic macrocyclic (MnII) complexes that possesses SOD enzymatic activity has been synthesized, which has the same activity as native SOD but can significantly cross the BBB (Salvemini et al., 1999). A SOD mimetic complex has been shown to significantly protect against the apoptotic cell death that occurs in astroglia that was incubated with supernatants of HIV-1 infected human macrophages. This effect was accompanied by a reduction of MDA concentration in astroglial cells and by a reduction of nitrotyrosine staining in these cells, showing that the effect of this mimetic complex occurred via reduction of ROS formation, and in turn, could reduce the neurodegenerative processes that occur in neuroAIDS (Mollace et al., 2001).

Many clinical trials on HIV-1 dementia have centered on drugs that block receptors or are antagonists to the neurotoxic chemokines and cytokines released from activated microglia, macrophages, and astrocytes. These drugs, including nimodipine (L-type calcium channel antagonist), peptide T (possible chemokine receptor blocker), selegiline and deprenyl (monoamine oxidase-B inhibitors), lexipafant (platelet-activating factor antagonist), and CPI-1189 (TNF antagonist), indirectly act as antioxidants by blocking the downstream effects of these neurotoxic agents that usually result in an increase of ROS, RNS, and neuronal death (Turchan et al., 2003).

The importance of micronutrients in the prevention and treatment of childhood infections is well known, and evidence is emerging that micronutrient interventions may also affect HIV-1 transmission and progression. To clarify this issue, Friis (2006) reviewed evidences on the role of micronutrient supplementation in HIV-1 transmission and progression. The author concluded that interventions to improve micronutrient intake and status could contribute to a reduction in the magnitude and impact of the global HIV-1 epidemic. However, more research is needed before specific recommendations can be made. Fawzi et al (2005) underscored that poor nutrition and HIV-1 related adverse health outcomes contribute to a vicious cycle that may be slowed down by using nutritional interventions, including vitamins and minerals. Among children, periodic supplementation with vitamin A starting at six months of age has been shown to be beneficial in reducing mortality and morbidity among both HIV-1-infected and uninfected children. Limited data exist on the role of other nutrient supplements among children. Among HIV-1 infected adults, the safety and the efficacy of vitamin A supplements need further study, although adequate dietary intake of this essential nutrient is recommended. Multivitamin supplements were efficacious in reducing adverse pregnancy outcomes and early childhood infections, and is currently provided to HIV-1 infected pregnant women in many programs. The efficacy of such supplements among HIV-1 negative pregnant women needs further study. Daily multivitamin supplements were found to reduce HIV-1 disease progression among men and women and could be provided to adults in early stages of HIV-1 disease to prolong the time before antiretroviral therapy.

In order to assess whether micronutrient supplements are effective and safe in reducing mortality and morbidity in adults and children with HIV-1 infection, 30 randomized controlled trials were selected that compared the effects of micronutrient supplements (vitamins, trace elements, and combinations of these) with other supplements, placebo or no treatment on mortality, morbidity, pregnancy outcomes, immunologic indicators, and anthropometric measures in HIV-1 infected adults and children (Irlam et al, 2005, 2010). Any adverse effects of supplementation were recorded in 30 trials involving 22,120 participants: 20 trials of single supplements (vitamin A, vitamin D, zinc, selenium) and 10 of multiple micronutrients. Eight trials were undertaken in child populations. The results of this meta-analysis showed that multiple micronutrient supplements reduced morbidity and mortality in HIV-1 infected pregnant women and their offspring and also improved early child growth in one large randomized controlled trial in Africa. Additional research is needed to determine if these are generalisable findings. Vitamin A supplementation is beneficial and safe in HIV-1 infected children, but further evidence is needed to establish if supplementation confers similar benefits in HIV-1 infected adults. Zinc is safe in HIV-1 infected adults and children. It may have similar benefits in HIV-1 infected children and adults, and uninfected children with diarrhea, as it does in HIV-1 uninfected children. Further trials of single supplements (vitamin

D, zinc, and selenium) are required to build the evidence base. The long-term clinical benefits, adverse effects, and optimal formulation of multiple micronutrient supplements require further investigation in individuals with diverse disease status.

The exogenous supply of antioxidants using novel and more-specific molecules that scavenge free radical might allow further advances in understanding the processes that underlie the pathogenesis of HIV-1 infection and thus might represent the basis for novel and potentially efficient strategies in the complementary treatment of neurological, endothelium, and cardiovascular diseases associated with the HIV-1 infection.

9. Conclusion

There is clear evidence that the gp120 and Tat HIV-1 proteins and antiretroviral drugs directly and indirectly induce oxidative stress. Damage-induced by oxidative stress in endothelial cells and neurons may be correlated with an increase in the risk of cardiovascular disease and dementia, respectively, in HIV-1 infected patients. Although differences may exists to the relative contribution and mechanisms of toxicity, the preponderance of clinical and experimental data suggest roles for both of these factors in the context of HIV-1 infection. In assessing cardiovascular risk, it is important to take into account potential contributions from both infection and therapy. To various degrees, multiple HIV-1 viral proteins and antiretroviral drugs activate cell signaling cascades, induce oxidative stress, disturb mitochondrial function, alter gene expression, and impair lipid metabolism. These changes occur in endothelial cells, in vascular muscle cells, macrophages, adipocytes, and in neuronal cells.

The main changes that have been reported by *in vivo* and *in vitro* studies are the increase of the LPO, protein oxidation, and NO metabolites, decrease in the individual antioxidants defenses such as vitamin C, vitamin E, GSH, catalase, selenium, and zinc. In addition, the total status antioxidant is also impaired in HIV-1 infected individuals. NO cannot be rigidly classified as an anti-inflammatory or pro-inflammatory molecule, but it can be considered a true inflammatory mediator. It has been also reported that oxidative stress in HIV-1 infected individuals is associated with increase of DNA fragmentation in lymphocytes, reduction of glutathione peroxidase, and an increase in SOD activity in erythrocytes.

The better knowledge of the ways in which HIV-1 proteins and antiretroviral drugs interact with each other and with the host cells, mainly the endothelial, the neuronal, and immune system cells, may contribute to discover new approaches to be associated with the antiretroviral therapies in order to prevent cardiovascular diseases and neurological disorders in HIV-1 infected individuals.

10. References

Adamson, D.C.; Wildemann, B.; Sasaki, M.; Glass, J.D.; McArthur, J.C.; Christov, V.I.; Dawson, T.M. & Dawson, V.L. (1996). Immunologic NO synthase: elevation in severe AIDS dementia and induction by HIV-1 gp 41. *Science*, Vol. 274, No. 5294, pp. 1917-1921, ISSN 0036-8075.

Barbul, A.; Lazzarou, S.A.; Efron, D.T.; Wasserkrug, H.L. & Efron, G. (1990). Arginine enhances would healing and lymphocyte immune responses in humans. *Surgery*, Vol.108, pp. 331-337, ISSN 0039-6060.

Beckman, J.S. & Koppenol, W.H. (1996). Nitric oxide, superoxide, and peroxynitrite: the good, the bad, ad ugly. *The American Journal of Physiology*, Vol.271, pp. C1424-C1437, ISSNJ 0002-9513.

Beherns, G.; Dejam, A.; Schmidt, H.; Balks, H.J.; Braasbant, G. & Körner, T. (1999). Impaired glucose tolerance, beta cell function and lipid metabolism in HIV patients under treatment with protease inhibitors. *AIDS*, Vo.13, pp. F63-F67, ISSN 0269-9370.

Beutler, E. (1989). Nutritional and metabolic aspects of glutathione. *Annual Review of Nutrition*, Vol.9, pp.287-302, ISSN 0199-9885.

Blenis, J. (1993). Signal transduction via the MAP kinases: proceed at your own RSK. *Proceedings of National Academy of Sciences USA*, Vol. 90, pp. 5889-5892, ISSN 0027-8424.

Blond, D.; Raoul, H.; Le Grand, R. & Dormont, D. (2000). Nitric oxide synthesis enhances human immunodeficiency virus replication in primary human macrophages. *Journal of Virology*, Vol.74, No.19, pp. 8904-9812, ISSN 0022-528X.

Bodgan, C. (2001). Nitric oxide and the immune response. *Nature Immunology*, Vol.2, pp. 907-916, ISSN 1529-2908.

Buhl, R.; Jaffe, H.A.; Holroyd, K.J.; Wells, F.B.; Mastrangeli, A.; Saltini, C.; Cantin, A.M. & Crystal, R.G. (1989). Systemic glutathione deficiency in symptom-free HIV-seropositive individuals. *The Lancet*, Vol. 2, No. 8675, pp. 1294-1298, ISSN 0099-5355.

Butterfield, D.A.; Castegna, A.; Lauderback, C.M. & Drake, J. (2002). Evidence that amyloid beta-peptide-induced lipid peroxidation and its sequelae in Alzheimer's disease brain contribute to neuronal death. *Neurobiology of Aging*, Vol.32, pp.655-664, ISSN 0197-4580.

Butterfield, D.A. & Stadman, E. R. (1997). Protein oxidation processes in aging brain. *Advances in Cell Aging and Gerontology*, Vol. 2, pp.161-191, ISSN 1566-3125.

Cairoli, E.; Scott-Algara, D.; Pritsch, O.; Dighiero, G. & Cayota, A. (2008). HIV-1 induced decrease of nitric oxide production and inducible nitric oxide synthase expression during *in vivo* and *in vitro* infection. *Clinical Immunology*, Vol.127, pp. 26-33, ISSN 1521-6616.

Carr, A.; Samaras, K.; Chilsom, D.J. & Cooper, D.A. (1998). Pathogenesis of HIV-1 protease inhibitor-associated peripheral lipodystrophy, hyperlipidemia, and insulin resistance. *The Lancet*, Vol.351, pp. 1881-1883, ISSN 0099-5355.

Chai, H.; Zhou, W.; Lin, P.; Lumsden, A.; Yao, Q. & Chen, C. (2005a). Ginsenosides block HIV protease inhibitor ritonavir-induced vascular dysfunction of porcine coronary arteries. *American Journal of Physiology - Heart and Circulatory Physiology*, Vol. 288, No.6, pp. H2965-2971, ISSN 0363-6135.

Chai, H.; Yan, S.; Lin, P.; Lumsden, A.B.; Yao, Q. & Chen, C. (2005b). Curcumin blocks HIV protease inhibitor ritonavir-induced vascular dysfunction in porcine coronary arteries. *Journal of the American College of Surgeons*, Vol. 200, No. 6, pp. 820-830, ISSN 1072-7515.

Christeff, N.; Melchior, J.C.; de Truchis, P.; Perronne, C.; Nunez, E.A. & Gougeon, M.L. (1999). Lipodystrophy defined by a clinical score in HIV-infected men on highly antiretroviral therapy: correlation between dyslipidemia and steroid hormone alterations. *AIDS*, Vo.13, pp. 2251-2260, ISSN 0269-9370.

Concklin, B.S.; Fu, W.; Lin, P.H.; Lumsden, A.B.; Yao, Q. & Chen, C. (2004). HIV protease inhibitor ritonavir decreases endothelium-dependent vasorelaxation and increases superoxide in porcine arteries. *Cardiovascular Research*, Vol. 63, No.1, pp.168-175, ISSN 0008-6363.

Coopper, D.; Heera, J.; Goodrich, J.; Tawadrous, M.; Saag, M.; Dejesus, E.; Clumeck, N.; Walmsley, S.; Ting, N.; Coakley, E.; Reeves, J.D.; Reyes-Teran, G.; Westby, M.; Van Der Ryst, E.; Ive, P.; Mohapi, L.; Mingrone, H.; Horban, A.; Hackman, F.; Sullivan, J. & Mayer, H. (2010). Maraviroc versus efavirenz, both in combination with zidovudine-lamivudine, for the treatment of antiretroviral-naïve subjects with CCR5-tropic HIV-1 infection. *Journal of Infectious Diseases*, Vo. 201, No.6, pp. 803-813, ISSN 0022-1899.

Cossarizza, A. & Moyle, G. (2004). Antiretroviral nucleoside and nucleotide analogues and mitochondria. *AIDS*, Vol. 18, No. 2, pp. 137-151, ISSN 0269-9370.

Coyle, J.T. & Putfarcken, P. (1993). Oxidative stress, glutamate, and neurodegenerative disorders. *Science*, Vol. 262, pp. 689-695, ISSN 0036-8075.

Das, U.N.; Podma, M.; Sogar, P.S.; Ramesh, G. & Koratkar, R. (1990). Stimulation of free radical generation in human leucocytes by various agents including tumor necrosis factor is a calmodulin-dependent process. *Biochemical and Biophysical Research Communications*, Vol. 167, No.3, pp. 1030–1036, ISSN 0006-291X.

Dawson, V.L;. Dawson, T.M.; Uhl, G.R. & Snyder, S.H. (1993). Human immunodeficiency virus type 1 coat protein neurotoxicity mediated by nitric oxide in primary cortical cultures. *Proceedings of National Academy of Sciences USA*, Vol.90, pp. 3256-3259, ISSN 0027-8424.

Day, B.J; & Lewis, W. (2004). Oxidative stress in NRTI-induced toxicity: evidence from clinical experience and experiments *in vitro* and *in vivo*. *Cardiovascular Toxicology*, Vol. 4, No. 3, pp. 207-216, ISSN 1530-7905.

De La Asunción, J.; Del Olmo, M.L.; Sastre, J.; Millán, A.; Pellín, A.; Pallardó, F.V. & Viña, J. (1998). AZT treatment induces molecular and ultrastructural oxidative damage to muscle mitochondria. Prevention by antioxidant vitamins. *The Journal of Clinical Investigation*, Vol. 102, No. 1, pp. 4-9, ISSN 0021-9738.

De La Fuente, M.; Miquel, J.; Catalán, M.P.; Victor, V.M. & Guayerbas, N. (2002). The amount of thiolic antioxidant ingestion related to improve several immune functions is higher in aged than in adult mice. *Free Radical Biology & Medicine*, Vol. 36, pp. 119-126, ISSN 0891-5849.

Droge, W.; Eck, H.P.; Gmunder, H. & Mihm, S. (1991). Modulation of lymphocytes functions and immune responses by cysteine and cysteine derivatives. *The American Journal of Medicine Supplements*, Vol. 91, No.3C, pp. 140S-144S, ISSN 0002-9343.

Emery, S. & Winston, A. (2009). Raltegravir: a new choice in HIV and new chance for research. *Lancet*, Vol.374, pp. 764-766, ISSN 0099-5355.

Estrada, V & Portilla KJ. (2011). Dyslipidemia related to antiretroviral therapy. *AIDS Reviews*, Vol.13, pp. 49-56, ISSN 0269-9370.

Evans, T.G; Rasmussen, K.; Wiebke, G. & Hibbs, J.B. (1994) Nitric oxide synthesis in patients with advanced HIV infection. *Clinical and Experimental Immunology*, Vol. 97, pp. 83-86, ISSN 0009-9104.

Favier, A.; Sappey, C.; Leclerc, P.; Faure, P. & Micoud, M. (1994). Antioxidant status and lipid peroxidation in patients infected with HIV. *Chemico-Biological Interactions*, Vol. 91, pp. 165-180, ISSN 0009-2797.

Fawzi, W.; Msamanga, G.; Spiegelman, D. & Hunter, D.J. (2005). Studies of vitamins and minerals and HIV transmission and disease progression. *The Journal of Nutrition*, Vol. 135, No. 4, pp. 938-944, ISSN 0022-3166.

Fu, W.;Chai, H.; Yao, Q. & Chen, C. (2005). Effects of HIV protease inhibitor ritonavir on vasomotor function and endothelial nitric oxide synthase expression. *Journal of Acquired immune Deficiency Syndromes*, Vol.39, No.2, pp. 152-158, ISSN 1525-4135.

Gil, L.; Tarinas, A.; Hernádez, D.; Riverón, B.V.; Pérez, D.; Tápanes, R.; Capo, V. & Pérez, J. (2010). Altered oxidative stress indexes related to disease progression marker in human immunodeficiency virus infected patients with antiretroviral therapy. *Biomedicine and Pharmacotherapy*, (in press), ISSN 0753-3322.

Gil, L.; Martínez, G.; González, I.; Tarinas, A.; Álvarez, A.; Giuliani, A.; Molina, R.; Tápanes, R.; Pérez, J. & León, O.S. (2003). Contribution to characterization of oxidative stress in HIV/AIDS patients. *Pharmacological Research*, Vol.47, pp.217-224, ISSN 1043-6618.

Greene, W.C. (1991). The molecular biology of human immunodeficiency virus type 1 infection. *The New England Journal of Medicine*, Vol. 324, pp. 308-317, ISSN 0028-4793.

Greenspan, H.C. & Aruoma, O. (1994). Could oxidative stress initiate programmed cell death in HIV infection? A role from plant derived metabolites having synergistic antioxidant activity. *Chemico-Biological Interactions*, Vol.143, pp.145-148, ISSN 0009-2797.

Greenwood, A.J.; Highes, J.; Wallace, G.; Seed, P.; Stanford, M.R. & Graham, E.M. (1998). Soluble intercellular adhesion molecule-1 (sICAM-1) and vascular cell adhesion molecule -1 (sVCAM-1) in patients with HIV/AIDS does not appear to correlate with cytomegalovirus retinitis. *International Journal of STD & AIDS*, Vol.9, No.11, pp.713-714, ISSN 0956-4624.

Groeneveld, P.H.P.; Kroon, F.P.; Nibbering, P.H.; Bruisten, S.M.; Van Swieten, P. & Van Furth, R. (1996). Increased production of nitric oxide correlates with viral load and activation of mononuclear phagocytes in HIV-infected patients. *Scandinavian Journal of Infectious Diseases*, Vol.28, pp. 341-345, ISSN 0036-5548.

Guevara, I.; Iwanejko, J.; Dembińska-Kieć, A.; Pankiewicz, J.; Wanat, A.; Anna, P.; Gołabek, I.; Bartuś, S.; Malczewska-Malec, M. & Szczudlik, A. (1998). Determination of nitrite/nitrate in human biological material by the simple Griess reaction. *Clinica Chimica Acta*, Vol. 274, No.2, pp. 177-188, ISSN 0009-8981.

Gunnett, C.A.; Heistad, D.D. & Faraci, F.M. (2003). Gene-targeted mice reveal a critical role for inducible nitric oxide synthase in vascular dysfunction during diabetes. *Stroke*, Vol. 34, pp. 2970-2974, ISSN 0039-2499.

Halliwell, B. & Gutteridge JMC. (1999). Detection of free radicals and others reactive species: trapping and fingerprinting. In: *Free Radical in Biology and Medicine*. Halliwell, B. & Gutteridge, J.M.C. (editors), pp 351-429, Oxford University Press 3th ed, ISBN, Oxford, UK, ISBN 0198500459 (Hbk),. ISBN 0198500440 (Pbk).

Hamdy, O. Lifestyle modification and endothelial function in obese subjects. (2005). *Expert Review of Cardiovascular Therapy*, Vol.3, pp.231-241, ISSN 1477-9072.

Herzenberg, L.A.; De Rosa, S.C.; Dubs, J.G.; Roederer M, Anderson MT, Ela SW, Deresinski SC, Herzenberg LA. (1997). Glutathione deficiency is associated with impaired survival in HIV disease. *Proceedings of National Academy of Science USA*, Vol. 94, No.5, pp. 1967-1972. ISSN 0027-8424.

Hill, A.; Sawyer, W. & Gazzard, B. (2009). Effects of first-line use of nucleoside analogues, efavirenz, and ritonavir boosted protease inhibitors on lipid levels. *HIV Clinical Trials*, Vol. 10, pp. 1-12, ISSN 1528-4336.

Holt, P.G.; Oliver, J.; Bilyk, N. McMenamin C, McMenamin PG, Kraal G, Thepen T. (1993). Downregulation of the antigen presenting cell function(s) of pulmonary dendritic cells *in vivo* by resident alveolar macrophages. *Journal of Experimental Medicine*, Vol. 177, No.2, pp. 397-407, ISSN 0022-1007.

Hua, L.L.; Liu, J.S.H.; Brosnan, C.F. & Lee, C.C. (1998). Selective inhibition of human glial inducible nitric oxide synthase by interferon-beta implications for multiple sclerosis. *Annals of Neurology*, Vol. 43, No.3, pp. 384-387, ISSN 1531-8249.

Hulgan T, Morrow J, D'Aquila RT, Raffanti S, Morgan M, Rebeiro P, Haas DW. (2004). Oxidative stress is increased during treatment of human immunodeficiency virus infection. *Clinical Infectious Diseases*, Vol. 4, No. 3, pp. 207-216, ISSN 1058-4838.

Irlam, J.H; Visser, M.M.; Rollins, N.N. & Siegfried, N. (2010). Micronutrient supplementation in children and adults with HIV infection. *Cochrane Database Systematic Reviews*, Vol. 12, pp. CD003650, ISSN 1469-493X.

Irlam, J.H.; Visser, M.E.; Rollins, N. & Siegfried, N. (2005). Micronutrient supplementation in children and adults with HIV infection. *Cochrane Database Systematic Reviews*, Vol. 4, pp. CD003650, ISSN 1469-493X.

Israel, N. & Gougerot-Pocidalo, M.A. (1997). Oxidative stress in human immunodeficiency virus infection. *Cellular and Molecular Life Sciences*, Vol. 53, pp. 864-870, ISSN1420-682X.

Janssen, R.S.; Nwanyamwu, O.C.; Selk, R.M. & Stehr-Green, J.K. (1992). Epidemiology of human immunodeficiency virus encephalopathy in the United States. *Neurology*, Vol.42, pp. 1472-1476, ISSN 0028-3878.

Jimenez, J.L.; Gonzalez-Nicolas, J.; Alvarez, S. Fresno M, Muñoz-Fernández MA. (2001). Regulation of human immunodeficiency virus type 1 replication in human T lymphocytes by nitric oxide. *The Journal of Virology*, Vol. 75, pp. 4655-4663, ISSN 0022-538X.

Jordão Júnior, AA; Figueiredo JF, Silveira S; Junqueira-Franco MV & Vannucchi H. (1998). Urinary excretion of vitamin A and thiobarbituric acid reactive substance in AIDS patients. *Revista do Hospital das Clínicas da Faculdade de Medicina de São Paulo*, Vol. 53, No.1, pp.11-15, ISSN 0041-8781.

Kalebic, T.; Kinter, A.; pol, G.; Anderson, M.E.; Meister, A. & Fauci, A.S. (1991). Suppression of human immunodeficiency virus expression in chronically infected monocytic cells by glutathione, glutathione ester, and N-acetylcysteine. *AIDS*, Vol. 6, pp. 815-819, ISSN 0269-9370.

Kim, R.J.; Wilson,C.G.; Wabitsch, M.; Lazar MA, Steppan CM. (2006). HIV protease inhibitor specific alterations in human adipocyte differentiation and metabolism. *Obesity*, Vol.14, No.6, pp. 949-1002, ISSN 1930-7381.

Kline, E.R. & Sutliff, R.L. (2008). The roles of HIV-1 proteins and antiretroviral drug therapy in HIV-1-associated endothelial dysfunction. *Journal of Investigative Medicine*, Vol. 56, No. 5, pp. 752-769, ISSN 1081-5589.

Koutkia, P. & Grinspoon, S. (2003). HIV-associated lipodystrophy: pathogenesis, prognosis, treatment, and controversies. *Annual Review of Medicine*, Vol. 55, pp.303-317, ISSN.

Kumar, G.N.; Dykstra, J.; Roberts. E;M.; Jayanti, V.K.; Hickman, D.; Uchic, J.; Yao, Y.; Surber, B.; Thomas, S. & Granneman, G.R. (1999). Potent inhibition of the cytochrome P450 3A-mediated human liver microsomal metabolism of a novel HIV protease inhibitor by ritonavir: a positive drug-drug interaction. *Drug Metabolism and Disposition*, Vol. 27, No. 8, pp. 902-908, ISSN 0056-9556.

Lamas, S.; Pérez-Sala, D. & Moncada, S. (1998). Nitric oxide: from discovery to the clinic. *Trends in Pharmacological Sciences*, Vol. 19, No.11, pp. 436-438, ISSN 0165-6147.

Lander, H.M.; Sehaipal, P.; Levine, D.M. & Novogrodsky, A. (1993). Activation of human peripheral blood mononuclear cells by nitric oxide-generating compounds. *The Journal of Immunology*, Vol.150, pp.1509-1516, ISSN 0022-1767.

Lewis W. (2003). Mitochondrial dysfunction and nucleoside reverse transcriptase inhibitor therapy: experimental clarifications and persistent clinical question. *Antiviral Research*, Vol.58, No. 3, pp.189-197, ISSN0166-3542.

Li, R.; Wang, W.Q.; Zhang, H.; Yang, X.; Fan, Q.; Christopher, T.A.; Lopez, B.L.; Tao, L.; Goldstein, B.J.; Gao, F. & Ma, X.L. (2007). Adiponectin improves endothelial function in hyperlipidemic rats by reducing oxidative/nitrative stress and differential regulation of eNOS/iNOS activity. *American Journal of Physiology, Endocrinology and Metabolism*, Vol.293, No.6, pp. E1703-E1708.

Mandas, A.; Iorio, E.L.; Congiu, M.G.; Balestrieri, C.; Mereu, A.; Cau, D.; Dessi, S. & Curreli, N. (2009). Oxidative imbalance in HIV-1 infected patients treated with antiretroviral therapy. *Journal of Biomedicine & Biotechnology* , Vol. 2009, pp.749575, ISSN 1110-7243.

Mannick, J.B. (1995). The antiviral role of nitric oxide. *Research Immunology*, Vol.146, pp. 693-697, ISSN 0923-2494.

Martinez, E.; Larrouse, M.; Libre, J. Gutiérrez F, Saumoy M, Antela A, Knobel H, Murillas J, Berenguer J, Pich J, Pérez I, Gatell JM & SPIRAL Study Group. (2010). Substitution of raltegravir for ritonavir-boosted protease inhibitors in HIV-infected patients: the SPIRAL study. *AIDS*, Vol. 24, No.11, pp. 1697-1707, ISSN 0269-9370

McDermid, J.M.; Lalonde, R.G.; Gray-Donald, K.; Baruchel, S. & Kubow, S. (2002). Association between dietary antioxidant intake and oxidative stress in HIV-seropositive and HIV-seronegative men and women. *Journal of Acquired Immune Deficiency Syndrome*, Vol. 29, No. 2, pp. 158-164, ISSN 1525-4135.

Meyer, L.; Rabaud, C.; Ziegler, O.; May, T. & Drouin, P. (1998). Protease inhibitors, diabetes mellitus and blood lipids. *Diabetes & Metabolism*, Vol.24, pp. 547-549, ISSN 1262-3636.

Mollace, V. & Nistico, G. (1995). Release of nitric oxide from astroglial cells: a key mechanism in neuroimmune disorders. *Advances in Neuroimmunology*, Vol. 5, pp. 421-430, ISSN 0960-5428.

Moncada, S. et al. (1991). Nitric oxide: Physiology, pathophysiology and pharmacology. *Pharmacological Reviews*, Vol. 43, pp. 109-142, ISSN 0031-6997.

Mondal, D.; Pradhan, I.; Ali, M. & Agrawal, K.C. (2004). HAART drugs induce oxidative stress in human endothelial cells and increase endothelial recruitment of mononuclear cells: exacerbation by inflammatory cytokines and amelioration by antioxidants. *Cardiovascular Toxicology*, Vol. 4, No. 3, pp. 287-302, ISSN 1530-7905.

Mossalayi, M.D.; Becherel, P.A. & Debre, P. (1999). Critical role of nitric oxide during the apoptosis of peripheral blood leukocytes from patients with AIDS. *Molecular Medicine*, Vol. 5, pp. 812-819, ISSN 1076-1551.

Nathan, C. (1007). Inducible nitric oxide synthase: what difference does it make? *The Journal of Clinical Investigation*, Vol. 100, pp. 2417-2423, ISSN 0021-9738.

Navarro-Gonzalvez,J.A.; Garcia-Benayas, C. & Arenas, J. (1998). Semi-automated measurement of nitrate in biological fluids. *Clinical Chemistry*, Vol.44, pp. 679-681, ISSN 0009-9147.

Ngondi, J.L.; Oben, J.; Etame, L.H.; Forkah, D.M. & Mbanya, D. (2006). The effect of different combination therapies on oxidative stress markers in HIV infected patients in Cameroon. *AIDS Research Therapy*, Vol.3, pp.19, ISSN 1742-6405.

Ogunro, P.S.; Ogungbamigbe, T.O.; Ajala, M.O. & Egbewale, B.E. (2005). Total antioxidant status and lipid peroxidation in HIV-1 infected patients in a rural area of south western Nigeria. *African Journal of Medicine and Medical Sciences*, Vol. 34, No.3, pp221-225, ISSN 0309-3913.

Petit, J.M.; Doung, M.; Duvillard, L.; Florentin, E.; Portier, H.; Lizard, G.; Brun, J.M.; Gambert, P. & Verges, B. (2002). LDL-receptors expression in HIV-infected patients: relations to antiretroviral therapy, hormonal status, and presence of lypodystrophy. *European Journal of Clinical Investigation*, Vol.32, pp. 354-359, ISSN 0014-2972.

Pietraforte, D.; Tritarelli, E.; Testa, U. & Minetti, M. (1994). Gp 120 HIV envelope glycoprotein increases the production of nitric oxide in human monocyte-derived macrophages. *Journal of Leukocyte Biology*, Vol. 55, pp.175-182, ISSN 0741-5400.

Pocernich, C.B.; Sultana, R.; Mohmmad-Abdul, H.; Nath, A. & Butterfield, A. (2005). HIV-dementia, Tat-induced oxidative stress, and antioxidant therapeutic considerations. *Brain Research Reviews*, Vol. 50, pp.14-26,ISSN 0165-0173.

Radi, R. (2004). Nitric oxide, oxidants, and protein tyrosine nitration. *Proceedings of the National Academy of Sciences USA*, Vol. 101, pp. 4003-4008, ISSN 0027-8424.

Rayyes, O.A.; Wallmark, A. & Floren, C.H. (1996). Cyclosporine inhibits catabolism of low-density lipoprotein in HEPG2 cells by about 25%. *Hepatology*, Vol.24, pp. 613-619, ISSN 0270-9139.

Repetto, M.; Reides, C.; Gomez, M.L.; Costa, M.; Griemberg, G. & Llesuy, S. (1006). Oxidative stress in blood of HIV patients. *Clinical Chimica Acta*, Vol. 255, pp. 107-117, ISSN 0009-8981.

Roederer, M.F.; Staal, J.T.; Anderson, M.; Rabin, R.; Raju, P.A.; Herzenberg, L.A. & Herzenberg, L.A. (1993). Dysregulation of leukocytes glutathione in AIDS. *Annals of New York Academy of Sciences*, Vol.677, pp. 113-125, ISSN 0077-8923.

Schöndorf, T.; Maiworm, A.; Emmison, N.; Forst, T. & Pfützner, A. (2005). Biological background and role of adiponectin as marker for insulin resistance and cardiovascular risk. *Clinical Laboratory*, Vol.51, pp. 489-494, ISSN 1433-6510.

Schwarz, K.B. (1996). Oxidative stress during viral infection: a review. *Free Radical Biology & Medicine*, Vol. 21, No. 5, pp.641-649, ISSN 0891-5849.

Seigneur, M.; Constans, J.; Blann A.; Renard, M.; Pellegrin, J.L.; Amiral, J.; Boisseau, M. & Conri, C. (1997). Soluble adhesion molecules and endothelial cell damage in HIV infected patients. *Thrombosis and Haemostasis*, Vol.77, No.4, pp. 646-649, ISSN 0340-6245.

Shankar, S.S. & Dube, M.P. (2004). Clinical aspects of endothelial dysfunction associated with human immunodeficiency virus infection and antiretroviral agents. *Cardiovascular Toxicology*, No.4, pp.261-269, ISSN 1530-7905.

Smyth, M.J. (1991). Glutathione modulates activation-dependent proliferation of human peripheral blood lymphocyte populations without regulating their activated function. *The Journal of Immunology*, Vol.146, pp. 1921-1927, ISSN 0022-1767.

Sprietsma, J.E. (1997). Zinc-controlled Th1/Th2 switch significantly determines development of disease. *Medical Hypotheses*, Vol. 49, pp.1-14, ISSN 0306-9877.

Stehbens, W.E. (2004). Oxidative stress in viral hepatitis and AIDS. *Experimental and Molecular Pathology*, Vol.77, pp.121-132, ISSN 0014-4800.

Stein, J.H.; Klein, M.A.; Bellehumeur, J.L.; McBride, P.E.; Wiebe, D.A.; Otvos, J.D. & Sosman JM. (2001). Use of human immunodeficiency virus-1 protease inhibitors is associated with atherogenic lipoprotein changes and endothelial dysfunction. *Circulation*, Vol.104, No.3, pp.257-262, ISSN 0009-7322.

Suresh, D.R.; Annam, V.;, Pratibha, K. & Prasad, B.V.M. (2009). Total antioxidant capacity – a novel early biochemical marker of oxidative stress in HIV infected individuals. *Journal of Biomedical Science*, Vol.16, pp.61-64, ISSN 1021-7770

Tao, L.; Gao, E.; Jiao, X.; Yuan, Y.; Li, S.; Christopher, T.A.; Lopez, B.L.; Koch, W.; Chan, L.; Goldstein, B.J. & Ma, X.L. (2007). Adiponectin cardioprotection after myocardial ischemia/reperfusion involves the reduction of oxidative/nitrative stress. *Circulation*, Vol.115, No.11, pp.1408-1416, ISSN 0009-7322.

Torre, D.; Ferrario, G.; Speranza, F.; Martegani, R. & Zeroli, C. (1996a). Increased levels of nitrite in the sera of children infected with human immunodeficiency virus type 1. *Clinical Infectious Diseases*, Vol. 22, pp.650-653, ISSN 1058-4838.

Torre, D.; Ferrario, G.; Speranza, F.; Orani, A.; Fiori, G.P. & Zeroli, C. (1996b). Serum concentrations of nitrite in patients with HIV-1 infection. *Journal of Clinical Pathology*, Vol.49, pp.574-576, ISSN 0021-9746.

Torre, D.; Pugliese, A. & Speranza, F. (2002). Role of nitric oxide in HIV-1 infection: friend or foe. *Lancet Infectious Diseases*, Vol. 2, pp.273-280, ISSN 1473-3099.

Touzet, O. & Philips, A. (2010). Resveratrol protects against protease inhibitor-induced reactive oxygen species production, reticulum stress and lipid raft perturbation. *AIDS*, Vol. 24, No. 10, pp. 1437-1447, ISSN 0269-9370.

Tran, H.; Robinson, S.; Mikhailenko, I. & Strickland, D.K. (2003). Modulation of the LDL receptor and LPR levels by HIV protease inhibitors. *Journal of Lipid Research*, Vol. 44, No.10, pp. 1859-1969, ISSN 0022-2275.

Turchan, J.; Sactor, N.; Wojna, V.; Conant, K. & Nath, A. (2003). Neuroprotective therapy for HIV dementia. *Current HIV Research*, Vol.1, pp. 373-383, ISSN 1570-162X.

UNAIDS - Joint United Nations Programme on HIV/AIDS. AIDS epidemic update. December, 2007. Available in : <http://www.unaids.org/hivaidsinfo/statistics/fact_sheets/pdfs/brazil_em.pdf> . Access in January 30, 2008.

Walli, R.; Herfort, O.; Michl, G.M.;Demant , T. ; Jägr, H. & Dietele, C. (1998) Treatment with protease inhibitors associated with peripheral insulin resistance and impaired oral glucose tolerance in HIV-1 infected patients. *AIDS*, Vol.12, F167-F173, ISSN 0269-9370.

Wanchu, A.; Rana, S.V.; Pallikkuth, S. & Sachdeva, R.K. (2009). Oxidative Stress in HIV-Infected Individuals: A Cross-Sectional Study. *AIDS Research and Human Retroviruses*, Vol.25, No.12, pp.1307-1311, ISSN 0889-2229.

Wang, X.; Chai, H.; Yao, Q. & Chen, C. (2007). Molecular mechanisms of HIV protease inhibitor-induced endothelial dysfunction. *Journal of Acquired Immune Deficiency Syndromes*, Vol.44, No.5, pp.493-499, ISSN 1525-4135.

Westendorp, M.O.; Frank, R.; Ochsenbauer, C.; Stricker, K.; Dhein, J.; Walczak, H, Debatin, K.M. & Krammer, P.H. (1995). Sensitization of T cells to CD95-mediated apoptosis by HIV-1 Tat and gp 120. *Nature*, Vol.375, pp. 497-500, ISSN 0028-0836.

Witko-Sarsat, V.; Friedlander, M.; Nguyen-Khoa, T.; Capeillere-Blandin, C.; Nguyen, A.T.; Canteloup, S.; Dayer, J.M.; Jungers, P.; Drüeke, T. & Descamps-Latscha, B. (1998). Advanced oxidation protein products as novel mediators of inflammation and monocyte activation in chronic renal failure. *The Journal of Immunology*, Vol. 161, pp. 2524-2532, ISSN 0022-1767.

Wolf, K.; Tsakiris, D.A.; Weber, R.; Erb, P.; Battegay, M. & Swiss HIV Cohort Study. (2002). Antiretroviral therapy reduces markers of endothelial and coagulation activation in patients infected with human immunodeficiency virus type 1. *Journal of Infectious Diseases*, Vol. 185, No.4, pp. 456-462, ISSN 0022-1899

Worm, S.; Sabin, C.; Weber, R. , Reiss, P.; El-Sadr, W.; Dabis, F.; De Wit, S.; Law, M.; Monforte, A.D.; Friis-Møller, N.; Kirk, O.; Fontas, E.; Weller, I.; Phillips, A. & Lundgren, J. (2010). Risk of myocardial infarction in patients with HIV infection exposed to specific individuals antiretroviral drugs from the 3 major drug classes: the data collection on adverse events of anti-HIV drugs (D.A.D) study. *Journal of Infectious Diseases*, Vol. 201, No.3, pp. 318-330, ISSN 0022-1899.

Xu, A.; Yin, S.; Wong, I.; Chan, K.W. & Lam, K.S. (2004). Adiponectin ameliorated dyslipidemia induced by the human immunodeficiency virus protease inhibitor ritonavir in mice. *Endocrinology*, Vol. 145, No.2, pp. 487-494, ISSN 0013-7227.

Yamaguchi, Y.; Yoshikawa, N.; Kagota, S.; Nakamura, K.; Haginaka, J. & Kunitomo, M. (2006). Elevated circulating levels of markers of oxidative-nitrative stress and inflammation in a genetic rat model of metabolic syndrome. *Nitric Oxide*, Vol.15, pp. 380-386, ISSN 1089-8603.

Yano, S.;Yano, N.; Rodriguez, N.; Baek, J.H.; Que, X.; Yamamura, Y. & Kim, S.J. (1998). Suppression of intracellular hydrogen peroxide generation and catalase levels in $CD8^+$ T lymphocytes from HIV+ individuals. *Free Radical Biology & Medicine*, Vol. 24, No.2, pp. 349-359, ISSN 0891-5849.

Zangerle, R.; Fuchs, D.; Reibnegger, G.; Werner-Felmayer, G.; Gallati, H.; Wachter, H. & Werner, E.R. (1995). Serum nitrite plus nitrate in infection with human immunodeficiency virus type 1. *Immunobiology*, Vol. 193, No.1, pp. 59-70, ISSN 0171-2985.

3

HIV Toxins: Gp120 as an Independent Modulator of Cell Function

Leonor Huerta and César N. Cortés Rubio
Instituto de Investigaciones Biomédicas, Universidad Nacional Autónoma de México
México

1. Introduction

Current notions on the pathogenesis of the HIV-induced disease sustain that progressive immunodeficiency results from a combination of the cell cytotoxicity produced by infection and replication of the virus in the target cells, mainly immune system cells, and of the indirect, harmful effects mediated by two main mechanisms: a sustained, chronic activation of the immune system that turns into immune dysfunction with the progressive degradation of lymphoid tissues, and the immunoregulatory and toxic properties of extracellular viral proteins on bystander cells (Choudhary et al., 2007; Moir et al., 2011). Bystander, non infected cells that show altered function and death, include cells with null or low expression of the CD4 receptor, such as $CD8^{+}$ T and B lymphocytes, dendritic cells, neurons and tumor cells.

The HIV-1 Gp120 protein has properties that maintain resemblance with animal toxins. Active forms of free Gp120 can be found at nanomolar concentrations in the plasma of a considerable proportion of HIV infected individuals (Rychert et al., 2010; Gilbert et al., 1991; Santosuosso et al., 2009). A number of in vitro and in vivo activities have been described for the extracellular form of this molecule, indicating that it may contribute to deregulation of immune function and damage to several tissues during HIV infection. Activation, apoptosis, chemotaxis and impaired cellular function are the most frequently reported effects of Gp120 in the absence of HIV infection. Gp120 interacts with chemokine receptors (mainly CXCR4 and CCR5) which are expressed by different cells and tissues, besides the immune system, thus providing a range of possible target cells for toxic effects. However, the high structural variability of Gp120, absorption by host's glycan-binding compounds, and the complexity of the regulation processes involved in chemokine receptor function, have made difficult to asses the actual significance of the free form of this molecule for AIDS pathogenesis. On the other hand, soluble Gp120 or peptides derived of active portions of the molecule may be considered as potential therapeutic agents to target undesirable cells, i.e., tumor cells.

This article provides a review of the main factors influencing the biological outcome of the interaction of the soluble form of Gp120 with cells and tissues, and a selection of recent literature illustrating the diversity of the effects induced by this molecule.

2. Structure-function and evolutionary considerations

The HIV Env protein is synthesized in the form of the gp160 precursor, which processing and folding occur through what is known as the secretory pathway: the Env precursor protein (gp160) is co-translationally translocated into the endoplasmic reticulum (ER), where 10 disulfide bonds are formed and the molecule starts to fold. Glycosylation of most of the approximately 30 potential N-linked glycosylation sites, with around 25 of them located in the Gp120 region (Zhang et al., 2004), also occurs co-translationally in the ER. Disulfide bond formation and glycosylation, along with interaction with the lectin chaperones calnexin and calreticulin, allows the proper final folding of the gp160 precursor (Earl et al., 1991; Otteken et al., 1996). Then, the molecule forms trimers and is transported to the Golgi complex, where the cleavage into the surface (Gp120) and transmembrane (Gp41) subunits is carried out. Cleavage of the precursor by host proteases generates the N-terminal hydrophobic fusion peptide of Gp41. Gp120 and Gp41 are kept joined by non-covalent interactions on the surface of infected cells and virions.

Binding to cell membranes and disruption of the lipid bilayer integrity are the basic functional properties of the HIV Env complex. Env mediates the fusion of biological membranes that allows the entry of the virus nucleocapsid into target cells, as well as the fusion of infected with non-infected cells. Env-mediated membrane fusion is involved in virus entry, cell-to-cell transmission of virus particles, and syncytia formation. Membrane fusion is a multi-step process which is conducted by Gp120/Gp41 heterotrimers and involves: a) binding of Gp120 to the CD4 receptor on the cell surface, an interaction that is favored by adhesion molecules (Cantin et al., 1997, Bastiani et al., 1997); b) conformational rearrangements allowing Gp120 to interact with a coreceptor molecule, mainly CCR5 and CXCR4; c) projection of a trimer formed by the extended chains of the Gp41 ectodomain; d) insertion of the Gp41 amino-terminal hydrophobic ends, the fusion peptides, into the target membrane and the subsequent packing of the Gp41 molecule into a 6-helix bundle, a structure which formation provides the free energy necessary for membrane fusion (Jones et al., 1998; Melikyan et al., 2000; Sattentau & Moore, 1991; Sullivan et al., 1998; Trkola et al., 1996; Wu et al., 1996; Wyatt & Sodroski, 1998).

Gp120 oligosaccharide moieties greatly influence Gp120 folding, processing, and intracellular transport (Stansell & Desrosiers, 2010), and the ability of the virus to escape from host neutralizing antibodies. N-linked glycosylation sites are main targets of neutralizing antibodies, which exert selective pressure on the viral surface. Thus, it has been postulated that the evolving glycan shield is a mechanism to avoid elimination of the infection by the humoral immune response (Wei et al., 2003; Canducci et al, 2009). Instead, it has been frequently observed that the enzymatic removal of Gp120 oligosaccharides does not greatly affect the interaction of Gp120 with CD4 (Bahraoui et al., 1992; Fenouillet et al., 1989). However, glycosylation is necessary for the acquisition of the proper folding of Gp120 in the ER required for interaction with CD4 (Li et al., 1993). On the other hand, glycans play an important role in the usage of CXCR4 and CCR5 (Polzer et al., 2002; Ogert et al., 2001; Bandres et al., 1998).

Env share a number of structural and biological characteristics with pore-forming protein toxins from widely separated phyla such as bacteria, plants, cnidaria and mammals (Iacovache, et al., 2008): they undergo extensive post-translational modifications, are specific for susceptible structures (acceptor sites), have an hetero-oligomer structure, they tend to aggregate, show variable toxic efficiency among different cell types, act through their pore-forming activity (in conjunction with Gp41), have neurotoxic effects, and present considerable and continuous genetic variation (Butzke & Luch, 2010; Suput, 2009; Kristan et al., 2009). Particularly, a striking similitude exists among the mechanism of pore formation of the Env complex and that of the pore-forming toxins such as the actinoporins, the sea anemone toxins: 1) attachment of toxin to the cell surface through recognition of specific cellular membrane components; 2) transfer of the N-terminal segment to the lipid-water interface; 3) oligomerization of the toxin on the cell surface followed by the insertion of multiple α-helices monomeres into the membrane to form an ion conductive channel (Kristan et al., 2009; Edwards & Hessinger 2000; Butzke & Luch, 2010). As in the case of Env, the N-terminal portion of the toxin is essential for the final pore formation step (Kristan 2009). Finally, membrane-binding and pore-forming functions relay on different domains in both Env and animal pore-forming toxins.

Early works reported sequence homology between a short portion of Gp120 and the putative actives sites of the snake neurotoxin alpha-bungarotoxin and the rabies virus glycoprotein (Neri et al., 1990; Bracci & Neri, 1995), which interact with the mammals' nicotinic acetylcholine receptor, a member of the ligand-gated ion channel proteins. Later, it was found that Gp120 can bind to the acetylcholine binding site of the nicotinic receptor and the binding can be inhibited by an albumin-conjugated peptide encompassing the 160-170 amino acids of Gp120 (Bracci et al., 1997), which belong to a relatively conserved region of the Gp120 V2 loop. Gp120 can act as competitive antagonist of the nicotinic acetycholine receptors. Although the overall structure of the snake neurotoxins consists of a low molecular weight protein with three beta-strands with finger-like loops (Pawlak et al., 2006; Ackermann et al., 1998), and thus it is quite different to that of Gp120 and the rabies glycoprotein (both belonging to the Class I fusion proteins), the homologous sequence was located in a loop structure in both viral proteins and the snake neurotoxin, suggesting an evolutionary convergence towards the appropriate acetylcholine receptor binding structure.

3. The CXCR4 and CCR5 chemokine receptors

In principle, the biological effects of the interaction of Gp120 with CXCR4 and CCR5 may be conditioned by events similar to those regulating the coreceptor activity after interaction with their corresponding natural ligands. This section presents a general review of the characteristics of these receptors and the main extracellular events regulating their function. Comprehensive reviews of the regulatory pathways involved in CXCR4 and CCR5 signaling can be found elsewhere (Busillo & Benovic 2007; Kucia et al., 2005; Oppermann, 2004; Wu & Yoder, 2009).

CXCR4 and CCR5 belong to the super family of the seven-transmembrane G-protein coupled receptors (GPCRs). CXCR4 has SDF-1 as its sole natural ligand, whereas CCR5 can interact with several chemokines, mainly CCL5, CCL3, CCL4, CCL8 and CCL14 (RANTES, MIP-1alpha, MIP-1beta, MCP-2, and CC-1, respectively). Ligand binding triggers phosphorylation at various sites of the intracellular domains, which act as signals for migration, activation and transcription. Like for others GPCRs, ligand binding induces receptor desensitization and internalization to avoid prolonged activation, followed by degradation or recycling (Marchese et al., 2008). In addition, chemokine receptors can also be subjected to "heterologous desensitization", i.e., inhibition of receptor function by signaling processes triggered by ligand binding to an unrelated GPCR. Thus, cross heterologous desensitization of T cell functions can be induced by CCR5 and CXCR4 ligands, resulting in mutual interference with cellular signaling, adhesion and chemotaxis (Hecht et al., 2003). In another example, it has been shown that activation of toll-like receptor 2 (TLR2) negatively regulates CCR5 on human blood monocytes, inhibiting monocyte migration after pathogen recognition (Fox et al., 2011). On the other hand, it is clear that that signaling through CD4 by the CD4 ligand interleukin-16 (IL-16) desensitizes the chemokine receptors CCR5, CXCR4, and CXCR3 (Rahangdale et al., 2006; Van Drenth et al., 2000).

CXCR4 is expressed by many tissues and cell types, such as T leukocytes, progenitor cells in the bone morrow, endothelial (Murdoch et al., 1999) and epithelial cells (lung, retina, intestine), and tumor cells. In the brain, CXCR4 has been found in the endothelial cells forming the blood-brain barrier, microglia, neurons, and astrocytes (Berger et al., 1999; Edinger et al., 1997). CXCR4 is important for lymphocyte trafficking and recruitment of lymphocytes and monocytes at sites of inflammation, and plays a role in cell proliferation, organogenesis and vascularization. On the other hand, CCR5 is expressed on resting T-cells with a memory/effector phenotype, monocytes, macrophages and immature dendritic cells (Blanpain et al., 2002). Differentiation of monocytes to macrophages is accompanied by an increase of the CCR5 expression (Kaufmann et al., 2001). Increased CCR5 expression has been found to be induced by interferon-alpha (IFN-alpha) in thymus implants infected by the R5 HIV (Stoddart et al., 2010). Expression of CCR5 in T $CD4^+$ cells is particularly high in mucosa-associated lymphoid tissues (MALT), where the fraction of $CCR5^+$ CD4+ T cells is >50%. It is known that signaling through CCR5 is significantly involved in the induction of an immunological hyporesponsive state that leads to oral tolerance to high doses of antigen (DePaolo et al., 2004) and prevents uncontrolled postinfarction inflammation of myocardium in mice (Dobaczewski et al., 2010). Anti-inflammatory properties of $CCR5^+$ mononuclear cells have been related to the expression of high levels of IL-10 and their ability to recruit $CD4^+$/$foxp3^+$ regulatory T cells (Tregs) (Dobaczewski et al., 2010).

The expression of CXCR4 on the cell surface is increased by several cytokines (IL-4, IL-2, IL-7, IL-10, IL-5, TGF-1), as well as by fibroblast and vascular growth factors, whereas it is reduced by others, mainly those pro-inflammatory cytokines (TNF-alpha, INF-gamma, and IL-1-beta). However this pattern is not absolute and it is thought that mixed signals regulate de expression of CXCR4 signaling in different circumstances (reviewed in Busillo & Benovic 2007). On the other hand, sensitization of CXCR4 (priming to low concentrations of SDF) through its translocation to lipid rafts during inflammatory responses has also been described (Wysoczynski et al., 2005).

Membrane events participating in the regulation of CXCR4 and CCR5 function include dimerization as well as extensive downregulation by endocytosis and/or macropinocytosis. In addition, proteases released by neutrophils cleavage the N-terminus extracellular portion of CXCR4, avoiding ligand interaction (Hezareh et al., 2004; Lévesque et al., 2003).

In the last decade, the CXCR4-SF-1 axis has been increasingly involved in the generation, progression and metastasis of a variety of tumors, so that the expression of CXCR4 is currently considered an important biomarker for identification of the metastatic potential of primary tumors and a potential therapeutic target (Nimmagadda et al., 2010; Muller et al., 2001). CXCR4 was found to be one of the few genes which elevated over expression and function was associated to high osteolytic bone metastatic activity of human breast cancer cells in immunodeficient mice (Kang et al., 2003). In addition, CXCR4 is expressed on normal tissue-committed stem cells, which are currently considered a potential source of transformed cells. There are evidences that the CXCR4-SDF-1 axis can mediate locomotion, chemotaxis, adhesion, and even proliferation and survival of these cells, as well as the secretion of matrix proteases by different cell types (Fernandis et al., 2004; Janowska-

Wieczorek et al., 2000; Spiegel et al., 2004). Studies using RNA interference (RNAi) to reduce the expression of CXCR4 in animal models, have found that this treatment readily reduce growth and inhibits metastasis in a number of tumors, like breast and prostate cancer (Liang et al., 2005; Wang et al., 2011), melanoma (Kim et al., 2010), and neuroblastoma (Wang et al., 2006).

4. In vitro and in vivo effects of extracellular Gp120 on cell function

Although Gp120 interaction with CD4 can induce signaling events in many cell types, a number of effects that were originally attributed to the Gp120-CD4 interaction have been recently found to be explained by binding and signaling events mediated mainly by CXCR4 and CCR5. It should be noted, however, that although signaling intermediates recruited by Gp120 and the natural chemokine receptor ligands are usually the same, the ability of Gp120 to activate those signal transduction pathways may depend on the cell activation status. In general, activated cells are more sensitive to the activity of Gp120 than resting cells (Kinet et al., 2002; Weissman et al., 1997; Schols & De Clercq, 1996).

Gp120 signaling through CXCR4 triggers intracellular events facilitating infection by the HIV. Recently, it was found that Gp120 increases the dynamics of actin by activating cofilin, an actin-depolymerizing factor, which promotes the movement of the viral preintegration complex toward the centre of the cytoplasm. CXCR4-mediated actin rearrangement markedly facilitates viral infection of resting T cells (Yoder et al., 2008). Similarly, CXCR4 signaling after interaction with Gp120 is involved in a variety of other activation events in T cells and macrophages (Table 1). Likewise, it is well known that Gp120 exerts chemotactic effects on T, dendritic cells (DC), and monocyte/macrophages (Table 1). Conversely, it has been also reported that Gp120 can inhibit migration of T (Trushin et al., 2010) and B cells (Badr et al., 2005). It has been suggested that reprogramming of the $CD4^+$ T-cell migration behavior induced by Gp120 may provides a mechanism for lymphadenopathy during HIV infection (Green et al., 2009).

A study using oligonucleotide microarrays showed that tropism of Gp120 for the CCR5 and CXCR4 receptors, along with the cell activation status, are related to the Gp120 biological activity. R5 and X4 HIV envelopes (CCR5 and CXCR4-tropic Gp120, respectively) were found to induce distinct gene expression profiles in primary peripheral blood mononuclear cells (Cicala et al., 2006a). In this study, both R5 and X4 Gp120 activated genes associated with cell proliferation and protein tyrosine kinases, although R5 envelopes were more pronounced in their capacity to activate the p38 mitogen-activated protein kinase (p38 MAPK) cascade. In addition, R5 Gp120 exclusively activated a subset of genes in the resting $CD4^+$ T cell population derived from viremic individuals. p38 is activated in macrophages, neutrophils, and T cells by numerous extracellular mediators of inflammation, including chemoattractants, cytokines, chemokines, and bacterial lipopolysaccharide. Functional responses involving p38 include respiratory burst activity, chemotaxis, granular exocytosis, adherence and apoptosis (Ono & Han, 2000). Activation of p38 kinase has also been associated with HIV replication (Muthumani et al., 2004) and thus, it is proposed that R5 envelopes induce genes that may facilitate replication of virus in resting $CD4^+$ T cells, contributing to the establishment and/or maintenance of viral reservoirs, and the productive infection at mucosal surfaces, favoring transmission (Cicala et al., 2006a). Other studies also shown that R5 and X4 Gp120 can activate NFATs and induce their translocation into the nucleus. Translocation of NFATs is an important signal for HIV transcription, given that the HIV long terminal repeat (LTR) contains NFATs binding sites which are able to enhance transcription of viral genes (Cron et al., 2000; Cicala et al., 2006b; Kinoshita et al., 1998; Williams & Greene, 2007).

Cell	Mayor finding	Mechanism or concurrent events	Receptor involved	Reference
CD4+ T cell lines	Signal transduction	Protein tyrosine kinase Pyk2 phosphorylation-dependent cell growth, survival and differentiation.	CXCR4 CCR5	Davis et al., 1997
T cell lines	Gp120-CXCR4 co-internalization, cell signaling, and chemotaxis	Translocation of Gp120 and CXCR4 into early endosomes. CD4-independent phosphorylation of Pyk2.	CXCR4	Misse et al., 1999
CD4+ T cell line	Anergy	Inhibition of T cell activation and signaling through the TCR by Gp120/anti- Gp120 complexes, probably by sequestering p56 (lck) to the cytoskeleton.	CD4	Goldman et al., 1997
CHO cell line	Ca2+ mobilization	Coreceptor and CD4-dependent Ca2+ fluxing.	CXCR4 CCR5	Melar et al., 2007
CD4+ T cells, kidney epithelial cell lines and blood CD4+ lymphocytes	Apoptosis and viral replication	Caspase 8 dependent NF-kappaB activation and enhanced HIV replication.	N.D.*	Bren et al., 2009
Intestinal cell line	Functional alterations resembling HIV enteropathy	Activation of GPR15/Bob, presumably in a GalCer-rich membrane subdomain involving PKC activation. Microtubule disruption, perturbation of the transepithelial electrical resistance and decrease of glucose absorption.	GPR15/ Bob GalCer CXCR4	Maresca et al., 2003
Human hepatocyte cell lines and primary hepatocytes	Apoptosis	Gia protein signaling, and independent of caspase cascade activation.	CXCR4	Vlahakis et al., 2003
Blood CD4+ T lymphocytes	Apoptosis	Activation of caspases 3 and 6	CD4	Cicala et al., 2000
Blood CD4+ T lymphocytes	Apoptosis	Activation of the proapoptotic p38 protein	CXCR4	Trushin et al., 2007
Blood CD4+ T lymphocytes	Anergy	Diminished production of IL-2 and IL-4 and reduction of the proliferative responses of stimulated cells Production of high amounts of IL-10, INFγ and TNF-α of unstimulated cells.	CD4	Schols et al., 1996
Blood CD4+ T lymphocytes	Anergy	Dysregulation of the IL-2/IL-2R signal transduction pathway	CD4	Kryworuchko et al., 2003

Cell	Mayor finding	Mechanism or concurrent events	Receptor involved	Reference
Umbilical cord blood CD4+ T lymphocytes	HIV-1 replication in non-dividing cells	Activation of PKCε and its upstream effector PI3K/Akt, involved in HIV-1 replication. Enhancing of expression of the cellular Tat cofactors Tat-Sf1 and SPT5.	CXCR4	Missè et al., 2005
Blood CD4+T lymphocytes	Chemotaxis	Chemotaxis	CCR5	Weissman et al., 1997
Blood CD4+ T lymphocytes	Chemotaxis	CD4-independent signaling through CXCR4 in CD4+ and CD8+ T cells.	CXCR4	Iyengar et al., 1999
Blood CD4+ T lymphocytes	Chemotaxis of unstimulated CD4+ T cells.	Activation of major G protein-dependent pathways: calcium mobilization, phosphoinositide-3 kinase, and Erk-1/2 MAPK activation.	CXCR4	Balabanian et al., 2004
Blood CD4+ T lymphocytes	Inhibition of SDF-1α-induced chemotaxis	Actin cytoskeleton rearrangements Lck-dependent phosphorylation and inactivation of cofilin, a cellular depolymerizing factor.	CD4	Trushin et al., 2010
Blood CD4+ T lymphocytes	NFAT nuclear translocation in resting cells	Facilitation of viral replication in resting cells.	CD4 CCR5 CXCR4	Cicala et al., 2006
Blood CD4+ T lymphocytes	Activation of LFA-1	Binding of gp120 to α4β, an integrin mediating migration of lymphocytes to gut-associated lymphoid tissue, activates LFA-1, favoring formation of virological synapses.	Integrin α4β7	Arthos et al., 2008
Blood resting CD4+ T lymphocytes	Induction of actin dynamics in resting CD4+ T cells	Activation of the cellular actin depolymerizing factor cofilin, which promotes the movement of the viral preintegration complex to the nucleous.	CXCR4	Yoder et al., 2008
Blood CD4+ and CD8+ T lymphocytes	Apoptosis	Reduction of the expression of the proto-oncogene Bcl-2 with induction of apoptosis in CD4+ but not in CD8+ T cells.	CD4	Hashimoto et al., 1997
Blood CD8+ T lymphocytes	Apoptosis dependent of macrophage activation	Activation of macrophages for enhanced expression of TNF and TNFRII. Apoptosis was mediated by the interaction between macrophage TNF-α and the TNFRII on CD8+ T.	CXCR4	Herbein et al., 1998
Blood CD8+ T lymphocytes	Anergy	Synthesis of high amounts of IL-10 by unstimulated PBMC. Reduction of activation and proliferation of CD8+ T cells.	CD4	Schols et al., 1996
Blood CD4+ and CD8+ T lymphocytes	Chemotaxis	CD4-independent signaling.	CXCR4	Iyengar et al., 1999

Cell	Mayor finding	Mechanism or concurrent events	Receptor involved	Reference
PBMCs and monocyte-derived macrophages (MDMs)	Transcriptional program conducive to productive HIV infection.	Modulation of ~300 genes. Induction of the expression of cytokines, chemokines, kinases, and transcription factors associated with antigen-specific T cell activation but not cell proliferation.	N.D.	Cicala et al., 2002
Blood monocytes	Anergy	Induction of IL-10 production	CD4	Schols et al., 1996
Blood monocytes and MDMs	Production of β chemokines	Enhancement of MCP-1, MIP-1β, and RANTES secretion by primary monocytes/ macrophages but not by THP-1 and U937 cells.	CCR5 CXCR4	Fantuzzi et al., 2001
Blood monocytes and MDMs	Aberrant activation	Pertussis toxin-insensitive signal transduction, activation of Ca2+ channels and Pyk2 and MAPK pathways Secretion of the MIP-1β and MCP-1 chemoattractants.	CCR5 CXCR4	Del Corno et al., 2001
MDMs	Production of pro-inflammatory cytokines	Release of pro-inflammatory cytokines. Activation of multiple protein kinases like the Src family kinase Lyn, PI3K and Pyk2.	CCR5	Cheung et al., 2008
Immature DCs derived from monocytes	Migration	Migration of dendritic cells mediated by a novel pathway involving phosphorylation of Pyk2 and activation of the p38 MAP kinase.	CCR5	Anand et al., 2009
Tonsil primary naïve and memory B cells	Apoptosis and inhibition of B cell chemotaxis.	Gp120-induced cleavage of CD62L by a mechanism dependent on matrix metalloproteinase 1 and 3, CD4, CXCR4, G!i, and p38 MAPK. Increase of CD95-mediated apoptosis.	CXCR4 CCR5	Badr et al., 2005
Rat hippocampal neurons	Apoptosis and necrosis	Activation of NMDA receptors with increase of neuronal calcium concentration. Impairment of neuronal calcium homeostasis was prevented by TGF-β1.	NMDA receptors	Meucci et al., 1996
Rat hippocampal neurons	Increase of intracellular calcium concentration.	Dramatic and persistent release of calcium from intracellular stores.	N.D.	Medina et al., 1999
Human neuroblastoma cells	Neurotoxicity Necrosis	Increment of intracellular calcium induced increased cyclooxygenase and 5-lipoxygenase activity. Membrane lipoperoxidation and mitochondrial uncoupling.	CXCR4	Maccarrone et al., 2002
Rat hippocampal neurons	Neurotoxicity and apoptosis	Activation of JNK	N.D.	Bodner et al., 2002

Cell	Mayor finding	Mechanism or concurrent events	Receptor involved	Reference
Rat cerebellar granule cells	Neurotoxicity	Signaling through CXCR4.	CXCR4	Bachis et al., 2004
Rodent dorsal root ganglia and sensory neurons	Neurotoxicity, axonal degeneration and apoptosis	Activation of the mitochondrial caspase pathway.	CXCR4 CCR5	Melli et al., 2006
Rat microglia	Neurotoxicity	Enhancing of outward potassium currents via CXCR4 and cAMP-dependent PKA signaling.	CXCR4	Xu et al., 2011
Rat and human neurons Human monocytes	Neuronal death and monocyte activation	Gp120 and Tat induction of phosphorylation of MLK3 (MAP3K11).	N.D.	Ziye et al., 2006
Rat cerebellar cells	Apoptosis	Caspase-3-mediated apoptosis.	CXCR4	Bachis et al., 2006
Human astroglia	Glutamine metabolism dysfuntion and apoptosis	Imbalanced glutamine synthetase activity accompanied by generation of free radicals.	N.D.	Visalli et al., 2007
Human neuroblastoma cell line differentiated into neurons. Fetal rat neurons	Apoptosis	Pretreatment with platelet-derived growth factor BB reduced gp120-associated neurotoxicity and rescued neurite outgrowth.	N.D.	Peng et al., 2008
Rat brain endothelial cell line	Oxidative stress	Induction of decreased levels of intracellular GSH (reduced glutathione), GPx (glutathione peroxidase), and GR (glutathione reductase) and increased levels of MDA (malondialdehyde)	N.D.	Price et al., 2005
Rat lung metastasis of mammary adenocarcinoma cells.	Tumor retention and enhancing of metastasis	Infusion of Gp120 into the brain enhanced tumor metastasis. Blocked by antagonists of IL-1.	N.D.	Hodgson et al., 1998
Prostate cancer tumor in SCID mice	Apoptosis and inhibition of tumor growth	Tumor regression associated with significant decreases in CD44, CD34, and LYVE-1 and increases in caspase 3 and 9.	CXCR4	Singh et al., 2009
Rats pituitary cells	Supression of growth hormone (GH) release	Gp120 also supressed GHRH release by pituitary cells in vitro. Loss of body weight in chronically treated animals.	GHRH receptor	Mulroney et al., 1998
Rat neuronal progenitor cells from HIV/gp120-transgenic mice	Inhibition of proliferation	Arrests of cell cycle in G1 trough signaling by the p38 MAPK.	CXCR4 CCR5	Okamoto et al., 2007

Cell	Mayor finding	Mechanism or concurrent events	Receptor involved	Reference
Rat brain endothelial cells	Cytotoxicity	Reduction of the expression of ICAM-1- and laminin. Lipidperoxidation.	N.D.	Louboutin et al., 2010
PBMCs in SCID mice	Reprogramming of the CD4+ T-cell migratory behavior	Enhancing of sensitivity to CCL20 and CCL21 and inhibition of migration in response to sphingosine-1-phosphate. Increased accumulation of cells in lymph nodes with a reciprocal decrease in blood and spleen.	CD4	Green et al., 2009

* Not determined

Table 1. *In vitro* and *in vivo* effects of soluble gp120

In addition to activation for proliferation, Gp120 can exert a diversity of potent effects in immune system cells in vitro, being apoptosis the most frequently reported, although anergy, and induction of proinflammatory cytokine production are also well known effects. An early review of the influence of Gp120 on the immune system was carried out by Chirmule and Pahwa in 1996 (see reference). Table 1 shows recent studies about the effect of Gp120 on immune system cells, confirming early findings and adding new effects, particularly those related to the induction or inhibition of chemotaxis, and the role of Gp120/anti-Gp120 immune complexes on depletion of bystander lymphocytes. Table 1 also shows the receptor implicated in each case.

Apoptosis is the event more frequently attributed to the interaction of Gp120 with CD4 and coreceptor molecules. The importance of Gp120-mediated apoptosis for AIDS pathogenesis was assessed in an early study performed on lymph-node cell suspensions prepared from three HIV-positive patients. Free Gp120 colabeled with both apoptotic and normal $CD4^+$ T lymphocytes, although it was more often identified on apoptotic than on normal $CD4^+$ T lymphocytes but not on $CD8^+$ T lymphocytes or B cells. HIV particles were not found associated either with normal or apoptotic lymphocytes. This study pointed out that free Gp120 can bind to $CD4^+$ T cells in lymph nodes of HIV-infected individuals and potentially mark them for premature death by apoptosis (Sunila et al., 1997).

Holm and cols., demonstrated that the affinity of native, virion-associated Gp120, for the CD4 and CXCR4 or CCR5 receptors was important for induction of apoptosis on primary human $CD4^+$ T cells with an activated phenotype. In this study, virions expressing a mutant Gp120 defective for CD4 binding induced apoptosis, whereas mutants defective for CXCR4 binding did not. These observations indicated that the Gp120-CD4 interaction did not induce apoptosis, but seems to promote it by enhancing the exposure of the CXCR4 binding site on Gp120 (Holm et al., 2004). Gp120 expressed by *env*-transfected, non-infected cells, also induced CXCR4-dependent apoptosis in umbical cord $CD4^+$ $CXCR4^+$ cells; apoptosis was inhibited by SDF-1 (Roggero et al., 2001).

As for virion-associated Gp120, studies performed with recombinant Gp120 showed that Gp120 induced apoptosis through Fas-dependent and Fas-independent mechanisms and that not all lymphocytes were equally sensitive (reviwed in Cicala et al., 2000). Induction of apoptosis by soluble Gp120 was characterized by Thrushin and cols., whose shown that binding of soluble Gp120 to CD4 facilitate apoptosis of primary human CD4+ T cells, but that it was caused primordially by the Gp120-CXCR4 interaction, since apoptosis was prevented by the CXCR4 inhibitor AMD3100 and by the anti-CXCR4 antibody 12G5 (Trushin et al., 2007). Similarly, soluble Gp120-induced apoptosis mediated by CXCR4 was demonstrated in adult human hepatocytes, which lack CD4 (Vlahakis et al., 2003). Binding of Gp120 to CXCR4 is also able to induce apoptosis of CD8+ T cells by upregulating the expression of TNF and TNF-receptor II on interacting CD8+ T cells and macrophages (Herbein, et al., 1998). Thus, the expression of CXCR4 or CCR5 may restrict the cell sensitivity to Gp120 and explain the differential response of T cells subsets.

Recent studies have shown that the expression of CXCR4 on cancer cells makes them susceptible to apoptosis induced by the HIV-1 envelope. Endo et al. (2008) observed that apoptosis of breast cancer cell lines induced by HIV-1 particles was dependent on Gp120 and CXCR4 but not CD4. In addition, a Gp120 mutant with low CD4 binding ability induced apoptosis in breast cancer cells but not in T-cells. Importantly, conformational heterogeneity of CXCR4 in breast cancer cells in comparison with CXCR4 in T cells was related to the ability of Gp120 to induce apoptosis mediated by CXCR4 (Endo et al., 2008, 2010). Likewise, it has been shown that the Gp120-CXR4 interaction mediated apoptosis of prostate cancer cell lines but not of normal prostatic epithelial cells (Singh et al., 2009).

Anergy is a state of inhibition of proliferation and/or effector functions normally induced in T cells after encounter with antigen; the cell stay alive and functional inactivation is reversible upon antigen removal. It is induced by incomplete stimulation though the TCR and co-stimulatory molecules, and by the normal stimulation in the presence of IL-10 (Schwartz, 2003). Studies addressing the anergic effect of Gp120 use activation with anti-CD3 or mitogen-activation to simulate the effect of antigen stimulation. The contribution of anergy to the reduced immune function induced by X4 Gp120 in peripheral blood lymphocytes (PBMC) was early described by Schols and De Clercq (Schols & De Clercq, 1996). The addition of low concentrations of Gp120 was able to inhibit the proliferative response and the production of interleukin-2 (IL-2) and interleukin-4 (IL-4) in PBMC previously stimulated with an anti-CD3 antibody and concanavalin-A. In contrast, Gp120 induced the production of high amounts of IL-10, gamma interferon (IFN-g), and tumor necrosis factor alpha (TNF-a) in unstimulated PBMC. The induction of IL-10 by Gp120 was found to be important for the inhibitory effect of Gp120 on PBMC proliferation. Thus, X4 Gp120 can reduce the function of T lymphocytes by directly inducing anergy or by stimulation of the production of anergy-inducer immunosupressive cytokines. Importantly, the activation status played an important role in the cytokine pattern induced by Gp120 in PBMC (Schols & De Clercq, 1996).

Evidence of the participation of chemokine receptors in the induction of anergy by Gp120 has been obtained in studies of the long-lasting hypo-responsiveness to antigen stimulation caused by Gp120 in naive T lymphocytes. Gp120 was found to induce anergy by stimulating the activity of the cyclic adenosine monophosphate (cAMP)-dependent protein kinase A (PKA), which causes the progressive accumulation of the phosphorylated form of the cAMP-responsive element binding, a pathway which is also activated by the ligation of CXCR4 by SDF-1 (Masci et al., 2003).

It should be noted that although there is an association between circulating Gp120 and the induction of proinflammatory and immunoregulatory cytokines like IL-6, IL-10, and TNF-alpha in some HIV infected individuals (Rychert et al., 2010), this effect can not be necessarily induced by direct cell interaction with Gp120, since cytokines could be induced also by deposition of Gp120-anti-Gp120 immune complexes, which has been associated with disease progression (Daniel et al., 2001; Gerencer et al., 1998).

Evidences indicate that Gp120, Tat and Nef may be largely involved in the events allowing the initial entry of HIV into the brain and in the injury and apoptosis of neurons. HIV gains entry into the brain at the asymptomatic stage of the infection trough infected circulating monocytes or as free virus. It is thought that entry is favored by a subclinical, early loss of the functional integrity of tight junctions of the brain endothelium, the brain blood barrier (BBB) (Strazza et al., 2011; Annunziata, 2003). Once in the brain, monocytes can repopulate the resident macrophage population and become a productive source of virus, extending the infection to microglia, astrocytes and endothelial cells, where it can establish a protected reservoir and give rise to the production of cytokines and chemokines (An et al., 1999). Inflammatory soluble factors like IL-1 and TNF-alpha, along with high amounts of viral proteins like Gp120, Tat and Nef, likely released by a particular kind of monocytes ($CD14^{low}CD16^{+}$) (Thieblemont et al., 1995), may cause a continuous activation of the brain endothelium, leading to the attraction and diapedesis of more virus and activated cells. Increased numbers of $CD14^{low}CD16^{+}$ monocytes in the circulation associates with HIV-associated neurocognitive disorders (HAND) (Thieblemont et al., 1995; reviewed in Gras & Kaul, 2010) and are abundant in brain autopsies from patients with HIV encephalitis (Fisher-Smith et al, 2001).

Perturbation of the brain blood barrier (BBB) may be induced by the HIV non-productive infection of brain endothelial cells by micropinocytosis or adsorptive endocytosis of the virus mediated by Gp120 (Banks et al., 2001). The transit of free virions by a paracellular route favored by TNF-alpha has been also observed (Fiala et al., 1997). Another explanation is the increase of BBB permeability by the activity of viral proteins. It has been found that soluble forms of Tat, Nef and Gp120 proteins, which circulate in the blood of HIV infected patients, alter the expression of cell junction proteins and thus disrupt the integrity of the BBB (reviewed in Toborek et al., 2005; Kanmogne et al., 2005). Gp120 is also able to increase monocyte migration through a brain microendothelial cells monolayer and to reduce the transendothelial electric resistance (Kanmogne et al., 2007). The presence of functional CD4 and chemokine receptors on discrete regions of brain microvessels derived from children has been demonstrated (Stins et al., 2004). In the presence of interferon (IFN)-gamma, children brain microvessels, but not adult brain microvessels, suffer cytotoxicity induced by Gp120. The effect associated with an increase of the expression levels of CCR3 and CCR5 induced by IFN-gamma. Several Gp120 peptides and RANTES, but not SDF-1, inhibited the Gp120 cytotoxic effect. Authors also showed that Gp120-mediated endothelial cell cytotoxicity involved the p38 MAPK pathway. Thus, a blood-brain barrier dysfunction induced by Gp120 in the brain of HIV-1-infected children may explain the higher incidence of HAND in this population (Khan et al., 2007).

Besides its potential role in BBB damage, chemokine receptors have been involved in direct and indirect Gp120-induced neuronal damage. Macrophages and microglia, the resident immunocompetent phagocytic cells in the brain, are the main cellular reservoirs of HIV in the central nervous system. Activated microglia produces free radicals and proinflammatory cytokines and chemokines which can damage neurons. Gp120 and Tat activates human fetal microglia in vitro, the resident phagocytes of the brain, to induce the expression of CD40 and MHC class II, and the secretion of inflammatory mediators, like cytokines, chemokines, and neurotoxins favoring the recruitment of cell from the circulation (reviwed in D'Aversa et al., 2005). The progressive increase in the immune activation with increased expression of cytokines is suggested to cause neuropathological changes and neuronal and axonal damage. A recent report shows that Gp120 is able to activate rat microglia and cause neurotoxicity by inducing an increase in the expression of the voltage-gated K^+ channels (K_V), enhancing the cell outward K^+ currents. The Gp120-associated enhancement of K^+ current was blocked by a CXCR4 receptor antagonist or a specific protein kinase A (PKA) inhibitor. This data suggest that interaction of Gp120 with CXCR4 may underlay the microglia activation leading to neurotoxin production and neuronal apoptosis (Xu et al., 2011). In other study, Gp120-mediated neurotoxicity was found to involve signaling trough the p38 MAPK in macrophages, microglia and neuronal cells. Gp120-mediated p38 MAPK activation and neuronal death was prevented by CCL4 (MIP-1beta), one of the CCR5 ligands (Medders et al., 2010). On the other hand, soluble Tat is able to cross the BBB and to induce the production of chemoattractive factors by astrocytes and monocytes (mainly MCP-1, which is considered one of the most important chemokines in HIV infection and HAND), and the expression of CCR5 on monocytes (Weiss et al., 1999).

5. Relevance of extracellular Gp120 to HIV pathogenesis

It is known that molecular diversity produce a variety of ligand-receptor interactions, which in turn, induce signaling events that diverge from the optimal agonist effect (Edwards & Evavold, 2011). Thus, an important issue to be considered in the studies of the biological activity of Gp120 is its extreme heterogeneity at the amino acid sequence and glycosylation levels. A survey of the HIV sequences contained in Los Alamos database in the year 2000 showed that, of 566 full-length Gp120 protein sequences, protein lengths varied from 484 to 543 amino acids because of the insertions and deletions found in hypervariable regions. Main factors contributing to Env variation are: base-substitution due a lack of proofreading during the reverse transcription of the HIV genome, large insertions and deletions, and recombination. These processes are accelerated by the viral high replication rate, the rapid viral turnover and the pressure to change imposed for the immune response of the HIV infected individuals (Korber et al., 2001). Many of substitutions at the hypervariable regions of Gp120, as well as insertions and deletions involve glycosylation sites, so that the number of N-linked glycosylation sites ranges from 18 to 33 (Korber et al., 2001).

Another source of Gp120 molecular variation is the non-uniform content of carbohydrate units. The addition of oligosaccharides and oligomerization of the Gp160 precursor are both co-translational events that take place in the ER (reviewed by Land & Braakman 2001). It is known that incomplete or "immature" glycosylation is present in trimeric Gp120, due to steric limitations imposed to the glycan-modifying enzymes in the Golgi apparatus. Numerous Gp120 glycosylation variants can be produced even within a single cell population, as has been shown in the H9 lymphoblastoid cell line (Pal et al., 1993; Mizuochi et al., 1990). Instead, recombinant monomeric Gp120 is believed to contain fully mature glycans (Eggink et al., 2010; Binley et al., 2010). Thus, monomeric and native, trimeric Gp120 derived from virus and infected cells, may differ in their pattern of glycosylation (Means & Desrosiers, 2000; Mizuochi 1990). A recent study of the expression of a model oligomeric Gp120 showed that N-glycosylation of varied depending on the cell type used for expression (Raska et al., 2010). Cell-dependent addition of oligosaccharides may explain the observation that HIV laboratory strains exposed a higher proportion of high-mannose glycans that HIV primary isolates (Astoul et al., 2000).

The actual amount of Gp120 in tissues and fluids of the HIV infected individual is another important consideration regarding the role of free Gp120 in AIDS pathogenesis. The Gp120 Env subunit can shed from viral particles and infected cells in vitro to adopt a water-soluble form (McKeating et al., 1991; Smith-Franklin et al., 2002; Layne et al., 1992; Schneider et al., 1986). As described in the previous section of this review, a myriad of biological activities has been described for soluble Gp120, and thus the potential of this molecule to account for a significant portion of the physiological dysfunction observed during the HIV-1 infection is considerable. However, few studies have estimated the extension of the presence of Gp120 in the organism of HIV-infected subjects. Gp120 has been detected in the circulation of about on third of HIV-infected subjects at concentrations of 4-130 pM (Rychert et al., 2010) and 2-20 pM (Gilbert et al., 1991) in early and chronic HIV-infected subjects, respectively. A different study by Oh and cols. (1992) reported a higher concentration in plasma, although the methodology used has been questioned (Klasse & Moore, 2004). The amount of Gp120 bound to tissues can be relevant to the understanding of the dynamics of this molecule in the body. A recent study by Santosuosso and cols. (2009) showed that concentration of Gp120 in secondary lymphoid tissues obtained from autopsies of HIV-infected subjects can be high (up to 9007 pg/ml, or 75 pM), even when Gp120 is not detected in plasma. Although a distinction among the amount of soluble Gp120 and virus or cell-associated Gp120 was not clear in this study, it was shown that Gp120 can accumulate in lymphoid tissues early in the HIV infection, and that levels of viral protein in these tissues can exceed significantly those found in plasma.

The presence of physiologically significant amounts of soluble Gp120 in vivo is still a matter of debate. Klasse and More (2004) have discussed several factors that may limit the effective concentration of Gp120 in fluids and tissues, like the capture of Gp120 by antibodies and serum lectins (Daniel et al., 1998), and the absorption of Gp120 by proteoglycans on cell surfaces (Mbemba et al., 1999;). The soluble mannose binding lectin (MBL), a innate immunity molecule present in the human serum, is able to capture HIV particles probably through the high-mannose glycosylation sites of the Gp120/Gp41 complex (Saifuddin et al., 2000). It has been proposed that MBL can participate in the clearance of HIV, since it activates complement and opzonise particles for binding to phagocytic cells (Mass et al., 1998; Pastinen et al., 1998). Soluble Gp120 could be also cleared or inactivated by MBL.

6. Conclusion

Gp120 is a molecule with remarkable properties, some of which are related to a probable evolutionary relationship with animal toxins, and others to its interaction and adaptation to the human immunological and physiological environment. The Gp120 primary role in viral entry using CD4 and chemokine receptors, allow it to induce signaling events which final outcome depends on the particular cell physiological status, thus leading to activation, altered function or death. The high mutation rate of the *env* gene, combined with a rapid replication and viral turnover rates and the pressure to change imposed for the immune response, allow HIV (and the secreted Gp120 molecule) to extent its range of functional capabilities and cellular tropism. Along with other viral proteins such as Nef and Tat, which also have a spectrum of biological effects as soluble proteins, Gp120 may be an important mediators of the bystander $CD4^{+}$-T-cell death and chronic inflammation that are hallmark of the disease leading to AIDS.

In the recent years, the interaction of Gp120 with chemokine receptors, enabled by the initial interaction with CD4, as been identified as the origin of many of the effects of Gp120 on the function of immune system cells and other tissues. By reviewing the recent literature, a general picture emerges that indicate that properties of Gp120 strongly associate with its chemokine receptor specificity and the activation status of the target cells. R5 Gp120 is able to activate resting cells, where X4 Gp120 seems to induce mainly anergy and apoptosis. On the other hand, X4 Gp120 is able to enhance the activation phenotype in cells that have been previously stimulated. A proper understanding of the influence of cell status on the effect of particular forms of Gp120 on cell viability and function is necessary to get an integrated view of the significance of free Gp120 for the HIV disease.
Several studies indicate that CD4 is not required for apoptosis of tumor cells induced by Gp120, since it can be mediated by CXCR4. In particular, the importance of CXCR4 expression for development and metastasis of breast cancer cells has been demonstrated, as well as for the Gp120-mediated apoptosis of these cells. Interestingly, HIV infected individuals do not present an increased incidence of this type of tumor, whereas they develop others (Amir et al., 2000; Herida et al., 2003; Pantanowitz & Dezube, 2001). Although other factors may determine this effect, participation of Gp120 can not be discarded. The complex structure and variability of Gp120 provides a substrate for the search of active molecules targeting chemokine receptor-expressing tumor cells.

7. References

Ackermann, E., Ang, E., Kanter, J., Tsigelny, I., & Taylor, P. (1998). Identification of pairwise interactions in the alpha-neurotoxin-nicotinic acetylcholine receptor complex through double mutant cycles. *The Journal of Biological Chemistry*, Vol. 273, No. 18, (May 1998), pp.10958-10964, ISSN 0021-9258

Amir, H., Kaaya, E., Kwesigabo, G., & Kiitinya, J. (2000). Breast cancer before and during the AIDS epidemic in women and men: a study of Tanzanian Cancer Registry Data 1968 to 1996. *Journal of the National Medical Association,* Vol.96, No. 6, (Jun 2000), pp. 301-3055, ISSN 0027-9684

An, S., Groves, M., Gray, F., & Scaravilli, F. (1999). Early entry and widespread cellular involvement of HIV-1 DNA in brains of HIV-1 positive asymptomatic individuals. *Journal of Neuropathology & Experimental Neurology*, Vol. 58, No.11, (Nov 1999), pp. 1156-1162, ISSN 0022-3069

Anand, A., Prasad, A., Bradley, R., Deol, Y., Nagaraja, T., Ren, X., Terwilliger, E., & Ganju, R. (2009). HIV-1 gp120-induced migration of dendritic cells is regulated by a novel kinase cascade involving Pyk2, p38 MAPkinase, and LSP1. *Blood*, Vol. 114, No. 17, (2009), pp. 3588-3600, ISSN 0006-4971

Annunziata, P. (2003). Blood-brain barrier changes during invasion of the central nervous system by HIV-1. Old and new insights into the mechanism. *Journal of Neurology,* Vol. 250, No. 8, (Aug 2003), pp.901-906, ISSN 0340-5354

Arthos, J., Cicala, C., Martinelli, E., Macleod, K., Van Ryk, D., Wei, D., Xiao, Z., Veenstra, T., Conrad, T., Lempicki, R., McLaughlin, S., Pascuccio, M., Gopaul, R., McNally, J., Cruz, C., Censoplano, N., Chung, E., Reitano, K., Kottilil, S., Goode, D., & Fauci, A. (2008). HIV-1 envelope protein binds to and signals through integrin α4β7, the gut mucosal homing receptor for peripheral T cells. *Nature Immunology,* Vol. 9, No. 3, (March 2008), pp. 301–309, ISSN 1529-2908

Astoul, C., Peumans, W., Van Damme, E., & Rougé, P. (2000). Accessibility of the High-Mannose Glycans of Glycoprotein gp120 from Human Immunodeficiency Virus Type 1 Probed by in Vitro Interaction with Mannose-Binding Lectins. *Biochemical and Biophysical Research Communications,* Vol. 274, No. 2, (August 2000), pp. 455-460, ISSN 0006-291X

Bachis, A., & Mocchetti, I. (2004). The Chemokine Receptor CXCR4 and Not the N-Methyl-D-Aspartate Receptor Mediates gp120 Neurotoxicity in Cerebellar Granule Cells. *Journal of Neuroscience Research,* Vol.75, No.1, (2004), pp.75–82, ISSN 0360-4012

Bachis, A., & Mocchetti, I.(2006). Semisynthetic sphingoglycolipid LIGA20 is neuroprotective against human immunodeficiency virus-gp120-mediated apoptosis. *Journal of Neuroscience Research,* Vol.83, No.5, (2006), pp.890–896, ISSN 0360-4012

Badr, G., Borhis, G., Treton, D., Moog, C., Garraud, O., & Richard, Y. (2005). HIV type 1 glycoprotein 120 inhibits human B cell chemotaxis to CXC chemokine ligand (CXCL) 12, CC chemokine ligand (CCL) 20, and CCL21. *The Journal of Immunology,* Vol. 175, No. 1, (Jul 2005), pp. 302-310, ISSN 0022-1767

Bahraoui, E., Benjouad, A., Guetard, D., Kolbe, H., Gluckman, J., & Montagnier, L. (1992). Study of the interaction of HIV-1 and HIV-2 envelope glycoproteins with the CD4 receptor and role of N-glycans. *AIDS Research and Human Retroviruses,* Vol. 8, No. 5, (May 1992), pp.565-573, ISSN 0889-2229

Balabanian, K., Harriague, J., Décrion, C., Lagane, B., Shorte, S., Baleux, F., Virelizier, J., Arenzana-Seisdedos, F., & Chakrabarti, L. (2004). CXCR4-Tropic HIV-1 Envelope Glycoprotein Functions as a Viral Chemokine in Unstimulated Primary CD4+ T Lymphocytes. *The Journal of Immunology,* Vol.173, No.12, (2004), pp. 7150–7160, ISSN 0022-1767

Bandres, J., Wang, Q., O'Leary, J., Baleaux, F., Amara, A., Hoxie, J., Zolla-Pazner, S., & Gorny, M. (1998). Human immunodeficiency virus (HIV) envelope binds to CXCR4 independently of CD4, and binding can be enhanced by interaction with soluble CD4 or by HIV envelope deglycosylation. *The Journal of Virology,* Vol. 72, No.3, (Mar 1998), pp. 2500-2504, ISSN 0022-538X

Banks, W., Freed, E., Wolf, K., Robinson, S., Franko, M., & Kumar V. (2001). Transport of human immunodeficiency virus type 1 pseudoviruses across the blood-brain barrier: role of envelope proteins on adsorptive endocytosis. *The Journal of Virology,* Vol. 75, No.10, (May 2001), pp. 4681–4691, ISSN 0022-538X

Bastiani, L., Laal, S., Kim, M., & Zolla-Pazner, S. (1997). Host cell-dependent alterations in envelope components of human immunodeficiency virus type 1 virions. *The Journal of Virology,* Vol. 71, No. 5, (May 1997), pp. 3444-3450, ISSN 0022-538X

Berger, O., Gan, X., Gujuluva, C., Burns, A., Sulur, G., Stins, M., Way, D., Witte, M., Weinand, M., Said, J., Kim, K., Taub, D., Graves, M., & Fiala, M. (1999). CXC and CC chemokine receptors on coronary and brain endothelia. *Molecular Medicine,* Vol. 5, No. 12, (Dec 1999), pp. 795-805, ISSN 1076-1551

Binley, J., Ban, Y., Crooks, E., Eggink, D., Osawa, K., Schief, W., & Sanders, R., (2010). Role of complex carbohydrates in human immunodeficiency virus type 1 infection and resistance to antibody neutralization. *The Journal of Virology,* Vol. 84, No.11, (Jun 2010), pp. 5637-5655, ISSN 0022-538X

Blanpain, C., Libert, F., Vassart, G., & Parmentier, M. (2002). CCR5 and HIV infection. *Receptors Channels,* Vol. 8, No. 1, (2002), pp.19–31, ISSN 1060-6823

Bodner, A., Maroney, A., Finn, J., Ghadge, G., Roos, R., & Miller, R. (2002).Mixed lineage kinase 3 mediates gp120IIIB-induced neurotoxicity. *Journal of Neurochemistry*, Vol.82, No.6, (2002), pp.1424–1434, ISSN 0022-3042

Bracci, L., & Neri, P.(1995). Molecular mimicry between the rabies virus and human immunodeficiency virus. *Archives of Pathology & Laboratory Medicine*, Vol.119, No. 5, (May 1995), pp. 391-393, ISSN 0003-9985

Bracci, L., Ballas, S., Spreafico, A., & Neri, P. (1997). Molecular mimicry between the rabies virus glycoprotein and human immunodeficiency virus-1 GP120: cross-reacting antibodies induced by rabies vaccination. *Blood*, Vol. 90 , No. 9, (Nov 1997), pp. 3623-3628, ISSN: 0006-4971

Bren, G., Trushin, S., Whitman, J., Shepard, B., & Badley, A. (2009). HIV gp120 Induces, NF-kB Dependent, HIV Replication that Requires Procaspase 8. *PLoS One*, Vol.4, No.3, (2009), p.e4875, ISSN 1932-6203

Busillo, J., & Benovic, J. (2007). Regulation of CXCR4 signaling. *Biochimica et Biophysica Acta* , Vol. 1768, No. 4, (Apr 2007), pp. 952-963, ISSN 0005-2736

Butzke, D., & Luch, A. (2010). High-molecular weight protein toxins of marine invertebrates and their elaborate modes of action. *EXS*, Vol.100, (2010), pp.213-232, ISSN 1023-294X

Canducci, F., Marinozzi, M., Sampaolo, M., Berrè, S., Bagnarelli, P., Degano, M., Gallotta, G., Mazzi, B., Lemey, P., Burioni, R., & Clementi, M. (2009). Dynamic features of the selective pressure on the human immunodeficiency virus type 1 (HIV-1) gp120 CD4-binding site in a group of long term non progressor (LTNP) subjects. *Retrovirology*, Vol.6, No.1, (Jan 2009), p. 4, ISSN. 1742-4690

Cantin, R., Fortin, J., Lamontagne, G., & Tremblay, M. (1997). The acquisition of host-derived major histocompatibility complex class II glycoproteins by human immunodeficiency virus type 1 accelerates the process of virus entry and infection in human T-lymphoid cells. *Blood*, Vol.90, No. 3, (1997), pp. 1091-1100, ISSN. 0006-4971

Cheung, R., Ravyn, V., Wang, L., Ptasznik, A., & Collman, R. (2008). Signaling Mechanism of HIV-1 gp120 and Virion-Induced IL-1β Release in Primary Human Macrophages. *The Journal of Immunology*, Vol.180, No.10, (2008), pp. 6675–6684, ISSN 0022-1767

Chirmule, N., & Pahwa, S. (1996). Envelope glycoproteins of human immunodeficiency virus type 1: profound influences on immune functions. *Microbiological Reviews*, Vol.60, No.2, (Jun 1996), pp. 386-406, ISSN 0146-0749

Choudhary, S., Vrisekoop, N., Jansen, C., Otto, S., Schuitemaker, H., Miedema, F., & Camerini, D. (2007). Low Immune Activation despite High Levels of Pathogenic Human Immunodeficiency Virus Type 1 Results in Long-Term Asymptomatic Disease. *The Journal of Virology*, Vol.81, No.16, (Aug 2007), pp. 8838-8842, ISSN 0022-538X

Cicala, C., Arthos, J., Rubbert, A., Selig, S., Wildt, K., Cohen, O., & Fauci, A. (2000). HIV-1 envelope induces activation of caspase-3 and cleavage of focal adhesion kinase in primary human CD4(+) T cells. *Proceedings of the National Academy of Sciences*, Vol. 97, No.3, (Feb 2000), pp. 1178-1183, ISSN 0027-8424

Cicala, C., Arthos, J., Selig, S., Dennis, G. Jr., Hosack, D., Van Ryk, D., Spangler, M., Steenbeke, T., Khazanie, P., Gupta, N., Yang, J., Daucher, M., Lempicki, R., & Fauci, A. (2002). HIV envelope induces a cascade of cell signals in non-proliferating target cells that favor virus replication. *Proceedings of the National Academy of Sciences*, Vol.99, No.14, (2002), pp.9380-9385, ISSN 0027-8424

Cicala, C., Arthos, J., Martinelli, E., Censoplano, N., Cruz, C., Chung, E., Selig, S., Van Ryk, D., Yang, J., Jagannatha, S., Chun, T., Ren, P., Lempicki, R., & Fauci, A. (2006a). R5 and X4 HIV envelopes induce distinct gene expression profiles in primary peripheral blood mononuclear cells. *Proceedings of the National Academy of Sciences*, Vol.103, No.10, (Mar 2006), pp. 3746-3751, ISSN 0027-8424

Cicala, C., Arthos, J., Censoplano, N., Cruz, C., Chung, E., Martinelli, E., Lempicki, R., Natarajan, V., VanRyk, D., Daucher, M., & Fauci, A. (2006b). HIV-1 gp120 induces NFAT nuclear translocation in resting CD4+ T-cells. *Virology*, Vol. 345, No. 1, (2006), pp. 105-114, ISSN 0042-6822.

Cron, R., Bartz, S., Clausell, A., Bort, S., Klebanoff, S., & Lewis, D. (2000). NFAT1 enhances HIV-1 gene expression in primary human CD4 T cells.*Clinical Immunology*, Vol.94, No.3, (Mar 2000), pp. 179-191, ISSN 1521-6616

Daniel, V., Süsal, C., Weimer, R., Zipperle, S., Kröpelin, M., Melk, A., Zimmermann, R., Huth-Kühne, A., & Opelz, G. (1998). Association of viral load in plasma samples of HIV-infected hemophilia patients with autoantibodies and gp120-containing immune complexes on CD4+ lymphocytes. *Immunology Letters*, Vol.60, No.2-3, (Feb 1998), pp. 179-187, ISSN 0165-2478

Daniel, V., Süsal, C., Weimer, R., Zimmermann, R., Huth-Kühne, A., & Opelz, G. (2001). Association of immune complexes and plasma viral load with CD4+ cell depletion, CD8+ DR+ and CD16+ cell counts in HIV+ hemophilia patients. Implications for the immunopathogenesis of HIV-induced CD4+ lymphocyte depletion. *Immunology Letters*, Vol.76, No.2, (Mar 2001), pp. 69-78, ISSN 0165-2478

D'Aversa, T., Eugenin, E., & Berman, J. (2005). NeuroAIDS: contributions of the human immunodeficiency virus-1 proteins Tat and gp120 as well as CD40 to microglial activation. *Journal of Neuroscience Research*, Vol.81, No.3, (Aug 2005), pp. 436-446, ISSN 0360-4012

Davis, C., Dikic, I., Unutmaz, D., Hill, C., Arthos, J., Siani, M., Thompson, D., Schlessinger, J., & Littman, D. (1997). Signal transduction due to HIV-1 envelope interactions with chemokine receptors CXCR4 or CCR5. *The Journal of Experimental Medicine*, Vol.186, No.10, (Nov 1997), pp.1793-1798, ISSN 0022-1007

Del Corno, M., Liu, Q., Schols, D., Clercq, E., Gessani, S., Freedman, B., & Collman, R. (2001). HIV-1 gp120 and chemokine activation of Pyk2 and mitogen-activated protein kinases in primary macrophages mediated by calcium-dependent, pertussis toxin-insensitive chemokine receptor signaling. *Blood*, Vol.98, No.10, (2001), pp. 2909-2916, ISSN 0006-4971

DePaolo, R., Lathan, R., & Karpus, W. (2004). CCR5 Regulates High Dose Oral Tolerance by Modulating CC Chemokine Ligand 2 Levels in the GALT. *The Journal of Immunology*, Vol.173, No.1, (2004), pp. 314-320, ISSN 0022-1767

Dobaczewski, M., Xia, Y., Bujak, M., Gonzalez-Quesada, C., & Frangogiannis, N. (2010). CCR5 Signaling Suppresses Inflammation and Reduces Adverse Remodeling of the Infarcted Heart, Mediating Recruitment of Regulatory T Cells. *The American Journal of Pathology*, Vol.176, No.5, (May 2010), pp. 2177–2187, ISSN 0002-9440

Earl, P., Moss, B., & Doms, R. (1991). Folding, interaction with GRP78-BiP, assembly, and transport of the human immunodeficiency virus type 1 envelope protein. *The Journal of Virology*, Vol.65, No.4, (Apr 1991), pp. 2047-2055, ISSN 0022-538X

Edinger, A., Mankowski, J., Doranz, B., Margulies, B., Lee, B., Rucker, J., Sharron, M., Hoffman, T., Berson, J., Zink, M., Hirsch, V., Clements, J., & Doms, R. (1997). CD4-independent, CCR5-dependent infection of brain capillary endothelial cells by a neurovirulent simian immunodeficiency virus strain. *Proceedings of the National Academy of Sciences,* Vol.94, No.26, (1997), pp.14742-14747, ISSN 0027-8424

Edwards, L., & Hessinger, D. (2000). Portuguese man-of-war (Physalia physalis) venom induces calcium influx into cells by permeabilizing plasma membranes. *Toxicon,* Vol.38, No.8, (2000), pp. 1015–1028, ISSN 0041-0101

Edwards, L., & Evavold, B. (2011). T cell recognition of weak ligands: roles of signaling, receptor number, and affinity. *Immunologic Research,* Vol.50, No.1, (May 2011), pp. 39-48, ISSN 1559-0755

Eggink, D., Melchers, M., Wuhrer, M., Van Montfort, T., Dey, A., Naaijkens, B., David, K., Le Douce, V., Deelder, A., Kang, K., Olson, W., Berkhout, B., Hokke, C., Moore, J., & Sanders, R. (2010). Lack of complex N-glycans on HIV-1 envelope glycoproteins preserves protein conformation and entry function. *Virology,* Vol.401, No.2, (Jun 2010), pp. 236-247, ISSN 0042-6822

Endo, M., Inatsu, A., Hashimoto, K., Takamune, N., Shoji, S., & Misumi, S. (2008). Human immunodeficiency virus-induced apoptosis of human breast cancer cells via CXCR4 is mediated by the viral envelope protein but does not require CD4. *Current HIV Research,* Vol.6, No.1, (Jan 2008), pp. 34-42, ISSN 1570-162X

Endo, M., Gejima, S., Endo, A., Takamune, N., Shoji, S., & Misumi, S. (2010). Treatment of breast cancer cells with proteasome inhibitor lactacystin increases the level of sensitivity to cell death induced by human immunodeficiency virus type 1. *Biological & Pharmaceutical Bulletin,* Vol.33, No.11, (2010), pp. 1903-1906, ISSN 0918-6158

Fantuzzi, L., Canini, I., Belardelli, F., & Gessani, S. (2001). HIV-1 gp120 Stimulates the Production of β-Chemokines in Human Peripheral Blood Monocytes Through a CD4-Independent Mechanism. *The Journal of Immunology,* Vol.166, No.9, (2001), pp. 5381–5387, ISSN 0022-1767

Fenouillet, E., Clerget-Raslain, B., Gluckman, J., Guétard, D., Montagnier, L., & Bahraoui, E. (1989). Role of N-linked glycans in the interaction between the envelope glycoprotein of human immunodeficiency virus and its CD4 cellular receptor. Structural enzymatic analysis. *The Journal of Experimental Medicine,* Vol.169, No.3, (1989), pp. 807-822, ISSN 0022-1007

Fernandis, A., Prasad, A., Band, H., Klösel, R., & Ganju, R. (2004). Regulation of CXCR4-mediated chemotaxis and chemoinvasion of breast cancer cells. *Oncogene,* Vol.23, No.1, (Jan 2004), pp.157-167, ISSN 0950-9232

Fiala, M., Looney, D., Stins, M., Way, D., Zhang, L., Gan, X., Chiappelli, F., Schweitzer, E., Shapshak, P., Weinand, M., Graves, M., Witte, M., & Kim, K. (1997). TNF-alpha opens a paracellular route for HIV-1 invasion across the bloodbrain barrier. *Molecular Medicine*, Vol.3, No.8, (1997), pp. 553–564, ISSN 1076-1551

Fischer-Smith, T., Croul, S., Sverstiuk, A., Capini, C., L'Heureux, D., Regulier, E., Richardson, M., Amini, S., Morgello, S., Khalili, K., & Rappaport, J. (2001). CNS invasion by CD14+/CD16+ peripheral blood-derived monocytes in HIV dementia: perivascular accumulation and reservoir of HIV infection. *Journal of Neurovirology,* Vol.7, No.6, (2001), pp. 528–541, ISSN 1355-0284

Fox, J., Letellier, E., Oliphant, C., & Signoret, N. (2011). TLR2-dependent pathway of heterologous down-modulation for the CC chemokine receptors 1, 2, and 5 in human blood monocytes. *Blood,* Vol.117, No.6, (2011), pp.1851-1860, ISSN 0006-4971

Gerencer, M., Burek, V., Crowe, B., Barrett, N., & Dorner, F. (1998). The role of complement and gp120-specific antibodies in virus lysis and CD4+ T cell depletion in HIV-1-

infected patients. *Microbial Pathogenesis* , Vol.25, No.5, (1998), pp.253-266, ISSN 0882-4010

Gilbert, M., Kirihara, J., & Mills, J. (1991). Enzyme-linked immunoassay for human immunodeficiency virus type 1 envelope glycoprotein 120. *Journal of Clinical Microbiology*, Vol.29, No.1, (Jan 1991), pp.142-147, ISSN 0095-1137

Goldman, F., Crabtree, J., Hollenback, C., & Koretzky, G. (1997). Sequestration of p56(lck) by gp120, a model for TCR desensitization. *The Journal of Immunology*, Vol. 158, No. 5, (1997), pp. 2017-2024, ISSN 0022-1767

Gras, G., & Kaul, M. (2010). Molecular mechanisms of neuroinvasion by monocytes-macrophages in HIV-1 infection. *Retrovirology*, Vol.7, (Apr 2010), p. 30, ISSN 1742-4690

Green, D., Center, D., & Cruikshank, W. (2009). Human Immunodeficiency Virus Type 1 gp120 Reprogramming of CD4+ T-Cell Migration Provides a Mechanism for Lymphadenopathy. *Journal of Virology*, Vol.83, No.11, (Jun 2009), pp. 5765-5772, ISSN 0022-538X

Hashimoto, F., Oyaizu, N., Kalyanaraman, V., & Pahwa, S. (1997). Modulation of Bcl-2 protein by CD4 cross-linking: a possible mechanism for lymphocyte apoptosis in human immunodeficiency virus infection and for rescue of apoptosis by interleukin-2. *Blood*, Vol.90, No.2, (Jul 1997), pp. 745-753, ISSN 0006-4971

Hecht, I., Cahalon, L., Hershkoviz, R., Lahat, A., Franitza, S., & Lider, O. (2003). Heterologous desensitization of T cell functions by CCR5 and CXCR4 ligands: inhibition of cellular signaling, adhesion and chemotaxis. *International Immunology*, Vol. 15, No.1, (2003), pp. 29-38, ISSN 0953-8178

Herbein, G., Mahlknecht, U., Batliwalla, F., Gregersen, P., Pappas, T., Butler, J., O'Brien, W., & Verdin, E. (1998). Apoptosis of CD8+ T cells is mediated by macrophages through interaction of HIV gp120 with chemokine receptor CXCR4. *Nature*, Vol.395, No.6698, (Sep 1998), pp.189-194, ISSN 0028-0836

Herida, M., Mary-Krause, M., Kaphan, R., Cadranel, J., Poizot-Martin, I., Rabaud, C., Plaisance, N., Tissot-Dupont, H., Boue, F., Lang, J., Costagliola, D. (2003). Incidence of non-AIDS-defining cancers before and during the highly active antiretroviral therapy era in a cohort of human immunodeficiency virus-infected patients. *Journal of Clinical Oncology*, Vol.21, No.18, (Sep 2003), pp. 3447-3453, ISSN 1527-7755

Hezareh, M., Moukil, M., Szanto, I., Pondarzewski, M., Mouche, S., Cherix, N., Brown, S., Carpentier, J., & Foti, M. (2004). Mechanisms of HIV receptor and co-receptor down-regulation by prostratin: role of conventional and novel PKC isoforms.*Antiviral Chemistry & Chemotherapy* , Vol.15, No.4, (Jul 2004), pp.207-222, ISSN 0956-3202

Hodgson, D., Yirmiya, R., Chiappelli, F., & Taylor, A. (1998). Intracerebral HIV glycoprotein gp120. enhances tumor metastasis via centrally released interleukin-1. *Brain Research*, Vol.781, No.1-2, (1998), pp. 244–251, ISSN 0006-8993.

Holm, G., Zhang, C., Gorry, P., Peden, K., Schols, D., De Clercq, E., Gabuzda, D. (2004). Apoptosis of bystander T cells induced by human immunodeficiency virus type 1 with increased envelope/receptor affinity and coreceptor binding site exposure. *The Journal of Virology*, Vol.78, No.9, (May 2004), pp. 4541-4551, ISSN 0022-538X

Iacovache, I., Van der Goot, F., & Pernot, L. (2008). Pore formation: An ancient yet complex form of attack. *Biochimica et Biophysica Acta*, Vol.1778, No.7-8, (2008), pp.1611–1623, ISSN 0005-2736

Iyengar, S., Schwartz, D., & Hildreth, J. (1999). T Cell-Tropic HIV gp120 Mediates CD4 and CD8 Cell Chemotaxis through CXCR4 Independent of CD4: Implications for HIV Pathogenesis. *The Journal of Immunology*, Vol.162, No.10, (1999), pp. 6263-6267, ISSN 0022-1767

Janowska-Wieczorek, A., Marquez, L., Dobrowsky, A., Ratajczak, M., & Cabuhat, M. (2000). Differential MMP and TIMP production by human marrow and peripheral blood CD34(+) cells in response to chemokines. *Experimental Hematology*, Vol.28, No.11, (Nov 2000), pp.1274-1285, ISSN 0301-472X

Jones, P., Korte, T., & Blumenthal, R. (1998). Conformational changes in cell surface HIV-1 envelope glycoproteins are triggered by cooperation between cell surface CD4 and co-receptors. *The Journal of Biological Chemistry*, Vol.273, No.1, (1998), pp. 404–409, ISSN 0021-9258

Kang, Y., Siegel, P., Shu, W., Drobnjak, M., Kakonen, S., Cordón-Cardo, C., Guise, T., Massagué, J. (2003). A multigenic program mediating breast cancer metastasis to bone. *Cancer Cell*, Vol. 3, No. 6, (2003), pp. 537-549, ISSN 1535-6108

Kanmogne, G., Primeaux, C., & Grammas, P. (2005). HIV-1 gp120 proteins alter tight junction protein expression and brain endothelial cell permeability: implications for the pathogenesis of HIV-associated dementia. *Journal of Neuropathology & Experimental Neurology*, Vol.64, No.6, (Jun 2005), pp. 498-505, ISSN 0022-3069

Kanmogne, G., Schall, K., Leibhart, J., Knipe, B., Gendelman, H., & Persidsky, Y. (2007). HIV-1 gp120 compromises blood-brain barrier integrity and enhances monocyte migration across blood-brain barrier: implication for viral neuropathogenesis. *Journal of Cerebral Blood Flow & Metabolism*, Vol.27, No.1, (Jan 2007), pp. 123-134, ISSN 0271-678X

Kaufmann, A., Salentin, R., Gemsa, D., & Sprenger, H. (2001). Increase of CCR1 and CCR5 expression and enhanced functional response to MIP-1α during differentiation of human monocytes to macrophages. *Journal of Leukocyte Biology*, Vol.69, No.2, (2001), pp. 248-252, ISSN 0741-5400

Khan, N., Di Cello, F., Stins, M., & Kim, K. (2007). Gp120-mediated cytotoxicity of human brain microvascular endothelial cells is dependent on p38 mitogen-activated protein kinase activation. *Journal of Neurovirology*, Vol.13, No.3, (Jun 2007), pp. 242-251, ISSN 1355-0284

Kim, M., Koh, Y., Kim, K., Koh, B., Nam, D., Alitalo, K., Kim, I., & Koh, G. (2010). CXCR4 signaling regulates metastasis of chemoresistant melanoma cells by a lymphatic metastatic niche. *Cancer Research*, Vol.70, No.24, (2010), pp. 10411-10421, ISSN 0008-5472

Kinet, S., Bernard, F., Mongellaz, C., Perreau, M., Goldman, F., & Taylor, N. (2002). Gp120-mediated induction of the MAPK cascade is dependent on the activation state of CD4(+) lymphocytes. *Blood*, Vol.100, No.7, (Oct 2002), pp. 2546-2553, ISSN 0006-4971

Kinoshita, S., Chen, B., Kaneshima, H., & Nolan, G. (1998). Host control of HIV-1 parasitism in T cells by the nuclear factor of activated T cells. *Cell*, Vol.95, No.5, (Nov 1998), pp. 595-604, ISSN 0092-8674

Klasse, P., & Moore, J. (2004). Is there enough gp120 in the body fluids of HIV-1-infected individuals to have biologically significant effects?. *Virology*, Vol.323, No.1, (May 2004), pp.1-8, ISSN 0042-6822

Korber, B., Gaschen, B., Yusim, K., Thakallapally, R., Kesmir, C., & Detours, V. (2001). Evolutionary and immunological implications of contemporary HIV-1 variation. *British Medical Bulletin,* Vol.58, (2001), pp.19–42, ISSN 0007-1420

Kristan, K., Viero, G., Dalla Serra, M., Macek, P., & Anderluh, G. (2009). Molecular mechanism of pore formation by actinoporins. *Toxicon,* Vol.54, No.8, (Dec 2009), pp. 1125-1134, ISSN 0041-0101

Kryworuchko, M., Pasquier, V., & Thèze, J. (2003). Human immunodeficiency virus-1 envelope glycoproteins and anti-CD4 antibodies inhibit interleukin-2-induced Jak/STAT signaling in human CD4 T lymphocytes. *Clinical & Experimental Immunology,* Vol. 131, No.3, (2003), pp. 422–427, ISSN 0009-9104

Kucia, M., Reca, R., Miekus, K., Wanzeck, J., Wojakowski, W., Janowska-Wieczorek, A., Ratajczak, J., & Ratajczak, M. (2005).Trafficking of normal stem cells and metastasis of cancer stem cells involve similar mechanisms: pivotal role of the SDF-1-CXCR4 axis. *Stem Cells,* Vol.23, No.7, (2005), pp.879-894, ISSN 1066-5099

Land, A., & Braakman, I. (2001). Folding of the human immunodeficiency virus type 1 envelope glycoprotein in the endoplasmic reticulum. *Biochimie,* Vol.83, No.8, (Aug 2001), pp. 783-790, ISSN 0300-9084

Layne, S., Merges, M., Dembo, M., Spouge, J., Conley, S., Moore, J., Raina, J., Renz, H., Gelderblom, H., & Nara, P. (1992). Factors underlying spontaneous inactivation and susceptibility to neutralization of human immunodeficiency virus. *Virology,* Vol.189, No.2, (1992), pp. 695-714, ISSN 0042-6822

Lévesque, J., Hendy, J., Takamatsu, Y., Simmons, P., & Bendall, L. (2003). Disruption of the CXCR4/CXCL12 chemotactic interaction during hematopoietic stem cell mobilization induced by GCSF or cyclophosphamide. *The Journal of Clinical Investigation,* Vol.111, No.2, (Jan 2003), pp.187–196, ISSN 0021-9738

Li, Y., Luo, L., Rasool, N., & Kang, C. (1993). Glycosylation is necessary for the correct folding of human immunodeficiency virus gp120 in CD4 binding. *The Journal of Virology,* Vol.67, No.1, (Jan 1993), pp. 584-588, ISSN 0022-538X

Liang, Z., Yoon, Y., Votaw, J., Goodman, M., Williams, L., & Shim, H. (2005). Silencing of CXCR4 blocks breast cancer metastasis. *Cancer Research,* Vol.65, No.3, (Feb 2005), pp. 967-971, ISSN 0008-5472

Louboutin, J., Reyes, B., Agrawal, L., Maxwell, C., Van Bockstaele, E., & Strayer, D. (2010). Blood–brain barrier abnormalities caused by exposure to HIV-1 gp120 -Protection by gene delivery of antioxidant enzymes. *Neurobiology of Disease,* Vol.38, No.2, (2010), pp. 313–325, ISSN 0969-9961

Maas, J., De Roda Husman, A., Brouwer, M., Krol, A., Coutinho, R., Keet, I., Van Leeuwen, R., & Schuitemaker, H. (1998). Presence of the variant mannose binding lectin alleles associated with slower progression to AIDS. Amsterdam Cohort Study. *AIDS.,* Vol.12, No.17, (1998), pp. 2275-2280, ISSN 0269-9370

Maccarrone, M., Navarra, M., Catani, V., Corasaniti, T., Bagetta, G., & Finazzi-Agro, A. (2002). Cholesterol-dependent modulation of the toxicity of HIV-1 coat protein gp120 in human neuroblastoma cells. *Journal of Neurochemistry,* Vol. 82, No.6, (2002), pp. 1444–1452, ISSN 0022-3042

Marchese, A., Paing, M., Temple, B., &Trejo, J.(2008). G protein-coupled receptor sorting to endosomes and lysosomes. *Annual Review of Pharmacology and Toxicology* , Vol.48, (2008), pp. 601–629, ISSN 0362-1642

Maresca, M., Mahfoud, R., Garmy, N., Kotler, D., Fantini, J., & Clayton, F. (2003). The virotoxin model of HIV-1 enteropathy: involvement of GPR15/Bob and galactosylceramide in the cytopathic effects induced by HIV-1 gp120 in the HT-29-D4 intestinal cell line. *Journal of Biomedical Science*, Vol.10, No.1, (Jan-Feb 2003), pp. 156-166, ISSN 1021-7770

Masci, A., Galgani, M., Cassano, S., De Simone, S., Gallo, A., De Rosa, V., Zappacosta, S., & Racioppi, L.(2003). HIV-1 gp120 induces anergy in naive T lymphocytes through. CD4-independent protein kinase-A-mediated signaling. *Journal of Leukocyte Biology*, Vol.74, No.6, (2003), pp. 1117–1124, ISSN 0741-5400

Mbemba, E., Benjouad, A., Saffar, L., & Gattegno, L.(1999). Glycans and proteoglycans are involved in the interactions of human immunodeficiency virus type 1 envelope glycoprotein and of SDF-1alpha with membrane ligands of CD4(+) CXCR4(+) cells. *Virology*, Vol. 265, No.2, (Dec 1999), pp. 354-364, ISSN 0042-6822

McKeating, J., McKnight, A., & Moore, J. (1991). Differential loss of envelope glycoprotein gp120 from virions of human immunodeficiency virus type 1 isolates: effects on infectivity and neutralization. *The Journal of Virology*,Vol.65, No.2, (Feb 1991), pp. 852-860, ISSN 0022-538X

Means, R., & Desrosiers, R. (2000). Resistance of native, oligomeric envelope on simian immunodeficiency virus to digestion by glycosidases. *The Journal of Virology*, Vol.74, No.23, (Dec 2000), pp. 11181-11190, ISSN 0022-538X

Medders, K., Sejbuk, N., Maung, R., Desai, M., & Kaul, M. (2010). Activation of p38 MAPK is required in monocytic and neuronal cells for HIV glycoprotein 120-induced neurotoxicity. *The Journal of Immunology*, Vol.185, No.8, (Oct 2010), pp. 4883-4895, ISSN 0022-1767

Medina, I., Ghose, S., & Ben-Ari, Y. (1999). Mobilization of intracellular calcium stores participates in the rise of [Ca21]i and the toxic actions of the HIV coat protein gp120. *European Journal of Neuroscience*, Vol. 11, No. 4, (1999), pp. 1167–1178, ISSN 0953-816X

Melar, M., Ott, D., & Hope, T. (2007). Physiological levels of virion-associated human immunodeficiency virus type 1 envelope induce coreceptor-dependent calcium flux. *The Journal of Virology*, Vol. 81, No.4, (2007), pp.1773-1785, ISSN 0022-538X

Melikyan, G., Markosyan, R., Hemmati, H., Delmedico, M., Lambert, D., & Cohen, F.(2000). Evidence that the transition of HIV-1 gp41 into a six-helix bundle, not the bundle configuration, induces membrane fusion. *The Journal of Cell Biology*, Vol. 151, No.2, (2000), pp.413–423, ISSN 0021-9525

Melli, G., Keswani, S., Fischer, A., Chen, W., & Hoke, A. (2006). Spatially distinct and functionally independent mechanisms of axonal degeneration in a model of HIV-associated sensory neuropathy. *Brain*, Vol.129, No.5, (2006), pp.1330–1338, ISSN 0006-8950

Meucci, O., & Miller, R. (1996). gp120-induced neurotoxicity in hippocampal pyramidal neuron cultures: protective action of TGF-beta1. *The Journal of Neuroscience*, Vol.16, No.13, (1996), pp. 4080–4088, ISSN 0270-6474

Missé, D., Cerutti, M., Noraz, N., Jourdan, P., Favero, J., Devauchelle, G., Yssel, H., Taylor, N., & Veas, F. (1999). A CD4-Independent Interaction of Human Immunodeficiency Virus-1 gp120 With CXCR4 Induces Their Cointernalization, Cell Signaling, and T-Cell Chemotaxis. *Blood*, Vol. 93, No. 8, (1999), pp. 2454-2462, ISSN 0006-4971

Missé, D., Gajardo, J., Oblet, C., Religa, A., Riquet, N., Mathieu, D., Yssel, H., & Veas, F. (2005). Soluble HIV-1 gp120 enhances HIV-1 replication in non-dividing CD4+ T cells, mediated via cell signaling and Tat cofactor overexpression. *AIDS*, Vol.19, No.9, (Jun 2005), pp. 897-905, ISSN 0269-9370

Mizuochi, T., Matthews, T., Kato, M., Hamako, J., Titani, K., Solomon, J., & Feizi, T.(1990). Diversity of oligosaccharide structures on the envelope glycoprotein gp 120 of human immunodeficiency virus 1 from the lymphoblastoid cell line H9. Presence of complex-type oligosaccharides with bisecting N-acetylglucosamine residues. *The Journal of Biological Chemistry,* Vol.265, No.15, (May 1990), pp. 8519-8524, ISSN 0021-9258

Moir, S., Chun, T., & Fauci, A. (2011). Pathogenic Mechanisms of HIV Disease. *Annual Review Of Pathology* ,Vol.6, (2011), pp. 223-248, ISSN 1553-4014

Muller, A., Homey, B., Soto, H., Ge, N., Catron, D., Buchanan, M., McClanahan, T., Murphy, E., Yuan, W., Wagner, S., Barrera, J., Mohar, A., Verastegui, E., & Zlotnik, A. (2001). Involvement of chemokine receptors in breast cancer metastasis. *Nature,* Vol.410, No.6824, (2001), pp.50-56, ISSN 0028-0836

Mulroney, S., McDonnell, K., Pert, C., Ruff, M., Resch, Z., Samson, W., & Lumpkin, M. (1998). HIV gp120 inhibits the somatotropic axis: a possible GH-releasing hormone receptor mechanismfor the pathogenesis of AIDS wasting. *Proceedings of the National Academy of Sciences,* Vol.95, No.4, (Feb 1998), pp.1927-1932, ISSN 0027-8424

Murdoch, C., Monk, P., & Finn, A. (1999). CXC chemokine receptor expression on human endothelial cells. *Cytokine,* Vol.11, No.9, (1999), pp. 704–712, ISSN 1043-4666

Muthumani, K., Wadsworth, S., Dayes, N., Hwang, D., Choo, A., Abeysinghe, H., Siekierka, J., & Weiner, D. (2004). Suppression of HIV-1 viral replication and cellular pathogenesis by a novel p38/JNK kinase inhibitor. *AIDS.*, Vol.18, No.5, (Mar 2004), pp.739-748, ISSN 0269-9370

Neri, P., Bracci, L., Rustici, M., & Santucci, A.(1990). Sequence homology between HIV gp120, rabies virus glycoprotein, and snake venom neurotoxins. Is the nicotinic acetylcholine receptor an HIV receptor?. *Archives of Virology,* Vol.114, No.3-4, (1990), pp. 265-269, ISSN 0304-8608

Nimmagadda, S., Pullambhatla, M., Stone, K., Green, G., Bhujwalla, Z., & Pomper, M. (2010). Molecular imaging of CXCR4 receptor expression in human cancer xenografts with [64Cu]AMD3100 positron emission tomography. *Cancer Research,* Vol.70, No.10, (May 2010), pp. 3935-3944, ISSN 0008-5472

Ogert, R., Lee, M., Ross, W., Buckler-White, A., Martin, M., & Cho, M. (2001). N-linked glycosylation sites adjacent to and within the V1/V2 and the V3 loops of dualtropic human immunodeficiency virus type 1 isolate DH12 gp120 affect coreceptor usage and cellular tropism. *The Journal of Virology,* Vol.75, No.13, (Jul 2001), pp. 5998-6006, ISSN 0022-538X

Oh, S., Cruikshank, W., Raina, J., Blanchard, G., Adler, W., Walker, J., & Kornfeld, H.(1992). Identification of HIV-1 envelope glycoprotein in the serum of AIDS and ARC patients. *Journal of Acquired Immune Deficiency Syndromes,*Vol.5, No.3, (1992), pp.251-256, ISSN 0894-9255

Okamoto, S., Kang, Y., Brechtel, C., Siviglia, E., Russo, R., Clemente, A., Harrop, A., Mckercher, S., Kaul, M., & Lipton, R. (2007). HIV/gp120 decreases adult neural progenitor cell proliferation via checkpoint kinase-mediated cell cycle withdrawal and G1 Arrest. *Cell Stem Cell,* Vol.1, No.2, (2007), pp. 230-236, ISSN 1934-5909

Ono, K., & Han, J. (2000). The p38 signal transduction pathway: activation and function. *Cell Signal,* Vol.12, No.1, (2000), pp. 1-13, ISSN 0898-6568

Oppermann, M. (2004). Chemokine receptor CCR5: insights into structure, function, and regulation. *Cellular Signalling* ,Vol.16, No. 11, (November 2004), pp. 1201-1210, ISSN 0898-6568

Otteken, A., Earl, P., & Moss, B. (1996). Folding, assembly, and intracellular trafficking of the human immunodeficiency virus type 1 envelope glycoprotein analyzed with monoclonal antibodies recognizing maturational intermediates. *The Journal of Virology*, Vol.70, No.6, (Jun 1996), pp.3407-3415, ISSN 0022-538X

Pal, R., Di Marzo Veronese, F., Nair, B., Rittenhouse, S., Hoke, G., Mumbauer, S., & Sarngadharan, M.(1993). Glycoprotein of human immunodeficiency virus type 1 synthesized in chronically infected Molt3 cells acquires heterogeneous oligosaccharide structures. *Biochemical and Biophysical Research Communications*, Vol.196, No.3, (Nov 1993), pp.1335-1342, ISSN 0006-291X

Pantanowitz, L., Dezube, B. (2001). Breast cancer in women with HIV/AIDS. *The Journal of the American Medical Association*,Vol.285, No.24, (2001), pp. 3090-3091, ISSN 0098-7484

Pastinen, T., Liitsola, K., Niini, P., Salminen, M., & Syvanen, A. (1998). Contribution of the CCR5 and MBL genes to susceptibility to HIV type 1 infection in the Finnish population. *AIDS Research and Human Retroviruses*, Vol.14, No.8, (1998), pp. 695-698, ISSN 0889-2229

Pawlak, J., Mackessy, S., Fry, B., Bhatia, M., Mourier, G., Fruchart-Gaillard, C., Servent, D., Ménez, R., Stura, E., Ménez, A., & Kini, R. (2006). Denmotoxin, a three-finger toxin from the colubrid snake Boiga dendrophila (Mangrove Catsnake) with bird-specific activity. *The Journal of Biological Chemistry*, Vol.281, No.39, (Sep 2006), pp. 29030-29041, ISSN 0021-9258

Peng, F., Dhillon, N., Callen, S., Yao, H., Bokhari, S., Zhu, X., Baydoun, H., & Buch, S. (2008). Platelet-Derived Growth Factor Protects Neurons against Gp120- Mediated Toxicity. *Journal of Neurovirology*, Vol.14, No.1, (2008), pp. 62–72, ISSN 1355-0284

Polzer, S., Dittmar, M., Schmitz, H., & Schreiber, M. (2002). The N-linked glycan g15 within the V3 loop of the HIV-1 external glycoprotein gp120 affects coreceptor usage, cellular tropism, and neutralization. *Virology*, Vol. 304, No.1, (2002), pp. 70-80, ISSN 0042-6822

Price, O., Ercal, N., Nakaoke, R., & Banks, W. (2005). HIV-1 viral proteins gp120 and Tat induce oxidative stress in brain endothelial cells. *Brain Research*, Vol.1045, No.1-2, (2005), pp. 57–63, ISSN 0006-8993

Rahangdale, S., Morgan, R., Heijens, C., Ryan, T., Yamasaki, H., Bentley, E., Sullivan, E., Center, D., & Cruikshank. W. (2006). Chemokine receptor CXCR3 desensitization by IL-16/CD4 signaling is dependent on CCR5 and intact membrane cholesterol. *The Journal of Immunology*, Vol.176, No.4, (2006), pp. 2337-2345, ISSN 0022-1767

Raska, M., Takahashi, K., Czernekova, L., Zachova, K., Hall, S., Moldoveanu, Z., Elliott, M., Wilson, L., Brown, R., Jancova, D., Barnes, S., Vrbkova, J., Tomana, M., Smith, P., Mestecky, J., Renfrow, M., & Novak, J.(2010). Glycosylation patterns of HIV-1 gp120 depend on the type of expressing cells and affect antibody recognition. *The Journal of Biological Chemistry*, Vol.285, No.27, (Jul 2010), pp. 20860-20869. ISSN 0021-9258

Roggero, R., Robert-Hebmann, V., Harrington, S., Roland, J., Vergne, L., Jaleco, S., Devaux, C., & Biard-Piechaczyk, M. (2001). Binding of human immunodeficiency virus type 1 gp120 to CXCR4 induces mitochondrial transmembrane depolarization and cytochrome *c*-mediated apoptosis independently of Fas signaling. *The Journal of Virology*, Vol.75, No.16, (2001), pp.7637-7650, ISSN 0022-538X

Rychert, J., Strick, D., Bazner, S., Robinson, J., & Rosenberg, E. (2010). Detection of HIV gp120 in plasma during early HIV infection is associated with increased proinflammatory and immunoregulatory cytokines. *AIDS Research and Human Retroviruses*, Vol.26, No.10, (Oct 2010), pp.1139-1145, ISSN 1931-8405

Saifuddin, M., Hart, M., Gewurz, H., Zhang, Y., & Spear, G.(2000). Interaction of mannose-binding lectin with primary isolates of human immunodeficiency virus type 1. *Journal of General Virology*, Vol.81, No.4, (Apr 2000), pp. 949-955, ISSN 0022-1317

Santosuosso, M., Righi, E., Lindstrom, V., Leblanc, P., & Poznansky, M.(2009). HIV-1 envelope protein gp120 is present at high concentrations in secondary lymphoid organs of individuals with chronic HIV-1 infection. *Journal of Infectious Diseases*, Vol.200, No.7, (Oct 2009), pp. 1050-1053, ISSN 0022-1899

Sattentau, Q., & Moore, J. (1991). Conformational changes induced in the human immunodeficiency virus envelope glycoprotein by soluble CD4 binding, *The Journal of Experimental Medicine*, Vol.174, No.2, (1991), pp. 407–415, ISSN 0022-1007

Schneider, J., Kaaden, O., Copeland, T., Oroszlan, S., & Hunsmann, G. (1986). Shedding and interspecies type sero-reactivity of the envelope glycopolypeptide gp120 of the human immunodeficiency virus. *Journal of General Virology*, Vol.67, No.11, (1986), pp.2533-2538, ISSN 0022-1317

Schols, D., De Clercq, E.(1996). Human immunodeficiency virus type 1 gp120 induces anergy in human peripheral blood lymphocytes by inducing interleukin-10 production. *The Journal of Virology*, Vol.70, No.8, (1996), pp. 4953-4960, ISSN 0022-538X

Schwartz, R.(2003). T cell anergy. *Annual Review of Immunology*, Vol.21, (2003), pp. 305–334, ISSN 0732-0582

Singh, S., Bond, V., Powell, M., Singh, U., Bumpers, H., Grizzle, W., & Lillard, J.(2009). CXCR4-gp120-IIIB interactions induce caspase-mediated apoptosis of prostate cancer cells and inhibit tumor growth. *Molecular Cancer Therapeutics*, Vol.8, No.1, (Jan 2009), pp. 178-184, ISSN 1535-7163

Smith-Franklin, B., Keele, B., Tew, J., Gartner, S., Szakal, A., Estes, J., Thacker, T., & Burton, G.(2002). Follicular dendritic cells and the persistence of HIV infectivity: the role of antibodies and Fc gamma receptors. *The Journal of Immunology*, Vol.168, No.5, (Mar 2002), pp. 2408-2414, ISSN 0022-1767

Spiegel, A., Kollet, O., Peled, A., Abel, L., Nagler, A., Bielorai, B., Rechavi, G., Vormoor, J., & Lapidot, T.(2004) Unique SDF-1-induced activation of human precursor-B ALL cells as a result of altered CXCR4 expression and signaling. *Blood*, Vol.103, No.8, (Apr 2004), pp. 2900-2907, ISSN 0006-4971

Stansell, E., & Desrosiers, R. (2010). Functional Contributions of Carbohydrate on AIDS Virus Glycoprotein. *Yale Journal of biology and medicine*, Vol. 83, No.4, (2010), pp.201-208, ISSN 1551-4056

Stins, M., Pearce, D., Choi, H., Di Cello, F., Pardo, C., & Kim, K. (2004). CD4 and chemokine receptors on human brain microvascular endothelial cells, implications for human immunodeficiency virus type 1 pathogenesis. *Endothelium*, Vol.11, No.5-6, (2004), pp. 275-284, ISSN 1062-3329

Stoddart, C., Keir, M., & McCune, J. (2010). IFN-alpha-induced upregulation of CCR5 leads to expanded HIV tropism in vivo. *PLoS Pathogens*, Vol.6, No.2, (Feb 2010), pp. e1000766, ISSN 1553-7366

Strazza, M., Pirrone, V., Wigdahl, B., & Nonnemacher, M. (2011). Breaking down the barrier: The effects of HIV-1 on the blood-brain barrier. *Brain Research* , Vol.1399, (Jul 2011), pp. 96-115, ISSN 1872-6240

Sullivan, N., Sun, Y., Sattentau, Q., Thali, M., Wu, D., Denisova, G., Gershoni, J., Robinson, J., Moore, J., & Sodroski, J.(1998). CD4-induced conformational changes in the human immunodeficiency virus type 1 gp120 glycoprotein: consequences for virus entry and neutralization. *The Journal of Virology*, Vol. 72, No. 6, (1998), pp. 4694–4703, ISSN 0022-538X

Sunila, I., Vaccarezza, M., Pantaleo, G., Fauci, A., & Orenstein, J. (1997). gp120 is present on the plasma membrane of apoptotic CD4 cells prepared from lymph nodes of HIV-1-infected individuals: an immunoelectron microscopic study. *AIDS.*, Vol.11, No.1, (Jan 1997), pp. 27-32, ISSN 0269-9370

Suput, D.(2009). In vivo effects of cnidarian toxins and venoms. *Toxicon*, Vol.54, No.8, (2009), pp. 1190-1200, ISSN 0041-0101

Thieblemont, N., Weiss, L., Sadeghi, H., Estcourt, C., & Haeffner-Cavaillon, N. (1995). CD14lowCD16high: a cytokine-producing monocyte subset which expands during human immunodeficiency virus infection. *European Journal of Immunology*, Vol.25, No.12, (1995), pp.3418–3424, ISSN 0014-2980

Toborek, M., Lee, Y., Flora, G., Pu, H., András, I., Wylegala, E., Hennig, B., & Nath, A.(2005). Mechanisms of the blood-brain barrier disruption in HIV-1 infection. *Cellular and Molecular Neurobiology*, Vol.25, No.1, (Feb 2005), pp.181-199, ISSN 0272-4340

Trkola, A., Dragic, T., Arthos, J., Binley, J., Olson, W., Allaway, G., Cheng-Mayer, C., Robinson, J., Maddon, P., & Moore, J.(1996). CD4-dependent, antibody-sensitive interactions between HIV-1 and its co-receptor CCR-5. *Nature*, Vol.384, No.6605, (1996), pp.184–187, ISSN 0028-0836

Trushin, S., Algeciras-Schimnich, A., Vlahakis, S., Bren, G., Warren, S., Schnepple, D., & Badley, A. (2007). Glycoprotein 120 binding to CXCR4 causes p38-dependent primary T cell death that is facilitated by, but does not require cell-associated CD4. *The Journal of Immunology*, Vol.178, No.8, (2007), pp. 4846-4853, ISSN 0022-1767

Trushin, S., Bren, G., & Badley, A. (2010). CXCR4 Tropic HIV-1 gp120 Inhibition of SDF-1α-Induced Chemotaxis Requires Lck and is Associated with Cofilin Phosphorylation. *The Open Virology Journal*, Vol. 4, (Jun 2010), pp.157-62, ISSN 1874-3579

Van Drenth, C., Jenkins, A., Ledwich, L., Ryan, T., Mashikian, M., Brazer, W., Center, D., & Cruikshank, W. (2000). Desensitization of CXC chemokine receptor 4, mediated by IL-16/CD4, is independent of p56lck enzymatic activity. *The Journal of Immunology*, Vol.165, No.11, (2000), pp. 6356-6363, ISSN 0022-1767

Visalli, V., Muscoli, C., Sacco, I., Sculco, F., Palma, E., Costa, N., Colica, C., Rotiroti, D., & Mollace, V. (2007). N-acetylcysteine prevents HIV gp 120-related damage of human cultured astrocytes: correlation with glutamine synthase dysfunction.*BMC Neuroscience*, Vol.8, No.1, (2007), p.106, ISSN 1471-2202

Vlahakis, S., Villasis-Keever, A., Gomez, T., Bren, G., & Paya, C. (2003). Human immunodeficiency virus-induced apoptosis of human hepatocytes via CXCR4. *Journal of Infectious Diseases*, Vol.188, No.10, (2003), pp. 1455-1460, ISSN 1537-6613

Wang, Q., Diskin, S., Rappaport, E., Attiyeh, E., Mosse, Y., Shue, D., Seiser, E., Jagannathan, J., Shusterman, S., & Bansal, M. (2006). Integrative genomics identifies distinct molecular classes of neuroblastoma and shows that multiple genes are targeted by regional alterations in DNA copy number. *Cancer Research*, Vol.66, No.12, (2006), pp. 6050-6062, ISSN 0008-5472

Wang, Q., Diao, X., Sun, J., & Chen, Z. (2011). Regulation of VEGF, MMP-9, and metastasis by CXCR4 in a prostate cancer cell line. *Cell Biology International*, Vol.35, No.9, (Feb 2011), pp. 897-904, ISSN 1095-8355

Wei, X., Decker, J., Wang, S., Hui, H., Kappes, J., Wu, X., Salazar-Gonzalez, J., Salazar, M., Kilby, J., Saag, M., Komarova, N., Nowak, M., Hahn, B., Kwong, P., & Shaw, G. (2003). Antibody neutralization and escape by HIV-1. *Nature,* Vol.422, No.6929, (2003), pp. 307-312, ISSN 0028-0836

Weiss, J., Nath, A., Major, E., & Berman, J.(1999). HIV-1 Tat induces monocyte chemoattractant protein-1-mediated monocyte transmigration across a model of the human blood-brain barrier and up-regulates CCR5 expression on human monocytes. *The Journal of Immunology,* Vol.163, No.5, (1999), pp. 2953-2959, ISSN 0022-1767

Weissman, D., Rabin, R., Arthos, J., Rubbert, A., Dybul, M., Swofford, R., Venkatesan, S., Farber, J., & Fauci, A. (1997). Macrophage-tropic HIV and SIV envelope proteins induce a signal through the CCR5 chemokine receptor. *Nature,* Vol.389, No.6654, (1997), pp. 981-985, ISSN 0028-0836

Williams, S., & Greene, W.(2007). Regulation of HIV-1 latency by T-cell activation. *Cytokine,* Vol.39, No.1, (Jul 2007) , pp. 63-74, ISSN 1043-4666

Wu, L., Gerard, N., Wyatt, R., Choe, H., Parolin, C., Ruffing, N., Borsetti, A., Cardoso, A., Desjardin, E., Newman, W., Gerard, C., & Sodroski, J. (1996). CD4-induced interaction of primary HIV-1 gp120 glycoproteins with the chemokine receptor CCR-5, *Nature,* Vol.384, No.6605, (1996), pp. 179–183, ISSN 0028-0836

Wu, Y., & Yoder, A. (2009). Chemokine coreceptor signaling in HIV-1 infection and pathogenesis. *PLoS Pathogens,* Vol.5, No.12, (Dec 2009), p., ISSN 1553-7366

Wyatt, R., & Sodroski, J.(1998). The HIV-1 envelope glycoproteins: fusogens, antigens, and immunogens, *Science,* Vol.280, No.5371, (1998), pp.1884–1888, ISSN 0036-8075

Wysoczynski, M., Reca, R., Ratajczak, J., Kucia, M., Shirvaikar, N., Honczarenko, M., Mills, M., Wanzeck, J., Janowska-Wieczorek, A., & Ratajczak, M. (2005). Incorporation of CXCR4 into membrane lipid rafts primes homing-related responses of hematopoietic stem/progenitor cells to an SDF-1 gradient. *Blood,* Vol.105, No.1, (Jan 2005), pp.40-48, ISSN 0006-4971

Xu, C., Liu, J., Chen, L., Liang, S., Fujii, N., Tamamura, H., & Xiong, H. (2011). HIV-1 gp120 enhances outward potassium current via CXCR4 and cAMP-dependent protein kinase a signaling in cultured rat microglia. *Glia,* Vol.59, No.6, (Mar 2011), pp.997-1007, ISSN 1098-1136

Yoder, A., Yu, D., Dong, L., Iyer, S., Xu, X., Kelly, J., Liu, J., Wang, W., Vorster, P., Agulto, L., Stephany, D., Cooper, J., Marsh, J., & Wu, Y.(2008). HIV Envelope-CXCR4 Signaling Activates Cofilin to Overcome Cortical Actin Restriction in Resting CD4 T Cells. *Cell,* Vol.134, No.5, (2008), pp. 782–792, ISSN 0092-8674

Zhang, M., Gaschen, B., Blay, W., Foley, B., Haigwood, N., Kuiken, C., & Korber, B.(2004). Tracking global patterns of *N*-linked glycosylation site variation in highly variable viral glycoproteins: HIV, SIV, and HCV envelopes and influenza hemagglutinin. *Glycobiology,* Vol.14, No.12, (2004), pp. 1229-1246, ISSN 0959-6658

Ziye, S., Fan, S., Sniderhan, L., Reisinger, E., Litzburg, A., Schifitto, G., Gelbard, H., Dewhurst, S., & Maggirwar, S. (2006). Inhibition of Mixed Lineage Kinase 3 Prevents HIV-1 Tat-Mediated Neurotoxicity and Monocyte Activation. *The Journal of Immunology,* Vol.177, No.1, (2006), pp.702-711, ISSN 0022-1767

4

HIV Recombination and Pathogenesis – Biological and Epidemiological Implications

Nitin K. Saksena[1], Katherine A. Lau[2], Dominic E. Dwyer[3] and Bin Wang[1]
[1]*Retroviral Genetics Division, Centre for Virus Research, Westmead Millennium Institute, The University of Sydney, Sydney*
[2]*Perinatal Medicine Group, Kolling Institute of Medical Research, Royal North Shore Hospital, St Leonards, NSW, Sydney*
[3]*Department of Virology, Institute for Clinical Pathology and Medical Research, Sydney*
Australia

1. Introduction

1.1 The origin, evolution and distribution of HIV: Introduction of HIV into the human population

There are several lines of evidence, which suggest that HIV-1 and HIV-2 originated from primates and were introduced into the human population via cross-species transmission events (Sharp et al., 1995). The viral genome structure of the simian form of the virus, simian immunodeficiency virus (SIV) is very similar to that of HIV (Huet et al., 1990), and phylogenetic relatedness has been established (Gao et al., 1999; Hirsch et al., 1989). SIV has been shown to infect primates that live in geographical areas where HIV is endemic (Gao et al., 1999; Hirsch et al., 1989), and possible routes of transmission, such as the butchering of primates for food and keeping monkeys as pets, have been proposed (Gao et al., 1999).

A natural primate host for HIV-1 has been proposed however there still remains some controversy. Strains of SIV (SIVcpz) from the chimpanzee Pan troglodytes troglodytes, phylogenetically cluster closer to HIV-1 strains than many other characterized SIV strains (Gao et al., 1999). However there is still a moderate amount of diversity between SIVcpz and HIV-1, and the prevalence of SIV infections in wild chimpanzees is low. There are three major groups within HIV-1, M (main), O (outlier) and N (new, or 'non-O non-M'). Each of the three groups of HIV-1 share a common branch with SIVcpz strains, but do not diverge from a common stem with SIVcpz, suggesting that they each arose from different cross-species transmissions (Gao et al., 1999; Thomson et al., 2002b). To support the idea that P.t. troglodytes is the natural reservoir of HIV, the HIV-1 N group was shown to be a recombinant between diverse viral strains within the HIV/SIVcpz group, suggesting an ancestral recombination in this sub-species of chimpanzee (Gao et al., 1999; Garcia et al., 1999).

It is thought that the HIV-1 M group originated in the Democratic Republic of Congo, as an extremely high genetic diversity is seen within the region (Vidal et al., 2000) and the earliest confirmed HIV-1 infection was found there in a stored serum sample from 1959 (Zhu et al.,

1998). Based on sequence analysis of the HIV-1 M group, it was estimated that these strains arose from a common ancestor in about 1931 (Korber et al., 2000).

Unlike HIV-1, the origin of HIV-2 is more definitive. The discovery of a form of SIV in sooty mangabeys (SIVsm) which is nearly identical to HIV-2, and which is found in these primates from the area where HIV-2 circulates in humans, provides very strong evidence that HIV-2 came from these primates (Gao et al., 1992). At present, there are eight designated groups of HIV-2, A-H, which are analogous to the HIV-1 groups (M, N and O) although, groups C-H have only been identified in single individuals (Chen et al., 1997; Damond et al., 2004). All groups of HIV-2 are believed to have arisen from individual cross-species transmission events from sooty mangabeys (Chen et al., 1996). Analysis conducted with HIV-2 strains from subtypes A and B, dated a recent common ancestor to around 1940 and 1945 respectively (Lemey et al., 2003).

Currently, there are 33 million people living with HIV/AIDS globally with 16,000 new infections happening every day (UNAIDS 2010) (**Figure 1**). As the acquired immune deficiency syndrome (AIDS) pandemic enters its third decade, the number of people living with human immunodeficiency virus (HIV) infection continues to increase. Although the HIV/AIDS epidemic was recognized in Southeast Asia later than elsewhere, local risk behaviors have allowed the epidemic to expand rapidly. Today, injecting drug use (IDU) accounts for up to 70% of HIV-1 transmission in many Asian countries, including China, Indonesia, Malaysia, Myanmar, Eastern India and Vietnam (Saksena et al., 2005). Also, there is ample evidence that heterosexual transmission through commercial sex workers has increased over the last few years (Saksena et al., 2005).

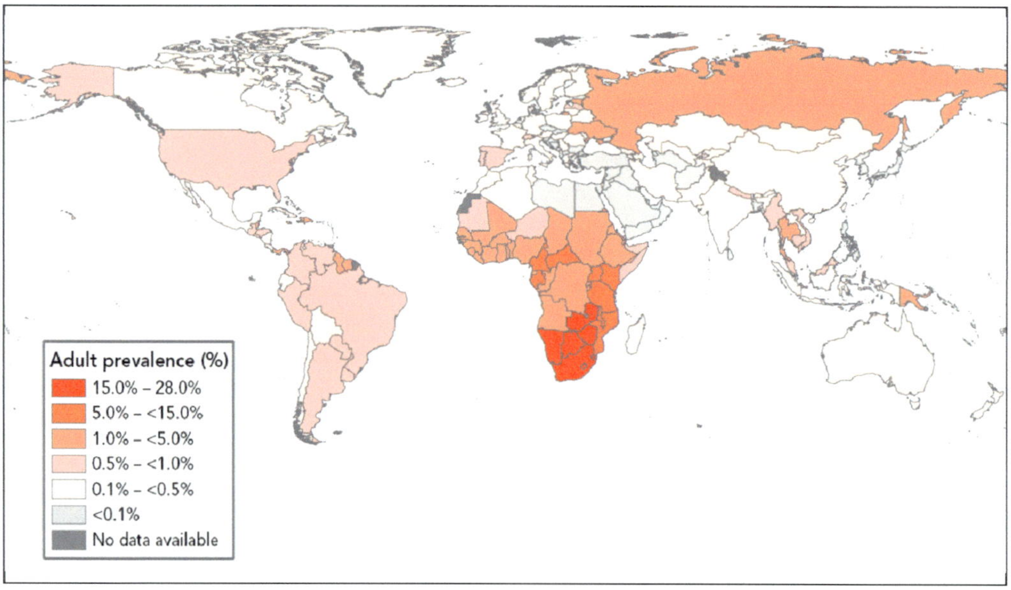

Fig. 1. Estimation of global adult prevalence in 2007, with an approximately 33 million of people living with HIV. Diagram source: UNAIDS, 2008: Report on the global AIDS epidemic.

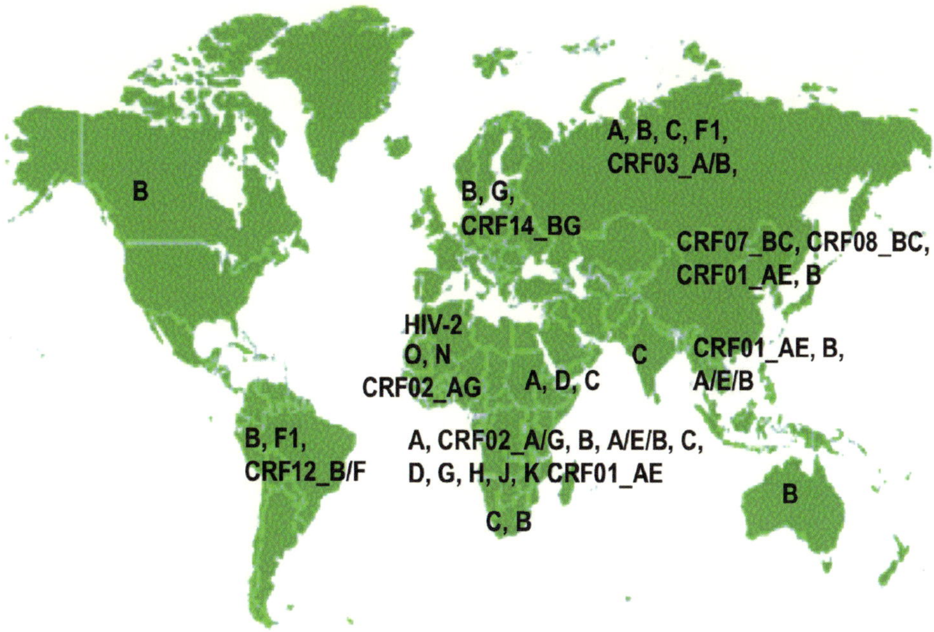

Fig. 2. Map showing the global dispersal of diverse HIV subtypes (represented by single letter codes) and their replacement by circulating recombinant forms (CRFs).

2. Genetic diversity in HIV: Recombination – A unique trait for the continuation of viral progeny

One of the major hallmarks of HIV infection is high genetic diversity. This high genetic diversity in HIV-1 is attributed to the infidelity of its reverse transcriptase enzyme, which leads to high rates of mutation [Preston et al., 1988] and rapid viral variant turnover in patients-termed quasispecies [Ho et al., 1995 and Wei et al., 1995]. This quasispecies or the swarm of viral variants is a powerful asset of HIV in creating recombinants with superior ability to survive, evade and infect in vivo. In addition, the subtypic diversity within HIV-1 M group also provides the virus with a wider selection of strains to recombine with and disperse effectively by creating creating virulent forms. Currently, major subtypes are being replaced by circulating recombinant forms (CRFs), the evidence of which can be seen in **figure 2**.

The HIV-1 M group can be divided into 9 subtypes (A-D, F-H, J and K), and some subtypes are further broken down into subsubtypes, according to their topologies within phylogenetic trees. There is possibly a 10th subtype, L, for which 2 full-length sequences have been identified (Mokili et al., 2002). All of these subtypes can be found in Africa, where they are thought to have originated (Thomson et al., 2002b). Other continents have a variety of subtypes circulating, resulting in an uneven representation of the subtypes. Based on the amino acid sequence of the env region, each subtype is separated by approximately 25-30% genetic distance (Robertson et al., 1999; Thomson et al., 2002b). Subtypes A and F can be further broken down into subsubtypes, A1-A4 and F1 and F2 (Vidal et al., 2006). Technically subtypes B and D are closely related and could be classified together as sub-subtypes, however they are generally still mentioned separately for consistency (Lal et al., 2005). In addition, within subtypes there are clusters that represent strains from different geographical locations, such as subtype B strains from Thailand, which are referred to as B′ or Thai B (Kalish et al., 1995). These clusters most likely arose due to the initial introduction of only a small number of strains into a particular region, and their subsequent diversification and spread (known as a founder effect) (Thomson et al., 2002b). In addition to the nine subtypes of HIV-1, there exists circulating recombinant forms (CRFs), which are mosaic viruses of two or more HIV-1 subtypes. To be classified as a CRF, an inter-subtype recombinant virus must be isolated from at least two (preferably three) unlinked individuals and sequenced in full (Carr et al., 1998). Currently 34 CRFs have been recognized, with 26 described in detail (Los Alamos HIV Database) (**Figure 6**). These CRFs now include second generation CRFs such as CRF09_cpx and CRF15_01B, which is contain the primary CRFs CRF02_AG and CRF01_AE respectively. Regions within CRFs that cannot be classified as a known subtype are designated U for unknown, and a CRF comprised of more than two subtypes is denoted by cpx for complex (Peeters, 2000; Robertson et al., 1999). The first CRF identified was CRF01_AE, and was originally classified as subtype E, before it was designated a recombinant (CRF01_AE has subtype A gag and pol regions and a subtype E env) (Gao et al., 1996), and interestingly a full-length subtype E virus has not been identified, possibly indicating that the gag and pol regions were lost through an ancestral recombination event (Gao et al., 1996).

Recombination is common in HIV and it uses recombination in order to acquire viral fitness, virulence and ability to evade the host immune system. Recombination occurs as a result of the low affinity binding of RT, which is necessary for the strand transfers of reverse transcription to occur. As HIV carries two copies of its viral RNA, during reverse transcription both of these can serve as templates to generate the provirus. If the two copies of RNA encapsulated with a virion are distinct, and are both used during reverse transcription, then the resulting provirus will be a recombinant. Thus the first requirement for recombination is a dually infected cell, which can give rise to a heterozygous virion, which carries two distinct copies of RNA. Once a heterozygous virion is formed recombination then occurs upon infection of a new cell (**Figure 3**). The theories behind how recombination occurs at the molecular level can be divided into two groups, recombination that occurs during the synthesis of the minus-strand DNA and that which occurs during the synthesis of the plus-strand DNA. Each theory has its own explanation and some supporting experimental evidence, implying that both mechanisms can occur (Hu and Temin, 1990b).

3. Heterozygous virions and their formation

A requirement for the generation of recombinant HIV genomes is a heterozygous virion, that is, a virion with two non-identical RNA strands (Hu and Temin, 1990a; Weiss et al., 1973). Heterozygous virions are generated in individual cells which are infected with two or more different viral variants, which integrate their proviral genome, and generate new full length viral RNA.

As packaging of the viral RNA is not selective for specific RNA copies (D'Souza and Summers, 2005), a heterozygous virus can be formed, by encapsidation of an RNA copy from each viral variant. Heterozygous virions can then infect other cells and recombination between the two co-packaged viral RNAs can occur during reverse transcription (Duesberg, 1968). (**Figure 3**). The different viral RNAs can come from variants within the viral quasispecies, or from other HIV strains or subtypes, if the patient has a dual infection.

Multiple infection of a single cell with HIV can occur simultaneously or sequentially. There is some debate regarding the sequential infection, as once a cell is infected, HIV downregulates the CD4 and CCR5 receptor molecules (Michel et al., 2005), and therefore simultaneous infection may be the primary mechanism involved. Interestingly, a study by Dang et al. (2004) showed that dual infections of cells occurs at a much higher rate than predicted by chance, in both a T cell line, and primary T cells, regardless of how the virus was transmitted. In a follow up study it was also shown that coreceptor differences were not a barrier to recombination, as viruses using different co-receptors, CCR5 or CXCR4 also exhibited rates of double infection that were higher than predicted from a random distribution (Chen et al., 2005). Likewise, other studies have also shown co-infection of cells to be common, which implies that opportunities for recombination are favoured (Jung et al., 2002).

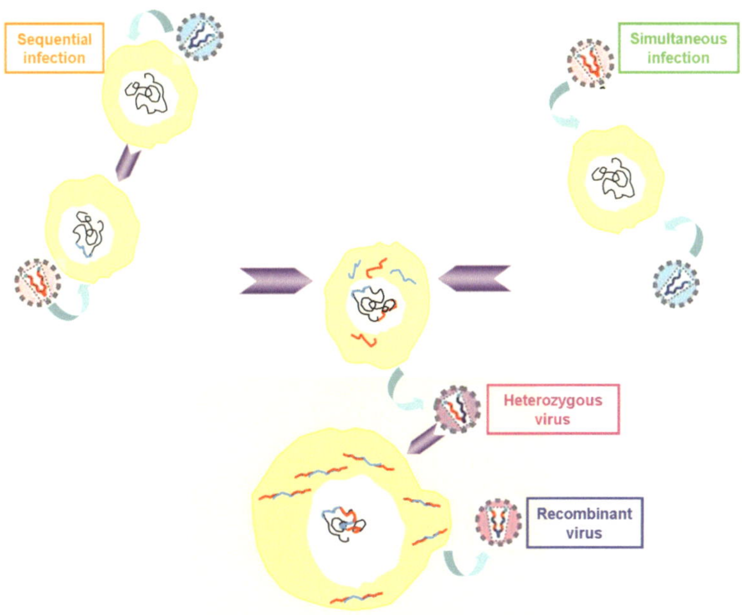

Fig. 3. HIV dual infection of a cell, heterozygous virion formation and recombination. Modified from: Najera et al. (2002).

3.1 Minus-strand recombination

There have been several studies addressing minus-strand recombination, and it has been shown to occur frequently, with an average of three crossovers occurring per replication cycle (Yu et al., 1998).

The first mechanism proposed to account for recombination was the forced copy-choice model (Coffin, 1979), and was based on evidence that suggested the genomic RNA of retroviruses is fragmented. A break in the RNA would halt reverse transcription and consequently force the reverse transcriptase to switch to the second copy of RNA in order to continue synthesis, that is, a strand transfer event would occur (Hu and Temin, 1990b). In order for this to take place, the RT enzyme must be transferred to a homologous region on the second RNA copy. This model assumes therefore that recombination occurs during minus-strand synthesis, and is comparable to the minus-strand strong stop strand transfer that occurs during reverse transcription (Negroni and Buc, 2001) (**Figure 4**). However, no studies have been able to establish a firm connection between strand switching and the frequency of RNA breaks. Further, experiments have shown that a strand break is not necessary for a template switch (Hu and Temin, 1990b). Consequently, the minus-strand exchange model was proposed which suggests that the low processivity (loose adherence to the RNA template) of RT causes strand transfers (Coffin, 1979; Yu et al., 1998). It has also been shown that obstacles to reverse transcription, causing the enzyme to pause, can trigger a strand transfer (Wu et al., 1995). In addition, studies have also suggested that secondary structures of the RNA templates could also increase template switching without a pause, by bringing the two templates into close proximity (Balakrishnan et al., 2001) (**Figure 4**).

3.2 Plus-strand recombination

Recombination that occurs during the synthesis of the positive strand of DNA is referred to as the strand displacement assimilation model (Hu and Temin, 1990b). This model suggests that both copies of viral RNA are transcribed to produce two minus-strand DNA copies. Synthesis of plus-strand DNA is initially discontinuous, and internally initiated fragments occur eg. at the cPPT (Hsu and Taylor, 1982). Therefore, it has been proposed that an internally initiated fragment can be displaced by an elongating upstream DNA fragment, and this can cause the internally initiated fragment to dissociate and re-anneal to the complementary region of the second minus-strand DNA. The resulting double stranded DNA will have a mismatched region and mismatch DNA repair will then correct the sequence differences (Hu and Temin, 1990b) (**Figure 4**). Two positive strands of RNA, which may contain breaks. During minus-strand synthesis, the RT can switch to the other template at a break.

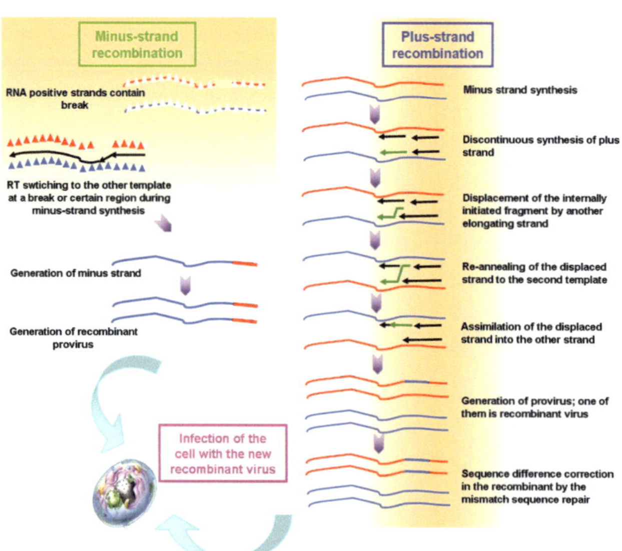

Fig. 4. Model of retrovirus recombination: minus-strand recombination (forced-copy choice) and plus-strand recombination (strand displacement assimilation).

4. The global distribution of HIV-1 subtypes and CRFs

Across the globe there is an uneven representation of the HIV-1 M group subtypes (**Figure 2**), along with the presence of diverse subtypes and its CRFs in Asia (**Figure 5**). This uneven distribution is thought to have arisen partially due to a founder effect, where one subtype is introduced into a region by a single or a few individuals from which the epidemic radiates out (Korber et al., 2000). Subtype A is currently divided in to four sub-subtypes: A1-A4. Subsubtype A1 is one of the more common variants and is found throughout Western, Central and Eastern Africa and Eastern Europe, and two CRF forms containing subtype A1 (CRF02_AG and CRF03_AB) are also widely spread in these regions (Andersson et al., 1999; Bobkov et al., 2004; Dowling et al., 2002; Steain et al., 2005). Subtype A (sub-subtypes 1 and 2) strains are highly predominant in Kenya, with one study showing 93% of all strains found in the region being subtype A or a recombinant containing subtype A (Dowling et al., 2002). In addition, CRF01_AE is one of the major strains found in Thailand and Southeast Asia (McCutchan et al., 1992; Tovanabutra et al., 2004). Subsubtype A2 was first identified from sequences originating in the Democratic Republic of Congo and Cyprus (Gao et al., 2001), and is now also found in Kenya (Visawapoka et al., 2006). In addition, there have been 2 recognised CRF forms, CRF16_A2D and CRF21_A2D, both of which were also identified in Kenya (Visawapoka et al., 2006). CRF16_A2D has also achieved a global spread and has been identified in Korea and Argentina (Gomez-Carrillo et al., 2004). Subsubtype A3 has only been recently described (Meloni et al., 2004a), and has thus far only been identified in areas of West and Central Africa (Meloni et al., 2004a; Meloni et al., 2004b). Similarly subsubtype A4 is a relatively new strain, and has only been identified within the Democratic Republic of Congo (Vidal et al., 2006).

Subtype B is the most common subtype in Australia, as well as the USA, and Western and Central Europe (de Oliveira et al., 2000; Essex, 1999; Herring et al., 2003). It is also found in South America, where CFR012_BF also circulates (Montano et al., 2005), Thailand (B′ strains), with CRF15_01B (Tovanabutra et al., 2001), China, with CRF07_BC and CRF08_BC (Saksena et al., 2005), Spain with CRF14_BG (Delgado et al., 2002) and Eastern Europe with CRF03_AB (Liitsola et al., 1998). This subtype was one of the first to spread globally, however generally seems to be on the decline, with the wider spread of other subtypes and intersubtype recombinants (Soares et al., 2005; Tatt et al., 2004).

Subtype C is currently the most prevalent subtype. It is found circulating widely through South Africa, East Africa and India (Bessong et al., 2005) and to a lesser extent in South America, Eastern Europe and Chine (Saksena et al., 2005; Soares et al., 2005). It has been suggested that strains of subtype C possess some selective advantage due to its rapid dispersal across the globe that has been seen in recent years (Walker et al., 2005).

Subtype D is found across most of Africa, particularly East African countries, where in Uganda it has been reported as a predominating strain (Harris et al., 2002). It has also been reported in other continents, though usually as a minor variant (Tatt et al., 2004). In addition, subtype D is frequently a component of unique intersubtype recombinants, from Kenya and other East African countries (Steain et al., 2005), and it has been suggested that recombinants between subtypes A and D are selected for in dually infected patients (Songok et al., 2004). Subsubtype F1 is found in South America and Europe, whereas subtype F strains from Africa (eg Cameroon) more commonly belong to subsubtype F2 (Laukkanen et al., 2000). Subtype F also forms part of CRF12_BF, which has become widespread across South America, and more recently as a part of CRF17_BF, CRF28_BF and CRF29_BF, which have also been identified in South America (De Sa Filho et al., 2006; Hierholzer et al., 2002).

CRF05_DF has also been reported in Europe, although is thought to have arisen in Africa (Casado et al., 2003; Laukkanen et al., 2000).

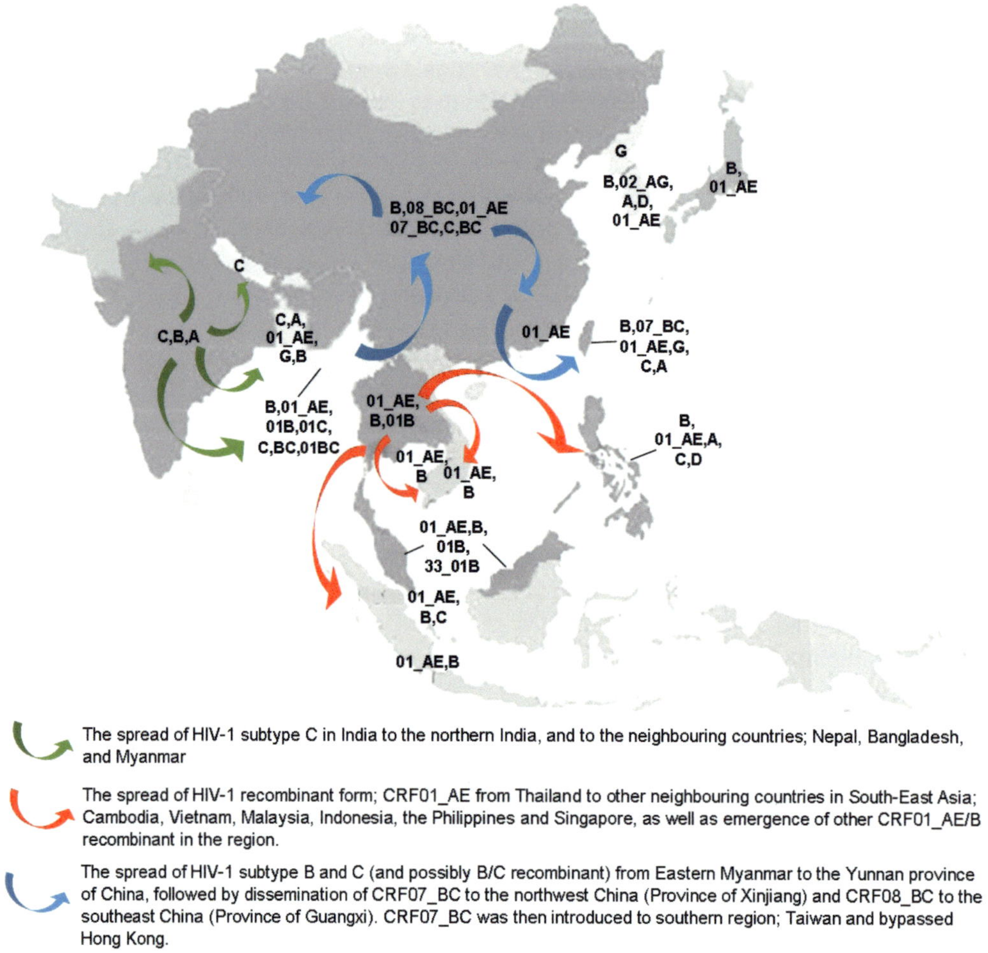

Fig. 5. The complex HIV-1 genetic diversity and the spread of the predominant HIV-1 strains in Asia. Distribution of different HIV-1 subtypes and CRFs (demonstrated in descending order; from the most to the least prevalent strain) in major Asian countries, including subtypes A; B; C; D; G, CRFs such as 01_AE, CRF01_AE; 02_AG, CRF02_AG; 07_BC, CRF07_BC; 08_BC, CRF08_BC; 33_01B, CRF33_01B and other HIV-1 recombinant forms: BC, B/C inter-subtype recombinant; 01B, CRF01_AE/B; 01C, CRF01_AE/C and 01BC, CRF01_AE/B/C. The three different routes of spread for subtype C, CRF01_AE as well as subtype B, C and B/C recombinants are highlighted in green, red and blue, respectively. Diagram source: Lau *et al.* (2007).

Subtype G has been reported across Africa, and parts of Europe (Esteves et al., 2003; Gutierrez et al., 2004; Parreira et al., 2005; Yang et al., 2005a), however it is its CRF02_AG that has had the greater impact. This strain is currently the most prevalent CRF and is found predominantly across West and Central Africa (Mamadou et al., 2003). CRF14_BG, as well as other G recombinants are also found in Spain and neighbouring regions (Perez-Alvarez et al., 2003). Subtypes H, J and K have had only a minor impact on the HIV epidemic and are generally only found in small numbers across West and Central Africa (Mokili et al., 1999; Thomson et al., 2002b; Vidal et al., 2000; Yang et al., 2005a). The remaining CRFs are also found in varying proportions, usually each within a distinct geographical region. Whole spectrum of emerging and well-established CRFs have been identified, which are listed in **Figure 6**.

5. Dual infections and recombination of HIV

The magnitude of genetic diversity in a host relates to the size of the viral population, the extent of replication, the mutation and recombination rates and the selective pressures placed on the virus (Saksena et al., 2001). Overall the divergence between the circulating HIV strains within a single individual and the original infecting strain/s is thought to increase by around 1% per year in early infection (Shankarappa et al., 1999). Thus, within an individual a heterogeneous viral population exists which has been termed a 'quasispecies'. Within an individual this viral diversity can reach as 15% (Lukashov and Goudsmit, 1997). The reasons behind such viral diversity include a fast turnover of virions, approximately 109 new virions are produced each day (Ho et al., 1995), and the low fidelity of reverse transcriptase. Reverse transcriptase lacks a proof-reading function, meaning that any nucleotides that are mis-incorporated during DNA synthesis are not corrected (Battula and Loeb, 1976). Studies have shown the mutation rate of HIV RT to be 3.4 x 10-5 mutations per base pair per cycle, which is relatively high compared to other retroviruses (Mansky and Temin, 1995). However, as the rate of recombination, 3-9 crossovers per round of replication (Jetzt et al., 2000), exceeds the mutation rate, recombination is the largest contributing factor in viral evolution (Bocharov et al., 2005).

Intra-strain recombination between variants within the viral quasispecies, as well as inter-strain/intersubtype recombination, increases genetic diversity and thereby increases the chance of survival for the virus. Recombination can generate strains capable of evading the host's immune system, strains that are resistant to one or more antiretroviral drugs, or that can replicate faster and more efficiently (Steain et al., 2004). It can also result in the formation of novel genes (Sharp et al., 1996). Recombination can also be a repair mechanism for HIV, allowing viral replication to continue in the presence of a break in a strand of RNA. However, recombination can also result in the emergence of less fit viral strains, as it can break-up favourable combinations of genes and therefore is not always advantageous for the virus (Bretscher et al., 2004).

Studies have shown that multidrug resistant viruses emerge rapidly in the presence of two drugs, due to recombination between strains that were each resistant to a single drug (Moutouh et al., 1996). In vivo, this could allow the emergence of strains that are resistant to many different classes of drugs, and recently intrapatient recombination leading to a multidrug resistant strain has been reported (Weiser et al., 2005). Further, selective pressure placed on the pol region in the presence of anti-retroviral drugs, does not need to be carried across the entire genome as recombination could occur between strains with diverse gag and env regions with an escape mutant in the pol region (Charpentier et al., 2006). Similarly, a study of two patients by van Rij et al. (2003) observed that after the emergence of X4 utilising strains, the R5 and X4 gp120 envelope sequences diverged from each other, whereas the respective gag p17 regions did not. Thus it was proposed that recombination was occurring between the two strains in vivo.

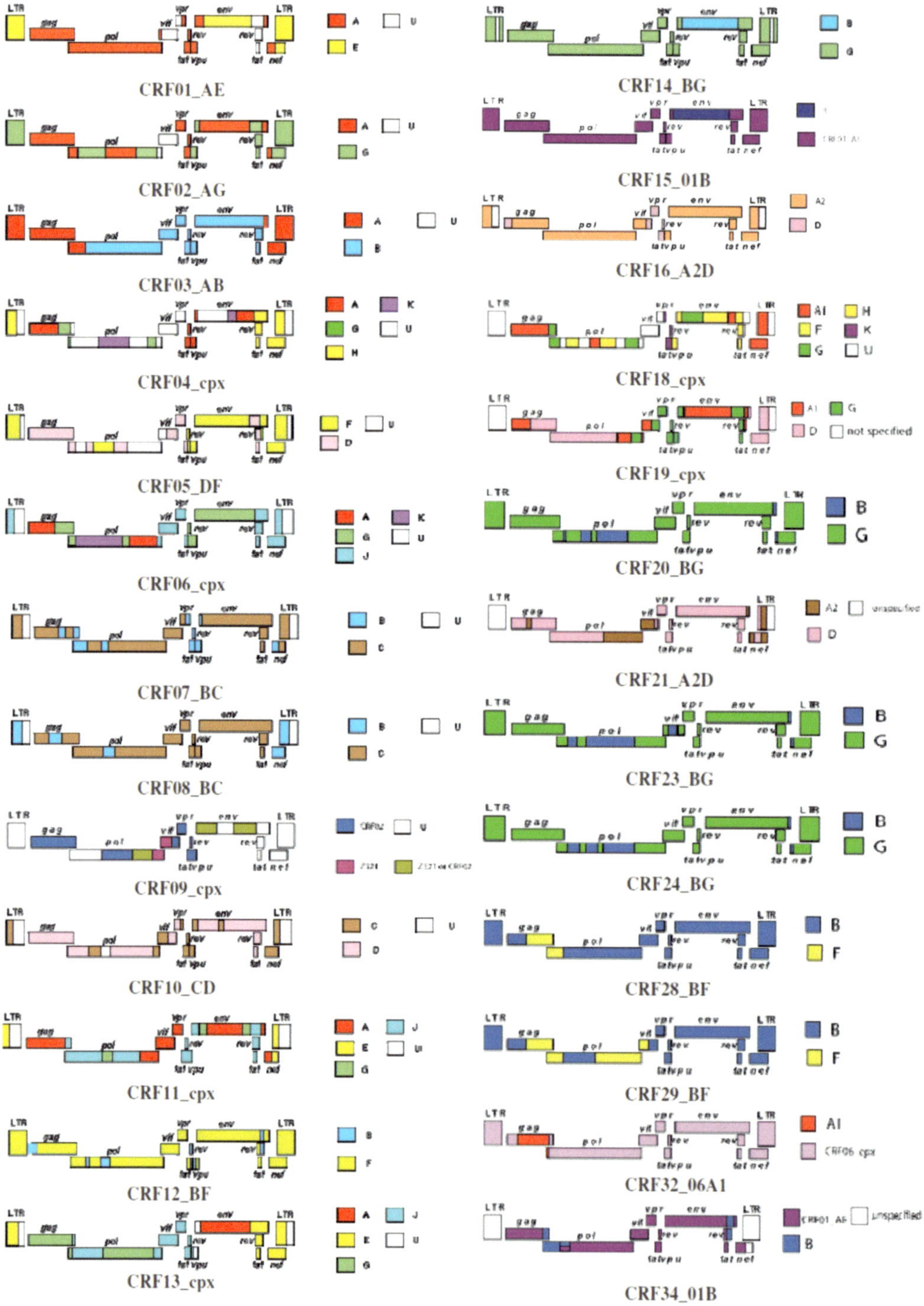

Fig. 6. Schematic representation of the genomic organization of the described CRF genomes. Adapted from the Los Alamos National Laboratory HIV Database (2006b).

Recombination may also produce virus strains that are more successfully transmitted either via sexual contact or perinatal transmission, possibly by increasing the strains affinity for a particular tissue type. A study in Buenos Aires by Thomson et al. (2002b), showed that recombinant viruses predominated in IDUs and heterosexually infected women, whereas subtype B viral strains were more common in men, both heterosexually and homosexually infected (Gao et al., 1996). Studies have also shown that inter-subtype recombinants were more likely to be transmitted via breast milk than subtype C in Tanzania (Koulinska et al., 2006). Further, in Southeast Asia, CRF01_AE was spread much more rapidly than subtype B, which was also present in the area. In addition, no type E gag or pol gene has been found which may suggest that the recombinant CRF01_AE virus was more viable and consequently the pure type E was eliminated by selective pressures

6. HIV co-infection and superinfection: Pathogenic implications

It is widely recognised that a single individual can become infected with more than one HIV-1 subtype or strain i.e. they harbour a dual infection (Gottlieb et al., 2004; Wang et al., 2000). This circumstance is possible via superinfection or coinfection. In superinfection, new infection takes place with a divergent HIV-1 or HIV-2 strain in already infected individuals. In contrast, coinfection is a concomitant exposure to diverse HIV strains prior to seroconversion, and therefore before the immune system has mounted a response (Steain et al., 2004).

For the majority of patients that have been characterized as being infected with two or more HIV strains, it has generally been assumed that the infections occurred within a very short period of time, if not simultaneously. This is because it was originally thought that establishment of infection with HIV would provide some immunity against re-infection, and that the decrease in the expression of CD4 molecules would make superinfection unlikely (Benson et al., 1993). Furthermore, a study by Otten et al. (1999) examined HIV-2 infection in Pig-tailed Macaques and found that a secondary infection could only be established in the first 2-4 weeks after the initial infection.

However, there are to date at least 10 papers examining patients with evidence of superinfection (Chohan et al., 2005; McCutchan et al., 2005; Smith et al., 2005). These include one patient with a triple infection who was thought to have acquired an additional 2 strains through superinfection (van der Kuyl et al., 2005). It was also initially hypothesised that if superinfections were occurring that they would be the result of intravenous inoculation of the virus, with a high dose exposure. However of the reported superinfections, several were acquired via sexual exposures, including heterosexual contact (Chohan et al., 2005).

Many of these papers documenting superinfection note that upon acquisition of a second virus, patients tend to experience a more rapid disease progression, with an increase in plasma viral load and a concomitant decrease in CD4+ T cell count (Smith et al., 2005; van der Kuyl et al., 2005). Superinfection has also been reported to lead to recombination between the two infecting strains (McCutchan et al., 2005). For these reasons HIV-infected individuals should be warned that safe-sex practices are still necessary even between sero-concordant couples, to prevent superinfection and the associated disease progression (Steain et al., 2004).

Now that superinfection has been demonstrated, it is unknown if these are rare cases or if superinfection is a more common event that is not always detected, and may in part provide some explanation for the large number of recombinant strains seen globally. In cases where the second infecting strain is of the same subtype, the differences between the strains may be attributed to the normal quasispecies variation seen within a patient, and therefore may not be recognized as superinfections. Thus in cases where superinfection is detected it is likely to be intersubtype related and thus any quantification of superinfections may be an underestimation (Steain et al., 2004).

It is important to screen for dual infections, as such patients can provide an ideal setting for examining biological and molecular interactions between two viral strains in vivo. Wang et al. (2000), reported the case of a patient who was co-infected with two divergent forms of subtype B, which appeared to be acting in synergy. The two strains were able to segregate based on a differential tropism for monocytes and macrophages. While one of the strains appeared to dominate when co-cultured in peripheral blood mononuclear cells (PBMCs), it was discovered that this strain was only able to productively infect PBMCs when the second viral strains was present, indicating a potential synergistic effect between the two viral strains. In addition, a greater cytopathic effect was observed when the two strains where co-cultured, further supporting the idea that a synergistic association of these two viral strains resulted in greater pathogenicity. The patient had acquired the infections via intravenous drug use and progressed rapidly to AIDS, dying within 5 years of infection. This case demonstrates that distinct biological differences exist between strains of the same subtype, and that two strains are able to act in synergy.

7. CRFs and pathogenic implications: Asia the "hotbed" of CRFs

The highly unequal geographic distribution of viral variants is the result of the global variation in the HIV-1 strains, the dynamic nature of the HIV-1 epidemic, and the accidental epidemiologic transmissions. The recombinant HIV-1 strains have been reported from almost all geographic regions of the globe where multiple HIV-1 subtypes have been circulating. Despite this, few HIV-1 geographic "recombination hotspots" have been identified around the world, such as central Myanmar [Vidal et al., 2005], Yunnan province of China [Saksena et al., 2005], Argentina [Renjifo et al., 2001], Brazil [Ball et al., 2003], East Africa [Yang et al., 2003,Renjifo et al., 2004] and more recently Cuba [Wu et al., 2001]. While the predominant viral forms in the global HIV epidemic are subtypes A and C [UNAIDS/WHO, 2006], a different and even more complex HIV genetic diversity has been found in Asia. The HIV spread and its epidemiology in Asia are interesting and closely related to the routes of spread of the epidemic. This is evident from the distribution of subtype C (Figure 5), which was found primarily in India and Africa, and is now spreading to Northern India, Myanmar, and Thailand [Eshleman et al., 2005]. Although the biological aspects that explain this high rate of infection remain unclear, subtype C has dominated the HIV-1 epidemic in India and accounts for almost 97% of infections. Apart from the predominant subtype C, the A/C and B/C inter-subtype recombinants have also been recently identified in North-eastern India [Peeters et al., 2000]. Emergence of A/C recombinants is also consistent with the epidemic observed in Bangladesh [Sanders-Nuell et al., 2007], from where triple recombinants between subtypes A, C and G have been recently reported. Also, it is established that the spread of subtypes B and C, as well as B/C recombinants occurred through the drug route from Eastern Myanmar into Yunnan province of China and moving to north and west into Xinjiang province of China (Figure 5).

While other recombinants account for only 4% of the total HIV-1 infection in South and Southeast Asia, the CRF01_AE has been found to be responsible for 84% of all HIV-1 infections. CRF01_AE, which was originally identified in Thailand appears to circulate in major parts of Asia, particularly Southeast Asia (Figure 5 and 6). Together, CRF01_AE and other recombinants account for nearly 89%, the highest across the world [Hemelaar et al., 2006]. Since the beginning of HIV pandemic in the last two decades until recently, changes in HIV-1 subtype distribution in Asia have been overwhelming. In Asian countries, the HIV-1 prevalence has been high from the late 1980s to 1990s, with subtype B" (known as the Thai variant of subtype B) being the predominant strain and was most frequently observed amongst IDU [Weniger et al., 1991; Nerurkar et al., 1997]. Concurrently in Thailand and other areas, CRF01_AE was introduced independently in commercial sex workers [Ou et al., 1993]. Interestingly in the last decade, a gradual yet evident spread of the Thai variant of CRF01_AE was witnessed in many countries of Asia [Nerurkar et al., 1996]. It was later observed that CRF01_AE takes over in the HIV-1 epidemic in Southeast Asia, even among IDUs in Thailand, Cambodia, and Vietnam [Nerurkar et al., 1996]. Likewise, countries such as Indonesia and Malaysia demonstrate the predominance of CRF01_AE and subtype B prior to the year 2000.

8. Inter-CRF recombination and its possible epidemiologic implications

Among all the HIV-1 subtypes distributed in Asia, CRF01_AE is reported to play a considerably important role in its epidemic [Hemelaar et al., 2006]. The HIV epidemiology in Asia is bound to be more complex as other recombinant forms are introduced from neighbouring geographic regions, along with the continuing emergence of novel second and third generation recombinant forms of CRF01_AE in this region. Geographic regions known as recombination hotspots in Asia, including Myanmar and Yunnan province of China appear to have varied and complex forms of HIV-1 recombinants, which emerge continually. Between 2002 and 2004, a novel inter-CRF recombinant has been identified in Yangon, Myanmar, which also appears to be a second class of HIV-1 inter-CRF recombinants comprised of CRF01_AE and CRF07_BC [Takebe et al., 2006]. Other Asian region, for instance Macao has first identified the circulation of CRF12_BF (prevalent in Brazil) among the IDUs, although CRF01_AE has always being the major HIV-1 strain [Chan et al., 2007a]. This suggests the epidemiologically associated transmission of the current HIV-1 infection in the region and gives clues to the possible initiation of the emergence of novel inter-CRF recombinants between CRF01_AE and CRF12_BF. Concurrently in Macao, a diverse form of HIV-1 recombinant has been recently full-length characterized and comprised of CRF12_BF, CRF14_BG and subtype G [Chan et al., 2007b].

As the result of the co-circulation of subtypes B and C, two CRFs; CRF07_BC and CRF08_BC have emerged in the Yunnan province of China [Piyasirisilp et al., 2000]. An ongoing evolution and emergence of novel recombinant forms of HIV are anticipated in this region, while these two CRFs continue to co-circulate with "pure" subtypes B and C, along with other URF in Yunnan [Yang et al., 2002]. It is predicted that more new recombinant strains between these two CRFs will continue to emerge [Peeters et al., 2000]. With the extensive variability in recombinant breakpoints and crossover points in China, a possible emergence of second and third generation recombinant CRF will continue to give rise to more HIV-1 variants. A recent study has identified approximately 12% of HIV-1 strains found among the IDUs in Southeast Yunnan to be the diverse forms of inter-CRF recombinants between CRF07_BC and CRF08_BC [Chan et al., 2007]. This further provides a good insight into inter-CRF recombinants, and only time will tell regarding epidemiologic.

9. HIV fitness in vivo and in vitro as a consequence of recombination

Fitness is a parameter defining the replicative adaptation of an organism to its environment [Domingo et al., 1997] as a consequence of the interaction of a multitude of viral and host factors [Quinones-Mateu et al., 2006; Nijhuis et al., 1999]. Within a given viral „quasispecies", each clone possesses a fitness denoting to the selection of the viral properties (e.g. activity and stability) in a particular environment. Under a certain selective pressure in a defined microenvironment, viral replication will take place to encode virus that replicates at high rates [331]. Thus, one or more strains possessing better viral properties within a given quasispecies will be positively selected, while unfit variants will be negatively eliminated [331]. The HIV-1 viral factors that affect viral fitness are mainly the biological processes in the virus life cycle: cell entry, genome replication, protein synthesis and processing, and particle assembly and release from cells. The survival of the fittest form of HIV-1 recombinant leads to further viral evolution in a complex population, suggesting a continuous evolving of HIV-1 dynamics, mainly attributed to an incessant process of growth, competition and selection.

As a result of high mutation rate of HIV-1, wide range of sequence possibilities is created. While sometimes it resulted in non-replicative viruses, others may possess varying degree of fitness. Recombinant viruses may have some advantages over the parental strain and thus, may possess important genetic variability for HIV-1 pathogenesis, transmission, diagnosis, treatment and vaccine development. It is undeniable that different biological properties of diverse subtypes will possibly result in transmissibility and pathogenicity variation. During early infection, most subtypes conform to the non-syncytium-inducing CCR5 receptor usage phenotype. However, towards the late infection, these subtypes will shift to the syncytium-inducing CXCR4 receptor usage phenotype. This is true for most but subtype C and D viruses, which do not follow this pattern [336]. In terms of transmission, several studies of vertical transmission have suggested that the maternal HIV-1 subtype is likely to play a role while others disregard this perception [Yang et al., 2003; Tapia et al., 2003].

What is yet to be known is the consistent role of the subtype-associated differences in the efficiency of transmission via different routes. While some studies have reported that subtype D is associated with faster disease progression compared with subtype A [Condra et al., 1995], others have denied the possibilities that HIV genetic subtype determines the rate of disease progression [Alaeus et al., 1999]. Findings of these studies are inconsistent, due to the difference in the study design (sample size, duration of clinical follow-up and the use of surrogate markers of progression) as well as other virus, host and environmental factors. Previous work has also suggested possible biological differences among the HIV-1 subtypes [Jeeninga et al., 2000]. It was reported that the long terminal repeat (LTR) region of CRF01_AE (the predominant HIV-1 strain in Asia) is much more potent in vitro than the subtype B LTR. When a recombinant CRF01_AE/B virus was constructed in vitro, it exhibited an intense replication advantage compared to the parental subtype B. This indicated that restrained differences in the LTR promoter activity can exert a significant impact on viral replication kinetics. A recent profound analysis was done by Kozaczynska et al. [Kozaczynska et al., 2007] to describe the study over time of HIV-1 isolates in a patient twice superinfected with HIV-1; an initial infection with a subtype B1 strain, followed by first superinfection with a subtype B2 strain and then with CRF01_AE. Again, the LTR of CRF01_AE was found to possess a higher promoter activity, although this was not reflected in the plasma viral load differences. It is remarkable that the later-arriving viruses (strain B2 and CRF01_AE) replicated at much higher levels in blood compared with the first infecting virus B1. Except for the excessive recombination between both subtype B strains, there was only minimal evidence that the different HIV-1 strains found in the patient appeared to influence the evolution of each other. While HIV-1 has been constantly exposed to host immune system for eradication of the virus, its replication relies profoundly on host cell machinery. Thus, the HIV-1 fitness is said to be closely related to the host environment (e.g. cellular receptors, intracellular factors and host defence mechanism). Viral diversity gives important impact in the determination of viral load, as well as viral diagnosis. Therefore, HIV-1 diagnosis test, which includes HIV-1 immunoassays have to be competent in detecting all known group M subtypes [Koch et al.,]. Other viral load measurements assays have to be reliable too, for instance polymerase chain reaction-based assays for quantification of the HIV-1 RNA from all known genetic variants of HIV-1 [Swanson et al., 2005].

Genotypic or phenotypic variations within different subtypes are somehow related to any differences in ex vivo fitness. Troyer et a.l [Troyer et al., 2005] provided evidence that increased viral fitness in vivo may be related to a concomitant increase in HIV-1 diversity, and thus serves as a crucial factor in determining disease progression. Furthermore, HIV-1 strains that display viral properties that increase their fitness, for instance subtype C isolates appear to have an extra or third nuclear factor-kappa B (NFκB) element in the long-terminal repeat (LTR). This would enhance transcription in the presence or absence of HIV-1 Tat protein [Hunt et al., 2006]. Another study showed that in comparison to subtype B, subtype C possesses an increased protease activity, and thus augmented cleavage of peptide substrates and possibly improved viral fitness [Velazquez et al., 2001]. Therefore, it is proposed that the increased replicative capacity of subtype C over other HIV-1 subtype isolates suggests its dominance in HIV-1 epidemic. However, in another pair-wise competition study by Arien et al. [Arien et al., 2005] to establish the „pathogenic fitness" (or virulence) of HIV in PBMCs, subtype C seems to have lower fitness when competed with other HIV-1 group M (subtypes A, B, D and CRF01_AE). These viruses were classified as using either CCR5 or the CXCR4 co-receptor for entry and were competed against the same phenotype to determine the fitness (based on > 2000 competitions). In the same study, it was reported that all HIV-1 group M viruses have a greater fitness than HIV-2 and HIV-1 group O showed the lowest fitness. Thus, with the exception of subtype C, this fitness order seems to reflect the prevalence of HIV in the human population and also the proposed rates of transmission efficiency. It has been reported in 2003 that the CCR5 HIV-1 subtype C isolates were at least 100-fold less fit than any other group M HIV-1 isolates [Ball et al., 2003]. Throughout the disease, subtype C isolates was predicted as preferentially CCR5-tropic and non-syncytium-inducing (NSI). This has absolute difference in infections with isolates of other HIV-1 subtypes, whereby the viruses switch from CCR5 to CXCR4 co-receptor entry during later stage of the disease. Other ex vivo [Ball et al., 2003] and in vivo study [Walker et al., 2005] has implied that subtype C is efficiently transmitted but is less virulent in comparison with other HIV-1 group M isolates. However, among all HIV strains, HIV-1 group M seems to be more virulent and transmissible. It is believed that its progenitor might have been „fitter" for human infection and more adaptive, even after going through the rapid evolution and passage. By contrast, HIV-2 and HIV-1 groups O and N might have limited expansion in the human population, possibly due to poor host adaptation and transmission efficiencies, although the exact reasons for their poor transmissibility and active establishment in human populations have remained unclear and speculative.

Viral fitness is generally defined as the ability of the virus to replicate within the host and is therefore dependant on host and viral factors [Weber et al., 2003]. Recombination is thought to increase viral fitness. In an HIV-1 recombinant-related fitness study by Njai et al. [Njai et al., 2006], CRF02_AG isolates demonstrated a higher ex vivo replicative fitness compared to subtypes A and G from the same geographic region in Cameroon, irrespective of the level of CD4+ count and co-receptor tropism. A similar study by Konings et al. [Vijay et al., 2008] showed a 1.4 to 1.9 times higher replication rate increase in the CRF02_AG strains, in contrast to its progenitor subtypes A and G; an adaptation which implies its broader spread and predominance in West Central Africa. A computer simulation has been developed that mimic the HIV genomic diversification within an infected individual and elucidate the influence of recombination [Vijay et al., 2008]. This study has shown that recombination increases viral fitness regardless of the size of the effective population. In light of these results, it is likely that HIV-1 recombination events in Asia can also contribute to the emergence of viruses for instance, the widespread CRF01_AE/B inter-subtype recombinants with a biological edge in their host. In vitro studies of the viral fitness and interactions between different viral strains have been assessed with limitation, as only viral replication capacity, defined as "intrinsic capacity of virus to replicate in an ideal environment" [Weber et al., 2003] can be studied in the absence of host selection pressures. As a result, viral replication capacities are compared in vitro between two or more HIV-1 strains in dual infection cultures. This can be achieved by establishing a competition assay, whereby primary strains or recombinant viruses are competed against laboratory strains or parental isolates. In general, two HIV-1 strains are allowed to replicate concurrently for a designated period of time, or as an alternative, HIV-1 recombinant viruses, which are unable to produce new infectious virions are used in a single cycle growth assay, to limit the replication to a single cycle. The experiment is analysed through the measurement of the proportion of each of the initial strains to give a relative replication capacity at the end of the assay. Few studies have taken this approach in order to compare a number of different HIV-1 strains including drug resistance mutants [Weber et al., 2003,Van Maarseveen et al., 2006], isolates from HIV-progressors versus LTNPs [Arien et al., 2005], variable subtypes, as well as different HIV-1 groups or HIV-1 versus HIV-2. To date, none of these studies have been performed on the currently emerging CRF01_AE/B inter-subtype recombinants from Malaysia, particularly CRF33_01B. It is therefore important and urgent to identify and understand the biological advantages of these new HIV-1 forms, which presumably will take over the predominance in HIV-1 epidemic in Malaysia.

10. Anti-HIV therapy, drug resistance and its dissemination: An example of China

In global terms, over the past 15 years the treatment of HIV-1 infection has evolved significantly. In North America and Western Europe, no effective therapy existed until the development and availability of zidovudine (ZDV, AZT) in 1987. In 2005, there are now 26 commercially available antiviral agents (both RT inhibitors [NRTI and NNRTI] and protease inhibitors) to treat HIV-1-infected individuals.

ARV treatment of HIV-1-infected patients in China fell behind that of most developed countries. While highly active antiretroviral therapy (HAART) became widely used in North America and Western Europe in 1996, China was still debating whether or not HIV/AIDS would become a huge epidemic there, despite the large number of IDUs testing positive in the southwest province of Yunnan and almost all provinces reporting HIV cases. In 1998, facing the rapid upsurge in HIV-1 incidence nation-wide, the Chinese government made a concerted effort to strategize the "Middle and Long-term Programming for the Prevention and Control of AIDS" in China. A year later in 1999, several small clinical trails were initiated in Beijing primarily for safety and efficacy testing, sponsored largely by international pharmaceutical companies. The drug regimen tested then consisted of Combivir plus either Indinavir or Abacavir. This small-scale trial period (1999-2001) can be regarded as the first phase of ARV treatment in China.

The second treatment phase started when the cost of imported drugs used for HAART declined significantly and more patients could afford the medications (2001-2003). The population of Chinese patients undergoing therapy for HIV increased, especially in economically developed areas such as Beijing and Shanghai. However, the number of clinical doctors trained to administer these drugs did not expand. Many patients did not have the opportunity to receive comprehensive care, including standardized immunologic and virologic assessments prior to treatment and regularly scheduled follow-up interviews. Some patients judged the efficacy of the medication by a moderation of their symptoms, and consequently decreased their dosage or stopped taking the medicine altogether, without the consent of a physician. Of the patients who initiated treatment in this period, an estimated 25-30 % stopped taking medicine after only one or two months. Whether or not the other patients were able to persist with treatment and return for follow-up interviews is still to be determined.

The third phase of treatment (2003-present) began with the availability of low-priced domestically manufactured and imported generic anti-HIV drugs. This has been undeniably the most beneficial phase in increasing the number of individuals receiving gratis treatment. Nation-wide free ARV treatment started in 2003, part of the China CARES program, consisting of 51 model sites with plans to further expand to 127 counties. However, the bigger hurdle for this ambitious plan has been again the critical shortage of properly trained doctors, nurses and community care workers. Some patients were so anxious to begin taking medicine for HIV that they obtained the necessary drugs without a doctor's prescription. As a consequence, lacking professional guidance and clinical supervision, they used the medicines improperly, leading to the development of a drug resistant virus. In addition, as generic HIV drugs entered the Chinese market from developing countries, some patients began taking medicine without any medical assessment before treatment, and without choosing to register for interviews during treatment. Furthermore, severe side effects associated with generic ARV produced in China led to a large number of patients stopping medication entirely or becoming unwilling to follow doctors' advice and suggestions. As the incidence of HIV infection rises in China, it is anticipated that problems associated with the abuse of ARV will only escalate. It is therefore expected that drug resistant HIV-1 strains will emerge leading to their high prevalence and transmission over time.

A number of studies in other countries have shown that the prevalence of viruses with drug resistance mutations in acutely or recently infected persons varies between 10 to 20% [Boden et al., 1999; Grant et al., 2002; Little et al., 2002]. Research examining the prevalence and genetic features of drug-resistance strains at national level is lacking in China. Several major institutes in China are combining forces to carry-out genetic studies on viruses collected before and after nation-wide free ARV treatment. Based on preliminary data, it is fairly clear that the prevalence of drug-resistant strains were extremely rare before year 2000.

Between year 2001 and 2003, however, drug-resistant strains began to emerge and in some areas the prevalence is as high as 5%. Beginning in 2004, there was a significant increase in the prevalence of drug-resistant drugs across entire China, coinciding with the nation-wide free ARV treatment. Some areas have reported 20-30% drug-resistant strains specifically against NNRTI (unpublished data), and some areas were reported to have as high as 60% drug-resistant strains. The significant increase in the prevalence of drug-resistance could be due to the selection of the cohort and the time from transmission to resistance testing. However, it has clearly shown that resistance tests should be recommended routinely for patients with new infection.

The widespread use of antiretroviral drugs has led to the development and subsequent transmission of drug-resistant HIV-1 and the transmission of drug-resistant viruses has been documented through vertical, sexual, and parenteral routes [Erice et al., 1993; Masquelier et al., 1993; Veenestra et al., 1995]. Patients who are infected with drug-resistant HIV-1 and initiate antiretroviral therapy show poorer treatment responses than patients who are infected with wild-type (WT) viruses [Grant et al., 2002; Little et al., 2002]. Also, in the absence of selection pressures exerted by drugs, some transmitted drug-resistance mutations may persist for months before reversion to a more replication-competent variant. Even when these drug resistant mutations are no longer detectable by population-based nucleotide-sequence, they can persist in the reservoir of latently infected CD4+ memory T cells and may rapidly reemerge under the selective pressure provided by antiretroviral treatment [Wong et al., 1997; Finzi et al., 1997]. In subjects who acquired drug-resistant virus during primary infection, plasma HIV RNA is not suppressed as readily by potent antiretroviral therapy. The slower response to the treatment and the limited viral suppression may facilitate the selection of variants with greater drug resistance.

Thus, given the current spread and changing trends in HIV epidemiology in China, it is extremely urgent to understand the prevalence of drug-resistant strains in China and its changing patterns over time. Otherwise, we will face insurmountable challenges in tailoring our ARV regimens to elicit optimal therapeutic responses. In addition, the recombination between drug resistance HIV-1 strains in the Asia-pacific can cause epidemiologic shift, which may eventually compromise effective drug treatments currently available in these countries, including China. Since, at present, China and India are the economic hubs of Asia the human trafficking may lead to effective dispersal of such recombinant viruses. Therefore, well-coordinated international approaches are needed for surveillance and monitoring of the emergence of new drug resistance recombinant viruses.

11. Conclusions

It is hard to predict how the future of HIV epidemic will shape-up, since a number of complicating factors appear to unfold, including the possible effects of government intervention and unexpected changes (for the better or for the worse) in the behavior of affected populations. However, it is likely that the number of HIV infections is now on the rise, it is expected that the total number of HIV infections in China and India will surpass rest of the world, if no effective countermeasures are taken. Nonetheless, recombination between HIV-1 strains in geographical areas where multiple subtypes circulate will continue to shape future HIV epidemic through the generation of fitter strains capable of transmitting and dispersing in human populations fatser. China, India and other developing countries provide the right medium for this scenario. These countries stand at a critical juncture to prevent widespread of HIV transmission from the high-risk groups to the general population. Comprehensive approaches are necessary, integrating prevention and treatment efforts. Government, NGO, and international organizations bear responsibility to stop this epidemic in China. Scientific communities and pharmaceutical companies both inside and outside China need to work jointly to develop more potent anti-HIV drugs and therapeutics to inhibit viral replication and reduce HIV transmission. We have seen clear evidence in favor of evolution of complex second and third generation recombinant viruses. Continued monitoring and surveillance of these viruses is needed, if an HIV vaccine is to be developed. Moreover, concerted efforts by joint ventures between the state and the private sector are highly needed for developing an HIV vaccine for the ultimate control of HIV and its spread in the most populous nation of the world.

12. References

Alaeus A, Lidman K, Bjorkman A, Giesecke J, Albert J. Similar rate of disease progression among individuals infected with HIV-1 genetic subtypes A-D. (1999) AIDS. May 28;13(8):901-7.

Andersson S, Norrgren H, Dias F, Biberfeld G and Albert J. (1999). Molecular characterization of human immunodeficiency virus (HIV)-1 and -2 in individuals from guinea-bissau with single or dual infections: predominance of a distinct HIV-1 subtype A/G recombinant in West Africa. Virology. 262(2): 312-20.

Arien KK, Abraha A, Quinones-Mateu ME, Kestens L, Vanham G, Arts EJ. The replicative fitness of primary human immunodeficiency virus type 1 (HIV-1) group M, HIV-1 group O, and HIV-2 isolates. (2005) J Virol. Jul;79(14):8979-90.

Arien KK, Troyer RM, Gali Y, Colebunders RL, Arts EJ, Vanham G. Replicative fitness of historical and recent HIV-1 isolates suggests HIV-1 attenuation over time. (2005)AIDS Oct 14;19(15):1555-64.

Balakrishnan M, Fay PJ and Bambara RA. (2001). The kissing hairpin sequence promotes recombination within the HIV-I 5' leader region. J Biol Chem. 276(39): 36482-92.

Ball SC, Abraha A, Collins KR, Marozsan AJ, Baird H, Quinones-Mateu ME, Penn-Nicholson A, Murray M, Richard N, Lobritz M, et al. (2003). Comparing the ex vivo fitness of CCR5-tropic human immunodeficiency virus type 1 isolates of subtypes B and C. J Virol. 77(2): 1021-38.

Ball SC, Abraha A, Collins KR, Marozsan AJ, Baird H, Quinones-Mateu ME, et al. Comparing the ex vivo fitness of CCR5-tropic human immunodeficiency virus type 1 isolates of subtypes B and C. (2003) J Virol. Jan;77(2):1021-38.

Battula N and Loeb LA. (1976). On the fidelity of DNA replication. Lack of exodeoxyribonuclease activity and error-correcting function in avian myeloblastosis virus DNA polymerase. J Biol Chem. 251(4): 982-6.

Benson RE, Sanfridson A, Ottinger JS, Doyle C and Cullen BR. (1993). Downregulation of cell-surface CD4 expression by simian immunodeficiency virus Nef prevents viral super infection. J Exp Med. 177(6): 1561-6.

Bessong PO, Larry Obi C, Cilliers T, Choge I, Phoswa M, Pillay C, Papathanasopoulos M and Morris L. (2005). Characterization of human immunodeficiency virus type 1 from a previously unexplored region of South Africa with a high HIV prevalence. AIDS Res Hum Retroviruses. 21(1): 103-9.

Bobkov AF, Kazennova EV, Selimova LM, Khanina TA, Ryabov GS, Bobkova MR, Sukhanova AL, Kravchenko AV, Ladnaya NN, Weber JN, et al. (2004). Temporal trends in the HIV-1 epidemic in Russia: predominance of subtype A. J Med Virol. 74(2): 191-6.

Bocharov G, Ford NJ, Edwards J, Breinig T, Wain-Hobson S and Meyerhans A. (2005). A genetic-algorithm approach to simulating human immunodeficiency virus evolution reveals the strong impact of multiply infected cells and recombination. J Gen Virol. 86(Pt 11): 3109-18.

Boden, D., et al., HIV-1 drug resistance in newly infected individuals. Jama, 1999. 282:1135-41.

Bretscher MT, Althaus CL, Muller V and Bonhoeffer S. (2004). Recombination in HIV and the evolution of drug resistance: for better or for worse? Bioessays. 26(2): 180-8.

Carr JK, Foley BT, Leitner T, Salminen M, Korber B and McCutchan F. (1998). Reference Sequences Representing the Principal Genetic Diversity of HIV-1 in the Pandemic. In Human Retroviruses and AIDS 1998. Korber B, KC, Foley B, Hahn B, McCutchan F, Mellors JW, and Sodroski J. Los Alamos, NM, Theoretical Biology and Biophysics Group. III-10-19.

Casado G, Thomson MM, Delgado E, Sierra M, Vazquez-De Parga E, Perez- Alvarez L, Ocampo A and Najera R. (2003). Near full-length genome characterization of an HIV type 1 CRF05_DF virus from Spain. AIDS Res Hum Retroviruses. 19(8): 719-25.

Chan DP, Tsui SK, Ip P, Lee S, Lam C, Lau I, et al. Analysis of the full-length genome sequence of HIV-1 BF recombinant from an injection drug user in Macao. 4th International AIDS Society conference; 2007; Sydney, Australia.

Chan DP, Tsui SK, Ip P, Lee S, Lam C, Lau I, et al. Identification of a cluster of HIV-1 CRF12_BF in a population of injection drug users in Macao. 4th International AIDS Society conference; 2007; Sydney, Australia.

Chan DP, Tsui SK, Ip P, Lee S, Lam C, Lau I, et al. Identification of a cluster of HIV-1 CRF12_BF in a population of injection drug users in Macao. 4th International AIDS Society conference; 2007; Sydney, Australia.

Charpentier C, Nora T, Tenaillon O, Clavel F and Hance AJ. (2006). Extensive recombination among human immunodeficiency virus type 1 quasispecies makes an important contribution to viral diversity in individual patients. Journal of Virology. 80(5): 2472-82.

Chen Z, Luckay A, Sodora DL, Telfer P, Reed P, Gettie A, Kanu JM, Sadek RF, Yee J, Ho DD, et al. (1997). Human immunodeficiency virus type 2 (HIV-2) seroprevalence and characterization of a distinct HIV-2 genetic subtype from the natural range of simian immunodeficiency virus-infected sooty mangabeys. J Virol. 71(5): 3953-60.

Chen Z, Telfier P, Gettie A, Reed P, Zhang L, Ho DD and Marx PA. (1996). Genetic characterization of new West African simian immunodeficiency virus SIVsm: geographic clustering of household-derived SIV strains with human immunodeficiency virus type 2 subtypes and genetically diverse viruses from a single feral sooty mangabey troop. J Virol. 70(6): 3617-27.

Chohan B, Lavreys L, Rainwater SM and Overbaugh J. (2005). Evidence for frequent reinfection with human immunodeficiency virus type 1 of a different subtype. J Virol. 79(16): 10701-8.

Coffin JM. (1979). Structure, replication, and recombination of retrovirus genomes: some unifying hypotheses. J Gen Virol. 42(1): 1-26.

Condra JH, Schleif WA, Blahy OM, Gabryelski LJ, Graham DJ, Quintero JC, et al. In vivo emergence of HIV-1 variants resistant to multiple protease inhibitors. (1995) Nature. Apr 6;374(6522):569-71.

D'Souza V and Summers MF. (2005). How retroviruses select their genomes. Nat Rev Microbiol. 3(8): 643-55.

Damond F, Worobey M, Campa P, Farfara I, Colin G, Matheron S, Brun-Vezinet F, Robertson DL and Simon F. (2004). Identification of a highly divergent HIV type 2 and proposal for a change in HIV type 2 classification. AIDS Res Hum Retroviruses. 20(6): 666-72.

Dang Q, Chen J, Unutmaz D, Coffin JM, Pathak VK, Powell D, KewalRamani VN, Maldarelli F and Hu WS. (2004). Nonrandom HIV-1 infection and double infection via direct and cell-mediated pathways. Proc Natl Acad Sci U S A. 101(2): 632-7.

De Sa Filho DJ, Sucupira MC, Caseiro MM, Sabino EC, Diaz RS and Janini LM. (2006). Identification of two HIV type 1 circulating recombinant forms in Brazil. AIDS Res Hum Retroviruses. 22(1): 1-13.

Delgado E, Thomson MM, Villahermosa ML, Sierra M, Ocampo A, Miralles C, Rodriguez-Perez R, Diz-Aren J, Ojea-de Castro R, Losada E, et al. (2002).

Domingo E, Holland JJ. RNA virus mutations and fitness for survival. (1997). Annu Rev Microbiol;51:151-78.

Dowling WE, Kim B, Mason CJ, Wasunna KM, Alam U, Elson L, Birx DL, Robb ML, McCutchan FE and Carr JK. (2002). Forty-one near full-length HIV-1 sequences from Kenya reveal an epidemic of subtype A and A-containing recombinants. AIDS. 16(13): 1809-20.

Duesberg PH. (1968). Physical properties of Rous Sarcoma Virus RNA. Proc Natl Acad Sci U S A. 60(4): 1511-8.

Erice, A., et al., Brief report: primary infection with zidovudine-resistant human immunodeficiency virus type 1. N Engl J Med, 1993. 328:1163-5.

Esteves A, Parreira R, Piedade J, Venenno T, Franco M, Germano de Sousa J, Patricio L, Brum P, Costa A and Canas-Ferreira WF. (2003). Spreading of HIV- 1 subtype G and envB/gagG recombinant strains among injecting drug users in Lisbon, Portugal. AIDS Res Hum Retroviruses. 19(6): 511-7.

Finzi, D., et al., Identification of a reservoir for HIV-1 in patients on highly active antiretroviral therapy. Science, 1997. 278:1295-300.

Gao F, Bailes E, Robertson DL, Chen Y, Rodenburg CM, Michael SF, Cummins LB, Arthur LO, Peeters M, Shaw GM, et al. (1999). Origin of HIV-1 in the chimpanzee Pan troglodytes troglodytes. Nature. 397(6718): 436-41.

Gao F, Vidal N, Li Y, Trask SA, Chen Y, Kostrikis LG, Ho DD, Kim J, Oh MD, Choe K, et al. (2001). Evidence of two distinct subsubtypes within the HIV-1 subtype A radiation. AIDS Res Hum Retroviruses. 17(8): 675-88.

Gao F, Yue L, White A, Pappas B, Barchue J, Hanson A, Greene B, Sharp P, Shaw G and Hahn B. (1992). Human infection by genetically diverse SIVSM-related HIV-2 in west Africa. Nature. 358(6386): 495-9.

Garcia PM, Kalish LA, Pitt J, Minkoff H, Quinn TC, Burchett SK, Kornegay J, Jackson B, Moye J, Hanson C, et al. (1999). Maternal levels of plasma human immunodeficiency virus type 1 RNA and the risk of perinatal transmission. Women and Infants Transmission Study Group. N Engl J Med. 341(6): 394-402.

Gomez-Carrillo M, Quarleri JF, Rubio AE, Carobene MG, Dilernia D, Carr JK and Salomon H. (2004). Drug resistance testing provides evidence of the globalization of HIV type 1: a new circulating recombinant form. AIDS Research & Human Retroviruses. 20(8): 885-8.

Gottlieb GS, Nickle DC, Jensen MA, Wong KG, Grobler J, Li F, Liu SL, Rademeyer C, Learn GH, Karim SS, et al. (2004). Dual HIV-1 infection associated with rapid disease progression. Lancet. 363(9409): 619-22.

Grant, R.M., et al., Time trends in primary HIV-1 drug resistance among recently infected persons. Jama, 2002. 288:181-8.

Gutierrez M, Tajada P, Alvarez A, De Julian R, Baquero M, Soriano V and Holguin A. (2004). Prevalence of HIV-1 non-B subtypes, syphilis, HTLV, and hepatitis B and C viruses among immigrant sex workers in Madrid, Spain. J Med Virol. 74(4): 521-7.

Harris ME, Serwadda D, Sewankambo N, Kim B, Kigozi G, Kiwanuka N, Phillips JB, Wabwire F, Meehen M, Lutalo T, et al. (2002). Among 46 near full length HIV type 1 genome sequences from Rakai District, Uganda, subtype D and AD recombinants predominate. AIDS Res Hum Retroviruses. 18(17): 1281-90.

Hemelaar J, Gouws E, Ghys PD, Osmanov S. Global and regional distribution of HIV-1 genetic subtypes and recombinants in 2004. (2006) AIDS. Oct 24;20(16):W13-23.

Hierholzer J, Montano S, Hoelscher M, Negrete M, Hierholzer M, Avila MM, Carrillo MG, Russi JC, Vinoles J, Alava A, et al. (2002). Molecular Epidemiology of HIV Type 1 in Ecuador, Peru, Bolivia, Uruguay, and Argentina. AIDS Res Hum Retroviruses. 18(18): 1339-50.

Hirsch VM, Olmsted RA, Murphey-Corb M, Purcell RH and Johnson PR. (1989). An African primate lentivirus (SIVsm) closely related to HIV-2. Nature. 339(6223): 389-92.

Ho DD, Neumann AU, Perelson AS, Chen W, Leonard JM, Markowitz M. Rapid turnover of plasma virions and CD4 lymphocytes in HIV-1 infection. Nature 1995; 373:123-126.

Hsu TW and Taylor JM. (1982). Effect of aphidicolin on avian sarcoma virus replication. J Virol. 44(2): 493-8.

Hu WS and Temin HM. (1990a). Genetic consequences of packaging two RNA genomes in one retroviral particle: pseudodiploidy and high rate of genetic recombination. Proc Natl Acad Sci U S A. 87(4): 1556-60.

Hu WS and Temin HM. (1990b). Retroviral recombination and reverse transcription. Science. 250(4985): 1227-33.

Huet T, Cheynier R, Meyerhans A, Roelants G and Wain-Hobson S. (1990). Genetic organization of a chimpanzee lentivirus related to HIV-1. Nature. 345(6273): 356-9.

Hunt PW, Harrigan PR, Huang W, Bates M, Williamson DW, McCune JM, et al. Prevalence of CXCR4 Tropism among Antiretroviral-Treated HIV-1-Infected Patients with Detectable Viremia. (2006) J Infect Dis. Oct 1;194(7):926-30.

Jeeninga RE, Hoogenkamp M, Armand-Ugon M, de Baar M, Verhoef K, Berkhout B. Functional differences between the long terminal repeat transcriptional promoters of human immunodeficiency virus type 1 subtypes A through G. (2000) J Virol. Apr;74(8):3740-51.

Jetzt AE, Yu H, Klarmann GJ, Ron Y, Preston BD and Dougherty JP. (2000). High rate of recombination throughout the human immunodeficiency virus type 1 genome. J Virol. 74(3): 1234-40.

Jung A, Maier R, Vartanian JP, Bocharov G, Jung V, Fischer U, Meese E, Wain- Hobson S and Meyerhans A. (2002). Multiply infected spleen cells in HIV patients. Nature. 418(6894): 144.

Kalish ML, Baldwin A, Raktham S, Wasi C, Luo CC, Schochetman G, Mastro TD, Young N, Vanichseni S, Rubsamen-Waigmann H, et al. (1995). The evolving molecular epidemiology of HIV-1 envelope subtypes in injecting drug users in Bangkok, Thailand: implications for HIV vaccine trials. AIDS. 9(8): 851-7.

Koch WH, Sullivan PS, Roberts C, Francis K, Downing R, Mastro TD, et al. Evaluation of United States-licensed human immunodeficiency virus immunoassays for detection of group M viral variants. (2001) J Clin Microbiol. Mar;39(3):1017-20.

Konings FA, Burda ST, Urbanski MM, Zhong P, Nadas A, Nyambi PN. Human immunodeficiency virus type 1 (HIV-1) circulating recombinant form 02_AG (CRF02_AG) has a higher in vitro replicative capacity than its parental subtypes A and G.(2006) J Med Virol. May;78(5):523-34.

Korber B, Muldoon M, Theiler J, Gao F, Gupta R, Lapedes A, Hahn BH, Wolinsky S and Bhattacharya T. (2000). Timing the ancestor of the HIV-1 pandemic strains. Science. 288(5472): 1789-96.

Koulinska IN, Ndung'u T, Mwakagile D, Msamanga G, Kagoma C, Fawzi W, Essex M and Renjifo B. (2001). A new human immunodeficiency virus type 1 circulating recombinant form from Tanzania. AIDS Res Hum Retroviruses. 17(5): 423-31.

Kozaczynska K, Cornelissen M, Reiss P, Zorgdrager F, van der Kuyl AC. HIV-1 sequence evolution in vivo after superinfection with three viral strains. (2007) Retrovirology. Aug 23;4(1):59.

Lal RB, Chakrabarti S and Yang C. (2005). Impact of genetic diversity of HIV-1 on diagnosis, antiretroviral therapy & vaccine development. Indian J Med Res. 121(4): 287-314.

Lau KA, Wang B, Saksena NK. (2007). Emerging trends of HIV epidemiology in Asia. AIDS Rev. Oct-Dec;9(4):218-29. Review.

Laukkanen T, Carr JK, Janssens W, Liitsola K, Gotte D, McCutchan FE, Op de Coul E, Cornelissen M, Heyndrickx L, van der Groen G, et al. (2000). Virtually full-length subtype F and F/D recombinant HIV-1 from Africa and South America. Virology. 269(1): 95-104.

Lemey P, Pybus OG, Wang B, Saksena NK, Salemi M and Vandamme AM. (2003). Tracing the origin and history of the HIV-2 epidemic. Proc Natl Acad Sci U S A. 100(11): 6588-92.

Liitsola K, Tashkinova I, Laukkanen T, Korovina G, Smolskaja T, Momot O, Mashkilleyson N, Chaplinskas S, Brummer-Korvenkontio H, Vanhatalo J, et al. (1998). HIV-1 genetic subtype A/B recombinant strain causing an explosive epidemic in injecting drug users in Kaliningrad. AIDS. 12(14): 1907-19.

Little, S.J., et al., Antiretroviral-drug resistance among patients recently infected with HIV. N Engl J Med, 2002. 347:385-94.

Lukashov VV and Goudsmit J. (1997). Evolution of the human immunodeficiency virus type 1 subtype-specific V3 domain is confined to a sequence space with a fixed distance to the subtype consensus. J Virol. 71(9): 6332-8.

Mamadou S, Vidal N, Montavon C, Ben A, Djibo A, Rabiou S, Soga G, Delaporte E, Mboup S and Peeters M. (2003). Emergence of complex and diverse CRF02- AG/CRF06-cpx recombinant HIV type 1 strains in Niger, West Africa. AIDS Res Hum Retroviruses. 19(1): 77-82.

Mansky LM and Temin HM. (1995). Lower in vivo mutation rate of human immunodeficiency virus type 1 than that predicted from the fidelity of purified reverse transcriptase. J Virol. 69(8): 5087-94.

Masquelier, B., et al., Primary infection with zidovudine-resistant HIV. N Engl J Med, 1993. 329:1123-4.

McCutchan FE, Hegerich PA, Brennan TP, Phanuphak P, Singharaj P, Jugsudee A, Berman PW, Gray AM, Fowler AK and Burke DS. (1992). Genetic variants of HIV-1 in Thailand. AIDS Res Hum Retroviruses. 8(11): 1887-95.

McCutchan FE, Hoelscher M, Tovanabutra S, Piyasirisilp S, Sanders-Buell E, Ramos G, Jagodzinski L, Polonis V, Maboko L, Mmbando D, et al. (2005). Indepth analysis of a heterosexually acquired human immunodeficiency virus type 1 superinfection: evolution, temporal fluctuation, and intercompartment dynamics from the seronegative window period through 30 months post-infection. J Virol. 79(18): 11693-704.

Meloni ST, Kim B, Sankale JL, Hamel DJ, Tovanabutra S, Mboup S, McCutchan FE and Kanki PJ. (2004a). Distinct human immunodeficiency virus type 1 subtype A virus circulating in West Africa: sub-subtype A3. J Virol. 78(22): 12438-45.

Meloni ST, Sankale JL, Hamel DJ, Eisen G, Gueye-Ndiaye A, Mboup S and Kanki PJ. (2004b). Molecular epidemiology of human immunodeficiency virus type 1 sub-subtype A3 in Senegal from 1988 to 2001. J Virol. 78(22): 12455-61.

Michel N, Allespach I, Venzke S, Fackler OT and Keppler OT. (2005). The Nef protein of human immunodeficiency virus establishes superinfection immunity by a dual strategy to downregulate cell-surface CCR5 and CD4. Curr Biol. 15(8): 714-23.

Mokili JL, Rogers M, Carr JK, Simmonds P, Bopopi JM, Foley BT, Korber BT, Birx DL and McCutchan FE. (2002). Identification of a novel clade of human immunodeficiency virus type 1 in Democratic Republic of Congo. AIDS Res Hum Retroviruses. 18(11): 817-23.

Moutouh L, Corbeil J and Richman DD. (1996). Recombination leads to the rapid emergence of HIV-1 dually resistant mutants under selective drug pressure. Proc Natl Acad Sci U S A. 93(12): 6106-11.

Negroni M and Buc H. (2001). Mechanisms of retroviral recombination. Annu Rev Genet. 35: 275-302.

Nerurkar VR, Nguyen HT, Dashwood WM, Hoffmann PR, Yin C, Morens DM, et al. HIV type 1 subtype E in commercial sex workers and injection drug users in southern Vietnam. (1996) AIDS Res Hum Retroviruses. Jun 10;12(9):841-3.

Nijhuis M, Schuurman R, de Jong D, Erickson J, Gustchina E, Albert J, et al. Increased fitness of drug resistant HIV-1 protease as a result of acquisition of compensatory mutations during suboptimal therapy. (1999) AIDS. Dec 3;13(17):2349-59.

Njai HF, Gali Y, Vanham G, Clybergh C, Jennes W, Vidal N, et al. The predominance of Human Immunodeficiency Virus type 1 (HIV-1) circulating recombinant form 02 (CRF02_AG) in West Central Africa may be related to its replicative fitness. (2006) Retrovirology. Jul 3;3(1):40.

Otten RA, Ellenberger DL, Adams DR, Fridlund CA, Jackson E, Pieniazek D and Rayfield MA. (1999). Identification of a window period for susceptibility to dual infection with two distinct human immunodeficiency virus type 2 isolates in a Macaca nemestrina (pig-tailed macaque) model. J Infect Dis. 180(3): 673-84.

Ou CY, Takebe Y, Weniger BG, Luo CC, Kalish ML, Auwanit W, et al. Independent introduction of two major HIV-1 genotypes into distinct high-risk populations in Thailand. (1993). Lancet. May 8;341(8854):1171-4.

Parreira R, Padua E, Piedade J, Venenno T, Paixao MT and Esteves A. (2005). Genetic analysis of human immunodeficiency virus type 1 nef in Portugal: subtyping, identification of mosaic genes, and amino acid sequence variability. J Med Virol. 77(1): 8-16.

Peeters M. (2000). Recombinant HIV sequences: Their role in the global epidemic. In HIV Sequence Compendium 2000. Kuiken CL, Foley B, Hahn B et al.. Los Alamos, Theoretical Biology and Biophysics Group, Los Alamos National Laboratory, NM. 39-54.

Perez-Alvarez L, Carmona R, Munoz M, Delgado E, Thomson MM, Contreras G, Pedreira JD, Rodriguez Real R, Vazquez de Parga E, Medrano L, et al. (2003). High incidence of non-B and recombinant HIV-1 strains in newly diagnosed patients in Galicia, Spain: study of genotypic resistance. Antivir Ther. 8(4): 355-60.

Piyasirisilp S, McCutchan FE, Carr JK, Sanders-Buell E, Liu W, Chen J, et al. A recent outbreak of human immunodeficiency virus type 1 infection in southern China was initiated by two highly homogeneous, geographically separated strains, circulating recombinant form AE and a novel BC recombinant. (2000). J Virol. Dec;74(23):11286-95.

Preston BD, Poiesz BJ, Loeb LA. Fidelity oh HIV-1 reverse transcriptase. Science 1988; 242:1168-1171.

Quinones-Mateu ME, Arts EJ. Virus fitness: concept, quantification, and application to HIV population dynamics. (2006) Curr Top Microbiol Immunol ;299:83-140.

Quinones-Mateu ME, Ball SC, Marozsan AJ, Torre VS, Albright JL, Vanham G, et al. A dual infection/competition assay shows a correlation between ex vivo human immunodeficiency virus type 1 fitness and disease progression. (2000) J Virol. Oct;74(19):9222-33.

Renjifo B, Fawzi W, Mwakagile D, Hunter D, Msamanga G, Spiegelman D, Garland M, Kagoma C, Kim A, Chaplin B, et al. (2001). Differences in perinatal transmission among human immunodeficiency virus type 1 genotypes. J Hum Virol. 4(1): 16-25.

Renjifo B, Gilbert P, Chaplin B, Msamanga G, Mwakagile D, Fawzi W, Group TVaHS and Essex M. (2004). Preferential in-utero transmission of HIV-1 subtype C as compared to HIV-1 subtype A or D. AIDS. 18(12): 1629-1636.

Robertson DL, Anderson J, P., Bradac JA, Carr JK, Foley B, Funkhouser RK, Gao F, Hahn BH, Kuiken C, Learn GH, et al. (1999). HIV-1 Nomenclature Proposal. In Human Retroviruses and AIDS 1999. Kuiken, CL, Foley, B, Hahn, B et al. . Los Alamos,

NM., Theoretical Biology and Biophysics Group, Los Alamos National Laboratory.: 492-505.

Saksena NK, Wang B and Dyer WB. (2001). Biological and Molecular Mechanisms in Progression of HIV Disease. AIDS reviews. 3(3): 133-44.

Saksena NK, Wang B, Steain MC, Yang RG and Zhang LQ. (2005). Snapshot of HIV pathogenesis in China. Cell Res. 15(11-12): 953-61.

Sanders-Buell E, Saad MD, Abed AM, Bose M, Todd CS, Strathdee SA, Botros BA, Safi N, Earhart KC, Scott PT, Michael N, McCutchan FE. (2007). A nascent HIV type 1 epidemic among injecting drug users in Kabul, Afghanistan is dominated by complex AD recombinant strain, CRF35_AD. (2007). AIDS Res Hum Retroviruses. Jun;23(6):834-9. Erratum in: AIDS Res Hum Retroviruses. 2007 Jul;23(7):953-4.

Sharp PM, Bailes E, Stevenson M, Emerman M and Hahn BH. (1996). Gene acquisition in HIV and SIV. Nature. 383(6601): 586-7.

Sharp PM, Robertson DL and Hahn BH. (1995). Cross-species transmission and recombination of 'AIDS' viruses. Philos Trans R Soc Lond B Biol Sci. 349(1327): 41-7.

Smith DM, Wong JK, Hightower GK, Ignacio CC, Koelsch KK, Daar ES, Richman DD and Little SJ. (2004). Incidence of HIV superinfection following primary infection. JAMA. 292(10): 1177-8.

Soares EA, Martinez AM, Souza TM, Santos AF, Da Hora V, Silveira J, Bastos FI, Tanuri A and Soares MA. (2005). HIV-1 subtype C dissemination in southern Brazil. AIDS. 19 Suppl 4(4): S81-6.

Songok EM, Lihana RW, Kiptoo MK, Genga IO, Kibaya R, Odhiambo F, Kobayashi K, Ago Y, Ndembi N, Okoth F, et al. (2003). Identification of env CRF-10 among HIV variants circulating in rural western Kenya. AIDS Res Hum Retroviruses. 19(2): 161-5.

Steain MC, Wang B, Dwyer DE and Saksena NK. (2004). HIV-1 co-infection, superinfection and recombination. Sexual Health. 1(4): 239-250.

Steain MC, Wang B, Yang C, Shi YP, Nahlen B, Lal RB and Saksena NK. (2005). HIV type 1 sequence diversity and dual infections in Kenya. AIDS Res Hum Retroviruses. 21(10): 882-5.

Swanson P, de Mendoza C, Joshi Y, Golden A, Hodinka RL, Soriano V, et al. Impact of human immunodeficiency virus type 1 (HIV-1) genetic diversity on performance of four commercial viral load assays: LCx HIV RNA Quantitative, AMPLICOR HIV-1 MONITOR v1.5, VERSANT HIV-1 RNA 3.0, and NucliSens HIV-1 QT. (20035)J Clin Microbiol. Aug;43(8):3860-8.

Takebe Y. Inter-CRF Recombinants: A New Class of HIV-1 Recombinants and Its Epidemiological Implications. 13th Conference on Retroviruses and Opportunistic Infections; 2006; Denver, Colorado, USA.

Tapia N, Franco S, Puig-Basagoiti F, Menendez C, Alonso PL, Mshinda H, et al. Influence of human immunodeficiency virus type 1 subtype on mother-to-child transmission. (2003) J Gen Virol. Mar;84(Pt 3):607-13.

Tatt ID, Barlow KL, Clewley JP, Gill ON and Parry JV. (2004). Surveillance of HIV- 1 subtypes among heterosexuals in England and Wales, 1997-2000. J Acquir Immune Defic Syndr. 36(5): 1092-9.

Thomson MM, Perez-Alvarez L and Najera R. (2002b). Molecular epidemiology of HIV-1 genetic forms and its significance for vaccine development and therapy. Lancet Infect Dis. 2(8): 461-71.

Tovanabutra S, Beyrer C, Sakkhachornphop S, Razak MH, Ramos GL, Vongchak T, Rungruengthanakit K, Saokhieo P, Tejafong K, Kim B, et al. (2004). The changing molecular epidemiology of HIV type 1 among northern Thai drug users, 1999 to 2002. AIDS Res Hum Retroviruses. 20(5): 465-75.

Tovanabutra S, Polonis V, De Souza M, Trichavaroj R, Chanbancherd P, Kim B, Sanders-Buell E, Nitayaphan S, Brown A, Robb MR, et al. (2001). First CRF01_AE/B recombinant of HIV-1 is found in Thailand. AIDS. 15(8): 1063-5.

Troyer RM, Collins KR, Abraha A, Fraundorf E, Moore DM, Krizan RW, et al. Changes in human immunodeficiency virus type 1 fitness and genetic diversity during disease progression. (2005) J Virol.Jul;79(14):9006-18.

UNAIDS. (2010). AIDS-epidemic update 2010. From http://www.unaids.org/epi/2010/index.asp.

Van der Kuyl AC, Kozaczynska K, van den Burg R, Zorgdrager F, Back N, Jurriaans S, Berkhout B, Reiss P and Cornelissen M. (2005). Triple HIV-1 infection. New England Journal of Medicine. 352(24): 2557-9.

van Maarseveen NM, Huigen MC, de Jong D, Smits AM, Boucher CA, Nijhuis M. A novel real-time PCR assay to determine relative replication capacity for HIV-1 protease variants and/or reverse transcriptase variants. (2006) J Virol Methods. May;133(2):185-94.

van Rij RP, Worobey M, Visser JA and Schuitemaker H. (2003). Evolution of R5 and X4 human immunodeficiency virus type 1 gag sequences in vivo: evidence for recombination. Virology. 314(1): 451-9.

Veenstra, J., et al., Transmission of zidovudine-resistant human immunodeficiency virus type 1 variants following deliberate injection of blood from a patient with AIDS: characteristics and natural history of the virus. Clin Infect Dis, 1995. 21:556-60.

Velazquez-Campoy A, Todd MJ, Vega S, Freire E. Catalytic efficiency and vitality of HIV-1 proteases from African viral subtypes. (2001) Proc Natl Acad Sci U S A. May 22;98(11):6062-7.

Vidal N, Mulanga C, Bazepeo SE, Lepira F, Delaporte E and Peeters M. (2006). Identification and molecular characterization of subsubtype A4 in central Africa. AIDS Res Hum Retroviruses. 22(2): 182-7.

Vidal N, Peeters M, Mulanga-Kabeya C, Nzilambi N, Robertson D, Ilunga W, Sema H, Tshimanga K, Bongo B and Delaporte E. (2000). Unprecedented degree of human immunodeficiency virus type 1 (HIV-1) group M genetic diversity in the Democratic Republic of Congo suggests that the HIV-1 pandemic originated in Central Africa. J Virol. 74(22): 10498-507.

Vijay NN, Vasantika, Ajmani R, Perelson AS, Dixit NM. Recombination increases human immunodeficiency virus fitness, but not necessarily diversity. (2008) J Gen Virol. Jun;89(Pt 6):1467-77.

Visawapoka U, Tovanabutra S, Currier JR, Cox JH, Mason CJ, Wasunna M, Ponglikitmongkol M, Dowling WE, Robb ML, Birx DL, et al. (2006). Circulating and unique recombinant forms of HIV type 1 containing subsubtype A2. AIDS Res Hum Retroviruses. 22(7): 695-702.

Walker PR, Pybus OG, Rambaut A and Holmes EC. (2005). Comparative population dynamics of HIV-1 subtypes B and C: subtype-specific differences in patterns of epidemic growth. Infect Genet Evol. 5(3): 199-208.

Walker PR, Pybus OG, Rambaut A, Holmes EC. Comparative population dynamics of HIV-1 subtypes B and C: subtype-specific differences in patterns of epidemic growth. (2005) Infect Genet Evol. Apr;5(3):199-208.

Wang B, Lal RB, Dwyer DE, Miranda-Saksena M, Boadle R, Cunningham AL and Saksena NK. (2000). Molecular and biological interactions between two HIV- 1 strains from a coinfected patient reveal the first evidence in favor of viral synergism. Virology. 274(1): 105-19.

Weber J, Rangel HR, Chakraborty B, Tadele M, Martinez MA, Martinez-Picado J, et al. A novel TaqMan real-time PCR assay to estimate ex vivo human immunodeficiency virus type 1 fitness in the era of multi-target (pol and env) antiretroviral therapy. (2003) J Gen Virol. Aug;84(Pt 8):2217-28.

Wei X, Ghosh SK, Taylor ME, Johnson VA, Emini EA, Deutsch P, et al. Viral dynamics in human immunodeficiency virus type 1 infection. Nature 1995; 373:117-122.

Weiss RA, Mason WS and Vogt PK. (1973). Genetic recombinants and heterozygotes derived from endogenous and exogenous avian RNA tumor viruses. Virology. 52(2): 535-52.

Weniger BG, Limpakarnjanarat K, Ungchusak K, Thanprasertsuk S, Choopanya K, Vanichseni S, et al. The epidemiology of HIV infection and AIDS in Thailand. (1991) AIDS;5 Suppl 2:S71-85.

Wong, J.K., et al., Recovery of replication-competent HIV despite prolonged suppression of plasma viremia. Science, 1997. 278:1291-5.

Wu W, Blumberg BM, Fay PJ and Bambara RA. (1995). Strand transfer mediated by human immunodeficiency virus reverse transcriptase in vitro is promoted by pausing and results in mis-incorporation. J Biol Chem. 270(1): 325-32.

Wu Y and Marsh JW. (2003). Early transcription from nonintegrated DNA in human immunodeficiency virus infection. J Virol. 77(19): 10376-82.

Yang C, Li M, Newman RD, Shi YP, Ayisi J, van Eijk AM, et al. Genetic diversity of HIV-1 in western Kenya: subtype-specific differences in mother-to-child transmission. (2003) AIDS. Jul 25;17(11):1667-74.

Yang C, Li M, Newman RD, Shi YP, Ayisi J, van Eijk AM, Otieno J, Misore AO, Steketee RW, Nahlen BL, et al. (2003a). Genetic diversity of HIV-1 in western Kenya: subtype-specific differences in mother-to-child transmission. AIDS. 17(11): 1667-74.

Yang C, Li M, Shi YP, Winter J, van Eijk AM, Ayisi J, Hu DJ, Steketee R, Nahlen BL and Lal RB. (2004). Genetic diversity and high proportion of intersubtype recombinants among HIV type 1-infected pregnant women in Kisumu, western Kenya. AIDS Res Hum Retroviruses. 20(5): 565-74.

Yang R, Xia X, Kusagawa S, Zhang C, Ben K, Takebe Y. On-going generation of multiple forms of HIV-1 intersubtype recombinants in the Yunnan Province of China. (2002) AIDS. Jul 5;16(10):1401-7.

Yu H, Jetzt AE, Ron Y, Preston BD and Dougherty JP. (1998). The nature of human immunodeficiency virus type 1 strand transfers. J Biol Chem. 273(43): 28384-91.

Zhu T, Korber BT, Nahmias AJ, Hooper E, Sharp PM and Ho DD. (1998). An African HIV-1 sequence from 1959 and implications for the origin of the epidemic. Nature. 391(6667): 594-7.

5

Insulin-Like Growth Factor System in HIV/AIDS: A Structure Based Approach to the Design of New Therapeutics

Monalisa Swain, Harsha Balaram and Hanudatta S. Atreya
Indian institute of Science, India

1. Introduction

One of the important regulators for growth and development of the human body is the endocrine system. The endocrine system is composed of glands that secrete hormones into the circulatory system, which are then distributed throughout the body, regulating the function of tissues and maintaining homeostasis. Among these hormones are the insulin-like growth factors (IGF), similar in molecular structure to insulin and playing an important role in cell growth, proliferation, differentiation (LeRoith & Roberts, 2003).

A complex network of molecules, including its binding proteins, proteases and receptors, which together comprise the 'IGF system', modulates the biological function of the IGFs. This system comprises the following components (Figure 1): (i) Two peptide hormones, IGF-1 and -2, (ii) type 1 and type 2 IGF receptors, (iii) six IGF-binding proteins (IGFBP; numbered 1-6) and (iv) IGFBP proteases. IGF-1 and -2 are small signalling peptides (~7.5 kDa) that stimulate action by binding to specific cell surface receptors (IGF-1R) evoking subsequent response inside the cell. Six soluble IGF binding proteins, the IGFBPs, which range in size from 22-31 kDa and share overall sequence and structural homology with each other, regulate the activity of the IGFs. IGFBPs bind strongly to IGFs (K_D ~ 300-700 pM) to ensure that the majority of circulating IGF in the blood stream is sequestered and at the tissue level inhibit the action of IGFs by blocking their access to the receptors. Proteolysis of the IGFBPs dissociates IGFs from the complex, enabling them to bind and activate the cell surface receptors (Figure 1). In tissues, IGFs form a binary complex with IGFBPs, whereas circulating IGFs are associated in ternary complexes containing IGFBP-3 (and IGFBP-5) and a third protein known as the acid-labile subunit (ALS). The ternary complex has a molecular mass of 150 kDa. The most abundant IGF-binding protein in the circulation is IGFBP-3 followed by IGFBP-2.

In recent years, the IGF system in general and IGFBPs in particular have become the focus as clinically important targets of cancer therapeutics (Chan et al., 1998; Harrison et al., 1996; LeRoith & Roberts, 2003; Ma et al., 1999; Rosenzweig & Atreya, 2010; Wu et al., 2004; Yu et al., 1999). Different strategies have been proposed to inhibit cancer growth by blocking IGF-I-R binding and function (recently reviewed by (Rosenzweig & Atreya, 2010)). In this regard, the therapeutic potential of the IGFBPs in inhibiting IGF-1/IGF-2 activity and thereby inhibiting cancer cell growth has been demonstrated. Notably, the IGFBPs do not bind insulin and thus do not interfere with insulin-insulin receptor interactions.

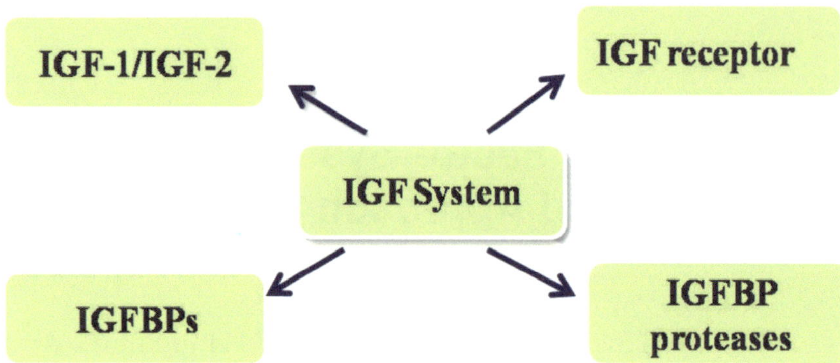

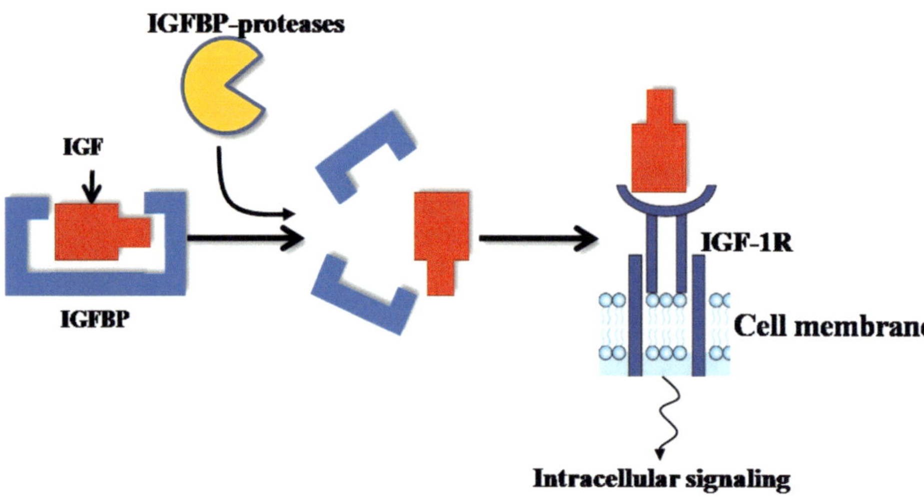

Fig. 1. Illustration of the IGF-system and its components.

1.1 IGF-binding proteins (IGFBPs)

While extensive studies have been carried out on the role of IGFs in different biological systems and under diseased conditions, a molecular-level understanding of IGF-IGFBP interactions is lacking. The three-dimensional (3D) structures have not yet been determined for any of the full-length IGFBPs. Based on sequence analysis, it is now understood that all IGFBPs contain three structural domains of nearly equal size (Firth & Baxter, 2002; Krywicki & Yee, 1992; LeRoith & Roberts, 2003; Rosenzweig, 2004). The N-and C-terminal domains are highly conserved in sequence across the IGFBPs. They contain 16-18 cysteine residues, forming 8-9 disulfide bonds. Their disulphide bonding indicates that the IGFBPs are thyroglobulin type-1 domain homologues. In recent years, structural studies have been carried out on individual domains in IGFBP-1, -2, -4, -5 and -6 (Kalus et al., 1998; Kibbey et al., 2006; Kuang et al., 2006; Sala et al., 2005; Sitar et al., 2006; Siwanowicz et al., 2005). Studies involving site directed mutagenesis have identified key residues in IGFBPs that are required for binding the IGFs (Clemmons, 2001). These studies have also revealed that both

the N- and C-terminal domains in IGFBPs are essential for IGF-1/2 binding (Clemmons, 2001; Kibbey et al., 2006; Siwanowicz et al., 2005). The central 'linker' domain which is structurally disordered has been proposed to be site where most of the post-translational modifications take place. This is also the region where proteases act to cleave the IGFBPs.
IGFBP levels are regulated by proteolysis following their secretion from the cell, which dissociates the IGFBP-IGF complex resulting in an increase in IGF-1/2 available for interacting with the IGF-1R (Bunn & Fowlkes, 2003) (Figure 1). This is evidenced from the differential effects of IGFBP-3 in tumor vs. normal prostate cells, wherein IGF-1 bio-availability is increased via IGFBP proteolysis (Miyamoto et al., 2004).

1.2 Role of IGF system in HIV & AIDS

1.2.1 Involvement of growth hormone/IGF axis in AIDS

In addition to its involvement in various cancers, the IGF-system has also been implicated in diabetes, uremic cachexia, muscle wasting in congestive heart failure (CHF), aging, human immunodeficiency virus (HIV), acquired immunodeficiency syndrome (AIDS), and AIDS cachexia (Hambrecht et al., 2002). It is now well understood that the growth hormone (GH)/IGF axis is significantly affected in HIV and AIDS patients (Meininger & Grinspoon, 2001). Patients with HIV infection or AIDS are known to have multiple growth hormone (GH)/IGF axis related defects which include: abnormal GH secretion, profound decrease in serum levels of IGF- I and IGF- II, abnormal post-translational modifications of IGF binding proteins, increased concentration of IGFBP-2 and reduced IGFBP-1/-3 concentration (Meininger & Grinspoon, 2001). In patients with AIDS wasting syndrome acquired GH resistance has been found to result in increased GH concentrations which occurs as a function of weight loss and loss of lean body mass. Conversely in patients with HIV lipodystrophy syndrome GH concentrations are reduced due to increased abdominal visceral adiposity. The GH/IGF axis has also been implicated in HIV associated osteopenia in patients with HIV-1-infection but without any symptoms of AIDS-associated wasting (Stagi et al., 2004). Thus, due to its significant role IGF levels are closely monitored in HIV/AIDS patients and help to track disease progression (see review by Congote 2005).

1.2.2 Role of IGF-binding proteins in HIV & AIDS

In addition to changes in IGF levels, the concentration of IGFBPs has also been observed to vary in patients with AIDs or HIV infection compared to healthy individuals. It has been observed that the levels of IGFBP-3 decrease whereas those of IGFBP-1 and -2 increase in HIV/AIDS patients (Congote, 2005). The levels of IGF-1/2 and those of IGFBP-1, -2 and -3 in HIV-infected children and adults vary throughout the course of the disease. Administration of GH significantly increases the levels of IGFBP-3 in all HIV infected patients except for patients with AIDS wasting (Mynarcik et al., 1999). Disease progression is associated with decrease IGF-2 levels and increase in IGFBP-2 & IGFBP-3 protease activity, infact IGFBP-2 levels are one of the first parameters to increase after HIV infection, before the development of AIDS (Helle et al., 2001) . The elevated IGFBP-3 protease activity is somewhat restored in patients undergoing antiretroviral therapy treatment (Helle et al., 2001). The proteolysis of IGFBP-3 causes IGF to be released, which is captured by IGFBP-2. It has been hypothesized that the low IGF and high IGFBP-2 levels found in HIV infection may contribute to enhanced lymphocyte apoptosis. This may in turn lead to immune dysfunction in patients. In another study, IGFBP-1 was observed to be highly phosphorylated and IGFBP-3 ternary complexes were formed with reduced ability in AIDS patients with wasting (Frost et al., 1996; Gelato & Frost, 1997).

1.3 IGF-system in treatment of HIV & AIDS

Given the significant role played by GH, IGFs and IGFBPs in HIV and AIDs, different approaches for treatment based on the GH/IGF-system have been proposed. We discuss here the two approaches, which underscore the importance of this system.

1.3.1 Treatment with growth hormone

In our body carbohydrates are the main source of energy needed for survival. Insufficient carbohydrate intake causes the body to burn the reserved fats followed by burning the muscle for energy which leads to loss of lean body mass (LBM). Muscle wasting or Wasting Syndrome (WS) is the most frequent problem in the patients with HIV infection and results in significant loss of body mass (Dudgeon et al., 2006). There are a variety of reasons why patients continue to lose weight, including: loss of appetite, increased metabolism, altered hormone levels, increased cytokine production which produces more fats than proteins. This is further aggravated by different drugs which cause nausea resulting in decreased food intake by patients and poor nutrient absorption which are necessary to maintain body mass. HIV-associated adipose redistribution syndrome (HARS) is an HIV-associated disorder characterized by excess truncal fat, including visceral adipose tissue (VAT). Muscle wasting, and particularly loss of metabolically active lean tissue, contributes to increased mortality, accelerated disease progression, and impairment of strength and functional status. The effect of treatment with protein anabolic agents, including GH, IGF-I, testosterone, nandrolonedecanoate, oxandrolone, and oxymetholone, have been studied in patients with HIV associated wasting. These studies have demonstrated that this treatment can increase lean body mass (LBM) and in some cases provide functional benefits and improvements in quality of life (Mulligan & Schambelan, 2002; Spinola-Castro et al., 2008). The immunologic effects of recombinant human growth hormone (rhGH), recombinant human insulin-like growth factor-1 (IGF-1), or their combination, in patients with moderately advanced HIV infection has been studied. The treatment with a combination of rhGH/rhIGF-1 and low dose of rhGH is reasonably well tolerated, resulting in increased body weight and modest improvements in HIV-specific immune function (Lee et al., 1996; Nguyen et al., 1998). Patients treated with rhGH sustain losses in VAT and truncal fat with no effect on subcutaneous fat in the abdomen or limbs. It has also been observed that non-high-density lipoprotein cholesterol (non-HDL-C) decreases significantly with rhGH treatment (Grunfeld et al., 2007).

1.3.2 Treatment with IGF-1 and IGF: IGFBP complexes

The observation that improved muscle mass, but not linear growth is associated with normalized IGF-1 concentration suggests that IGF-1 may be a potential therapeutic strategy to improve lean body mass in HIV-infected children (Chantry et al., 2008). Treatment with low dose recombinant IGF-1 produces significant, but transient, nitrogen retention. Alternate routes of IGF-1 administration or co-administration with GH prevents attenuation of IGF-1 action (Lieberman et al., 1994). However, administration of IGF-1 has its own set of problems. It causes lowering of glucose levels, which restricts its dosage, and thereby it's anabolic potential. Further, high levels of IGF-1 are warning signs for the increased risk of malignancy. In the case of cancer cachexia, which includes muscle wasting and anorexia, the growth of the tumor is associated with increased IGF-1 levels.

Interestingly, it was found that administration of IGF-I in complex with IGFBP-3, but not free IGF-I, is a potent stimulator of muscle protein synthesis in rats with chronic under nutrition (Zdanowicz & Teichberg, 2003). In contrast to free IGF-1, significantly higher dosage levels can be used. Administration of IGF-1 in this form increases the bioavailability of IGF-1. Moreover, a high dosage level of this complex does not result in hypoglycemic condition owing to the fact that IGF-1/IGFBP-3 complex does not interact with the insulin receptor. In the case of cancer cachexia, the IGF-1/IGFBP-3 complex fails to alter tumor growth, but improves the tumor-host nutritional state by improving food intake, attenuating weight loss and improving glucose metabolism (Wang et al., 2000). Thus treatment with IGF-1/IGFBP-3 complex seems to be a promising approach to improve whole-body glucose uptake and glucose tolerance, while increasing hepatic glucose production (Congote, 2005; Rao et al., 2010).

1.4 Structural studies of IGFBP-IGF interactions for developing potent therapeutics

In order to improve the efficacy of treatment involving the administration of IGF-1/IGFBP-3 complex discussed above, it is important to understand the structural aspects of IGF-IGFBP interactions. Such studies help in enhancing the binding affinity of IGF-1 to IGFBP-3 and also aid in engineering IGFBPs to be protease resistant. We discuss below a thermodynamic approach that we have adopted to study IGF-IGFBP interactions. This brings out the utility of such studies in designing new forms of IGFBPs with enhanced IGF binding affinity thereby serving as potent therapeutics.

1.4.1 Structural characterization of IGFBP-2 and its fragments

While structures of individual domains are known, 3D structures of full-length IGFBPs and/or their complex with IGF-1 have not yet been determined. This has been due to the difficulty in expressing full-length IGFBPs at milligram quantity levels required for X-ray-crystallography or NMR spectroscopy. All IGFBPs contain 16-18 cysteines bridged by disulphide bonds, which makes them difficult to be expressed in bacterial systems. These proteins thus tend to precipitate inside bacterial cells resulting in inclusion bodies. We recently reported the first high-yield expression and structural characterization of functional full-length recombinant human IGFBP-2 (rhIGFBP-2) in *E. Coli* (Swain et al., 2010a). Figure 2 shows the 2D [^{15}N-^{1}H] NMR spectrum of bacterially expressed IGFBP-2. A good dispersion of peaks seen in the spectrum indicates a well-folded conformation of the protein. The secondary structural content estimated based on the NMR spectrum was found to be consistent with those observed in the individual domains.

In cysteine rich proteins, a key requirement is to conserve the pattern of intra-molecular disulphide bonds required for the protein function. Often scrambling (mis-pairing) of disulphide bonds result during purification resulting in heterogeneity of conformations. In our study, we employed an efficient denaturing-refolding protocol. This involved first denaturing the protein in presence of the a reducing agent such as β-mercaptoethanol or DTT followed by slow removal of the denaturing agent and the reducing agent through dialysis resulting in a unique pattern of intra-molecular disulphide bonds. This is evident from the single set of peaks seen in the 2D NMR spectrum shown in Figure 2 (Swain et al., 2010a).

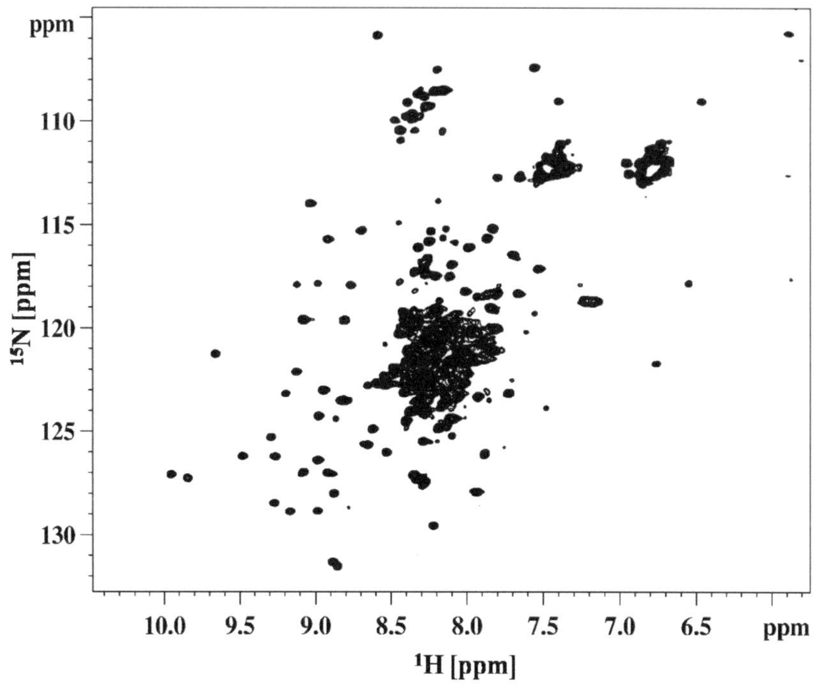

Fig. 2. Two dimensional [^{15}N-^{1}H] HSQC NMR spectrum of full length hIGFBP-2 (33 kDa) which correlates the polypeptide backbone ^{15}N chemical shift with its directly attached ^{1}H. The spectrum was acquired at 288 K at ^{1}H resonance frequency of 700 MHz with a ~1 mM sample concentration. A good dispersion of peaks indicates a well-folded conformation of the protein.

In order to understand the mechanistic aspects of IGF-IGFBP interactions, we have undertaken the study of different domains and fragments of IGFBP-2. Biochemical studies reveal that removal of 41 residues (249-289) from the C-terminal tail of full-length hIGFBP-2 (hereafter denoted as IGFBP-$2_{249-289}$) significantly increases the rate of IGF dissociation, in turn abolishing the ability of the truncated protein to effectively bind IGF (Kibbey et al., 2006). Wild type IGFBP-2 $_{249-289}$ contains two cysteines. However, due to an artifact of cloning full length IGFBP-2 and subsequently the C-terminal polypeptide IGFBP-$2_{249-289}$, our recombinant species all have an additional cysteine at position 281. This resulted in three cysteines in IGFBP-2 $_{249-289}$ raising the possibility of forming dimers or higher order aggregates. In the presence of reducing agents such as β-mercaptoethanol (which are known to reduce disulphide bonds) the protein remained as a monomer. However, upon removal of β-mercaptoethanol by dialysis and/or ultrafiltration, it was found that the polypeptide self-assembled spontaneously into soluble nanotubes several micrometers long (Swain et al., 2010b) (see Figure 3). These tubular structures were studied using different biophysical techniques such as transmission electron microscopy (TEM), NMR spectroscopy, fluorescence and circular dichroism (CD). The observation that formation/dissociation of such nanotubes is reversible (they exchange between monomeric and polymeric forms in presence/absence of reducing agents) and their high mechanical stability due to covalent interaction between the individual components offers new avenues for designing novel IGFBP-based self-assembling nanotubes for biomedical applications.

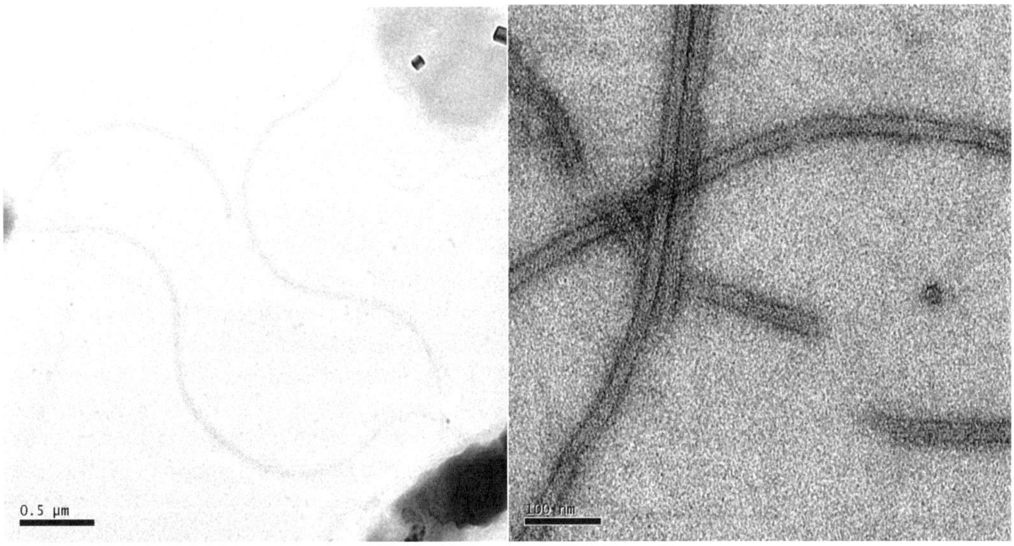

Fig. 3. TEM images of IGFBP-$2_{249-289}$ nanotubes under non-reducing conditions

1.4.2 IGFBP-2 as a biomarker for monitoring disease progression

Bacterial expression of functional full length human IGFBP-2 opens up new avenues to carry out structure-based functional studies in this protein family. One promising application is to generate/engineer antibodies against human IGFBP-2 and use it for detection of IGFBP-2 in HIV/AIDS patients. As mentioned above, it is now established that IGFBP-2 levels are significantly elevated in HIV/AIDS patients (Congote, 2005) and hence IGFBP-2 can be used a bio-marker for diagnosing or tracking the progression of this disease. In recent years, several bio-markers have been proposed or developed for monitoring HIV infection. These include: CD4 count (Smurzynski et al., 2010), TNF-alpha receptor type 2 as a useful serum marker for metabolic dysfunction (Gelato et al., 2002), fibroblast growth factor-21 (FGF21) (Domingo et al., 2010), levels of iron bound and iron-related proteins in urine to identify HIV-infected children at risk of developing HIVAN and HIV-HUS (Soler-Garcia et al., 2009), plasma levels of high sensitivity C reactive protein (hsCRP), interleukin-6 (IL-6), intercellular adhesion molecule-1 (ICAM-1) (Padilla et al., 2011), vascular cell adhesion molecule-1 (sVCAM-1) and plasminogen activator inhibitor-1 (PAI-1) (Padilla et al., 2011). Elements of the IGF system have also been found to be promising bio-markers. However, the detection of proteins by antibodies is the most efficient and sensitive method. This will serve to detect/monitor variations in IGFBP-2 levels in patients with HIV/AIDS. Further, once the structural details of IGFBP2-IGFBP-2 antibody interactions are defined, the antibodies can be engineered to have tight binding to IGFBP-2 which in turn will enhance the sensitivity of IGFBP-2 detection.

1.4.3 Structural features of IGF-IGFBP interactions

Structural studies of individual domains of the IGFBPs in free and complexed form with IGF-1 has provided considerable insights into their interactions (Kalus et al., 1998; Kibbey et al., 2006; Kuang et al., 2006; Sala et al., 2005; Sitar et al., 2006; Siwanowicz et al., 2005). As mentioned above, IGFBPs contain three structural domains of nearly equal size (these are denoted as N-terminal, middle or L-domain and C-terminal domains, respectively). It is now established that both N- and C-domains in IGFBPs are involved in binding IGF-1 with the central domain structurally disordered. High-resolution 3D structures are available for the following IGFBP domains in uncomplexed form: (i) N-terminal domain of IGFBP-1, (ii) C-terminal domain of IGFBP-2, (iii) N-terminal domain of IGFBP-5 and (iv) C-terminal domain of IGFBP-6. In IGF-bound form, structures are available for N-terminal domain of IGFBP-4 and -5 and C-terminal domain of IGFBP-1.

The relative affinities of IGFs vary for the different IGFBPs with IGFBP-1,3,4 having higher affinities for IGF-1 compared to IGF-2 and vice-versa for IGFBP-2,5,6 (Kiefer et al., 1992; Roghani et al., 1991). The salient features of these structural interactions are: (i) the individual domains of different IGFBPs are similar in structure with root mean square deviation (RMSD) < 2-3 Å; (ii) the structures of N- and C-domains of IGFBPs in free and in complex with IGFs are similar indicating that the domains do no undergo a significant conformational change upon binding; (iii) there is a cooperativity between the N- and C-domains of IGFBPs in binding IGF (Kuang et al., 2007). That is, binding of IGF-1 to one of the domains enhances its binding to the other domain. This is presumably due to conformation change or stabilization of IGF-1 upon binding to one domain, which renders its conformation suitable for binding the other domain; (iv) the individual domains bind IGFs with much lower affinity than the full-length protein; (v) the IGF-receptor binding sites of IGFs are masked upon binding IGFBPs. This explains why IGFs do not bind the receptor in IGFBP bound form; (vi) upon binding IGFBP the structurally flexible or disordered regions of IGFs are stabilized. Figure 4 illustrates the mode of IGF binding to IGFBP along with structures of N- and C-domains of IGFBP-5 and IGFBP-1, respectively, in complexed and uncomplexed forms.

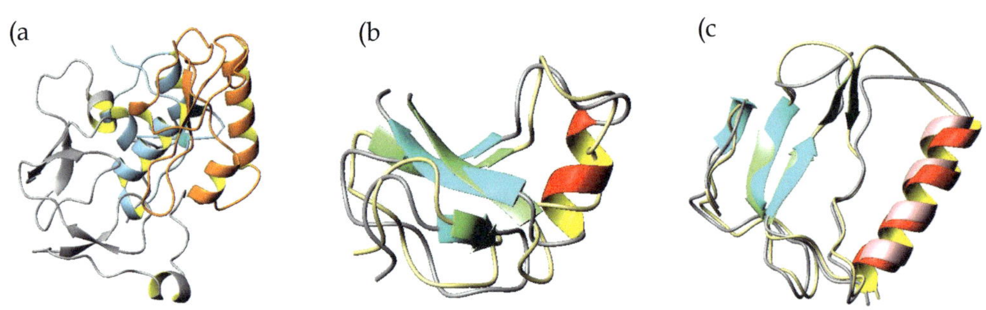

Fig. 4. Three-dimensional structures of IGFBPs in complexed and uncomplexed forms. (a) A ternary complex consisting of the N-domain of IGFBP-4 (orange), C-domain of IGFBP-4 (grey) bound to IGF-1 (light blue). The two domains clasp IGF-1 binding it tightly and blocking its interaction with IGF-1 receptor. (b) Superimposition of 3D the structures of the N-terminal domain of IGFBP-5 in complex and uncomplexed form (RMSD = 1.9Å) and (c) Superimposition of the 3D structures of the C-terminal domain of IGFBP-1 in complex and uncomplexed form (RMSD = 1.3 Å). The low RMSD values indicate that the conformation of IGFBPs do not change significantly upon binding IGF-1.

1.4.4 Improving IGF-IGFBP interaction

One of the goals of our work is to engineer IGFBPs in order to improve their IGF binding affinity. This will be useful in therapeutics discussed above, which involves the administration of IGF-IGFBP complex rather than free IGF-1 alone. Towards this end, we have carried out structure-based thermodynamic studies of IGFBP in complex with IGF-1 to evaluate the extent of change in stability of the protein complex upon mutation of key residues in IGFBP. The residues chosen were those that have been verified experimentally to be involved in binding IGFs. A large body of work has been carried out in the past wherein different site-specific mutants, deletion mutants and/or truncated forms of the IGFBPs have been tested for their IGF-1 binding activities (Clemmons, 2001). Many of these residues are known to be conserved across all six IGFBPs. With this information in hand, our objective is to map on the 3D structures of IGFBP mutations that are known to destabilize IGF-IGFBP interactions.

In recent years, computational methods have been proposed to design specific mutants with enhanced ligand binding affinity (Sammond et al., 2007). These are structure-based methods that systematically predict single mutations at protein-protein interfaces which enhance binding affinities. This is based on the hypothesis that increasing the buried hydrophobic surface area or reducing buried hydrophilic surface area leads to enhanced affinity if steric clashes are avoided and all polar groups buried in the core of the protein have a hydrogen bond partner. In the 3D structures of IGFBPs in complex with IGF-1, we mutated residues, which are known to be involved in binding IGF-1, and evaluated the resulting change in thermodynamic stability (via free-energy change). We observed that mutation of residues important for binding IGF-1 increases the free energy of the complex resulting in the de-stabilization and weakening of IGF-IGFBP interaction. This implies that thermodynamic stability of the IGF-IGFBP complex can be used as an indicator of IGF-1 binding affinity. The study was carried out in 3 stages: first, the change in free energy of the IGF-IGFBP complex upon mutation of residues in IGFBP was predicted. This was carried out using the program I-MUTANT (Capriotti et al., 2005). Next, based on these results, the structure of the complex containing residues in IGFBP that resulted in lowering or increasing the stability of the complex was structurally modeled using the software ROSETTA-DOCK (Lyskov & Gray, 2008). Finally, the modeled structures were subjected to energy minimization followed by 10 ns MD simulations using the program GROMACS (Van der Spoel et al., 2005). In order to understand the structural basis of increased or decreased thermodynamic stability of the IGF-IGFBP complex, the hydrophobic and polar surface areas accessible were evaluated using the program NACCSESS (Hubbard et al.,1993). Two protein complexes of IGFBP with IGF-1 and two uncomplexed forms of the same protein were used for the analysis namely, IGFBP5 N- terminal and IGFBP1 C-terminal having PDB ID 1H59, 1BOE (representing the complexed form) and 2DSQ, 1ZT3 (representing the uncomplexed form), respectively. These two proteins were chosen due to the fact that high-resolution structures of IGF-bound and unbound forms are currently only available for these proteins.

1.4.4.1 Energy calculations

Using I-MUTANT 2.0, each residue within the predicted binding sites and conserved regions of N- and C-domain of IGFBP-4 and IGFBP-1, respectively, was mutated to the 19 other possible amino acids at that position and the change in free energy for each mutation was identified based on the ΔΔG value (defined below) predicted by the software. Based on this, 5 residues from the N-domain of IGFBP5 and 2 residues from the IGFBP1 that gave the highest number of stable predictions among all the 19 possible substitutions were identified. The free energy calculations were done as follows:

$$\text{Overall}\Delta\Delta G\,(\text{mutation}) = [\Delta\Delta G\,(\text{mutation})]_{complex} - [\Delta\Delta G\,(\text{mutation})]_{uncomplexed}$$

ΔΔG (mutation) is in general the free energy change of a given structure (complexed or uncomplexed) upon mutation of a given residue. The value of ΔΔG (mutation) either in complex or uncomplexed form (indicated in the subscript above) was obtained from I-MUTANT 2.0 by specifying the desired residue to be mutated. Thus, the overall ΔΔG (mutation) for a desired mutation depends on the free energies of both complexed and uncomplexed forms. A positive value of the overall ΔΔG (mutation) indicates that the particular mutation stabilizes the complex, whereas a negative value for the overall ΔΔG (mutation) indicates de-stabilization.

Figure 5 shows an example of two mutations (one in the N-domain of IGFBP-5 and the second in the C-domain of IGFBP-1), which show de-stabilization upon mutation to any of the other 19 amino acids. This indicates that these residues are very important for binding and mutation of these residues lowers IGF-binding affinity. The lowering of binding strengths upon mutation of these residues has been verified experimentally in the past. For instance L-70 was mutated to Glu in one study (Imai et al., 2000) and C226 was mutated to Tyr in another study (Brinkman et al., 1991). Since cysteines are highly conserved across IGFBPs and are involved in extensive intra-molecular disulphide bonds, their mutation to any other amino acid causes a reduction of IGF-1 binding. This is corroborated by the thermodynamics analysis presented here.

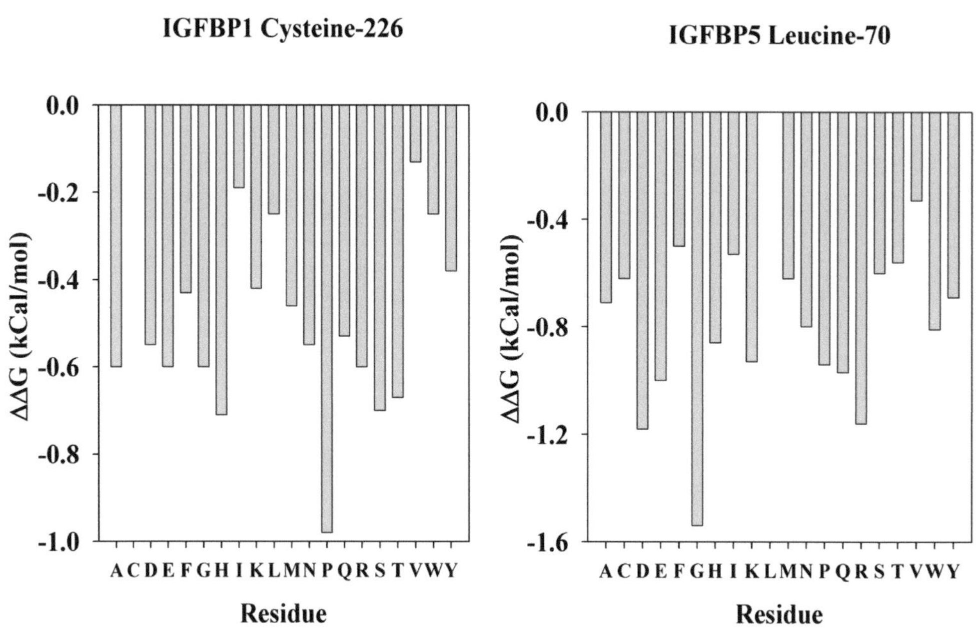

Fig. 5. Thermodynamic analysis of mutations in IGFBP which cause de-stabilization or weakening of the IGF-IGFBP complex. The ΔΔG (mutation) values (defined above) are shown for two residues: L-70 of IGFBP-5 and C-226 of IGFBP-5 which are highly conserved across all IGFBPs and involved in binding IGF-1. Their mutation to any of the other 19 amino acid types results in de-stabilization of the interaction of IGFBP with IGF-1. Thus, these residues are important for binding IGF-1.

Figure 6 illustrates mutation of residue G-57 of the N-domain of IGFBP-5, resulting in enhancement of binding with IGF. Thus, if carried out this mutation will strengthen the IGF-IGFBP complex.

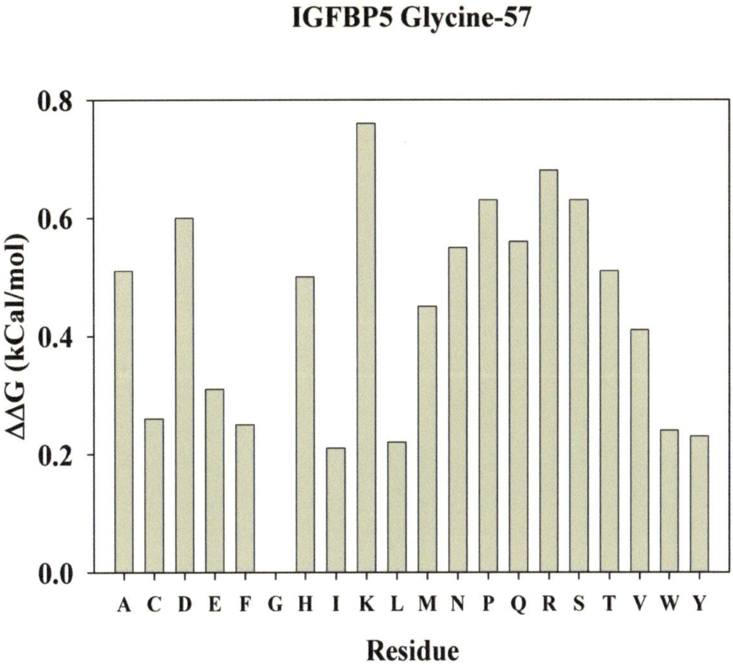

Fig. 6. Thermodynamic analysis of mutations in IGFBP which enhance IGF-IGFBP interactions. The ΔΔG (mutation) values (defined above) are shown for G57 of IGFBP-5. Its mutation to several of the other 19 amino acid types results in increased stabilization of the IGF-IGFBP complex.

1.4.4.2 Structural basis for increase/decrease IGF-binding affinity in mutant IGFBP

In order to understand the structural basis of our findings above, the structure of IGF-IGFBP complex containing the mutations (L70Q and G57K) were constructed using ROSETTA-DOCK software and subjected to energy minimization and MD simulations. The solvent accessible areas of hydrophobic residues at the interface were then evaluated as follows:

$$\begin{aligned}&\text{Exposed hydrophobic surface area at interface}\\&=\left[\text{Exposed hydrophobic surface area of IGF}-1\right]+\\&\left[\text{Exposed hydrophobic surface area of IGFBP}\right]-\\&\left[\text{Exposed hydrophobic surface area of IGF}-\text{IGFBP Complex}\right]\end{aligned}$$

In general, a large exposure of hydrophobic surface area in the binding interface of two proteins (that is, an increase in solvent accessibility of non-polar residues) is known to result in destabilization of protein interactions (Jones et al., 2008; Sammond et al., 2007; Vallone et al., 1998). On the other hand, decreases in hydrophobic surface area at the binding interface upon mutation indicates that the complex formed is more stable than the wild type. Figure 7 shows the result of analyzing the solvent accessible areas of the two mutations described above.

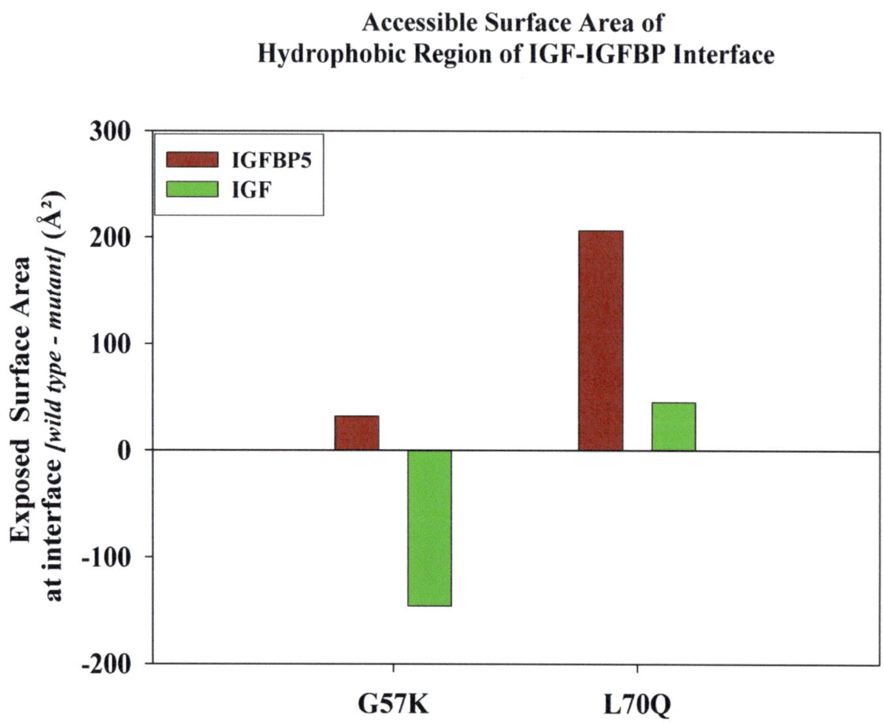

Fig. 7. The change in hydrophobic surface area of the IGF-IGFBP-5 interfaces upon mutation. G57K is a stabilizing mutation for the IGF-IGFBP-5 complex due to a large decrease in non-polar surface area at the interface for IGF-1. On the other hand, the L70Q mutation renders the IGF-IGFBP complex unstable due to a large exposure of hydrophobic surface area in IGFBP-5.

In the case of L70Q mutation, the exposed hydrophobic surface areas of both IGFBP-5 and IGF-1 are increased at the interface. This together results in weakening of the complex and hence the IGF-binding affinity of IGFBP-5 is reduced. In the case of G57K, the exposed surface area of IGF-1 at the interface is reduced considerably while that of IGFBP-5 increases slightly. Significantly, the overall change in surface areas is favorable for enhanced binding of IGF-1 with IGFBP-5. This underscores the importance of thermodynamic studies in evaluating ligand binding affinities in this class of proteins.

2. Conclusion

AIDS is a debilitating disease with more than 25 million people having succumbed since the start of the epidimic. In order to combat this disease, multiple approaches have been proposed and needs to be taken. New findings related to diagnosis and disease progression continue to emerge. A key finding in the past decade, which is now well established, is the involvement of the hormonal peptides IGF-1 and IGF-2 and the IGF-binding proteins in various stages of the disease with different manifestations. The IGF system in general has been extensively studied in this context. While the system is complex in nature with many different proteins interacting to form a regulatory network, the key players have been the IGFs themselves and their binding proteins, the IGFBPs. The recent finding that administration of IGF-1: IGFBP-3 complexes improves whole body glucose uptake is a promising step towards treatment of HIV-associated wasting. In this context, it is important to understand the structural basis of IGF-IGFBP interactions in general, which has been elusive due to the difficulty in producing functional human IGFBPs in large quantities. In our laboratory, we have been successful for the first time in producing bacterially expressed human IGFBP-2 in soluble, functional and monomeric form. This opens up new avenues to study IGF-IGFBP interactions at the atomic level. Further, human IGFBP-2 antibodies can now be generated and used for detection of IGFBP-2 in HIV patients. High-resolution structural studies of IGF in complex with IGFBP will help us to design improved IGFBP species with improve interactions and enhanced binding affinity. All six IGFBPs in the human body are similar in nature as far as their interaction with IGF is concerned. Thus, findings from one IGFBP may be extended to other IGFBPs as well. The available structures of individual domains of IGFBPs are thus very helpful and will aid in future unraveling in detail, of the modes of the interaction of the full length proteins with the IGFs. Efforts are underway in this direction in our laboratory. While much work still needs to be done, the light at the end of tunnel is getting brighter.

3. Acknowledgements

The facilities provided by NMR Research Centre at IISc supported by Department of Science and Technology (DST), India is gratefully acknowledged. HSA acknowledges support from DST-SERC research award. MS acknowledges fellowship from Council of Scientific and Industrial Research (CSIR) This project is in collaboration with Prof. S. A. Rosenzweig, Medical University of South Carolina, USA and Prof. P. Kondaiah, MRDG, Indian Institute of Science, Bangalore.

4. References

Brinkman, A.; Kortleve, D. J.; Zwarthoff, E. C. & Drop, S. L. S. (1991). Mutations in the c-terminal part of insulin-like growth factor (IGF)-binding protein-1 result in dimer formation and loss of IGF binding capacity. *Molecular Endocrinology,* Vol. 5, pp. 987-994, ISSN 0888-8809

Bunn, R. C. & Fowlkes, J. L. (2003). Insulin-like growth factor binding protein proteolysis. *Trends in Endocrinology and Metabolism,* Vol. 14, pp. 176-181, ISSN 1043-2760

Capriotti, E.; Fariselli, P. & Casadio, R. (2005). I-Mutant2.0: predicting stability changes upon mutation from the protein sequence or structure. *Nucleic Acids Research,* Vol. 33, pp. W306-W310, ISSN 0305-1048

Chan, J. M.; Stampfer, M. J.; Giovannucci, E.; Gann, P. H.; Ma, J.; Wilkinson, P.; Hennekens, C. H. & Pollak, M. (1998). Plasma insulin-like growth factor I and prostate cancer risk: A prospective study. *Science,* Vol. 279, pp. 563-566, ISSN 0036-8075

Chantry, C. J.; Hughes, M. D.; Alvero, C.; Cervia, J. S.; Hodge, J.; Borum, P.; Moye, J. & Team, P. (2008). Insulin-like growth factor-1 and lean body mass in HIV-infected children. *Jaids-Journal of Acquired Immune Deficiency Syndromes,* Vol. 48, pp. 437-443, ISSN 1525-4135

Clemmons, D. R. (2001). Use of mutagenesis to probe IGF-binding protein structure/function relationships. *Endocrine Reviews,* Vol. 22, pp. 800-817, ISSN 0163-769X

Congote, L. F. (2005). Monitoring insulin-like growth factors in HIV infection and AIDS. *Clinica Chimica Acta,* Vol. 361, pp. 30-53, ISSN 0009-8981

Domingo, P.; Gallego-Escuredo, J. M.; Domingo, J. C.; Gutierrez, M. D.; Mateo, M. G.; Fernandez, I.; Vidal, F.; Giralt, M. & Villarroya, F. (2010). Serum FGF21 levels are elevated in association with lipodystrophy, insulin resistance and biomarkers of liver injury in HIV-1-infected patients. *Aids,* Vol. 24, pp. 2629-2637, ISSN 0269-9370

Dudgeon, W. D.; Phillips, K. D.; Carson, J. A.; Brewer, R. B.; Durstine, J. L. & Hand, G. A. (2006). Counteracting muscle wasting in HIV-infected individuals. *Hiv Medicine,* Vol. 7, pp. 299-310, ISSN 1464-2662

Firth, S. M. & Baxter, R. C. (2002). Cellular actions of the insulin-like growth factor binding proteins. *Endocrine Reviews,* Vol. 23, pp. 824-854, ISSN 0163-769X

Frost, R. A.; Fuhrer, J.; Steigbigel, R.; Mariuz, P.; Lang, C. H. & Gelato, M. C. (1996). Wasting in the acquired immune deficiency syndrome is associated with multiple defects in the serum insulin-like growth factor system. *Clinical Endocrinology,* Vol. 44, pp. 501-514, ISSN 0300-0664

Gelato, M. C. & Frost, R. A. (1997). IGFBP-3 - Functional and structural implications in aging and wasting syndromes. *Endocrine,* Vol. 7, pp. 81-85, ISSN 0969-711X

Gelato, M. C.; Mynarcik, D. & McNurlan, M. A. (2002). Soluble tumour necrosis factor alpha receptor 2, a serum marker of resistance to the anabolic actions of growth hormone in subjects with HIV disease. *Clinical Science,* Vol. 102, pp. 85-90, ISSN 0143-5221

Grunfeld, C.; Thompson, M.; Brown, S. J.; Richmond, G.; Lee, D.; Muurahainen, N. & Kotler, D. P. (2007). Recombinant human growth hormone to treat HIV-associated adipose redistribution syndrome - 12-Week induction and 24-week maintenance therapy. *Jaids-Journal of Acquired Immune Deficiency Syndromes,* Vol. 45, pp. 286-297, ISSN 1525-4135

Hambrecht, R.; Schulze, P. C.; Gielen, S.; Linke, A.; Mobius-Winkler, S.; Yu, J. T.; Kratzsch, J.; Baldauf, G.; Busse, M. W.; Schubert, A.; Adams, V. & Schuler, G. (2002). Reduction of insulin-like growth factor-1 expression in the skeletal muscle of noncachectic patients with chronic heart failure. *Journal of the American College of Cardiology,* Vol. 39, pp. 1175-1181, ISSN 0735-1097

Harrison, L. E.; Blumberg, D.; Berman, R.; Ng, B.; Hochwald, S.; Brennan, M. F. & Burt, M. (1996). Effect of human growth hormone on human pancreatic carcinoma growth, protein, and cell cycle kinetics. *Journal of Surgical Research,* Vol. 61, pp. 317-322, ISSN 0022-4804

Helle, S. I.; Ueland, T.; Ekse, D.; Froland, S. S.; Holly, J. M. P.; Lonning, P. E. & Aukrust, P. (2001). The insulin-like growth factor system in human immunodeficiency virus infection: Relations to immunological parameters, disease progression, and antiretroviral therapy. *Journal of Clinical Endocrinology & Metabolism,* Vol. 86, pp. 227-233, ISSN 0021-972X

Hubbard, S. J. & Thoronton, J. M. (1993). Computer program, Department of Biochemistry and Molecular biology, University College London

Imai, Y.; Moralez, A.; Andag, U.; Clarke, J. B.; Busby, W. H. & Clemmons, D. R. (2000). Substitutions for hydrophobic amino acids in the N-terminal domains of IGFBP-3 and-5 markedly reduce IGF-I binding and alter their biologic actions. *Journal of Biological Chemistry,* Vol. 275, pp. 18188-18194, ISSN 0021-9258

Jones, D. S.; Silverman, A. P. & Cochran, J. R. (2008). Developing therapeutic proteins by engineering ligand-receptor interactions. *Trends in Biotechnology,* Vol. 26, pp. 498-505, ISSN 0167-7799

Kalus, W.; Zweckstetter, M.; Renner, C.; Sanchez, Y.; Georgescu, J.; Grol, M.; Demuth, D.; Schumacher, R.; Dony, C.; Lang, K. & Holak, T. A. (1998). Structure of the IGF-binding domain of the insulin-like growth factor-binding protein-5 (IGFBP-5): Implications for IGF and IGF-I receptor interactions. *EMBO Journal,* Vol. 17, pp. 6558-6572, ISSN 0261-4189

Kibbey, M. M.; Jameson, M. J.; Eaton, E. M. & Rosenzweig, S. A. (2006). Insulin-like growth factor binding protein-2: Contributions of the C-terminal domain to insulin-like growth factor-1 binding. *Molecular Pharmacology,* Vol. 69, pp. 833-845, ISSN 0026-895X

Kiefer, M. C.; Schmid, C.; Waldvogel, M.; Schlapfer, I.; Futo, E.; Masiarz, F. R.; Green, K.; Barr, P. J. & Zapf, J. (1992). Characterization of recombinant human insulin-like growth factor binding protein-4, protein-5, and protein-6 produced in yeast. *Journal of Biological Chemistry,* Vol. 267, pp. 12692-12699, ISSN 0021-9258

Krywicki, R. F. & Yee, D. (1992). The insulin-like growth factor family of ligands, receptors, and binding-proteins. *Breast Cancer Research and Treatment,* Vol. 22, pp. 7-19, ISSN 0167-6806

Kuang, Z. H.; Yao, S. G.; Keizer, D. W.; Wang, C. C.; Bach, L. A.; Forbes, B. E.; Wallace, J. C. & Norton, R. S. (2006). Structure, dynamics and heparin binding of the C-terminal domain of insulin-like growth factor-binding protein-2 (IGFBP-2). *Journal of Molecular Biology,* Vol. 364, pp. 690-704, ISSN 0022-2836

Kuang, Z. H.; Yao, S. G.; McNeil, K. A.; Thompson, J. A.; Bach, L. A.; Forbes, B. E.; Wallace, J. C. & Norton, R. S. (2007). Cooperativity of the N- and C-terminal domains of insulin-like growth factor (IGF) binding protein 2 in IGF binding. *Biochemistry,* Vol. 46, pp. 13720-13732, ISSN 0006-2960

Lee, P. D. K.; Pivarnik, J. M.; Bukar, J. G.; Muurahainen, N.; Berry, P. S.; Skolnik, P. R.; Nerad, J. L.; Kudsk, K. A.; Jackson, L.; Ellis, K. J. & Gesundheit, N. (1996). A randomized, placebo-controlled trial of combined insulin-like growth factor I and low dose growth hormone therapy for wasting associated with human immunodeficiency virus infection. *Journal of Clinical Endocrinology & Metabolism,* Vol. 81, pp. 2968-2975, ISSN 0021-972X

LeRoith, D. & Roberts, C. T. (2003). The insulin-like growth factor system and cancer. *Cancer Letters,* Vol. 195, pp. 127-137, ISSN 0304-3835

Lieberman, S. A.; Butterfield, G. E.; Harrison, D. & Hoffman, A. R. (1994). Anabolic effects of recombinant insulin-like growth factor-1 in cachexia patients with the acquired-immunodeficiency-syndrome. *Journal of Clinical Endocrinology & Metabolism,* Vol. 78, pp. 404-410, ISSN 0021-972X

Lyskov, S. & Gray, J. J. (2008). The RosettaDock server for local proteinprotein docking. *Nucleic Acids Research,* Vol. 36, pp. W233-W238, ISSN 0305-1048

Ma, J.; Pollak, M. N.; Giovannucci, E.; Chan, J. M.; Tao, Y. Z.; Hennekens, C. H. & Stampfer, M. J. (1999). Prospective study of colorectal cancer risk in men and plasma levels of insulin-like growth factor (IGF)-I and IGF-binding protein-3. *Journal of the National Cancer Institute,* Vol. 91, pp. 620-625, ISSN 0027-8874

Meininger, G. & Grinspoon, S. (2001). Regulation of the growth hormone/insulin-like growth factor-I axis in HIV disease. *Endocrinologist,* Vol. 11, pp. 188-195, ISSN 1051-2144

Miyamoto, S.; Yano, K.; Sugimoto, S.; Ishii, G.; Hasebe, T.; Endoh, Y.; Kodama, K.; Goya, M.; Chiba, T. & Ochiai, A. (2004). Matrix metalloproteinase-7 facilitates insulin-like growth factor bioavailability through its proteinase activity on insulin-like growth factor binding protein 3. *Cancer Research,* Vol. 64, pp. 665-671, ISSN 0008-5472

Mulligan, K. & Schambelan, M. (2002). Anabolic treatment with GH, IGF-I, or anabolic steroids in patients with HIV-associated wasting. *International Journal of Cardiology,* Vol. 85, pp. 151-159, ISSN 0167-5273

Mynarcik, D. C.; Frost, R. A.; Lang, C. H.; DeCristofaro, K.; McNurlan, M. A.; Garlick, P. J.; Steigbigel, R. T.; Fuhrer, J.; Ahnn, S. & Gelato, M. C. (1999). Insulin-like growth factor system in patients with HIV infection: Effect of exogenous growth hormone administration. *Journal of Acquired Immune Deficiency Syndromes,* Vol. 22, pp. 49-55, ISSN 1077-9450

Nguyen, B. Y.; Clerici, M.; Venzon, D. J.; Bauza, S.; Murphy, W. J.; Longo, D. L.; Baseler, M.; Gesundheit, N.; Broder, S.; Shearer, G. & Yarchoan, R. (1998). Pilot study of the immunologic effects of recombinant human growth hormone and recombinant insulin-like growth factor in HIV-infected patients. *Aids,* Vol. 12, pp. 895-904, ISSN 0269-9370

Padilla, S.; Masia, M.; Garcia, N.; Jarrin, I.; Tormo, C. & Gutierrez, F. (2011). Early changes in inflammatory and pro-thrombotic biomarkers in patients initiating antiretroviral therapy with abacavir or tenofovir. *Bmc Infectious Diseases,* Vol. 11, pp. ISSN 1471-2334

Rao, M. N.; Mulligan, K.; Tai, V.; Wen, M. J.; Dyachenko, A.; Weinberg, M.; Li, X. J.; Lang, T.; Grunfeld, C.; Schwarz, J. M. & Schambelan, M. (2010). Effects of Insulin-Like Growth Factor (IGF)-I/IGF-Binding Protein-3 Treatment on Glucose Metabolism and Fat Distribution in Human Immunodeficiency Virus-Infected Patients with Abdominal Obesity and Insulin Resistance. *Journal of Clinical Endocrinology & Metabolism,* Vol. 95, pp. 4361-4366, ISSN 0021-972X

Roghani, M.; Lassarre, C.; Zapf, J.; Povoa, G. & Binoux, M. (1991). 2 Insulin-like growth-factor (IGF)-binding proteins are responsible for the selective affinity for IGF-II if cerebrospinal-fluid binding-protein. *Journal of Clinical Endocrinology & Metabolism,* Vol. 73, pp. 658-666, ISSN 0021-972X

Rosenzweig, S. A. (2004). What's new in the IGF-binding proteins? *Growth Hormone & Igf Research,* Vol. 14, pp. 329-336, ISSN 1096-6374

Rosenzweig, S. A. & Atreya, H. S. (2010). Defining the pathway to insulin-like growth factor system targeting in cancer. *Biochemical Pharmacology,* Vol. 80, pp. 1115-1124, ISSN 0006-2952

Sala, A.; Capaldi, S.; Campagnoli, M.; Faggion, B.; Labo, S.; Perduca, M.; Romano, A.; Carrizo, M. E.; Valli, M.; Visai, L.; Minchiotti, L.; Galliano, M. & Monaco, H. L. (2005). Structure and properties of the C-terminal domain of insulin-like growth factor-binding protein-1 isolated from human amniotic fluid. *Journal of Biological Chemistry,* Vol. 280, pp. 29812-29819, ISSN 0021-9258

Sammond, D. W.; Eletr, Z. M.; Purbeck, C.; Kimple, R. J.; Siderovski, D. P. & Kuhlman, B. (2007). Structure-based protocol for identifying mutations that enhance protein-protein binding affinities. *Journal of Molecular Biology,* Vol. 371, pp. 1392-1404, ISSN 0022-2836

Sitar, T.; Popowicz, G. M.; Siwanowicz, I.; Huber, R. & Holak, T. A. (2006). Structural basis for the inhibition of insulin-like growth factors by insulin-like growth factor-binding proteins. *Proceedings of the National Academy of Sciences of the United States of America,* Vol. 103, pp. 13028-13033, ISSN 0027-8424

Siwanowicz, I.; Popowicz, G. M.; Wisniewska, M.; Huber, R.; Kuenkele, K. P.; Lang, K.; Engh, R. A. & Holak, T. A. (2005). Structural basis for the regulation of insulin-like growth factors by IGF binding proteins. *Structure,* Vol. 13, pp. 155-167, ISSN 0969-2126

Smurzynski, M.; Wu, K. L.; Benson, C. A.; Bosch, R. J.; Collier, A. C. & Koletar, S. L. (2010). Relationship Between CD4(+) T-Cell Counts/HIV-1 RNA Plasma Viral Load and AIDS-Defining Events Among Persons Followed in the ACTG Longitudinal Linked Randomized Trials Study. *Jaids-Journal of Acquired Immune Deficiency Syndromes,* Vol. 55, pp. 117-127, ISSN 1525-4135

Soler-Garcia, A. A.; Johnson, D.; Hathout, Y. & Ray, P. E. (2009). Iron-Related Proteins: Candidate Urine Biomarkers in Childhood HIV-Associated Renal Diseases. *Clinical Journal of the American Society of Nephrology,* Vol. 4, pp. 763-771, ISSN 1555-9041

Spinola-Castro, A. M.; Siviero-Miachon, A. A.; Da Silva, M. T. N. & Guerra-Junior, G. (2008). The use of growth hormone to treat endocrine-metabolic disturbances in Acquired Immunodeficiency Syndrome (Aids) patients. *Arquivos Brasileiros De Endocrinologia E Metabologia,* Vol. 52, pp. 818-832, ISSN 0004-2730

Stagi, S.; Bindi, G.; Galluzzi, F.; Galli, L.; Salti, R. & de Martino, M. (2004). Changed bone status in human immunodeficiency virus type 1 (HIV-1) perinatally infected children is related to low serum free IGF-1. *Clinical Endocrinology,* Vol. 61, pp. 692-699, ISSN 0300-0664

Swain, M.; Slomiany, M. G.; Rosenzweig, S. A. & Atreya, H. S. (2010a). High-yield bacterial expression and structural characterization of recombinant human insulin-like growth factor binding protein-2. *Archives of Biochemistry and Biophysics,* Vol. 501, pp. 195-200, ISSN 0003-9861

Swain, M.; Thirupathi, R.; Krishnarjuna, B.; Eaton, E. M.; Kibbey, M. M.; Rosenzweig, S. A. & Atreya, H. S. (2010b). Spontaneous and reversible self-assembly of a polypeptide fragment of insulin-like growth factor binding protein-2 into fluorescent nanotubular structures. *Chemical Communications,* Vol. 46, pp. 216-218, ISSN 1359-7345

Vallone, B.; Miele, A. E.; Vecchini, P.; Chiancone, E. & Brunori, M. (1998). Free energy of burying hydrophobic residues in the interface between protein subunits. *Proceedings of the National Academy of Sciences of the United States of America,* Vol. 95, pp. 6103-6107, ISSN 0027-8424

Van der Spoel, D.; Lindahl, E.; Hess, B.; Groenhof, G.; Mark, A. E. & Berendsen, H. J. C. (2005). GROMACS: Fast, flexible, and free. *Journal of Computational Chemistry,* Vol. 26, pp. 1701-1718, ISSN 0192-8651

Wang, W.; Iresjo, B. M.; Karlsson, L. & Svanberg, E. (2000). Provision of rhIGF-I/IGFBP-3 complex attenuated development of cancer cachexia in an experimental tumor model. *Clinical Nutrition,* Vol. 19, pp. 127-132, ISSN 0261-5614

Wu, X. F.; Zhao, H.; Do, K. A.; Johnson, M. M.; Dong, Q.; Hong, W. K. & Spitz, M. R. (2004). Serum levels of insulin growth factor (IGF-I) and IGF-binding protein predict risk of second primary tumors in patients with head and neck cancer. *Clinical Cancer Research,* Vol. 10, pp. 3988-3995, ISSN 1078-0432

Yu, H.; Spitz, M. R.; Mistry, J.; Gu, J.; Hong, W. K. & Wu, X. F. (1999). Plasma levels of insulin-like growth factor-I and lung cancer risk: a case-control analysis. *Journal of the National Cancer Institute,* Vol. 91, pp. 151-156, ISSN 0027-8874

Zdanowicz, M. M. & Teichberg, S. (2003). Effects of insulin-like growth factor-1/binding protein-3 complex on muscle atrophy in rats. *Experimental Biology and Medicine,* Vol. 228, pp. 891-897, ISSN 1535-3702

6

Cellular Restriction Factors: Exploiting the Body's Antiviral Proteins to Combat HIV-1/AIDS

Jenna N. Kelly, Jessica G.K. Tong, Clayton J. Hattlmann,
Matthew W. Woods and Stephen D. Barr
*The University of Western Ontario London,
Canada*

1. Introduction

1.1 Overview of HIV-1/AIDS therapies

In 1983, when researchers first isolated HIV-1 from an AIDS patient, few imagined that it foretold a worldwide pandemic (Broder & Gallo, 1984, Barre-Sinoussi et al., 1983). More than 25 years later, 65 million people have been infected with HIV-1; nearly half of these people have died of AIDS, and despite many scientific advances we are still without an efficacious vaccine (Merson, 2006). The majority of HIV-1 infections and deaths have occurred in developing countries, with sub-Saharan Africa accounting for over 38 million HIV-1 infections alone. Sadly, the number of new infections currently exceeds our ability to treat everyone infected with the virus, and in the hardest-hit countries the social and economic backlash has been profound.

After HIV-1 was isolated, a blood test to screen patients and the blood supply quickly followed, as did research on its structure and pathogenesis. Many assumed that a vaccine would be available in a few years, and excitement increased further with the licensing of the first effective drug against HIV-1, zidovudine (AZT) (Fischl et al., 1987). However, researchers soon discovered that the virus was highly resilient, and HIV-1 quickly developed resistance to AZT (Poli et al., 1989, Richman et al., 1994). Over the next few years, a number of new antiretroviral drugs were developed that attacked the virus in different ways, and it was at this time that a new approach to therapy ensued. Highly active antiretroviral therapy (HAART) combined three or more different drugs to reduce HIV-1 replication, and significantly improved the prognosis of HIV-1-infected individuals (Richman et al., 2009). However, HAART was not a cure, and many patients were resistant to at least one of the antiretroviral drugs. In addition, the drugs were highly toxic, making adherence to treatment difficult.

During this time, the vaccine field was also hard at work, trying to develop a safe and effective HIV-1 vaccine. Most initial vaccine approaches focused on the HIV-1 envelope protein (gp120), and aimed to induce an antibody response to gp120. AIDSVAX was the first vaccine candidate of this type, and was developed by a U.S. pharmaceutical company called VaxGen (Flynn et al., 2005, Pitisuttithum et al., 2006). An alternative approach, developed by Merck, aimed to induce a T-cell response to HIV-1 using a recombinant adenovirus vector expressing HIV-1 Gag, Pol and Nef proteins (Shiver et al., 2002). Unfortunately, results from both of these trials were disappointing, and neither approach provided protection from HIV-1 infection (Buchbinder et al., 2008, McElrath et al., 2008). Moreover, the Merck vaccine actually seemed to suppress the immune response, due to pre-existing immunity to the adenovirus vector (Priddy et al., 2008, Roberts et al., 2006).

The third and largest trial was recently performed in Thailand, and aimed to induce both a T-cell and antibody response to HIV-1. In the study, 16,000 Thai men and women received either placebo or vaccine injections, and were subsequently monitored for HIV-1 infection over a 3 year period (Rerks-Ngarm et al., 2009). The vaccine group received injections of a recombinant canarypox vector vaccine ALVAC-HIV (Sanofi Pasteur), plus booster injections of a recombinant gp120 subunit vaccine AIDSVAX B/E (Global Solutions for Infectious Diseases). Results from this trial showed a modest benefit among vaccine recipients, with a vaccine efficacy of 26-30%. However, vaccination did not affect the levels of viremia or CD4+ T cell counts of infected individuals, and many were disappointed with the results (Rerks-Ngarm et al., 2009).

Over the last decade, several host proteins have been identified that are capable of inhibiting HIV-1 replication (Figure 1). These so-called 'cellular-restriction factors' are a new arm of the innate immune system, and inhibit stages of the HIV-1 lifecycle that are not targeted by current AIDS therapies. Our understanding of how cellular restriction factors target HIV-1 replication is far from compete, but research in this area may provide a new avenue for future AIDS therapies (Barr, 2010).

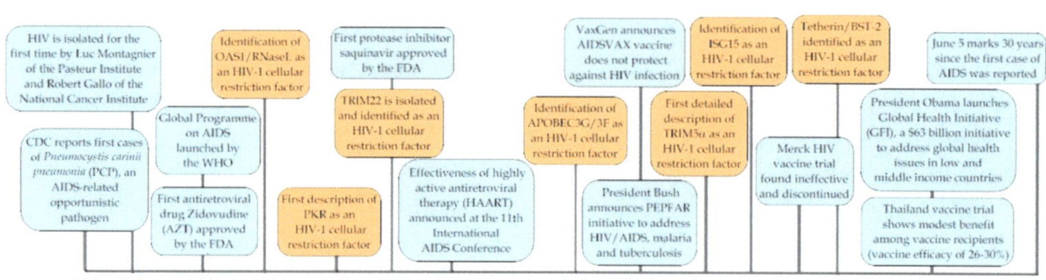

Fig. 1. HIV-1/AIDS timeline. Timeline documenting major events in the HIV-1/AIDS pandemic, as well as the identification of several key HIV-1 cellular restriction factors.

1.2 Cellular restriction factors

Cellular restriction factors are host proteins that can inhibit specific steps in the lifecycle of a virus. The concept of cellular restriction factors first emerged in the 1970's, when researchers identified strains of inbred mice that were resistant to Friend murine leukemia virus (MLV)-induced leukemia (Lilly, 1967, Pincus et al., 1971). Interestingly, these studies showed that mice with certain 'Friend virus susceptibility' (Fv) loci, could inhibit MLV replication *in vitro* and were subsequently resistant to leukemia. The *Fv1* and *Fv4* genes were particularly interesting, and were later shown to encode host proteins that resembled virus components. The *Fv1* gene encoded a protein that was similar to an endogenous retroviral Gag protein, and was shown to inhibit a post-entry stage of MLV replication (Ikeda et al., 1985). In contrast, the *Fv4* gene encoded a protein that resembled *env* (envelope) sequences in a specific strain of MLV, which obstructed binding of wild-type MLV to target cells (Pryciak & Varmus, 1992).

Since these discoveries, several new cellular restriction factors have been identified, including a number of factors that restrict HIV-1 replication (Chakrabarti & Simon, 2010). Many of these restriction factors are up-regulated in response to type I interferons (IFNs), which are typically activated in the presence of viruses by pattern recognition receptors (PRRs), such as Toll-like receptors or retinoic acid induced gene (RIG)-like receptors (Kumagai et al., 2008). Following secretion, type I IFNs bind to the interferon α/β receptor (IFNAR) on the cell surface and induce signalling through the Janus Kinases/Signal Transducers and Activators of Transcription (Jak/Stat) pathway. This leads to the activation of hundreds of IFN-responsive genes that restrict viral replication, including cellular restriction factors (Baum & Garcia-Sastre, 2010) (Figure 2).

Type I IFNs potently inhibit early and late stages of the HIV-1 lifecycle, and systemic administration of IFNα reduces HIV-1 plasma viremia *in vivo* (Meylan et al., 1993, Tavel et al., 2010). During viral infection, plasmacytoid dendritic cells (pDCs) are the main producers of IFNα, however the capacity of pDCs to produce IFNα is impaired during acute HIV-1 infection, and this DC subtype appears to be depleted in chronic HIV-1 infection (Borrow & Bhardwaj, 2008, Soumelis et al., 2001). In addition, the HIV-1 accessory proteins Vpr and Vif can degrade interferon regulatory factor 3 (IRF-3), which plays a critical role in type I IFN induction (Okumura et al., 2008). Since cellular restriction factors are the 'effector' proteins of the IFN response, differences in the ability of pDCs to produce IFNα may contribute to differences in HIV-1 replication and disease progression among patients. Understanding the molecular mechanisms behind these HIV-1 restriction factors, may lead to the development of drugs that mimic or promote their activities.

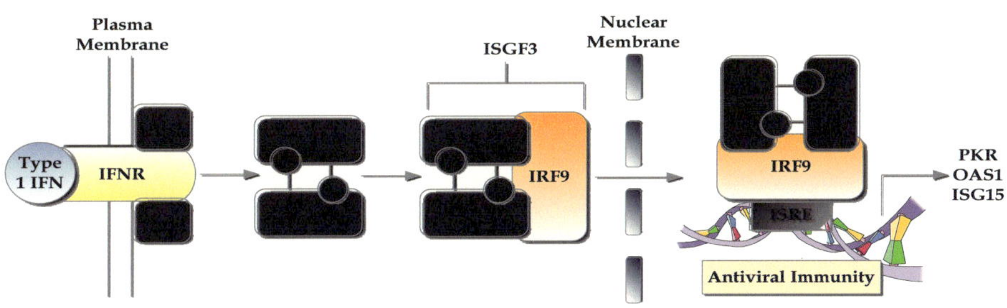

Fig. 2. The interferon response. Interferon (IFN) binds to the interferon receptor at the plasma membrane, activating the Janus Kinases/Signal Transducers and Activators of Transcription (Jak/Stat) pathway. This results in the up-regulation of hundreds of IFN-responsive genes, including cellular restriction factors that prevent HIV-1 replication.

1.3 The HIV-1 lifecycle

The HIV-1 lifecycle offers a multitude of steps that can be targeted by cellular HIV-1 restriction factors (Figure 3). The lifecycle begins when the HIV-1 envelope protein (gp120) binds to the host cell via its CD4 receptor, and following a conformational change, it binds to either the CXCR4 or CCR5 chemokine co-receptor (Deng et al., 1996). This interaction facilitates viral and cell membrane fusion, which is followed by the release of the viral core into the cell cytoplasm. In the cytoplasm, the HIV-1 capsid protein is lost in a process called uncoating, and the single-stranded RNA genome is reverse-transcribed into double-stranded cDNA. Reverse transcription is carried out by the virion-associated reverse transcriptase enzyme, and precedes the formation of the multimeric pre-integration complex. This complex, which consists of both host and viral proteins, is transported along microtubules to the nucleus, where the HIV-1 integrase enzyme facilitates integration of the viral cDNA into the host genome. Following integration, HIV-1 transcription occurs from the 5′ long terminal repeat (LTR) promoter, and leads to the synthesis of spliced HIV-1 RNA and unspliced HIV-1 genomic RNA. The RNA is exported into the cytoplasm where the main structural protein of HIV-1, the Gag polyprotein, is translated along with other viral proteins. The Gag protein oligomerizes and traffics to the cell membrane, where it forms higher-order structures and assembles into virions with other viral proteins. Cellular proteins are also involved in assembly, particularly Tsg101 and AIP1/ALIX, which participate in the budding and release of immature, non-infectious virions from the cell membrane (Garrus et al., 2001, Strack et al., 2003). As budding occurs, the Gag protein is cleaved into its four structural domains (matrix, capsid, nucleocapsid and p6) by the viral protease, generating mature infectious viral particles that are released from the cell membrane (Ganser-Pornillos et al., 2008, Ono, 2009). The following sections review the main HIV-1 cellular restriction factors in the order of their point of attack in the lifecycle, beginning with capsid uncoating and ending with viral release.

2. Lifecycle target: HIV-1 capsid uncoating

2.1 TRIM5α

2.1.1 TRIM5α: History and background

For years, researchers have been aware of a barrier to HIV-1 infection in Old world monkey (OWM) cells, however they have only recently begun to understand the nature of it. Early in the AIDS epidemic, the discovery that the host-range of HIV-1 was limited to humans and apes suggested that other primates may have an internal mechanism to combat HIV-1 infection (Alter et al., 1984, Gajdusek et al., 1985, Lusso et al., 1988). A large number of mammalian cell lines were tested for susceptibility to HIV-1 infection, including cells derived from humans, OWMs (monkeys of African and Asian origin) and New world monkeys (NWM) (monkeys of Central and South American origin) (Hofmann et al., 1999). Interestingly, HIV-1 replication was blocked in most OWM-derived cell lines and one species of NWM, the Owl monkey. Because of its initial definition as a genetic barrier to lentiviral infection, the restriction factor was originally named lentivirus susceptibility factor-1 (Lv-1) (Cowan et al., 2002).

TRIM5α was not identified as the protein responsible for the OWM block until it was isolated during a cDNA screen of HIV-1 resistant rhesus macaque cells. In the study, a cDNA library was created from HIV-1 resistant rhesus macaque cells and the cDNA clones from this library were transduced into an HIV-1 sensitive human cell line (HeLa) (Stremlau et al., 2004). The human cells were then challenged with HIV-1 and screened for resistant clones, which identified the rhesus orthologue of TRIM5α (rhTRIM5α). Excitingly, around the same time, TRIM5α was also linked to the HIV-1 block in Owl monkey cells; however, the Owl monkey version of *TRIM5α* encoded a TRIM5α-cyclophilin A fusion protein (Sayah et al., 2004). Cyclophilin A (CypA) was previously shown to bind to the HIV-1 capsid protein and promote HIV-1 replication in human cells; however, in Owl monkey cells CypA seemed to restrict HIV-1 (Luban, 2007, Sokolskaja & Luban, 2006). The discovery of a TRIM5α-CypA fusion protein explained these results and indicated that CypA may target TRIM5α-CypA to incoming HIV-1 capsid proteins.

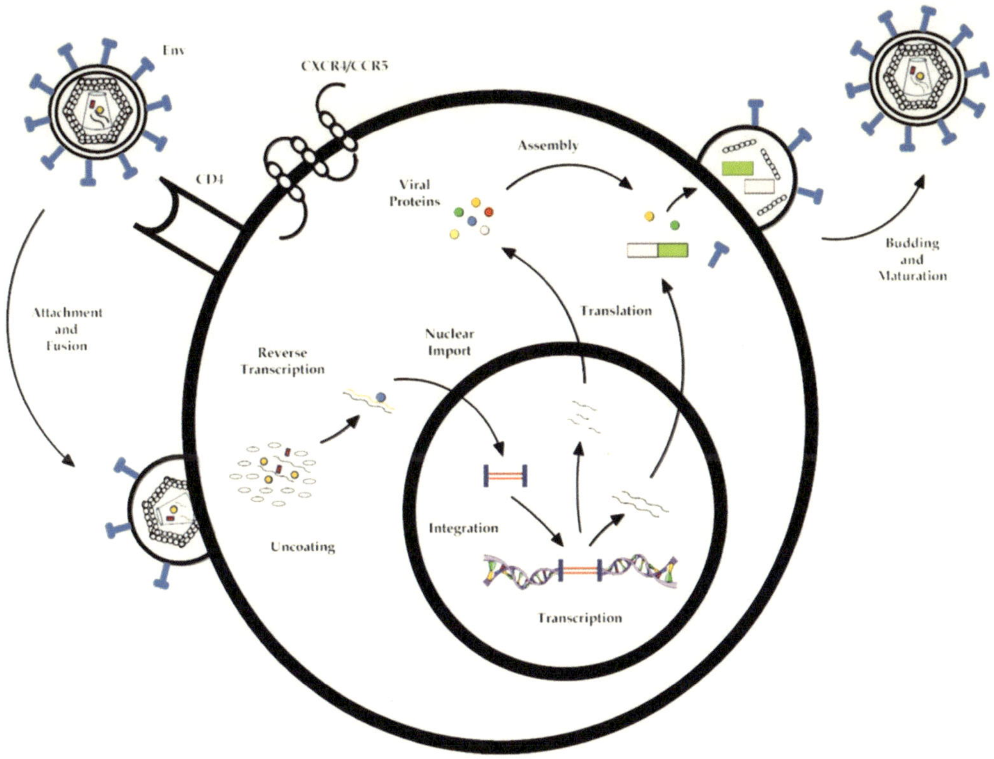

Fig. 3. The HIV-1 lifecycle. The HIV-1 envelope protein (Env) binds to the CD4+ receptor and CXCR4/CCR5 co-receptor on the host cell. The viral core is released into the cytoplasm, where the RNA genome is reverse-transcribed into double-stranded cDNA. The cDNA is imported into the nucleus, where it integrates into the host genome. The viral genes are transcribed and the RNA is exported to the cytoplasm, where it is translated into protein. The viral proteins traffic to the membrane where they assemble and bud out of the host cell.

2.1.2 TRIM5α: Structure and function

TRIM5α belongs to the tripartite motif-containing (TRIM) family of proteins, of which there are currently 77 identified members (Nisole et al., 2005). Although the *TRIM5* gene gives rise to several isoforms through differential splicing, TRIM5α is the only isoform with potent anti-HIV-1 activity. All TRIM proteins have a conserved RBCC motif, which consists of a RING domain, one or two B-box domains and a predicted coiled-coil region. The majority of TRIM proteins, including TRIM5α, have a C-terminal B30.2 domain. The **R**eally **I**nteresting **N**ew **G**ene (RING) domain has intrinsic E3 ligase activity, and together with an E1 activating enzyme and an E2 conjugating enzyme it can transfer ubiquitin or ubiquitin-like molecules to target proteins (Ozato et al., 2008). This modification can alter a protein's half-life, subcellular localization or interaction with other proteins. Importantly, two RING domain cysteine residues (C15 and C18) are essential for the E3 ligase activity of the RING domain (C15 and C18). These two residues are also required by rhTRIM5α for restricting HIV-1 replication (Diaz-Griffero et al., 2006).

The function of the B-box domain remains largely uncharacterized; however, it is an interesting domain because it is unique to TRIM proteins. Deletion of the B-box domain of TRIM5α eliminates the ability of TRIM5α to restrict HIV-1, suggesting that this domain is critical for TRIM5α-mediated restriction (Stremlau et al., 2004, Javanbakht et al., 2005, Li & Sodroski, 2008, Perez-Caballero et al., 2005). In addition, it was recently shown that the B-box domain promotes HIV-1 capsid binding by mediating higher-order self-association (Li & Sodroski, 2008). The coiled-coil region is involved in protein-protein interactions and more specifically, it is thought to mediate TRIM5α oligomer formation. It has been proposed that oligomer formation is important for positioning the B30.2 domain of TRIM5α for optimal HIV-1 capsid binding and accordingly, TRIM5α coiled-coil mutants fail to restrict HIV-1 (Perez-Caballero et al., 2005, Javanbakht et al., 2006). Finally, the specificity and interspecies variability of TRIM5α is found in the B30.2 domain. Sequence analysis has shown a significant amount of interspecies variability within the B30.2 domain of both NWM and OWM, especially on several variable loops that are thought to form the binding surface for HIV-1 capsid recognition (Ohkura et al., 2006, Woo et al., 2006, Yao et al., 2006).

2.1.3 TRIM5α-mediated HIV-1 restriction

To date, rhTRIM5α is the earliest-acting HIV-1 restriction factor and targets virus replication immediately after HIV-1 entry into target cells. Several studies have shown that rhTRIM5α blocks reverse transcription and nuclear import of viral cDNA. The mechanisms underlying this restriction are thought to include: sequestration of the virus core in the cytoplasm, modification of the virus core leading to degradation, or interference in the trafficking of the preintegration complex (Bieniasz, 2004, Chatterji et al., 2006, Stremlau et al., 2006). The most favoured mechanism involves rhTRIM5α binding to the viral core and disrupting the normal uncoating process of the core (Figure 4). This binding involves the recognition of specific sequences

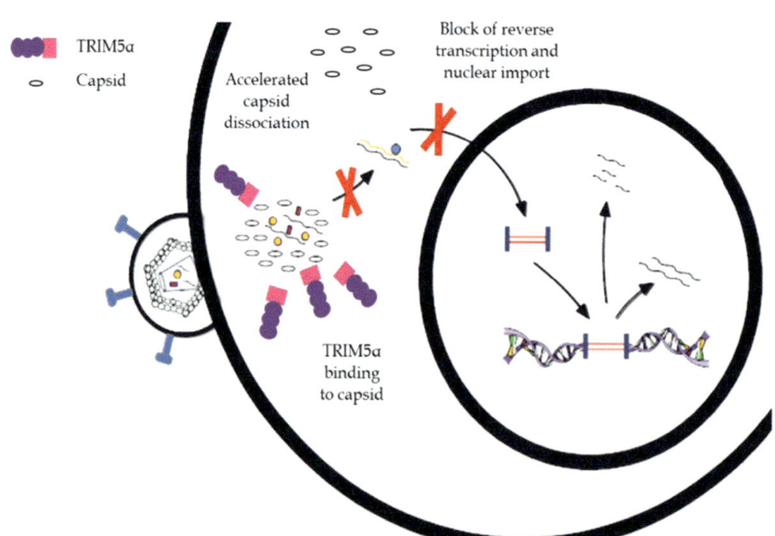

Fig. 4. TRIM5α-mediated HIV-1 restriction. RhTRIM5α binds to incoming HIV-1 capsid proteins via its B30.2 domain, causing them to rapidly dissociate and prematurely disassemble. This leads to a block in HIV-1 reverse transcription and inhibits nuclear import of viral cDNA, restricting further propagation of the virus.

on the HIV-1 capsid by the B30.2 domain of rhTRIM5α and subsequent block at the level of reverse transcription. Interestingly, human TRIM5α (huTRIM5α) only modestly inhibits HIV-1 replication and substitution of a single amino acid (R332) in its B30.2 domain enables it to restrict HIV-1 as potently as rhTRIM5α (Yap et al., 2005).

3. Lifecycle target: HIV-1 reverse transcription

3.1 APOBEC3

3.1.1 APOBEC3: Structure and function

The human apolipoprotein B mRNA-editing catalytic polypeptide-like 3 (APOBEC3) family is part of a larger family of APOBEC cytidine deaminases, capable of converting cytosine to uracil in RNA or DNA. The APOBEC3 family is found on chromosome 22 and contains seven members (A-H), which are believed to be the result of multiple duplication events (Conticello et al., 2005). Interestingly, APOBEC3 proteins appear to be under positive selective pressure, possibly as a defence against endogenous retroelements, and have been shown to have antiviral activity against a variety of viruses, including murine leukemia virus, human T-lymphotropic virus, simian immunodeficiency virus and the recently discovered Xenotropic Murine leukemia virus-Related Virus (XMRV) (Sawyer et al., 2004, Sawyer et al., 2004, Groom et al., 2010, Groom et al., 2010, Aguiar & Peterlin, 2008, Niewiadomska & Yu, 2009). In addition, all seven members have been implicated in HIV-1 restriction, however APOBEC3F/G are the best studied and appear to be the most potent restrictors (Hultquist & Harris, 2009).

Before APOBEC3 proteins were specifically identified, it was discovered that HIV-1 clones with the accessory protein Vif deleted were capable of replicating in certain cell lines. These cells were termed "permissive cells", and included HeLa, HEK 293T, SupT1 and CEM-SS lines. In other cells, such as primary human T-lymphocytes or macrophages, or the H9 and CEM T cell lines, virions produced from Vif-deficient strains were up to 1,000 times less infectious compared to virions from wild-type strains (Gabuzda et al., 1992). Cell fusion experiments revealed that this "non-permissive" phenotype was dominant, and comparison of the related CEM T and CEM-SS cell lines revealed a 1.5 kb cDNA segment expressed in CEM T cells that was not produced in CEM-SS cells (Madani & Kabat, 1998, Sheehy et al., 2002, Simon et al., 1998). This protein, termed CEM15 and later renamed APOBEC3G (A3G), was shown to be suppressed by Vif, thus resulting in productive infection of non-permissive cells with wild-type HIV-1 (Sheehy et al., 2002).

3.1.2 APOBEC3-mediated HIV-1 restriction

In the absence of Vif, A3G is packaged into newly formed virions and blocks HIV-1 replication after infection of a new cell. Two mechanisms of HIV-1 inhibition have been reported for A3G: 1) the production of hyper-mutated viral DNA and 2) decreased accumulation of viral DNA (Figure 5) (Anderson & Hope, 2008, Bishop et al., 2008, Lecossier et al., 2003, Mangeat et al., 2003, Simon & Malim, 1996). During reverse transcription, A3G induces cytidine deamination (C→U mutations) in the negative strand of newly synthesized viral cDNA. The latter results in G→A hyper-mutated viral DNA and increases the probability of producing premature stop codons or mutated, non-functional viral proteins. Interestingly, cytidine deamination also recruits cellular uracil-DNA glycosylases that cleave off the uracil side chain as part of the base-excision repair pathway. The resulting abasic site may then prevent plus-strand DNA synthesis or lead to degradation of viral DNA by endonucleases (Klarmann et al., 2003, Yang et al., 2007). However, there is some controversy over the degree to which APOBEC3-mediated cytidine deamination contributes to reduced accumulation of HIV-1 DNA, and it has been reported that the HIV-1 accessory protein Vpu induces the degradation of certain cellular uracil-DNA glycosylases (Schrofelbauer et al., 2005). Furthermore, loss of certain uracil-DNA glycosylases does not appear to affect APOBEC3 restriction of HIV-1, and similar results have been obtained for A3G restriction of other viruses (Kaiser & Emerman, 2006, Nguyen et al., 2007). Nevertheless, this does not rule out the possible involvement of other glycosylases, and additional studies will be required to fully elucidate the effects of APOBEC3 cytidine deaminase activity on HIV-1 replication.

Cytidine deaminase mutants of both A3F and A3G still retain a degree of anti-HIV-1 activity, and both proteins have been shown to affect the initiation of reverse transcription by interfering with $tRNA_3^{Lys}$ binding to viral RNA. In addition, A3G has been shown to inhibit both plus and minus strand transfer RNA integration and DNA elongation during reverse transcription (Hultquist & Harris, 2009). Interestingly, endogenous A3G in resting naive and memory CD4+ T cells may inhibit newly infecting virus, contributing to the known resistance of quiescent T cells to HIV-1 infection (Chiu et al., 2005, Muckenfuss et al., 2006). In this model, A3G can exist in two forms: an inactive high molecular mass complex (HMM) in activated T cells or an enzymatically active low molecular mass form (LMM) in resting T cells. Since A3G can interfere with multiple steps of reverse transcription, this hypothesis is consistent with infection of resting T cells, in which cDNA synthesis is initiated, but the viral genome is not completely reverse transcribed.

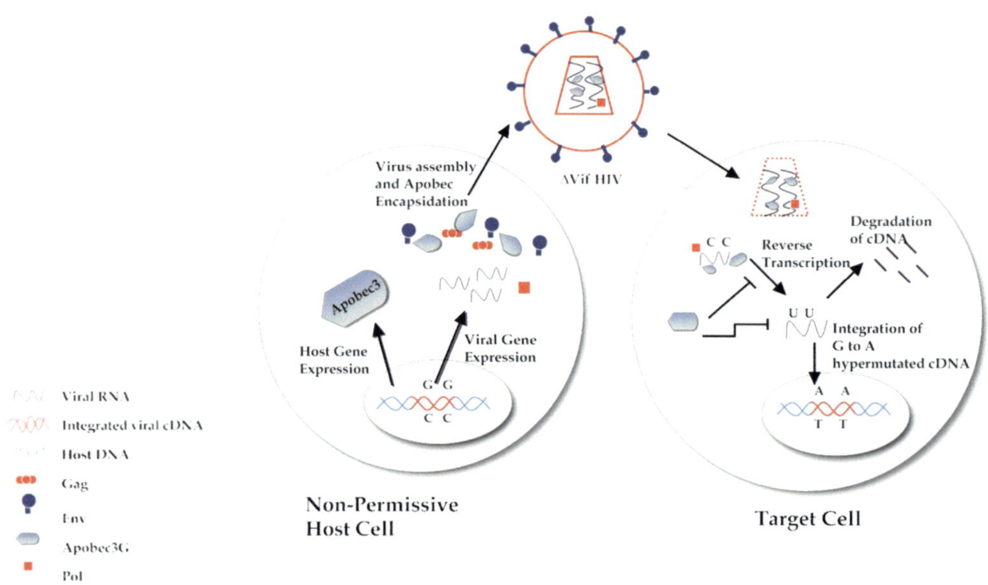

Fig. 5. APOBEC3G-mediated restriction of Vif-deficient HIV-1. APOBEC3G (A3G) is packaged into newly formed virions and interferes with viral replication upon infection of new cells. A3G directly interferes with reverse transcription, resulting in decreased amounts of viral cDNA. In addition, A3G acts as a cytidine deaminase, inducing C→U mutations in minus-strand viral cDNA. This leads to base excision by cellular uracil-DNA glycosylases or uracil bases are replaced with thymine, resulting in extensiveG→A hypermutations in the viral genome.

In recent years, the resting T cell theory has received criticism, mainly because several results in the original work were not repeatable. However, it should be noted that many results were still repeatable including the presence of LMM/HMM in resting/activated T cells and the enzymatically active nature of LMM forms (Chiu et al., 2005). Furthermore, it was observed that factors such as IL-2 and IL-15 both increase susceptibility of resting T cells to HIV-1 infection and induce a shift of A3G organization from LMM to HMM forms, suggesting that these results may warrant further investigation. In addition, several APOBEC3 proteins appear to have cytidine deaminase-independent antiviral activity against Hepatitis B virus, Adeno-associated virus, and a number of retroelements, further supporting the existence of a cytidine deaminase-independent antiviral mechanism (Bogerd et al., 2006, Chen et al., 2006, Stenglein & Harris, 2006, Turelli et al., 2004). As such, the extent to which cytidine deaminase-dependent or -independent functions contribute to the antiviral activity of APOBEC3 proteins against HIV-1 requires further elucidation.

3.1.3 Countermeasures to APOBEC3-mediated HIV-1 restriction

Vif restores HIV-1 infectivity by inducing the degradation of APOBEC3 proteins (Conticello et al., 2003, Marin et al., 2003, Sheehy et al., 2003). Vif and APOBEC3 proteins physically interact with each other, and these interactions are specific, however they differ depending on the APOBEC3 member being targeted (Niewiadomska & Yu, 2009). Vif also contains several conserved elements that allow it to form a complex with certain cellular proteins. Specifically, the SLQxLA motif in Vif interacts with ElonginC, allowing the recruitment of ElonginB and Cul5, which bind Vif through another conserved motif. Rbc1 is also recruited to the complex, creating an E3 ligase capable of polyubiquitinating APOBEC3 proteins and targeting them for 26S proteasomal degradation (Figure 6) (Kobayashi et al., 2005, Mehle et al., 2004,

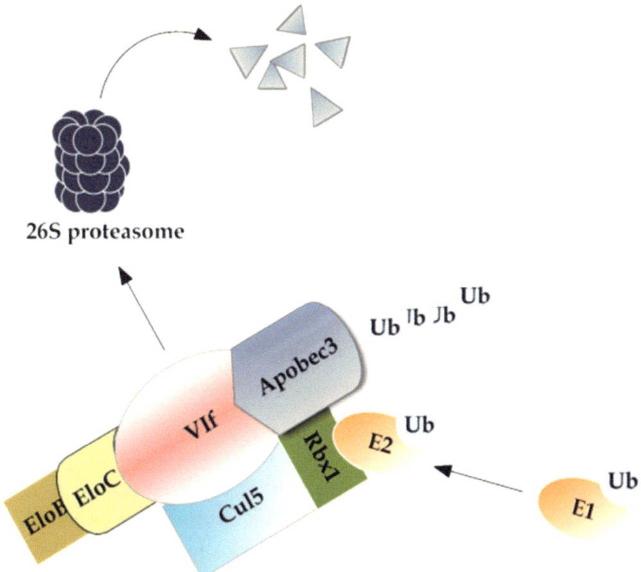

Fig. 6. Vif-mediated degradation of APOBEC3. Vif interacts with cellular factors to create a Skp1-cullin-F-box (SCF)-like complex that polyubiquitinates and degrades APOBEC3 molecules. Vif binds Cullin5 (Cul5) through two conserved motifs and other cellular factors, forming a scaffold for other E3 ligase components.

Yu et al., 2003). Interestingly, one report suggests that Vif instead of A3G is actually polyubiquitinated, possibly to serve as a way to transport A3G to the 26S proteasome for degradation (Dang et al., 2008). However, mutated and modified forms of Vif that are still capable of degrading A3G are unable to restore viral infectivity (Mehle et al., 2004, Kao et al., 2007). Thus, Vif may also inhibit A3G through degradation-independent mechanisms. Possible theories include a competitive inhibition model, where Vif binds to a common target, preventing A3G packaging, or that Vif inactivates A3G by inducing the formation of high molecular mass complexes (Goila-Gaur & Strebel, 2008, Goila-Gaur et al., 2008).

3.1.4 APOBEC3: Effects on HIV-1 replication *in vivo*

The extent to which APOBEC3 proteins are functional during HIV-1 infection *in vivo* is a highly contested topic. One report has observed the presence of extensive G→A hypermutation in virus samples collected from one HIV-1 long-term non-progressor (Wang et al., 2003)(Kao et al., 2007)(Kao et al., 2007)(Kao et al., 2007)(Kao et al., 2007)(Kao et al., 2007)(Kao et al., 2007)(Kao et al., 2007). Although this may suggest a role for APOBEC3 in controlling infection, it appears to be the only reported case, and thus the effects of APOBEC3 may have been secondary to some other mechanism of control. Still, it is possible that APOBEC3 proteins are more functional in certain patients/infections than in others. There are reports of both significant correlations and lack of correlation, between hypermutation and reduced viral load/higher CD4+ cell counts (Land et al., 2008, Piantadosi et al., 2009, Ulenga et al., 2008). Though hypermutation-independent mechanisms may exist, other groups have shown a negative correlation between A3G mRNA expression levels and HIV-1 viremia, and a positive correlation between A3G mRNA levels and CD4+ cell counts (Ulenga et al., 2008, Vazquez-Perez et al., 2009). Furthermore, it was shown that A3F/G mRNA levels post-infection are higher in patients with low viral set points than in patients with high viral set points, and higher in seronegative patients compared to healthy controls. Nevertheless, another group observed no correlation between A3F/G mRNA levels and viremia or CD4+ cell counts (Cho et al., 2006). Although conflicting reports exist, these may, in part, be explained by varying levels of APOBEC3 mRNA between donors (Koning et al., 2009). More detailed studies into both APOBEC3 expression and activity at the host level, in addition to correlation with disease progression, will be required to further elucidate its relationship to HIV-1 infection.

4. Lifecycle target: HIV-1 RNA

4.1 PKR

4.1.1 PKR: Structure and function

Protein kinase R (PKR) is constitutively expressed in human cells as an inactive monomer. In the presence of double-stranded RNA (dsRNA), which forms the genetic material of some viruses, PKR forms a dimer and phosphorylates itself to become active (Dey et al., 2005, Garcia et al., 2007). Activation of PKR is also possible through type I IFN signalling, and PKR is upregulated in the presence of IFNs. PKR contains a N-terminal dsRNA binding domain (dsRBD), which is made up of two dsRBD motifs and can bind to dsRNA as short as 30bp (Figure 1) (Lemaire et al., 2008). Dimerization relies strongly on the dsRBD, and studies deleting this domain show impaired dimerization as well as lack of PKR activation (Cosentino et al., 1995). In addition to its dsRBD, PKR contains a C-terminal kinase domain that has intrinsic phosphotransferase activity. This function hinges on a key lysine residue at position 296, without which the kinase domain is inactive (Sadler et al., 2009).

4.1.2 PKR-mediated inhibition of HIV-1 transcription

Upon activation, PKR inhibits HIV-1 replication through a number of different mechanisms. One mechanism involves phosphorylation of the enzyme RNA Helicase A (RHA), which has been shown to enhance HIV-1 transcriptional activity and binds to the HIV-1 trans-activation response (TAR) element (Fujii et al., 2001, Jeang & Yedavalli, 2006). The HIV-1 TAR element is required for trans-activation of the viral promoter and binds to the viral trans-activator of transcription (Tat) protein. This interaction greatly increases transcription of viral genes from the HIV-1 promoter, and results in the production of many full-length HIV-1 transcripts. The TAR element is an unusual stem-loop RNA structure that is located at the 5′ end of all HIV-1 mRNAs (Adelson et al., 1999, Nagai et al., 1997). PKR recognizes TAR RNA as dsRNA, and it binds to the upper bulge of the lower stem-loop structure using both of its dsRNA binding motifs (Carpick et al., 1997, Kim et al., 2006).

Like PKR, RHA contains a dsRBD with two dsRNA binding motifs, which are required for TAR recognition and binding (Fujii et al., 2001). A lysine residue at position 236 of RHA is essential for TAR binding (Fujii et al., 2001, Jeang & Yedavalli, 2006). Recently, PKR has been shown to phosphorylate the dsRBD of RHA; a modification that depends on lysine 296 of the PKR protein (Sadler et al., 2009). Phosphorylation of RHA by PKR seems to inhibit RHA-TAR binding, which in turn decreases the levels of HIV-1 mRNA transcripts (Sadler et al., 2009).

4.1.3 PKR-mediated inhibition of HIV-1 translation

Upon activation, PKR inhibits HIV-1 replication through a number of different mechanisms. The most widely researched pathway occurs through PKR-mediated phosphorylation of the alpha subunit of the eukaryotic initiation factor 2 (eIF2α), a key regulator of protein synthesis (Figure 7) (Dey et al., 2005, Rojas et al., 2010). In eukaryotic cells, eIF2α bound to GTP mediates the formation of a trimeric complex with methionine transfer RNA (met-tRNA). This complex leads to met-tRNA binding to the 40S ribosomal subunit, and allows for the initiation of translation (Rojas et al., 2010, Nallagatla et al., 2011). However, phosphorylation of eIF2α by PKR prevents the eIF2α-GTP interaction and eliminates the formation of the trimeric complex, thus inhibiting translation of all mRNA, including viral mRNA (Nallagatla et al., 2011).

The HIV-1 trans-activation response (TAR) element is required for trans-activation of the viral promoter and binds to the viral trans-activator of transcription (Tat) protein. This interaction greatly increases viral gene expression from the HIV-1 promoter by inducing chromatin remodelling and by recruiting elongation-competent transcriptional complexes onto the viral LTR. The TAR element is an unusual stem-loop RNA structure that is located at the 5′ end of all HIV-1 mRNAs (Adelson et al., 1999, Nagai et al., 1997). PKR recognizes TAR RNA as dsRNA, and it binds to the upper bulge of the lower stem-loop structure using both of its dsRNA binding motifs (Carpick et al., 1997, Kim et al., 2006). This leads to activation of PKR and phosphorylation of eIF2α, which subsequently inhibits protein translation (Nallagatla et al., 2011, Roy et al., 1991)

4.1.4 Countermeasures to PKR-mediated HIV-1 restriction

Although *in vitro* studies have shown that PKR can inhibit HIV-1 replication, *in vivo* models of infection fail to exhibit viral restriction. Interestingly, low levels of dsRNA have been shown to have beneficial effects on PKR activation; however, higher levels of dsRNA

(greater than a 1:1 ratio of dsRNA:PKR) may actually inhibit PKR activity (Chu et al., 1998, Hunter et al., 1975). During the initial stages of HIV-1 infection, low levels of TAR RNA (dsRNA) are produced and this leads to PKR activation (Lemaire et al., 2008). Conversely, in later stages of viral replication (when Tat-TAR binding enhances transcription), much more TAR RNA (dsRNA) is generated, which seems to inhibit PKR activity (Lemaire et al., 2008, Hunter et al., 1975, Clerzius et al., 2011, Manche et al., 1992). It has been proposed that high concentrations of dsRNA cause PKR to bind dsRNA as a monomer, which inhibits PKR dimerization and subsequent activation (Manche et al., 1992, Cole, 2007).
PKR activation is also interrupted by the HIV-1 Tat protein. Tat binds to the HIV-1 TAR element and in doing so, masks TAR recognition by PKR and inhibits PKR activation (Cai et al., 2000). Furthermore, Tat binds to PKR directly and therefore competes for PKR binding with eIF2α (Brand et al., 1997). There is a high degree of sequence homology between the Tat and eIF2α binding sites in PKR, which leads to a decrease in eIF2α phosphorylation (Cai et al., 2000, Brand et al., 1997). In addition, Tat binding to PKR inhibits autophosphorylation, possibly by inhibiting PKR dimerization, which is necessary for its antiviral activity (Cai et al., 2000, Brand et al., 1997). There is also evidence that phosphorylation of Tat by PKR at several key amino acids (S62, T64, S68) actually enhances Tat's ability to initiate transcription; however, the precise mechanism of transcriptional enhancement is not yet clear (Endo-Munoz et al., 2005).

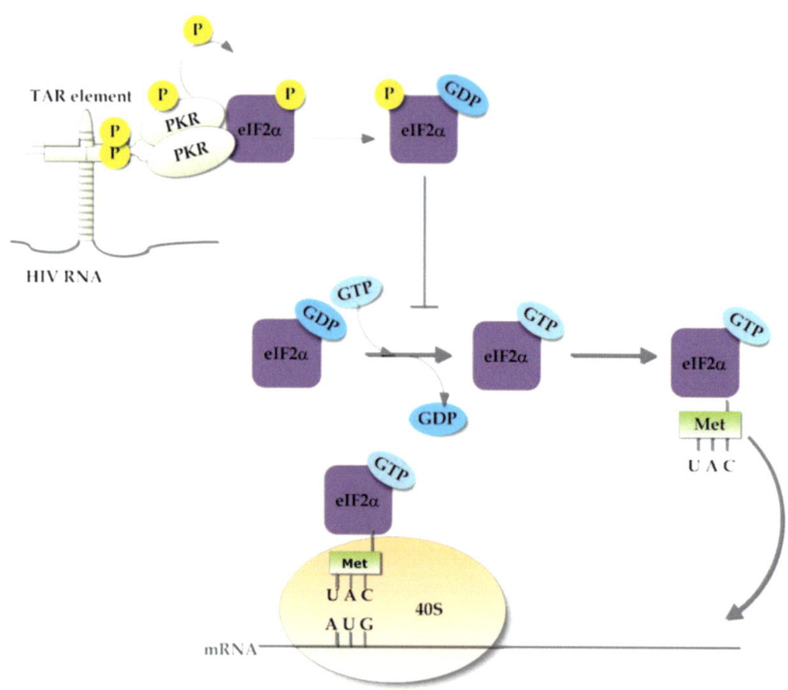

Fig. 7. PKR-mediated inhibition of HIV-1 protein translation. PKR recognizes the HIV-1 TAR element (dsRNA) and dimerizes and phosphorylates itself to become active. Active PKR phosphorylates eIF2α, preventing guanine nucleotide exchange and eIF2α activation. Inactive eIF2α is unable to transfer methionine-tRNA to the 40S ribosome for mRNA translation, and protein translation is inhibited.

4.2 TRIM22

4.2.1 TRIM22: Structure and function

Tripartite motif-containing protein 22 (TRIM22) was originally isolated during a search for IFN-induced genes in Daudi cells, and is located at chromosomal position 11p15, immediately adjacent to the TRIM5α gene (Tissot & Mechti, 1995). Similar to TRIM5α, TRIM22 belongs to the TRIM family of proteins and is upregulated in response to Type I and Type II IFNs (Bouazzaoui et al., 2006). TRIM22 expression is altered by multiple cytokines and viral antigens/infections, including Hepatitis B virus, encephalomyocarditis virus, and HIV-1 (Gao et al., 2009, Gao et al., 2009, Eldin et al., 2009). TRIM22 may also play a role in cellular processes such as cell differentiation/proliferation, as it is a known p53 target gene and has been suggested to have potential anti-proliferative functions (Obad et al., 2004, Obad et al., 2007).

To date, several studies have addressed the effect of TRIM22 on HIV-1 replication. TRIM22 expression was first shown to reduce HIV-1 transcription from a luciferase reporter construct under control of the HIV-1 long terminal repeat promoter (LTR) (Tissot & Mechti, 1995). Although this report did not follow up these observations in the context of full-length, replication competent HIV-1, it was fundamental in identifying TRIM22 as a potential HIV-1 restriction factor. Eleven years later, TRIM22 expression was shown to be increased in response to *ex vivo* HIV-1 infection of primary monocyte-derived macrophages, a biological target of HIV-1 (Bouazzaoui et al., 2006). In addition, overexpression of TRIM22 restricted HIV-1 infection by 70-90% and prevented the formation of syncytia. In 2008, TRIM22 was confirmed to be a potent effector of the IFN response against HIV-1 infection, and two different methods of TRIM22-mediated late-stage HIV-1 restriction were observed: one dependent on, and a second independent of, the HIV-1 Gag polyprotein (Barr et al., 2008).

4.2.2 TRIM22-mediated inhibition of HIV-1 transcription

It has since been confirmed that TRIM22 is capable of restricting HIV-1 mediated transcription (Kajaste-Rudnitski et al., 2011). Different clones of the U937 promonocytic cell line have previously been identified to be either permissive or nonpermissive to HIV-1 replication (Franzoso et al., 1994). Examination of multiple IFN-induced restriction factors revealed that only TRIM22 was present in nonpermissive clones and absent in permissive clones. LTR-driven transcription between permissive and nonpermissive clones was examined using a reporter construct expressing luciferase under control of the HIV-1 LTR. Basal transcription levels were decreased 7-10 fold in nonpermissive clones, but recovered to levels observed in permissive cells when shRNA was used to knockdown TRIM22 expression. Furthermore, LTR-driven transcription was decreased in permissive cells transduced with TRIM22, suggesting that the constitutive expression of TRIM22 is responsible for the restrictive phenotype observed in nonpermissive clones (Kajaste-Rudnitski et al., 2011). Reduced LTR-driven luciferase expression and HIV-1 replication were also observed in A3.01 cells (T cell line) expressing TRIM22, further supporting the effects of TRIM22 on HIV-1 infection in critical cell targets (Kajaste-Rudnitski et al., 2011).

TRIM22 appears to strongly target basal transcription from the HIV-1 LTR. In further experiments using LTR-driven luciferase constructs, TRIM22 had no effect on transcription when cells were transfected with a plasmid encoding the HIV-1 Tat protein (Kajaste-Rudnitski et al., 2011). Although statistical significance was not reached, this may be due to the effects of exogenously provided Tat masking the efficacy of TRIM22. It should also be noted that all direct evidence to date of TRIM22 inhibiting HIV-1 transcription has been through the use of LTR-driven reporter constructs. It will be important to test the effects of TRIM22 on replication-competent HIV-1, which will provide a more natural scenario of virus transcription, Tat-induction, and possible effects of other HIV-1 accessory proteins.

4.2.3 TRIM22-mediated effects on HIV-1 replication *in vivo*

Interestingly, there is evidence to support a role for TRIM22 as an anti-HIV effector *in vivo*. A study monitoring gene expression in high-risk HIV-1 negative individuals detected a positive correlation between TRIM22 expression and increased control of HIV-1 infection (Singh et al., 2011). It was observed that IFNβ and TRIM22 levels in peripheral blood mononuclear cells (PBMCs) were increased in patients after HIV-1 infection. In addition, infected patients expressing higher TRIM22 levels exhibited significantly lower viral loads and significantly higher CD4+ T cell counts, suggesting that TRIM22 may play a role in controlling HIV-1 infection. Surprisingly, a significant inverse correlation was observed between the closely related, IFN-inducible TRIM5α protein and IFNβ expression (Singh et al., 2011). TRIM22 and TRIM5α have been under positive selection episodically for approximately 23 million years; however, these two genes have evolved in a mutually exclusive manner, with only one being selected for in a given primate lineage (Sawyer et al., 2007). Since human TRIM5α has little to no inhibitory effect on HIV-1 replication compared to the potent inhibitory effects of rhesus TRIM5α, it is possible that human TRIM22 has evolved to compensate for the loss of antiretroviral activity of human TRIM5α.

5. Lifecycle target: HIV-1 protein

5.1 OAS1/RNaseL

5.1.1 OAS1/RNaseL-mediated inhibition of HIV-1 translation

Similar to PKR, 2′5′ oligoadenylate synthetase 1 (OAS1) senses viral infection by recognizing dsRNA, and is constitutively expressed in an inactive monomeric form (Sadler et al., 2009). However, unlike PKR, OAS1 recognizes dsRNA in the absence of a dsRBD. Exactly how OAS1 recognizes dsRNA without this domain remains unclear (Kodym et al., 2009, Marie et al., 1990, Sadler & Williams, 2008). Once OAS1 is activated by dsRNA, it forms a tetramer, which converts ATP molecules into 2′5′ oligoadenylates (2-5A) (Marie et al., 1990, Hovanessian, 2007). These 2-5As are strong inducers of an enzyme called RNaseL. By binding to the N-terminus of RNaseL, 2-5As activate the ribonuclease activity of RNaseL, which then degrades single-stranded RNA (ssRNA) by cleaving the phosphodiester bonds of uracil rich sequences to produce products with 3′ monophosphate and 5′ hydroxyl termini (Chakrabarti et al., 2011, Malathi et al., 2007). This leads to a reduction in mRNA translation and induces the RIG-I and/or MDA5 pathways, which are positive regulators of interferon signalling and the antiviral response (Figure 8) (Malathi et al., 2007).
The HIV-1 TAR element (dsRNA) is sufficient for OAS1 recognition and activation, and OAS1-TAR binding leads to 2-5A production, RNaseL recognition, cleavage of HIV-1 transcripts and inhibition of protein translation (Maitra et al., 1994). Interestingly, Jurkat T cells that overexpress RNaseL show a substantial decrease in HIV-1 mRNA production, as well as a 1000-fold decrease in HIV-1 replication two weeks post-infection (Maitra & Silverman, 1998). In addition, overexpression of RNaseL leads to accelerated HIV-induced apoptotic cell death, possibly through Fas-Fas ligand-mediated signalling (Maitra & Silverman, 1998). In contrast, cells devoid of RNaseL are unable to restrict HIV-1 replication, highlighting the importance of this pathway in cellular restriction of virus replication.

5.1.2 Countermeasures to OAS1/RNaseL-mediated HIV-1 restriction

Overexpression studies have shown that OAS1/RNaseL-mediated HIV-1 restriction is possible; however, when RNaseL is expressed at biologically relevant levels, HIV-1 can inhibit this pathway. The HIV-1 Tat protein sequesters the TAR element *in vivo*, thus preventing OAS1-TAR binding and RNaseL activation (Schroder et al., 1990b). It is possible that this pathway is responsible for the low levels of mRNA production during the initial stages of HIV-1 infection; however, as Tat expression increases, activation of the OAS1/RNaseL pathway decreases and the production of HIV-1 mRNA rises significantly. In addition, cells that contain latent virus may be kept under control by the OAS1/RNaseL pathway. Nevertheless, the ability of cells to endocytose Tat from other apoptotic cells may lead to trans-activation of the TAR element and HIV-1 mRNA production in these latently infected cells (Schroder et al., 1990b, Frankel & Pabo, 1988).

Although PKR and OAS1/RNaseL are potent HIV-1 restriction factors *in vitro*, the HIV-1 Tat protein is an effective viral countermeasure *in vivo*. Research on these restriction factors however, does provide insight into future therapeutics that may target the HIV-1 Tat protein, or overpower Tat for TAR binding. *In vitro* studies have already shown that shRNA directed against Tat or a TAR RNA decoy can provide long-term inhibition of HIV-1 replication; however, these studies must still be confirmed *in vivo* (Li et al., 2005).

5.2 TRIM22

5.2.1 TRIM22-mediated HIV-1 restriction

Interestingly, TRIM22 appears to restrict HIV-1 replication by multiple mechanisms. TRIM22 has been shown to be an integral part of IFNβ-mediated HIV-1 restriction, and its expression can restrict HIV-1 replication in several transformed cell lines. In cell lines such as human osteosarcoma (HOS) and HeLa, TRIM22 restricts the release of virus, but has little to no effect on intracellular levels of the HIV-1 structural protein Gag. Conversely, in the osteosarcoma cell lines U2OS and 143B, TRIM22 expression not only restricts the release of virus, but also prevents the intracellular accumulation of Gag protein (Barr et al., 2008). The presence of different mechanisms in different cell lines, and the fact that multiple localizations for TRIM22 have been observed, suggests that there are many complex details of TRIM22 function that remain to be discovered (Figure 9).

Further investigation of the mechanism of TRIM22-induced restriction in HOS cells revealed that TRIM22 likely interferes with intracellular trafficking of the HIV-1 Gag protein (Barr et al., 2008). Of note, Gag is both necessary and sufficient for budding and release of virus particles. This property allows Gag, in the absence of other viral proteins, to assemble and bud from the cell membrane, resulting in the production of non-infectious, virus-like particles (VLP). Importantly, TRIM22 expression was shown to inhibit the release of VLPs and prevent accumulation of Gag at the cell membrane, a step that is critical for virus assembly. These effects were dependent on the E3 ubiquitin ligase activity of TRIM22.

5.3 TRIM5α

5.3.1 TRIM5α-mediated HIV-1 restriction

RhTRIM5α was originally shown to target incoming HIV-1 capsid proteins, thus inhibiting early stages of HIV-1 replication (see Section 2.1). For this reason, it was initially assumed that rhTRIM5α didn't affect late stages of HIV-1 replication. However, subsequent research showed that it could also restrict HIV-1 through rapid degradation of the Gag polyprotein, the main structural component of HIV-1 (Sakuma et al., 2007). Treatment of cells

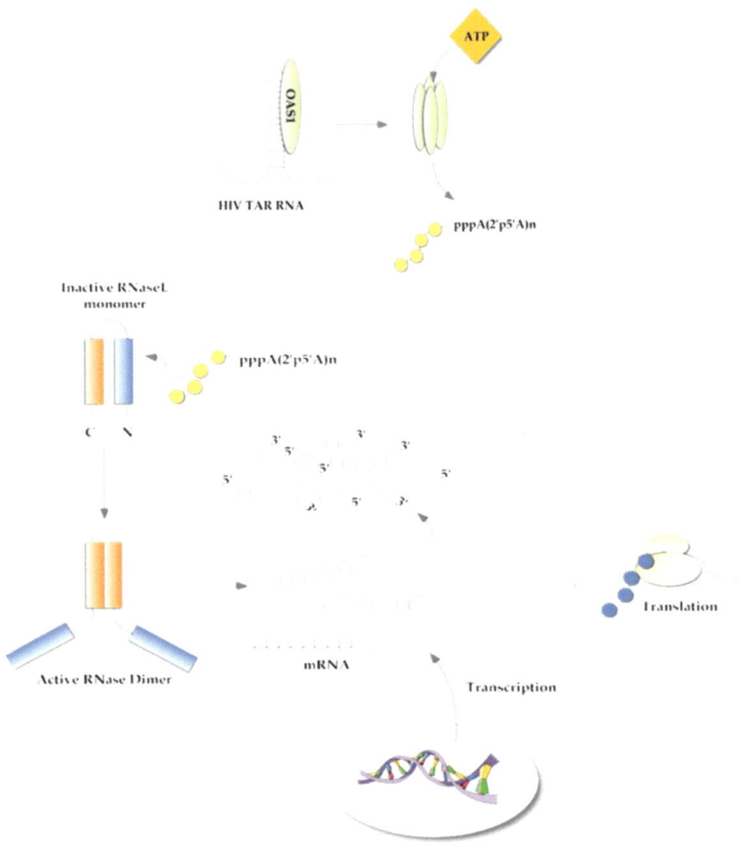

Fig. 8. OAS1/RNaseL-mediated inhibition of HIV-1 protein translation. Following recognition of the HIV-1 TAR element (dsRNA), OAS1 forms a tetramer whose catalytic activity turns ATP molecules into 2'5'oligoadenylates (2-5As). The 2-5As activate the RNaseL enzyme, which leads to its dimerization and stimulates it to cleave ssRNA (such as mRNA). Cleavage of mRNA by RNaseL results in the inhibition of protein translation, including the translation of viral proteins.

with the proteasome inhibitors MG132 and MG115 did not restore HIV-1 Gag protein stability, suggesting that late restriction by rhTRIM5α occurs independently of the ubiquitin/proteasome system. Interestingly, similar to early-stage restriction, the human orthologue of rhTRIM5α did not restrict late stages of HIV-1 replication (Sakuma et al., 2007, Sakuma et al., 2007, Sakuma et al., 2010).

Unlike early-stage rhTRIM5α-mediated restriction, the B30.2 domain was dispensable for Gag degradation. However, two amino acids in the coiled-coil domain (M133 and T146) and the E3 ligase activity of rhTRIM5α were required for late-stage restriction (Sakuma et al., 2010). It is possible that rhTRIM5α acts synergistically with other TRIM proteins or cell proteases to degrade the Gag polyprotein. For example, TRIM22 has been shown to affect late stages of HIV-1 replication and thus may be involved in rhTRIM5α-mediated restriction (Barr et al., 2008). Additional research will determine if other TRIM proteins are involved and help define the exact mechanism of late-stage rhTRIM5α-mediated restriction.

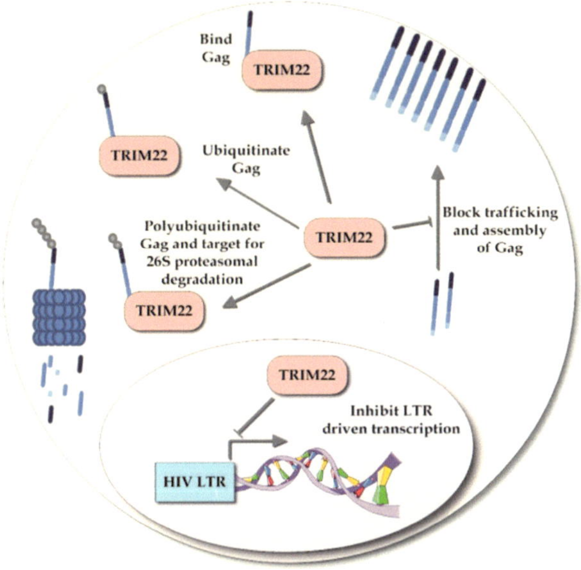

Fig. 9. Possible mechanisms of TRIM22-mediated HIV-1 restriction. TRIM22 prevents accumulation of the Gag polyprotein at the plasma membrane, and as such may bind directly to Gag. Alternatively, TRIM22 may mono-ubiquitinate or polyubiquitinate Gag. Experiments using LTR-luciferase reporter constructs have also shown that TRIM22 restricts transcription from the 5′ HIV-1 LTR.

6. Lifecycle target: HIV-1 budding

6.1 ISG15

Interferon-stimulated gene 15 (ISG15) is a ubiquitin-like protein (Ubl) that was first discovered in 1979, and is highly induced in the presence of IFN-α/β (Herrmann et al., 2007, Farrell et al., 1979). The ISG15 protein is composed of two ubiquitin-like domains that can modify substrate proteins similarly to ubiquitin (Jeon et al., 2010). In addition, the C-terminus of ISG15 contains the Gly-Gly motif which is required for ISG15 conjugation to target proteins. ISG15ylation requires the aid of an E1 activating protein, an E2 conjugating protein, and an E3 ligase protein. First, the ISG15-specific E1 activating protein, Ube1L, uses ATP to adenylate the Gly-Gly motif of ISG15. Ube1L then forms a thioester bond between its catalytic cysteine residue and the C-terminal Gly residue of ISG15. With the help of the E2 conjugating protein, UbcH8, and a substrate-specific E3 ligase, ISG15 forms a covalent bond with the ϵ-NH_2 of a substrate lysine residue (reviewed in (Kerscher et al., 2006)). Importantly, ISG15 is conjugated to both viral and host proteins, and can have an antiviral effect by altering the activity of substrate proteins required for viral propagation (Harty et al., 2009, Shi et al., 2010).

ISG15ylation has been implicated in restriction of HIV-1 replication at the budding stage of the HIV-1 lifecycle (Okumura et al., 2006, Pincetic et al., 2010). The HIV-1 Gag protein contains a late-budding or L domain that has a PTAP motif, and can interact with endosomal sorting complex required for transport (ESCRT)-I. Specifically, tumour susceptibility gene 101 (TSG101), a component of ESCRT-I, interacts with the PTAP motif on the HIV-1 Gag protein, and subsequently recruits ESCRT-II and ESCRT-III (VerPlank et al., 2001). ESCRT-III promotes viral budding and the recruitment of vacuolar protein sorting (Vps4), an ATPase that releases ESCRT factors from the membrane (reviewed in (Usami et al., 2009)(Williams & Urbe, 2007)). Interestingly, ISG15 has been shown to interrupt the interaction between TSG101 and the HIV-1 Gag protein; however, neither TSG101 nor HIV-1 Gag are directly modified with ISG15 (Okumura et al., 2006). ISG15 was also shown to interfere with the recruitment of Vps4 to the HIV-1 budding complex; however, the mechanism of this interruption has not yet been characterized. It is possible that charged multi-vesicular body protein CHMP-5, a component of ESCRT-III, prevents the recruitment of Vps4 as it was shown to be ISG15ylated (Pincetic et al., 2010). Further characterization of ISG15-mediated HIV-1 restriction is required to understand the antiviral effects of ISG15 on HIV-1 budding.

7. Lifecycle target: HIV-1 release

7.1 Tetherin

7.1.1 Tetherin: History and structure

For the past two decades, scientists have known that the HIV-1 Vpu protein is required for efficient release of virus particles (Gottlinger et al., 1993). HIV-1 particles lacking Vpu (HIVΔVpu) cannot release properly from certain cells; however, until recently the cause of this phenotype was unknown (Varthakavi et al., 2003). Tetherin (also known as BST-2 and CD317) was first suggested to be an antiviral protein in 2006, when it was shown to target the K5 protein of Kaposi's sarcoma-associated herpes virus (Bartee et al., 2006). A few years later, tetherin was identified as the causative agent of the HIVΔVpu phenotype when it was shown to inhibit the release of HIVΔVpu particles at the cell membrane of certain restrictive cells such as the HeLa cell line (Neil et al., 2008).

Tetherin is an interferon-induced, transmembrane protein that contains a short cytoplasmic N-terminus, a transmembrane region, an ectodomain, and a C-terminal glycosylphosphatidylinositol (GPI) anchor (Kupzig et al., 2003). Both the transmembrane region and the ectodomain are made from a single alpha helix, and the ectodomain contains an additional coiled-coil region. Tetherin exists as a homodimer, which is formed by disulphide bridges between the coiled-coil ectodomain regions of two tetherin proteins. Importantly, tetherin dimerization has been shown to be crucial for HIVΔVpu restriction (Andrew et al., 2009).

7.1.2 Tetherin-mediated restriction of HIV-1 release

Currently, the precise mechanism of tetherin-induced HIVΔVpu restriction is uncertain. Among the proposed models, two aspects seem to be consistent: 1) tetherin proteins form homodimers via the coiled-coil regions in their ectodomains and 2) the N- and C-terminus of tetherin are incorporated into the cell and/or viral membrane (Perez-Caballero et al., 2009). Tetherin homodimers localize to the cell membrane where they associate with HIV-1 Gag oligomers on lipid rafts (where budding of the virus occurs) (Neil et al., 2008, Nguyen & Hildreth, 2000). Details of the tethering mechanism underlying restriction are poorly understood. One favourable hypothesis involves the C-terminal GPI being anchored to the cell membrane and the N-terminal transmembrane region being associated with the Gag oliogomers of the budding virus. As budding occurs, the cell membrane-bound C-terminus tethers the budding virus to the cell via the virion-bound N-terminus (Perez-Caballero et al.,

2009). Conversely, the N-terminal transmembrane region of tetherin may anchor to the cell membrane whereas the GPI terminus may associate with the budding virus. Another plausible hypothesis is that one tetherin molecule binds to the cell membrane and another tetherin molecule binds to the budding virus. In this case, HIV-1 release would be inhibited by the interaction between coiled-coil regions in the tetherin dimer (Perez-Caballero et al., 2009) (Figure 10).

In spite of tetherin-induced restriction of HIVΔVpu virus, trapping virus at the membrane is not sufficient to prevent cell-to-cell transmission of HIV-1 (Casartelli et al., 2010, Kuhl et al., 2010). This binding leads to efficient cell-to-cell transmission of the virus. Interestingly, tetherin has also been shown to prevent HIV-1 transmission through this route. Specifically, tetherin appears to link budding HIV-1 particles together in a chain-like fashion, tethering them to the cell membrane in viral aggregates (Hammonds et al., 2010). The formation of these aggregates prevents HIV-1 transmission through the virological synapse, possibly because the aggregates cannot fuse properly to the target cells (Casartelli et al., 2010). It is possible that tetherin is incorporated into the budding virions and that this causes abnormal virus fusion to the target cell; however, more studies are needed to confirm the presence of tetherin in HIV-1 particles and further define its role in HIV-1 restriction at the virological synapse. Taken as a whole, current research suggests that tetherin may have two roles in HIV-1 restriction: tethering virus particles to the cell membrane and preventing cell-to-cell transmission of HIV-1 to uninfected target cells.

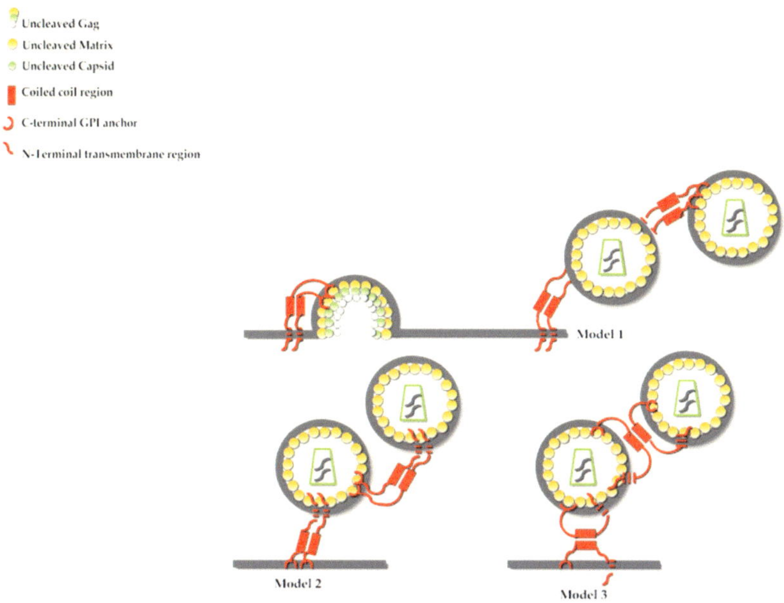

Fig. 10. Tetherin-induced inhibition of HIV-1 particle release. Each model centres on the dimerization of two tetherin molecules. In model 1, the N-terminal transmembrane regions of the tetherin dimer anchor to the cell surface and the C-terminal GPI domains associate with the budding virus. Model 2 is the opposite of model 1. In model 3, each tetherin molecule of the dimer associates with either only the budding virus or only the cell membrane, and HIV-1 restriction depends on the interaction between the coiled-coil regions.

7.1.3 Countermeasures to tetherin-mediated HIV-1 restriction

The HIV-1 Vpu protein has been shown to degrade tetherin, thus abolishing its anti-HIV-1 effects. Specifically, the transmembrane domain of Vpu can bind to tetherin, and this domain is necessary for Vpu localization to the cell membrane and subsequent association with tetherin (Kobayashi et al., 2011, Skasko et al., 2011, Vigan & Neil, 2010). Interestingly, mutating a single amino acid in the Vpu transmembrane domain (A18H) traps Vpu in the endoplasmic reticulum, where it is unable to translocate to the cell membrane or degrade tetherin (Skasko et al., 2011). Furthermore, it has recently been shown that four amino acids in the Vpu transmembrane domain (I34, L37, L41, and T45) are necessary for Vpu interaction with and antagonism of tetherin (Kobayashi et al., 2011). Mutational experiments with tetherin show that its transmembrane domain is also important for Vpu-tetherin interactions. Given this data, it is likely that Vpu and tetherin interact through their respective transmembrane domains and thus, that these domains are critical for Vpu-mediated tetherin degradation.

There are currently two major hypotheses for the mechanism of Vpu-mediated tetherin degradation. The first hypothesis involves tetherin degradation at a post-translational step, as there is no decrease in tetherin transcript levels in the presence of Vpu, but there is a decrease in protein expression (Douglas et al., 2009, Mangeat et al., 2009). It is possible that this degradation is mediated by Vpu binding to β-transducin repeat-containing protein (β-TrCP), which is a substrate adaptor for a multi-subunit E3 ligase complex and is able to interact with Vpu through its C-terminus. The consequence of Vpu binding to the β-TrCP-E3 ligase complex is the ubiquitination of cell surface proteins, including tetherin, on lysine residues at positions 18 and/or 21 (Mangeat et al., 2009, Guatelli, 2009, Iwabu et al., 2009, Pardieu et al., 2010). Tetherin ubiquitination leads to its endocytosis from the cell membrane and degradation through either the proteasomal or lysosomal degradation pathways (Douglas et al., 2009, Mitchell et al., 2009, Van Damme et al., 2008).

Tetherin degradation by Vpu and the β-TrCP-E3 ligase complex however, is insufficient to explain one interesting finding: Vpu constructs that contain mutations in the motif that recognizes β-TrCP can still partially, or in some cases totally, overcome tetherin-mediated HIV-1 restriction (Douglas et al., 2009, Mangeat et al., 2009, Mangeat et al., 2009, Mitchell et al., 2009, Miyagi et al., 2009). Thus, a second hypothesis has been proposed that involves tetherin degradation in late endosomal compartments. It has previously been shown that Vpu is distributed throughout the trans-golgi network, and that it can modulate tetherin cell surface expression by sequestering it intracellularly. Sequestration of tetherin prevents its anterograde trafficking to the cell membrane and subsequently delivers it to late endosomal compartments (Dube et al., 2010, Dube et al., 2010, Hauser et al., 2010). Of note, the specifics of this mechanism of Vpu-mediated degradation are still largely uncharacterized and further studies are needed to elucidate the details of this mechanism. However, taken together, current research suggests that there may be two mechanisms by which Vpu counteracts the antiviral activity of tetherin.

8. Conclusion

8.1 Pharmaceutical approach

In the future, it is probable that new HIV-1 therapies will be developed based on the actions of cellular restriction factors. Currently, many studies are focused on defining the molecular mechanisms of these factors; however, it is still unclear how this information will be used to create effective therapies. In the short-term, drug-based therapies are the most likely to be successful, and due to the constant development of HIV-1 resistance, new drugs are always needed. To date, there are 32 antiretroviral drugs approved by the FDA, and none of these drugs target the same steps in the HIV-1 lifecycle as cellular restriction factors. This makes restriction factors excellent candidates for drug design, specifically proteins such as TRIM22 or ISG15, which do not appear to be directly targeted by any HIV-1 proteins. With the development of any new HIV-1 drug, resistance is always a concern; however, identifying new stages of the HIV-1 lifecycle to antagonize may reduce viral replication enough to prevent escape mutants.

Alternatively, drugs targeting cellular restriction factor antagonists could be developed. For example, the HIV-1 Vif protein antagonizes APOBEC3 by marking it for proteasomal degradation (Yu et al., 2003). Inhibiting the interaction between APOBEC3 and Vif may prevent this degradation, and many studies have focused on identifying important interacting regions on both proteins (Chen et al., 2009, Huthoff & Malim, 2007, Yamashita et al., 2008). Unfortunately, many of the interacting regions on Vif differ depending on the specific APOBEC3 protein it is interacting with, and it is likely that three-dimensional structures of APOBEC3 proteins bound to Vif will be needed to effectively target this interaction (Russell et al., 2009, Tian et al., 2006). Despite these challenges, one small molecule antagonist of Vif was recently identified (RN-18) and shown to decrease levels of Vif protein *in vitro* (Nathans et al., 2008). It will be interesting to follow-up this research *in vivo*, and learn whether RN-18 has an effect on HIV-1 replication in infected individuals. Finally, another option to shield APOBEC3 from Vif involves designing a molecule that binds to APOBEC3 and prevents this interaction; however, this molecule would also have to preserve APOBEC3's antiviral function (Albin & Harris, 2010).

The HIV-1 Tat protein is another attractive drug target, since it is essential for HIV-1 replication and antagonizes two HIV-1 restriction factors (PKR and OAS1). For unknown reasons, Tat hasn't received much attention as a potential drug target, possibly because its actions are hard to re-create *in vitro*. However, inhibition of Tat potently inhibits HIV-1 replication, and further research in this area is certainly warranted. Drugs that target the HIV-1 Vpu protein could also be considered; however, because Vpu is not critical for HIV-1 replication *in vivo* it may not be an ideal candidate (Friborg et al., 1995, Terwilliger et al., 1989). Conversely, drugs that mimic the effects of tetherin, but are resistant to Vpu, may successfully reduce HIV-1 replication. In fact, an artificial Vpu-resistant tetherin protein was recently engineered; however, it has not yet been tested in clinical trials (Perez-Caballero et al., 2009). Inhibiting the action of host proteins that assist HIV-1 replication is another possibility. For example, cyclophilin A (CypA) is required for HIV-1 replication, and without Cyp A HIV-1 virions are not infectious (Sokolskaja & Luban, 2006, Thali et al., 1994). Small molecule inhibitors targeting Cyp A may block HIV-1 replication at the uncoating stage, and targeting a host protein avoids the problem of viral resistance. However, HIV-1 propagation in the absence of Cyp A may allow HIV-1 variants to evolve that no longer require Cyp A for replication.

8.2 Gene therapy approach

An alternative approach to HIV-1 therapy involves using cellular restriction factors in conjunction with gene therapy. In this approach, DNA encoding one or more cellular restriction factors is inserted into target cells to interfere with HIV-1 infection or replication.

One advantage of this approach is that cellular restriction factors are naturally expressed in human cells, and as such may be less toxic or immunogenic *in vivo* (Barr, 2010). Since there are no known viral countermeasures to TRIM22, Rhesus TRIM5α or ISG15, these proteins are currently the best candidates for gene therapy. Another possibility involves using molecular engineering to create modified restriction factors that are resistant to viral antagonists, making them more suitable candidates for gene therapy. For example, a human protein modeled after the TRIM5α-CypA fusion protein in Owl monkeys was recently engineered, and shown to block HIV-1 replication in primary $CD4^+$ T-cells and macrophages (Neagu et al., 2009). In addition, mice engrafted with inhibitor-expressing $CD4^+$ T-cells had decreased viremia and increased levels of $CD4^+$ T-cells. It is possible that this human TRIM5α-CypA protein could be used for gene therapy, and it is likely that it will be tested clinically in the near future.

Since many cellular restriction factors are IFN-inducible, they are not constitutively expressed in cells. As such, it is desirable to employ a gene therapy approach that mimics this pattern of expression. One interesting strategy involves creating a construct that contains restriction factor genes under the control of the HIV-1 LTR promoter. In this strategy, target cells are preloaded with the construct, and when HIV-1 infects these cells, Tat expression activates transcription of the LTR-fused restriction factor genes. Restriction factor expression reduces HIV-1 replication in infected cells, limiting further propagation of the virus. Notably, this approach has been successfully tested *in vitro* using the restriction factors PKR, OAS1 and ISG15; however, more experiments are needed to validate this strategy *in vivo*, and to test various construct delivery methods (Muto et al., 1999, Schroder et al., 1990a, Su et al., 1995). Gene therapy continues to be a promising approach for the treatment of HIV/AIDS; however, several problems need to be addressed before this technology can be fully realized. Some of these issues include, but are not limited to, increasing the stability of DNA and longevity of target cells, avoiding adverse immune responses, and targeting specific cells or tissues.

8.3 Additional approaches

8.3.1 Nanotechnology

Nanotechnology is revolutionizing many areas of medicine, particularly in the realm of drug delivery. With nanotechnology, it is now possible to target drugs to specific cells or tissues, a method that could be used to direct antiretroviral drugs to $CD4^+$ T-cells and macrophages (Farokhzad, 2008, Farokhzad & Langer, 2009). In addition, targeted antiviral delivery to the brain or other organs could ensure that drugs reach latent HIV-1 reservoirs (Vyas et al., 2006, Vyas et al., 2006, Amiji et al., 2006). The development of controlled-release delivery systems could also allow antiretroviral drugs to be released over longer times, and enhance their half-lives. For example, a new anti-HIV-1 drug called Rilpivirine was recently administered to dogs and mice in nanosuspensions (Baert et al., 2009). This resulted in the sustained release of the drug over 3 months in dogs and 3 weeks in mice, compared to a half-life of 38 hours for free drug. Importantly, this type of drug delivery system could have major implications in reducing antiretroviral toxicity and improving drug adherence. Thus, nanotechnology should be considered in the development of new antiretroviral drugs, including drugs that mimic the effects of cellular restriction factors.

In addition to improving antiretroviral therapies, there are ongoing efforts to apply nanotechnology to gene therapy. Early attempts in gene therapy for HIV/AIDS have used viral vectors as gene delivery systems, with some encouraging results (Li et al., 2005, Morris

& Rossi, 2006, Morris & Rossi, 2006, Lee et al., 2005, Lee et al., 2005). However, the use of viral vectors for gene delivery poses several potential problems such as toxicity, immunogenicity, and insertion mutagenesis. As such, the use of non-viral vectors for gene delivery must be further explored, and nanotechnology is one promising option (Lundin et al., 2009, Mintzer & Simanek, 2009). One example is the use of RNA interference (RNAi) for HIV/AIDS therapies. RNAi may have therapeutic potential in the treatment of HIV/AIDS; however, delivery of siRNA to specific cells continues to be a problem (Haasnoot et al., 2007, Haasnoot et al., 2007, Whitehead et al., 2009, Whitehead et al., 2009, Berkhout & ter Brake, 2009). Nanosuspensions of siRNA are currently being tested in humans for cancer treatment, and have recently entered Phase I clinical trials (Davis, 2009). If this technique is successful, it could be applied to cellular restriction factor-based HIV/AIDS gene therapy. For example, nanosuspensions of siRNA could be targeted to HIV-1-infected cells to knockdown the viral mRNA of restriction factor antagonists, such as Vif, Tat and Vpu. This would increase the antiviral activity of restriction factors, specifically reducing HIV-1 replication in infected cells. Alternatively, DNA from one or more cellular restriction factors could be delivered to HIV-1 infected cells using nanotechnology platforms. This may provide a safe and effective way to deliver cellular restriction factor genes to HIV-1 infected cells.

8.3.2 Zinc finger nucleases

Zinc finger nucleases (ZFN) have recently emerged as an important technology for gene modification, and there are several potential applications for ZFNs in HIV/AIDS therapy. ZFNs function by inducing a double-stranded break in a specific DNA sequence and generate the desired gene modification during DNA repair (Urnov et al., 2010). One of the main advantages of ZFNs is that the changes they make are both permanent and heritable, eliminating the need for persistent therapeutic intervention. For HIV-1, most ZFN research has focused on the manipulation of the human CCR5 gene, which encodes one of HIV-1's co-receptors and is required for viral entry into the host cell. Deletion of a 32-bp region from this gene (CCR5Δ32) results in a non-functional receptor, and people with this mutation are resistant to HIV-1 infection (Huang et al., 1996). Thus far, ZFN researchers have succeeded in deleting the 32-bp region from the human CCR5 gene, both in primary $CD4^+$ T-cells and hematopoietic stem cells (Bobis-Wozowicz et al., 2011, Lei et al., 2011, Perez et al., 2008). Furthermore, there are two Phase I clinical trials in progress testing the efficacy of *ex vivo* expansion and infusion of these modified cells in HIV-1 infected individuals (Urnov et al., 2010).

In addition to gene deletion, ZFNs have also been used successfully for gene correction (allele editing) and gene addition (Urnov et al., 2005, Urnov et al., 2005, Moehle et al., 2007). Both gene correction and addition may be useful for cellular restriction factor-based HIV-1 therapies; however, to date this has never been experimentally tested. For example, the addition of one or more cellular restriction factor genes to HIV-1 target cells may produce a 'super-restrictive' phenotype, whereby cells with multiple genes express higher levels of restriction factor proteins, thus increasing their capacity to fight HIV-1 infection. Several HIV-1 restriction factors have been shown to be more effective restrictors when expressed at higher levels. For example, higher expression of TRIM22 was recently shown to be correlated with lower levels of viremia and higher $CD4^+$ T-cell counts in HIV-1-infected individuals (Singh et al., 2011). Another possibility involves adding cellular restriction factor genes to hematopoietic stem cells, allowing the generation of 'super-restrictive' cells in all blood lineages (including macrophages and dendritic cells, which are often the first cells to encounter HIV-1 *in vivo*). However, many more studies need to be performed, particularly to identify any deleterious effects caused by amplified expression of cellular restriction factors.

8.3.3 Next-generation sequencing

Next-generation sequencing is another new and exciting technology that has potential applications in HIV/AIDS therapy. With this calibre of sequencing, it is now possible to read hundreds of DNA samples simultaneously, an approach that has helped researchers identify polymorphisms in different human genes. It is well known that people differ significantly in their susceptibility to HIV-1 infection and disease progression to AIDS, and polymorphisms in cellular restriction factors may contribute to these differences (Ball et al., 2007, Beyrer et al., 1999, Cao et al., 1995). For example, there is research suggesting that various polymorphisms in the TRIM5α and APOBEC3 genes contribute to HIV-1 disease progression; however, due to confounding reports further research is needed in this area (van Manen et al., 2008, van Manen et al., 2008, An et al., 2009, Goldschmidt et al., 2006, Harari et al., 2009, Valcke et al., 2006). In addition, polymorphisms in other cellular restriction factors may influence the clinical course of HIV-1 infection, but many of these factors have never been tested. In the future, it may be possible to generate an individual's cellular restriction factor polymorphism "blueprint"(Barr, 2010). This blueprint could help predict a person's susceptibility to HIV-1 infection and progression to AIDS, and may potentially lead to a more personalized HIV-1 treatment regime. Alternatively, with the advent of ZFN technology it may also be possible to "edit" multiple restriction factor genes (change disadvantageous polymorphisms to advantageous polymorphisms) to create an optimal cellular restriction factor blueprint *in vivo*, and better equip individuals to fight HIV-1 infection.

9. References

Adelson, M.E., Martinand-Mari, C., Iacono, K.T., Muto, N.F. & Suhadolnik, R.J. 1999, Inhibition of human immunodeficiency virus (HIV-1) replication in SupT1 cells transduced with an HIV-1 LTR-driven PKR cDNA construct, *European journal of biochemistry / FEBS*, vol. 264, no. 3, pp. 806-815.

Aguiar, R.S. & Peterlin, B.M. 2008, APOBEC3 proteins and reverse transcription, *Virus research*, vol. 134, no. 1-2, pp. 74-85.

Albin, J.S. & Harris, R.S. 2010, Interactions of host APOBEC3 restriction factors with HIV-1 in vivo: implications for therapeutics, *Expert reviews in molecular medicine*, vol. 12, pp. e4.

Alter, H.J., Eichberg, J.W., Masur, H., Saxinger, W.C., Gallo, R., Macher, A.M., Lane, H.C. & Fauci, A.S. 1984, Transmission of HTLV-III infection from human plasma to chimpanzees: an animal model for AIDS, *Science (New York, N.Y.)*, vol. 226, no. 4674, pp. 549-552.

Amiji, M.M., Vyas, T.K. & Shah, L.K. 2006, Role of nanotechnology in HIV/AIDS treatment: potential to overcome the viral reservoir challenge, *Discovery medicine*, vol. 6, no. 34, pp. 157-162.

An, P., Johnson, R., Phair, J., Kirk, G.D., Yu, X.F., Donfield, S., Buchbinder, S., Goedert, J.J. & Winkler, C.A. 2009, APOBEC3B deletion and risk of HIV-1 acquisition, *The Journal of infectious diseases,* vol. 200, no. 7, pp. 1054-1058.

Anderson, J.L. & Hope, T.J. 2008, APOBEC3G restricts early HIV-1 replication in the cytoplasm of target cells, *Virology,* vol. 375, no. 1, pp. 1-12.

Andrew, A.J., Miyagi, E., Kao, S. & Strebel, K. 2009, The formation of cysteine-linked dimers of BST-2/tetherin is important for inhibition of HIV-1 virus release but not for sensitivity to Vpu, *Retrovirology,* vol. 6, pp. 80.

Baert, L., van 't Klooster, G., Dries, W., Francois, M., Wouters, A., Basstanie, E., Iterbeke, K., Stappers, F., Stevens, P., Schueller, L., Van Remoortere, P., Kraus, G., Wigerinck, P. & Rosier, J. 2009, Development of a long-acting injectable formulation with nanoparticles of rilpivirine (TMC278) for HIV treatment, *European journal of pharmaceutics and biopharmaceutics : official journal of Arbeitsgemeinschaft fur Pharmazeutische Verfahrenstechnik e.V,* vol. 72, no. 3, pp. 502-508.

Ball, T.B., Ji, H., Kimani, J., McLaren, P., Marlin, C., Hill, A.V. & Plummer, F.A. 2007, Polymorphisms in IRF-1 associated with resistance to HIV-1 infection in highly exposed uninfected Kenyan sex workers, *AIDS (London, England),* vol. 21, no. 9, pp. 1091-1101.

Barr, S.D. 2010, Cellular HIV-1 restriction factors: a new avenue for AIDS therapy?, *Future Virology,* vol. 5, no. 4, pp. 417-433.

Barr, S.D., Smiley, J.R. & Bushman, F.D. 2008, The interferon response inhibits HIV particle production by induction of TRIM22, *PLoS pathogens,* vol. 4, no. 2, pp. e1000007.

Barre-Sinoussi, F., Chermann, J.C., Rey, F., Nugeyre, M.T., Chamaret, S., Gruest, J., Dauguet, C., Axler-Blin, C., Vezinet-Brun, F., Rouzioux, C., Rozenbaum, W. & Montagnier, L. 1983, Isolation of a T-lymphotropic retrovirus from a patient at risk for acquired immune deficiency syndrome (AIDS), *Science (New York, N.Y.),* vol. 220, no. 4599, pp. 868-871.

Bartee, E., McCormack, A. & Fruh, K. 2006, Quantitative membrane proteomics reveals new cellular targets of viral immune modulators, *PLoS pathogens,* vol. 2, no. 10, pp. e107.

Baum, A. & Garcia-Sastre, A. 2010, Induction of type I interferon by RNA viruses: cellular receptors and their substrates, *Amino acids,* vol. 38, no. 5, pp. 1283-1299.

Berkhout, B. & ter Brake, O. 2009, Towards a durable RNAi gene therapy for HIV-AIDS, *Expert opinion on biological therapy,* vol. 9, no. 2, pp. 161-170.

Beyrer, C., Artenstein, A.W., Rugpao, S., Stephens, H., VanCott, T.C., Robb, M.L., Rinkaew, M., Birx, D.L., Khamboonruang, C., Zimmerman, P.A., Nelson, K.E. & Natpratan, C. 1999, Epidemiologic and biologic characterization of a cohort of human immunodeficiency virus type 1 highly exposed, persistently seronegative female sex workers in northern Thailand. Chiang Mai HEPS Working Group, *The Journal of infectious diseases,* vol. 179, no. 1, pp. 59-67.

Bieniasz, P.D. 2004, Intrinsic immunity: a front-line defense against viral attack, *Nature immunology,* vol. 5, no. 11, pp. 1109-1115.

Bishop, K.N., Verma, M., Kim, E.Y., Wolinsky, S.M. & Malim, M.H. 2008, APOBEC3G inhibits elongation of HIV-1 reverse transcripts, *PLoS pathogens,* vol. 4, no. 12, pp. e1000231.

Bobis-Wozowicz, S., Osiak, A., Rahman, S.H. & Cathomen, T. 2011, Targeted genome editing in pluripotent stem cells using zinc-finger nucleases, *Methods (San Diego, Calif.)*, vol. 53, no. 4, pp. 339-346.

Bogerd, H.P., Wiegand, H.L., Hulme, A.E., Garcia-Perez, J.L., O'Shea, K.S., Moran, J.V. & Cullen, B.R. 2006, Cellular inhibitors of long interspersed element 1 and Alu retrotransposition, *Proceedings of the National Academy of Sciences of the United States of America*, vol. 103, no. 23, pp. 8780-8785.

Borrow, P. & Bhardwaj, N. 2008, Innate immune responses in primary HIV-1 infection, *Current opinion in HIV and AIDS*, vol. 3, no. 1, pp. 36-44.

Bouazzaoui, A., Kreutz, M., Eisert, V., Dinauer, N., Heinzelmann, A., Hallenberger, S., Strayle, J., Walker, R., Rubsamen-Waigmann, H., Andreesen, R. & von Briesen, H. 2006, Stimulated trans-acting factor of 50 kDa (Staf50) inhibits HIV-1 replication in human monocyte-derived macrophages, *Virology*, vol. 356, no. 1-2, pp. 79-94.

Brand, S.R., Kobayashi, R. & Mathews, M.B. 1997, The Tat protein of human immunodeficiency virus type 1 is a substrate and inhibitor of the interferon-induced, virally activated protein kinase, PKR, *The Journal of biological chemistry*, vol. 272, no. 13, pp. 8388-8395.

Broder, S. & Gallo, R.C. 1984, A pathogenic retrovirus (HTLV-III) linked to AIDS, *The New England journal of medicine*, vol. 311, no. 20, pp. 1292-1297.

Buchbinder, S.P., Mehrotra, D.V., Duerr, A., Fitzgerald, D.W., Mogg, R., Li, D., Gilbert, P.B., Lama, J.R., Marmor, M., Del Rio, C., McElrath, M.J., Casimiro, D.R., Gottesdiener, K.M., Chodakewitz, J.A., Corey, L., Robertson, M.N. & Step Study Protocol Team 2008, Efficacy assessment of a cell-mediated immunity HIV-1 vaccine (the Step Study): a double-blind, randomised, placebo-controlled, test-of-concept trial, *Lancet*, vol. 372, no. 9653, pp. 1881-1893.

Cai, R., Carpick, B., Chun, R.F., Jeang, K.T. & Williams, B.R. 2000, HIV-I TAT inhibits PKR activity by both RNA-dependent and RNA-independent mechanisms, *Archives of Biochemistry and Biophysics*, vol. 373, no. 2, pp. 361-367.

Cao, Y., Qin, L., Zhang, L., Safrit, J. & Ho, D.D. 1995, Virologic and immunologic characterization of long-term survivors of human immunodeficiency virus type 1 infection, *The New England journal of medicine*, vol. 332, no. 4, pp. 201-208.

Carpick, B.W., Graziano, V., Schneider, D., Maitra, R.K., Lee, X. & Williams, B.R. 1997, Characterization of the solution complex between the interferon-induced, double-stranded RNA-activated protein kinase and HIV-I trans-activating region RNA, *The Journal of biological chemistry*, vol. 272, no. 14, pp. 9510-9516.

Casartelli, N., Sourisseau, M., Feldmann, J., Guivel-Benhassine, F., Mallet, A., Marcelin, A.G., Guatelli, J. & Schwartz, O. 2010, Tetherin restricts productive HIV-1 cell-to-cell transmission, *PLoS pathogens*, vol. 6, no. 6, pp. e1000955.

Chakrabarti, A., Jha, B.K. & Silverman, R.H. 2011, New insights into the role of RNase L in innate immunity, *Journal of interferon & cytokine research : the official journal of the International Society for Interferon and Cytokine Research*, vol. 31, no. 1, pp. 49-57.

Chakrabarti, L.A. & Simon, V. 2010, Immune mechanisms of HIV control, *Current opinion in immunology*, vol. 22, no. 4, pp. 488-496.

Chatterji, U., Bobardt, M.D., Gaskill, P., Sheeter, D., Fox, H. & Gallay, P.A. 2006, Trim5alpha accelerates degradation of cytosolic capsid associated with productive HIV-1 entry, *The Journal of biological chemistry*, vol. 281, no. 48, pp. 37025-37033.

Chen, G., He, Z., Wang, T., Xu, R. & Yu, X.F. 2009, A patch of positively charged amino acids surrounding the human immunodeficiency virus type 1 Vif SLVx4Yx9Y motif influences its interaction with APOBEC3G, *Journal of virology,* vol. 83, no. 17, pp. 8674-8682.

Chen, H., Lilley, C.E., Yu, Q., Lee, D.V., Chou, J., Narvaiza, I., Landau, N.R. & Weitzman, M.D. 2006, APOBEC3A is a potent inhibitor of adeno-associated virus and retrotransposons, *Current biology : CB,* vol. 16, no. 5, pp. 480-485.

Chiu, Y.L., Soros, V.B., Kreisberg, J.F., Stopak, K., Yonemoto, W. & Greene, W.C. 2005, Cellular APOBEC3G restricts HIV-1 infection in resting CD4+ T cells, *Nature,* vol. 435, no. 7038, pp. 108-114.

Cho, S.J., Drechsler, H., Burke, R.C., Arens, M.Q., Powderly, W. & Davidson, N.O. 2006, APOBEC3F and APOBEC3G mRNA levels do not correlate with human immunodeficiency virus type 1 plasma viremia or CD4+ T-cell count, *Journal of virology,* vol. 80, no. 4, pp. 2069-2072.

Chu, W.M., Ballard, R., Carpick, B.W., Williams, B.R. & Schmid, C.W. 1998, Potential Alu function: regulation of the activity of double-stranded RNA-activated kinase PKR, *Molecular and cellular biology,* vol. 18, no. 1, pp. 58-68.

Clerzius, G., Gelinas, J.F. & Gatignol, A. 2011, Multiple levels of PKR inhibition during HIV-1 replication, *Reviews in medical virology,* vol. 21, no. 1, pp. 42-53.

Cole, J.L. 2007, Activation of PKR: an open and shut case?, *Trends in biochemical sciences,* vol. 32, no. 2, pp. 57-62.

Conticello, S.G., Thomas, C.J., Petersen-Mahrt, S.K. & Neuberger, M.S. 2005, Evolution of the AID/APOBEC family of polynucleotide (deoxy)cytidine deaminases, *Molecular biology and evolution,* vol. 22, no. 2, pp. 367-377.

Conticello, S.G., Harris, R.S. & Neuberger, M.S. 2003, The Vif protein of HIV triggers degradation of the human antiretroviral DNA deaminase APOBEC3G, *Current biology : CB,* vol. 13, no. 22, pp. 2009-2013.

Cosentino, G.P., Venkatesan, S., Serluca, F.C., Green, S.R., Mathews, M.B. & Sonenberg, N. 1995, Double-stranded-RNA-dependent protein kinase and TAR RNA-binding protein form homo- and heterodimers in vivo, *Proceedings of the National Academy of Sciences of the United States of America,* vol. 92, no. 21, pp. 9445-9449.

Cowan, S., Hatziioannou, T., Cunningham, T., Muesing, M.A., Gottlinger, H.G. & Bieniasz, P.D. 2002, Cellular inhibitors with Fv1-like activity restrict human and simian immunodeficiency virus tropism, *Proceedings of the National Academy of Sciences of the United States of America,* vol. 99, no. 18, pp. 11914-11919.

Dang, Y., Siew, L.M. & Zheng, Y.H. 2008, APOBEC3G is degraded by the proteasomal pathway in a Vif-dependent manner without being polyubiquitylated, *The Journal of biological chemistry,* vol. 283, no. 19, pp. 13124-13131.

Davis, M.E. 2009, The first targeted delivery of siRNA in humans via a self-assembling, cyclodextrin polymer-based nanoparticle: from concept to clinic, *Molecular pharmaceutics,* vol. 6, no. 3, pp. 659-668.

Deng, H., Liu, R., Ellmeier, W., Choe, S., Unutmaz, D., Burkhart, M., Di Marzio, P., Marmon, S., Sutton, R.E., Hill, C.M., Davis, C.B., Peiper, S.C., Schall, T.J., Littman, D.R. & Landau, N.R. 1996, Identification of a major co-receptor for primary isolates of HIV-1, *Nature,* vol. 381, no. 6584, pp. 661-666.

Dey, M., Cao, C., Dar, A.C., Tamura, T., Ozato, K., Sicheri, F. & Dever, T.E. 2005, Mechanistic link between PKR dimerization, autophosphorylation, and eIF2alpha substrate recognition, *Cell*, vol. 122, no. 6, pp. 901-913.

Diaz-Griffero, F., Li, X., Javanbakht, H., Song, B., Welikala, S., Stremlau, M. & Sodroski, J. 2006, Rapid turnover and polyubiquitylation of the retroviral restriction factor TRIM5, *Virology*, vol. 349, no. 2, pp. 300-315.

Douglas, J.L., Viswanathan, K., McCarroll, M.N., Gustin, J.K., Fruh, K. & Moses, A.V. 2009, Vpu directs the degradation of the human immunodeficiency virus restriction factor BST-2/Tetherin via a {beta}TrCP-dependent mechanism, *Journal of virology*, vol. 83, no. 16, pp. 7931-7947.

Dube, M., Roy, B.B., Guiot-Guillain, P., Binette, J., Mercier, J., Chiasson, A. & Cohen, E.A. 2010, Antagonism of tetherin restriction of HIV-1 release by Vpu involves binding and sequestration of the restriction factor in a perinuclear compartment, *PLoS pathogens*, vol. 6, no. 4, pp. e1000856.

Eldin, P., Papon, L., Oteiza, A., Brocchi, E., Lawson, T.G. & Mechti, N. 2009, TRIM22 E3 ubiquitin ligase activity is required to mediate antiviral activity against encephalomyocarditis virus, *The Journal of general virology*, vol. 90, no. Pt 3, pp. 536-545.

Endo-Munoz, L., Warby, T., Harrich, D. & McMillan, N.A. 2005, Phosphorylation of HIV Tat by PKR increases interaction with TAR RNA and enhances transcription, *Virology journal*, vol. 2, pp. 17.

Farokhzad, O.C. & Langer, R. 2009, Impact of nanotechnology on drug delivery, *ACS nano*, vol. 3, no. 1, pp. 16-20.

Farokhzad, O.C. 2008, Nanotechnology for drug delivery: the perfect partnership, *Expert opinion on drug delivery*, vol. 5, no. 9, pp. 927-929.

Farrell, P.J., Broeze, R.J. & Lengyel, P. 1979, Accumulation of an mRNA and protein in interferon-treated Ehrlich ascites tumour cells, *Nature*, vol. 279, no. 5713, pp. 523-525.

Fischl, M.A., Richman, D.D., Grieco, M.H., Gottlieb, M.S., Volberding, P.A., Laskin, O.L., Leedom, J.M., Groopman, J.E., Moldvan, D., Schooley, R.T. & al., e. 1987, The efficacy of azidothymidine (AZT) in the treatment of patients with AIDS and AIDS-related complex. A double-blind, placebo-controlled trial, *N.Engl.J.Med.*, vol. 317, pp. 185-191.

Flynn, N.M., Forthal, D.N., Harro, C.D., Judson, F.N., Mayer, K.H., Para, M.F. & rgp120 HIV Vaccine Study Group 2005, Placebo-controlled phase 3 trial of a recombinant glycoprotein 120 vaccine to prevent HIV-1 infection, *The Journal of infectious diseases*, vol. 191, no. 5, pp. 654-665.

Frankel, A.D. & Pabo, C.O. 1988, Cellular uptake of the tat protein from human immunodeficiency virus, *Cell*, vol. 55, no. 6, pp. 1189-1193.

Franzoso, G., Biswas, P., Poli, G., Carlson, L.M., Brown, K.D., Tomita-Yamaguchi, M., Fauci, A.S. & Siebenlist, U.K. 1994, A family of serine proteases expressed exclusively in myelo-monocytic cells specifically processes the nuclear factor-kappa B subunit p65 in vitro and may impair human immunodeficiency virus replication in these cells, *The Journal of experimental medicine*, vol. 180, no. 4, pp. 1445-1456.

Friborg, J., Ladha, A., Gottlinger, H., Haseltine, W.A. & Cohen, E.A. 1995, Functional analysis of the phosphorylation sites on the human immunodeficiency virus type 1

Vpu protein, *Journal of acquired immune deficiency syndromes and human retrovirology : official publication of the International Retrovirology Association,* vol. 8, no. 1, pp. 10-22.

Fujii, R., Okamoto, M., Aratani, S., Oishi, T., Ohshima, T., Taira, K., Baba, M., Fukamizu, A. & Nakajima, T. 2001, A Role of RNA Helicase A in cis-Acting Transactivation Response Element-mediated Transcriptional Regulation of Human Immunodeficiency Virus Type 1, *The Journal of biological chemistry,* vol. 276, no. 8, pp. 5445-5451.

Gabuzda, D.H., Lawrence, K., Langhoff, E., Terwilliger, E., Dorfman, T., Haseltine, W.A. & Sodroski, J. 1992, Role of vif in replication of human immunodeficiency virus type 1 in CD4+ T lymphocytes, *Journal of virology,* vol. 66, no. 11, pp. 6489-6495.

Gajdusek, D.C., Amyx, H.L., Gibbs, C.J.,Jr, Asher, D.M., Rodgers-Johnson, P., Epstein, L.G., Sarin, P.S., Gallo, R.C., Maluish, A. & Arthur, L.O. 1985, Infection of chimpanzees by human T-lymphotropic retroviruses in brain and other tissues from AIDS patients, *Lancet,* vol. 1, no. 8419, pp. 55-56.

Ganser-Pornillos, B.K., Yeager, M. & Sundquist, W.I. 2008, The structural biology of HIV assembly, *Current opinion in structural biology,* vol. 18, no. 2, pp. 203-217.

Gao, B., Duan, Z., Xu, W. & Xiong, S. 2009, Tripartite motif-containing 22 inhibits the activity of hepatitis B virus core promoter, which is dependent on nuclear-located RING domain, *Hepatology (Baltimore, Md.),* vol. 50, no. 2, pp. 424-433.

Garcia, M.A., Meurs, E.F. & Esteban, M. 2007, The dsRNA protein kinase PKR: virus and cell control, *Biochimie,* vol. 89, no. 6-7, pp. 799-811.

Garrus, J.E., von Schwedler, U.K., Pornillos, O.W., Morham, S.G., Zavitz, K.H., Wang, H.E., Wettstein, D.A., Stray, K.M., Cote, M., Rich, R.L., Myszka, D.G. & Sundquist, W.I. 2001, Tsg101 and the vacuolar protein sorting pathway are essential for hiv-1 budding, *Cell,* vol. 107, no. 1, pp. 55-65.

Goila-Gaur, R., Khan, M.A., Miyagi, E., Kao, S., Opi, S., Takeuchi, H. & Strebel, K. 2008, HIV-1 Vif promotes the formation of high molecular mass APOBEC3G complexes, *Virology,* vol. 372, no. 1, pp. 136-146.

Goila-Gaur, R. & Strebel, K. 2008, HIV-1 Vif, APOBEC, and intrinsic immunity, *Retrovirology,* vol. 5, pp. 51.

Goldschmidt, V., Bleiber, G., May, M., Martinez, R., Ortiz, M., Telenti, A. & Swiss HIV Cohort Study 2006, Role of common human TRIM5alpha variants in HIV-1 disease progression, *Retrovirology,* vol. 3, pp. 54.

Gottlinger, H.G., Dorfman, T., Cohen, E.A. & Haseltine, W.A. 1993, Vpu protein of human immunodeficiency virus type 1 enhances the release of capsids produced by gag gene constructs of widely divergent retroviruses, *Proceedings of the National Academy of Sciences of the United States of America,* vol. 90, no. 15, pp. 7381-7385.

Groom, H.C., Yap, M.W., Galao, R.P., Neil, S.J. & Bishop, K.N. 2010, Susceptibility of xenotropic murine leukemia virus-related virus (XMRV) to retroviral restriction factors, *Proceedings of the National Academy of Sciences of the United States of America,* vol. 107, no. 11, pp. 5166-5171.

Guatelli, J.C. 2009, Interactions of viral protein U (Vpu) with cellular factors, *Current topics in microbiology and immunology,* vol. 339, pp. 27-45.

Haasnoot, J., Westerhout, E.M. & Berkhout, B. 2007, RNA interference against viruses: strike and counterstrike, *Nature biotechnology,* vol. 25, no. 12, pp. 1435-1443.

Hammonds, J., Wang, J.J., Yi, H. & Spearman, P. 2010, Immunoelectron microscopic evidence for Tetherin/BST2 as the physical bridge between HIV-1 virions and the plasma membrane, *PLoS pathogens,* vol. 6, no. 2, pp. e1000749.

Harari, A., Ooms, M., Mulder, L.C. & Simon, V. 2009, Polymorphisms and splice variants influence the antiretroviral activity of human APOBEC3H, *Journal of virology,* vol. 83, no. 1, pp. 295-303.

Harty, R.N., Pitha, P.M. & Okumura, A. 2009, Antiviral activity of innate immune protein ISG15, *Journal of innate immunity,* vol. 1, no. 5, pp. 397-404.

Hauser, H., Lopez, L.A., Yang, S.J., Oldenburg, J.E., Exline, C.M., Guatelli, J.C. & Cannon, P.M. 2010, HIV-1 Vpu and HIV-2 Env counteract BST-2/tetherin by sequestration in a perinuclear compartment, *Retrovirology,* vol. 7, pp. 51.

Herrmann, J., Lerman, L.O. & Lerman, A. 2007, Ubiquitin and ubiquitin-like proteins in protein regulation, *Circulation research,* vol. 100, no. 9, pp. 1276-1291.

Hofmann, W., Schubert, D., LaBonte, J., Munson, L., Gibson, S., Scammell, J., Ferrigno, P. & Sodroski, J. 1999, Species-specific, postentry barriers to primate immunodeficiency virus infection, *Journal of virology,* vol. 73, no. 12, pp. 10020-10028.

Hovanessian, A.G. 2007, On the discovery of interferon-inducible, double-stranded RNA activated enzymes: the 2'-5'oligoadenylate synthetases and the protein kinase PKR, *Cytokine & growth factor reviews,* vol. 18, no. 5-6, pp. 351-361.

Huang, Y., Paxton, W.A., Wolinsky, S.M., Neumann, A.U., Zhang, L., He, T., Kang, S., Ceradini, D., Jin, Z., Yazdanbakhsh, K., Kunstman, K., Erickson, D., Dragon, E., Landau, N.R., Phair, J., Ho, D.D. & Koup, R.A. 1996, The role of a mutant CCR5 allele in HIV-1 transmission and disease progression, *Nature medicine,* vol. 2, no. 11, pp. 1240-1243.

Hultquist, J.F. & Harris, R.S. 2009, Leveraging APOBEC3 proteins to alter the HIV mutation rate and combat AIDS, *Future virology,* vol. 4, no. 6, pp. 605.

Hunter, T., Hunt, T., Jackson, R.J. & Robertson, H.D. 1975, The characteristics of inhibition of protein synthesis by double-stranded ribonucleic acid in reticulocyte lysates, *The Journal of biological chemistry,* vol. 250, no. 2, pp. 409-417.

Huthoff, H. & Malim, M.H. 2007, Identification of amino acid residues in APOBEC3G required for regulation by human immunodeficiency virus type 1 Vif and Virion encapsidation, *Journal of virology,* vol. 81, no. 8, pp. 3807-3815.

Ikeda, H., Laigret, F., Martin, M.A. & Repaske, R. 1985, Characterization of a molecularly cloned retroviral sequence associated with Fv-4 resistance, *Journal of virology,* vol. 55, no. 3, pp. 768-777.

Iwabu, Y., Fujita, H., Kinomoto, M., Kaneko, K., Ishizaka, Y., Tanaka, Y., Sata, T. & Tokunaga, K. 2009, HIV-1 accessory protein Vpu internalizes cell-surface BST-2/tetherin through transmembrane interactions leading to lysosomes, *The Journal of biological chemistry,* vol. 284, no. 50, pp. 35060-35072.

Javanbakht, H., Yuan, W., Yeung, D.F., Song, B., Diaz-Griffero, F., Li, Y., Li, X., Stremlau, M. & Sodroski, J. 2006, Characterization of TRIM5alpha trimerization and its contribution to human immunodeficiency virus capsid binding, *Virology,* vol. 353, no. 1, pp. 234-246.

Javanbakht, H., Diaz-Griffero, F., Stremlau, M., Si, Z. & Sodroski, J. 2005, The contribution of RING and B-box 2 domains to retroviral restriction mediated by monkey TRIM5alpha, *The Journal of biological chemistry,* vol. 280, no. 29, pp. 26933-26940.

Jeang, K.T. & Yedavalli, V. 2006, Role of RNA helicases in HIV-1 replication, *Nucleic acids research,* vol. 34, no. 15, pp. 4198-4205.

Jeon, Y.J., Yoo, H.M. & Chung, C.H. 2010, ISG15 and immune diseases, *Biochimica et biophysica acta,* vol. 1802, no. 5, pp. 485-496.

Kaiser, S.M. & Emerman, M. 2006, Uracil DNA glycosylase is dispensable for human immunodeficiency virus type 1 replication and does not contribute to the antiviral effects of the cytidine deaminase Apobec3G, *Journal of virology,* vol. 80, no. 2, pp. 875-882.

Kajaste-Rudnitski, A., Marelli, S.S., Pultrone, C., Pertel, T., Uchil, P.D., Mechti, N., Mothes, W., Poli, G., Luban, J. & Vicenzi, E. 2011, TRIM22 Inhibits HIV-1 Transcription Independently of Its E3-Ubiquitin Ligase Activity, Tat and NF-{kappa}B Responsive LTR Elements, *Journal of virology,* .

Kao, S., Goila-Gaur, R., Miyagi, E., Khan, M.A., Opi, S., Takeuchi, H. & Strebel, K. 2007, Production of infectious virus and degradation of APOBEC3G are separable functional properties of human immunodeficiency virus type 1 Vif, *Virology,* vol. 369, no. 2, pp. 329-339.

Kerscher, O., Felberbaum, R. & Hochstrasser, M. 2006, Modification of proteins by ubiquitin and ubiquitin-like proteins, *Annu Rev Cell Dev Biol,* vol. 22, pp. 159-180.

Kim, I., Liu, C.W. & Puglisi, J.D. 2006, Specific recognition of HIV TAR RNA by the dsRNA binding domains (dsRBD1-dsRBD2) of PKR, *Journal of Molecular Biology,* vol. 358, no. 2, pp. 430-442.

Klarmann, G.J., Chen, X., North, T.W. & Preston, B.D. 2003, Incorporation of uracil into minus strand DNA affects the specificity of plus strand synthesis initiation during lentiviral reverse transcription, *The Journal of biological chemistry,* vol. 278, no. 10, pp. 7902-7909.

Kobayashi, M., Takaori-Kondo, A., Miyauchi, Y., Iwai, K. & Uchiyama, T. 2005, Ubiquitination of APOBEC3G by an HIV-1 Vif-Cullin5-Elongin B-Elongin C complex is essential for Vif function, *The Journal of biological chemistry,* vol. 280, no. 19, pp. 18573-18578.

Kobayashi, T., Ode, H., Yoshida, T., Sato, K., Gee, P., Yamamoto, S.P., Ebina, H., Strebel, K., Sato, H. & Koyanagi, Y. 2011, Identification of amino acids in the human tetherin transmembrane domain responsible for HIV-1 Vpu interaction and susceptibility, *Journal of virology,* vol. 85, no. 2, pp. 932-945.

Kodym, R., Kodym, E. & Story, M.D. 2009, 2'-5'-Oligoadenylate synthetase is activated by a specific RNA sequence motif, *Biochemical and biophysical research communications,* vol. 388, no. 2, pp. 317-322.

Koning, F.A., Newman, E.N., Kim, E.Y., Kunstman, K.J., Wolinsky, S.M. & Malim, M.H. 2009, Defining APOBEC3 expression patterns in human tissues and hematopoietic cell subsets, *Journal of virology,* vol. 83, no. 18, pp. 9474-9485.

Kuhl, B.D., Sloan, R.D., Donahue, D.A., Bar-Magen, T., Liang, C. & Wainberg, M.A. 2010, Tetherin restricts direct cell-to-cell infection of HIV-1, *Retrovirology,* vol. 7, pp. 115.

Kumagai, Y., Takeuchi, O. & Akira, S. 2008, Pathogen recognition by innate receptors, *Journal of infection and chemotherapy : official journal of the Japan Society of Chemotherapy,* vol. 14, no. 2, pp. 86-92.

Kupzig, S., Korolchuk, V., Rollason, R., Sugden, A., Wilde, A. & Banting, G. 2003, Bst-2/HM1.24 is a raft-associated apical membrane protein with an unusual topology, *Traffic (Copenhagen, Denmark)*, vol. 4, no. 10, pp. 694-709.

Land, A.M., Ball, T.B., Luo, M., Pilon, R., Sandstrom, P., Embree, J.E., Wachihi, C., Kimani, J. & Plummer, F.A. 2008, Human immunodeficiency virus (HIV) type 1 proviral hypermutation correlates with CD4 count in HIV-infected women from Kenya, *Journal of virology*, vol. 82, no. 16, pp. 8172-8182.

Lecossier, D., Bouchonnet, F., Clavel, F. & Hance, A.J. 2003, Hypermutation of HIV-1 DNA in the absence of the Vif protein, *Science (New York, N.Y.)*, vol. 300, no. 5622, pp. 1112.

Lee, S.K., Dykxhoorn, D.M., Kumar, P., Ranjbar, S., Song, E., Maliszewski, L.E., Francois-Bongarcon, V., Goldfeld, A., Swamy, N.M., Lieberman, J. & Shankar, P. 2005, Lentiviral delivery of short hairpin RNAs protects CD4 T cells from multiple clades and primary isolates of HIV, *Blood*, vol. 106, no. 3, pp. 818-826.

Lei, Y., Lee, C.L., Joo, K.I., Zarzar, J., Liu, Y., Dai, B., Fox, V. & Wang, P. 2011, Gene Editing of Human Embryonic Stem Cells via an Engineered Baculoviral Vector Carrying Zinc-finger Nucleases, *Molecular therapy : the journal of the American Society of Gene Therapy*, .

Lemaire, P.A., Anderson, E., Lary, J. & Cole, J.L. 2008, Mechanism of PKR Activation by dsRNA, *Journal of Molecular Biology*, vol. 381, no. 2, pp. 351-360.

Li, M.J., Kim, J., Li, S., Zaia, J., Yee, J.K., Anderson, J., Akkina, R. & Rossi, J.J. 2005, Long-term inhibition of HIV-1 infection in primary hematopoietic cells by lentiviral vector delivery of a triple combination of anti-HIV shRNA, anti-CCR5 ribozyme, and a nucleolar-localizing TAR decoy, *Molecular therapy : the journal of the American Society of Gene Therapy*, vol. 12, no. 5, pp. 900-909.

Li, X. & Sodroski, J. 2008, The TRIM5alpha B-box 2 domain promotes cooperative binding to the retroviral capsid by mediating higher-order self-association, *Journal of virology*, vol. 82, no. 23, pp. 11495-11502.

Lilly, F. 1967, Susceptibility to two strains of Friend leukemia virus in mice, *Science (New York, N.Y.)*, vol. 155, no. 761, pp. 461-462.

Luban, J. 2007, Cyclophilin A, TRIM5, and resistance to human immunodeficiency virus type 1 infection, *Journal of virology*, vol. 81, no. 3, pp. 1054-1061.

Lundin, K.E., Simonson, O.E., Moreno, P.M., Zaghloul, E.M., Oprea, I.I., Svahn, M.G. & Smith, C.I. 2009, Nanotechnology approaches for gene transfer, *Genetica*, vol. 137, no. 1, pp. 47-56.

Lusso, P., Markham, P.D., Ranki, A., Earl, P., Moss, B., Dorner, F., Gallo, R.C. & Krohn, K.J. 1988, Cell-mediated immune response toward viral envelope and core antigens in gibbon apes (Hylobates lar) chronically infected with human immunodeficiency virus-1, *Journal of immunology (Baltimore, Md.: 1950)*, vol. 141, no. 7, pp. 2467-2473.

Madani, N. & Kabat, D. 1998, An endogenous inhibitor of human immunodeficiency virus in human lymphocytes is overcome by the viral Vif protein, *Journal of virology*, vol. 72, no. 12, pp. 10251-10255.

Maitra, R.K. & Silverman, R.H. 1998, Regulation of human immunodeficiency virus replication by 2',5'-oligoadenylate-dependent RNase L, *Journal of virology*, vol. 72, no. 2, pp. 1146-1152.

Maitra, R.K., McMillan, N.A., Desai, S., McSwiggen, J., Hovanessian, A.G., Sen, G., Williams, B.R. & Silverman, R.H. 1994, HIV-1 TAR RNA has an intrinsic ability to activate interferon-inducible enzymes, *Virology,* vol. 204, no. 2, pp. 823-827.

Malathi, K., Dong, B., Gale, M.,Jr & Silverman, R.H. 2007, Small self-RNA generated by RNase L amplifies antiviral innate immunity, *Nature,* vol. 448, no. 7155, pp. 816-819.

Manche, L., Green, S.R., Schmedt, C. & Mathews, M.B. 1992, Interactions between double-stranded RNA regulators and the protein kinase DAI, *Molecular and cellular biology,* vol. 12, no. 11, pp. 5238-5248.

Mangeat, B., Gers-Huber, G., Lehmann, M., Zufferey, M., Luban, J. & Piguet, V. 2009, HIV-1 Vpu neutralizes the antiviral factor Tetherin/BST-2 by binding it and directing its beta-TrCP2-dependent degradation, *PLoS pathogens,* vol. 5, no. 9, pp. e1000574.

Mangeat, B., Turelli, P., Caron, G., Friedli, M., Perrin, L. & Trono, D. 2003, Broad antiretroviral defence by human APOBEC3G through lethal editing of nascent reverse transcripts, *Nature,* vol. 424, no. 6944, pp. 99-103.

Marie, I., Svab, J., Robert, N., Galabru, J. & Hovanessian, A.G. 1990, Differential expression and distinct structure of 69- and 100-kDa forms of 2-5A synthetase in human cells treated with interferon, *The Journal of biological chemistry,* vol. 265, no. 30, pp. 18601-18607.

Marin, M., Rose, K.M., Kozak, S.L. & Kabat, D. 2003, HIV-1 Vif protein binds the editing enzyme APOBEC3G and induces its degradation, *Nature medicine,* vol. 9, no. 11, pp. 1398-1403.

McElrath, M.J., De Rosa, S.C., Moodie, Z., Dubey, S., Kierstead, L., Janes, H., Defawe, O.D., Carter, D.K., Hural, J., Akondy, R., Buchbinder, S.P., Robertson, M.N., Mehrotra, D.V., Self, S.G., Corey, L., Shiver, J.W., Casimiro, D.R. & Step Study Protocol Team 2008, HIV-1 vaccine-induced immunity in the test-of-concept Step Study: a case-cohort analysis, *Lancet,* vol. 372, no. 9653, pp. 1894-1905.

Mehle, A., Goncalves, J., Santa-Marta, M., McPike, M. & Gabuzda, D. 2004, Phosphorylation of a novel SOCS-box regulates assembly of the HIV-1 Vif-Cul5 complex that promotes APOBEC3G degradation, *Genes & development,* vol. 18, no. 23, pp. 2861-2866.

Merson, M.H. 2006, The HIV-AIDS pandemic at 25--the global response, *The New England journal of medicine,* vol. 354, no. 23, pp. 2414-2417.

Meylan, P.R., Guatelli, J.C., Munis, J.R., Richman, D.D. & Kornbluth, R.S. 1993, Mechanisms for the inhibition of HIV replication by interferons-alpha, -beta, and -gamma in primary human macrophages, *Virology,* vol. 193, no. 1, pp. 138-148.

Mintzer, M.A. & Simanek, E.E. 2009, Nonviral vectors for gene delivery, *Chemical reviews,* vol. 109, no. 2, pp. 259-302.

Mitchell, R.S., Katsura, C., Skasko, M.A., Fitzpatrick, K., Lau, D., Ruiz, A., Stephens, E.B., Margottin-Goguet, F., Benarous, R. & Guatelli, J.C. 2009, Vpu antagonizes BST-2-mediated restriction of HIV-1 release via beta-TrCP and endo-lysosomal trafficking, *PLoS pathogens,* vol. 5, no. 5, pp. e1000450.

Miyagi, E., Andrew, A.J., Kao, S. & Strebel, K. 2009, Vpu enhances HIV-1 virus release in the absence of Bst-2 cell surface down-modulation and intracellular depletion, *Proceedings of the National Academy of Sciences of the United States of America,* vol. 106, no. 8, pp. 2868-2873.

Moehle, E.A., Rock, J.M., Lee, Y.L., Jouvenot, Y., DeKelver, R.C., Gregory, P.D., Urnov, F.D. & Holmes, M.C. 2007, Targeted gene addition into a specified location in the human genome using designed zinc finger nucleases, *Proceedings of the National Academy of Sciences of the United States of America,* vol. 104, no. 9, pp. 3055-3060.

Morris, K.V. & Rossi, J.J. 2006, Lentiviral-mediated delivery of siRNAs for antiviral therapy, *Gene therapy,* vol. 13, no. 6, pp. 553-558.

Muckenfuss, H., Hamdorf, M., Held, U., Perkovic, M., Lower, J., Cichutek, K., Flory, E., Schumann, G.G. & Munk, C. 2006, APOBEC3 proteins inhibit human LINE-1 retrotransposition, *The Journal of biological chemistry,* vol. 281, no. 31, pp. 22161-22172.

Muto, N.F., Martinand, C., Adelson, M.E. & Suhadolnik, R.J. 1999, Inhibition of Replication of Reactivated Human Immunodeficiency Virus Type 1 (HIV-1) in Latently Infected U1 Cells Transduced with an HIV-1 Long Terminal Repeat-Driven PKR cDNA Construct, *J. Virol.,* vol. 73, pp. 9021-9028.

Nagai, K., Wong, A.H., Li, S., Tam, W.N., Cuddihy, A.R., Sonenberg, N., Mathews, M.B., Hiscott, J., Wainberg, M.A. & Koromilas, A.E. 1997, Induction of CD4 expression and human immunodeficiency virus type 1 replication by mutants of the interferon-inducible protein kinase PKR, *Journal of virology,* vol. 71, no. 2, pp. 1718-1725.

Nallagatla, S.R., Toroney, R. & Bevilacqua, P.C. 2011, Regulation of innate immunity through RNA structure and the protein kinase PKR, *Current opinion in structural biology,* vol. 21, no. 1, pp. 119-127.

Nathans, R., Cao, H., Sharova, N., Ali, A., Sharkey, M., Stranska, R., Stevenson, M. & Rana, T.M. 2008, Small-molecule inhibition of HIV-1 Vif, *Nature biotechnology,* vol. 26, no. 10, pp. 1187-1192.

Neagu, M.R., Ziegler, P., Pertel, T., Strambio-De-Castillia, C., Grutter, C., Martinetti, G., Mazzucchelli, L., Grutter, M., Manz, M.G. & Luban, J. 2009, Potent inhibition of HIV-1 by TRIM5-cyclophilin fusion proteins engineered from human components, *The Journal of clinical investigation,* vol. 119, no. 10, pp. 3035-3047.

Neil, S.J., Zang, T. & Bieniasz, P.D. 2008, Tetherin inhibits retrovirus release and is antagonized by HIV-1 Vpu, *Nature,* vol. 451, no. 7177, pp. 425-430.

Nguyen, D.H., Gummuluru, S. & Hu, J. 2007, Deamination-independent inhibition of hepatitis B virus reverse transcription by APOBEC3G, *Journal of virology,* vol. 81, no. 9, pp. 4465-4472.

Nguyen, D.H. & Hildreth, J.E. 2000, Evidence for budding of human immunodeficiency virus type 1 selectively from glycolipid-enriched membrane lipid rafts, *Journal of virology,* vol. 74, no. 7, pp. 3264-3272.

Niewiadomska, A.M. & Yu, X.F. 2009, Host restriction of HIV-1 by APOBEC3 and viral evasion through Vif, *Current topics in microbiology and immunology,* vol. 339, pp. 1-25.

Nisole, S., Stoye, J.P. & Saib, A. 2005, TRIM family proteins: retroviral restriction and antiviral defence, *Nat Rev Microbiol,* vol. 3, no. 10, pp. 799-808.

Obad, S., Olofsson, T., Mechti, N., Gullberg, U. & Drott, K. 2007, Expression of the IFN-inducible p53-target gene TRIM22 is down-regulated during erythroid differentiation of human bone marrow, *Leuk Res,* .

Obad, S., Brunnstrom, H., Vallon-Christersson, J., Borg, A., Drott, K. & Gullberg, U. 2004, Staf50 is a novel p53 target gene conferring reduced clonogenic growth of leukemic U-937 cells, *Oncogene*, vol. 23, no. 23, pp. 4050-4059.

Ohkura, S., Yap, M.W., Sheldon, T. & Stoye, J.P. 2006, All three variable regions of the TRIM5alpha B30.2 domain can contribute to the specificity of retrovirus restriction, *Journal of virology*, vol. 80, no. 17, pp. 8554-8565.

Okumura, A., Alce, T., Lubyova, B., Ezelle, H., Strebel, K. & Pitha, P.M. 2008, HIV-1 accessory proteins VPR and Vif modulate antiviral response by targeting IRF-3 for degradation, *Virology*, vol. 373, no. 1, pp. 85-97.

Okumura, A., Lu, G., Pitha-Rowe, I. & Pitha, P.M. 2006, Innate antiviral response targets HIV-1 release by the induction of ubiquitin-like protein ISG15, *Proc Natl Acad Sci U S A*, vol. 103, no. 5, pp. 1440-1445.

Ono, A. 2009, HIV-1 Assembly at the Plasma Membrane: Gag Trafficking and Localization, *Future virology*, vol. 4, no. 3, pp. 241-257.

Ozato, K., Shin, D.M., Chang, T.H. & Morse, H.C.,3rd 2008, TRIM family proteins and their emerging roles in innate immunity, *Nature reviews.Immunology*, vol. 8, no. 11, pp. 849-860.

Pardieu, C., Vigan, R., Wilson, S.J., Calvi, A., Zang, T., Bieniasz, P., Kellam, P., Towers, G.J. & Neil, S.J. 2010, The RING-CH ligase K5 antagonizes restriction of KSHV and HIV-1 particle release by mediating ubiquitin-dependent endosomal degradation of tetherin, *PLoS pathogens*, vol. 6, no. 4, pp. e1000843.

Perez, E.E., Wang, J., Miller, J.C., Jouvenot, Y., Kim, K.A., Liu, O., Wang, N., Lee, G., Bartsevich, V.V., Lee, Y.L., Guschin, D.Y., Rupniewski, I., Waite, A.J., Carpenito, C., Carroll, R.G., Orange, J.S., Urnov, F.D., Rebar, E.J., Ando, D., Gregory, P.D., Riley, J.L., Holmes, M.C. & June, C.H. 2008, Establishment of HIV-1 resistance in CD4+ T cells by genome editing using zinc-finger nucleases, *Nature biotechnology*, vol. 26, no. 7, pp. 808-816.

Perez-Caballero, D., Hatziioannou, T., Yang, A., Cowan, S. & Bieniasz, P.D. 2005, Human tripartite motif 5alpha domains responsible for retrovirus restriction activity and specificity, *J Virol*, vol. 79, no. 14, pp. 8969-8978.

Perez-Caballero, D., Zang, T., Ebrahimi, A., McNatt, M.W., Gregory, D.A., Johnson, M.C. & Bieniasz, P.D. 2009, Tetherin inhibits HIV-1 release by directly tethering virions to cells, *Cell*, vol. 139, no. 3, pp. 499-511.

Piantadosi, A., Humes, D., Chohan, B., McClelland, R.S. & Overbaugh, J. 2009, Analysis of the percentage of human immunodeficiency virus type 1 sequences that are hypermutated and markers of disease progression in a longitudinal cohort, including one individual with a partially defective Vif, *Journal of virology*, vol. 83, no. 16, pp. 7805-7814.

Pincetic, A., Kuang, Z., Seo, E.J. & Leis, J. 2010, The interferon-induced gene ISG15 blocks retrovirus release from cells late in the budding process, *Journal of virology*, vol. 84, no. 9, pp. 4725-4736.

Pincus, T., Hartley, J.W. & Rowe, W.P. 1971, A major genetic locus affecting resistance to infection with murine leukemia viruses. I. Tissue culture studies of naturally occurring viruses, *The Journal of experimental medicine*, vol. 133, no. 6, pp. 1219-1233.

Pitisuttithum, P., Gilbert, P., Gurwith, M., Heyward, W., Martin, M., van Griensven, F., Hu, D., Tappero, J.W., Choopanya, K. & Bangkok Vaccine Evaluation Group 2006,

Randomized, double-blind, placebo-controlled efficacy trial of a bivalent recombinant glycoprotein 120 HIV-1 vaccine among injection drug users in Bangkok, Thailand, *The Journal of infectious diseases,* vol. 194, no. 12, pp. 1661-1671.

Poli, G., Orenstein, J.M., Kinter, A., Folks, T.M. & Fauci, A.S. 1989, Interferon-alpha but not AZT suppresses HIV expression in chronically infected cell lines, *Science,* vol. 244, no. 4904, pp. 575-577.

Priddy, F.H., Brown, D., Kublin, J., Monahan, K., Wright, D.P., Lalezari, J., Santiago, S., Marmor, M., Lally, M., Novak, R.M., Brown, S.J., Kulkarni, P., Dubey, S.A., Kierstead, L.S., Casimiro, D.R., Mogg, R., DiNubile, M.J., Shiver, J.W., Leavitt, R.Y., Robertson, M.N., Mehrotra, D.V., Quirk, E. & Merck V520-016 Study Group 2008, Safety and immunogenicity of a replication-incompetent adenovirus type 5 HIV-1 clade B gag/pol/nef vaccine in healthy adults, *Clinical infectious diseases : an official publication of the Infectious Diseases Society of America,* vol. 46, no. 11, pp. 1769-1781.

Pryciak, P.M. & Varmus, H.E. 1992, Fv-1 restriction and its effects on murine leukemia virus integration in vivo and in vitro, *Journal of virology,* vol. 66, no. 10, pp. 5959-5966.

Rerks-Ngarm, S., Pitisuttithum, P., Nitayaphan, S., Kaewkungwal, J., Chiu, J., Paris, R., Premsri, N., Namwat, C., de Souza, M., Adams, E., Benenson, M., Gurunathan, S., Tartaglia, J., McNeil, J.G., Francis, D.P., Stablein, D., Birx, D.L., Chunsuttiwat, S., Khamboonruang, C., Thongcharoen, P., Robb, M.L., Michael, N.L., Kunasol, P., Kim, J.H. & MOPH-TAVEG Investigators 2009, Vaccination with ALVAC and AIDSVAX to prevent HIV-1 infection in Thailand, *The New England journal of medicine,* vol. 361, no. 23, pp. 2209-2220.

Richman, D.D., Margolis, D.M., Delaney, M., Greene, W.C., Hazuda, D. & Pomerantz, R.J. 2009, The challenge of finding a cure for HIV infection, *Science (New York, N.Y.),* vol. 323, no. 5919, pp. 1304-1307.

Richman, D.D., Meng, T.C., Spector, S.A., Fischl, M.A., Resnick, L. & Lai, S. 1994, Resistance to AZT and ddC during long-term combination therapy in patients with advanced infection with human immunodeficiency virus, *JAIDS,* vol. 7, pp. 135-138.

Roberts, D.M., Nanda, A., Havenga, M.J., Abbink, P., Lynch, D.M., Ewald, B.A., Liu, J., Thorner, A.R., Swanson, P.E., Gorgone, D.A., Lifton, M.A., Lemckert, A.A., Holterman, L., Chen, B., Dilraj, A., Carville, A., Mansfield, K.G., Goudsmit, J. & Barouch, D.H. 2006, Hexon-chimaeric adenovirus serotype 5 vectors circumvent pre-existing anti-vector immunity, *Nature,* vol. 441, no. 7090, pp. 239-243.

Rojas, M., Arias, C.F. & Lopez, S. 2010, Protein kinase R is responsible for the phosphorylation of eIF2alpha in rotavirus infection, *Journal of virology,* vol. 84, no. 20, pp. 10457-10466.

Roy, S., Agy, M., Hovanessian, A.G., Sonenberg, N. & Katze, M.G. 1991, The integrity of the stem structure of human immunodeficiency virus type 1 Tat-responsive sequence of RNA is required for interaction with the interferon-induced 68,000-Mr protein kinase, *Journal of virology,* vol. 65, no. 2, pp. 632-640.

Russell, R.A., Smith, J., Barr, R., Bhattacharyya, D. & Pathak, V.K. 2009, Distinct domains within APOBEC3G and APOBEC3F interact with separate regions of human immunodeficiency virus type 1 Vif, *Journal of virology,* vol. 83, no. 4, pp. 1992-2003.

Sadler, A.J., Latchoumanin, O., Hawkes, D., Mak, J. & Williams, B.R. 2009, An antiviral response directed by PKR phosphorylation of the RNA helicase A, *PLoS pathogens,* vol. 5, no. 2, pp. e1000311.

Sadler, A.J. & Williams, B.R. 2008, Interferon-inducible antiviral effectors, *Nature reviews.Immunology,* vol. 8, no. 7, pp. 559-568.

Sakuma, R., Ohmine, S. & Ikeda, Y. 2010, Determinants for the rhesus monkey TRIM5alpha-mediated block of the late phase of HIV-1 replication, *The Journal of biological chemistry,* vol. 285, no. 6, pp. 3784-3793.

Sakuma, R., Noser, J.A., Ohmine, S. & Ikeda, Y. 2007, Rhesus monkey TRIM5alpha restricts HIV-1 production through rapid degradation of viral Gag polyproteins, *Nat Med,* vol. 13, no. 5, pp. 631-635.

Sawyer, S.L., Emerman, M. & Malik, H.S. 2007, Discordant evolution of the adjacent antiretroviral genes TRIM22 and TRIM5 in mammals, *PLoS pathogens,* vol. 3, no. 12, pp. e197.

Sawyer, S.L., Emerman, M. & Malik, H.S. 2004, Ancient adaptive evolution of the primate antiviral DNA-editing enzyme APOBEC3G, *PLoS biology,* vol. 2, no. 9, pp. E275.

Sayah, D.M., Sokolskaja, E., Berthoux, L. & Luban, J. 2004, Cyclophilin A retrotransposition into TRIM5 explains owl monkey resistance to HIV-1, *Nature,* vol. 430, no. 6999, pp. 569-573.

Schroder, H.C., Ugarkovic, D., Merz, H., Kuchino, Y., Okamoto, T. & Muller, W.E. 1990a, Protection of HeLa-T4+ cells against human immunodeficiency virus (HIV) infection after stable transfection with HIV LTR-2',5'-oligoadenylate synthetase hybrid gene, *The FASEB journal : official publication of the Federation of American Societies for Experimental Biology,* vol. 4, no. 13, pp. 3124-3130.

Schroder, H.C., Ugarkovic, D., Wenger, R., Reuter, P., Okamoto, T. & Muller, W.E. 1990b, Binding of Tat protein to TAR region of human immunodeficiency virus type 1 blocks TAR-mediated activation of (2'-5')oligoadenylate synthetase, *AIDS Research and Human Retroviruses,* vol. 6, no. 5, pp. 659-672.

Schrofelbauer, B., Yu, Q., Zeitlin, S.G. & Landau, N.R. 2005, Human immunodeficiency virus type 1 Vpr induces the degradation of the UNG and SMUG uracil-DNA glycosylases, *Journal of virology,* vol. 79, no. 17, pp. 10978-10987.

Sheehy, A.M., Gaddis, N.C. & Malim, M.H. 2003, The antiretroviral enzyme APOBEC3G is degraded by the proteasome in response to HIV-1 Vif, *Nature medicine,* vol. 9, no. 11, pp. 1404-1407.

Sheehy, A.M., Gaddis, N.C., Choi, J.D. & Malim, M.H. 2002, Isolation of a human gene that inhibits HIV-1 infection and is suppressed by the viral Vif protein, *Nature,* vol. 418, no. 6898, pp. 646-50.

Shi, H.X., Yang, K., Liu, X., Liu, X.Y., Wei, B., Shan, Y.F., Zhu, L.H. & Wang, C. 2010, Positive regulation of interferon regulatory factor 3 activation by Herc5 via ISG15 modification, *Molecular and cellular biology,* vol. 30, no. 10, pp. 2424-2436.

Shiver, J.W., Fu, T.M., Chen, L., Casimiro, D.R., Davies, M.E., Evans, R.K., Zhang, Z.Q., Simon, A.J., Trigona, W.L., Dubey, S.A., Huang, L., Harris, V.A., Long, R.S., Liang, X., Handt, L., Schleif, W.A., Zhu, L., Freed, D.C., Persaud, N.V., Guan, L., Punt, K.S., Tang, A., Chen, M., Wilson, K.A., Collins, K.B., Heidecker, G.J., Fernandez, V.R., Perry, H.C., Joyce, J.G., Grimm, K.M., Cook, J.C., Keller, P.M., Kresock, D.S., Mach, H., Troutman, R.D., Isopi, L.A., Williams, D.M., Xu, Z., Bohannon, K.E., Volkin, D.B., Montefiori, D.C., Miura, A., Krivulka, G.R., Lifton, M.A., Kuroda, M.J., Schmitz, J.E., Letvin, N.L., Caulfield, M.J., Bett, A.J., Youil, R., Kaslow, D.C. &

Emini, E.A. 2002, Replication-incompetent adenoviral vaccine vector elicits effective anti-immunodeficiency-virus immunity, *Nature,* vol. 415, no. 6869, pp. 331-335.

Simon, J.H., Gaddis, N.C., Fouchier, R.A. & Malim, M.H. 1998, Evidence for a newly discovered cellular anti-HIV-1 phenotype, *Nature medicine,* vol. 4, no. 12, pp. 1397-1400.

Simon, J.H. & Malim, M.H. 1996, The human immunodeficiency virus type 1 Vif protein modulates the postpenetration stability of viral nucleoprotein complexes, *Journal of virology,* vol. 70, no. 8, pp. 5297-5305.

Singh, R., Gaiha, G., Werner, L., McKim, K., Mlisana, K., Luban, J., Walker, B.D., Karim, S.S., Brass, A.L., Ndung'u, T. & CAPRISA Acute Infection Study Team 2011, Association of TRIM22 with the type 1 interferon response and viral control during primary HIV-1 infection, *Journal of virology,* vol. 85, no. 1, pp. 208-216.

Skasko, M., Tokarev, A., Chen, C.C., Fischer, W.B., Pillai, S.K. & Guatelli, J. 2011, BST-2 is rapidly down-regulated from the cell surface by the HIV-1 protein Vpu: evidence for a post-ER mechanism of Vpu-action, *Virology,* vol. 411, no. 1, pp. 65-77.

Sokolskaja, E. & Luban, J. 2006, Cyclophilin, TRIM5, and innate immunity to HIV-1, *Curr Opin Microbiol,* vol. 9, no. 4, pp. 404-408.

Soumelis, V., Scott, I., Gheyas, F., Bouhour, D., Cozon, G., Cotte, L., Huang, L., Levy, J.A. & Liu, Y.J. 2001, Depletion of circulating natural type 1 interferon-producing cells in HIV-infected AIDS patients, *Blood,* vol. 98, no. 4, pp. 906-912.

Stenglein, M.D. & Harris, R.S. 2006, APOBEC3B and APOBEC3F inhibit L1 retrotransposition by a DNA deamination-independent mechanism, *The Journal of biological chemistry,* vol. 281, no. 25, pp. 16837-16841.

Strack, B., Calistri, A., Craig, S., Popova, E. & Gottlinger, H.G. 2003, AIP1/ALIX is a binding partner for HIV-1 p6 and EIAV p9 functioning in virus budding, *Cell,* vol. 114, no. 6, pp. 689-699.

Stremlau, M., Perron, M., Lee, M., Li, Y., Song, B., Javanbakht, H., Diaz-Griffero, F., Anderson, D.J., Sundquist, W.I. & Sodroski, J. 2006, Specific recognition and accelerated uncoating of retroviral capsids by the TRIM5alpha restriction factor, *Proc Natl Acad Sci U S A,* vol. 103, no. 14, pp. 5514-5519.

Stremlau, M., Owens, C.M., Perron, M.J., Kiessling, M., Autissier, P. & Sodroski, J. 2004, The cytoplasmic body component TRIM5alpha restricts HIV-1 infection in Old World monkeys, *Nature,* vol. 427, pp. 848-853.

Su, Y., Popik, W. & Pitha, P.M. 1995, Inhibition of human immunodeficiency virus type 1 replication by a Tat-activated, transduced interferon gene: targeted expression to human immunodeficiency virus type 1-infected cells, *Journal of virology,* vol. 69, no. 1, pp. 110-121.

Tavel, J.A., Huang, C.Y., Shen, J., Metcalf, J.A., Dewar, R., Shah, A., Vasudevachari, M.B., Follmann, D.A., Herpin, B., Davey, R.T., Polis, M.A., Kovacs, J., Masur, H. & Lane, H.C. 2010, Interferon-alpha produces significant decreases in HIV load, *Journal of interferon & cytokine research : the official journal of the International Society for Interferon and Cytokine Research,* vol. 30, no. 7, pp. 461-464.

Terwilliger, E.F., Cohen, E.A., Lu, Y.C., Sodroski, J.G. & Haseltine, W.A. 1989, Functional role of human immunodeficiency virus type 1 vpu, *Proceedings of the National Academy of Sciences of the United States of America,* vol. 86, no. 13, pp. 5163-5167.

Thali, M., Bukovsky, A., Kondo, E., Rosenwirth, B., Walsh, C.T., Sodroski, J. & Gottlinger, H.G. 1994, Functional association of cyclophilin A with HIV-1 virions, *Nature*, vol. 372, pp. 363-365.

Tian, C., Yu, X., Zhang, W., Wang, T., Xu, R. & Yu, X.F. 2006, Differential requirement for conserved tryptophans in human immunodeficiency virus type 1 Vif for the selective suppression of APOBEC3G and APOBEC3F, *Journal of virology*, vol. 80, no. 6, pp. 3112-3115.

Tissot, C. & Mechti, N. 1995, Molecular cloning of a new interferon-induced factor that represses human immunodeficiency virus type 1 long terminal repeat expression, *J Biol Chem*, vol. 270, no. 25, pp. 14891-14898.

Turelli, P., Mangeat, B., Jost, S., Vianin, S. & Trono, D. 2004, Inhibition of hepatitis B virus replication by APOBEC3G, *Science (New York, N.Y.)*, vol. 303, no. 5665, pp. 1829.

Ulenga, N.K., Sarr, A.D., Hamel, D., Sankale, J.L., Mboup, S. & Kanki, P.J. 2008, The level of APOBEC3G (hA3G)-related G-to-A mutations does not correlate with viral load in HIV type 1-infected individuals, *AIDS Research and Human Retroviruses*, vol. 24, no. 10, pp. 1285-1290.

Urnov, F.D., Rebar, E.J., Holmes, M.C., Zhang, H.S. & Gregory, P.D. 2010, Genome editing with engineered zinc finger nucleases, *Nature reviews.Genetics*, vol. 11, no. 9, pp. 636-646.

Urnov, F.D., Miller, J.C., Lee, Y.L., Beausejour, C.M., Rock, J.M., Augustus, S., Jamieson, A.C., Porteus, M.H., Gregory, P.D. & Holmes, M.C. 2005, Highly efficient endogenous human gene correction using designed zinc-finger nucleases, *Nature*, vol. 435, no. 7042, pp. 646-651.

Usami, Y., Popov, S., Popova, E., Inoue, M., Weissenhorn, W. & G Gottlinger, H. 2009, The ESCRT pathway and HIV-1 budding, *Biochemical Society transactions*, vol. 37, no. Pt 1, pp. 181-184.

Valcke, H.S., Bernard, N.F., Bruneau, J., Alary, M., Tsoukas, C.M. & Roger, M. 2006, APOBEC3G genetic variants and their association with risk of HIV infection in highly exposed Caucasians, *AIDS (London, England)*, vol. 20, no. 15, pp. 1984-1986.

Van Damme, N., Goff, D., Katsura, C., Jorgenson, R.L., Mitchell, R., Johnson, M.C., Stephens, E.B. & Guatelli, J. 2008, The interferon-induced protein BST-2 restricts HIV-1 release and is downregulated from the cell surface by the viral Vpu protein, *Cell host & microbe*, vol. 3, no. 4, pp. 245-252.

van Manen, D., Rits, M.A., Beugeling, C., van Dort, K., Schuitemaker, H. & Kootstra, N.A. 2008, The effect of Trim5 polymorphisms on the clinical course of HIV-1 infection, *PLoS pathogens*, vol. 4, no. 2, pp. e18.

Varthakavi, V., Smith, R.M., Bour, S.P., Strebel, K. & Spearman, P. 2003, Viral protein U counteracts a human host cell restriction that inhibits HIV-1 particle production, *Proceedings of the National Academy of Sciences of the United States of America*, vol. 100, no. 25, pp. 15154-15159.

Vazquez-Perez, J.A., Ormsby, C.E., Hernandez-Juan, R., Torres, K.J. & Reyes-Teran, G. 2009, APOBEC3G mRNA expression in exposed seronegative and early stage HIV infected individuals decreases with removal of exposure and with disease progression, *Retrovirology*, vol. 6, pp. 23.

VerPlank, L., Bouamr, F., LaGrassa, T.J., Agresta, B., Kikonyogo, A., Leis, J. & Carter, C.A. 2001, Tsg101, a homologue of ubiquitin-conjugating (E2) enzymes, binds the L domain in HIV type 1 Pr55(Gag), *Proc Natl Acad Sci U S A,* vol. 98, no. 1421332273, pp. 7724-779.

Vigan, R. & Neil, S.J. 2010, Determinants of tetherin antagonism in the transmembrane domain of the human immunodeficiency virus type 1 Vpu protein, *Journal of virology,* vol. 84, no. 24, pp. 12958-12970.

Vyas, T.K., Shah, L. & Amiji, M.M. 2006, Nanoparticulate drug carriers for delivery of HIV/AIDS therapy to viral reservoir sites, *Expert opinion on drug delivery,* vol. 3, no. 5, pp. 613-628.

Wang, B., Mikhail, M., Dyer, W.B., Zaunders, J.J., Kelleher, A.D. & Saksena, N.K. 2003, First demonstration of a lack of viral sequence evolution in a nonprogressor, defining replication-incompetent HIV-1 infection, *Virology,* vol. 312, no. 1, pp. 135-150.

Whitehead, K.A., Langer, R. & Anderson, D.G. 2009, Knocking down barriers: advances in siRNA delivery, *Nature reviews.Drug discovery,* vol. 8, no. 2, pp. 129-138.

Williams, R.L. & Urbe, S. 2007, The emerging shape of the ESCRT machinery, *Nature reviews.Molecular cell biology,* vol. 8, no. 5, pp. 355-368.

Woo, J.S., Imm, J.H., Min, C.K., Kim, K.J., Cha, S.S. & Oh, B.H. 2006, Structural and functional insights into the B30.2/SPRY domain, *The EMBO journal,* vol. 25, no. 6, pp. 1353-1363.

Yamashita, T., Kamada, K., Hatcho, K., Adachi, A. & Nomaguchi, M. 2008, Identification of amino acid residues in HIV-1 Vif critical for binding and exclusion of APOBEC3G/F, *Microbes and infection / Institut Pasteur,* vol. 10, no. 10-11, pp. 1142-1149.

Yang, B., Chen, K., Zhang, C., Huang, S. & Zhang, H. 2007, Virion-associated uracil DNA glycosylase-2 and apurinic/apyrimidinic endonuclease are involved in the degradation of APOBEC3G-edited nascent HIV-1 DNA, *The Journal of biological chemistry,* vol. 282, no. 16, pp. 11667-11675.

Yao, S., Liu, M.S., Masters, S.L., Zhang, J.G., Babon, J.J., Nicola, N.A., Nicholson, S.E. & Norton, R.S. 2006, Dynamics of the SPRY domain-containing SOCS box protein 2: flexibility of key functional loops, *Protein science : a publication of the Protein Society,* vol. 15, no. 12, pp. 2761-2772.

Yap, M.W., Nisole, S. & Stoye, J.P. 2005, A single amino acid change in the SPRY domain of human Trim5alpha leads to HIV-1 restriction, *Curr Biol,* vol. 15, no. 1, pp. 73-78.

Yu, X., Yu, Y., Liu, B., Luo, K., Kong, W., Mao, P. & Yu, X.F. 2003, Induction of APOBEC3G ubiquitination and degradation by an HIV-1 Vif-Cul5-SCF complex, *Science (New York, N.Y.),* vol. 302, no. 5647, pp. 1056-1060.

7

Retroviral Host Cell Factors: TRIM5, APOBEC3G and Cyclophilins

Ryuta Sakuma and Hiroaki Takeuchi
Department of Molecular Virology, Tokyo Medical and Dental University, Japan

1. Introduction

The conventional innate and adaptive immune systems are very effective at viral infections. However, for retroviral infections, there is another immune system that can recognize at multiple levels e.g. expression of internal host factors with antiviral activity. This is a component of viral recognition and subsequent restriction that has been called "intrinsic immunity"(Bieniasz, 2004). Intrinsic immunity can distinguish from innate and adaptive immunity, and it does not need to be induced by viral infections. Retrovirus replication has many steps in common with other retroviruses. Upon entry into the cytoplasm of target cells, some host factors are required for efficient retroviral replication cycle, and others act as restriction factors that block reverse transcription and ligation of viral cDNA to chromosomal DNA. Recently, several host factors have been identified such as the proline isomerase cyclophilin A (CypA), ApoB mRNA editing catalytic subunit (APOBEC) and tripartite motif protein 5 alpha (TRIM5α) against retrovirus infection. This review will focus on how these host factors modulate retroviral activity. It will then present our current understanding of the mechanism that may explain zoonotic transmission of retroviruses.

1.1 Fv1 and Fv4: Restriction factors that block infection by Friend-MLV in murine cells

The most intensively studied anti-cellular gene is Friend virus susceptibility (Fv) gene in laboratory mice. Fv1 and Fv4 were of special interest in Fv alleles because cultured murine cells containing them were resistant to infection by Friend murine leukemia virus (MLV)(Gardner et al., 1980; Hartley et al., 1970; Pincus et al., 1971; Rasheed and Gardner, 1983; Suzuki, 1975). Fv1-mediated restriction of MLV, for instance, is a well-studied representative of a class of restriction factors that act after membrane fusion, are highly virus-specific (Goff, 2004). Fv1 has two alleles, $Fv1^n$ and $Fv1^b$, targeting B- and N-tropic MLV, respectively (Rein et al., 1976). Fv4 was shown to encode an ecotropic MLV-like *env* gene and recent report showed that Fv4 inhibits infection by exerting dominant negative effect on MLV Env (Takeda and Matano, 2007). Although the precise mechanism of Fv1 restriction remains unclear, the important point is that the viral determinants for this type of restriction have been mapped to the capsid protein (MLV amino acid 110) and as a target of host factors that can modulate retroviral life cycle (Gautsch et al., 1978; Kozak and Chakraborti, 1996).

1.2 Ref1 and Lv1: Fv1-type restriction factors in human or primate cells

A host factor that belongs to the same category of Fv1-type restriction factors is Ref1 (restriction factor 1). Ref1 is expressed in human and other non-murine cells and imposes a similar restriction of Fv1 that is controlled by relationship between the same capsid residue (MLV CA 110) and Fv1 (Towers et al., 2000). The difference between Ref1 and Fv1 function is that Ref1 restricts retroviral replication at a step prior to reverse transcription while Fv1 seems to impose a post-reverse transcription block (Goff, 2004). Another restriction factor, lentivirus susceptibility factor 1 (Lv1), was found to be responsible for restricting HIV-1 and N-tropic MLV but not rhesus macaque simian immunodeficiency virus (SIVmac) replication in Old World monkey cells (Besnier et al., 2002; Cowan et al., 2002; Munk et al., 2002).

1.3 TRIM5α: Fv1-type host factor restricting HIV-1 in primate cells

Recently, the host protein which dictates Ref1 activity was identified as an α-isoform of rhesus macaque TRIM5α protein by the laboratory of Dr. Joseph Sodroski (Stremlau et al., 2004). TRIM5 is a member of the tripartite motif (TRIM) family of proteins, and has RING, B-box 2 and coiled-coil as common and conserved domains among the family and B30.2(PRYSPRY) domain on its c-terminal region (Nisole et al., 2005). Subsequently, the human and non-human primates homologues of TRIM5α were shown to explain restriction activity against retroviruses, N-MLV, and equine anemia virus (Hatziioannou et al., 2004b; Keckesova et al., 2004; Perron et al., 2004; Si et al., 2006; Song et al., 2005; Yap et al., 2004; Ylinen et al., 2005). Rhesus monkey TRIM5α has strong anti-HIV-1 activity, only modest restriction against SIVmac, and does not block MLV infection, whereas its human homologue does not active against HIV-1 infection.

TRIM5α recognizes incoming viral core, but not a monomeric capsid protein, thorough its B30.2(PRYSPRY) domain. B-box2 and coiled-coil domains are required for TRIM5α multimerization, and both coiled-coil and B30.2(PRYSPRY) domains are essential for viral core binding (Reymond et al., 2001; Stremlau et al., 2006). TRIM5α captures HIV-1 core at a very early step(s) after infection, immediately after the release of core into cytoplasm. To restrict HIV-1 infection and to recognize viral core, TRIM5α must be oligomerized through its B-box 2 and coiled-coil domains. Its RING domain has E3 ubiqutin ligase activity, and self-ubiqutination is occurred, then TRIM5α is quickly degraded. This quick degradation of TRIM5α is not necessary for post-entry restriction, since replacement of TRIM5α RING domain with the corresponding domain of TRIM21 which has lower self-ubiqutination activity and longer half life than TRIM5α didn't alter the antiviral activity. When TRIM5α was over expressed, cytoplasmic body is formed, and the cytoplasmic body is supposed to be required for its antiviral activity. During TRIM5α-mediated post-entry restriction, disassembly of viral core is induced too quickly and the accumulation of viral RT-products is reduced. MG132 treatment inhibits to induce quick-disassembly, but still HIV-1 infectivity was restricted. Two reports showed that TRIM5α could block not only viral cDNA accumulation but also the nuclear import of viral cDNA (Berthoux et al., 2004; Wu et al., 2006). Thus TRIM5α-mediated post-entry restriction is thought to have at least two phases: (i) TRIM5α induces quick-disassembly of viral core in a proteasome dependent manner and (ii) TRIM5α degrades HIV-1 cDNAs in a proteasome independent manner. The determinant of specificity and magnitude of the post-entry restriction lies on B30.2(PRYSPRY) domain. Recently, Pacheco *et al.* reported that new world monkey TRIM5α restricts foamy virus infection (Pacheco et al., 2010). Another consideration is the clinical significance of TRIM5α against acquired immunodeficiency syndrome (AIDS) in human. Moreover several reports showed that the efficacy of TRIM5α-mediated suppression of HIV-1 replication might interfere with disease progression of AIDS in humans (Cagliani et al., 2010; van Manen et al., 2008). Thus, TRIM5α-mediated restriction may occur multi step in retrovirus replication with the relationship between other host factor(s).

Recently, the lab of Dr. Yasuhiro Ikeda reported that rhesus macaque TRIM5α also inhibits HIV-1 production by inducing the degradation of a viral precursor Gag protein (Sakuma et al., 2007). To restrict HIV-1 production, amino acid residues in B-box 2 and coiled-coil domains dictated the specificity of the restriction. In the late restriction, the accumulation of HIV-1 RNA was not affected but the accumulation of precursor Gag was inhibited in an ubiqutine-proteasome independent manner. This TRIM5α-mediated late-restriction is still controversial (Zhang et al., 2008), yet it is presumable that TRIM5α restricts HIV-1 infection and production in two distinct mechanisms. Although TRIM5α restricts HIV-1 infection in broad range of cells, its late restriction depends on a cell line (Sakuma et al., 2007).

Here is another notable class of the TRIM family called TRIM-Cyp isolated from new wold monkeys (NWM). A report from the laboratory of Dr. Jeremy Luban demonstrated that owl monkey has TRIM-Cyp that restricts HIV-1 infection (Sayah et al., 2004). Although TRIM-Cyp has a cyclophilin A sequence in its C-terminal region instead of B30.2(PRYSPRY) domain that dictates the specificity and the magnitude of post entry restriction in OWM-TRIM5α-mediated post-entry restriction, it recognizes incoming core structure and restricts HIV-1 infection (Stremlau et al., 2006). Recently, TRIM-Cyp mRNA was also detected in a rhesus macaque cell, and over-expressed rhesus TRIM-Cyp restricts HIV-1 infection and production (Brennan et al., 2008; Dietrich et al., 2010; Sakuma et al., 2010; Wilson et al., 2008).

Not like other restriction factors, the counter part of TRIM5α-mediated restrictions is not accessory gene product of HIV-1, and human TRIM5α has just a modest restriction activity. NWM cell doesn't have TRIM5α, yet even without B30.2(PRYSPRY), TRIM5-Cyp can be a defense against viral infection. These evidences suggest that TRIM5α could be a key molecule to explain the species-species barrier. And if so, TRIM5α's dual antiviral activities can block the viral transmission even from closer species like to human from monkeys.

1.4 APOBEC: Enzymatic restriction factor that target retroviruses

Replication of HIV-1 in primary CD4+ T cells, monocyte and some immortalized T cell lines depends on the presence of HIV-1 accessory gene product, Vif (stands for virus infectivity factor)(Fisher et al., 1987; Strebel et al., 1987), and it works in a host cell-specific manner. Vif is required for enhanced HIV-1 replication in some cell types called non-permissive cells, in contrast HIV-1 replication is Vif-independent in permissive cells (Akari et al., 1992; Blanc et al., 1993; Borman et al., 1995; Fan and Peden, 1992; Gabuzda et al., 1992; Sakai et al., 1993; von Schwedler et al., 1993). Recently, some cytidine deaminases were identified as a new class of host restriction factors that target retroviruses such as HIV-1 or SIV (Cullen, 2006; Harris and Liddament, 2004). APOBEC3G (Apo3G), a member of the APOBEC family of cytidine deaminases, is the first identified enzymatic restriction factor and the determinant that makes cells permissive or non-permissive. Unlike TRIM5α nor Fv1, Apo3G does not exert its antiviral activity by targeting the viral capsid protein, but it has to be incorporated into a newly synthesized virion during a production step, and then inhibits virus replication by targeting single-stranded viral cDNA during an infection step. HIV-1 counteracts Apo3G with Vif expression. During the production of progeny virions, Vif binds to Apo3G and induces Apo3G's proteosomal degradation, resulting in the decreased steady-state levels of human Apo3G (hApo3G) (Yu et al., 2003).

There are several antiretroviral mechanisms of Apo3G against HIV-1 infection. First, Apo3G-containing virus can be resulted in a large number substitution that register as cytidine (C) to thymine (T) in a virus minus-strand during reverse transcription, resulting guanine (G) to adenine (A) mutations in a viral plus strand, known as 'G to A hypermutaion'(Harris et al., 2003; Lecossier et al., 2003; Mangeat et al., 2003; Mariani et al., 2003; Yu et al., 2004; Zhang et al., 2003). Second, Apo3G can inhibit tRNA annealing or tRNA processing during reverse transcription (Guo et al., 2006; Guo et al., 2007; Mbisa et al., 2007). Third, Apo3G inhibits DNA strand transfer or integration (Li et al., 2007; Luo et al., 2007; Mbisa et al., 2007). Although Apo3G has the most potent anti-HIV-1 activity among the APOBEC family of proteins, another member of the family, APOBEC3F (Apo3F) was shown to inhibit HIV-1 infection in the absence of Vif (Bishop et al., 2004a; Liddament et al., 2004; Wiegand et al., 2004; Zheng et al., 2004), whereas APOBEC3B (Apo3B) can inhibit HIV-1 infection in both the presence and absence of Vif (Bishop et al., 2004a; Doehle et al., 2005; Rose et al., 2005).

Although we can imagine the broad range of antiretroviral activity of APOBEC family because APOBEC proteins from non-human species can also inhibit HIV-1 infection (Bishop et al., 2004a; Bishop et al., 2004b; Cullen, 2006; Mariani et al., 2003; Wiegand et al., 2004), the Vif-Apo3G interaction is thought to be species specific (Mariani et al., 2003; Simon et al., 1998). Accordingly, hApo3G is insensitive to SIVagm Vif while african green monkey Apo3G (agmApo3G) is insensitive to HIV-1 Vif and the determinant of this species specificity depends on amino acid 128 of hApo3G and agmApo3G (Bogerd et al., 2004; Mangeat et al., 2004; Mariani et al., 2003; Schrofelbauer et al., 2004; Xu et al., 2004). However, such species specificity is not strictly controlled, for example a report from the laboratory of Klaus Strebel demonstrated that SIVagm Vif supported replication of SIVagm virus in the hApo3G-positive human A3.01 T cell line. Replication of *vif*-defective SIVagm in A3.01 cells was severely restricted, resulted in an accumulation of cytidine deaminase-induced G-to-A mutations in SIVagm genome (Takeuchi et al., 2005). Therefore, it is probable that SIV Vif has evolved to counteract hApo3G restriction and this might contribute zoonotic transmission of SIV.

Although the antiviral activity of Apo3G is clearly correlated with its deaminase activity (Iwatani et al., 2006; Mangeat et al., 2003; Navarro et al., 2005; Opi et al., 2006; Shindo et al., 2003; Zhang et al., 2003), some members of APOBEC family have additional anti-retrovirus activities that do not require catalytically activity of itself (Li et al., 2007; Luo et al., 2007). In fact, several reports showed that deaminase-defective Apo3G and Apo3F have antiviral activity, and some antiviral-inactive mutants of both Apo3G and Apo3F have cytidine deaminase activity (Bishop et al., 2006; Holmes et al., 2007; Newman et al., 2005; Shindo et al., 2003).

However, deaminase-defective Apo3G mutant with C288S/C291A substitutions did not show any anti-viral actibity and over-expression of the mutant could work as a dominant negative agent of wild-type Apo3G, suggesting a tightly-relationship between antiviral and deaminase activities (Miyagi et al., 2007; Opi et al., 2006). Recently, it was demonstrated that hApo3G has an intrinsic immune effect on viral DNA synthesis, which may account for cytidine deaminase-independent antiviral activity of Apo3G, and did not abort replication steps following reverse transcription (Iwatani et al., 2007). Therefore, precise mechanism of Apo3G-dependent restriction of retroviral infection still remains unclear.

1.5 Cyclophilin A: positive factor against retrovirus replication (or restriction factor?)

Cyclophilins are ubiquitous proteins and first identified as the target of cyclosporine A (CsA), an immunosuppressive reagent (Takahashi et al., 1989). CypA has proline-isomerase activity that catalyzes the cis-trans isomerization of proline residue (Fischer et al., 1989). The binding of cyclosporine A to cyclophilin A inhibits this isomerase activity (Takahashi et al., 1989). In retrovirus replication, CypA was found to bind HIV-1 capsid (CA) in the yeast two-hybrid system (Luban et al., 1993). The sequence Ala88-Gly89-Pro90-Ile91 of CA protein is the major fragment bound to the active site of CypA (Franke et al., 1994; Gamble et al., 1996; Zhao et al., 1997). Interestingly, The peptidyl-prolyl bond between Gly89 and Pro90 of the CA fragment has a trans conformation, in contrast to the cis conformation observed in other known CypA-peptide complexes (Bosco et al., 2002; Zhao et al., 1997), and Gly89 preceding Pro90 has an unfavorable backbone formation usually only adopted by glycine, suggesting that special Gly89-Pro90 sequence but not other Gly-Pro motif is required for the binding of CA protein to CypA. Therefore, CypA might be likely to act as a molecular chaperone but not a cis-trans isomerase (Zhao et al., 1997). However, one report showed that CypA does not only bind CA protein but also catalyzes efficiently cic-trans isomerization of Gly89-Pro90 peptidyl-prolyl bond (Bosco et al., 2002). The relationship between the Gly89-Pro90 bond and catalysis of cis-trans isomerization by CypA still remain unclear.

It has been well established that CypA promotes an early step of HIV-1 infection in human cells (Braaten et al., 1996a; Braaten et al., 1996c; Braaten and Luban, 2001; Franke and Luban, 1996; Franke et al., 1994; Hatziioannou et al., 2005; Sokolskaja et al., 2004; Thali et al., 1994). CypA is efficiently encapsidated into HIV-1 produced from infected cells through interaction with the CA domains of the Gag polyprotein and disruption of CypA incorporation into virions by CsA or HIV-1 Gag mutants caused a decrease in replication efficiency (Ackerson et al., 1998; Braaten et al., 1996a; Braaten and Luban, 2001; Bukovsky et al., 1997; Franke et al., 1994; Ott et al., 1995; Thali et al., 1994). It is still unclear how CypA is efficiently packaged into HIV-1 virion, but several report showed that both dimerization of CA and multimerization of CypA is required for efficient binding each other (Colgan et al., 1996; Javanbakht et al., 2007). Although CA-CypA interaction is required for infectivity, the important point is that CypA interacts with incoming HIV-1 cores in newly target cells than occurring as core assemble during HIV-1 budding from the virion producer cells, indicated that target cell CypA promotes HIV-1 infectivity (Kootstra et al., 2003; Sokolskaja et al., 2004; Towers et al., 2003).

CypA-dependent virus replication is only limited the retroviruses which encode CA that binds CypA. In fact, only those retroviruses are dependent upon CypA for replication (Braaten et al., 1996c; Franke and Luban, 1996; Franke et al., 1994; Luban et al., 1993; Thali et al., 1994). These observations suggested that CA-CypA interaction might contribute tropism determinants for retroviruses. HIV-1 infection in non-human primate cells inhibits prior to reverse transcription after virus entry (Besnier et al., 2002; Cowan et al., 2002; Hatziioannou et al., 2003; Himathongkham and Luciw, 1996; Hofmann et al., 1999; Munk et al., 2002; Shibata et al., 1995; Towers et al., 2003). This restriction is thought to be the same step in the retrovirus life cycle where CypA works (Braaten et al., 1996b). Indeed, Analysis of CypA-binding region of CA with chimeric viruses of HIV-1 and SIV showed the viral determinant for species-specificity (Berthoux et al., 2004; Bukovsky et al., 1997; Cowan et al., 2002;

Dorfman and Gottlinger, 1996; Hatziioannou et al., 2004a; Hatziioannou et al., 2006; Ikeda et al., 2004; Kamada et al., 2006; Kootstra et al., 2003; Owens et al., 2004; Owens et al., 2003; Sayah et al., 2004; Shibata et al., 1991; Shibata et al., 1995; Stremlau et al., 2004; Towers et al., 2003).

Human CypA is required for efficient HIV-1 infection but not SIV. There is no known role for CypA in SIV infection in human cells. Recently, the first report from the laboratory of Klaus Strebel showed that human CypA acts as restriction factor against SIV infection in human cells, and SIV Vif counteracts a CypA-imposed inhibition against SIV infection with exclusion of CypA from SIV vision (Takeuchi et al., 2007). This phenomenon could distinguish from the function of SIV Vif against hApo3G previously reported from same laboratory (Takeuchi et al., 2005) because they used human cells lacking detectable deaminase activity. This observation raised the possibility that SIV Vif is crucial for zoonotic transmission of SIV from monkey to human.

2. Conclusion

Viral replication requires a lot of host cell factors, whose species specificity may affect viral tropism. On the other hand, there exist host factors that restrict viral replication. The anti-viral system mediated by some of these restriction factors, termed intrinsic immunity, which is distinguished from the conventional innate and adaptive immunity has been indicated to play an important role in making species-specific barriers against viral infection. As discussed in this chapter, we describe the current progress in understanding of such restriction factors against retroviral replication, especially focusing on TRIM5α and APOBEC whose anti-retroviral effects have recently been recognized. Additionally, we mentioned CypA that is essential for HIV-1 replication in human cells and may affect viral tropism. Understanding of these host factors would contribute to identification of the determinants for viral tropism. Finally, understanding of the factors mediating intrinsic immunity may lead to the development of antiviral agents that can boost their potency and thereby lead to treatments for viral disease.

3. References

Ackerson, B., Rey, O., Canon, J., and Krogstad, P. (1998). Cells with high cyclophilin A content support replication of human immunodeficiency virus type 1 Gag mutants with decreased ability to incorporate cyclophilin A. *Journal of virology 72*, 303-308.

Akari, H., Sakuragi, J., Takebe, Y., Tomonaga, K., Kawamura, M., Fukasawa, M., Miura, T., Shinjo, T., and Hayami, M. (1992). Biological characterization of human immunodeficiency virus type 1 and type 2 mutants in human peripheral blood mononuclear cells. *Archives of virology 123*, 157-167.

Berthoux, L., Sebastian, S., Sokolskaja, E., and Luban, J. (2004). Lv1 inhibition of human immunodeficiency virus type 1 is counteracted by factors that stimulate synthesis or nuclear translocation of viral cDNA. *Journal of virology 78*, 11739-11750.

Besnier, C., Takeuchi, Y., and Towers, G. (2002). Restriction of lentivirus in monkeys. *Proceedings of the National Academy of Sciences of the United States of America 99*, 11920-11925.

Bieniasz, P.D. (2004). Intrinsic immunity: a front-line defense against viral attack. *Nature immunology 5*, 1109-1115.

Bishop, K.N., Holmes, R.K., and Malim, M.H. (2006). Antiviral potency of APOBEC proteins does not correlate with cytidine deamination. *Journal of virology 80*, 8450-8458.

Bishop, K.N., Holmes, R.K., Sheehy, A.M., Davidson, N.O., Cho, S.J., and Malim, M.H. (2004a). Cytidine deamination of retroviral DNA by diverse APOBEC proteins. *Curr Biol 14*, 1392-1396.

Bishop, K.N., Holmes, R.K., Sheehy, A.M., and Malim, M.H. (2004b). APOBEC-mediated editing of viral RNA. *Science* (New York, NY *305*, 645.

Blanc, D., Patience, C., Schulz, T.F., Weiss, R., and Spire, B. (1993). Transcomplementation of VIF- HIV-1 mutants in CEM cells suggests that VIF affects late steps of the viral life cycle. *Virology 193*, 186-192.

Bogerd, H.P., Doehle, B.P., Wiegand, H.L., and Cullen, B.R. (2004). A single amino acid difference in the host APOBEC3G protein controls the primate species specificity of HIV type 1 virion infectivity factor. *Proceedings of the National Academy of Sciences of the United States of America 101*, 3770-3774.

Borman, A.M., Quillent, C., Charneau, P., Dauguet, C., and Clavel, F. (1995). Human immunodeficiency virus type 1 Vif- mutant particles from restrictive cells: role of Vif in correct particle assembly and infectivity. *Journal of virology 69*, 2058-2067.

Bosco, D.A., Eisenmesser, E.Z., Pochapsky, S., Sundquist, W.I., and Kern, D. (2002). Catalysis of cis/trans isomerization in native HIV-1 capsid by human cyclophilin A. *Proceedings of the National Academy of Sciences of the United States of America 99*, 5247-5252.

Braaten, D., Aberham, C., Franke, E.K., Yin, L., Phares, W., and Luban, J. (1996a). Cyclosporine A-resistant human immunodeficiency virus type 1 mutants demonstrate that Gag encodes the functional target of cyclophilin A. *Journal of virology 70*, 5170-5176.

Braaten, D., Franke, E.K., and Luban, J. (1996b). Cyclophilin A is required for an early step in the life cycle of human immunodeficiency virus type 1 before the initiation of reverse transcription. *Journal of virology 70*, 3551-3560.

Braaten, D., Franke, E.K., and Luban, J. (1996c). Cyclophilin A is required for the replication of group M human immunodeficiency virus type 1 (HIV-1) and simian immunodeficiency virus SIV(CPZ)GAB but not group O HIV-1 or other primate immunodeficiency viruses. *Journal of virology 70*, 4220-4227.

Braaten, D., and Luban, J. (2001). Cyclophilin A regulates HIV-1 infectivity, as demonstrated by gene targeting in human T cells. *The EMBO journal 20*, 1300-1309.

Brennan, G., Kozyrev, Y., and Hu, S.L. (2008). TRIMCyp expression in Old World primates Macaca nemestrina and Macaca fascicularis. *Proceedings of the National Academy of Sciences of the United States of America 105*, 3569-3574.

Bukovsky, A.A., Weimann, A., Accola, M.A., and Gottlinger, H.G. (1997). Transfer of the HIV-1 cyclophilin-binding site to simian immunodeficiency virus from Macaca mulatta can confer both cyclosporin sensitivity and cyclosporin dependence. *Proceedings of the National Academy of Sciences of the United States of America 94*, 10943-10948.

Cagliani, R., Fumagalli, M., Biasin, M., Piacentini, L., Riva, S., Pozzoli, U., Bonaglia, M.C., Bresolin, N., Clerici, M., and Sironi, M. (2010). Long-term balancing selection maintains trans-specific polymorphisms in the human TRIM5 gene. *Hum Genet 128*, 577-588.

Colgan, J., Yuan, H.E., Franke, E.K., and Luban, J. (1996). Binding of the human immunodeficiency virus type 1 Gag polyprotein to cyclophilin A is mediated by the central region of capsid and requires Gag dimerization. *Journal of virology 70*, 4299-4310.

Cowan, S., Hatziioannou, T., Cunningham, T., Muesing, M.A., Gottlinger, H.G., and Bieniasz, P.D. (2002). Cellular inhibitors with Fv1-like activity restrict human and simian immunodeficiency virus tropism. *Proceedings of the National Academy of Sciences of the United States of America 99*, 11914-11919.

Cullen, B.R. (2006). Role and mechanism of action of the APOBEC3 family of antiretroviral resistance factors. *Journal of virology 80*, 1067-1076.

Dietrich, E.A., Jones-Engel, L., and Hu, S.L. (2010). Evolution of the antiretroviral restriction factor TRIMCyp in Old World primates. *PLoS One 5*, e14019.

Doehle, B.P., Schafer, A., and Cullen, B.R. (2005). Human APOBEC3B is a potent inhibitor of HIV-1 infectivity and is resistant to HIV-1 Vif. *Virology 339*, 281-288.

Dorfman, T., and Gottlinger, H.G. (1996). The human immunodeficiency virus type 1 capsid p2 domain confers sensitivity to the cyclophilin-binding drug SDZ NIM 811. *Journal of virology 70*, 5751-5757.

Fan, L., and Peden, K. (1992). Cell-free transmission of Vif mutants of HIV-1. Virology *190*, 19-29.

Fischer, G., Wittmann-Liebold, B., Lang, K., Kiefhaber, T., and Schmid, F.X. (1989). Cyclophilin and peptidyl-prolyl cis-trans isomerase are probably identical proteins. *Nature 337*, 476-478.

Fisher, A.G., Ensoli, B., Ivanoff, L., Chamberlain, M., Petteway, S., Ratner, L., Gallo, R.C., and Wong-Staal, F. (1987). The sor gene of HIV-1 is required for efficient virus transmission in vitro. *Science* (New York, NY *237*, 888-893.

Franke, E.K., and Luban, J. (1996). Inhibition of HIV-1 replication by cyclosporine A or related compounds correlates with the ability to disrupt the Gag-cyclophilin A interaction. *Virology 222*, 279-282.

Franke, E.K., Yuan, H.E., and Luban, J. (1994). Specific incorporation of cyclophilin A into HIV-1 virions. *Nature 372*, 359-362.

Gabuzda, D.H., Lawrence, K., Langhoff, E., Terwilliger, E., Dorfman, T., Haseltine, W.A., and Sodroski, J. (1992). Role of vif in replication of human immunodeficiency virus type 1 in CD4+ T lymphocytes. *Journal of virology 66*, 6489-6495.

Gamble, T.R., Vajdos, F.F., Yoo, S., Worthylake, D.K., Houseweart, M., Sundquist, W.I., and Hill, C.P. (1996). Crystal structure of human cyclophilin A bound to the amino-terminal domain of HIV-1 capsid. *Cell 87*, 1285-1294.

Gardner, M.B., Rasheed, S., Pal, B.K., Estes, J.D., and O'Brien, S.J. (1980). Akvr-1, a dominant murine leukemia virus restriction gene, is polymorphic in leukemia-prone wild mice. *Proceedings of the National Academy of Sciences of the United States of America 77*, 531-535.

Gautsch, J.W., Elder, J.H., Schindler, J., Jensen, F.C., and Lerner, R.A. (1978). Structural markers on core protein p30 of murine leukemia virus: functional correlation with Fv-1 tropism. *Proceedings of the National Academy of Sciences of the United States of America 75*, 4170-4174.

Goff, S.P. (2004). Genetic control of retrovirus susceptibility in mammalian cells. *Annual review of genetics 38*, 61-85.

Guo, F., Cen, S., Niu, M., Saadatmand, J., and Kleiman, L. (2006). Inhibition of formula-primed reverse transcription by human APOBEC3G during human immunodeficiency virus type 1 replication. *Journal of virology 80*, 11710-11722.

Guo, F., Cen, S., Niu, M., Yang, Y., Gorelick, R.J., and Kleiman, L. (2007). The interaction of APOBEC3G with human immunodeficiency virus type 1 nucleocapsid inhibits tRNA3Lys annealing to viral RNA. *Journal of virology 81*, 11322-11331.

Harris, R.S., Bishop, K.N., Sheehy, A.M., Craig, H.M., Petersen-Mahrt, S.K., Watt, I.N., Neuberger, M.S., and Malim, M.H. (2003). DNA deamination mediates innate immunity to retroviral infection. *Cell 113*, 803-809.

Harris, R.S., and Liddament, M.T. (2004). Retroviral restriction by APOBEC proteins. *Nat Rev Immunol 4*, 868-877.

Hartley, J.W., Rowe, W.P., and Huebner, R.J. (1970). Host-range restrictions of murine leukemia viruses in mouse embryo cell cultures. *Journal of virology 5*, 221-225.

Hatziioannou, T., Cowan, S., Goff, S.P., Bieniasz, P.D., and Towers, G.J. (2003). Restriction of multiple divergent retroviruses by Lv1 and Ref1. *The EMBO journal 22*, 385-394.

Hatziioannou, T., Cowan, S., Von Schwedler, U.K., Sundquist, W.I., and Bieniasz, P.D. (2004a). Species-specific tropism determinants in the human immunodeficiency virus type 1 capsid. *Journal of virology 78*, 6005-6012.

Hatziioannou, T., Perez-Caballero, D., Cowan, S., and Bieniasz, P.D. (2005). Cyclophilin interactions with incoming human immunodeficiency virus type 1 capsids with opposing effects on infectivity in human cells. *Journal of virology 79*, 176-183.

Hatziioannou, T., Perez-Caballero, D., Yang, A., Cowan, S., and Bieniasz, P.D. (2004b). Retrovirus resistance factors Ref1 and Lv1 are species-specific variants of TRIM5alpha. *Proceedings of the National Academy of Sciences of the United States of America 101*, 10774-10779.

Hatziioannou, T., Princiotta, M., Piatak, M., Jr., Yuan, F., Zhang, F., Lifson, J.D., and Bieniasz, P.D. (2006). Generation of simian-tropic HIV-1 by restriction factor evasion. *Science* (New York, NY *314*, 95.

Himathongkham, S., and Luciw, P.A. (1996). Restriction of HIV-1 (subtype B) replication at the entry step in rhesus macaque cells. *Virology 219*, 485-488.

Hofmann, W., Schubert, D., LaBonte, J., Munson, L., Gibson, S., Scammell, J., Ferrigno, P., and Sodroski, J. (1999). Species-specific, postentry barriers to primate immunodeficiency virus infection. *Journal of virology 73*, 10020-10028.

Holmes, R.K., Koning, F.A., Bishop, K.N., and Malim, M.H. (2007). APOBEC3F can inhibit the accumulation of HIV-1 reverse transcription products in the absence of hypermutation. Comparisons with APOBEC3G. *The Journal of biological chemistry 282*, 2587-2595.

Ikeda, Y., Ylinen, L.M., Kahar-Bador, M., and Towers, G.J. (2004). Influence of gag on human immunodeficiency virus type 1 species-specific tropism. *Journal of virology 78*, 11816-11822.

Iwatani, Y., Chan, D.S., Wang, F., Maynard, K.S., Sugiura, W., Gronenborn, A.M., Rouzina, I., Williams, M.C., Musier-Forsyth, K., and Levin, J.G. (2007). Deaminase-independent inhibition of HIV-1 reverse transcription by APOBEC3G. *Nucleic Acids Res.*

Iwatani, Y., Takeuchi, H., Strebel, K., and Levin, J.G. (2006). Biochemical activities of highly purified, catalytically active human APOBEC3G: correlation with antiviral effect. *Journal of virology 80,* 5992-6002.

Javanbakht, H., Diaz-Griffero, F., Yuan, W., Yeung, D.F., Li, X., Song, B., and Sodroski, J. (2007). The ability of multimerized cyclophilin A to restrict retrovirus infection. *Virology 367,* 19-29.

Kamada, K., Igarashi, T., Martin, M.A., Khamsri, B., Hatcho, K., Yamashita, T., Fujita, M., Uchiyama, T., and Adachi, A. (2006). Generation of HIV-1 derivatives that productively infect macaque monkey lymphoid cells. *Proceedings of the National Academy of Sciences of the United States of America 103,* 16959-16964.

Keckesova, Z., Ylinen, L.M., and Towers, G.J. (2004). The human and African green monkey TRIM5alpha genes encode Ref1 and Lv1 retroviral restriction factor activities. *Proceedings of the National Academy of Sciences of the United States of America 101,* 10780-10785.

Kootstra, N.A., Munk, C., Tonnu, N., Landau, N.R., and Verma, I.M. (2003). Abrogation of postentry restriction of HIV-1-based lentiviral vector transduction in simian cells. *Proceedings of the National Academy of Sciences of the United States of America 100,* 1298-1303.

Kozak, C.A., and Chakraborti, A. (1996). Single amino acid changes in the murine leukemia virus capsid protein gene define the target of Fv1 resistance. *Virology 225,* 300-305.

Lecossier, D., Bouchonnet, F., Clavel, F., and Hance, A.J. (2003). Hypermutation of HIV-1 DNA in the absence of the Vif protein. *Science* (New York, NY *300,* 1112.

Li, X.Y., Guo, F., Zhang, L., Kleiman, L., and Cen, S. (2007). APOBEC3G inhibits DNA strand transfer during HIV-1 reverse transcription. *The Journal of biological chemistry 282,* 32065-32074.

Liddament, M.T., Brown, W.L., Schumacher, A.J., and Harris, R.S. (2004). APOBEC3F properties and hypermutation preferences indicate activity against HIV-1 in vivo. *Curr Biol 14,* 1385-1391.

Luban, J., Bossolt, K.L., Franke, E.K., Kalpana, G.V., and Goff, S.P. (1993). Human immunodeficiency virus type 1 Gag protein binds to cyclophilins A and B. *Cell 73,* 1067-1078.

Luo, K., Wang, T., Liu, B., Tian, C., Xiao, Z., Kappes, J., and Yu, X.F. (2007). Cytidine deaminases APOBEC3G and APOBEC3F interact with human immunodeficiency virus type 1 integrase and inhibit proviral DNA formation. *Journal of virology 81,* 7238-7248.

Mangeat, B., Turelli, P., Caron, G., Friedli, M., Perrin, L., and Trono, D. (2003). Broad antiretroviral defence by human APOBEC3G through lethal editing of nascent reverse transcripts. *Nature 424,* 99-103.

Mangeat, B., Turelli, P., Liao, S., and Trono, D. (2004). A single amino acid determinant governs the species-specificsensitivity of APOBEC3G to Vif action. *The Journal of biological chemistry 279,* 14481-14483.

Mariani, R., Chen, D., Schrofelbauer, B., Navarro, F., Konig, R., Bollman, B., Munk, C., Nymark-McMahon, H., and Landau, N.R. (2003). Species-specific exclusion of APOBEC3G from HIV-1 virions by Vif. *Cell 114,* 21-31.

Mbisa, J.L., Barr, R., Thomas, J.A., Vandegraaff, N., Dorweiler, I.J., Svarovskaia, E.S., Brown, W.L., Mansky, L.M., Gorelick, R.J., Harris, R.S., *et al.* (2007). Human immunodeficiency virus type 1 cDNAs produced in the presence of APOBEC3G exhibit defects in plus-strand DNA transfer and integration. *Journal of virology 81*, 7099-7110.

Miyagi, E., Opi, S., Takeuchi, H., Khan, M., Goila-Gaur, R., Kao, S., and Strebel, K. (2007). Enzymatically active APOBEC3G is required for efficient inhibition of human immunodeficiency virus type 1. *Journal of virology 81*, 13346-13353.

Munk, C., Brandt, S.M., Lucero, G., and Landau, N.R. (2002). A dominant block to HIV-1 replication at reverse transcription in simian cells. *Proceedings of the National Academy of Sciences of the United States of America 99*, 13843-13848.

Navarro, F., Bollman, B., Chen, H., Konig, R., Yu, Q., Chiles, K., and Landau, N.R. (2005). Complementary function of the two catalytic domains of APOBEC3G. *Virology 333*, 374-386.

Newman, E.N., Holmes, R.K., Craig, H.M., Klein, K.C., Lingappa, J.R., Malim, M.H., and Sheehy, A.M. (2005). Antiviral function of APOBEC3G can be dissociated from cytidine deaminase activity. *Curr Biol 15*, 166-170.

Nisole, S., Stoye, J.P., and Saib, A. (2005). TRIM family proteins: retroviral restriction and antiviral defence. *Nature reviews 3*, 799-808.

Opi, S., Takeuchi, H., Kao, S., Khan, M.A., Miyagi, E., Goila-Gaur, R., Iwatani, Y., Levin, J.G., and Strebel, K. (2006). Monomeric APOBEC3G is catalytically active and has antiviral activity. *Journal of virology 80*, 4673-4682.

Ott, D.E., Coren, L.V., Johnson, D.G., Sowder, R.C., 2nd, Arthur, L.O., and Henderson, L.E. (1995). Analysis and localization of cyclophilin A found in the virions of human immunodeficiency virus type 1 MN strain. *AIDS research and human retroviruses 11*, 1003-1006.

Owens, C.M., Song, B., Perron, M.J., Yang, P.C., Stremlau, M., and Sodroski, J. (2004). Binding and susceptibility to postentry restriction factors in monkey cells are specified by distinct regions of the human immunodeficiency virus type 1 capsid. *Journal of virology 78*, 5423-5437.

Owens, C.M., Yang, P.C., Gottlinger, H., and Sodroski, J. (2003). Human and simian immunodeficiency virus capsid proteins are major viral determinants of early, postentry replication blocks in simian cells. *Journal of virology 77*, 726-731.

Pacheco, B., Finzi, A., McGee-Estrada, K., and Sodroski, J. (2010). Species-specific inhibition of foamy viruses from South American monkeys by New World Monkey TRIM5{alpha} proteins. *Journal of virology 84*, 4095-4099.

Perron, M.J., Stremlau, M., Song, B., Ulm, W., Mulligan, R.C., and Sodroski, J. (2004). TRIM5alpha mediates the postentry block to N-tropic murine leukemia viruses in human cells. *Proceedings of the National Academy of Sciences of the United States of America 101*, 11827-11832.

Pincus, T., Hartley, J.W., and Rowe, W.P. (1971). A major genetic locus affecting resistance to infection with murine leukemia viruses. I. Tissue culture studies of naturally occurring viruses. *The Journal of experimental medicine 133*, 1219-1233.

Rasheed, S., and Gardner, M.B. (1983). Resistance to fibroblasts and hematopoietic cells to ecotropic murine leukemia virus infection; an Akvr-1R gene effect. *International journal of cancer 31*, 491-496.

Rein, A., Kashmiri, S.V., Bassin, R.H., Gerwin, B.L., and Duran-Troise, G. (1976). Phenotypic mixing between N- and B-tropic murine leukemia viruses: infectious particles with dual sensitivity to Fv-1 restriction. *Cell 7,* 373-379.

Reymond, A., Meroni, G., Fantozzi, A., Merla, G., Cairo, S., Luzi, L., Riganelli, D., Zanaria, E., Messali, S., Cainarca, S., *et al.* (2001). The tripartite motif family identifies cell compartments. *The EMBO journal 20,* 2140-2151.

Rose, K.M., Marin, M., Kozak, S.L., and Kabat, D. (2005). Regulated production and anti-HIV type 1 activities of cytidine deaminases APOBEC3B, 3F, and 3G. *AIDS research and human retroviruses 21,* 611-619.

Sakai, H., Shibata, R., Sakuragi, J., Sakuragi, S., Kawamura, M., and Adachi, A. (1993). Cell-dependent requirement of human immunodeficiency virus type 1 Vif protein for maturation of virus particles. *Journal of virology 67,* 1663-1666.

Sakuma, R., Noser, J.A., Ohmine, S., and Ikeda, Y. (2007). Rhesus monkey TRIM5alpha restricts HIV-1 production through rapid degradation of viral Gag polyproteins. *Nature medicine 13,* 631-635.

Sakuma, R., Ohmine, S., and Ikeda, Y. (2010). Determinants for the rhesus monkey TRIM5alpha-mediated block of the late phase of HIV-1 replication. *The Journal of biological chemistry 285,* 3784-3793.

Sayah, D.M., Sokolskaja, E., Berthoux, L., and Luban, J. (2004). Cyclophilin A retrotransposition into TRIM5 explains owl monkey resistance to HIV-1. *Nature 430,* 569-573.

Schrofelbauer, B., Chen, D., and Landau, N.R. (2004). A single amino acid of APOBEC3G controls its species-specific interaction with virion infectivity factor (Vif). *Proceedings of the National Academy of Sciences of the United States of America 101,* 3927-3932.

Shibata, R., Kawamura, M., Sakai, H., Hayami, M., Ishimoto, A., and Adachi, A. (1991). Generation of a chimeric human and simian immunodeficiency virus infectious to monkey peripheral blood mononuclear cells. *Journal of virology 65,* 3514-3520.

Shibata, R., Sakai, H., Kawamura, M., Tokunaga, K., and Adachi, A. (1995). Early replication block of human immunodeficiency virus type 1 in monkey cells. *The Journal of general virology 76 (Pt 11),* 2723-2730.

Shindo, K., Takaori-Kondo, A., Kobayashi, M., Abudu, A., Fukunaga, K., and Uchiyama, T. (2003). The enzymatic activity of CEM15/Apobec-3G is essential for the regulation of the infectivity of HIV-1 virion but not a sole determinant of its antiviral activity. *The Journal of biological chemistry 278,* 44412-44416.

Si, Z., Vandegraaff, N., O'Huigin, C., Song, B., Yuan, W., Xu, C., Perron, M., Li, X., Marasco, W.A., Engelman, A., *et al.* (2006). Evolution of a cytoplasmic tripartite motif (TRIM) protein in cows that restricts retroviral infection. *Proceedings of the National Academy of Sciences of the United States of America 103,* 7454-7459.

Simon, J.H., Miller, D.L., Fouchier, R.A., Soares, M.A., Peden, K.W., and Malim, M.H. (1998). The regulation of primate immunodeficiency virus infectivity by Vif is cell species restricted: a role for Vif in determining virus host range and cross-species transmission. *The EMBO journal 17,* 1259-1267.

Sokolskaja, E., Sayah, D.M., and Luban, J. (2004). Target cell cyclophilin A modulates human immunodeficiency virus type 1 infectivity. *Journal of virology 78,* 12800-12808.

Song, B., Javanbakht, H., Perron, M., Park, D.H., Stremlau, M., and Sodroski, J. (2005). Retrovirus restriction by TRIM5alpha variants from Old World and New World primates. *Journal of virology 79*, 3930-3937.

Strebel, K., Daugherty, D., Clouse, K., Cohen, D., Folks, T., and Martin, M.A. (1987). The HIV 'A' (sor) gene product is essential for virus infectivity. *Nature 328*, 728-730.

Stremlau, M., Owens, C.M., Perron, M.J., Kiessling, M., Autissier, P., and Sodroski, J. (2004). The cytoplasmic body component TRIM5alpha restricts HIV-1 infection in Old World monkeys. *Nature 427*, 848-853.

Stremlau, M., Perron, M., Lee, M., Li, Y., Song, B., Javanbakht, H., Diaz-Griffero, F., Anderson, D.J., Sundquist, W.I., and Sodroski, J. (2006). Specific recognition and accelerated uncoating of retroviral capsids by the TRIM5alpha restriction factor. *Proceedings of the National Academy of Sciences of the United States of America 103*, 5514-5519.

Suzuki, S. (1975). FV-4: a new gene affecting the splenomegaly induction by Friend leukemia virus. *The Japanese journal of experimental medicine 45*, 473-478.

Takahashi, N., Hayano, T., and Suzuki, M. (1989). Peptidyl-prolyl cis-trans isomerase is the cyclosporin A-binding protein cyclophilin. *Nature 337*, 473-475.

Takeda, A., and Matano, T. (2007). Inhibition of infectious murine leukemia virus production by Fv-4 env gene products exerting dominant negative effect on viral envelope glycoprotein. *Microbes Infect.*

Takeuchi, H., Buckler-White, A., Goila-Gaur, R., Miyagi, E., Khan, M.A., Opi, S., Kao, S., Sokolskaja, E., Pertel, T., Luban, J., *et al.* (2007). Vif counteracts a cyclophilin A-imposed inhibition of simian immunodeficiency viruses in human cells. *Journal of virology 81*, 8080-8090.

Takeuchi, H., Kao, S., Miyagi, E., Khan, M.A., Buckler-White, A., Plishka, R., and Strebel, K. (2005). Production of infectious SIVagm from human cells requires functional inactivation but not viral exclusion of human APOBEC3G. *The Journal of biological chemistry 280*, 375-382.

Thali, M., Bukovsky, A., Kondo, E., Rosenwirth, B., Walsh, C.T., Sodroski, J., and Gottlinger, H.G. (1994). Functional association of cyclophilin A with HIV-1 virions. *Nature 372*, 363-365.

Towers, G., Bock, M., Martin, S., Takeuchi, Y., Stoye, J.P., and Danos, O. (2000). A conserved mechanism of retrovirus restriction in mammals. *Proceedings of the National Academy of Sciences of the United States of America 97*, 12295-12299.

Towers, G.J., Hatziioannou, T., Cowan, S., Goff, S.P., Luban, J., and Bieniasz, P.D. (2003). Cyclophilin A modulates the sensitivity of HIV-1 to host restriction factors. *Nature medicine 9*, 1138-1143.

van Manen, D., Rits, M.A., Beugeling, C., van Dort, K., Schuitemaker, H., and Kootstra, N.A. (2008). The effect of Trim5 polymorphisms on the clinical course of HIV-1 infection. *PLoS Pathog 4*, e18.

von Schwedler, U., Song, J., Aiken, C., and Trono, D. (1993). Vif is crucial for human immunodeficiency virus type 1 proviral DNA synthesis in infected cells. *Journal of virology 67*, 4945-4955.

Wiegand, H.L., Doehle, B.P., Bogerd, H.P., and Cullen, B.R. (2004). A second human antiretroviral factor, APOBEC3F, is suppressed by the HIV-1 and HIV-2 Vif proteins. *The EMBO journal 23*, 2451-2458.

Wilson, S.J., Webb, B.L., Ylinen, L.M., Verschoor, E., Heeney, J.L., and Towers, G.J. (2008). Independent evolution of an antiviral TRIMCyp in rhesus macaques. *Proceedings of the National Academy of Sciences of the United States of America 105*, 3557-3562.

Wu, X., Anderson, J.L., Campbell, E.M., Joseph, A.M., and Hope, T.J. (2006). Proteasome inhibitors uncouple rhesus TRIM5alpha restriction of HIV-1 reverse transcription and infection. *Proceedings of the National Academy of Sciences of the United States of America 103*, 7465-7470.

Xu, H., Svarovskaia, E.S., Barr, R., Zhang, Y., Khan, M.A., Strebel, K., and Pathak, V.K. (2004). A single amino acid substitution in human APOBEC3G antiretroviral enzyme confers resistance to HIV-1 virion infectivity factor-induced depletion. *Proceedings of the National Academy of Sciences of the United States of America 101*, 5652-5657.

Yap, M.W., Nisole, S., Lynch, C., and Stoye, J.P. (2004). Trim5alpha protein restricts both HIV-1 and murine leukemia virus. *Proceedings of the National Academy of Sciences of the United States of America 101*, 10786-10791.

Ylinen, L.M., Keckesova, Z., Wilson, S.J., Ranasinghe, S., and Towers, G.J. (2005). Differential restriction of human immunodeficiency virus type 2 and simian immunodeficiency virus SIVmac by TRIM5alpha alleles. *Journal of virology 79*, 11580-11587.

Yu, Q., Konig, R., Pillai, S., Chiles, K., Kearney, M., Palmer, S., Richman, D., Coffin, J.M., and Landau, N.R. (2004). Single-strand specificity of APOBEC3G accounts for minus-strand deamination of the HIV genome. *Nature structural & molecular biology 11*, 435-442.

Yu, X., Yu, Y., Liu, B., Luo, K., Kong, W., Mao, P., and Yu, X.F. (2003). Induction of APOBEC3G ubiquitination and degradation by an HIV-1 Vif-Cul5-SCF complex. *Science* (New York, NY *302*, 1056-1060.

Zhang, F., Perez-Caballero, D., Hatziioannou, T., and Bieniasz, P.D. (2008). No effect of endogenous TRIM5alpha on HIV-1 production. *Nature medicine 14*, 235-236; *author reply* 236-238.

Zhang, H., Yang, B., Pomerantz, R.J., Zhang, C., Arunachalam, S.C., and Gao, L. (2003). The cytidine deaminase CEM15 induces hypermutation in newly synthesized HIV-1 DNA. *Nature 424*, 94-98.

Zhao, Y., Chen, Y., Schutkowski, M., Fischer, G., and Ke, H. (1997). Cyclophilin A complexed with a fragment of HIV-1 gag protein: insights into HIV-1 infectious activity. *Structure 5*, 139-146.

Zheng, Y.H., Irwin, D., Kurosu, T., Tokunaga, K., Sata, T., and Peterlin, B.M. (2004). Human APOBEC3F is another host factor that blocks human immunodeficiency virus type 1 replication. *Journal of virology 78*, 6073-6076.

Part 2

From the Laboratory to the Clinic: HIV and the Immune System

8

HIV Without AIDS: The Immunological Secrets of Natural Hosts

Zachary Ende, Michelle Bonkosky and Mirko Paiardini
Emory University, Atlanta,
USA

1. Introduction

Human Immunodeficiency Virus (HIV) infection causes Acquired Immune Deficiency Syndrome (AIDS), while its ape and monkey progenitor Simian Immunodeficiency Virus (SIV) does not cause AIDS in its nonhuman primate natural reservoir hosts. Astonishingly, AIDS is avoided despite findings in a number of these host primate species indicating they too harbor high levels of virus replication that kills off CD4 T cells. These primate species that are so called "natural hosts" of SIV, essentially have HIV without ever getting AIDS.

The elucidation of the exact mechanisms allowing natural SIV hosts to avoid disease progression may prove decisive in the battle to understand HIV pathogenesis for the purpose of preventative or curative HIV and AIDS therapy. Comparative studies in natural and nonnatural hosts of lentiviral infections (i.e. HIV or SIV) have defined essential distinguishing features, opening up new avenues for possible therapeutic and preventative intervention.

In this chapter, we will describe recent and past breakthroughs that come from comparing lentiviral infections in AIDS-free natural hosts, to immunocompromised nonnatural hosts. In addition, we will discuss how the knowledge derived from the study of natural hosts may inform the design of novel therapies and vaccine strategies for HIV-infected humans.

1.1 A brief history of HIV

The observation in the late '70s and early '80s of a previously unrecognized adult-onset immunodeficiency associated with Kaposi's sarcoma (a skin cancer now known to be caused by Herpes Virus 8) and *Pneumocystis carinii* (a yeast-like fungus now known as *Pneumocystis jiroveci*) pneumonia signaled the beginning of one of the most devastating tragedies of modern times: the AIDS epidemic. Early epidemiological hypotheses on the etiologic agent of this disease included sexually transmitted pathogens as well as toxic "street" drugs (Centers for Disease Control (CDC), 1982; Harris et al., 1983). During these early years, basic and clinical researchers alike began furiously searching for the causes of AIDS, which culminated in 1983 with the discovery of the Human Immunodeficiency Virus (Barre-Sinoussi et al., 1983).

A series of studies in molecular virology and epidemiology conducted in subsequent years have delineated both the timing and geographical origin of the AIDS pandemic. The African city of Kinshasa (formerly known as Leopoldville), in the Democratic Republic of the Congo, is the place where the oldest known HIV-infected samples were discovered in a lymph node biopsy from 1960 and a blood-plasma sample from 1959 (Paul M Sharp & Beatrice H Hahn, 2008). In 1998, Zhu et al. estimated that HIV-1 originated in the 1940's or early 1950's, and also proposed that the split between HIV-1 and HIV-2 must have occurred considerably earlier (T. Zhu et al., 1998). Ten years later, Worobey et al. proposed the origin of HIV-1 to be anywhere from 1884-1933, a range corresponding to the rise of urban populations in the Leopoldville/Kinshasa area (Worobey et al., 2008). Collectively, these observations and models have refuted the controversial speculation that experimental polio vaccine formulations from the 1950's were responsible for the AIDS epidemic (Worobey et al., 2004). Subsequent studies indicated that HIV infection in humans arose from cross-species transmission of viruses that naturally infect African nonhuman primates (NHP), which are referred to as natural hosts for SIV (P M Sharp & B H Hahn, 2010). The next section will describe the different African nonhuman primates infected with SIV, focusing on those that infected giving rise to HIV-1 and HIV-2.

1.2 Introduction to natural hosts

At least 40 monkey species in Africa have been found to be naturally infected with species-specific strains of SIVs, and usually with a high prevalence. In the vast majority of cases the virus is designated by a three-letter abbreviation of the infected nonhuman primates (NHP) species name to differentiate between SIV strains (VandeWoude and Apetrei, 2006). For example, SIVcpz is the virus isolated from chimpanzees (*Pan troglodytes*), SIVsmm from sooty mangabeys (*Cercocebus atys*), SIVmnd from mandrills (*Mandrillus sphinx*), SIVagm from African green monkeys (AGM), and so on. The viruses that infect the different species of AGM are named SIVagm.ver (Vervet monkey), SIVagm.gri (Grivet monkey), SIVagm.sab (Green monkey), SIVagm.tan (Tantalus monkey). Table 1 lists the different African nonhuman primates infected with SIV.

These natural hosts for SIV represent an extremely large reservoir of lentiviruses potentially infecting other species. Phylogenetic analyses revealed that there have been cross-species transmissions of divergent viral strains since the beginning of the evolution of primate lentiviruses (Courgnaud et al., 2003; Hirsch, Dapolito, Goeken, & Campbell, 1995; P M Sharp & B H Hahn, 2010). For instance, HIV-2 emerged from the west African natural host sooty mangabey (*Cercocebus atys*) in at least eight cross-species events into the human population (Wertheim & Worobey, 2009), while the origins of HIV-1 have been more controversial. Four HIV-1 lineages originating in chimpanzees have been independently transmitted across species to infect humans, though one or two may have come via gorillas (P M Sharp & B H Hahn, 2010; Takehisa & Miura, 2010). Most HIV-1 isolates resemble viruses found in a chimpanzee subspecies (*Pan troglodytes troglodytes*) native to areas in and around Cameroon, Gabon and Equatorial Guinea, including the areas around Kinshasa (Gao et al., 1999; P M Sharp & B H Hahn, 2010). HIV-1 group M, responsible for a suggested 98% of the global epidemic, as well as rare groups N and O, are endemic in the aforementioned areas. Hunting chimpanzees for food, which is thought to be the method of cross-species transmission is also common in this central African region (Gao et al., 1999). In addition, the SIVs that have been isolated from Asian macaques, the most commonly used primate model of HIV infection, appear to have been transmitted from captive sooty mangabeys (reviewed in I. Pandrea, Sodora, Silvestri, & Apetrei, 2008).

Genus	Species/subspecies	Virus
African green monkeys (*Chlorocebus*)	Vervet monkey (*C. pygerythrus*) Grivet monkey (*C. aethiops*) Green monkey (*C. sabaeus*) Tantalus monkey (*C. tantalus*)	SIVagm.ver SIVagm.gri SIVagm.sab SIVagm.tan
Black and white colobus (*Colobus*)	Manted guereza (*C. guereza*) Western red colobus (*Piliocolobus badius)* Olive colobus (*Procolobus verus)*	SIVcol SIVwrc SIVolc
Chimpanzee (*Pan*)	Western chimpanzee (*P. troglodytes troglodytes*) Eastern chimpanzee (*P. troglodytes schweinfirthii*)	SIVcpz.ptt SIVcpz.pts
Guenons (*Cercopithecus*)	Sykes' monkey (*C. mitis*) L'Hoest monkey (*C. lhoesti*) Sun-tailed monkey (*C. solatus*) De Brazza monkey (*C. neglectus*) Mona (*C. mona*) Mustached monkey (*C. cephus*)	SIVsyk SIVlhoest SIVsun SIVdeb SIVmon SIVmus
Lophocebus	Black mangabey (*Lophocebus aterrimus*)	SIVbkm
Mandrills (*Mandrillus*)	Mandrill (*M. sphinx*) Drill (*M. leucophaeus*)	SIVmnd/SIVmnd2 SIVdrl
Talapoins (*Miopithecus*)	Angolan talapoin (*M. talapoin*)	SIVtal
White-eyelid mangabeys (*Cercocebus*)	Sooty mangabey (*C. atys*) Red-capped mangabey (*C. torquatus*)	SIVsmm SIVrcm

Table 1. Natural SIV hosts (reviewed on (VandeWoude & Apetrei, 2006))

Most of the naturally occurring SIVs do not cause disease in their natural hosts (Paiardini, et al., 2009); however, they can be highly pathogenic when replicating in nonnatural hosts, such as rhesus macaques and humans. Wild chimpanzee studies of SIV prevalence and pathogenicity, made possible by testing stool samples, have recently demonstrated that SIV positive chimpanzees die at a faster rate than their uninfected counterparts –a 9.8-15.6-fold increased death hazard) (Keele et al., 2009). While searching for the age and origins of the chimpanzee SIV, a major breakthrough came when it was noticed that the 5′ region of the chimpanzee SIV genome closely matches that found in red-capped mangabeys (*Cercocebus torquatus*), but the 3′ end closely resembles SIVs found in greater spot-nosed (*Cercopithecus nictitans*), mustached (*Cercopithecus cephus*) and mona monkeys (*Cercopithecus mona*). Based on these findings, SIV_{cpz} is thought to be a recombination of viruses ancestral to those found in red-capped mangabeys, mona, spot-nosed and mustached monkeys (Paul M Sharp, Shaw, & Beatrice H Hahn, 2005). The data suggest that chimpanzees have not evolved along with their own SIV for very long, and may represent a necessary evolutionary stage for the virus to enable cross-species transmission into humans. In a recent study, Worobey et al. established that SIV is at least 32,000 years old, based on Bioko Island geography and SIV relatedness of the various African nonhuman primates on the island. The authors conclude

that humans may have had previous encounters with this virus over time, and that natural hosts that show low pathogenicity to SIV have arisen likely as "a consequence of long-term host-virus coevolution" (P M Sharp & B H Hahn, 2010; Worobey et al., 2010) .
As above mentioned, and in obvious contrast with HIV infection in humans, which almost invariably leads to AIDS if left untreated, SIV infection in natural African NHP hosts is typically non-progressive. The infected animals live an apparently normal lifespan, without experiencing any signs of illness whether in the wild or captivity (Paiardini ann rev med). The fact that HIV causes a deadly disease in humans while its simian counterparts are virtually non-pathogenic in their natural hosts remains one of the fundamental mysteries of modern medicine, and it is widely recognized that the elucidation of the exact mechanisms allowing natural SIV hosts to avoid disease progression may prove critical in terms of HIV pathogenesis, therapy, and vaccines. Over the past few years, comparative studies in natural and nonnatural hosts of lentiviral infections have shed light on a number of critical distinguishing features.

2. Immunology and virology of HIV and SIV infections

2.1 Viral loads

2.1.1 Nonnatural hosts for HIV and SIV infections

As previously noted, HIV and SIV infections in humans and Asian macaques were generated from cross-species transmissions of viruses that naturally infect nonhuman primates in Africa. These primate lentiviruses replicate very efficiently *in vivo*, with the vast majority of HIV-infected humans and SIV-infected Asian macaques showing approximately 10^8 virions per milliliter of plasma during the acute phase of infection (Picker, 2006) (figure 1). Tracking SIV-infected macaques has been and continues to be indispensible for our understanding of virus kinetics at all stages of infection and in key tissues (i.e. gut and lymph node). Information obtained early in the infection process when virus replication begins and the adaptive immune response is underway, is vital to our ability to rationally design effective treatment and preventative strategies.
As the infection advances into the chronic phase, viral load in plasma declines and stabilizes to its "set point" (figure 1). This stage is reached once the immune system develops antibodies in an attempt to fight the virus. The behavior of the virus at set point is characterized by three major factors: (i) viral load remains relatively stable for several years; (ii) individuals who have a higher set point level have faster progression to AIDS; and (iii) shortly before the development of clinical AIDS, viral load increases. Despite declining levels of viral replication from peak viremia to set point, other factors persist, such as generalized immune activation, that play important roles in damaging a progressively dysfunctional immune system.

2.1.2 Natural hosts for SIV infections

Worth noting is the point that both in the acute and chronic phases of infection, the levels of plasma viremia are similar in HIV-infected humans and SIV-infected natural hosts, such as sooty mangabeys and African green monkeys (figure 1) (Picker, 2006) . The implication of the data is clear and extremely important: the presence of a cytophatic virus that replicates at high levels is not sufficient, by itself, to induce AIDS. In other words, additional factors are required for disease progression in HIV-infected humans and SIV-infected rhesus macaques.

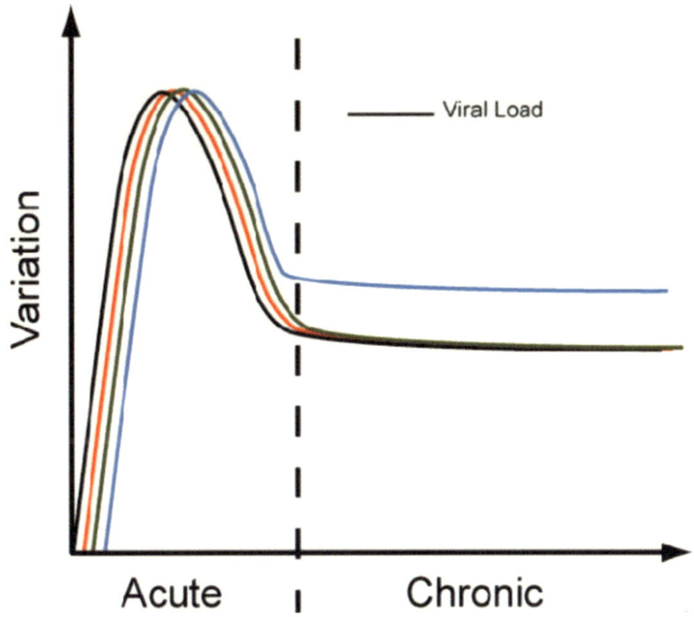

Fig. 1. Viral load in natural and nonnatural host species.
Natural host species (sooty mangabeys —, African green monkeys —) and nonnatural host species (humans —, rhesus macaques —) have similar levels of viremia in the acute and chronic phase of infection. Originally published in *Blood* Online. Brenchley JM & Paiardini M. Immunodeficiency lentiviral infections in natural and nonnatural hosts. *Blood*. Prepublished April 19, 2011; DOI:10.1182/blood-2010-12-325936.

2.2 CD4 T cell homeostasis

2.2.1 Nonnatural hosts for HIV and SIV infections

The depletion of CD4 T cells is the immunological hallmark of progressive HIV infection. The loss of circulating CD4 T cell numbers at levels below 200 cells/ml of blood coincides with onset of opportunistic infections. As such, a better understanding of the dynamics of CD4 T cell depletion is essential when studying the pathogenesis of HIV infection. Depletion of CD4 T cells from the peripheral blood is generally quite slow, with HIV-infected humans losing approximately 40 CD4 T cells per μl of blood per year during the chronic phase of infection (Moore, Keruly, Richman, Creagh-Kirk, & Chaisson, 1992).

The study of SIV-infected macaques has provided important information on the dynamics of CD4 T cell depletion, particularly in the early phase of infection and in anatomical locations difficult to study in HIV-infected humans. In particular, a series of influential studies have elucidated the early consequences of pathogenic HIV and SIV infections at the level of mucosal tissues, showing that the depletion of CD4 T cells is more rapid and severe at this site than in the peripheral blood or secondary lymphoid organs (figure 2) (Brenchley, Schacker, et al., 2004a; Douek, Mario Roederer, & Koup, 2009; Guadalupe et al., 2003; Haase, 2005; Mehandru et al., 2004; T Schneider et al., 1995; Veazey et al., 1998). Other observations underpin the reasons why the mucosal tissues undergo such stress: (i) the large majority of CD4 T cells located in the effector mucosal sites show a memory, activated, CCR5+

phenotype, (ii) the majority of newly transmitted HIV and SIV strains are CCR5-tropic, and (iii) primate lentiviruses preferentially infect activated CD4 T cells (Z. Zhang et al., 1999; Brenchley, Hill, et al., 2004b; Brenchley, Silvestri, & Douek, 2010; Veazey et al., 2000; Y . Zhang et al., 2000). As such, a large fraction of mucosal-resident CD4 T cells represent a highly susceptible target for virus replication, especially at a time when no antiviral adaptive immune response has yet been generated. Using the macaque SIV model, it was demonstrated that mucosal memory CD4+CCR5+ T cells are the earliest targets of the virus regardless of the route of infection (Veazey et al., 1998), and the majority (70-95%) of CD4 T cells in the jejunum, ileum, and colon are depleted in less than three weeks post infection (Li et al., 2005; Mattapallil et al., 2005). Due to the large surface area of the gastrointestinal (GI) tract, this severe loss of mucosal CD4 T cells during the acute phase of infection likely translates to depletion of most CD4 T cells within the body.

While there is a general consensus on the dramatic loss of mucosal CD4 T cells, the exact mechanisms accounting for this depletion are not completely clear, with evidence pointing in different directions. Direct virus-mediated killing of infected CD4 T cells is responsible for the earliest (within days of infection) loss of CD4 T cells (Mattapallil et al., 2005) and CD95-mediated activation induced cell death of uninfected bystander CD4 T cells (Li et al., 2005) accounts for the subsequent depletion (within weeks). Of note, recent studies comparing multiple GI sites have shown anatomic-specific differences in the extent of CD4 T cell loss in chronically SIV-infected rhesus macaques, with CD4 T cell depletion being more severe in the small intestine compared to the large intestine (L. D. Harris, Klatt, et al., 2010a). Due to the complexity of performing longitudinal mucosal collections and sampling multiple anatomic sites, similar comparative analysis has not, systematically, been performed in humans. Therefore it is debatable whether this phenomenon extends to HIV-infected individuals.

Based on these findings, a new model of AIDS pathogenesis has been proposed. That is to say, the early and complex dysfunction of the mucosal immune system induces a significant impairment of mucosal barrier integrity resulting in a series of pathogenic sequelae that become mostly apparent during chronic infection. The best characterized consequences of damage to the mucosal barrier are the translocation of microbial products from the intestinal lumen into systemic circulation, and the establishment of high levels of chronic immune activation. From this relatively new point of view, the depletion of CD4 T cells from mucosal tissues during acute HIV or SIV infection is a key determinant of disease progression [1, 49-52].

2.2.2 Natural hosts for SIV infection

One of the most peculiar features of natural hosts of SIV infection is their ability to preserve healthy levels of peripheral CD4 T cells, despite levels of plasma viremia similar or even higher than those described in HIV-infected individuals (Chakrabarti et al., 2000; Rey-Cuillé et al., 1998; Silvestri et al., 2003). For instance, approximately 90% of SIV-infected sooty mangabeys maintain CD4 T cell counts comparable to those observed in uninfected animals (Sumpter et al., 2007). This is a clear difference compared to the progressive depletion of circulating CD4 T cells that characterize pathogenic HIV and SIV infections in humans and rhesus macaques (figure 2).

Intriguingly, two recent studies aimed at investigating the kinetics of mucosal CD4 T cells during SIV infection of sooty mangabeys and African green monkeys (Gordon et al., 2007; I. V. Pandrea et al., 2007b) demonstrated that just like HIV-infected humans and SIV-infected rhesus macaques, SIV-infected sooty mangabeys manifest a rapid and severe depletion of mucosal CD4 T cells (figure 2). In the first study, Gordon et al. showed that memory CD4 T cells are rapidly and severely depleted from the mucosal sites (but not from peripheral blood or lymph nodes) of SIV infected sooty mangabeys, with kinetics remarkably similar to those observed during pathogenic SIVmac infection of macaques (Gordon et al., 2007). In the second study, Pandrea et al. observed a similar level of mucosal CD4 T cell depletion in African green monkeys compared to rhesus macaques during the acute phase of SIV infection (I. V. Pandrea et al., 2007b). Notably, the early loss of mucosal CD4 T cells does not progress further after reaching a stable plateau in sooty mangabeys and is followed by a partial recovery of these cells in African green monkeys—trends that contrast with that described in pathogenic HIV and SIV infections in humans and rhesus macaques where mucosal CD4 T cell depletion becomes increasingly more severe as disease progresses to AIDS.

Intriguingly, despite levels of CD4 T cells in the gut comparable to those described in HIV-infected humans who progress to AIDS, sooty mangabeys and African green monkeys maintain normal mucosal immune function, as indicated by the maintenance of an intact mucosal barrier, the complete absence of any increased susceptibility to infections, and the lack of microbial translocation (Brenchley, Price, Schacker, Asher, et al., 2006a; Estes et al., 2010; Gordon et al., 2007; I. V. Pandrea et al., 2007b). These findings raise an important question of how SIV-infected natural hosts maintain mucosal immunity and avoid progression to AIDS despite the loss of mucosal CD4 T cells. One might hypothesize that in sooty mangabeys, preservation of CD4 T cell homeostasis in the peripheral blood compensates for the loss of mucosal CD4 T cells, and is sufficient to maintain a functional immune system. This hypothesis, however, is not consistent with the observation that a fraction of naturally and experimentally infected sooty mangabeys experience a variable but significant (with animals showing <100 cells/ul blood) loss of CD4 T cell in blood and tissues, while still remaining healthy and AIDS-free (Milush et al., 2007; Mir, Gasper, Sundaravaradan, & Sodora, 2011; Sumpter et al., 2007; Taaffe et al., 2010). The evidence indicates that even a generalized depletion of CD4 T cells, per se, is not sufficient to induce progression to AIDS in natural hosts for SIV. This leaves unanswered the question of how SIV-infected sooty mangabeys can afford to lose CD4 T cells but maintain mucosal immunity and avoid progression to AIDS.

To answer this question, several, non-mutually exclusive mechanisms have been suggested in the past few years. One possibility is that the lack of other pathogenic factors, in particular chronic immune activation, protects the CD4 T cell depleted mucosa of sooty mangabeys (Mirko Paiardini et al., 2009b). An alternative possibility is that the immune system of natural hosts evolved to be less dependent on CD4 T cells, with other cell types carrying on the CD4 T cell helper functions. In particular, two recently published studies of sooty mangabeys and African green monkeys showed the presence of a significant fraction of that despite lacking CD4 expression, indeed act as CD4 T cells; this allows the immune system to maintain "classical" helper functions that otherwise would be lost (Milush et al., 2011, Beaumier et al., 2009). A third possibility is that despite being quantitatively similar, the depletion of CD4 T cells is qualitatively different in pathogenic and nonpathogenic lentiviral infections. This last possibility implies that natural hosts for SIV are able to preserve certain critical CD4 T cell subsets, in the context of generalized CD4 T cell depletion, sufficient for maintaining a functional immune system.

Two of these mechanisms, i.e. the lack of immune activation and the preservation of the homeostasis of selective CD4 T cell subsets, are described in more details in the next sections.

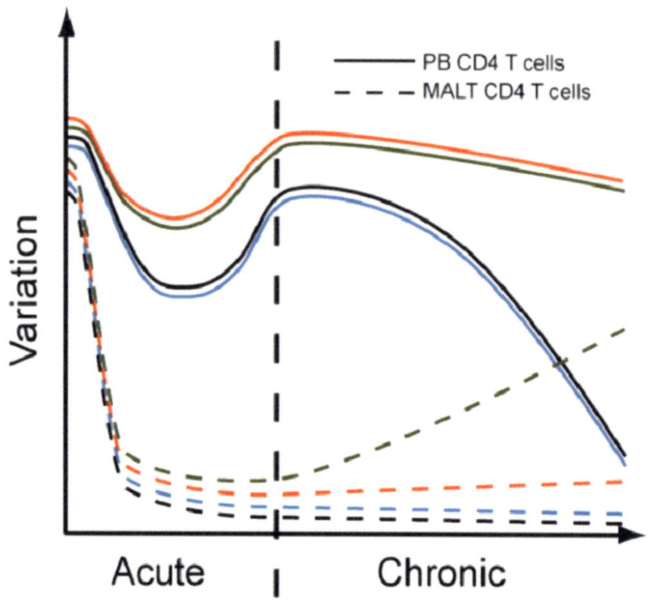

Fig. 2. CD4 T cell homeostasis in natural and nonnatural hosts.
In both pathogenic (humans —, rhesus macaques —) and nonpathogenic (sooty mangabeys — and African green monkeys —) HIV/SIV infection, CD4 T cells are rapidly lost in the mucosal associated lymphoid tissue (MALT, dotted lines). In contrast to pathogenic infection, CD4 T cells are generally preserved in the peripheral blood (PB, solid lines) of natural host species. Originally published in *Blood* Online. Brenchley JM & Paiardini M. Immunodeficiency lentiviral infections in natural and nonnatural hosts. *Blood*. Prepublished April 19, 2011; DOI:10.1182/blood-2010-12-325936.

3. Immune activation

3.1 Immune activation markers and their role as predictors of disease progression

The establishment of a state of chronic, generalized immune activation is a characteristic feature of pathogenic HIV infection in humans and SIV infection in macaques (Douek D Ann REv Med 2009; Sodora DL AIDS 2009). A large number of scientific evidence clearly shows that HIV infection is associated with high frequencies of numerous immune cell types, including CD4 and CD8 T cells, B cells, NK cells, and monocytes, that express markers of activation, proliferation, and apoptosis (reviewed in Sodora et al., 2008).

The strong association between immune activation and AIDS pathogenesis is well documented. A large 2006 study that took place over 20 years probing 2,801 treatment naïve HIV-1 infected patients concluded that only a small percent of CD4 loss variability could be attributed to HIV-1 RNA plasma viral loads, suggesting other factors, mainly immune activation, were likely responsible for CD4 T cell decline (Rodríguez et al., 2006). CD4 T cell recovery during antiretroviral treatment is mitigated when there are higher frequencies of CD4 and CD8 CD38+HLA-DR+ T cells (Hunt et al., 2003). Naïve CD8 T cells defined by

CD45RA and CD62L expression are lost in parallel with CD4 T cells, regardless of the stage of disease progression and despite rises in total numbers of CD8 T cells (M Roederer et al., 1995). Low levels of CD69, an early marker of activation, and increased T regulatory cells have been associated with HIV-resistant individuals (Card et al., 2009), along with low levels of HLA-DR+CD38+ CD4 T cells and Ki-67+ CD4 and CD8 T cells (Koning et al., 2005). Upon stimulation, activation markers CD80, CD86 and CD70 are increased in HIV infected patients (Wolthers et al., 1996). Other soluble activation markers have also been found in serum and plasma to be increased in HIV infected patients including beta$_2$-microglobulin (Grieco et al., 1984), IL-2 receptor (Sethi & Näher, 1986; Pizzolo et al., 1987), tumor necrosis factor (Reddy, Sorrell, Lange, & Grieco, 1988) tumor necrosis factor receptor II (Fahey et al., 1998) and others.

A recurrent trend in research focusing on immune activation is the consistent importance of CD38 as a marker of disease prognosis. CD38, otherwise known as cyclic ADP ribose hydrolase, is an ectoenzyme transmembrane glycoprotein that correlates with other cell activation markers and is associated with enhanced cell to cell adhesion, cytokine production and T-cell activation (Deeks et al., 2004). According to a Giorgi et al. study referenced over 330 times (ISI Web of Knowledge^{SM}), CD4 and CD8 T cell expression of CD38 is increased in clinically defined AIDS patients who survived less than 6 months versus those who survived greater than 18 months (J V Giorgi et al., 1999; Sandler et al., 2011). While the level of HIV RNA is a good predictor of disease progression early in infection, and CD4 T cell count is as good if not better later in infection, CD38 levels on CD8 T cells is a good early and late predictor (Janis V Giorgi et al., 2002). Activated CD8+CD38+CD45RO+ T cells predict CD4 T cell decline (Bofill et al., 1996), though CD8+HLA-DR+ cannot (J V Giorgi et al., 1993). An activation set-point measured by CD38 expression on CD4 and especially CD8 T cells arises early in infection and is relatively stable and able to predict subsequent CD4 T cell decline even without considering viral load (Deeks et al., 2004). Also, increased HLADR+CD38+ T cells in elite controllers with low plasma virus loads is associated with decreased CD4 counts (Hunt et al., 2008), in tune with the idea that T cell activation promotes HIV disease progression (Fahey et al., 1998).

Soluble markers of immune activation, that are more easily measurable than cellular activation, have also been shown to have prognostic value and predict HIV disease progression with comparable efficiency to CD4 counts and viral load measurements (Liu et al., 1997). In particular, neopterin, produced by macrophages upon IFNg stimulation (Melmed, Taylor, Detels, Bozorgmehri, & Fahey, 1989), beta$_2$-microglobulin for general lymphoid activation (Chitra, Bakthavatsalam, & Palvannan, 2011; Fahey et al., 1990), and soluble IL-2 receptor (Sethi & Näher, 1986) have all been shown to be elevated and predictive of disease progression to varying degrees (Fahey et al., 1998). Increased soluble CD14 levels, a marker of monocyte activation that also correlated with IL-6, C-reactive protein, serum amyloid A and D-dimer, independently predicts mortality in HIV patients (Sandler et al., 2011).

In summary, the HIV-associated immune activation (i) is characterized by high frequencies of numerous immune cell types expressing markers of activation, proliferation, and apoptosis; (ii) predicts the tempo of progression to AIDS independently from, and more accurately than viral load; (iii) strongly correlates with the efficacy of antiretroviral therapy (ART) in reconstituting the immune system of HIV-infected individuals. Although the benefits of being able to predict or modify the course of disease during acute HIV infection would likely be substantial, the value of immune activation biomarkers has largely been detected during chronic HIV infection due to the obvious constraints of human studies.

3.2 Causes and consequence of HIV-associated chronic immune activation

The causes of the chronic immune activation and subsequent immunopathogenesis in HIV infected patients is unsettled. Whether or not immunopathogenesis is mainly caused by the virus or the immune response to the virus has been the object of a long scientific debate. While some have focused on the virus and its direct cytophathicity by claiming "it's the virus stupid" (Cohen, 1993), others counterclaimed, "it's the immune system, stupid" (STEP perspective, 1999; Smith, 2006). Further studies in humans, natural hosts of SIV, rhesus macaque models of progressive infection and even mice models of immune activation have helped to clarify that the cause of HIV pathogenesis is multifactorial, with both viral and host factors contributing to progression to AIDS. Moreover, many arms of the immune system aside from infected CD4 T cells are dysregulated.

A particularly salient example of how immune activation alone damages the immune system comes from a transgenic mouse model of chronic immune activation triggered by CD27-CD70 costimulation. The mice showed uncanny familiarity with HIV disease without a virus present, with constant costimulation and TCR antigen stimulation leading to thymic involution, T cell turnover, loss of naïve T cell populations, and progressive inability of T cells to respond ex vivo upon stimulation (Tesselaar et al., 2003).

Possible explanations for HIV-associated chronic immune activation is a long list: gut damage and microbial translocation (Brenchley, Price, & Douek, 2006b), loss of T helper 17 (Th17) cells (Brenchley et al., 2008), loss of regulatory T cells (Hunt et al., 2011, Card et al., 2009), expansion and exhaustion of HIV-specific T cells (Khaitan & Unutmaz, 2011) decreased lymphopoiesis and increased depletion of central memory CD4 T cells (T_{CM}), both resulting in increases in homeostatic proliferation (Brenchley et al., 2010; Okoye et al., 2007; M Paiardini et al., 2009a; Picker et al., 2004; Sauce et al., 2011) and latent or newly acquired infections due to general immunodeficiency (Ford, Puronen, & Sereti, 2009).

In particular, special emphasis has been recently placed on the role played by the complex dysfunction of the mucosal immune system typical of pathogenic HIV and SIV infections in humans and rhesus macaques. The HIV-associated mucosal immune dysfunction is characterized by the loss of integrity of the mucosal barrier and the translocation of microbial products from the intestinal lumen into systemic circulation. Alexander and collaborators defined microbial translocation as "passage of both viable and nonviable microbes and microbial products, such as endotoxin across the intestinal barrier." They show that microbial translocation of microbes and microbial products occurred because of alterations in mucosal balance (Alexander et al., 1990).

Numerous evidences demonstrated the translocation of bacteria and bacterial products into the bloodstream in pathogenic HIV and SIV infections. Lipopolysacharides (LPS), which is excreted from gram-negative bacteria and act as an endotoxin, is one of the bacterial products that is translocated into the bloodstream and can therefore be used as an indicator of microbial translocation. Circulating LPS levels were increased in chronically HIV-infected individuals and SIV-infected rhesus macaques during the chronic phase of the disease, and LPS levels were associated with increased levels of soluble CD14, a marker of monocyte response to LPS (Brenchley, Price, Schacker, Asher, et al., 2006a). Of note, a recent case-control study demonstrated that soluble CD14 is an independent predictor of mortality in

HIV infection, with individuals falling in the highest quartile of sCD14 levels having a 6-fold higher risk of death than those in the lowest quartile, even after adjusting for inflammatory markers, CD4 T cell count, and HIV RNA level (Sandler et al., 2011). Moreover, another study demonstrated that microbial translocation was detected by the presence of 16S ribosomal DNA in 95% of untreated HIV-infected patients observed (Jiang et al., 2009). Interestingly, plasma LPS levels were found to be higher with drug abuse, or co-infection with hepatitis-c virus (HCV) (Ancuta et al., 2008).

Due to the immediacy of these events, and the fact that translocating products are bioactive in vivo, the gut breakdown and associated microbial translocation cascade has been thought to stoke the fire of, or at least contribute to, the establishment of high levels of innate and adaptive immune activation (Brenchley, Price, & Douek, 2006b; Douek et al., 2009). Evidence supporting this model comes from the fact that plasma levels of LPS are significantly increased, and correlate with the level of systemic immune activation in chronically HIV infected individuals and SIV infected rhesus macaques. Even uninfected CD4 T cells in the gut dive to extremely low numbers after just weeks of infection, as bacterial products rise in the blood of HIV infected patients. In a more recent study, Nowroozalizadeh and collaborators found elevated levels of plasma LPS in both individuals infected with HIV type 1 and HIV type 2. Furthermore, they showed that the severity of microbial translocation correlates with CD4 T cell count and viral load independently of HIV type, as well as with defective innate and mitogen responsiveness (Nowroozalizadeh et al., 2010).

Due to its broad impacts on several cell types of the innate and adaptive immune response, HIV-associated immune activation may damage the immune system in many different ways. Depletion of CD4 T cells in the gut and peripheral blood in the acute phase and beyond leads to vacancies in the T cell receptor repertoire that threatens immune resources normally in reserve to fight new, latent or mutating infections (Simons et al., 2008). Certain CD4 T cell specificities are preferentially lost. For instance, CD4 T cells specific for *Mycobacterium tuberculosis* (MTB) are lost quickly compared to those for CMV, likely due to lower expression of CCR5 ligand MIP-1b on MTB specific CD4 T cells (Geldmacher et al., 2010). Cytokines and other soluble factors (as described in the section about activation markers) are at dangerously abnormal levels. Th17, an IL-17 producing CD4 T cell subset critical for mucosal immunity are preferentially depleted (Brenchley et al., 2008). B cell dysfunction is also pronounced as HIV impacts activation states, hypergammaglobulinemia, exhaustion, and impaired antibody production against vaccination and infections (reviewed in Shen & Tomaras, 2011).

In spite of the large number of immune abnormalities that have been described, there are still unanswered questions about the exact mechanisms by which this virus causes progressive disease, possibly because so many constituents are impacted.

4. Depletion of Th17 cells and loss of mucosal barrier integrity

An important mechanism that appears to link loss of mucosal barrier integrity, microbial translocation and the establishment of immune activation is the preferential depletion of Th17 cells, a recently identified CD4 T cell subset that produce IL-17 and IL-22 and play a critical role in antimicrobial mucosal immunity. In particular, IL-17 and IL-22 (i) induce epithelial cells to express cytokines (i.e., IL-6 and GM-CSF), chemokines (i.e., IL-8, CXCL1, CXCL10, and CCL20) and metalloproteinases critical for the recruitment, activation and migration of neutrophils to areas of bacterial infection; (ii) promote the production of antimicrobial molecules, such as defensins; and (iii) regulate the integrity of the epithelial barrier by stimulating the proliferation and survival of GI enterocyte and the transcription of tight junction proteins (Aujla et al., 2008; Dandekar, George, & Bäumler, 2010; Guglani & Khader, 2010; Liang et al., 2006; Milner, Sandler, & Douek, 2010; Ouyang & Valdez, 2008; Romagnani, 2008; Zheng et al., 2008). Consistent with their important role in antimicrobial immunity, Th17 cells confer protection against several extracellular pathogens, such as *Candida albicans, Klebsiella pneumoniae, Citrobacter rodentium, Mycobacteria tuberculosis, Staphylococcus aureus, Bacteroides fragilis, Escherichia coli* (Huang, Na, Fidel, & Schwarzenberger, 2004; Khader et al., 2007; Ouyang & Valdez, 2008). Given the role of Th17 cells in mucosal immunity, and the observed mucosal immune dysfunction associated with HIV infection, we and others investigated the homeostasis of Th17 during pathogenic lentiviral infection, showing that Th17 cells are preferentially depleted in the gastrointestinal tracts of HIV-infected humans and SIV-infected macaques (Brenchley et al., 2008; Cecchinato et al., 2008; d'Ettorre, Mirko Paiardini, Ceccarelli, Silvestri, & Vullo, 2011; Favre et al., 2009; Gordon et al., 2010; Raffatellu et al., 2008). Moreover, Raffatellu and colleagues showed that in healthy SIV-negative rhesus macaques, the gene expression profile induced by S. typhimurium in ileal loops is dominated by Th17 responses, including the expression of IL-17 and IL-22; and severe depletion of mucosal Th17 cells in SIV-infected rhesus macaques resulted in an impaired mucosal barrier function and increased S. *typhimurium* dissemination (Raffatellu et al., 2008). Furthermore, loss of mucosal Th17 cells has been associated with increased systemic immune activation and disease progression in both HIV-infected humans and SIV-infected rhesus macaques (Cecchinato et al., 2008; Gordon et al., 2010; Hartigan-O'connor, Hirao, McCune, & Dandekar, 2011). Consistent with the model linking depletion of Th17 cells with compromised antimicrobial immunity, it has been shown that patients with dominant negative stat3 gene mutations, common in hyperimmunoglobulin E syndrome or the more biblical Job's syndrome, in which CD4 T cells are unable to differentiate into Th17 cells, are exquisitely susceptible to bacterial infections (Milner et al., 2008).

Collectively, these studies demonstrate that pathogenic HIV and SIV infections are associated with a preferential and sustained depletion of mucosal Th17 cells, the severity of which correlates with the structural and immunological maintenance of the mucosal barrier, the levels of immune activation, and progression to AIDS. These observations further elucidate the immunodeficiency of HIV disease and provide a mechanistic basis for the mucosal barrier breakdown that characterizes HIV infection.

5. Immunology of natural hosts for SIV

5.1 Absence of chronic immune activation

A very large body of evidence clearly demonstrated that, in sharp contrast with all the known models of pathogenic HIV infection, nonpathogenic SIV infection of natural hosts is characterized by the absence of high levels of chronic immune activation, assessed as the fraction of cells expressing markers of activation and proliferation, in the context of continuous virus replication (figure 3) (Mirko Paiardini et al., 2009b; Silvestri et al., 2003; Silvestri, Mirko Paiardini, I. Pandrea, Lederman, & Sodora, 2007). Consistent with their lower levels of immune activation, infected sooty mangabeys show no increase in lymphocyte apoptosis, lymph node structural damage, thymic involution, or loss of naïve T cell populations—all of which are normally attributed to chronic immune activation (Silvestri et al., 2003). Furthermore, naturally SIV-infected sooty mangabeys preserve the ability to properly regulate cell cycle progression when compared to SIV-infected macaques (Paiardini M JV 2006).

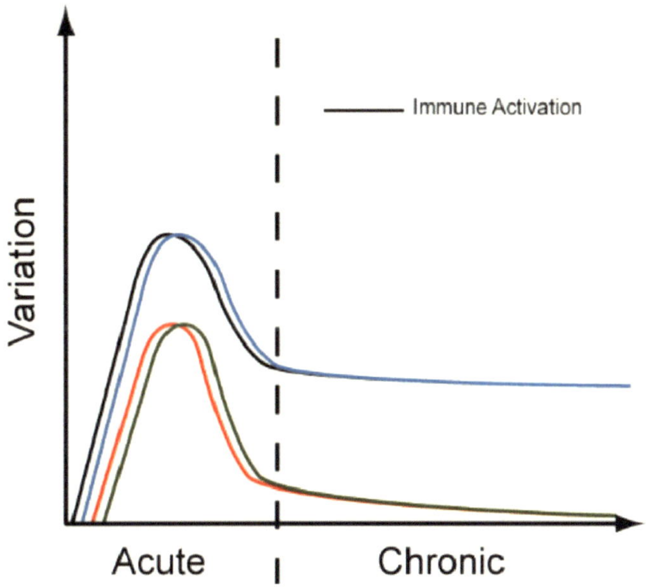

Fig. 3. Immune activation in natural and nonnatural hosts.
In contrast to pathogenic HIV/SIV infection (humans —, rhesus macaques —), nonpathogenic SIV infection in natural hosts (sooty mangabeys — and African green monkeys —) is associated with the resolution of immune activation during chronic infection. Originally published in *Blood* Online. Brenchley JM & Paiardini M. Immunodeficiency lentiviral infections in natural and nonnatural hosts. *Blood*. Prepublished April 19, 2011; DOI:10.1182/blood-2010-12-325936.

Interestingly, the consistently low levels of chronic immune activation in natural hosts does not result from intrinsically attenuated innate immune responses, but rather from active immuno-regulatory mechanisms that allow these animals to tune-down the immune response during the transition from the acute to the chronic phase of infection (figure 3). The initial studies of natural SIV infections were performed during chronic infection and were not able to inform early events. Indeed, more recent studies designed to characterize the acute phase of SIV infection consistently show that, as described for progressive infection, nonprogressive SIV infection is also associated with an early increase in T cell proliferation and activation (Gordon et al., 2007; Kornfeld et al., 2005; I. V. Pandrea et al., 2007b; Silvestri et al., 2005). This phenotype is very common among several natural hosts, even those less characterized than sooty mangabeys and African green monkeys. For instance, transient levels of immune activation have been described in Mandrills, in which CD4 and CD8 HLA-DR+ cells at first increase but then return to normal levels by day 60 post-infection (Onanga et al., 2006), as well as in Caribbean African green monkeys, which show a rapid increase in CD8 HLA-DR+ T cells and then a rapid return to baseline 2-3 weeks post-infection, while having no changes in CD4 HLA-DR+ T cell frequencies (Kornfeld et al., 2005; I. Pandrea et al., 2006). Furthermore, the rapid resolution of acute immune activation has also been shown at a genetic level in sooty mangabeys and African green monkeys from microarray data of early infection revealing that interferon stimulated genes are upregulated early in both natural and nonnatural hosts. Only natural hosts reduce their expression in blood and lymph nodes to near pre-infection levels in the acute to chronic phase transition (4-6 weeks), while macaques fail to resolve their early interferon stimulated gene response (Bosinger et al., 2009; Jacquelin et al., 2009; Lederer et al., 2009). Finally, immunohistochemical and immunofluorescent analyses recently demonstrated a robust IFN-α response in the lymph nodes of sooty mangabeys, African green monkeys, and rhesus macaques in the acute phase of SIV infection, which is later resolved only in mangabeys and African green monkeys (L. D. Harris, Tabb, et al., 2010b).

The finding that naturally SIV-infected sooty mangabeys do not experience elevated levels of chronic immune activation in the context of high levels of viral replication further confirms the association between chronic immune activation and disease progression, and highlights the clinical importance of defining the mechanisms accounting for the establishment of high levels of chronic activation, or lack thereof, in pathogenic and nonpathogenic lentiviral infections.

5.2 Preservation of Th17 cells and mucosal integrity

Homeostasis of mucosal Th17 cells is a feature that distinguishes pathogenic HIV/SIV infections of humans and rhesus macaques, where these cells are preferentially depleted, from nonprogressive SIV infection of sooty mangabeys and African green monkeys, wherein Th17 cells are preserved at healthy frequencies (Brenchley et al., 2008; Cecchinato et al., 2008; Favre et al., 2009; Hartigan-O'connor et al., 2011; Mirko Paiardini, 2010; Raffatellu et al., 2008).

As previously described, studies in natural hosts demonstrated that a significant depletion of mucosal CD4 T cells alone is not sufficient to cause AIDS (Gordon et al., 2007; I. V. Pandrea et al., 2007b), suggesting that preservation of a specific CD4 T cell subset may allow the maintenance of mucosal integrity in the context of generalized CD4 T cell depletion. An increasing number of experimental evidence suggests that Th17 cells represent this specific subset. Indeed, Th17 cells are depleted in all the known models of pathogenic HIV/SIV infection, and preserved in all the known models of nonprogressive HIV/SIV infection including natural hosts for SIV, human long-term non-progressors and rhesus macaque elite controllers (Brenchley et al., 2008; Cecchinato et al., 2008; Favre et al., 2009; Mirko Paiardini, 2010). Specifically, we showed that whereas human Th17 cells are preferentially diminished compared to IFNg secreting Th1 cells in the gastrointestinal tracts of HIV-infected people, sooty mangabey Th17 cells are maintained in blood and the gastrointestinal tract (Brenchley et al., 2008). Likewise, while pigtailed macaques lose most IL-17 producing CD4 T cells by day 10 post-infection, African green monkeys show no decline (Favre et al., 2009). Intriguingly, in nonprogressive infections of sooty mangabeys and African green monkeys preservation of healthy frequencies of Th17 cells is associated with maintenance of mucosal immunity, absence of microbial translocation and low levels of chronic immune activation (figure 4) (Brenchley, Price, Schacker, Asher, et al., 2006a). Finally, Th17 cells were measured in human long-term non-progressors (n=14) and were found to be at levels equivalent to uninfected controls and those successfully (i.e., viral loads <50 copies/mL) treated with antiretroviral therapy in the colon and peripheral blood (Ciccone et al., 2011).

To understand how natural hosts preserve Th17 cells and mucosal immunity might be central to the development of therapeutic interventions aimed at improving mucosal immunity in HIV-infected individuals. While the exact cause accounting for this phenotype

is still unclear, several non-mutually exclusive mechanisms have been proposed, including the increased susceptibility to HIV/SIV infection of Th17 cells and its CD4+CCR6+ and CD4+CD161+ T cell precursors (Gosselin et al., 2010; Kader et al., 2009; Monteiro et al., 2011; Prendergast et al., 2010) and the defective generation of Th17 cells in nonnatural versus natural hosts. Very recent and unpublished observations suggest that loss of CD4+IL-21+ T cells and CD103+ dendritic cells, with reduced availability of IL-21 or retinoic acid, respectively, may significantly contribute to Th17 cell depletion in SIV-infected rhesus macaques (Cervasi B et al, CROI 2011; Klatt N et al, Keystone 2011). Consistent with their important role in Th17 cell homeostasis, CD4+IL-21+ T cells and CD103+ dendritic cells are preserved in SIV-infected SM (Cervasi B et al, CROI 2011; Klatt N et al, Keystone 2011).
Collectively, these data indicate that by preserving the balance of IL-17 and IL-22 producing Th17 cells, natural hosts for SIV maintain mucosal barrier integrity and avoid the establishment of aberrant immune activation (figure 4). As such, the data suggest that differential regulation of Th17 cell homeostasis may be central in determining the pathogenic or nonpathogenic outcome of HIV and SIV infections in primates.

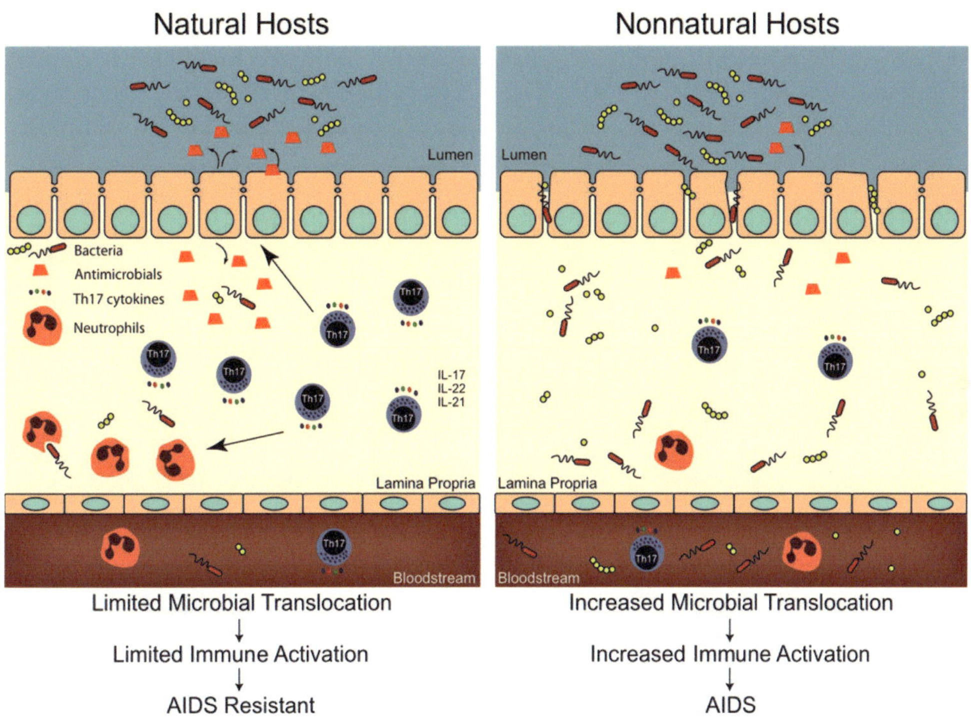

Fig. 4. Th17 cell homeostasis and mucosal immunity in natural and nonnatural hosts. Mucosal Th17 cells are preferentially depleted in nonnatural hosts (humans and RM) but preserved at healthy frequencies in natural hosts (sooty mangabeys and African green monkeys) for lentiviral infections. Th17 cells regulate antimicrobial immunity, i.e. recruiting neutrophils, maintaining tight junction integrity and stimulating antimicrobial molecule production. As such, the preservation of Th17 cells is one of the key factors limiting microbial translocation and chronic immune activation, thus contributing to the ability of natural hosts to remain AIDS-free. Adapted from (Mirko Paiardini, 2010).

5.3 Preservation of bone marrow based T cell renewal

As stated earlier, the mechanisms leading to CD4 T cell loss in HIV infection are multifactorial and still not completely defined. In addition to direct viral infection and bystander cell death, evidence has exhibited that insufficient T cell reconstitution may play a key role. Within the bone marrow, a major site of hematopoiesis and T cell proliferation, a suppression of function common in HIV-infected humans is associated with AIDS related neutropenia, thrombocytopenia and lymphopenia (Bain, 1997; Isgrò et al., 2005; Moses, Nelson, & Bagby, 1998; Silvestri et al., 2003).

Our group recently aimed to address the hypothesis that the preservation of bone marrow based proliferation and regeneration of T cells could be an important factor in regulating CD4 T cell homeostasis in progressive and nonprogressive lentiviral infections. To test this hypothesis, we utilized carboxyfluorescein diacetate succinimidyl ester (CFSE) labeling during in vitro stimulations, along with flow-cytometric intracellular measurements of the cell cycle marker Ki-67, to measure proliferation in sooty mangabeys and rhesus macaques; these assessments were performed also in the experimental setting of in vivo antibody-mediated CD4 or CD8 lymphocyte depletion (M Paiardini et al., 2009a). We discovered that SIV positive rhesus macaques have diminished proliferative capacity in bone marrow CD4 and CD8 T cells, while SIV positive SM had no decline compared to uninfected monkeys. Intriguingly, the rare subset of SIV-infected SM with low CD4 T cell count showed significantly lower levels of bone marrow proliferation when compared to SM that preserve the homeostasis of the CD4 T cell compartment (M Paiardini et al., 2009a). In addition, we found a correlation between Ki-67+ CD4 T cells and CD4 T cell count in the bone marrow but not in the peripheral blood (figure 5)(M Paiardini et al., 2009a).

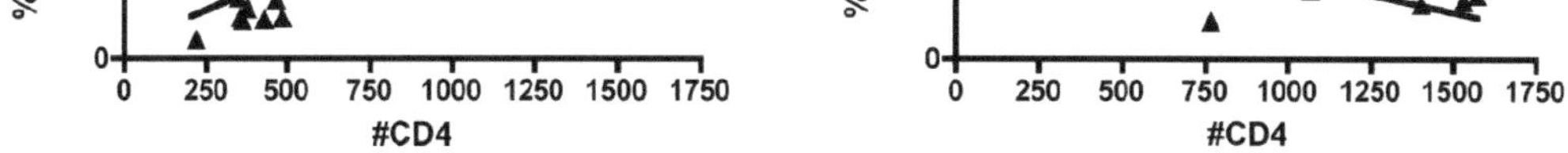

Fig. 5. Bone Marrow based CD4 T cell proliferation in sooty mangabeys.
In SIV-infected SM, blood CD4 T cell count correlates directly with the percentage of proliferating CD4 T cells in the bone marrow (BM, left panel) and inversely with the percentage of proliferating CD4 T cells in the peripheral blood (PB, right panel). This research was originally published in *Blood*. Paiardini M, *Blood*. 2009; *113*(3), 612-621. © the American Society of Hematology.

These findings suggest that the bone marrow is a major site of T cell proliferation in nonhuman primates, and the ability of SIV-infected sooty mangabeys to preserve the bone marrow based CD4 T cell proliferation is important for maintaining the homeostasis of the CD4 T cell compartment and avoiding progression to AIDS.

5.4 Lower expression of CCR5 on CD4 T cells

Another feature distinguishing natural and nonnatural hosts for lentiviral infections is the expression of CCR5, the main co-receptor used by HIV and SIV in vivo, to enter CD4 T cells. A comparative, cross sectional analysis of CCR5 expression in blood, lymph nodes and rectal biopsies obtained from several natural (sooty mangabeys, African green monkeys, and others) and nonnatural (human, rhesus macaques, and others) primate host species demonstrated that natural hosts for SIV infection consistently show a paucity of CD4 T cells expressing CCR5 (I. Pandrea et al., 2007a). This lower fraction of CD4 T cells expressing CCR5 was confirmed in both infected and uninfected animals, and in all sampled tissues, including those representing the major sites of viral replication (mucosa and lymph node) and CD4 T cell depletion (mucosa) during pathogenic HIV/SIV infection. Moreover, a five year longitudinal study of SIV-infected and uninfected sooty mangabeys showed stable median fractions (between 2-4%) of CD4 T cells expressing CCR5, independent of SIV (Taaffe et al., 2010). While this observation is very consistent and clear, its interpretation has been difficult, since naturally SIV-infected sooty mangabeys show levels of virus replication comparable to those of pathogenic infections. In an ongoing effort to better understand the pathophysiologic role of this decreased fraction of CCR5+ CD4 T cells in sooty mangabeys, we recently compared the levels and kinetics of CCR5 expression in sooty mangabey and rhesus macaque CD4 T cells, as well as the phenotype in their naïve, central memory, and effector memory subsets, following in vitro and in vivo activation. By doing this, we found CD4 T cells from sooty mangabeys failed to up-regulate CCR5 as do rhesus macaques in spite of activation and proliferation found to be equal in both species upon stimulation in vitro. Intriguingly, this phenomenon was more evident in CD4 T cells with a central-memory phenotype (T_{CM}), and associated with a markedly reduced susceptibility of these cells to SIV infection. Since recent findings indicated the depletion of CD4 T_{CM} cells as a critical step in the loss of CD4 T cell homeostasis and disease progression in SIV-infected rhesus macaques (Okoye et al., 2007; Picker et al., 2004), our recent data suggests that partial protection of CD4 T_{CM} cells from SIV infection is one mechanism contributing to maintenance of a healthy immune system and avoidance of progression to AIDS in SIV-infected sooty mangabeys (Paiardini et al., 2011).

6. How natural hosts may inform the design of novel vaccine and therapeutic approaches for HIV-infected humans

The pathogenesis of HIV infection results from a complex interaction between virus and host. Studies aimed at characterizing the virus-host interactions in natural hosts have led to important findings for understanding HIV pathogenesis in humans and, even more important, have many implications for new therapies and vaccines, giving us the opportunity to stop disease progression by understanding what nature has already discovered over millennia (Sodora et al., 2009). Table 2, along with the section above, summarizes several therapeutic approaches that could attempt to mimic the critical features of nonpathogenic infection in sooty mangabeys, which could be beneficial if included in the clinical management of HIV-infected humans.

1. *Targeting chronic immune activation to slow disease progression.* Considering that chronic immune activation is a key player in HIV pathogenesis, being associated with CD4 T cell depletion and the overall functionality of the immune system, and it

is absent in nonprogressive SIV infection of natural hosts, there is a strong rationale for introducing immune suppressive molecules in the treatment of HIV-infected individuals. In this context, it is important to note that in HIV-infected humans chronic immune activation is not fully resolved even in the setting of successful antiretroviral therapy (ART), and that this residual immune activation is considered the major cause for the increased "non-AIDS" morbidity and mortality observed in individuals undergoing long-term ART (Grund, Neuhaus, Phillips, INSIGHT SMART Study Group, 2009). Since the exact mechanisms and signaling pathways responsible for chronic immune activation in HIV-infected humans are still unclear, approaches have mostly focused on using drugs with a generic immune suppressive ability, such as Cyclosporin, Rapamycin, and Hydroxychloroquine, already in use for individuals with autoimmune disorders or recipients of transplants. Hydroxychloroquine, an antimalarial drug also used to reduce inflammation in rheumatoid arthritis and lupus, has already been shown to reduce the expression of the immune activation markers CD38, Ki-67 and HLA-DR on CD8 T-cells and to decrease viral loads in HIV infected patients (Murray et al., 2010, Sperber et al., 1995).

2. *Preserving Th17 cell homeostasis by increasing their differentiation and survival.* IL-21, a multifunctional cytokine that initiates the induction of Th17 cells (Korn et al., 2007; Nurieva et al., 2007; Yang et al., 2008) could be used to test the hypothesis that increased levels of Th17 cells will sure up gut permeability, thus preventing continuous microbial translocation and immune activation. The rationale for using this cytokine comes from several findings, including the following: (i) plasma levels of IL-21 are significantly decreased in HIV infected patients (Iannello et al., 2008); (ii) CD8 T cells producing IL-21 are increased in elite controllers, (Williams et al. 2011); (iii) circulating CD4 T cells expressing IL-21 are severely lost in pathogenic SIV infection of rhesus macaques, with the extent of this depletion being associated with that of Th17 cells (Cervasi B, CROI 2011),; (iv) CD4 T cells producing IL-21 are preserved at healthy frequencies in SIV-infected sooty mangabeys (Cervasi B, CROI 2011) ; (v) finally, IL-21 is already in clinical trials for the use against renal cell carcinoma and melanoma (Hashmi & Van Veldhuizen, 2010).
3. *Targeting of CCR5 expression.* Specifically targeting expression of CCR5 and other co-receptors for HIV may be critical in preventing AIDS. A unique bone marrow transplantation demonstrated the attainability of an HIV cure, despite the unusual and unrepeatable events that led to that cure: harsh chemotherapy, total body irradiation and an unlikely hematopoietic stem cell transplantation match of a homozygous CCR5Δ32 donor (Hütter, Nowak, Mossner, Ganepola, et al., 2009a). This case report of one patient has justifiably led to excitement about future therapies using CCR5Δ32 donors as well as other entry blocking strategies in HIV infection (Hütter, Thomas Schneider, & Thiel, 2009b). Other less strenuous methods to target CCR5 have been made possible by zinc finger nuclease-mediated gene disruption, maraviroc, small interfering RNA molecules, and a number of new molecular nanotechnologies (reviewed in Cannon & June, 2011). Data obtained in sooty mangabeys suggest that these treatments may be significantly enhanced upon targeting of CCR5 expression on CD4 T_{CM} cells specifically.

Feature of HIV or SIV infections	Natural hosts	Nonnatural hosts	Possible therapeutic intervention
Chronic immune activation	No	Yes	Immune modulators of activation
Progressive loss of peripheral CD4 T cells	No	Yes	CD4 T cell renewal strategies; IL-7 and other homeostatic cytokines
Mucosal Th17 cells	Preserved	Lost	Increase Th17 cell differentiation; IL-21 and other Th17-driving factors
Frequency of CD4+CCR5+ T cells	Very low	Normal	CCR5 blockade
Mucosal integrity	Preserved	Lost	Sure up mucosal boundaries

Table 2. Critical features distinguishing pathogenic from non nonpathogenic SIV infection in nonnatural and natural hosts, respectively. The last column includes general targets for intervention derived from studying natural hosts. These approaches mimic critical features of nonprogressive lentiviral infection and could improve the clinical management of HIV-infected humans.

7. Final remarks

We firmly believe that a comprehensive elucidation of how natural hosts for SIV have co-evolved to avoid disease progression is critical for understanding the mechanisms of AIDS pathogenesis in HIV-infected humans. The elucidation of these mechanisms may translate into major advances in prevention and therapy of HIV infection and AIDS.

8. References

Alexander, J. W., Boyce, S. T., Babcock, G. F., Gianotti, L., Peck, M. D., Dunn, D. L., Pyles, T., et al. (1990). The process of microbial translocation *Annals of surgery*, *212*(4), 496-510; discussion 511-2.

Ancuta, P., Kamat, A., Kunstman, K. J., Kim, E., Autissier, P., Wurcel, A., Zaman, T., et al. (2008). Microbial translocation is associated with increased monocyte activation and dementia in AIDS patients *PloS one*, *3*(6), e2516. doi:10.1371/journal.pone.0002516

Aujla, S. J., Chan, Y. R., Zheng, M., Fei, M., Askew, D. J., Pociask, D. A., Reinhart, T. A., et al. (2008). IL-22 mediates mucosal host defense against Gram-negative bacterial pneumonia *Nature medicine*, *14*(3), 275-281. doi:10.1038/nm1710

Bain, B. J. (1997). The haematological features of HIV infection *British journal of haematology*, *99*(1), 1-8.

Barré-Sinoussi, F., Chermann, J. C., Rey, F., Nugeyre, M. T., Chamaret, S., Gruest, J., Dauguet, C., et al. (1983). Isolation of a T-lymphotropic retrovirus from a patient at risk for acquired immune deficiency syndrome (AIDS) *Science (New York, N.Y.)*, *220*(4599), 868-871.

Bofill, M., Mocroft, A., Lipman, M., Medina, E., Borthwick, N. J., Sabin, C. A., Timms, A., et al. (1996). Increased numbers of primed activated CD8+CD38+CD45RO+ T cells predict the decline of CD4+ T cells in HIV-1-infected patients *AIDS (London, England)*, *10*(8), 827-834.

Bosinger, S. E., Li, Q., Gordon, S. N., Klatt, N. R., Duan, L., Xu, L., Francella, N., et al. (2009). Global genomic analysis reveals rapid control of a robust innate response in SIV-infected sooty mangabeys *The Journal of clinical investigation*, *119*(12), 3556-3572. doi:10.1172/JCI40115

Brenchley, J. M., Schacker, T. W., Ruff, L. E., Price, D. A., Taylor, J. H., Beilman, G. J., Nguyen, P. L., et al. (2004a). CD4+ T cell depletion during all stages of HIV disease occurs predominantly in the gastrointestinal tract *The Journal of experimental medicine*, *200*(6), 749-759. doi:10.1084/jem.20040874

Brenchley, J. M., Hill, B. J., Ambrozak, D. R., Price, D. A., Guenaga, F. J., Casazza, J. P., Kuruppu, J., et al. (2004b). T-cell subsets that harbor human immunodeficiency virus (HIV) in vivo: implications for HIV pathogenesis *Journal of virology*, *78*(3), 1160-1168.

Brenchley, J. M., Price, D. A., Schacker, T. W., Asher, T. E., Silvestri, G., Rao, S., Kazzaz, Z., et al. (2006a). Microbial translocation is a cause of systemic immune activation in chronic HIV infection *Nature medicine*, *12*(12), 1365-1371. doi:10.1038/nm1511

Brenchley, J. M., Paiardini, M., Knox, K. S., Asher, A. I., Cervasi, B., Asher, T. E., Scheinberg, P., et al. (2008). Differential Th17 CD4 T-cell depletion in pathogenic and nonpathogenic lentiviral infections *Blood*, *112*(7), 2826-2835. doi:10.1182/blood-2008-05-159301

Brenchley, J. M., Price, D. A., & Douek, D. C. (2006b). HIV disease: fallout from a mucosal catastrophe *Nature immunology*, *7*(3), 235-239. doi:10.1038/ni1316

Brenchley, J. M., Silvestri, G., & Douek, D. C. (2010). Nonprogressive and progressive primate immunodeficiency lentivirus infections *Immunity*, *32*(6), 737-742. doi:10.1016/j.immuni.2010.06.004

Cannon, P., & June, C. (2011). Chemokine receptor 5 knockout strategies *Current opinion in HIV and AIDS*, *6*(1), 74-79. doi:10.1097/COH.0b013e32834122d7

Card, C. M., McLaren, P. J., Wachihi, C., Kimani, J., Plummer, F. A., & Fowke, K. R. (2009). Decreased immune activation in resistance to HIV-1 infection is associated with an elevated frequency of CD4(+)CD25(+)FOXP3(+) regulatory T cells *The Journal of infectious diseases*, *199*(9), 1318-1322. doi:10.1086/597801

Cecchinato, V., Trindade, C. J., Laurence, A., Heraud, J. M., Brenchley, J. M., Ferrari, M. G., Zaffiri, L., et al. (2008). Altered balance between Th17 and Th1 cells at mucosal sites predicts AIDS progression in simian immunodeficiency virus-infected macaques *Mucosal immunology*, *1*(4), 279-288. doi:10.1038/mi.2008.14

Centers for Disease Control (CDC). (1982). A cluster of Kaposi's sarcoma and Pneumocystis carinii pneumonia among homosexual male residents of Los Angeles and Orange Counties, California *MMWR. Morbidity and mortality weekly report*, *31*(23), 305-307.

Cervasi B, Reyes-Aville E, Ende Z, Else J, Silvestri G, & Paiardini M. Differential Regulation of IL-21-producing CD4+ T Cells in Natural and Non-natural Hosts for SIV [abstract]. In: 18th Conference on Retroviruses and Opportunistic Infections, Boston, Feb 27-Mar 2, 2011 Abstract # 243.

Chakrabarti, L. A., Lewin, S. R., Zhang, L., Gettie, A., Luckay, A., Martin, L. N., Skulsky, E., et al. (2000). Normal T-cell turnover in sooty mangabeys harboring active simian immunodeficiency virus infection *Journal of virology, 74*(3), 1209-1223.

Chitra, P., Bakthavatsalam, B., & Palvannan, T. (2011). Beta-2 microglobulin as an immunological marker to assess the progression of human immunodeficiency virus infected patients on highly active antiretroviral therapy *Clinica chimica acta; international journal of clinical chemistry*. doi:10.1016/j.cca.2011.01.037

Ciccone, E. J., Greenwald, J. H., Lee, P. I., Biancotto, A., Read, S. W., Yao, M. A., Hodge, J. N., et al. (2011). CD4+ T Cells, Including Th17 and Cycling Subsets, are Intact in the Gut Mucosa of HIV-1 Infected Long-Term Non- Progressors *Journal of virology*. doi:10.1128/JVI.02643-10

Cohen, J. (1993, April 16). AIDS research. Keystone's blunt message: 'it's the virus, stupid' *Science (New York, N.Y.), 260*(5106), 292-293.

Courgnaud, V., Abela, B., Pourrut, X., Mpoudi-Ngole, E., Loul, S., Delaporte, E., & Peeters, M. (2003). Identification of a new simian immunodeficiency virus lineage with a vpu gene present among different cercopithecus monkeys (C. mona, C. cephus, and C. nictitans) from Cameroon *Journal of virology, 77*(23), 12523-12534.

d'Ettorre, G., Paiardini, Mirko, Ceccarelli, G., Silvestri, G., & Vullo, V. (2011). HIV-Associated Immune Activation: From Bench to Bedside *AIDS research and human retroviruses*. doi:10.1089/AID.2010.0342

Dandekar, S., George, M. D., & Bäumler, A. J. (2010). Th17 cells, HIV and the gut mucosal barrier *Current opinion in HIV and AIDS, 5*(2), 173-178. doi:10.1097/COH.0b013e328335eda3

Deeks, S. G., Kitchen, C. M. R., Liu, L., Guo, H., Gascon, R., Narváez, A. B., Hunt, P., et al. (2004). Immune activation set point during early HIV infection predicts subsequent CD4+ T-cell changes independent of viral load *Blood, 104*(4), 942-947. doi:10.1182/blood-2003-09-3333

Douek, D. C., Roederer, Mario, & Koup, R. A. (2009). Emerging concepts in the immunopathogenesis of AIDS *Annual review of medicine, 60*, 471-484. doi:10.1146/annurev.med.60.041807.123549

Estes, J. D., Harris, L. D., Klatt, N. R., Tabb, B., Pittaluga, S., Paiardini, M., Barclay, G. R., et al. (2010). Damaged intestinal epithelial integrity linked to microbial translocation in pathogenic simian immunodeficiency virus infections *PLoS pathogens, 6*(8). doi:10.1371/journal.ppat.1001052

Fahey, J. L., Taylor, J. M., Detels, R., Hofmann, B., Melmed, R., Nishanian, P., & Giorgi, J. V. (1990). The prognostic value of cellular and serologic markers in infection with human immunodeficiency virus type 1 *The New England journal of medicine, 322*(3), 166-172. doi:10.1056/NEJM199001183220305

Fahey, J. L., Taylor, J. M., Manna, B., Nishanian, P., Aziz, N., Giorgi, J. V., & Detels, R. (1998). Prognostic significance of plasma markers of immune activation, HIV viral load and CD4 T-cell measurements *AIDS (London, England), 12*(13), 1581-1590.

Favre, D., Lederer, S., Kanwar, B., Ma, Z., Proll, S., Kasakow, Z., Mold, J., et al. (2009). Critical loss of the balance between Th17 and T regulatory cell populations in pathogenic SIV infection *PLoS pathogens, 5*(2), e1000295. doi:10.1371/journal.ppat.1000295

Ford, E. S., Puronen, C. E., & Sereti, I. (2009). Immunopathogenesis of asymptomatic chronic HIV Infection: the calm before the storm *Current opinion in HIV and AIDS*, *4*(3), 206-214. doi:10.1097/COH.0b013e328329c68c

Gao, F., Bailes, E., Robertson, D. L., Chen, Y., Rodenburg, C. M., Michael, S. F., Cummins, L. B., et al. (1999). Origin of HIV-1 in the chimpanzee Pan troglodytes troglodytes *Nature*, *397*(6718), 436-441. doi:10.1038/17130

Geldmacher, C., Ngwenyama, N., Schuetz, A., Petrovas, C., Reither, K., Heeregrave, E. J., Casazza, J. P., et al. (2010). Preferential infection and depletion of Mycobacterium tuberculosis-specific CD4 T cells after HIV-1 infection *The Journal of experimental medicine*, *207*(13), 2869-2881. doi:10.1084/jem.20100090

Giorgi, J V, Liu, Z., Hultin, L. E., Cumberland, W. G., Hennessey, K., & Detels, R. (1993). Elevated levels of CD38+ CD8+ T cells in HIV infection add to the prognostic value of low CD4+ T cell levels: results of 6 years of follow-up. The Los Angeles Center, Multicenter AIDS Cohort Study *Journal of acquired immune deficiency syndromes*, *6*(8), 904-912.

Giorgi, J V, Hultin, L. E., McKeating, J. A., Johnson, T. D., Owens, B., Jacobson, L. P., Shih, R., et al. (1999). Shorter survival in advanced human immunodeficiency virus type 1 infection is more closely associated with T lymphocyte activation than with plasma virus burden or virus chemokine coreceptor usage *The Journal of infectious diseases*, *179*(4), 859-870. doi:10.1086/314660

Giorgi, Janis V, Lyles, R. H., Matud, J. L., Yamashita, T. E., Mellors, J. W., Hultin, L. E., Jamieson, B. D., et al. (2002). Predictive value of immunologic and virologic markers after long or short duration of HIV-1 infection *Journal of acquired immune deficiency syndromes*, *29*(4), 346-355.

Gordon, S. N., Klatt, N. R., Bosinger, S. E., Brenchley, J. M., Milush, J. M., Engram, J. C., Dunham, R. M., et al. (2007). Severe depletion of mucosal CD4+ T cells in AIDS-free simian immunodeficiency virus-infected sooty mangabeys *Journal of immunology (Baltimore, Md. : 1950)*, *179*(5), 3026-3034.

Gordon, S. N., Cervasi, B., Odorizzi, P., Silverman, R., Aberra, F., Ginsberg, G., Estes, J. D., et al. (2010). Disruption of intestinal CD4+ T cell homeostasis is a key marker of systemic CD4+ T cell activation in HIV-infected individuals *Journal of immunology (Baltimore, Md. : 1950)*, *185*(9), 5169-5179. doi:10.4049/jimmunol.1001801

Gosselin, A., Monteiro, P., Chomont, N., Diaz-Griffero, F., Said, E. A., Fonseca, S., Wacleche, V., et al. (2010). Peripheral blood CCR4+CCR6+ and CXCR3+CCR6+CD4+ T cells are highly permissive to HIV-1 infection *Journal of immunology (Baltimore, Md. : 1950)*, *184*(3), 1604-1616. doi:10.4049/jimmunol.0903058

Grieco, M. H., Reddy, M. M., Kothari, H. B., Lange, M., Buimovici-Klein, E., & William, D. (1984). Elevated beta 2-microglobulin and lysozyme levels in patients with acquired immune deficiency syndrome *Clinical immunology and immunopathology*, *32*(2), 174-184.

Grund, B., Neuhaus, J., Phillips, A., INSIGHT SMART Study Group. (2009). Relative risk of death in the SMART study *The Lancet infectious diseases*, *9*(12), 724-725. doi:10.1016/S1473-3099(09)70302-0

Guadalupe, M., Reay, E., Sankaran, S., Prindiville, T., Flamm, J., McNeil, A., & Dandekar, S. (2003). Severe CD4+ T-cell depletion in gut lymphoid tissue during primary human immunodeficiency virus type 1 infection and substantial delay in restoration following highly active antiretroviral therapy *Journal of virology, 77*(21), 11708-11717.

Guglani, L., & Khader, S. A. (2010). Th17 cytokines in mucosal immunity and inflammation *Current opinion in HIV and AIDS, 5*(2), 120-127. doi:10.1097/COH.0b013e328335c2f6

Haase, A. T. (2005). Perils at mucosal front lines for HIV and SIV and their hosts *Nature reviews. Immunology, 5*(10), 783-792. doi:10.1038/nri1705

Harris, C., Small, C. B., Klein, R. S., Friedland, G. H., Moll, B., Emeson, E. E., Spigland, I., et al. (1983). Immunodeficiency in female sexual partners of men with the acquired immunodeficiency syndrome *The New England journal of medicine, 308*(20), 1181-1184. doi:10.1056/NEJM198305193082001

Harris, L. D., Klatt, N. R., Vinton, C., Briant, J. A., Tabb, B., Ladell, K., Lifson, J., et al. (2010a). Mechanisms underlying γδ T-cell subset perturbations in SIV-infected Asian rhesus macaques *Blood, 116*(20), 4148-4157. doi:10.1182/blood-2010-05-283549

Harris, L. D., Tabb, B., Sodora, D. L., Paiardini, M., Klatt, N. R., Douek, D. C., Silvestri, G., et al. (2010b). Downregulation of robust acute type I interferon responses distinguishes nonpathogenic simian immunodeficiency virus (SIV) infection of natural hosts from pathogenic SIV infection of rhesus macaques *Journal of virology, 84*(15), 7886-7891. doi:10.1128/JVI.02612-09

Hartigan-O'connor, D. J., Hirao, L. A., McCune, J. M., & Dandekar, S. (2011). Th17 cells and regulatory T cells in elite control over HIV and SIV *Current opinion in HIV and AIDS, 6*(3), 221-227. doi:10.1097/COH.0b013e32834577b3

Hashmi, M. H., & Van Veldhuizen, P. J. (2010). Interleukin-21: updated review of Phase I and II clinical trials in metastatic renal cell carcinoma, metastatic melanoma and relapsed/refractory indolent non-Hodgkin's lymphoma *Expert opinion on biological therapy, 10*(5), 807-817. doi:10.1517/14712598.2010.480971

Huang, W., Na, L., Fidel, P. L., & Schwarzenberger, P. (2004). Requirement of interleukin-17A for systemic anti-Candida albicans host defense in mice *The Journal of infectious diseases, 190*(3), 624-631. doi:10.1086/422329

Hunt, P. W., Martin, J. N., Sinclair, E., Bredt, B., Hagos, E., Lampiris, H., & Deeks, S. G. (2003). T cell activation is associated with lower CD4+ T cell gains in human immunodeficiency virus-infected patients with sustained viral suppression during antiretroviral therapy *The Journal of infectious diseases, 187*(10), 1534-1543. doi:10.1086/374786

Hunt, P. W., Brenchley, J., Sinclair, E., McCune, J. M., Roland, M., Page-Shafer, K., Hsue, P., et al. (2008). Relationship between T cell activation and CD4+ T cell count in HIV-seropositive individuals with undetectable plasma HIV RNA levels in the absence of therapy *The Journal of infectious diseases, 197*(1), 126-133. doi:10.1086/524143

Hunt, P. W., Landay, A. L., Sinclair, E., Martinson, J. A., Hatano, H., Emu, B., Norris, P. J., et al. (2011). A low T regulatory cell response may contribute to both viral control and generalized immune activation in HIV controllers *PloS one, 6*(1), e15924. doi:10.1371/journal.pone.0015924

Hütter, G., Nowak, D., Mossner, M., Ganepola, S., Müssig, A., Allers, K., Schneider, T., et al. (2009a). Long-term control of HIV by CCR5 Delta32/Delta32 stem-cell transplantation *The New England journal of medicine, 360*(7), 692-698. doi:10.1056/NEJMoa0802905

Hütter, G., Schneider, Thomas, & Thiel, E. (2009b). Transplantation of selected or transgenic blood stem cells - a future treatment for HIV/AIDS *Journal of the International AIDS Society, 12*(1), 10. doi:10.1186/1758-2652-12-10

Iannello, A., Tremblay, C., Routy, J., Boulassel, M., Toma, E., & Ahmad, A. (2008). Decreased Levels of Circulating IL-21 in HIV-Infected AIDS Patients: Correlation with CD4 +T-Cell Counts. *Viral Immunology, 21*(3), 385-388. doi:10.1089/vim.2008.0025

Isgrò, A., Aiuti, A., Leti, W., Gramiccioni, C., Esposito, A., Mezzaroma, I., & Aiuti, F. (2005). Immunodysregulation of HIV disease at bone marrow level *Autoimmunity reviews, 4*(8), 486-490. doi:10.1016/j.autrev.2005.04.014

Jacquelin, B., Mayau, V., Targat, B., Liovat, A., Kunkel, D., Petitjean, G., Dillies, M., et al. (2009). Nonpathogenic SIV infection of African green monkeys induces a strong but rapidly controlled type I IFN response *The Journal of clinical investigation, 119*(12), 3544-3555. doi:10.1172/JCI40093

Jiang, W., Lederman, M. M., Hunt, P., Sieg, S. F., Haley, K., Rodríguez, B., Landay, A., et al. (2009). Plasma levels of bacterial DNA correlate with immune activation and the magnitude of immune restoration in persons with antiretroviral-treated HIV infection *The Journal of infectious diseases, 199*(8), 1177-1185. doi:10.1086/597476

Kader, M., Wang, X., Piatak, M., Lifson, J., Roederer, M., Veazey, R., & Mattapallil, J. J. (2009). Alpha4(+)beta7(hi)CD4(+) memory T cells harbor most Th-17 cells and are preferentially infected during acute SIV infection *Mucosal immunology, 2*(5), 439-449. doi:10.1038/mi.2009.90

Keele, B. F., Jones, J. H., Terio, K. A., Estes, J. D., Rudicell, R. S., Wilson, M. L., Li, Y., et al. (2009). Increased mortality and AIDS-like immunopathology in wild chimpanzees infected with SIVcpz *Nature, 460*(7254), 515-519. doi:10.1038/nature08200

Khader, S. A., Bell, G. K., Pearl, J. E., Fountain, J. J., Rangel-Moreno, J., Cilley, G. E., Shen, F., et al. (2007). IL-23 and IL-17 in the establishment of protective pulmonary CD4+ T cell responses after vaccination and during Mycobacterium tuberculosis challenge *Nature immunology, 8*(4), 369-377. doi:10.1038/ni1449

Khaitan, A., & Unutmaz, D. (2011). Revisiting immune exhaustion during HIV infection *Current HIV/AIDS reports, 8*(1), 4-11. doi:10.1007/s11904-010-0066-0

Klatt, Nichole. Short Talk: Mechanisms Underlying Damage to the Mucosal Barrier and Immune Activation after Pathogenic SIV Infection of Rhesus Macaques. Keystone Symposia, HIV Evolution, Genomics and Pathogenesis, March 20-25, 2011, Whistler, British Columbia.

Koning, F. A., Otto, S. A., Hazenberg, M. D., Dekker, L., Prins, M., Miedema, F., & Schuitemaker, H. (2005). Low-level CD4+ T cell activation is associated with low susceptibility to HIV-1 infection *Journal of immunology (Baltimore, Md. : 1950), 175*(9), 6117-6122.

Korn, T., Bettelli, E., Gao, W., Awasthi, A., Jäger, A., Strom, T. B., Oukka, M., et al. (2007). IL-21 initiates an alternative pathway to induce proinflammatory T(H)17 cells *Nature, 448*(7152), 484-487. doi:10.1038/nature05970

Kornfeld, C., Ploquin, M. J., Pandrea, I., Faye, A., Onanga, R., Apetrei, C., Poaty-Mavoungou, V., et al. (2005). Antiinflammatory profiles during primary SIV infection in African green monkeys are associated with protection against AIDS *The Journal of clinical investigation, 115*(4), 1082-1091. doi:10.1172/JCI23006

Lederer, S., Favre, D., Walters, K., Proll, S., Kanwar, B., Kasakow, Z., Baskin, C. R., et al. (2009). Transcriptional profiling in pathogenic and non-pathogenic SIV infections reveals significant distinctions in kinetics and tissue compartmentalization *PLoS pathogens, 5*(2), e1000296. doi:10.1371/journal.ppat.1000296

Li, Q., Duan, L., Estes, J. D., Ma, Z., Rourke, T., Wang, Y., Reilly, C., et al. (2005). Peak SIV replication in resting memory CD4+ T cells depletes gut lamina propria CD4+ T cells *Nature, 434*(7037), 1148-1152. doi:10.1038/nature03513

Liang, S. C., Tan, X., Luxenberg, D. P., Karim, R., Dunussi-Joannopoulos, K., Collins, M., & Fouser, L. A. (2006). Interleukin (IL)-22 and IL-17 are coexpressed by Th17 cells and cooperatively enhance expression of antimicrobial peptides *The Journal of experimental medicine, 203*(10), 2271-2279. doi:10.1084/jem.20061308

Liu, Z., Cumberland, W. G., Hultin, L. E., Prince, H. E., Detels, R., & Giorgi, J. V. (1997). Elevated CD38 antigen expression on CD8+ T cells is a stronger marker for the risk of chronic HIV disease progression to AIDS and death in the Multicenter AIDS Cohort Study than CD4+ cell count, soluble immune activation markers, or combinations of HLA-DR and CD38 expression *Journal of acquired immune deficiency syndromes and human retrovirology : official publication of the International Retrovirology Association, 16*(2), 83-92.

Mattapallil, J. J., Douek, D. C., Hill, B., Nishimura, Y., Martin, M., & Roederer, M. (2005). Massive infection and loss of memory CD4+ T cells in multiple tissues during acute SIV infection *Nature, 434*(7037), 1093-1097. doi:10.1038/nature03501

Mehandru, S., Poles, M. A., Tenner-Racz, K., Horowitz, A., Hurley, A., Hogan, C., Boden, D., et al. (2004). Primary HIV-1 infection is associated with preferential depletion of CD4+ T lymphocytes from effector sites in the gastrointestinal tract *The Journal of experimental medicine, 200*(6), 761-770. doi:10.1084/jem.20041196

Melmed, R. N., Taylor, J. M., Detels, R., Bozorgmehri, M., & Fahey, J. L. (1989). Serum neopterin changes in HIV-infected subjects: indicator of significant pathology, CD4 T cell changes, and the development of AIDS *Journal of acquired immune deficiency syndromes, 2*(1), 70-76.

Milner, J. D., Brenchley, J. M., Laurence, A., Freeman, A. F., Hill, B. J., Elias, K. M., Kanno, Y., et al. (2008). Impaired T(H)17 cell differentiation in subjects with autosomal dominant hyper-IgE syndrome *Nature, 452*(7188), 773-776. doi:10.1038/nature06764

Milner, J. D., Sandler, N. G., & Douek, D. C. (2010). Th17 cells, Job's syndrome and HIV: opportunities for bacterial and fungal infections *Current opinion in HIV and AIDS, 5*(2), 179-183. doi:10.1097/COH.0b013e328335ed3e

Milush, J. M., Reeves, J. D., Gordon, S. N., Zhou, D., Muthukumar, A., Kosub, D. A., Chacko, E., et al. (2007). Virally induced CD4+ T cell depletion is not sufficient to induce AIDS in a natural host *Journal of immunology (Baltimore, Md. : 1950), 179*(5), 3047-3056.

Milush, J. M., Mir, K. D., Sundaravaradan, V., Gordon, S. N., Engram, J., Cano, C. A., Reeves, J. D., et al. (2011). Lack of clinical AIDS in SIV-infected sooty mangabeys with significant CD4+ T cell loss is associated with double-negative T cells *The Journal of clinical investigation, 121*(3), 1102-1110. doi:10.1172/JCI44876

Mir, K. D., Gasper, M. A., Sundaravaradan, V., & Sodora, D. L. (2011). SIV infection in natural hosts: resolution of immune activation during the acute-to-chronic transition phase *Microbes and infection / Institut Pasteur, 13*(1), 14-24. doi:10.1016/j.micinf.2010.09.011

Monteiro, P., Gosselin, A., Wacleche, V. S., El-Far, M., Said, E. A., Kared, H., Grandvaux, N., et al. (2011). Memory CCR6+CD4+ T Cells Are Preferential Targets for Productive HIV Type 1 Infection Regardless of Their Expression of Integrin {beta}7 *Journal of immunology (Baltimore, Md. : 1950), 186*(8), 4618-4630. doi:10.4049/jimmunol.1004151

Moore, R. D., Keruly, J., Richman, D. D., Creagh-Kirk, T., & Chaisson, R. E. (1992). Natural history of advanced HIV disease in patients treated with zidovudine. The Zidovudine Epidemiology Study Group *AIDS (London, England), 6*(7), 671-677.

Moses, A., Nelson, J., & Bagby, G. C. (1998). The influence of human immunodeficiency virus-1 on hematopoiesis *Blood, 91*(5), 1479-1495.

Murray, S. M., Down, C. M., Boulware, D. R., Stauffer, W. M., Cavert, W. P., Schacker, T. W., Brenchley, J. M., et al. (2010). Reduction of immune activation with chloroquine therapy during chronic HIV infection *Journal of virology, 84*(22), 12082-12086. doi:10.1128/JVI.01466-10

Nowroozalizadeh, S., Månsson, F., da Silva, Z., Repits, J., Dabo, B., Pereira, C., Biague, A., et al. (2010). Microbial translocation correlates with the severity of both HIV-1 and HIV-2 infections *The Journal of infectious diseases, 201*(8), 1150-1154. doi:10.1086/651430

Nurieva, R., Yang, X. O., Martinez, G., Zhang, Y., Panopoulos, A. D., Ma, L., Schluns, K., et al. (2007). Essential autocrine regulation by IL-21 in the generation of inflammatory T cells *Nature, 448*(7152), 480-483. doi:10.1038/nature05969

Okoye, A., Meier-Schellersheim, M., Brenchley, J. M., Hagen, S. I., Walker, J. M., Rohankhedkar, M., Lum, R., et al. (2007). Progressive CD4+ central memory T cell decline results in CD4+ effector memory insufficiency and overt disease in chronic SIV infection *The Journal of experimental medicine, 204*(9), 2171-2185. doi:10.1084/jem.20070567

Onanga, R., Souquière, S., Makuwa, M., Mouinga-Ondéme, A., Simon, F., Apetrei, C., & Roques, P. (2006). Primary simian immunodeficiency virus SIVmnd-2 infection in mandrills (Mandrillus sphinx) *Journal of virology, 80*(7), 3301-3309. doi:10.1128/JVI.80.7.3301-3309.2006

Ouyang, W., & Valdez, P. (2008). IL-22 in mucosal immunity *Mucosal immunology, 1*(5), 335-338. doi:10.1038/mi.2008.26

Paiardini, Mirko. (2010). Th17 cells in natural SIV hosts *Current opinion in HIV and AIDS, 5*(2), 166-172. doi:10.1097/COH.0b013e328335c161

Paiardini, M, Cervasi, B., Engram, J. C., Gordon, S. N., Klatt, N. R., Muthukumar, A., Else, J., et al. (2009a). Bone marrow-based homeostatic proliferation of mature T cells in nonhuman primates: implications for AIDS pathogenesis. *Blood, 113*(3), 612-621. doi:10.1182/blood-2008-06-159442

Paiardini M, Cervasi B, Reyes-Aviles E, Micci L, Ortiz AM, Chahroudi A, Vinton C, Gordon SN, Bosinger SE, Francella N, Hallberg PL, Cramer E, Schlub T, Chan ML, Riddick NE, Collman RG, Apetrei C, Pandrea I, Else J, Munch J, Kirchhoff F, Davenport MP, Brenchley JM, Silvestri G. (2011). Low levels of SIV infection in sooty mangabey central memory CD4(+) T cells are associated with limited CCR5 expression Nature Medicine 17(7):830-6. doi: 10.1038/nm.2395

Paiardini, Mirko, Pandrea, I., Apetrei, C., & Silvestri, G. (2009b). Lessons learned from the natural hosts of HIV-related viruses *Annual review of medicine, 60*, 485-495. doi:10.1146/annurev.med.60.041807.123753

Pandrea, I., Apetrei, C., Dufour, J., Dillon, N., Barbercheck, J., Metzger, M., Jacquelin, B., et al. (2006). Simian immunodeficiency virus SIVagm.sab infection of Caribbean African green monkeys: a new model for the study of SIV pathogenesis in natural hosts *Journal of virology, 80*(10), 4858-4867. doi:10.1128/JVI.80.10.4858-4867.2006

Pandrea, I., Apetrei, C., Gordon, S., Barbercheck, J., Dufour, J., Bohm, R., Sumpter, B., et al. (2007a). Paucity of CD4+CCR5+ T cells is a typical feature of natural SIV hosts *Blood, 109*(3), 1069-1076. doi:10.1182/blood-2006-05-024364

Pandrea, I. V., Gautam, R., Ribeiro, R. M., Brenchley, J. M., Butler, I. F., Pattison, M., Rasmussen, T., et al. (2007b). Acute loss of intestinal CD4+ T cells is not predictive of simian immunodeficiency virus virulence *Journal of immunology (Baltimore, Md. : 1950), 179*(5), 3035-3046.

Pandrea, I., Sodora, D. L., Silvestri, G., & Apetrei, C. (2008). Into the wild: simian immunodeficiency virus (SIV) infection in natural hosts *Trends in immunology, 29*(9), 419-428. doi:10.1016/j.it.2008.05.004

Picker, L. J. (2006). Immunopathogenesis of acute AIDS virus infection *Current opinion in immunology, 18*(4), 399-405. doi:10.1016/j.coi.2006.05.001

Picker, L. J., Hagen, S. I., Lum, R., Reed-Inderbitzin, E. F., Daly, L. M., Sylwester, A. W., Walker, J. M., et al. (2004). Insufficient production and tissue delivery of CD4+ memory T cells in rapidly progressive simian immunodeficiency virus infection *The Journal of experimental medicine, 200*(10), 1299-1314. doi:10.1084/jem.20041049

Pizzolo, G., Vinante, F., Sinicco, A., Chilosi, M., Agostini, C., Perini, A., Zuppini, B., et al. (1987). Increased levels of soluble interleukin-2 receptor in the serum of patients with human immunodeficiency virus infection *Diagnostic and clinical immunology, 5*(4), 180-183.

Prendergast, A., Prado, J. G., Kang, Y., Chen, F., Riddell, L. A., Luzzi, G., Goulder, P., et al. (2010). HIV-1 infection is characterized by profound depletion of CD161+ Th17 cells and gradual decline in regulatory T cells *AIDS (London, England), 24*(4), 491-502. doi:10.1097/QAD.0b013e3283344895

Raffatellu, M., Santos, R. L., Verhoeven, D. E., George, M. D., Wilson, R. P., Winter, S. E., Godinez, I., et al. (2008). Simian immunodeficiency virus-induced mucosal interleukin-17 deficiency promotes Salmonella dissemination from the gut *Nature medicine, 14*(4), 421-428. doi:10.1038/nm1743

Reddy, M. M., Sorrell, S. J., Lange, M., & Grieco, M. H. (1988). Tumor necrosis factor and HIV P24 antigen levels in serum of HIV-infected populations *Journal of acquired immune deficiency syndromes, 1*(5), 436-440.

Rey-Cuillé, M. A., Berthier, J. L., Bomsel-Demontoy, M. C., Chaduc, Y., Montagnier, L., Hovanessian, A. G., & Chakrabarti, L. A. (1998). Simian immunodeficiency virus replicates to high levels in sooty mangabeys without inducing disease *Journal of virology, 72*(5), 3872-3886.

Rodríguez, B., Sethi, A. K., Cheruvu, V. K., Mackay, W., Bosch, R. J., Kitahata, M., Boswell, S. L., et al. (2006). Predictive value of plasma HIV RNA level on rate of CD4 T-cell decline in untreated HIV infection *JAMA : the journal of the American Medical Association, 296*(12), 1498-1506. doi:10.1001/jama.296.12.1498

It's the immune system, stupid. (1999). It's the immune system, stupid *STEP perspective, 99*(1), 5.

Roederer, M, Dubs, J. G., Anderson, M. T., Raju, P. A., Herzenberg, L. A., & Herzenberg, L. A. (1995). CD8 naive T cell counts decrease progressively in HIV-infected adults *The Journal of clinical investigation, 95*(5), 2061-2066. doi:10.1172/JCI117892

Romagnani, S. (2008). Human Th17 cells *Arthritis research & therapy, 10*(2), 206. doi:10.1186/ar2392

Sandler, N. G., Wand, H., Roque, A., Law, M., Nason, M. C., Nixon, D. E., Pedersen, C., et al. (2011). Plasma levels of soluble CD14 independently predict mortality in HIV infection *The Journal of infectious diseases, 203*(6), 780-790. doi:10.1093/infdis/jiq118

Sauce, D., Larsen, M., Fastenackels, S., Pauchard, M., Ait-Mohand, H., Schneider, L., Guihot, A., et al. (2011). HIV disease progression despite suppression of viral replication is associated with exhaustion of lymphopoiesis *Blood*. doi:10.1182/blood-2011-01-331306

Schneider, T, Jahn, H. U., Schmidt, W., Riecken, E. O., Zeitz, M., & Ullrich, R. (1995). Loss of CD4 T lymphocytes in patients infected with human immunodeficiency virus type 1 is more pronounced in the duodenal mucosa than in the peripheral blood. Berlin Diarrhea/Wasting Syndrome Study Group *Gut, 37*(4), 524-529.

Sethi, K. K., & Näher, H. (1986). Elevated titers of cell-free interleukin-2 receptor in serum and cerebrospinal fluid specimens of patients with acquired immunodeficiency syndrome *Immunology letters, 13*(4), 179-184.

Sharp, Paul M, & Hahn, Beatrice H. (2008). AIDS: prehistory of HIV-1 *Nature, 455*(7213), 605-606. doi:10.1038/455605a

Sharp, P M, & Hahn, B H. (2010). The evolution of HIV-1 and the origin of AIDS. *Philosophical Transactions of the Royal Society B: Biological Sciences, 365*(1552), 2487-2494. doi:10.1098/rstb.2010.0031

Sharp, Paul M, Shaw, G. M., & Hahn, Beatrice H. (2005). Simian immunodeficiency virus infection of chimpanzees *Journal of virology, 79*(7), 3891-3902. doi:10.1128/JVI.79.7.3891-3902.2005

Shen, X., & Tomaras, G. D. (2011). Alterations of the B-cell response by HIV-1 replication *Current HIV/AIDS reports, 8*(1), 23-30. doi:10.1007/s11904-010-0064-2

Silvestri, G., Sodora, D. L., Koup, R. A., Paiardini, M., O'Neil, S. P., McClure, H. M., Staprans, S. I., et al. (2003). Nonpathogenic SIV infection of sooty mangabeys is characterized by limited bystander immunopathology despite chronic high-level viremia *Immunity, 18*(3), 441-452.

Silvestri, G., Fedanov, A., Germon, S., Kozyr, N., Kaiser, W. J., Garber, D. A., McClure, H., et al. (2005). Divergent host responses during primary simian immunodeficiency virus SIVsm infection of natural sooty mangabey and nonnatural rhesus macaque hosts *Journal of virology, 79*(7), 4043-4054. doi:10.1128/JVI.79.7.4043-4054.2005

Silvestri, G., Paiardini, Mirko, Pandrea, I., Lederman, M. M., & Sodora, D. L. (2007). Understanding the benign nature of SIV infection in natural hosts *The Journal of clinical investigation, 117*(11), 3148-3154. doi:10.1172/JCI33034

Simons, B. C., Vancompernolle, S. E., Smith, R. M., Wei, J., Barnett, L., Lorey, S. L., Meyer-Olson, D., et al. (2008). Despite biased TRBV gene usage against a dominant HLA B57-restricted epitope, TCR diversity can provide recognition of circulating epitope variants *Journal of immunology (Baltimore, Md. : 1950), 181*(7), 5137-5146.

Smith, S. M. (2006). The pathogenesis of HIV infection: stupid may not be so dumb after all *Retrovirology, 3*, 60. doi:10.1186/1742-4690-3-60

Sodora, D. L., Allan, J. S., Apetrei, C., Brenchley, J. M., Douek, D. C., Else, J. G., Estes, J. D., et al. (2009). Toward an AIDS vaccine: lessons from natural simian immunodeficiency virus infections of African nonhuman primate hosts *Nature medicine, 15*(8), 861-865. doi:10.1038/nm.2013

Sodora, D. L., & Silvestri, G. (2008). Immune activation and AIDS pathogenesis *AIDS (London, England), 22*(4), 439-446. doi:10.1097/QAD.0b013e3282f2dbe7

Sumpter, B., Dunham, R., Gordon, S., Engram, J., Hennessy, M., Kinter, A., Paiardini, M., et al. (2007). Correlates of preserved CD4(+) T cell homeostasis during natural, nonpathogenic simian immunodeficiency virus infection of sooty mangabeys: implications for AIDS pathogenesis *Journal of immunology (Baltimore, Md. : 1950), 178*(3), 1680-1691.

Taaffe, J., Chahroudi, A., Engram, J., Sumpter, B., Meeker, T., Ratcliffe, S., Paiardini, M., et al. (2010). A five-year longitudinal analysis of sooty mangabeys naturally infected with simian immunodeficiency virus reveals a slow but progressive decline in CD4+ T-cell count whose magnitude is not predicted by viral load or immune activation *Journal of virology, 84*(11), 5476-5484. doi:10.1128/JVI.00039-10

Takehisa, J., & Miura, T. (2010). [The origin and evolution of HIV] *Nippon rinsho. Japanese journal of clinical medicine, 68*(3), 410-414.

Tesselaar, K., Arens, R., van Schijndel, G. M. W., Baars, P. A., van der Valk, M. A., Borst, J., van Oers, M. H. J., et al. (2003). Lethal T cell immunodeficiency induced by chronic costimulation via CD27-CD70 interactions *Nature immunology, 4*(1), 49-54. doi:10.1038/ni869

VandeWoude, S., & Apetrei, C. (2006). Going wild: lessons from naturally occurring T-lymphotropic lentiviruses *Clinical microbiology reviews, 19*(4), 728-762. doi:10.1128/CMR.00009-06

Veazey, R. S., DeMaria, M., Chalifoux, L. V., Shvetz, D. E., Pauley, D. R., Knight, H. L., Rosenzweig, M., et al. (1998). Gastrointestinal tract as a major site of CD4+ T cell depletion and viral replication in SIV infection *Science (New York, N.Y.), 280*(5362), 427-431.

Wertheim, J. O., & Worobey, M. (2009). Dating the age of the SIV lineages that gave rise to HIV-1 and HIV-2 *PLoS computational biology, 5*(5), e1000377. doi:10.1371/journal.pcbi.1000377

Williams LD, Bansal A, Sabbaj S, Heath SL, Song W, Tang J, Zajac AJ, Goepfert PA. (2011). Interleukin-21-producing HIV-1-specific CD8 T cells are preferentially seen in elite controllers. *Journal of virology*, 85(5), 2316-24. doi:10.1128/JVI.01476-10

Wolthers, K. C., Otto, S. A., Lens, S. M., Kolbach, D. N., van Lier, R. A., Miedema, F., & Meyaard, L. (1996). Increased expression of CD80, CD86 and CD70 on T cells from HIV-infected individuals upon activation in vitro: regulation by CD4+ T cells *European journal of immunology, 26*(8), 1700-1706. doi:10.1002/eji.1830260806

Worobey, M., Santiago, M. L., Keele, B. F., Ndjango, J. N., Joy, J. B., Labama, B. L., Dhed'A, B. D., et al. (2004). Origin of AIDS: contaminated polio vaccine theory refuted *Nature, 428*(6985), 820. doi:10.1038/428820a

Worobey, M., Gemmel, M., Teuwen, D. E., Haselkorn, T., Kunstman, K., Bunce, M., Muyembe, J., et al. (2008). Direct evidence of extensive diversity of HIV-1 in Kinshasa by 1960 *Nature, 455*(7213), 661-664. doi:10.1038/nature07390

Worobey, M., Telfer, P., Souquière, S., Hunter, M., Coleman, C. A., Metzger, M. J., Reed, P., et al. (2010). Island biogeography reveals the deep history of SIV *Science (New York, N.Y.), 329*(5998), 1487. doi:10.1126/science.1193550

Yang, L., Anderson, D. E., Baecher-Allan, C., Hastings, W. D., Bettelli, E., Oukka, M., Kuchroo, V. K., et al. (2008). IL-21 and TGF-beta are required for differentiation of human T(H)17 cells *Nature, 454*(7202), 350-352. doi:10.1038/nature07021

Zheng, Y., Valdez, P. A., Danilenko, D. M., Hu, Y., Sa, S. M., Gong, Q., Abbas, A. R., et al. (2008). Interleukin-22 mediates early host defense against attaching and effacing bacterial pathogens *Nature medicine, 14*(3), 282-289. doi:10.1038/nm1720

Zhu, T., Korber, B. T., Nahmias, A. J., Hooper, E., Sharp, P. M., & Ho, D. D. (1998). An African HIV-1 sequence from 1959 and implications for the origin of the epidemic *Nature, 391*(6667), 594-597. doi:10.1038/35400

(n.d.).

9

Immunotherapies and Vaccines

Hermancia S. Eugene and Ted M. Ross
University of Pittsburgh
United States

1. Introduction

Human Immunodeficiency Virus (HIV) was first isolated in 1983 by Barre-Sinoussi and Gallo in parallel at two independent institutions (Barre-Sinoussi, Chermann et al. 1983; Gallo, Sarin et al. 1983). The following year, HIV was established as the causative agent of Acquired Immunodeficiency Syndrome (AIDS). Given such a monumental discovery, there were expectations that an effective vaccine or treatment was not far from being marketed. Unfortunately these expectations have yet to become reality and HIV has become a global epidemic. In 2010, the World Health Organization (WHO) reported that 33.3 million individuals worldwide were living with HIV/AIDS (World Health Organization 2009). The discovery of HIV as the causative agent of AIDS stimulated many areas of basic virological and immunological research. Researchers continue to stress the need for more integrated approaches for development of HIV antiviral treatments and vaccines. In this chapter, the viral and immune challenges, criteria for evaluating clinical studies, candidate therapies and vaccines will be reviewed.

1.1 Viral and immune challenges

Several factors have contributed to the delay of HIV vaccines and therapeutics. These factors can be grouped into two main categories; 1) intrinsic viral characteristics and 2) viral and host interactions. The intrinsic viral properties of HIV, such as rapid replication and virus mutation, virus recombination and viral integration have been obstacles in drug and vaccine development (Aaron N. Endsley 2008; Montagnier 2010). One of the major problems in HIV vaccine development is the high sequence variability of viral isolates (Monteiro, Alcantara et al. 2009; Cuevas, Fernandez-Garcia et al. 2010). The classification of HIV into clades is covered in the HIV nomenclature proposal now found on the Los Alamos HIV Sequence database website (Robertson, Anderson et al. 2000). A major contributor to the high variability of the virus is the lack of proof reading activity present in the viral polymerase (reverse transcriptase) combined with rapid replication rate. Such a combination allows for emergence of viral isolates that can evade the immune response elicited to older viral sequences. The constant escape from immune surveillance results in a constant need for "catch up" by the immune response. Another reason for increase variability is the ability of the virus to genetically recombine (Brown, Peters et al. 2011). Due to the possibility of superinfection, viruses from different clades can be present in the same cell during replication and may result in recombinant viruses. For example, a virus classified A/E has an envelope derived from a clade A virus and Gag proteins derived from a clade E virus.

The other major viral property that works against effective of therapy and viral clearance is viral integration. HIV contains a viral integrase responsible for integration of the HIV provirus into the DNA of an infected cell (Delelis, Carayon et al. 2008). Provirus integration is an essential part of replication (Engelman, Englund et al. 1995). This integrated viral DNA results in both establishment of viral reservoirs in the host and disruption of the immune responses against the infecting virus (Finzi, Blankson et al. 1999; Miedema 2008; Carter, Onafuwa-Nuga et al. 2010; Virgin and Walker 2010). These viral reservoirs are a source of actively replicating viruses in individuals who have controlled infection and have undetectable levels of virus(Wong, Hezareh et al. 1997; Chun, Nickle et al. 2008; Lerner, Guadalupe et al. 2011). Authors Siliciano J.D and Siliciano,R F discuss HIV reservoirs and how they contribute to the lack of virus eradication and the need for continuous HAART therapy by HIV infected individuals to prevent virus rebound (Siliciano and Siliciano 2004).

The lack of a defined correlate(s) of protection for HIV is a major obstacle in vaccine and therapeutic development. Humoral immune responses were initially proposed as a correlate of protection. Studies in experimental animals have shown that passively administering anti-HIV antibodies results in protection from infection (Prince, Reesink et al. 1991; Putkonen, Thorstensson et al. 1991; Emini, Schleif et al. 1992). The first prophylaxis vaccine to enter phase III trials, AIDSVAX by VaxGen, induced antibodies to HIV vaccine components but vaccine was not efficacious (Ltd. 2003). The failure of the initial studies has not changed the viewpoint of everyone on the role of humoral responses as the correlate of protection. The antigens used in these studies, monomeric gp120 and monomeric gp160, are not the functional unit of the HIV envelope. The HIV envelope is trimeric on the surface of the virus particle. Studies using trimeric envelope immunogens have been used to improve the humoral responses (Nkolola, Peng et al. 2010; Sundling, Forsell et al. 2010; Sundling, O'Dell et al. 2010). Also, the recent vaccine trial in Thailand, has provided some data to support the possibility that humoral responses may be the HIV correlate of protection (Rerks-Ngarm, Pitisuttithum et al. 2009).

Many investigators are designing preventative vaccines for HIV that induces cellular response (Nanjundappa, Wang et al. 2011; Ranasinghe, Eyers et al. 2011; Sistigu, Bracci et al. 2011). Data from preclinical studies, as well as infected individuals, showed that an effective cellular response was able to control viral replication and resulted in reduce progression to diseases (Wilson, Keele et al. 2009; Streeck and Nixon 2010). Coming off the heels of failed humorally-driven trials, the certainty of developing a preventative vaccine is questioned and some in the field believed that preventing progression to disease to be a viable alternate focus. Vaccines aimed at eliciting cellular responses for preventing infection or disease progression have also not been successful. In 2007, the Merck HIV vaccine trial used adenovirus to deliver HIV genes *gag, pol* and *nef* .The trial was stopped after intermediate data analysis showed no supportive evidence to continue (Sekaly 2008). It appears that pre-existing immune responses to the adenovirus may have increased susceptibility to infection. Other alternative theories of the immune correlates of HIV/AIDS protection need to be considered. The immune correlate(s) for preventing infection and prevention of disease symptoms (*i.e.* control of infection) may be different (Jose Esparza 1996). In the case of preventative vaccines, an effective initial response to the virus is needed. At the time of the initial assault, the immune system is not dysfunctional. In contrast, during HIV therapy the immune system is in a state of dysregulation due to the constant tug of war with the virus infection. HIV infection causes a dysregulation of the immune response (Kuhrt, Faith et al.

2010; Sabado, O'Brien et al. 2010; Kolte, Gaardbo et al. 2011). Therefore, the HIV immunotherapeutic field does not only have to establish the correlate for preventing disease progression but has to overcome the immune dysfunction caused by the viral infection. The moderate success of the Thailand study and the failure of the STEP trial have brought into question both humoral and cellular immunity as the correlates of protection. New vaccine designs are now aimed at inducing both of humoral and cellular responses. The key to overcoming these obstacles faced by drug and vaccine development is continued research not only in terms of treatment, but also basic research of HIV and human immunology.

1.2 Evaluation of immunotherapies and vaccines in human trials

Since there is a lack of protective correlate(s), standardized evaluation of clinical responses is needed to develop preventative AIDS vaccines and improved immunotherapies (Pantaleo and Koup 2004). Usually, when a correlate of protection is lacking, a vaccine's ability to provide clinical benefit by reducing mortality and morbidity gives precedent for licensing. Due to the availability of an FDA approved therapy, HAART, any therapy that will be approved is compared to benefits given by HAART. HAART reduces viral loads and restores some level of CD4+T cells in individuals that benefit from therapy. In a clinical setting, the hallmarks or surrogate markers of efficacy are reduction in viral loads and increase in the number of CD4+ T cells (Peto 1996; Peters 2000). While CD4 +T cells increase during HAART therapy leads to better prognosis of disease. Recent Proleukin (rIL-2) clinical trials, SILCAAT and ESPRIT volunteers showed increase in CD4 +T cells but the time to disease progression was not increased. These results have brought into question the validity of increase CD4+T cells as a readout for better disease outcome (Peters and Samuel 2010). The composition of the CD4+ T cell population recovered after therapy was evaluated at the end of the study to determine if the increase CD4+ T cells population was any different from populations seen after HAART therapy. Other T cells have also come into light in the last few years, Th17 cells and cells that secret IL-21 may play a role in the non-disease progression seen in African green monkeys and Sooty Mangabeys (Ciccone, Greenwald et al. 2011; Hartigan-O'Connor, Hirao et al. 2011; Milush, Mir et al. 2011). These trends are also being reported in long- term non-progressors and elite controllers (Hartigan-O'Connor, Hirao et al. 2011; Salgado, Rallun et al. 2011; Salgado, RallÛn et al. 2011). Results in animal studies have shown the possible role of Th17 cells in the gut mucosa in reduced bacterial translocation and slower disease progression (Cecchinato, Trindade et al. 2008; Maloy and Kullberg 2008; Hofer and Speck 2009).

There is a lack of consensus on the hallmarks or surrogate markers for preventative vaccine trials. The ideal standard for a preventative HIV vaccine would be sterilizing protection. Sterilizing protection is complete protection from HIV infection, no detectable HIV at any time and no transmission of HIV. In 2007 an NIH workshop on vaccine efficacy resulted in a reported by Follman et al. which stated three parameters for evaluating HIV vaccine efficacy(Follmann, Duerr et al. 2007). The three parameters for evaluating vaccine efficacy are 1) reduction in risk of acquiring HIV 2) the reduction in cumulative risk of progressing to AIDS from the time of infection to diagnosis and 3) reduction in the risk of transmission of HIV to others. Vaccine endpoints are based on years of clinical studies (Peto 1996; Follmann, Duerr et al. 2007; MacLachlan, Mayer et al. 2009). Preclinical (usually NHP) studies have established surrogate markers for vaccine efficacy. Thus far, the most relevant marker identified as a determinant of disease outcome is the reduction of plasma HIV genome RNA levels following infection (Lavreys, Baeten et al. 2006). The viral set point is a consistent marker for determining disease progression; i.e. the higher the viral set point, the more likely a patient will progress to AIDS (Lavreys, Baeten et al. 2006; Kelley, Barbour et al. 2007) The levels of CD4+T cells in the blood of infected individuals can also act as a surrogate of disease progression (Chouquet, Autran et al. 2002). However, the correlation between CD4+ T cell levels in the blood and disease progression becomes more significant closer to the onset of AIDS. Modeling studies have concluded that a reduction in blood viral titers of 1-1.5 $\log_{10}$ compared to peak infection leads to a significantly positive impact on progression to disease (Davenport, Ribeiro et al. 2004). The other aspect to a preventative vaccine is reduction of viral load leading to reduce transmission. A vaccine that results in a reduction in the rate or probability of transmission would have a positive impact on the HIV global epidemic. In the absence of a sterilizing vaccine, to have a vaccine, that not only lowers viral set point, but also reduces transmission rate would be beneficial (Gurunathan, Habib et al. 2009).

2. Immunotherapies

2.1 Highly Active Antiviral Therapy (HAART)

Two years after the discovery of the causative agent of AIDS, the first sign of possible treatment was reported in 1985 with the development of the first antiretroviral compound (Mitsuya, Weinhold et al. 1985). This compound was called Retrovir (zidovudine, AZT) and became the first drug in the family of nucleoside reverse transcriptase inhibitors (NRTI). AZT targets the reverse transcription process of HIV's replication cycle. Since AZT, several NRTI and other families of drugs targeting the replication cycle of HIV have been discovered. As of 2010, the FDA has licensed twenty-five antiretroviral drugs. These drugs can be grouped based on the mode of action and are placed into one of the following groups: nucleoside reverse transcriptase inhibitors (NRTI), nucleotide reverse transcriptase inhibitor (NtRTI), non-nucleoside reverse transcriptase inhibitor (NNRTI), protease inhibitor (PI), co-receptor inhibitor (CRI), integrase inhibitor (INI), and fusion inhibitor (FI) (De Clercq 2010). Figure 1 highlights licensed drugs and the mode of action of each group of drugs.

In 1996, the first use of combination drug therapy was attempted using a protease inhibitor that was combined with an NRTI (Gulick, Mellors et al. 1997). Combinational therapy confirmed that there was a longer period of undetectable or reduced viral loads as well as recovery of CD4+T cells in the blood. Combination therapy or HAART is now the treatment of choice for HIV infected individuals and results in various clinical outcomes (Greenbaum, Wilson et al. 2008; Crabtree-Ramirez, Villasis-Keever et al. 2010). Individuals on HAART need to be monitored at all times to ensure the combinational therapy is effective and does not result in viral mutants. Individuals on HAART will need their treatment regimen adjusted upon development of viral resistance (Paci, Martini et al. 2011; Von Kleist, Menz et al. 2011). In addition to viral resistance, HAART is highly toxic to patients resulting in reduced patient compliance (John, Moore et al. 2001; Kronenberg, Riehle et al. 2001). Moreover, HAART treatment is expensive and therefore people living in developing countries have less access to drugs even though these are the locations where the epidemic is greatest. Based on surveys and clinical research the WHO has identified factors that need to be considered to determine HAART treatment in an adult

(World Health Organization 2006) : 1) suitability of drug combination, 2) licensing of drugs by national regulatory department and recommended dose, 3) toxicity profile of the drug, 4) availability of laboratory monitoring, 5) potential of maintenance and adherence to treatment , 6) prevalence of co-existing infections (*e.g.* Tuberculosis), 7) child bearing age, 8) availability of local and international manufacturers, and 9) price and effectiveness of drug.

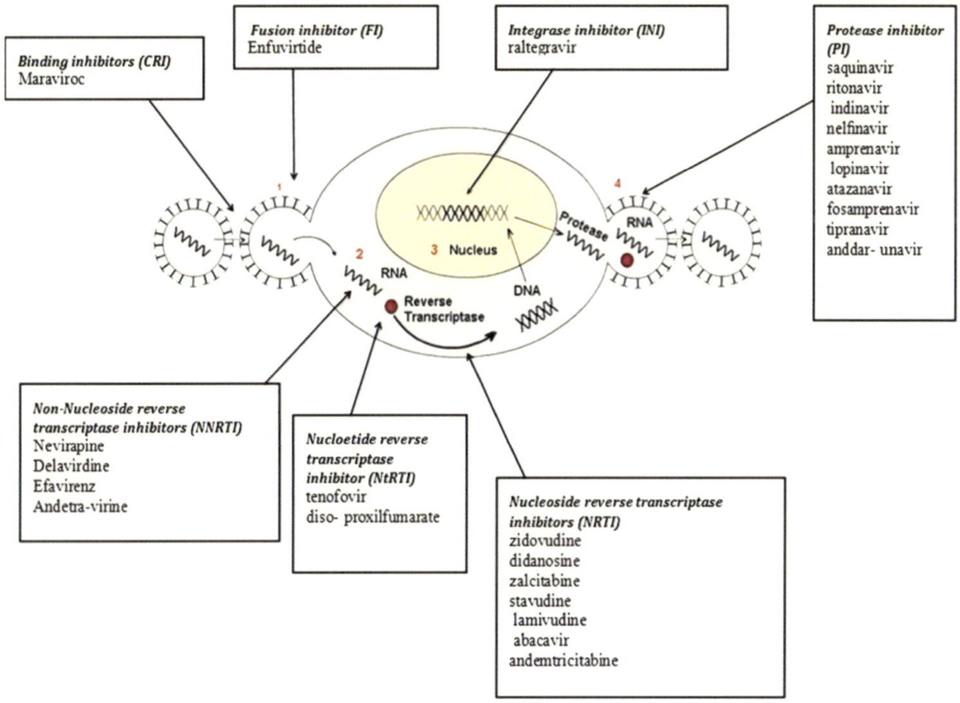

Stages of replication cycle where drugs act: 1) Receptor binding and membrane fusion, 2) RNA genome reverse transcribed into DNA, 3) Provirus integration, 4) Virion egress and maturation.

Fig. 1. Diagram showing the licensed antiretroviral HIV drugs and the step in the replication cycle they act on.

One of the complications that an individual can experience on HAART is immune reconstitution inflammatory syndrome (IRIS) (Letang, Miro et al. 2011). IRIS is seen in individuals recovering from immunodeficiency. Criteria for IRIS 1) Response to antiviral therapy by: viral loads >1 log10/ml decrease in RNA level 2) clinical deterioration of inflammatory of infectious condition upon antiviral treatment and 3) symptoms cannot be alleviated by: clinical course of treatment, medication side effects or toxicity, treatment failure or complete non adherence (Tappuni 2011). IRIS is also recorded in individuals with HIV co-infections such as tuberculosis (Lin, Lai et al. 2010). Additionally, individuals on HAART develop other diseases such as cardiac and metabolic complications that are affiliated with aging (Broder 2010). The side effects of HAART treatment and limited availability in HIV endemic areas are the drive for development of new immunotherapies for HIV.

2.2 Expanding HIV therapy from HAART

During HIV infection, the immune system does provide a defense aimed at eradicating the infection. This mounted immune response is insufficient and allows the viral infection to impair the immune system and persist. The use of therapeutics in infected individuals is aimed at overcoming the immune systems impairment to allow for viral control leading to decrease progression to AIDS. Human studies of long term non-progressor and elite progressors have observed a slower progression to disease in these individuals (Rodes, Toro et al. 2004; Okulicz and Lambotte 2011). Long term non-progressors are characterized based on absence of disease, low viral loads, and stable or increasing CD4 T cells.(Paroli, Propato et al. 2001). There is great need for drugs and vaccine strategies that reduce viral loads in infected individuals. Development of an effective HIV therapy needs to incorporate the knowledge that the immune system of an infected individual is dysfunctional. Figure 2 below simplifies the current knowledge of immune dysfunction and pathogenesis of HIV infection and table1(Fernandez, Lim et al. 2009). Immune dysfunction has been identified in Lymphocytes (T and B cells), NK cells, macrophages and even cytokine secretion.

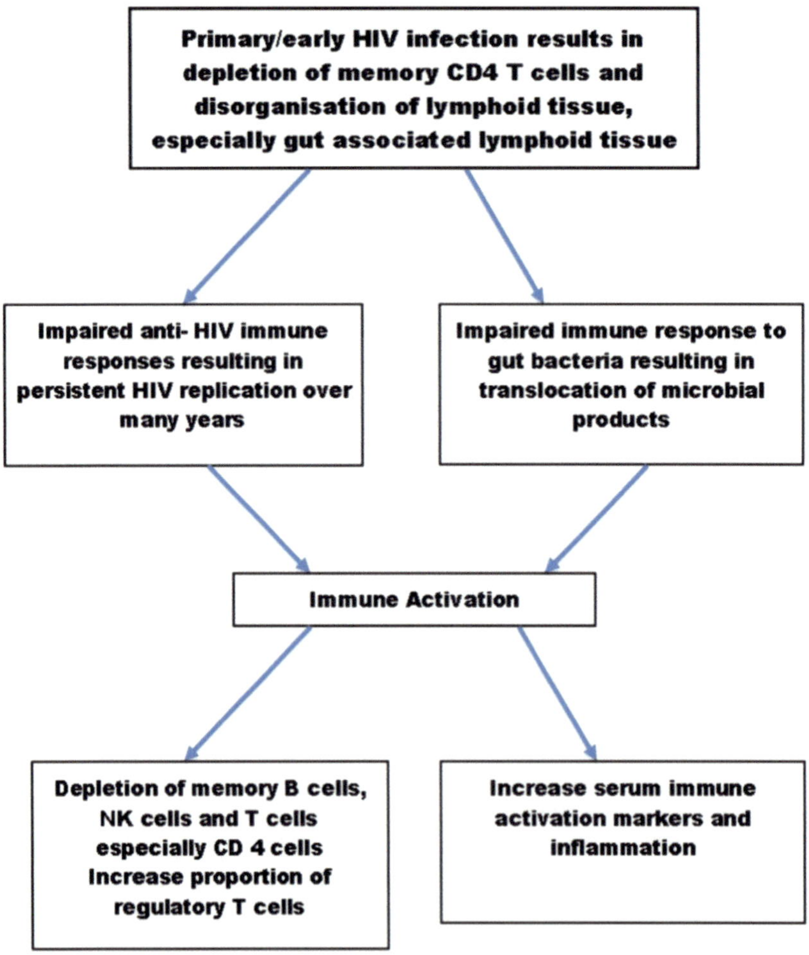

Fig. 2. Pathogenesis of immune dysfunction associated with HIV (Fernandez, Lim et al. 2009)

Dysfunction	References
The frequency of CD+ T cells infected by HIV in vivo is too low to account for the CD4 T cell loss	(Chun, Carruth et al. 1997),(Douek, Brenchley et al. 2002)
Most apoptotic CD4+T cells in peripheral blood and lymph nodes of patients with chronic HIV infection are infected HIV	(Finkel, Tudor-Williams et al. 1995)
Naïve CD8+T cells, memory B and NK cells as well as CD4+T cells decline in HIV infection	(D'Orsogna, Krueger et al. 2007),(Fauci, Mavilio et al. 2005),
SIV-infected macaques exhibit a persistently activated immune system and rapidly progress to AIDS, while SIV-infected sooty mangabeys show normal T cell division rates and do not progress to AIDS.	(M Roederer 1995)
HIV-2 infection is associated with lower levels of immune activation, which may explain the slower decline of CD4+Tcells compared with HIV-1 infection	(Michel, Balde et al. 2000)
In mice, TLR7 stimulation unrelated to a virus infection induces immune activation and immunopathology similar to that in HIV infection	(Baenziger, Heikenwalder et al. 2009)

Table 1. Evidence of dysfunction of the immune system of HIV infected individuals (Fernandez, Lim et al. 2009)

Current experimental therapies are grouped based on components and or modes of action, such as the HIV viral proteins targeted, the components of the immune system effected, fusion inhibitors, viral inhibitors, and HIV regulatory protein inhibitors, (Kilby 1999; Peters 2000; Pett 2009). Examples of these can be seen in Table 2.

Type of Immunotherapy	Examples
HIV Viral Protein	Remune, rgp160 (VaxSyn), rgp120, p24VLP, ALVAC1452
Components of Immune Systems	rIL-2, rIL-7, primed dendritic cells
Fusion inhibitors	T-20, T-1249
Viral inhibitors HIV regulatory protein inhibitors	sCD4 , Indinavir, nevirapine
DNAzymes	DzV3-9

Table 2. Some examples of Immunotherapies

HIV viral proteins used for immunotherapy include the viral envelope protein, core protein (Gag), reverse transcriptase, tat, nef, polymerase, as well as the whole killed virus (Tsoukas, Raboud et al. 1998; Gorse, Simionescu et al. 2006; Ensoli, Bellino et al. 2010). Viral proteins have been delivered as recombinant proteins, DNA vaccines, on virus-like-particles or in viral vectors (Buonaguro, Tornesello et al. 2009; Rosenberg, Graham et al. 2010). CD8+ T cells with cytolytic activity appeared to control viral titers in both non-human primate models, as well as infected individuals with HIV (O'Connell, Bailey et al. 2009). In an effort to induce more cytotoxic T lytic (CTL) responses viral vectors, such as canarypox virus and DNA vaccination, were implemented (Kutscher, Allgayer et al. 2010; Rosario, Bridgeman et al. 2010). One example of the use of recombinant canarypox virus vaccine to deliver viral proteins is the vaccine VCP1452 (ALVAC1452). ALVAC1452 was used to carry the HIV-1 genes: gag, pol, env and nef.

2.3 Remune

Remune, is a whole killed virus with a clade A envelope and a clade G gag depleted of gp120 administered in conjunction with incomplete Freund's adjuvant. This vaccine was shown to be safe and resulted in a maintenance of CD4+T cells in volunteers in a two year follow up study (Sukeepaisarncharoen, Churdboonchart et al. 2001). Remune clinical trial is covered in detail in the article by Fernandez -Cruz et al (Fernandez-Cruz, Navarro et al. 2003). The gp120 component of the virus was removed in an effort to present the more conserved antigens to induce T cell responses. In phase II clinical trials this vaccine was combined with HAART, where Remune was administered intramuscularly every 3 months. Trial participants had a mean CD4+T cell count of 586 cells /mm^3 and a mean viral load of 953 RNA copies /ml. Peripheral blood mononuclear cells (PBMC) were collected from trial participants. Following stimulation with Env gp120 depleted virus or recombinant Gag p24, PBMCs proliferate was observed in vaccine volunteers compared to a negative control group that was vaccinated against Candida. In addition, there was proliferation following HIV-specific antigen proliferation in isolated CD8+T, CD4+T and NK cells. Predominantly, memory CD4+T and CD8+T proliferated to HIV antigen stimulation.
Remune / HAART combination therapy entered phase III trials, but it was terminated after an intermediate evaluation of the data showed no significant benefit of Remune to the individuals receiving the therapeutic vaccine (Moss, Wallace et al. 1999). Additional studies using only Remune elicited significant increases in CD4+ T cells and reduced viral loads following vaccination (Fernandez-Cruz, Navarro et al. 2003). However, Remune /ALVAC did not elicit significant increases in the cytotoxic T cell activity or enhanced CD4+ T cell compared to ALVAC alone. (Angel, Routy et al. 2011). Remune did not meet criteria for evaluation by the FDA as an Immunotherapy. Although these studies with Remune did not result in licensing, these studies contributed to the knowledge of the field with a better appreciation that increases in specific T cell responses measured by *in vitro* assays do not always correlate with the efficacy of vaccination. Since increase in CD4+ T cells numbers do not correlate with better prognosis better surrogates or immune markers of vaccine efficacy are needed.

2.4 Proleukin (recombinant IL-2/rIL-2)

Another form of immunotherapy being investigated for HIV is the use of components of the immune system, including cytokines, innate cells, or T cells (Pett 2009). Investigation of cytokine levels identified IL-2 to be reduced in HIV infected individuals with greatest reduction seen in individuals who progress to disease. (Lane and Fauci 1985; Kannanganat, Kapogiannis et al. 2007). IL-2 is known to be a T cell derived cytokine needed for stimulation of cell proliferation and enhancement of cytolytic activity (Malek and Castro 2010). In the early 20th century, recombinant IL-2 (rIL-2) was administered to individuals with high and low CD4+T cell counts and low viral loads either intravenously or subcutaneously. IL-2 administration resulted in an increased numbers of CD4+T cell counts, which may be clinically beneficial especially in late stage disease (Arno, Ruiz et al. 1999; Davey, Chaitt et al. 1999; Levy, Capitant et al. 1999). Two rIL-2 trials called SILCAAT and ESPRIT is covered by the report of Peters B. and Samuel M(Peters and Samuel 2010) .

The rIL-2, termed Proleukin, was given subcutaneously in both these studies. The SILCAAT trial was designed for late stage HIV infected volunteers as defined by CD4+T cells between 50 and 299 cells/mm^3 and the ESPRIT trial was designed for early stage infected individuals, defined by CD4+T cells counts above 300 cells /mm^3 (Committee 2009). The endpoints for both trials were effect of treatment on disease progression and death. HAART was administered alone or in combination with Proleukin. There was a significant increase in CD4+T cell numbers in patients treated with the combination of HAART/Proleukin compared to HAART alone. Over a period of 7-8 years, there was an increase in cell numbers. Nonetheless, this increase did not translate to clinical benefits since there was not a reduction in incidence to AIDS or length of time to AIDS in individuals who received HAART/Proleukin versus HAART alone. Further analysis of these results showed that these up-regulated CD4+T cells following HAART/Proleukin treatment were different from CD4+T cells activated by HAART alone. The HAART/Proleukin treatment resulted in increased numbers of naïve and central memory CD4+T cells. Treatment with HAART alone resulted in increase of effector memory CD4+T cells. Fewer regulatory T cells were present with the HAART alone versus HAART/Proleukin treatment. Furthermore, Proleukin treatment resulted in toxicity in some individuals. Even though the Proleukin treatment increased CD4+T cell numbers, a surrogate maker for vaccine efficacy, the level of toxicity of this drug does not justify its use (Peters and Samuel 2010). Similar to the Remune trials, the use of Proleukin increased CD4+T cells a surrogate marker for vaccine efficacy. The discovery of cytokines linked to HIV immune dysfunction continue. Therefore, the use of interleukins as therapies both directly and as adjuvants need to be carefully considered (Clerici 2010).

In addition to cytokines, other immune system components were investigated as immunotherapies. One such immune component is serum Gc factor the precursor for macrophage activating factor (MAF) (Mosser 2003). During HIV infection, gp120 prevents deglycosylation of Gc factor affecting production of MAF and results in lack of macrophage activation (Nobuto Yamamoto 2009). The use of serum Gc factor as a therapy is a potent macrophage activator and has no side effects in humans (Mosser 2003; Yamamoto, Ushijima et al. 2009). Another immune component being used is dendritic cells (DC). Dendritic cells (DC) are potent professional antigen presenting cells and are ideal for priming T cells for cytotoxic activity (Van Gulck 2010). DC primed with HIV specific antigens stimulates T cells that can destroy HIV infected cells. In addition to DC primed T cells, direct use of T cells as therapy is being investigated. The use of genetically engineered T cells with modified CCR5 receptors demonstrate that these strategies increase CD4+T cells with engineered T cells/HAART compared to HAART alone (Gulick, Lalezari et al. 2008). As seen in previous studies, the populations of CD4+T cells increased need to be investigated as increase in CD4+T cells may not lead to better disease outcome.

Pharmacological compounds are another area of HIV therapeutic development. New targets of HV therapeutics is covered in a review by Jiang, Yan; Liu, Xinyong; De Clercq, Erik (Jiang 2011).These compounds target different stages of HIV replication cycle including viral entry, reverse transcription and viral exit. Most of the compounds initially developed were targeted at reverse transcriptase and fall under the categories of NRTI and NNRTI. Additional compounds have been developed that target other viral proteins and parts of the replication cycle. There are now compounds that target the HIV receptor CD4, the coreceptors CCR5 and CXCR4, integration of virus into the host genome, and viral membrane fusion (Latinovic, Le et al. ; Ferain, Hoveyda et al. 2011).

2.5 Enfurvirtide (T20)

One of the initial fusion proteins to enter clinical trials was called T20 (Kilby 1999). Following receptor/co-receptor binding, the viral envelope mediates fusion of the cell and viral membrane via the gp41 domain of the HIV envelope. The gp41 heptad repeat sequence is responsible for membrane fusion and is highly conserved between viruses of all clades. A therapy targeted at the fusion domain should overcome the challenge of virus diversity. Initial peptides DP107 and DP178 corresponding to the heptad repeat sequences were found to inhibit viral infectivity in cell culture (Wild, Oas et al. 1992; Wild, Shugars et al. 1994). To further support the theory that disruption of the fusion domain leads to lack of virus infectivity, mutations in the supercoil/heptad repeat region was performed. These mutant viruses could not infect permissive cells. The next step in development of this drug was determining the concentration needed in vivo to inhibit membrane fusion. Based on the DP178 peptide a 36 amino acid peptide was formulated and called T20. This peptide was confirmed to have inhibitory activity *in vitro*. After *in vitro* studies, dosing and safety studies were performed using T20 followed by clinical trials using this fusion inhibitor (Wild, Greenwell et al. 1993).

Sixteen HIV-infected adult volunteers were given T20 intravenously for 14 days (Kilby, Hopkins et al. 1998). Subjects were chosen based upon CD4+ T cell counts greater or equal to 100 cells/mm^3 and viral loads of 10,000 or more copies of RNA/ml of plasma. All participants were newly infected and not on therapy or were using antiretroviral therapy but ceased treatment for the trial. People were given 3mg to 100mg intravenous doses. No participants reported any adverse effects or toxicity. A few individuals had elevated temperatures and mild headaches. The drug had a half-life of 1.83 hours. Overall, there was a significant decrease in RNA plasma levels, with the fusion peptide can decrease viral infectivity and indirectly reduce viral load.

In a follow up study, increasing doses of T20 over time were used (Kilby, Lalezari et al. 2002). Volunteers with viral loads greater than 5000 copies of RNA/ml of plasma were placed on T20 therapy. Volunteers received either intermittent injection or were fitted with a device to allow for continuous drug infusion instead of intravenous dosing. The trial took place over 28 days of outpatient treatment. Adverse effects were seen in some individuals fitted with the infusion device. The pump used in treatment had frequent alarming caused tender nodules under the skin when infusion took place. Because of this side effect some individuals were taken off the pump and changed to the injection arm of the study. In the case of toxicity one individual withdrew from the study on that basis. Following 28 days of treatment, there was a dose-dependent decline in RNA levels. The best results were seen in individuals receiving intermediate dose of 30mg of T20. Potential T20 resistant-viruses showed the development of multiple point mutations in the present of T20 treatment. Therefore, several conclusion were made: 1) a more user friendly outpatient devise is needed for administering treatment, 2) understanding and characterizing possible resistant virus need to be carefully monitored and 3) correct combination of other antiretroviral therapies and fusion inhibitors need to be considered.

T20 was moved to a large phase III clinical trial performed in the United States (TORO1) and Europe/Australia (TORO2) (Joly, Jidar et al. 2010) . TORO1 consisted of 491 individuals who had more than 6 months of therapy including NRTI, NNRTI or protease inhibitors.

TORO 2 enrolled 504 volunteers with patients having had treatment with one or more of the same groups of antiretroviral (NTRI, NNRTI and PI). Volunteers in both studies had viral loads greater than 5000 copies/ml of plasma. Patients were treated with 90mg of T20 with HAART therapy or therapy alone. After 48 weeks, there was a significant drop in viral loads in the T20 plus antiretroviral therapy versus the antiretroviral treatment alone. The volunteers in the T20/HAART arm of the study had a 2-fold increase in CD4+ T cells counts from baseline compared to HAART alone that lasted greater than 96 weeks. At that point all individuals in the study were placed on T20/HAART. However the responses of the individuals originally on HAART alone never reached the levels of the individuals who received T20/HAART. This outcome indicated that T20 should be given early in treatment. T20 is now called Enfuvirtide and has been licensed by the FDA as the first fusion inhibitor to be used for HIV therapy.

This positive step forward in the immunotherapy field fuels the continuous research to find better and safer HIV immunotherapies. Other therapies being investigated include HIV frameshift efficiency modulators, DNAzymes and the theory of alloimmunity. The first two therapies are still early in development. Alloimmunity was observed in a NHP study where animals were protected from virus challenge. After investigation it was concluded that the protection observed because the virus was grown in human PBMCs (Langlois, Weinhold et al. 1992). The use of alloimmunity in the field of HIV vaccines has expanded since the initial finding. Thomas Lehner et al published a report covering discussions during a NIH workshop on the use of alloimmunity as a strategy for HIV vaccines (Lehner, Shearer et al. 2000)

3. Prophylaxis

Some of the earliest HIV/AIDS vaccines were based upon the envelope protein of the virus (Lasky, Groopman et al. 1986; Arthur, Pyle et al. 1987; Redfield, Birx et al. 1991). Soluble portion of envelope (gp120) or the entire gp160 envelope protein was used as recombinant proteins to vaccinate humans and induce a humoral response (Wintsch, Chaignat et al. 1991; Pincus, Messer et al. 1993). HIV envelope subunit vaccines elicited neutralizing antibody responses following vaccination without toxic side effect in human volunteers. The first phase III clinical trial in pursuit of an effective HIV vaccine was done by VaxGen using their vaccine called AIDSVAX and consisted of a bivalent subunit recombinant gp120 envelope proteins (Francis DP 1998).

3.1 Vaxgen (AIDSVAX B/B and B/E) vaccine clinical trial

After showing protection in chimpanzee after homologous and heterologous challenges, the Vaxgen vaccine moved into clinical trials. The primate study was not very well powered and complete protection was not achieved in a suboptimal HIV animal model (Berman, Gregory et al. 1990). The initial VaxGen studies were done with a monovalent vaccine either from the HIV strain MN or IIIB (Migasena, Suntharasamai et al. 2000). Both these envelopes were from lab adapted virus strains. The recombinant proteins envelope MN and IIIB gp120s were produced in engineered bacteria. The phase I and II clinical trials showed that AIDSVAX was well tolerated with irritation just at site of injection. Six individuals acquired HIV during the trial. The vaccine that was sent into phase III clinical trial was bivalent with both clade B envelopes MN and IIIB in an effort to deal with virus diversity. The vaccine trials took place in the US with a total of 5000 at-risk women and homosexual men and parallel studies were conducted in Thailand with intravenous drug users (Francis DP 1998). The vaccines were tailored to the trial sites. In the US, the vaccine consisted of envelopes from clade B. The Thailand vaccine was made from envelopes from clade B and E. Trials were powered to determine efficacy and were scheduled for three years allowing for long-term follow up. The endpoints designated for the trials were infection as measured by seroconversion and viral load as measured by polymerase chain reaction. In 2003, VaxGen reported the failure of its vaccine trial (Profile 2003). There was no significant decrease in infection in individuals who received the vaccine when all individuals were considered. However, the company reported that the vaccine was more immunogenic and produced higher levels of antibody responses in Black and Asian volunteers. Because of this finding, the AIDSVAX was included in a future study in combination with ALVAC-HIV-vCP1521 in Thailand.

Since the beginning of the VaxGen trials, HIV prophylaxis vaccines designed to elicit humoral response have increased in sophistication. Vaccine designs used to induce effective neutralizing antibodies is covered in a review by Vaine et al.(Vaine, Lu et al. 2009). Vaccine designs include use of envelopes with variable loops deleted, glycosylation mutated, eptitope grafting, envelope trimers and centralized sequences. Our lab has been involved in studies to increase antibody response to envelope. The initial studies performed used the molecular adjuvant in combination with sgp120 to increase antibody titers (Green, Montefiori et al. 2003). Results from that study showed that DNA vaccination with sgp120 linked to three copies of C3d efficiently increase antibody tiers in rabbits compared to non-C3d constructs. This work was expanded to link C3d3 to a more native envelope structure. Trimerize envelopes stabilized by the bacteriophage fibritin and linked to C3d showed better cross neutralizing titers to primary isolates compared to trimers without C3d. Both groups of mice vaccinated with envelope trimers with and without C3d induced high anti-envelope responses (Bower, Yang et al. 2004). Our lab has also used virus-like particles (VLP) in an effort to present envelope in its native form(Young, Smith et al. 2004). Responses of mice vaccinated with the HIV VLP when compared to soluble gp120 or trimers had higher envelope titers and broader immune responses (McBurney, Young et al. 2007). The VLP induced both mucosal and systemic responses.

In parallel with developing vaccines to eliciting antibody responses vaccines aimed at eliciting T cell responses were being developed (Egan, Pavlat et al. 1995). Both animal and human studies have indicated that CD8+T cells were linked to reduce viral load and led to development of vaccines aimed at producing the ideal cellular responses (Asquith and McLean 2007). Several viral vectors have been used to elicit cellular responses to HIV proteins including poxvirus vectors, vaccinia virus vectors, adenovirus vectors, alphaviruses vectors, avipoxvirus vectors, poliovirus vectors and rhabdovirus vectors (Polo and Dubensky 2002). Viral vectors allow for 1) high production levels of antigens directly into cells, 2) potential adjuvant effect on the immune response given the viral nature of the system and 3) the particular characteristic allows for efficient uptake of vaccine by professional antigen presenting cells to stimulate the immune response. Viral vectors can be mucosal adjuvants. Mucosal stimulation is an asset in HIV vaccine development as most infection takes place via the mucosa (Chenine, Siddappa et al. 2010). There is a major disadvantage to viral vectors, the possibility of pre-existing immunity may lead to adverse effects and reduced immune response directed at the vaccine antigens (Gudmundsdotter, Nilsson et al. 2009; Pine, Kublin et al. 2011). Other strategies that have been investigated for inducing a cellular response include using various vaccine regimens. One of the vaccine regimens that had proved successful in primates to stimulate a cellular response is a DNA prime followed by protein or viral vector boost (Barnett, Burke et al. 2010; Jaoko, Karita et al. 2010; Keefer, Frey et al. 2011).

3.2 Merck clinical trial

The Merck vaccine consisted of three recombinant adenoviral vectors of different serotype expressing the genes *gag, pol and nef* (Shiver, Fu et al. 2002). Preclinical trials in macaques vaccinated with the modified Ad5 expressing gag, pol and nef showed immunogenicity. When monkeys were challenge with SHIV and SIVmac239, animals had reduced viral loads. Further analysis identified the animal's HLA type as a major factor in the outcome of vaccination and efficacy seen. With reduced viral loads in the primate model after challenge the vaccine was moved into clinical trials. During clinical trials phase I and II the vaccine was safe and induce cellular immune responses measured by interferon gamma enzyme-linked assay. Interferon gamma enzyme-linked assay (INF gamma ELISPOT) used is the standardize assay for cellular responses in a vaccine setting. STEP phase III trial enrolled a total of 3,000 healthy individuals. The endpoints for the STEP trial as with the VaxGen study were infection and viral load. Each volunteer received three injections of the three genes and received vaccinations two and three 6 months apart from each other. The STEP trial was stop after analysis of data collected from the ongoing study. The study was stopped due to the results pointing to increase rate of infectivity in vaccine groups. This outcome was unexpected as the volunteers in the vaccine arm of the study had quality cellular responses. Quality cellular responses were defined by moderate to high total INF gamma producing cells ELISPOT and the CD8+T cells generated were polyfunctional by ICS staining after stimulation with HIV antigens. The polyfunctional nature of the CD8+T cells was thought to be needed for the ideal response to viral load (Betts and Harari 2008; Hanke 2008). However, the STEP results had an additional element that complicated the outcome. Volunteers who had pre-existing immunity to Ad5 had a trend for higher rates of infectivity (Sekaly 2008).The failure of the STEP trial brought into scrutiny both the use of viral vectors and cellular responses as a correlate of protection. To overcome the hurdle of pre-existing immunity ways to modifying vector delivery and engineering vectors has been under investigation.

After the failure of the STEP vaccine trial, the results of the next phase III vaccine trial was of great interest. The vaccine components had a potential for inducing both cellular and humoral responses. Inducing both humoral and cellular responses to HIV antigens had been investigated as early as 1986 when recombinant vaccinia virus was used to delivery envelope gp41 and gpIIO induced both humoural and cellular responses in macaques (Zarling, Morton et al. 1986).

3.3 ALVAC and AIDSVAX clinical trial

The ALVAC and AIDSVAX clinical trial in Thailand enrolled 16402 healthy men and women between the ages of 18-30 years into the study(Rerks-Ngarm, Pitisuttithum et al. 2009). The ALVAC vaccine contains a clade E envelope and a gag/pol from clade B. The AIDSVAX vaccine is the B/E vaccine covered in the previous section. The vaccine trial covered multiple centers and the individuals were randomized into placebo or vaccine groups. Vaccine groups received four injection of the canarypox virus vector vaccine ALVAC, followed by two boost injections with the AIDSVAX B/E recombinant gp120. The endpoints for the trials were HIV infection and early viral loads after the first 6 months and every 6 months thereafter for 3 years. Measurement of cellular immunogenicity was done by interferon gamma ELISPOT and intracellular cytokine staining (ICS) for antigens gag and envelope. Humoral responses were measured for binding antibodies to various gp120 envelopes and p24 (gag core). T cell responses via ELISPOT showed a 19.7 % in vaccinated individuals 6 months after the final vaccination. In addition greater cytokine responses were measured in the CD4+ T cells of vaccinated individuals. Binding antibodies to the envelopes MN and A244 present in the vaccine were similar and had a GMT-1 of 31,207 and 14588 respectively. There were only mild to moderate adverse effects mainly at the site of injection as in preliminary studies. When it came to trial endpoints there was no significant difference in viral loads of individuals who got infected whether or not they got the vaccine. Nonetheless there was a silver lining, the study recorded a 31.3% protection rate using a 95%confidence interval. This outcome resulted in ripples across the world. This was the first time any efficacy was reported in an HIV vaccine trial. However, a study did not result in the elucidation of a correlate of protection for HIV. The only immune parameter measured that should any potential as a correlate of protection was antibody binding to envelopes. This vaccine trial infused a new hope into the HIV vaccine field, showing that protection from infection was possible.

Besides establishing correlates of protection the HIV vaccine field has other hurdles to overcome. These challenges include (Moutsopoulos, Nares et al. 2007)vaccine design to overcoming variability and induce the appropriate immune response at the mucosal surface. The two main strategies being used to overcome virus variability are using centralized sequence usually based on envelopes of one or multiple clades, mosaic antigens and polyvalent vaccines consisting of multiple genes of HIV from one or multiple clades (McBurney and Ross 2008) (Santra, Korber et al. 2008; McElrath and Haynes 2010). Our lab have used consensus envelopes in an effort to expand HIV immune responses breath when compared to monovalent vaccines or a polyvalent primary envelope VLP mixture (McBurney and Ross 2009). In a review by Gao F et al. the use of centralized envelopes (consensus, center of the tree and ancestral) to induce HIV specific immune responses is covered (Gao 2007). The use of the centralized immunogens resulted in a superior breadth of cellular and humoral immune response (Kothe, Li et al. 2006; Liao, Sutherland et al. 2006; Kothe, Decker et al. 2007; Santra, Korber et al. 2008). In regard to generating mucosal immunity different vaccine strategies including vaccination at oral or vaginal in primates and use of adjuvants are being investigated to establish protective immune response at the mucosa (Peters, Peng et al. 2003; Duerr 2010; Sui, Zhu et al. 2010). To better direct the mucosal vaccine development investigation of the immune environment during infection and what is needed to prevent infection is being done (Gurney, Elliott et al. 2005; Moutsopoulos, Nares et al. 2007; Burgener, Boutilier et al. 2008; Schulbin, Bode et al. 2008).

4. Moving forward

Collaborative efforts between basic research, pharmacology, vaccinology and immunology are moving the HIV search for treatment forward. Trials aimed at investigating new drugs and therapeutic vaccines are being done worldwide (Choudhary and Margolis 2011). WHO and world governments continue to devote money to clinical trials for potential preventative measures in an effort to curb the HIV/AIDS global epidemic. The phase II and III clinical trials of preventative vaccines sponsored by National Institute of Allergy and

Infectious Diseases (NIAID) are ran by different clinical networks. The clinical networks include: 1) AIDS clinical trials groups, 2) HIV prevention trials network, 3) HIV vaccine trials Network 4) International maternal pediatric Adolescent AIDS Clinical trials, 5) International network of strategic initiatives in global HIV trials and 6) Microbicide trials network volunteers. Ongoing clinical trials can be found at the AIDSinfo website (http://www.aidsinfo.nih.gov/Vaccines).

In therapeutic research, studies are expanding to include drugs targeted at eliminating viral reservoirs (Huelsmann, Hofmann et al. 2011; Kovochich, Marsden et al. 2011). Follow up studies of individuals on HAART are being done to evaluating health and treatment efficacy (Mahdavi, Malyuta et al. 2010; Torti, d'Arminio-Monforte et al. 2011). Findings from these evaluations will be use to better treatments and evaluate possible side effects of long term drug use (Boyd and Hill 2010; Kranzer, Lewis et al. 2010; Shapiro, Hughes et al. 2010; Shrestha, Sudenga et al. 2010). Another area of HIV therapy receiving increase attention is the use and effectiveness of HAART in individuals with cancer and bacterial/virus co-infections such as tuberculosis, HPV (Crane, Sirivichayakul et al. 2010; Hermans, Kiragga et al. 2010; Minkoff, Zhong et al. 2010).

New strategies or modification of old strategies are being used for vaccine development as more knowledge of the virus and the immune response to the virus continue to be dissected. Table 3 shows vaccine strategies used over the years and their limitations. One example is seen in a paper by Somogyi, E., J. Xu, et al where a VLP is used to present 15 antigens(Somogyi, Xu et al. 2011). While this vaccine is design for therapeutic purposes the platform could be applied to prophylaxis vaccines as well. As with therapeutics, clinical trials for preventative vaccines are continuous taking place. The trials that are currently being done by HIV vaccine network can be found at http://www.hvtn.org/science/trials.html.

Vaccine Design	**Limitations**
Live, attenuated virus	Pathogenicity in vaccines
Inactivated viruses with adjuvants	Restricted specificity of neutralizing antibodies, absence of CTLs
Recombinant envelope protein	No neutralizing antibodies for patient isolates of HIV-1; absence of CTLs
Plasmid DNA	Limited immunogenicity in humans
Live, recombinant vectors: Poxviruses Vaccinia MVA, NYVAC Canary pox	Dissemination in immunosuppressed vaccines Limited experience in humans Limited immunogenicity in humans at achievable dosages
Gene-deleted adenovirus	Pre-existing immunity to adenovirus may limit immunogenicity
Alphaviruses, adeno-associated virus	Limited experience in humans
Envelope subunit immunogens	No elicitation of neutralizing antibodies

Table 3. HIV-1 vaccine design adapted from" Strategies for an HIV vaccine" by Norman L. Letvin (Letvin 2002)

Besides the strategies seen in the table prophylaxis treatment being investigated are topical microbicides, combination therapy of vaccines and microbicides and the use of antivirals as preventative treatment (PrEP) (Chirenje, Marrazzo et al. 2010; Mayer and Venkatesh 2010; Brinckmann, da Costa et al. 2011; Oh, Price et al. 2011). In areas where women are prohibited from use of condoms the use of effective microbicides would allow these women to protect themselves from infection. In the case of microbicides time of application is an essential part of evaluation.

The use of antiviral as post exposure treatment for healthcare workers is also under investigation. PrEP has been expanded to other individuals, including men who have sex with men. A national clinical trial was completed and results of trial were reported this year (2011). The PrEP was safe and resulted in partial efficiency in reducing HIV acquisition (DK Smith 2011). One concern of PrEP is the development of drug resistant viruses due to therapy prior to infection (Abbas, Hood et al. 2011).

The war against HIV continues to be fought with scientific innovation together with continued funding from both government and private agencies. With such continued efforts the road to epidemic control and /eradication may be closer than it was over twenty- five years ago.

5. References

Aaron N. Endsley, N. N. S., Rodney J.Y. Ho (2008). "Combining Drug and Immune Therapy: A Potential Solution to Drug Resistance and Challenges of HIV Vaccines?" Current HIV Research 6: 401-410.

Abbas, U. L., G. Hood, et al. (2011). "Factors Influencing the Emergence and Spread of HIV Drug Resistance Arising from Rollout of Antiretroviral Pre-Exposure Prophylaxis (PrEP)." PLoS ONE 6(4): e18165.

Angel, J. B. a., J.-P. b. Routy, et al. (2011). "A randomized controlled trial of HIV therapeutic vaccination using ALVAC with or without Remune." AIDS 25(6): 731-739.

Arno, A., L. Ruiz, et al. (1999). "Efficacy of Low-Dose Subcutaneous Interleukin-2 to Treat Advanced Human Immunodeficiency Virus Type 1 in Persons with ,©Ω250/Œ°L CD4 T Cells and Undetectable Plasma Virus Load." Journal of Infectious Diseases 180(1): 56-60.

Arthur, L. O., S. W. Pyle, et al. (1987). "Serological responses in chimpanzees inoculated with human immunodeficiency virus glycoprotein (gp120) subunit vaccine." Proceedings of the National Academy of Sciences 84(23): 8583-8587.

Asquith, B. and A. R. McLean (2007). "In vivo CD8+ T cell control of immunodeficiency virus infection in humans and macaques." Proceedings of the National Academy of Sciences 104(15): 6365-6370.

Baenziger, S., M. Heikenwalder, et al. (2009). "Triggering TLR7 in mice induces immune activation and lymphoid system disruption, resembling HIV-mediated pathology." Blood 113(2): 377-388.

Barnett, S. W., B. Burke, et al. (2010). "Antibody-Mediated Protection against Mucosal Simian-Human Immunodeficiency Virus Challenge of Macaques Immunized with Alphavirus Replicon Particles and Boosted with Trimeric Envelope Glycoprotein in MF59 Adjuvant." J. Virol. 84(12): 5975-5985.

Barre-Sinoussi, F., J. C. Chermann, et al. (1983). "Isolation of a T-Lymphotropic Retrovirus from a Patient at Risk for Acquired Immune Deficiency Syndrome (AIDS)." Science 220(4599): 868-871.

Berman, P. W., T. J. Gregory, et al. (1990). "Protection of chimpanzees from infection by HIV-1 after vaccination with recombinant glycoprotein gp120 but not gp160." Nature 345(6276): 622-625.

Betts, M. R. and A. Harari (2008). "Phenotype and function of protective T cell immune responses in HIV." Current Opinion in HIV and AIDS 3(3): 349-355 310.1097/COH.1090b1013e3282fbaa1081.

Bower, J. F., X. Yang, et al. (2004). "Elicitation of Neutralizing Antibodies with DNA Vaccines Expressing Soluble Stabilized Human Immunodeficiency Virus Type 1 Envelope Glycoprotein Trimers Conjugated to C3d." J. Virol. 78(9): 4710-4719.

Boyd, M. A. and A. M. Hill (2010). "Clinical Management of Treatment-Experienced, HIV/AIDS Patients in the Combination Antiretroviral Therapy Era." PharmacoEconomics 28: 17-34 10.2165/11587420-000000000-000000000.

Brinckmann, S., K. da Costa, et al. (2011). "Rational design of HIV vaccines and microbicides: report of the EUROPRISE network annual conference 2010." Journal of Translational Medicine 9(1): 40.

Broder, S. (2010). "The development of antiretroviral therapy and its impact on the HIV-1/AIDS pandemic." Antiviral Research 85(1): 1-18.

Brown, R. J. P., P. J. Peters, et al. (2011). "Inter-compartment recombination of HIV-1 contributes to env intra-host diversity and modulates viral tropism and senstivity to entry inhibitors." J. Virol.: JVI.00131-00111.

Buonaguro, L., M. L. Tornesello, et al. (2009). "Short Communication: Limited Induction of IL-10 in PBMCs from HIV-Infected Subjects Treated with HIV-VLPs." AIDS Research and Human Retroviruses 25(8): 819-822.

Burgener, A., J. Boutilier, et al. (2008). "Identification of Differentially Expressed Proteins in the Cervical Mucosa of HIV-1-Resistant Sex Workers." Journal of Proteome Research 7(10): 4446-4454.

Carter, C. C., A. Onafuwa-Nuga, et al. (2010). "HIV-1 infects multipotent progenitor cells causing cell death and establishing latent cellular reservoirs." Nat Med 16(4): 446-451.

Cecchinato, V., C. J. Trindade, et al. (2008). "Altered balance between Th17 and Th1 cells at mucosal sites predicts AIDS progression in simian immunodeficiency virus-infected macaques." Mucosal Immunol 1(4): 279-288.

Chenine, A. L., N. B. Siddappa, et al. (2010). "Relative Transmissibility of an R5 Clade C Simian- Human Immunodeficiency Virus Across Different Mucosae in Macaques Parallels the Relative Risks of Sexual HIV-1 Transmission in Humans via Different Routes." Journal of Infectious Diseases 201(8): 1155-1163.

Chirenje, Z. M., J. Marrazzo, et al. (2010). "Antiretroviral-based HIV prevention strategies for women." Expert Review of Anti-infective Therapy 8(10): 1177-1186.

Choudhary, S. K. and D. M. Margolis (2011). "Curing HIV: Pharmacologic Approaches to Target HIV-1 Latency." Annual Review of Pharmacology and Toxicology 51(1): 397-418.

Chouquet, C., B. Autran, et al. (2002). "Correlation between breadth of memory HIV-specific cytotoxic T cells, viral load and disease progression in HIV infection." AIDS 16(18): 2399-2407.

Chun, T.-W., L. Carruth, et al. (1997). "Quantification of latent tissue reservoirs and total body viral load in HIV-1 infection." Nature 387(6629): 183-188.

Chun, T.-W., D. C. Nickle, et al. (2008). "Persistence of HIV in Gut-Associated Lymphoid Tissue despite Long-Term Antiretroviral Therapy." Journal of Infectious Diseases 197(5): 714-720.

Ciccone, E. J., J. H. Greenwald, et al. (2011). "CD4+ T Cells, Including Th17 and Cycling Subsets, are Intact in the Gut Mucosa of HIV-1 Infected Long-Term Non-Progressors." J. Virol.: JVI.02643-02610.

Clerici, M. a. b. (2010). "Beyond IL-17: new cytokines in the pathogenesis of HIV infection." Current Opinion in HIV & AIDS 5(2): 184-188.

Committee, T. I. E. S. G. a. S. S. (2009). "Interleukin-2 Therapy in Patients with HIV Infection." New England Journal of Medicine 361(16): 1548-1559.

Crabtree-Ramirez, B., A. Villasis-Keever, et al. (2010). "Effectiveness of Highly Active Antiretroviral Therapy (HAART) Among HIV-Infected Patients in Mexico." AIDS Research and Human Retroviruses 26(4): 373-378.

Crane, M., S. Sirivichayakul, et al. (2010). "No Increase in Hepatitis B Virus (HBV)-Specific CD8+ T Cells in Patients with HIV-1-HBV Coinfections following HBV-Active Highly Active Antiretroviral Therapy." J. Virol. 84(6): 2657-2665.

Cuevas, M. T., A. Fernandez-Garcia, et al. (2010). "Short Communication: Biological and Genetic Characterization of HIV Type 1 Subtype B and Nonsubtype B Transmitted Viruses: Usefulness for Vaccine Candidate Assessment." AIDS Research and Human Retroviruses 26(9): 1019-1025.

D'Orsogna, L. J. a., R. G. b. Krueger, et al. (2007). "Circulating memory B-cell subpopulations are affected differently by HIV infection and antiretroviral therapy." AIDS 21(13): 1747-1752.

Davenport, M. P., R. M. Ribeiro, et al. (2004). "Predicting the Impact of a Nonsterilizing Vaccine against Human Immunodeficiency Virus." J. Virol. 78(20): 11340-11351.

Davey, R. T., D. G. Chaitt, et al. (1999). "A Randomized Trial of High-versus Low-Dose Subcutaneous Interleukin-2 Outpatient Therapy for Early Human Immunodeficiency Virus Type 1 Infection." Journal of Infectious Diseases 179(4): 849-858.

De Clercq, E. (2010). "Antiretroviral drugs." Current Opinion in Pharmacology 10(5): 507-515.

Delelis, O., K. Carayon, et al. (2008). "Integrase and integration: biochemical activities of HIV-1 integrase." Retrovirology 5(1): 114.

DK Smith, M., RM Grant, MD, PJ Weidle, PharmD, A Lansky, PhD, J Mermin, MD, KA Fenton, MD, PhD, National Center for HIV/AIDS, Viral Hepatitis, STD, and TB Prevention, CDC. (2011). Interim guidance: preexposure prophylaxis for the prevention of HIV infection in men who have sex with men. MMWR Weekly, Centers for Disease Control and Prevention (CDC). 60: 65-68.

Douek, D. C., J. M. Brenchley, et al. (2002). "HIV preferentially infects HIV-specific CD4+ T cells." Nature 417(6884): 95-98.

Duerr, A. (2010). "Update on mucosal HIV vaccine vectors." Current Opinion in HIV and AIDS 5(5): 397-403 310.1097/COH.1090b1013e32833d32832e32839.

Egan, M. A., W. A. Pavlat, et al. (1995). "Induction of Human Immunodeficiency Virus Type 1 (HIV-1)-Specific Cytolytic T Lymphocyte Responses in Seronegative Adults by a Nonreplicating, Host-Range-Restricted Canarypox Vector (ALVAC) Carrying the HIV-1MN env Gene." Journal of Infectious Diseases 171(6): 1623-1627.

Emini, E. A., W. A. Schleif, et al. (1992). "Prevention of HIV-1 infection in chimpanzees by gpl20 V3 domain-specific monoclonal antibody." Nature 355(6362): 728-730.

Engelman, A., G. Englund, et al. (1995). "Multiple effects of mutations in human immunodeficiency virus type 1 integrase on viral replication." J. Virol. 69(5): 2729-2736.

Ensoli, B., S. Bellino, et al. (2010). "Therapeutic Immunization with HIV-1 Tat Reduces Immune Activation and Loss of Regulatory T-Cells and Improves Immune Function in Subjects on HAART." PLoS ONE 5(11): e13540.

Fauci, A. S., D. Mavilio, et al. (2005). "NK cells in HIV infection: Paradigm for protection or targets for ambush." Nat Rev Immunol 5(11): 835-843.

Ferain, T., H. R. Hoveyda, et al. (2011). "Agonist-induced internalization of CCR5 as a mechanism to inhibit HIV replication." Journal of Pharmacology and Experimental Therapeutics.

Fernandez, S., A. Lim, et al. (2009). "Immune activation and the pathogenesis of HIV disease: implications for therapy.(LEADING ARTICLE)(Report)." Journal of HIV Therapy 14(3): 52(55).

Fernandez-Cruz, E., J. Navarro, et al. (2003). "The potential role of the HIV-1 immunogen (Remune¬Æ) as a therapeutic vaccine in the treatment of HIV infection." Expert Review of Vaccines 2(6): 739-752.

Fernandez-Cruz, E., J. n. Navarro, et al. (2003). "The potential role of the HIV-1 immunogen (Remune¬Æ) as a therapeutic vaccine in the treatment of HIV infection." Expert Review of Vaccines 2(6): 739-752.

Finkel, T. H., G. Tudor-Williams, et al. (1995). "Apoptosis occurs predominantly in bystander cells and not in productively infected cells of HIV- and SIV-infected lymph nodes." Nat Med 1(2): 129-134.

Finzi, D., J. Blankson, et al. (1999). "Latent infection of CD4+ T cells provides a mechanism for lifelong persistence of HIV-1, even in patients on effective combination therapy." Nat Med 5(5): 512-517.

Follmann, D. P., A. M. D. P. M. P. H. H. Duerr, et al. (2007). "Endpoints and Regulatory Issues in HIV Vaccine Clinical Trials: Lessons From a Workshop." JAIDS Journal of Acquired Immune Deficiency Syndromes 44(1): 49-60.

Francis DP, G. T., McElrath MJ, Belshe RB, Gorse GJ, Migasena S, Kitayaporn D, Pitisuttitham P, Matthews T, Schwartz DH, Berman PW (1998). "Advancing AIDSVAX to phase 3. Safety, immunogenicity, and plans for phase 3." AIDS Res Hum Retroviruses. 14(Suppl 3): S325-331.

Gallo, R. C., P. S. Sarin, et al. (1983). "Isolation of Human T-Cell Leukemia Virus in Acquired Immune Deficiency Syndrome (AIDS)." Science 220(4599): 865-867.

Gao, F. L., Hua-Xin; Hahn, Beatrice H.; Letvin, Norman L.; Korber, Bette T.; Haynes, Barton F. (2007). "Centralized HIV-1 Envelope Immunogens and Neutralizing Antibodies." Current HIV Research 5: 572-577.

Gorse, G. J., R. E. Simionescu, et al. (2006). "Cellular Immune Responses in Asymptomatic Human Immunodeficiency Virus Type 1 (HIV-1) Infection and Effects of Vaccination with Recombinant Envelope Glycoprotein of HIV-1." Clin. Vaccine Immunol. 13(1): 26-32.

Green, T. D., D. C. Montefiori, et al. (2003). "Enhancement of Antibodies to the Human Immunodeficiency Virus Type 1 Envelope by Using the Molecular Adjuvant C3d." J. Virol. 77(3): 2046-2055.

Greenbaum, A. H., L. E. Wilson, et al. (2008). "Effect of age and HAART regimen on clinical response in an urban cohort of HIV-infected individuals." AIDS 22(17): 2331-2339 2310.1097/QAD.2330b2013e32831883f32831889.

Gudmundsdotter, L., C. Nilsson, et al. (2009). "Recombinant Modified Vaccinia Ankara (MVA) effectively boosts DNA-primed HIV-specific immune responses in humans despite pre-existing vaccinia immunity." Vaccine 27(33): 4468-4474.

Gulick, R. M., J. Lalezari, et al. (2008). "Maraviroc for Previously Treated Patients with R5 HIV-1 Infection." New England Journal of Medicine 359(14): 1429-1441.

Gulick, R. M., J. W. Mellors, et al. (1997). "Treatment with Indinavir, Zidovudine, and Lamivudine in Adults with Human Immunodeficiency Virus Infection and Prior Antiretroviral Therapy." New England Journal of Medicine 337(11): 734-739.

Gurney, K. B., J. Elliott, et al. (2005). "Binding and Transfer of Human Immunodeficiency Virus by DC-SIGN+ Cells in Human Rectal Mucosa." J. Virol. 79(9): 5762-5773.

Gurunathan, S., R. E. Habib, et al. (2009). "Use of predictive markers of HIV disease progression in vaccine trials." Vaccine 27(14): 1997-2015.

Hanke, T. (2008). "STEP trial and HIV-1 vaccines inducing T-cell responses." Expert Review of Vaccines 7: 303-309.

Hartigan-O'Connor, D. J., L. A. Hirao, et al. (2011). "Th17 cells and regulatory T cells in elite control over HIV and SIV." Current Opinion in HIV and AIDS 6(3): 221-227 210.1097/COH.1090b1013e32834577b32834573.

Hermans, S. M., A. N. Kiragga, et al. (2010). "Incident Tuberculosis during Antiretroviral Therapy Contributes to Suboptimal Immune Reconstitution in a Large Urban HIV Clinic in Sub-Saharan Africa." PLoS ONE 5(5): e10527.

Hofer, U. and R. Speck (2009). "Disturbance of the gut-associated lymphoid tissue is associated with disease progression in chronic HIV infection." Seminars in Immunopathology 31(2): 257-266.

Huelsmann, P., A. Hofmann, et al. (2011). "A suicide gene approach using the human pro-apoptotic protein tBid inhibits HIV-1 replication." BMC Biotechnology 11(1): 4.

Jaoko, W., E. Karita, et al. (2010). "Safety and Immunogenicity Study of Multiclade HIV-1 Adenoviral Vector Vaccine Alone or as Boost following a Multiclade HIV-1 DNA Vaccine in Africa." PLoS ONE 5(9): e12873.

Jiang, Y. L., Xinyong; De Clercq, Erik (2011). "New Therapeutic Approaches Targeted at the Late Stages of the HIV-1 Replication Cycle." Current Medicinal Chemistry 18: 16-28.

John, M., C. B. Moore, et al. (2001). "Chronic hyperlactatemia in HIV-infected patients taking antiretroviral therapy." AIDS 15(6): 717-723.

Joly, V., K. Jidar, et al. (2010). "Enfuvirtide: from basic investigations to current clinical use." Expert Opinion on Pharmacotherapy 11(16): 2701-2713.

Jose Esparza, W. L. H., Saladin Osmanov (1996). "HIV Vaccine Development." AIDS 10(suppl): S123-S132.

Kannanganat, S., B. G. Kapogiannis, et al. (2007). "Human Immunodeficiency Virus Type 1 Controllers but Not Noncontrollers Maintain CD4 T Cells Coexpressing Three Cytokines." J. Virol. 81(21): 12071-12076.

Keefer, M. C., S. E. Frey, et al. (2011). "A phase I trial of preventive HIV vaccination with heterologous poxviral-vectors containing matching HIV-1 inserts in healthy HIV-uninfected subjects." Vaccine 29(10): 1948-1958.

Kelley, C. F., J. D. Barbour, et al. (2007). "The Relation Between Symptoms, Viral Load, and Viral Load Set Point in Primary HIV Infection." JAIDS Journal of Acquired Immune Deficiency Syndromes 45(4): 445-448 410.1097/QAI.1090b1013e318074ef318076e.

Kilby, J. M. (1999). "Therapeutic potential of blocking HIV entry into cells: focus on membrane fusion inhibitors." Expert Opinion on Investigational Drugs 8(8): 1157-1170.

Kilby, J. M., S. Hopkins, et al. (1998). "Potent suppression of HIV-1 replication in humans by T-20, a peptide inhibitor of gp41-mediated virus entry." Nat Med 4(11): 1302-1307.

Kilby, J. M., J. P. Lalezari, et al. (2002). "The Safety, Plasma Pharmacokinetics, and Antiviral Activity of Subcutaneous Enfuvirtide (T-20), a Peptide Inhibitor of gp41-Mediated Virus Fusion, in HIV-Infected Adults." AIDS Research and Human Retroviruses 18(10): 685-693.

Kolte, L., J. C. Gaardbo, et al. (2011). "Dysregulation of CD4+CD25+CD127lowFOXP3+ regulatory T cells in HIV-infected pregnant women." Blood 117(6): 1861-1868.

Kothe, D. L., J. M. Decker, et al. (2007). "Antigenicity and immunogenicity of HIV-1 consensus subtype B envelope glycoproteins." Virology 360(1): 218-234.

Kothe, D. L., Y. Li, et al. (2006). "Ancestral and consensus envelope immunogens for HIV-1 subtype C." Virology 352(2): 438-449.

Kovochich, M., M. D. Marsden, et al. (2011). "Activation of Latent HIV Using Drug-Loaded Nanoparticles." PLoS ONE 6(4): e18270.

Kranzer, K., J. J. Lewis, et al. (2010). "Treatment Interruption in a Primary Care Antiretroviral Therapy Program in South Africa: Cohort Analysis of Trends and Risk Factors." JAIDS Journal of Acquired Immune Deficiency Syndromes 55(3): e17-e23 10.1097/QAI.1090b1013e3181f1275fd.

Kronenberg, A., H. M. Riehle, et al. (2001). "Liver failure after long-term nucleoside antiretroviral therapy." The Lancet 358(9283): 759-760.

Kuhrt, D., S. A. Faith, et al. (2010). "Evidence of Early B-Cell Dysregulation in Simian Immunodeficiency Virus Infection: Rapid Depletion of Naive and Memory B-Cell Subsets with Delayed Reconstitution of the Naive B-Cell Population." J. Virol. 84(5): 2466-2476.

Kutscher, S., S. Allgayer, et al. (2010). "MVA-nef induces HIV-1-specific polyfunctional and proliferative T-cell responses revealed by the combination of short- and long-term immune assays." Gene Ther 17(11): 1372-1383.

Lane, H. C. and A. S. Fauci (1985). "Immunologic Abnormalities in the Acquired Immunodeficiency Syndrome." Annual Review of Immunology 3(1): 477-500.

Langlois, A. J., K. J. Weinhold, et al. (1992). "Detection of Anti-Human Cell Antibodies in Sera from Macaques Immunized with Whole Inactivated Virus." AIDS Research and Human Retroviruses 8(9): 1641-1652.

Lasky, L., J. Groopman, et al. (1986). "Neutralization of the AIDS retrovirus by antibodies to a recombinant envelope glycoprotein." Science 233(4760): 209-212.

Latinovic, O. a., N. a. Le, et al. "Synergistic inhibition of R5 HIV-1 by maraviroc and CCR5 antibody HGS004 in primary cells: implications for treatment and prevention." AIDS.

Lavreys, L., J. M. Baeten, et al. (2006). "Higher Set Point Plasma Viral Load and More-Severe Acute HIV Type 1 (HIV-1) Illness Predict Mortality among High-Risk HIV-1,ÄìInfected African Women." Clinical Infectious Diseases 42(9): 1333-1339.

Lehner, T., G. M. Shearer, et al. (2000). "Alloimmunization as a Strategy for Vaccine Design against HIV/AIDS." AIDS Research and Human Retroviruses 16(4): 309-313.

Lerner, P., M. Guadalupe, et al. (2011). "The Gut Mucosal Viral Reservoir in HIV-Infected Patients Is Not the Major Source of Rebound Plasma Viremia following Interruption of Highly Active Antiretroviral Therapy." J. Virol. 85(10): 4772-4782.

Letang, E., J. M. Miro, et al. (2011). "Incidence and Predictors of Immune Reconstitution Inflammatory Syndrome in a Rural Area of Mozambique." PLoS ONE 6(2): e16946.

Letvin, N. L. (2002). "Strategies for an HIV vaccine." The Journal of Clinical Investigation 110(1): 15-27.

Levy, Y., C. Capitant, et al. (1999). "Comparison of subcutaneous and intravenous interleukin-2 in asymptomatic HIV-1 infection: a randomised controlled trial." The Lancet 353(9168): 1923-1929.

Liao, H.-X., L. L. Sutherland, et al. (2006). "A group M consensus envelope glycoprotein induces antibodies that neutralize subsets of subtype B and C HIV-1 primary viruses." Virology 353(2): 268-282.

Lin, J.-N., C.-H. Lai, et al. (2010). "Immune reconstitution inflammatory syndrome presenting as chylothorax in a patient with HIV and Mycobacterium tuberculosis coinfection: a case report." BMC Infectious Diseases 10(1): 321.

Ltd., A. I. (2003). "HIV gp120 Vaccine - VaxGen: AIDSVAX(TM), AIDSVAX(TM) B/B, AIDSVAX(TM) B/E, HIV gp120 Vaccine - Genentech, HIV gp120 Vaccine AIDSVAX - VaxGen, HIV Vaccine AIDSVAX - VaxGen." Drugs in R&D 4(4): 249-253.

M Roederer, J. G. D., M T Anderson, P A Raju, L A Herzenberg, and L A Herzenberg (1995). "CD8 naive T cell counts decrease progressively in HIV-infected adults." J Clin Invest. 95(5): 2061-2066.

MacLachlan, E., K. H. Mayer, et al. (2009). "The Potential Role of Biomarkers in HIV Preventive Vaccine Trials." JAIDS Journal of Acquired Immune Deficiency Syndromes 51(5): 536-545 510.1097/QAI.1090b1013e3181adcbbe.

Mahdavi, S., R. Malyuta, et al. (2010). "Treatment and disease progression in a birth cohort of vertically HIV-1 infected children in Ukraine." BMC Pediatrics 10(1): 85.

Malek, T. R. and I. Castro (2010). "Interleukin-2 Receptor Signaling: At the Interface between Tolerance and Immunity." Immunity 33(2): 153-165.

Maloy, K. J. and M. C. Kullberg (2008). "IL-23 and Th17 cytokines in intestinal homeostasis." Mucosal Immunol 1(5): 339-349.

Mayer, K. H. and K. K. Venkatesh (2010). "Chemoprophylaxis for HIV Prevention: New Opportunities and New Questions." JAIDS Journal of Acquired Immune Deficiency Syndromes 55: S122-S127 110.1097/QAI.1090b1013e3181fbcb1094c.

McBurney, S. P. and T. M. Ross (2008). "Viral sequence diversity: challenges for AIDS vaccine designs." Expert Review of Vaccines 7(9): 1405-1417.

McBurney, S. P. and T. M. Ross (2009). "Human immunodeficiency virus-like particles with consensus envelopes elicited broader cell-mediated peripheral and mucosal immune responses than polyvalent and monovalent Env vaccines." Vaccine 27(32): 4337-4349.

McBurney, S. P., K. R. Young, et al. (2007). "Membrane embedded HIV-1 envelope on the surface of a virus-like particle elicits broader immune responses than soluble envelopes." Virology 358(2): 334-346.

McElrath, M. J. and B. F. Haynes (2010). "Induction of Immunity to Human Immunodeficiency Virus Type-1 by Vaccination." Immunity 33(4): 542-554.

Michel, P., A. T. Balde, et al. (2000). "Reduced Immune Activation and T Cell Apoptosis in Human Immunodeficiency Virus Type 2 Compared with Type 1: Correlation of T Cell Apoptosis with Œ≤2 Microglobulin Concentration and Disease Evolution." Journal of Infectious Diseases 181(1): 64-75.

Miedema, F. (2008). "A brief history of HIV vaccine research: stepping back to the drawing board?" AIDS 22(14): 1699-1703.

Migasena, S., P. Suntharasamai, et al. (2000). "AIDSVAX¬Æ (MN) in Bangkok Injecting Drug Users: A Report on Safety and Immunogenicity, Including Macrophage-Tropic Virus Neutralization." AIDS Research and Human Retroviruses 16(7): 655-663.

Milush, J. M., K. D. Mir, et al. (2011). "Lack of clinical AIDS in SIV-infected sooty mangabeys with significant CD4+ T cell loss is associated with double-negative T cells." The Journal of Clinical Investigation 121(3): 1102-1110.

Minkoff, H., Y. Zhong, et al. (2010). "Influence of Adherent and Effective Antiretroviral Therapy Use on Human Papillomavirus Infection and Squamous Intraepithelial Lesions in Human Immunodeficiency Virus,ÄìPositive Women." Journal of Infectious Diseases 201(5): 681-690.

Mitsuya, H., K. J. Weinhold, et al. (1985). "3'-Azido-3'-deoxythymidine (BW A509U): an antiviral agent that inhibits the infectivity and cytopathic effect of human T-lymphotropic virus type III/lymphadenopathy-associated virus in vitro." Proceedings of the National Academy of Sciences 82(20): 7096-7100.

Montagnier, L. (2010). "25†years after HIV discovery: Prospects for cure and vaccine." Virology 397(2): 248-254.

Monteiro, J. P., L. C. J. Alcantara, et al. (2009). "Genetic variability of human immunodeficiency virus-1 in Bahia state, Northeast, Brazil: High diversity of HIV genotypes." Journal of Medical Virology 81(3): 391-399.

Moss, R. B., M. R. Wallace, et al. (1999). "Phenotypic Analysis of Human Immunodeficiency Virus (HIV) Type 1 Cell-Mediated Immune Responses after Treatment with an HIV-1 Immunogen." Journal of Infectious Diseases 180(3): 641-648.

Mosser, D. M. (2003). "The many faces of macrophage activation." Journal of Leukocyte Biology 73(2): 209-212.

Moutsopoulos, N. M., S. Nares, et al. (2007). "Tonsil Epithelial Factors May Influence Oropharyngeal Human Immunodeficiency Virus Transmission." The American Journal of Pathology 171(2): 571-579.

Nanjundappa, R. H., R. Wang, et al. (2011). "GP120-specific exosome-targeted T cell-based vaccine capable of stimulating DC- and CD4+ T-independent CTL responses." Vaccine 29(19): 3538-3547.

Nkolola, J. P., H. Peng, et al. (2010). "Breadth of Neutralizing Antibodies Elicited by Stable, Homogeneous Clade A and Clade C HIV-1 gp140 Envelope Trimers in Guinea Pigs." J. Virol. 84(7): 3270-3279.

Nobuto Yamamoto, N. U., and Yoshihiko Koga (2009). "Immunotherapy of HIV-Infected Patients With Gc Protein-Derived Macrophage Activating Factor (GcMAF)." Journal of Medical Virology 81: 16-26.

O'Connell, K. A., J. R. Bailey, et al. (2009). "Elucidating the elite: mechanisms of control in HIV-1 infection." Trends in Pharmacological Sciences 30(12): 631-637.

Oh, C., J. Price, et al. (2011). "Inhibition of HIV-1 infection by aqueous extracts of Prunella vulgaris L." Virology Journal 8(1): 188.

Okulicz, J. F. and O. Lambotte (2011). "Epidemiology and clinical characteristics of elite controllers." Current Opinion in HIV and AIDS 6(3): 163-168 110.1097/COH.1090b1013e328344f328335e.

Paci, P., F. Martini, et al. (2011). "Timely HAART initiation may pave the way for a better viral control." BMC Infectious Diseases 11(1): 56.

Pantaleo, G. and R. A. Koup (2004). "Correlates of immune protection in HIV-1 infection: what we know, what we don't know, what we should know." Nat Med 10(8): 806-810.

Paroli, M., A. Propato, et al. (2001). "The immunology of HIV-infected long-term non-progressors--a current view." Immunology Letters 79(1-2): 127-129.

Peters, B. S. (2000). "HIV immunotherapeutic vaccines." Antiviral Chemistry & Chemotherapy 11(5): 311-320.

Peters, B. S. and M. Samuel (2010). "Implications of the SILCAAT and ESPRIT trials and the future for HIV immunotherapy.(LEADING ARTICLE)(human immunodeficiency virus)(enhanced suppression of the platelet IIb/IIIa receptor with integrilin therapy)(study of interleukin-2 in people with low CD4+ T cell counts on active anti-human immunodeficiency virus therapy)(Report)." Journal of HIV Therapy 15(1): 15(13).

Peters, C., X. Peng, et al. (2003). "The Induction of HIV Gag-Specific CD8+ T Cells in the Spleen and Gut-Associated Lymphoid Tissue by Parenteral or Mucosal

Immunization with Recombinant Listeria monocytogenes HIV Gag." The Journal of Immunology 170(10): 5176-5187.

Peto, T. (1996). "Surrogate markers in HIV disease." Journal of Antimicrobial Chemotherapy 37(suppl B): 161-170.

Pett, S. L. (2009). "Immunotherapies in HIV-1 infection." Current Opinion in HIV & AIDS 4(3): 188-193.

Pincus, S. H., K. G. Messer, et al. (1993). "Differences in the antibody response to human immunodeficiency virus-1 envelope glycoprotein (gp160) in infected laboratory workers and vaccinees." The Journal of Clinical Investigation 91(5): 1987-1996.

Pine, S. O., J. G. Kublin, et al. (2011). "Pre-Existing Adenovirus Immunity Modifies a Complex Mixed Th1 and Th2 Cytokine Response to an Ad5/HIV-1 Vaccine Candidate in Humans." PLoS ONE 6(4): e18526.

Polo, J. M. and T. W. Dubensky (2002). "Virus-based vectors for human vaccine applications." Drug Discovery Today 7(13): 719-727.

Prince, A. M., H. Reesink, et al. (1991). "Prevention of HIV Infection by Passive Immunization with HIV Immunoglobulin." AIDS Research and Human Retroviruses 7(12): 971-973.

Profile, A. R. D. (2003). "HIV gp120 Vaccine - VaxGen: AIDSVAX(TM), AIDSVAX(TM) B/B, AIDSVAX(TM) B/E, HIV gp120 Vaccine - Genentech, HIV gp120 Vaccine AIDSVAX - VaxGen, HIV Vaccine AIDSVAX - VaxGen." Drugs in R&D 4(4): 249-253.

Putkonen, P., R. Thorstensson, et al. (1991). "Prevention of HIV-2 and SIVsm infection by passive immunization in cynomolgus monkeys." Nature 352(6334): 436-438.

Ranasinghe, C., F. Eyers, et al. (2011). "A comparative analysis of HIV-specific mucosal/systemic T cell immunity and avidity following rDNA/rFPV and poxvirus-poxvirus prime boost immunisations." Vaccine 29(16): 3008-3020.

Redfield, R. R., D. L. Birx, et al. (1991). "A Phase I Evaluation of the Safety and Immunogenicity of Vaccination with Recombinant gp160 in Patients with Early Human Immunodeficiency Virus Infection." New England Journal of Medicine 324(24): 1677-1684.

Rerks-Ngarm, S., P. Pitisuttithum, et al. (2009). "Vaccination with ALVAC and AIDSVAX to Prevent HIV-1 Infection in Thailand." New England Journal of Medicine 361(23): 2209-2220.

Robertson, D. L., J. P. Anderson, et al. (2000). "HIV-1 Nomenclature Proposal." Science 288(5463): 55.

Rodes, B., C. Toro, et al. (2004). "Differences in disease progression in a cohort of long-term non-progressors after more than 16 years of HIV-1 infection." AIDS 18(8): 1109-1116.

Rosario, M., A. Bridgeman, et al. (2010). "Long peptides induce polyfunctional T cells against conserved regions of HIV-1 with superior breadth to single-gene vaccines in macaques." European Journal of Immunology 40(7): 1973-1984.

Rosenberg, E. S., B. S. Graham, et al. (2010). "Safety and Immunogenicity of Therapeutic DNA Vaccination in Individuals Treated with Antiretroviral Therapy during Acute/Early HIV-1 Infection." PLoS ONE 5(5): e10555.

Sabado, R. L., M. O'Brien, et al. (2010). "Evidence of dysregulation of dendritic cells in primary HIV infection." Blood 116(19): 3839-3852.

Salgado, M., N. I. Rallun, et al. (2011). "Long-term non-progressors display a greater number of Th17 cells than HIV-infected typical progressors." Clinical Immunology 139(2): 110-114.

Salgado, M., N. I. RallÛn, et al. (2011). "Long-term non-progressors display a greater number of Th17 cells than HIV-infected typical progressors." Clinical Immunology 139(2): 110-114.

Santra, S., B. T. Korber, et al. (2008). "A centralized gene-based HIV-1 vaccine elicits broad cross-clade cellular immune responses in rhesus monkeys." Proceedings of the National Academy of Sciences 105(30): 10489-10494.

Schulbin, H., H. Bode, et al. (2008). "Cytokine Expression in the Colonic Mucosa of Human Immunodeficiency Virus-Infected Individuals before and during 9 Months of Antiretroviral Therapy." Antimicrob. Agents Chemother. 52(9): 3377-3384.

Sekaly, R.-P. (2008). "The failed HIV Merck vaccine study: a step back or a launching point for future vaccine development?" The Journal of Experimental Medicine 205(1): 7-12.

Shapiro, R. L., M. D. Hughes, et al. (2010). "Antiretroviral Regimens in Pregnancy and Breast-Feeding in Botswana." New England Journal of Medicine 362(24): 2282-2294.

Shiver, J. W., T.-M. Fu, et al. (2002). "Replication-incompetent adenoviral vaccine vector elicits effective anti-immunodeficiency-virus immunity." Nature 415(6869): 331-335.

Shrestha, S., S. Sudenga, et al. (2010). "The impact of highly active antiretroviral therapy on prevalence and incidence of cervical human papillomavirus infections in HIV-positive adolescents." BMC Infectious Diseases 10(1): 295.

Siliciano, J. D. and R. F. Siliciano (2004). "A long-term latent reservoir for HIV-1: discovery and clinical implications." Journal of Antimicrobial Chemotherapy 54(1): 6-9.

Sistigu, A., L. Bracci, et al. (2011). "Strong CD8+ T cell antigenicity and immunogenicity of large foreign proteins incorporated in HIV-1 VLPs able to induce a Nef-dependent activation/maturation of dendritic cells." Vaccine 29(18): 3465-3475.

Somogyi, E., J. Xu, et al. (2011). "A plasmid DNA immunogen expressing fifteen protein antigens and complex virus-like particles (VLP+) mimicking naturally occurring HIV." Vaccine 29(4): 744-753.

Streeck, H. and D. F. Nixon (2010). "T Cell Immunity in Acute HIV-1 Infection." Journal of Infectious Diseases 202(Supplement 2): S302-S308.

Sui, Y., Q. Zhu, et al. (2010). "Innate and adaptive immune correlates of vaccine and adjuvant-induced control of mucosal transmission of SIV in macaques." Proceedings of the National Academy of Sciences 107(21): 9843-9848.

Sukeepaisarncharoen, W., V. Churdboonchart, et al. (2001). "Long-term follow-up of HIV-1-infected Thai patients immunized with Remune monotherapy." HIV Clinical Trials 2(5): 391-398.

Sundling, C., M. N. E. Forsell, et al. (2010). "Soluble HIV-1 Env trimers in adjuvant elicit potent and diverse functional B cell responses in primates." The Journal of Experimental Medicine 207(9): 2003-2017.

Sundling, C., S. O'Dell, et al. (2010). "Immunization with Wild-Type or CD4-Binding-Defective HIV-1 Env Trimers Reduces Viremia Equivalently following Heterologous Challenge with Simian-Human Immunodeficiency Virus." J. Virol. 84(18): 9086-9095.

Tappuni, A. R. (2011). "Immune Reconstitution Inflammatory Syndrome." Advances in Dental Research 23(1): 90-96.

Torti, C., A. d'Arminio-Monforte, et al. (2011). "Long-term CD4+ T-cell count evolution after switching from regimens including HIV nucleoside reverse transcriptase inhibitors (NRTI) plus protease inhibitors to regimens containing NRTI plus non-NRTI or only NRTI." BMC Infectious Diseases 11(1): 23.

Tsoukas, C. M., J. Raboud, et al. (1998). "Active Immunization of Patients with HIV Infection: A Study of the Effect of VaxSyn, a Recombinant HIV Envelope Subunit Vaccine, on Progression of Immunodeficiency." AIDS Research and Human Retroviruses 14(6): 483-490.

Vaine, M., S. Lu, et al. (2009). "Progress on the Induction of Neutralizing Antibodies Against HIV Type 1 (HIV-1)." BioDrugs 23(3): 137-153 110.2165/00063030-200923030-200900001.

Van Gulck, E. F. V. T., Viggo; N. Berneman, Zwi; Vanham, Guido (2010). "Role of Dendritic Cells in HIV-Immunotherapy." Current HIV Research 8(4): 310-322.

Virgin, H. W. and B. D. Walker (2010). "Immunology and the elusive AIDS vaccine." Nature 464(7286): 224-231.

Von Kleist, M., S. Menz, et al. (2011). "HIV Quasispecies Dynamics during Pro-Active Treatment Switching: Impact on Multi-Drug Resistance and Resistance Archiving in Latent Reservoirs." PLoS ONE 6(3): e18204.

Wild, C., T. Greenwell, et al. (1993). "A Synthetic Peptide from HIV-1 gp41 Is a Potent Inhibitor of Virus-Mediated Cell,ÄîCell Fusion." AIDS Research and Human Retroviruses 9(11): 1051-1053.

Wild, C., T. Oas, et al. (1992). "A Synthetic Peptide Inhibitor of Human Immunodeficiency Virus Replication: Correlation between Solution Structure and Viral Inhibition." Proceedings of the National Academy of Sciences of the United States of America 89(21): 10537-10541.

Wild, C. T., D. C. Shugars, et al. (1994). "Peptides Corresponding to a Predictive Œ±-Helical Domain of Human Immunodeficiency Virus Type 1 gp41 are Potent Inhibitors of Virus Infection." Proceedings of the National Academy of Sciences of the United States of America 91(21): 9770-9774.

Wilson, N. A., B. F. Keele, et al. (2009). "Vaccine-Induced Cellular Responses Control Simian Immunodeficiency Virus Replication after Heterologous Challenge." J. Virol. 83(13): 6508-6521.

Wintsch, J., C.-L. Chaignat, et al. (1991). "Safety and Immunogenicity of a Genetically Engineered Human Immunodeficiency Virus Vaccine." Journal of Infectious Diseases 163(2): 219-225.

Wong, J. K., M. Hezareh, et al. (1997). "Recovery of Replication-Competent HIV Despite Prolonged Suppression of Plasma Viremia." Science 278(5341): 1291-1295.

World Health Organization, W. (2006). ANTIRETROVIRAL THERAPY FOR HIV Infection in adults and adolescents: Recommendations for a public health approach W. H. A. Programme, World Health Organization 1-134.

World Health Organization , W. (2009). "Global summary of the AIDS epidemic." Retrieved 02.11.2011, 2011, from http://www.who.int/hiv/data/2009_global_summary.png.

Yamamoto, N., N. Ushijima, et al. (2009). "Immunotherapy of HIV-infected patients with Gc protein-derived macrophage activating factor (GcMAF)." Journal of Medical Virology 81(1): 16-26.

Young, K. R., J. M. Smith, et al. (2004). "Characterization of a DNA vaccine expressing a human immunodeficiency virus-like particle." Virology 327(2): 262-272.

Zarling, J. M., W. Morton, et al. (1986). "T-cell responses to human AIDS virus in macaques immunized with recombinant vaccinia viruses." Nature 323(6086): 344-346.

10

HIV Envelope-Specific Antibody and Vaccine Efficacy

Egidio Brocca-Cofano, Peng Xiao and Marjorie Robert-Guroff
Vaccine Branch, National Cancer Institute, Bethesda, USA

1. Introduction

Following transmission, the human immunodeficiency virus (HIV) initiates persistent infection by integrating into the genome of host cells. To date it has not been possible to clear these cells by anti-viral or immune therapy, during either active or latent infection. This makes design of an efficacious HIV vaccine exceedingly difficult, since complete prevention of infection, or "sterilizing immunity", is required. As cellular immunity targets already infected cells, humoral immune responses which can prevent initial infection by means of anti-envelope neutralizing antibodies have been a prime focus of vaccine development. In proof of concept studies, passive administration of potent neutralizing antibodies has prevented infection of non-human primates by intravenous and mucosal routes (Mascola et al., 1999; Baba et al., 2000; Mascola et al., 2000; Parren et al., 2001), validating the research focus on neutralizing antibody induction. However, the task of designing an envelope vaccine is complicated by the extreme variability among HIV isolates, the propensity for neutralization escape resulting from immune pressure exerted by induced antibodies, conformational features of the HIV envelope which make immunogen design difficult, and additional envelope characteristics which effectively hide areas of vulnerability which might ordinarily be antibody targets. There are several excellent recent reviews covering the issue of broadly neutralizing antibodies (Mascola & Montefiori, 2010; Walker & Burton, 2010; Zolla-Pazner & Cardozo, 2010; McElrath & Haynes, 2010) and it is not the intent of this review to reproduce that information. Rather, we will briefly summarize some of the salient issues and approaches, and then discuss more extensively non-neutralizing anti-envelope antibodies.

Broadly neutralizing antibodies are difficult to elicit by vaccination. But the HIV envelope protein is quite immunogenic, and an array of non-neutralizing antibodies is induced by both natural infection and vaccination. Through use of sensitive new methods, these antibodies have exhibited several functional activities associated with protection. In serum these include antibody-dependent cellular cytotoxicity (ADCC) (Weinhold, 1990) and antibody-dependent cell mediated viral inhibition (ADCVI) (Forthal et al., 2006). Secretory antibodies have also been associated with protection via mechanisms such as transcytosis inhibition (Bomsel et al., 1998). Augmented by high avidity and recall memory responses which improve their efficacy, these antibody activities can contribute in varying degrees to vaccine-induced protective efficacy. The main thrust of this review will be to examine these non-neutralizing antibody responses in HIV and SIV infection and following vaccination, to describe how they may contribute to protection, and to summarize their potential utility amidst the array of additional immune protective mechanisms available to the host, including innate, cellular, and mucosal immunity.

2. Neutralizing antibodies

The variability of the HIV envelope is notorious. The envelope exhibits a 30% difference in amino acid sequence between the 9 clades designated A - K, omitting E and I (Korber et al., 2001). Envelope diversity within clades can be as high as 20% (Mascola & Montefiori, 2010). Therefore the goal of eliciting anti-envelope antibodies able to broadly recognize and protect against this spectrum of isolates is daunting. In fact it is difficult to induce broadly neutralizing antibodies by vaccination. Most that arise are relatively weak and only able to neutralize the most sensitive or easy to neutralize "Tier I" isolates (Mascola et al., 2005; Seaman et al., 2010). Yet recent publications document development of cross-reactive neutralizing antibodies during HIV infection (Sather et al., 2009) with 20 to 34% of HIV-infected individuals possessing significant breadth (Simek et al., 2009; Doria-Rose et al., 2010). That vaccine induction of broadly neutralizing antibodies is a realistic goal is also illustrated by the isolation of a handful of naturally elicited antibodies that recognize a wide spectrum of HIV isolates. These include b12, an monoclonal antibody selected by random reassortment of a phage library which recognizes the CD4 binding site of the HIV envelope (Burton et al., 1994); 2G12, a monoclonal antibody that recognizes carbohydrate moieties (Trkola et al., 1996) on the silent face of the envelope; and monoclonal antibodies 2F5 and 4E10 that target the membrane-proximal external region (MPER) of the viral envelope transmembrane protein (Muster et al., 1993; Zwick et al., 2001). Additionally, the V3 region of the external envelope protein gp120, originally believed to elicit only type-specific neutralizing antibodies, has been shown to elicit broader responses. A panel of V3 monoclonal antibodies including 447-52D was recently reported to exhibit significant cross-clade neutralizing activity (Hioe et al., 2010). The basis for this breadth may be the conserved structural elements in the V3 loop which provide for its essential function as part of the binding region to chemokine co-receptors and which outweigh the inherent variability of the amino acid sequence in importance (Almond et al., 2010; Jiang et al., 2010). Portions of the V3 and V2 loops comprise a novel quaternary epitope, recognized only as part of the native trimer. Monoclonal antibody 2909, the first such described human antibody, is potent but relatively strain specific (Gorny et al., 2005). In contrast, the recently identified monoclonals PG9 and PG16 (Walker et al., 2009) also recognize quarternary epitopes, but differ by exhibiting great neutralization breadth, attributed to dependence on an asparagine-linked carbohydrate moiety at residue 160 in the V2 loop. The 2909 antibody recognizes a lysine at this position (Zolla-Pazner & Cardozo, 2010).

New methods of high-throughput monoclonal antibody cloning and screening have facilitated isolation of several additional broadly neutralizing antibodies (Scheid et al., 2009; Corti et al., 2010). To date VRC01, a CD4 binding site antibody, has shown the greatest breadth, neutralizing 91% of tested HIV isolates, representative of all major HIV clades (Wu et al., 2010). Structural knowledge of the HIV envelope, computer-assisted protein design, and state-of-the-art methods for memory B cell sorting and single cell PCR facilitated its isolation. It is hoped that similar new methodologies can lead to design of an appropriate vaccine component able to elicit neutralizing antibody breadth.

2.1 Development of neutralizing antibodies in natural infection

While a significant percentage of HIV-infected individuals with chronic disease have a degree of neutralizing antibody breadth, a much smaller percentage are able to neutralize across all HIV clades (Simek et al., 2009). Long-term non-progressors have rather poor neutralizing antibody responses. Rather potent neutralizing activity seems to require a lengthy time period of sustained viremia and development of strong binding avidity, suggesting that antigen persistence and antibody maturation are needed for development of a broad response (Sather et al., 2009). Neutralizing antibodies develop very slowly in HIV-infected individuals. Antibodies with specificity for gp41 appear first at around 13 days post-infection and anti-gp120 antibodies at around day 28 (Tomaras et al., 2008). However, neutralizing antibodies appear later, usually months after infection, and thus do not appear to control viremia (Aasa-Chapman et al., 2004; Gray et al., 2007). This slow development reflects, at least in part, the same obstacles facing vaccine-induction of a neutralizing antibody response: conformational and carbohydrate masking of critical epitopes; homology of some epitopes with self proteins, leading to polyreactive antibodies that are subject to immune tolerance; and envelope variability leading to immune selective pressure and viral escape (McElrath and Haynes, 2010). Later in the course of disease, loss of CD4 help and B cell dysfunction exacerbates the poor neutralizing antibody development (Alter and Moody, 2010).

2.2 Improved envelope immunogen design

In addition to improved envelope design based on increasing knowledge of the structure of the HIV envelope, other approaches have attempted to better expose critical conserved epitopes on envelope immunogens. These have included deletion of variable loops to expose otherwise hidden regions of the envelope; alteration of glycosylation patterns to prevent masking; preparation of trimeric forms of the envelope to mimic the natural structure on the surface of the virion, and introduction of critical epitopes on other scaffolds for better presentation to the immune system (Hu and Stamatatos, 2007). These alterations have had varying degrees of success, although none has induced the breadth and potency of neutralizing antibody response needed for a highly effective vaccine. It is hoped that continued improvements in envelope immunogens fostered by greater knowledge of envelope structure and understanding of the natural process of broadly neutralizing antibody induction will achieve the desired goal.

3. Non-neutralizing antibodies

The RV144 phase III trial in Thailand which assessed an ALVAC-recombinant prime/Env protein boost regimen, showed only modest efficacy, protecting 31% of vaccinated individuals in the intent-to-treat group (Rerks-Ngarm et al., 2009). Nevertheless, this outcome provided the first evidence that development of a safe and effective preventive HIV vaccine is possible. This study also highlighted the need to better understand immune correlates of protection associated with decreased HIV acquisition. The RV144 vaccine components have induced a broad constellation of immune responses, including T-cell-line adapted neutralizing antibody (Nitayaphan et al., 2004), antibody-dependent cell-mediated cytotoxicity (Karnasuta et al., 2005), and CD4+ and CD8+ T cell responses, but clear immune correlates have not been defined. Currently in order to combat the extensive genomic diversity of HIV both strong cellular and humoral immune responses are believed necessary for a successful vaccine (Amanna & Slifka, 2010; Benmira et al., 2010). However, as strong cellular immunity was not elicited in the majority of RV144 vaccinees, humoral immunity is believed to have contributed to the protection against HIV acquisition. As the vaccine regimen did not elicit antibodies able to neutralize primary HIV isolates, the focus of research has shifted to the potential for non-neutralizing antibodies to mediate protection. Neutralizing antibodies are able to prevent infection of susceptible cells; however, once a cell is infected it is difficult to imagine a role for neutralizing antibodies (Battle-Miller et al., 2002). Other antibody functions such as ADCC and ADCVI working together with innate effector cells provide a means to target and kill virus infected cells (Fig. 1A). Such mechanisms could control or possibly eradicate the small foci of infected cells that form in the lamina propria after viral transmission and prior to systemic spread of the virus (Fig. 1B; Haase, 2005).

3.1 ADCC

ADCC bridges innate and adaptive immunity. It involves effector cells able to mediate cell lysis, target cells expressing cell surface antigen, and specific antibody that recognizes the cell surface antigen and activates effector cells via interaction with Fc receptors. The interaction between the Fc domain of the antibody and the corresponding receptor on effector cells triggers a series of events that lead to the destruction of the infected cell via cytotoxic granules (perforin, granzyme) or a death-receptor-dependent pathway (Fas/Fas ligand; TNF/TNFR) (de Saint Basile et al., 2010; Chavez-Galan et al., 2009).

Most ADCC responses described in the literature are directed against the envelope protein (Env) (Ahmad & Menezes, 1996; Baum et al., 1996; Alsmadi & Tilley, 1998), although Nef (Yamada et al., 2004) and Tat (Florese et al., 2009) have also been shown to be ADCC targets. Additionally, a recent study in chronically infected subjects reported that Pol is an ADCC target, but this Pol-specific ADCC activity did not correlate with delayed HIV progression (Isitman et al., 2010). Moreover, the *pol* gene encodes internal proteins, so it is possible that the Pol-specific ADCC activity observed was targeting by-stander cells that had scavenged dead-cell debris. Despite the potential efficacy of ADCC, little is known about specific epitopes recognized by antibodies able to mediate ADCC. Epitopes recognized by both anti-Env and anti-Nef antibodies that mediate ADCC have been described (Alsmadi et al., 1997; Yamada et al., 2004; Los Alamos National Laboratory Molecular Immunology Database). As discussed below, anti-Env antibodies that mediate ADCC have been associated with protection, however, whether anti-Nef or anti-Tat antibodies have an impact on natural infection is not known.

Effector cells that mediate ADCC are not major histocompatibility complex restricted, and multiple subpopulations of peripheral blood mononuclear cells (PBMCs) are involved in mediating ADCC function. NK cells, γδ T cells, neutrophils, monocytes, and macrophages all express the Fc receptor that can engage antibodies (Forthal & Moog, 2009). A large number of these cells are always present in peripheral tissues, in contrast to memory B and T cells in lymphoid tissue which require activation for neutralizing antibody or T cell functions. Since HIV infection rapidly spreads during the first 2 weeks after transmission, the significant time advantage provided, for example, by pre-existing vaccine-elicited antibody and Fc receptor-bearing cells, may facilitate better control of viremia. IgG1 and IgG3 are the most common IgG isotypes to mediate ADCC via strong interaction with the Fc-binding receptor CD16/FcγRIII expressed mainly on NK cells (Niwa et al., 2005).

Traditionally, ADCC killing was assessed using assays in which target cells were labeled with radioactive isotopes such as ^{51}Chromium. Disadvantages of this method include difficulty labeling certain cell types, low assay sensitivity and high spontaneous chromium release resulting in high background values (Volgmann et al., 1989). Several flow cytometry-based alternatives have recently circumvented the problems associated with radioactive labeling of target cells in cytotoxicity assays (Wilkinson et al., 2001; Gomez-Roman et al., 2006a; Stratov et al., 2008; Chung et al., 2009). These assays have provided greater ease of use and importantly greater sensitivity, facilitating investigation of the role of ADCC activity in natural infection and vaccine-induced protection.

3.1.1 HIV-specific ADCC responses in natural infection

Over the past 20 years, the dogma that T cells and neutralizing antibodies are protective immune correlates for many vaccines led to lack of interest in the ADCC mechanism. However the gradual accumulation of evidence from natural infection and vaccine studies supporting a protective role for ADCC has stimulated studies of this immune response. A number of early studies documented the induction of ADCC antibodies during HIV infection (Lyerly et al., 1987; Rook et al., 1987; Ojo-amaize et al., 1987). A potential role for ADCC in modulating the course of HIV infection was eventually suggested based on studies showing an inverse association between ADCC antibody levels and clinical stage of the disease. Baum et al, (1996) presented strong evidence that higher titers of antibodies mediating ADCC correlated with a successful host defense against HIV-1, and Forthal et al., (2001a) reported an inverse association between ADCC activity and plasma viremia. Higher ADCC activity has also been correlated with slower disease progression in children (Ljunggren et al., 1990; Broliden et al., 1993). More recently, ADCC activity has been demonstrated in cervical lavage fluids of HIV-infected women (Battle-Miller et al., 2002), and associated with lower genital HIV RNA loads (Nag et al., 2004). Elite controllers also have higher ADCC antibody titers than viremic individuals, whereas neutralizing antibody activity tends to be higher in viremic individuals (Lambotte et al., 2009). Nevertheless, not all studies have concluded that ADCC plays a role in protective efficacy (Dalgleish et al., 1990; Lifson et al., 1991; Chuenchitra et al., 2003). The conflicting results reflect the complexity of the virus-host interaction and elements that contribute to the ADCC response, including the integrity of the host immune system, extent of viremia, level and affinity of antibodies induced, and functionality of effector cells.

3.1.2 ADCC responses in non-human primate models

Non-human primate studies have stimulated interest in the ADCC mechanism and its role in protective efficacy. ADCC activity has been correlated with delayed disease progression in SIV infected macaques (Banks et al., 2002). Additional convincing evidence has come from pre-clinical vaccine studies. A replicating adenovirus type 5 host range mutant (Ad5hr)-SIV recombinant prime/SIV gp120 protein boost regimen was shown to elicit potent protection against an intrarectal SIV_{mac251} challenge (Patterson et al., 2004). The vaccine did not induce antibodies able to neutralize primary SIV_{mac251}, however, the reduced acute viremia was significantly correlated with anti-envelope binding antibodies that mediated ADCC against SIV_{mac251}-infected cells (Gomez-Roman et al., 2005). Subsequent studies, one involving a comparison of Ad5hr-SIV recombinant priming via the upper respiratory tract versus the oral route followed by SIV gp120 boosting and SIV_{mac251}

challenge, and another involving a comparison of Ad5hr-recombinant priming with and without subsequent envelope protein boosting followed by challenge with the chimeric virus $SHIV_{89.6P}$, again showed significant correlations of ADCC activity with reduced acute viremia (Hidajat et al., 2009; Xiao et al., 2010). The latter study also revealed a correlation of ADCC activity with reduced chronic viremia. The importance of antibody maturation in induction of the functional antibody responses was indicated by the significant correlation of ADCC-mediating antibodies with binding antibody avidity.

The non-human primate model provides a good mimic for exploration of vaccine strategies and immune mechanisms. For example, passive antibody transfer studies can directly explore the ability of antibodies to mediate protection. Binley et al. (2000) observed that passive infusion of IgG to rapid and normal progressor SIV_{mac251} infected animals caused small and transient reductions in plasma viremia by a mechanism that was inconsistent with virus neutralization but which could have been effector cell mediated, implicating ADCC. In contrast, infusion of IgG possessing high titers of anti-Env antibodies able to mediate ADCC had no effect on viral loads following two sequential oral challenges of neonatel macaques with SIV_{mac251} (Florese et al., 2006). In both these studies, high viral loads may have contributed to negligible protective effects. Further, the neonatal macaque study may have been compromised by low levels and poorly functioning effector cells in the baby animals. An improved experimental design using repetitive low dose challenge might yield more significant results.

Passive transfer of monoclonal antibodies has proven more informative in elucidating mechanisms of antibody-mediated protection. An elegant study by Hessell et al. (2007) using the neutralizing b12 monoclonal antibody and a mutant unable to bind the Fc receptor and complement, showed that protection from a $SHIV_{SF162P3}$ challenge mediated by the b12 antibody was in part due to Fc-mediated effects. A follow-on study using low-titered b12, mutant antibody, and low-dose repeated $SHIV_{SF162P3}$ challenge, supported a contribution of effector function to the delayed acquisition observed (Hessell et al., 2009).

As illustrated by the b12 monoclonal, neutralizing antibodies may also mediate ADCC activity via their Fc domain. However, all ADCC mediating antibodies do not necessarily possess neutralizing activity. A neutralizing antibody must target a specific region of the viral envelope, whereas antibodies that mediate ADCC are required only to recognize an exposed target epitope on the surface of the infected cell. Antibodies elicited in chimpanzees to an HIV clade B immunization regimen were able to mediate ADCC killing of clade A, B, C, and AE env-expressing target cells (Gomez-Roman et al., 2006). Therefore, in addition to the ability to rapidly respond, the ADCC effector mechanism can provide the breadth of antibody recognition believed necessary for protective efficacy.

The extent to which the ADCC mechanism contributes to vaccine-induced protection is not yet clarified. A definitive conclusion will perhaps come from immune correlates identified in human clinical vaccine trials. To date only a few such trials have evaluated ADCC activity. Goepfert et al. (2007) reported that Env-specific ADCC activity, correlated with binding antibodies, was detected in most individuals that received a candidate AIDS vaccine containing gp120. Further, as mentioned above, a phase II human trial in Thailand has shown induction of ADCC mediating antibodies (Karnasuta et al., 2005). The role of these antibodies in the protection against HIV acquisition seen in the RV144 trial which used similar immunogens is currently being actively explored.

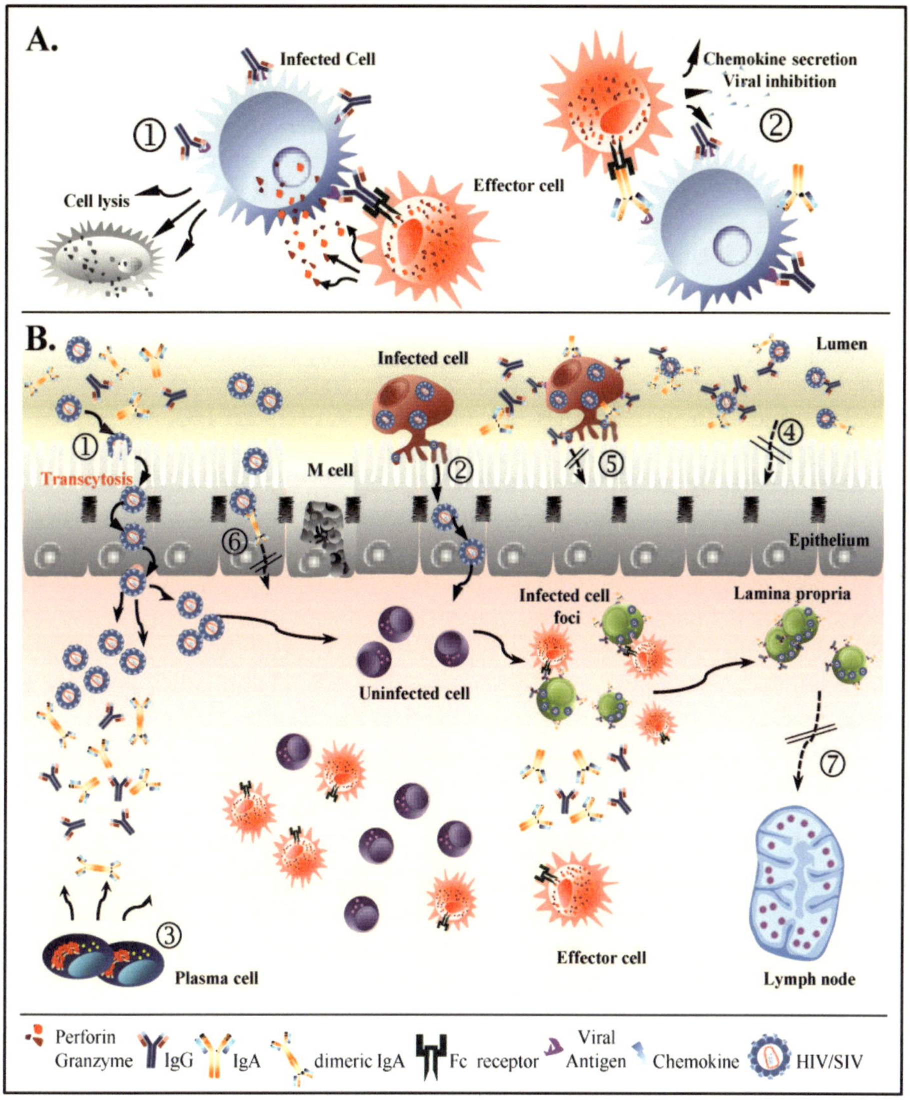

Fig. 1. **Control of viral infection by non-neutralizing antibodies. A. ADCC and ADCVI.** (1)Fc receptors on effector cells recognize the Fc domain of antibody bound to antigen on infected cells, inducing release of cytotoxic granules and cell lysis via ADCC. (2) Activation of effector cells may lead to production of chemokines and cytokines and viral inhibition by ADCVI. **B. A mucosal surface with a single layer of columnar epithelium**. Viral transmission may occur by transcytosis of cell-free (1) or cell-associated virus (2). T cells, effector cells (macrophages, monocytes, NK cells, γδ T-cells, neutrophils) and plasma cells are present in the lamina propria. Mucosal antibodies, secreted by plasma cells (3), may block infection by neutralizing virus (4), or by blocking transcytosis of cell-associated (5) or cell-free virus (6). Antibodies can mediate ADCC and ADCVI to eradicate or control infected cell foci, blocking dissemination of virus to lymph nodes (7).

3.2 ADCVI

Like ADCC, ADCVI requires antibody that forms a bridge between an infected target cell and an FcγR-bearing effector cell (Forthal et al., 2001). However, ADCVI is a broader activity not restricted to target cell lysis, as with ADCC. Rather it encompasses several mechanisms by which viral replication following target cell infection is inhibited. These may include ADCC activity, but also noncytolytic mechanisms of virus control, such as secretion of inhibitory chemokines (Fig. 1A), or FcγR-mediated phagocytosis of immune complexes. The readout in ADCVI assays is the percentage of virus inhibition due to effector cells together with a test antibody relative to a negative control antibody. This biological endpoint allows assessment of ADCVI against any lentiviral strain able to infect cells. As the ADCVI assay uses heat-inactivated serum, complement activities do not play a role (Forthal & Landucci, 1998). Overall, ADCVI is a measure of the combined ability of antibody and effector cells to inhibit the spread of virus infection (Forthal et al., 2001; Forthal & Moog, 2009). Both polyclonal and monoclonal antibodies can mediate ADCVI. Intact IgG, not just the F(ab')2 portion is required (Forthal et al., 2006), emphasizing the importance of Fc-Fc receptor interactions in mediating the functional activity.

3.2.1 ADCVI during HIV infection

ADCVI has been associated with reduction in viremia during HIV infection. In HIV-infected individuals, systemic non-neutralizing antibodies appear early during acute infection, generally before a neutralizing antibody response (Sawyer et al., 1990). Not surprisingly, in individuals with acute HIV infection, non-neutralizing ADCVI antibodies appeared as early as the first week after onset of symptoms or the first month after HIV exposure (Forthal et al., 2001). ADCVI activity became more potent as the viral load fell (in the absence of antiretroviral therapy), resulting in an inverse relationship between ADCVI activity and acute plasma viremia, suggesting a protective effect. Importantly, ADCVI antibodies appeared to be broadly reactive with different HIV strains. The demonstration of an association between non-neutralizing but functional antibodies able to mediate ADCVI activities and protection is noteworthy and timely, in view of the recent outcome of the RV144 phase IIb vaccine trial in Thailand as discussed above. A previous study of serum samples from the Vax004 trial which evaluated gp120 vaccines similar to those used for boosting in RV144 revealed an inverse correlation between the HIV infection rate of vaccinated individuals and vaccine-elicited ADCVI antibody activity (Forthal et al., 2007). Although this trial did not result in protection, the results support the hypothesis that similar functional antibody activities may have contributed to protection in the RV144 trial. Taken together, these observations have renewed interest in defining the mechanisms of FcγR-mediated protection by ADCC and ADCVI.

3.2.2 ADCVI in rhesus macaque models

In support of a protective role for ADCVI, significant correlations between ADCVI activity mediated by vaccine-induced antibodies and decreased acute viremia have been reported in both SIV and SHIV rhesus macaque models (Florese et al., 2009; Hidajat et al., 2009; Xiao et al., 2010). Further, passive infusion of anti-SIV immune serum with strong ADCVI activity to newborn rhesus macaques prevented infection from an oral SIV_{mac251} challenge (Forthal et al., 2006). A recent study showed that vaccine-elicited antibody mediated ADCVI activity that was recalled 4 weeks post-challenge. This post-challenge activity was correlated with reduced chronic phase viremia (Xiao et al., 2010) suggesting a broader role for ADCVI in controlling viral replication over the course of disease rather than impacting only early post-transmission viral spread. In this same study, a negative correlation between ADCVI activity 4 weeks post-challenge and neutralizing antibody titer 8 weeks post challenge was observed which became progressively weaker over time, and disappeared by 24 weeks post-challenge. The ADCVI assay evaluates viral inhibition in the presence of serum plus effector cells, and subtracts inhibition observed with serum in the absence of effector cells. This latter inhibition is attributed to neutralizing antibody. Therefore, the inverse correlation between the two activities might indicate that both neutralizing and non-neutralizing antibodies were mediating ADCVI. Neutralizing monoclonal antibodies are known to mediate ADCVI activity (Hessell et al., 2007). Development of *de novo* neutralizing antibody depends on the presence of sufficient viral antigen to drive the antibody response. The inverse relationship between ADCVI and the more slowly developing neutralizing antibody may reflect control of viremia by ADCVI and/or other immune mechanisms at the expense of strong neutralizing antibody induction due to a reduced viral burden. The complexity of the *in vivo* situation makes the relationships between functional antibody activities and viral burden difficult to resolve.

4. Secretory antibody

Mucosal surfaces are the major site for HIV entry. Therefore, an effective HIV vaccine may require the presence of antibodies able to prevent infection at mucosal sites. IgA antibodies are the most prevalent at mucosal surfaces, and might contribute to protection by one or more mechanisms including classical neutralization, but also non-neutralizing activities such as immune exclusion involving mucus entrapment and clearance, ADCC discussed above, and inhibition of HIV transcytosis across the epithelial cell barrier (Fig. 1B; Kozlowski and Neutra, 2003). Study of HIV-exposed but uninfected individuals (so called highly-exposed, seronegative; or HEPS), has shown the presence of functional HIV-specific IgA at mucosal surfaces of these individuals (Miyazawa et al., 2009; Lopalco, 2004), implicating the antibody in resistance to HIV infection.

Several vaccine approaches have been evaluated in non-human primates for the ability to elicit viral-specific IgA antibodies at genital/rectal sites. These have included tonsillar immunizations with replication-defective SIV (Vagenas et al., 2009), administration of DNA vaccines intranasally or rectally, followed by boosting with MVA recombinants (Bertley et al., 2004; Wang et al., 2004), intradermal or intramuscular administrations of DNA vaccines together with GM-CSF DNA or CCL27 DNA as adjuvants (Lai et al., 2007; Kraynyak et al., 2010) vaginal delivery of trimeric HIV envelope together with Carbopol gel (Cranage et al., 2011), upper respiratory track immunization with replication-competent Ad-recombinants followed by intramuscular boosting with envelope protein (Florese et al., 2009; Hidajat et al., 2009; Xiao et al., 2010), and intramuscular plus intranasal immunization with a gp41 subunit vaccine delivered on virosomes (Bomsel et al., 2011). These have had varying degrees of success in consistently eliciting mucosal IgA antibodies. Only a few studies, however, have investigated functionality of vaccine-elicited IgA as discussed below. Immune exclusion is difficult to assess in vitro due to the necessity for a mucus barrier, but neutralizing, ADCC, and ADCVI activities can be evaluated. Transcytosis inhibition seems especially relevant for mucosal protection.

4.1 Transcytosis inhibition

HIV-1 transmission mainly occurs through exposure of mucosal surfaces to HIV-infected fluids, such as semen, cervicovaginal fluid, saliva, colostrum, and breast milk (Pope and Haase, 2003). A key entry event is translocation of virus across the epithelium. In rectal, intestinal, colonic, and endocervical mucosa, the epithelium is made up of a single layer of polarized, columnar epithelial cells with tight junctions separating the cells into the apical domain, which faces the lumen, and the basolateral domain, which faces the serosal side and the internal milieu (Bomsel, 1997). In contrast, ectocervical and vaginal epithelium is composed of pluristratified epithelial cells that lack a polarized plasma membrane and tight junctions, allowing intraepithelial dendritic cells and Langerhans cells to diffuse into the epithelium (Bomsel and Alfsen, 2003). Depending on the site of infection, several mechanisms for HIV-1 transmission across mucosal epithelia have been proposed, including columnar epithelial cell transcytosis, direct infection of epithelial cells, and dendritic/Langerhans cell transport (Bomsel & David, 2002; Shattock et al., 2000).

The major type of HIV transcytosis is cell-associated (Bomsel & Alfsen, 2003), generated by cell-cell contact of virally-infected cells with apical epithelial cell surfaces. It is a rapid, efficient, and nondegradative process in which virus is transported from the apical to the basolateral surface of polarized epithelial cells. Cell-free virus transcytosis is also possible but inefficient (Bobardt et al., 2007; Bomsel, 1997). Rather than fusion and infection, interactions between viral components, including gp41 (Alfsen et al., 2001), gp120 (Bobardt et al., 2007), and gp160 (Hocini et al., 1997), and host epithelial cell surface molecules, such as glycosphingolipid galactosyl-ceramide (GalCer) (Alfsen & Bomsel, 2002; Meng et al., 2002), an important component of endocytotic "raft" membrane microdomains, the coreceptor CCR5 (Bomsel et al., 2007), and the heparin sulfate proteoglycan attachment receptor, agrin (Alfsen et al., 2005), lead to transcytosis of the virus across the epithelial barrier and its trapping by submucosal dendritic cells which disseminate it to target $CD4^+$ T cells.

Immunoglobulin A (IgA) and immunoglobulin G (IgG) anti-HIV antibodies have been detected in nearly all external secretions. Although mucosal IgG may interfere with viral infection in tissues underlying mucosal epithelia and secondary lymphoid tissues, mucosal IgA is thought to best protect mucosal surfaces (Pope and Haase, 2003). HIV-1 entry via transcytosis *in vitro* can be inhibited by dimeric IgA (dIgA) isolated from HIV-1-infected subjects (Bomsel et al., 1998), secretory IgA specific for gp41 (Alfsen et al., 2001), and mucosal and serum IgA from HIV-1-exposed seronegative individuals (Devito et al., 2000). Recently, transcytosis inhibition of both SIV and SHIV by vaccine-elicited mucosal antibodies has been evaluated in pre-clinical studies in non-human primates. In rhesus macaques, mucosal priming with replication-competent Ad-HIV or SIV recombinants followed by intramuscular boosting with envelope protein elicited antibodies in rectal secretions able to inhibit SIV and SHIV transcytosis *in vitro* (Hidajat et al., 2009; Xiao et al., 2010). Importantly, a significant correlation between transcytosis inhibition and reduced chronic viremia was seen in the study by Xiao et al. (2010) suggesting that mucosal IgA present in the submucosa may play a role in viremia control during the course of infection. However, the strongest evidence to date for a contribution of transcytosis inhibition to vaccine-elicited protection was recently reported by Bomsel et al. (2011). Following intramuscular plus intranasal immunization with gp41 subunit immunogens on virosomes, 4 out of 5 rhesus macaques were protected from $SHIV_{SF162P3}$ acquisition following repetitive low-dose challenge, whereas all controls became infected. The protected macaques had gp41-specific vaginal IgA that mediated transcytosis inhibition, and vaginal IgG that had neutralizing and/or ADCC activity. Both the transcytosis inhibition and ADCC activity were significantly inversely correlated with acute viremia. Of particular interest, sera from these macaques lacked anti-HIV activity in neutralization, ADCC, and transcytosis inhibition assays, suggesting that the IgG with protective activity was locally produced. A similar suggestion was reported in the study of Xiao et al. (2010).

5. Antibody avidity

In addition to functionality, the overall quality of an antibody response largely determines its effectiveness. Antibody avidity, a measure of the strength of the binding interaction between an antigen with multiple antigenic determinants and multivalent antibodies (Siegrist et al., 2004), is one characteristic which contributes to efficacy. It develops in germinal centers following somatic hypermutation of immunoglobulin genes and selection of B cells for high affinity binding to antigen (Berek et al., 1991; French et al., 1989; Griffiths et al., 1984). Thus, this antibody maturation process is dependent on both time and antigen exposure. The importance of antibody avidity has been shown in studies associating low antibody avidity with poor protective efficacy of an RSV vaccine (Delgado et al., 2009). In contrast, high-avidity neutralizing (Barnett et al., 2010) and non-neutralizing (Zhao et al., 2009; Xiao et al., 2010) HIV-1 Env-specific antibodies have been inversely correlated with reduced SHIV viremia following challenge. Importantly, in the Xiao et al. (2010) study, significant correlations were seen between antibody avidity and both functional antibody activities: ADCC and ADCVI, both also correlated with reduced viremia. The results overall suggest that antibody maturation following vaccination is associated with better functional antibody activity.

6. The role of memory B cells in vaccine-mediated immunity

A critical feature of protective humoral immunity is memory. The success of vaccination depends on the differentiation of naïve B cells into plasma cells and memory B cells. Plasma cells are terminally differentiated and continuously secrete antibody without requiring further antigenic stimulation. In contrast, memory B cells represent an important second line of immune defense that is initiated if pre-existing antibody levels are too low to prevent infection or if an invading pathogen is able to circumvent the pre-existing antibody response. Memory B cells do not actively secrete antibody but instead maintain their immunoglobulin in the membrane-bound form, which together with Igα and Igβ form the antigen-specific B cell receptor. Following exposure to the initial antigen these cells become fully activated, proliferate, and differentiate into antibody secreting cells (ASC) (Ahmed & Gray, 1996; McHeyzer-Williams & McHeyzer-Williams, 2005; Pierce & Liu, 2010). Little is understood about the regulation of vaccine-induced humoral immunity. Differentiation of memory B cells into short-lived plasma cells is dependent on the presence of antigen (Dorner & Radbruch, 2007; Cagigi, et al., 2008). In contrast, long-lived antibody responses generated by viral infections or vaccinations are not dependent on the continuous presence of memory B cells but are rather produced by long-lived plasma cells that reside in the bone marrow and do not require antigen for continued production of antibody (Dorner & Radbruch, 2007; Radbruch et al., 2006). In fact, vaccine-induced B cell memory is maintained for more than 50 years after smallpox vaccination (Crotty et al., 2003), whereas antibody

responses to tetanus toxoid and diphtheria vaccines have half-lives of 11 and 19 years, respectively (Amanna et al., 2007).
Memory B cell and serum antibody levels do not always correlate. This lack of correlation implies that the serum antibody level is maintained by long-lived plasma cells in the bone marrow and not by memory B cells circulating in the blood. However, in one of the first studies to examine the frequency of specific memory B cells in humans (Bonsignori et al., 2009), plasma antibody and memory B cell responses to HIV-1 envelope were compared in a group of chronic HIV-1 infected individuals and in volunteers vaccinated in the VAX004 clinical trial (Gilbert et al., 2005). A significant correlation between blood anti-Env memory B cells levels and plasma anti-Env antibody titers was found in both chronic HIV-1 infection and after vaccination with rgp120, suggesting that plasma antibody was maintained predominantly by short-lived memory B cells. Additionally, the half-life of anti-Env antibodies was shorter than those for influenza and tetanus toxoid, demonstrating that the HIV-1 envelope does not elicit long-lived B cell memory to the degree of other antigens. This outcome is not surprising for the HIV-infected cohort, as B-cell dysfunction, including loss of memory B cell subsets has been well-documented in HIV and SIV infection (Cagigi et al., 2008; Kuhrt et al., 2010a; Shen & Tomaras, 2011). However, the reasons for impaired memory induction in vaccinees is not well understood, and may include immune suppression due to binding of gp120 to CD4 or binding of carbohydrates to mannose receptors on dendritic cells and B cells (Bonsignori et al., 2009).
SIV and SHIV non-human primate models have been very valuable in HIV vaccine development. Human memory B cells have been extensively studied (Bonsignori et al., 2009; Crotty et al., 2004; Bernasconi et al., 2002), but only recently have rhesus macaque memory B cell studies been undertaken (Douagi et al., 2010; Kuhrt et al., 2010). We have recently shown induction of SIV and HIV Env-specific IgG and IgA ASC in rhesus macaques following priming with replicating Ad-SIV or HIV recombinants and boosting with SIV or HIV envelope protein (Brocca-Cofano et al., 2011). Env-specific IgG and IgA specific activities were correlated with several antibody activities, including ADCC, ADCVI, and/or transcytosis inhibition, indicating that maturation of antibody responses is critical for improved functionality. Further, IgG and IgA memory B cells post challenge were inversely correlated with chronic viremia indicating that vaccine-induced memory B cells were recalled and influenced disease outcome. That memory B cells should exhibit a protective role is not surprising in view of the reported association between loss of memory B cells and rapid disease progression in both HIV and SIV infection (Titanji et al., 2006; Titanji et al., 2010). Our induction of strong anti-envelope memory B cell responses by vaccination (Brocca-Cofano et al., 2011) may reflect use of a replicating vector to prime immune responses followed by envelope boosting. The combined approach may have provided both the antigen persistence and time necessary to allow antibody maturation.

7. Conclusion

Antibodies are key to host defense and critical for HIV vaccine design. Antibodies that recognize conserved epitopes and broadly neutralize virus can prevent infection. Once infection has occurred, other antibodies that interact with viral antigens expressed on the infected cell surface are needed to eliminate initial foci, or control subsequent systemic spread of the virus. Fc receptor-bearing effector cells, such as NK cells, can mediate killing of infected cells by ADCC and/or ADCVI activities. The latter can also inhibit viral replication. Mucosal antibodies that block viral entry through mechanisms such as transcytosis inhibition help control viral transmission and spread. As summarized here, maturation of vaccine-induced antibody responses is necessary for optimal function. Both antibody avidity and memory are directly associated with functional activity and control of viremia. An HIV/AIDS vaccine should be able to induce both cellular and humoral immunity. Regarding the latter, the success of a vaccine will depend on stimulating the production of mature high-titered antibodies with sufficiently broad reactivity to protect against HIV and SIV encounters. The path to induction of protective anti-envelope antibodies will come from understanding the B cell regulatory pathway of specific antibody production and from design of optimal immunogens. Coordination between human vaccine clinical trials and nonhuman primate vaccine challenge studies is essential to advance new vaccine concepts and accelerate the pace of HIV-1 vaccine efficacy trials.

8. Acknowledgement

This work was supported by the Intramural Research Program of the National Institutes of Health, National Cancer Institute.

9. References

Aasa-Chapman, M.M., Hayman, A., Newton, P., Cornforth, D., Williams, I., Borrow, P., Balfe, P., & McKnight, A. (2004). Development of the antibody response in acute HIV-1 infection. *AIDS* 18, 371-381.

Ahmad, A., & Menezes, J. (1996). Antibody-dependent cellular cytotoxicity in HIV infections. *FASEB Journal* 10, 258-266.

Ahmed, R., & Gray, D. (1996). Immunological memory and protective immunity: understanding their relation. *Science* 272, 54-60.

Alfsen, A. & Bomsel, M. (2002). HIV-1 gp41 envelope residues 650-685 exposed on native virus act as a lectin to bind epithelial cell galactosyl ceramide. *Journal of Biological Chemistry* 277, 25649-25659.

Alfsen, A., Iniguez, P., Bouguyon, E., & Bomsel, M. (2001). Secretory IgA specific for a conserved epitope on gp41 envelope glycoprotein inhibits epithelial transcytosis of HIV-1. *Journal of Immunology* 166, 6257-6265.

Alfsen, A., Yu, H., Magerus-Chatinet, A., Schmitt, A., & Bomsel, M. (2005). HIV-1-infected blood mononuclear cells form an integrin- and agrin-dependent viral synapse to induce efficient HIV-1 transcytosis across epithelial cell monolayer. *Molecular Biology of the Cell* 16, 4267-4279.

Almond, D., Kimura, T., Kong, X., Swetnam, J., Zolla-Pazner, S., & Cardozo, T. (2010). Structural conservation predominates over sequence variability in the crown of HIV type 1's V3 loop. *AIDS Research and Human Retroviruses*, 26, 717-723.

Alsmadi, O., Herz, R., Murphy, E., Pinter, A., & Tilley, S.A. (1997). A novel antibody-dependent cellular cytotoxicity epitope in gp120 is identified by two monoclonal antibodies isolated from a long-term survivor of human immunodeficiency virus type 1 infection. *Journal of Virology* 71, 925-933.

Alsmadi, O., & Tilley, S.A. (1998). Antibody-dependent cellular cytotoxicity directed against cells expressing human immunodeficiency virus type 1 envelope of primary or laboratory-adapted strains by human and chimpanzee monoclonal antibodies of different epitope specificities. *Journal of Virology* 72, 286-293.

Alter, G. & Moody, A. (2010). The humoral response to HIV-1: new insights, renewed focus. *The Journal of Infectious Diseases* 202, S315-S322.

Amanna, I.J., Carlson, N.E., & Slifka, M.K. (2007). Duration of humoral immunity to common viral and vaccine antigens. *New England Journal of Medicine* 357, 1903-1815.

Amanna, I.J., & Slifka, M.K. (2010). Contributions of humoral and cellular immunity to vaccine-induced protection in humans. *Virology* 411, 206-215.

Baba, T.W., Liska, V., Hofmann-Lehmann, R., Vlasak, J., Xu, W., Ayehunie, S., Cavacini, L.A., Posner, M.R., Katinger, H., Stiegler, G., Bernacky, B.J., Rizvi T.A., Schmidt, R., Hill, L.R., Keeling, M.E., Lu, Y., Wright, J.E., Chou, T-C., & Ruprecht, R.M. (2000). Human neutralizing monoclonal antibodies of the IgG1 subtype protect against mucosal simian-human immunodeficiency virus infection. *Nature Medicine* 6, 200-206.

Banks, N.D., Kinsey, N., Clements, J., & Hildreth, J.E.K. (2002). Sustained antibody-dependent cell-mediated cytotoxicity (ADCC) in SIV-infected macaques correlates with delayed progression to AIDS. *AIDS Research and Human Retroviruses* 18, 1197-1205.

Barnett, S.W., Burke, B., Sun, Y., Kan, E., Legg, H., Lian, Y., Bost, K., Zhou, F., Goodsell, A., Zur Megede, J., Polo, J., Donnelly, J., Ulmer, J., Otten, G.R., Miller, C.J., Vajdy, M., & Srivastava, I.K. (2010). Antibody-mediated protection against mucosal simian-human immunodeficiency virus challenge of macaques immunized with alphavirus replicon particles and boosted with trimeric envelope glycoprotein in MF59 adjuvant. *Journal of Virology* 84, 5975-5985.

Battle-Miller, K., Eby, C.A., Landay, A.L., Cohen, M.H., Sha, B.E., & Baum, L.L. (2002). Antibody-dependent cell-mediated cytotoxicity in cervical lavage fluids of human immunodeficiency virus type 1--infected women. *Journal of Infectious Diseases* 185, 439-447.

Baum, L.L., Cassutt, K.J., Knigge, K., Khattri, R., Margolick, J., Rinaldo, C., Kleeberger, C.A., Nishanian, P., Henrard, D.R., & Phair, J. (1996). HIV-1 gp120-specific antibody-dependent cell-mediated cytotoxicity correlates with rate of disease progression. *Journal of Immunology* 157, 2168-2173.

Benmira, S., Bhattacharya, V., & Schmid, M.L. (2010). An effective HIV vaccine: A combination of humoral and cellular immunity? *Current HIV Research* 8, 441-449.

Berek, C., Berger, A., & Apel, M. (1991). Maturation of the immune response in germinal centers. *Cell* 67, 1121-1129.

Bernasconi, N.L., Traggiai, E., & Lanzavecchia, A. (2002). Maintenance of serological memory by polyclonal activation of human memory B cells. *Science* 298, 2199-2202.

Bertley, F.M.N., Kozlowski, P.A., Wang, S., Chappelle, J., Patel, J., Sonuyi, O., Mazzara, G., Montefiori, D., Carville, A., Mansfield, K.G., & Aldovini, A. (2004). Control of simian/human immunodeficiency virus viremia and disease progression after IL-2-augmented DNA-modified vaccinia virus Ankara nasal vaccination in nonhuman primates. *Journal of Immunology* 172, 3745-3757.

Binley, J.M., Clas, B., Gettie, A., Vesanen, M., Montefiori, D.C., Sawyer, L., Booth, J., Lewis, M., Marx, P.A., Bonhoeffer, S., & Moore, J.P. (2000). Passive infusion of immune serum into simian immunodeficiency virus-infected rhesus macaques undergoing a rapid disease course has minimal effect on plasma viremia. *Virology* 270, 237-249.

Bobardt, M.D., Chatterji, U., Selvarajah, S., Van der Schueren, B., David, G., Kahn, B., & Gallay, P.A. (2007). Cell-free human immunodeficiency virus type 1 transcytosis through primary genital epithelial cells. *Journal of Virology* 81, 395-405.

Bomsel, M. (1997). Transcytosis of infectious human immunodeficiency virus across a tight human epithelial cell line barrier. *Nature Medicine* 3, 42-47.

Bomsel, M., & Alfsen, A. (2003). Entry of viruses through the epithelial barrier: pathogenic trickery. *Nature Reviews Molecular and Cellular Biology* 4, 57-68.

Bomsel, M., & David, V. (2002). Mucosal gatekeepers: selecting HIV viruses for early infection. *Nature Medicine* 8, 114-116.

Bomsel, M., Heyman, M., Hocini, H., Lagaye, S., Belec, L., Dupont, C., & Desgranges, C. (1998). Intracellular neutralization of HIV transcytosis across tight epithelial barriers by anti-HIV envelope protein dIgA or IgM. *Immunity* 9, 277-287.

Bomsel, M., Pastori, C., Tudor, D., Alberti, C., Garcia, S., Ferrari, D., Lazzarin, A., & Lopalco, L. (2007). Natural mucosal antibodies reactive with first extracellular loop of CCR5 inhibit HIV-1 transport across human epithelial cells. *AIDS* 21:13-22.

Bomsel, M., Tudor, D., Drillet, A., Alfsen, A., Ganor, Y., Roger, M., Mouz, N., Amacker, M., Chalifour, A., Diomede, L., Devillier, G., Cong, Z., Wei, Q., Gao, H., Qin, C., Yang, G., Zurbriggen, R., Lopalco, L., & Fleury, S. (2011). Immunization with HIV-1 gp41 subunit virosomes induces mucosal antibodies protecting nonhuman primates against vaginal SHIV challenges. *Immunity* 34, 269-280.

Bonsignori, M., Moody, M.A., Parks, R.J., Holl, T.M., Kelsoe, G., Hicks, C.B., Vandergrift, N., Tomaras, G.D., & Haynes, B.F. (2009). HIV-1 envelope induces memory B cell responses that correlate with plasma antibody levels after envelope gp120 protein vaccination or HIV-1 infection. *Journal of Immunology* 183, 2708-2717.

Brocca-Cofano, E., McKinnon, K., Demberg, T., Venzon, D., Hidajat, R., Xiao, P., Daltabuit-Test, M., Patterson, L.J., & Robert-Guroff, M. (2011). Vaccine-elicited SIV and HIV envelope-specific IgA and IgG memory B cells in rhesus macaque peripheral blood correlate with functional antibody responses and reduced viremia. *Vaccine* In press.

Broliden, K., Sievers, E., Tovo, P.A., Moschese, V., Scarlatti, G., Broliden, P.A., Fundaro, C., & Rossi, P. (1993). Antibody-dependent cellular cytotoxicity and neutralizing activity in sera of HIV-1-infected mothers and their children. *Clinical and Experimental Immunology* 93, 56-64.

Burton, D.R., Pyati, J., Koduri, R., Sharp, S.J., Thornton, G.B., Parren, P.W.H.I., Sawyer, L.S.W., Hendry, R.M., Dunlop, N., Nara, P.L., Lamacchia, M., Garratty, E., Stiehm, E.R., Bryson, Y.J., Cao, Y., Moore, J.P., Ho, D.D., & Barbas, C.F., III. (1994). Efficient neutralization of primary isolates of HIV-1 by a recombinant human monoclonal antibody. *Science* 266, 1024-1027.

Cagigi, A., Nilsson, A., De Milito, A., & Chiodi, F. (2008). B cell immunopathology during HIV-1 infection: lessons to learn for HIV-1 vaccine design. *Vaccine* 26, 3016-3025.

Chavez-Galan, L., Arenas-Del Angel, M.C., Zenteno, E., Chavez, R., & Lascurain, R. (2009). Cell death mechanisms induced by cytotoxic lymphocytes. *Cellular & Molecular Immunology* 6, 15-25.

Chuenchitra, T., Wasi, C., Louisirirojchanakul, S., Nitayaphan, S., Sutthent, R., Cox, J.H., de Souza, M.S., Brown, A.E., Birx, D.L., & Polonis, V.R. (2003). Longitudinal study of humoral immune responses in HIV type 1 subtype CRF01_AE (E)-infected Thai patients with different rates of disease progression. *AIDS Research and Human Retroviruses* 19, 293-305.

Chung, A.W., Rollman, E., Center, R.J., Kent, S.J., & Stratov, I. (2009). Rapid degranulation of NK cells following activation by HIV-specific antibodies. *Journal of Immunology* 182, 1202-1210.

Corti, D., Langedijk, J.P., Hinz, A., Seaman, M.S., Vanzetta, F., Fernandez-Rodriguez, B.M., Silacci, C., Pinna, D., Jarrossay, D., Balla-Jhagjhoorsingh, S., Willems, B., Zekveld, M.J., Dreja, H., O'Sullivan, E., Pade, C., Orkin C., Jeffs, S.A., Montefiori, D.C., Davis, D., Weissenhorn, W., McKnight, A., Heeney, J.L., Sallusto, F., Sattentau, Q.J., Weiss, R.A., & Lanzavecchia, A. (2010). Analysis of memory B cell responses and isolation of novel monoclonal antibodies with neutralizing breadth from HIV-1-infected individuals. *PLoS One* 5, e8805.

Cranage, M.P., Fraser, C.A., Cope, A., McKay, P.F., Seaman, M.S., Cole, T., Nahmoud, A.N., Hall, J., Giles, E., Voss, G., Page, M., Almond, N., & Shattock, R.J. (2011). Antibody responses after intravaginal immunization with trimeric HIV-1_{CN54} clade C gp140 in Carbopol gel are augmented by systemic priming or boosting with an adjuvanted formulation. *Vaccine* 29, 1421-1430.

Crotty, S., Aubert, R.D., Glidewell, J., & Ahmed, R. (2004). Tracking human antigen-specific memory B cells: a sensitive and generalized ELISPOT system. *Journal of Immunological Methods* 286, 111-122.

Crotty, S., Felgner, P., Davies, H., Glidewell, J., Villarreal, L., & Ahmed, R. (2003). Cutting edge: long-term B cell memory in humans after smallpox vaccination. *Journal of Immunology* 171, 4969-4973.

Dalgleish, A., Sinclair, A., Steel, M., Beatson, D., Ludlam, C., & Habeshaw, J. (1990). Failure of ADCC to predict HIV-associated disease progression or outcome in a haemophiliac cohort. *Clinical and Experimental Immunology* 81, 5-10.

Delgado, M.F., Coviello, S., Monsalvo, A.C., Melendi, G.A., Hernandez, J.Z., Batalle, J.P., Diaz, L., Trento, A., Chang, H.Y., Mitzner, W., Ravetch, J., Melero, J.A., Irusta, P.M., & Polack, F.P. (2009). Lack of antibody affinity maturation due to poor Toll-like receptor stimulation leads to enhanced respiratory syncytial virus disease. *Nature Medicine* 15, 34-41.

De Saint Basile, G., Menasche, G., & Fischer, A. (2010). Molecular mechanisms of biogenesis and exocytosis of cytotoxic granules. *Nature Reviews Immunology* 11, 568–579.

Devito, C., Broliden, K., Kaul, R., Svensson, L., Johansen, K., Kiama., P, Kimani, J., Lopalco, L., Piconi, S., Bwayo, J.J., Plummer, F., Clerici, M., & Hinkula, J. (2000). Mucosal and plasma IgA from HIV-1-exposed uninfected individuals inhibit HIV-1 transcytosis across human epithelial cells. *Journal of Immunology* 165, 5170-5176.

Doria-Rose, N.A., Klein, R.M., Daniels, M.G., O'Dell, S., Nason, M., Lagedes, A., Bhattacharya, T., Migueles, S.A., Wyatt, R.T., Korber, B.T., Mascola, J.R., & Connors, M. (2010). Breadth of human immunodeficiency virus-specific neutralizing activity in sera: clustering analysis and association with clinical variables. *Journal of Virology* 84, 1631-1636.

Dorner, T. & Radbruch, A. (2007). Antibodies and B cell memory in viral immunity. *Immunity* 27, 384-392.

Douagi, I., Forsell, M.N.E., Sundling, C., O'Dell, S., Feng, Y., Dosenovic, P., Li, Y., Seder, R., Loré, K., Mascola, J.R., Wyatt, R.T., & Hedestam, G.B.K. (2010) Influence of novel CD4 binding-defective HIV-1 envelope glycoprotein immunogens on neutralizing antibody and T-cell responses in nonhuman primates. *Journal of Virology* 84, 1683-1695.

Florese, R.H., Demberg, T., Xiao, P., Kuller, L., Larsen, K., Summers, L.E., Venzon, D., Cafaro, A., Ensoli, B., & Robert-Guroff, M. (2009). Contribution of nonneutralizing vaccine-elicited antibody activities to improved protective efficacy in rhesus macaques immunized with Tat/Env compared with multigenic vaccines. *Journal of Immunology* 182, 3718-3727.

Florese, R.H., Van Rompay, K.K., Aldrich, K., Forthal, D.N., Landucci ,G., Mahalanabis, M., Haigwood, N., Venzon, D., Kalyanaraman, V.S., Marthas, M.L., & Robert-Guroff, M. (2006). Evaluation of passively transferred, nonneutralizing antibody-dependent cellular cytotoxicity-mediating IgG in protection of neonatal rhesus macaques against oral SIVmac251 challenge. *Journal of Immunology* 177, 4028-4036.

Forthal, D.N., Gilbert, P.B., Landucci, G., & Phan, T. (2007). Recombinant gp120 vaccine-induced antibodies inhibit clinical strains of HIV-1 in the presence of Fc receptor-bearing effector cells and correlate inversely with HIV infection rate. *Journal of Immunology* 178, 6596-6603.

Forthal, D.N., & Landucci, G. (1998). In vitro reduction of virus infectivity by antibody-dependent cell-mediated immunity. *Journal of Immunological Methods* 220, 129-138.

Forthal, D.N., Landucci, G., Cole, K.S., Marthas, M., Becerra, J.C., & Van Rompay, K. (2006). Rhesus macaque polyclonal and monoclonal antibodies inhibit simian immunodeficiency virus in the presence of human or autologous rhesus effector cells. *Journal of Virology* 80, 9217-9225.

Forthal, D.N., Landucci, G., & Daar, E.S. (2001). Antibody from patients with acute human immunodeficiency virus (HIV) infection inhibits primary strains of HIV type 1 in the presence of natural-killer effector cells. *Journal of Virology* 75, 6953-6961.

Forthal, D.N., Landucci, G., & Keenan, B. (2001a). Relationship between antibody-dependent cellular cytotoxicity, plasma HIV type 1 RNA, and CD4+ lymphocyte count. *AIDS Research and Human Retroviruses* 17, 553-561.

Forthal, D.N., & Moog, C. (2009). Fc receptor-mediated antiviral antibodies. *Current Opinion in HIV AIDS* 4, 388-393.

French, D.L., Laskov, R., Scharff M.D. (1989). The role of somatic hypermutation in the generation of antibody diversity. *Science* 244, 1152-1157.

Gilbert, P.B., Peterson, M.L., Follmann, D., Hudgens, M.G., Francis, D.P., Gurwith, M., Heyward, W.L., Jobes, D.V., Popovic, V., Self, S.G., Sinangil, F., Burke, D., & Berman, P.W. (2005). Correlation between immunologic responses to a recombinant glycoprotein 120 vaccine and incidence of HIV-1 infection in a phase 3 HIV-1 preventive vaccine trial. *Journal of Infectious Diseases* 191, 666-677.

Goepfert, P.A., Tomaras, G.D., Horton, H., Montefiori, D., Ferrari, G., Deers, M., Voss, G., Koutsoukos, M., Pedneault, L., Vandepapeliere, P., McElrath, M.J., Spearman, P., Fuchs, J.D., Koblin, B.A., Blattner, W.A., Frey, S., Baden, L.R., Harro, C., Evans, T., & the NIAID HIV Vaccine Trials Network. (2007). Durable HIV-1 antibody and T-cell responses elicited by an adjuvanted multi-protein recombinant vaccine in uninfected human volunteers. *Vaccine* 25, 510-518.

Gomez-Roman, V.R. , Florese, R.H., Patterson, L.J., Peng, B., Venzon, D., Aldrich, K., & Robert-Guroff, M. (2006). A simplified method for the rapid fluorometric assessment of antibody-dependent cell-mediated cytotoxicity. *Journal of Immunological Methods* 308, 53-67.

Gomez-Roman, V.R., Florese, R.H., Peng, B., Montefiori, D., Kalyanaraman, V.S., Venzon, D., Srivastava, I., Barnett, S.W., & Robert-Guroff, M. (2006). An adenovirus-based HIV subtype-B prime/boost vaccine regimen elicits antibodies mediating broad antibody-dependent cellular cytotoxicity against non-subtype-B strains. *Journal of Acquired Immune Deficiency Syndromes* 43, 270-277.

Gomez-Roman, V.R., Patterson, L.J., Venzon, D., Liewehr, D., Aldrich, K., Florese, R., & Robert-Guroff, M. (2005). Vaccine-elicited antibodies mediate antibody-dependent cellular cytotoxicity correlated with significantly reduced acute viremia in rhesus macaques challenged with SIVmac251. *Journal of Immunology* 174, 2185-2189.

Gorny, M.K., Stamatatos, L., Volsky, B., Revesz, K., Williams, C., Wang, X., Cohen, S., Staudinger, R., & Zolla-Pazner, S. (2005). Identification of a new quaternary neutralizing epitope on human immunodeficiency virus type 1 virus particles. *Journal of Virology* 79, 5232-5237.

Gray, E.S., Moore, P.L., Choge, I.A., Decker, J.M., Bibollet-Ruche, F., Li, H., Leseka, N., Treurnicht, F., Mlisana, K., Shaw, G.M., Karim, S.S., Williamson, C., & Morris, L. (2007). Neutralizing antibody responses in acute human immunodeficiency virus type 1 subtype C infection. *Journal of Virology* 81, 6187-6196.

Griffiths, G.M., Berek, C., Kaartinen, M., & Milstein, C. (1984). Somatic mutation and the maturation of immune response to 2-phenyl oxazolone. *Nature* 312, 271-275.

Haase, A.T. (2005). Perils at mucosal front lines for HIV and SIV and their hosts. *Nature Reviews Immunology* 5, 783-792.

Hessell A.J., Hangartner, L., Hunter, M., Havenith, C.E.G., Beurskens, F.J., Bakker, J.M., Lanigan, C.M.S., Landucci, G., Forthal, D.N., Parren, P.W.H.I., Marx, P.A., & Burton, D.R. (2007). Fc receptor but not complement binding is important in antibody protection against HIV. *Nature* 449, 101-105.

Hessell, A.J., Poignard, P., Hunter, M., Hangartner, L., Tehrani, D.M., Bleeker, W.K., Parren, P.W.H.I., Marx, P.A., & Burton, D.R. (2009). Effective, low-titer antibody protection against low-dose repeated mucosal SHIV challenge in macaques. *Nature Medicine* 15, 951-955,

Hidajat, R., Xiao, P., Zhou, Q., Venzon, D., Summers, L.E., Kalyanaraman, V.S., Montefiori, D.C., & Robert-Guroff, M. (2009). Correlation of vaccine-elicited systemic and mucosal nonneutralizing antibody activities with reduced acute viremia following intrarectal simian immunodeficiency virus SIVmac251 challenge of rhesus macaques. *Journal of Virology* 83, 791-801.

Hioe, C.E., Wrin, T., Seaman, M.S., Yu, X., Wood, B., Self, S., Williams, C., Gorny, M.K., & Zolla-Pazner, S. Anti-V3 monoclonal antibodies display broad neutralizing activities against multiple HIV-1 subtypes. *PLoS One* 5, e10254.

Hocini, H., Belec, L., Iscaki, S., Garin, B., Pillot, J., Becquart, P., & Bomsel, M. (1997). High-level ability of secretory IgA to block HIV type 1 transcytosis: contrasting secretory IgA and IgG responses to glycoprotein 160. *AIDS Research and Human Retroviruses* 13,1179-1185.

Hu, S-L. & Stamatatos, L. (2007). Prospects of HIV Env modification as an approach to HIV vaccine design. *Current HIV Research* 5, 507-513.

Isitman, G., Chung, A.W., Navis, M., Kent, S.J., & Stratov, I. (2010). Pol as a target for antibody dependent cellular cytotoxicity responses in HIV-1 infection. *Virology* 412, 110-116.

Jiang, X., Burke, V., Totrov, M., Williams, C., Cardozo, T., Gorny, M.K., Zolla-Pazner, S., & Kong, X. (2010). Conserved structural elements in the V3 crown of HIV-1 gp120. *Nature Structural & Molecular Biology* 17, 955-962.

Karnasuta, C., Paris, R.M., Cox, J.H., Nitayaphan, S., Pitisuttithum, P., Thogncharoen, P., Brown, A.E., Gurunathan, S., Tartaglia, J., Heyward, W.L., McNeil, J.G., Birx, D.L., de Souza, M.S., & TAVEG Thai AIDS Vaccine Evaluation Group, Thailand. (2005). Antibody-dependent cell-mediated cytotoxic responses in participants enrolled in a phase I/II ALVAC-HIV/AIDSVAX B/E prime-boost HIV-1 vaccine trial in Thailand. *Vaccine* 23, 2522-2529.

Korber, B., Gaschen, B., Yusim K., Thakallapally, R., Kesmir, C., & Detours, V. (2001). Evolutionary and immunological implications of contemporary HIV-1 variation. *British Medical Bulletin* 58, 19-42.

Kozlowski, P.A. & Neutra, M.R. (2003). The role of nucosal immunity in prevention of HIV transmission. *Current Molecular Medicine* 3, 217-228.

Kraynyak, K.A., Kutzler, M.A., Cisper, N.J., Khan, A.S., Draghia-Akli, R., Sardesal, N.Y., Lewis, M.G., Yan, J., & Weiner, D.B. (2010). Systemic immunization with CCL27/CTACK modulates immune responses at mucosal sites in mice and macaques. *Vaccine* 28, 1942-1951.

Kuhrt, D., Faith, S., Hattemer, A., Leone A., Sodora, D., Picker, L., Borghesi, L., & Cole, K.S. (2010). Naive and memory B cells in the rhesus macaque can be differentiated by surface expression of CD27 and have differential responses to CD40 ligation. *Journal of Immunological Methods* 363, 166-176.

Kuhrt, D., Faith, S.A., Leone, A., Rohankedkar, M., Sodora, D.L., Picker, L.J., & Cole, K.S. (2010a). Evidence of early B-cell dysregulation in simian immunodeficiency virus infection: rapid depletion of naïve and memory B-cell subsets with delayed reconstitution of the naïve B-cell population. *Journal of Virology* 84, 2466-2476.

Lai, L., Vodros, D., Kozlowski, P.A., Montefiori, D.C., Wilson, R.L., Akerstrom, V.L., Chennareddi, L., Yu, T., Kannanganat, S., Ofielu, L., Villinger, F., Wyatt, L.S., Moss, B., Amara, R.R., & Robinson, H.L. (2007). GM-CSF DNA: an adjuvant for higher avidity IgG, rectal IgA, and increased protection against the acute phase of a SHIV-89.6P challenge by a DNA/MVA immunodeficiency virus vaccine. *Virology* 369, 153-167.

Lambotte, O., Ferrari, G., Moog, C., Yates, N..L, Liao, H-X., Parks, R.J., Hicks, C.B., Owzard, K., Tomaras, G.D., Montefiori, D.C., Haynes, B.F., & Delfraissy, J-F. (2009). Heterogeneous neutralizing antibody and antibody-dependent cell cytotoxicity responses in HIV-1 elite controllers. *AIDS* 23, 897-906.

Lifson, A.R., Buchbinder, S.R., Sheppard, H.W., Mawle, A.C., Wilber, J.C., Stanley, M., Hart C.E., Hessol, N.A., & Holmberg, S.D. (1991). Long-term human immunodeficiency virus infection in asymptomatic homosexual and bisexual men with normal CD4+ lymphocyte counts: immunologic and virologic characteristics. *Journal of Infectious Diseases* 163, 959-965.

Ljunggren, K., Moschese, V., Broliden, P.A., Giaquinto, C., Quinti, I., Fenyö, E.M., Wahren, B., Rossi, P., and Jondal, M. (1990). Antibodies mediating cellular cytotoxicity and neutralization correlate with a better clinical stage in children born to human immunodeficiency virus-infected mothers. *Journal of Infectious Diseases* 161,198-202.

Lopalco, L. (2004). Humoral immunity in HIV-1 exposure: cause or effect of HIV resistance? *Current HIV Research* 2, 127-139.

Lyerly, H.K., Reed, D.L., Matthers, T.J., Langlois, A.J., Ahearne, P.A., Petteway, S.R., Jr., & Weinhold, K.J. (1987). Anti-GP 120 antibodies from HIV seropositive individuals mediate broadly reactive anti-HIV ADCC. *AIDS Research and Human Retroviruses* 3, 409-422.

Mascola, J.R., D'Souza, P., Gilbert, P., Hahn, B.H., Haigwood, N.L., Morris, L., Petropoulos, C.J., Polonis, V.R., Sarzotti M., & Montefiori, D.C. (2005). Recommendations for the design and use of standard virus panels to assess neutralizing antibody responses elicited by candidate human immunodeficiency virus type 1 vaccines. *Journal of Virology* 79, 10103-10107.

Mascola, J.R., Lewis, M.G., Stiegler, G., Harris, D., VanCott, T.C., Hayes, D., Louder, M.K., Brown, C.R., Sapan, C.V., Frankel S.S., Lu, Y., Robb, M.L., Katinger, H., & Birx, D.L. (1999). Protection of macaques against pathogenic simian/human immunodeficiency virus 89.6PD by passive transfer of neutralizing antibodies. *Journal of Virology* 73, 4009-4018.

Mascola, J.R. & Montefiori, D.C. (2010). The role of antibodies in HIV vaccines. *Annual Review of Immunology* 28, 412-444.

Mascola, J.R., Stiegler, G., VanCott, T.C., Katinger, H., Carpenter, C.B., Hanson, C.E., Beary, H., Hayes, D., Frankel, S.S., Birx, D.L., & Lewis, M.G. (2000). Protection of macaques against vaginal transmission of a pathogenic HIV-1/SIV chimeric virus by passive infusion of neutralizing antibodies. *Nature Medicine* 5, 207-210.

McElrath, M.J. & Haynes, B.F. (2010). Induction of immunity to human immunodeficiency virus type-1 by vaccination. *Immunity* 33, 542-554.

McHeyzer-Williams, L.J., & McHeyzer-Williams, M.G. (2005). Antigen-specific memory B cell development. *Annual Review of Immunology* 23, 487-513.

Meng, G., Wei, X., Wu, X., Sellers, M.T., Decker, J.M., Moldoveanu, Z., Orenstein, J.M., Graham, M.F., Kappes, J.C., Mestecky, J., Shaw, G.M., & Smith, P.D. (2002). Primary intestinal epithelial cells selectively transfer R5 HIV-1 to CCR5+ cells. *Nature Medicine* 8, 150-156.

Miyazawa, M., Lopalco, L., Mazzotta, F., Caputo, S.L., Veas, F., & Clerici, M., for the ESN Study Group. (2009). The "immunologic advantage" of HIV-exposed seronegative individuals. *AIDS* 23, 161-175.

Muster, T., Steindl, F., Purtscher, M., Trkola, A., Klima, A., Himmler, G., Ruker, F., & Katinger, H. (1993). A conserved neutralizing epitope on gp41 of human immunodeficiency virus type 1. *Journal of Virology* 67, 6642-6647.

Nag, P., Kim, J., Sapiega, V., Landay, A.L., Bremer, J.W., Mestecky, J., Reichelderfer, P., Kovacs, A., Cohn, J., Weiser, B., & Baum, L.L. (2004). Women with cervicovaginal antibody-dependent cell-mediated cytotoxicity have lower genital HIV-1 RNA loads. *Journal of Infectious Diseases* 190, 1970-1978.

Nitayaphan, S., Pitisuttithum, P., Karnasuta, C., Eamsila, C., de Souza, M., Morgan, P., Polonis, V., Benenson, M., VanCott, T., Ratto-Kim, S., Kim, J., Thapinta, D., Garner,

R., Bussaratid, V., Singharaj, P., el Habib, R., Gurunathan, S., Heyward, W., Birx, D., McNeil, J., & Brown, A.E., for the Thai AIDS Vaccine Evaluation Group. (2004). Safety and immunogenicity of an HIV subtype B and E prime-boost vaccine combination in HIV-negative Thai adults. *The Journal of Infectious Diseases* 190, 702-706.

Niwa, R., Natsume, A., Uehara, A., Wakitani, M., Iida, S., Uchida, K., Satoh, M., & Shitara, K. (2005). IgG subclass-independent improvement of antibody-dependent cellular cytotoxicity by fucose removal from Asn297-linked oligosaccharides. *Journal of Immunological Methods* 306, 151-160.

Ojo-Amaize, E.A., Nishanian, P., Keith, D.E., Jr, Houghton, R.L., Heitjan, D.F., Fahey, J.L., & Giorgi, J.V. (1987). Antibodies to human immunodeficiency virus in human sera induce cell-mediated lysis of human immunodeficiency virus-infected cells. *Journal of Immunology* 139, 2458-2463.

Parren, P.W.H.I., Marx, P.A., Hessell, A.J., Luckay, A., Harouse J., Cheng-Mayer, C., Moore, J.P., & Burton, D.R. (2001). Antibody protect smacaques against vaginal challenge with a pathogenic R5 simian/human immunodeficiency virus at serum levels giving complete neutralization in vitro. *Journal of Virology* 75, 8340-8347.

Patterson, L.J., Malkevitch, N., Venzon, D., Pinczewski, J., Gómez-Román, V.R., Wang, L., Kalyanaraman, V.S., Markham, P.D., Robey, F.A., & Robert-Guroff, M. (2004). Protection against mucosal simian immunodeficiency virus SIV(mac251) challenge by using replicating adenovirus-SIV multigene vaccine priming and subunit boosting. *Journal of Virology* 78, 2212-2221.

Pierce, S.K., & Liu, W. (2010). The tipping points in the initiation of B cell signalling: how small changes make big differences. *Nature Reviews Immunology* 10, 767-777.

Pope, M., & Haase, A.T. (2003). Transmission, acute HIV-1 infection and the quest for strategies to prevent infection. *Nature Medicine* 9, 847-852.

Radbruch, A., Muehlinghaus, G., Luger, E.O., Inamine, A., Smith, K.G., Dörner, T., & Hiepe, F. (2006).Competence and competition: the challenge of becoming a long-lived plasma cell. *Nature Reviews Immunology* 6, 741-750.

Rerks-Ngarm, S., Pitisuttithum, P., Nitayaphan, S., Kaewkungwal, J., Chiu, J., Paris, R., Premsri, N., Namwat, C., de Souza, M., Adams, E., Benenson, M., Gurunathan, S., Tartaglia, J., McNeil, J.G., Francis, D.P., Stablein, D., Birx, D.L., Chunsuttiwat, S., Khamboonruang, C., Thongcharoen, P., Robb, M.L., Michael, N.L., Kunasol, P., & Kim, J.H. for the NOPH-TAVEG Investigators. (2009). Vaccination with ALVAC and AIDSVAX to prevent HIV-1 infection in Thailand. *New England Journal of Medicine* 361 2209-2220.

Rook, A.H., Lane, H.C., Folks, T., McCoy, S., Alter, H., & Fauci, A.S. (1987). Sera from HTLV-III/LAV antibody-positive individuals mediate antibody-dependent cellular cytotoxicity against HTLV-III/LAV-infected T cells. *Journal of Immunology* 138, 1064-1067.

Sather, D.N., Armann, J., Ching, L.K., Mavrantoni, A., Sellhorn, G., Caldwell, Z., Yu, X., Wood, B., Self, S., Kalams, S., & Stamatatos, L. (2009). Factors associated with the development of cross-reactive neutralizing antibodies during human immunodeficiency virus type 1 infection. *Journal of Virology* 83, 757-769.

Sawyer, L.A., Katzenstein, D.A., Hendry, R.M., Boone, E.J., Vujcic, L.K., Williams, C.C., Zeger, S.L., Saah, A.J., Rinaldo, C.R., Jr., Phair, J.P., Giorgi, J.V., & Quinnan, G.V., Jr.

(1990). Possible beneficial effects of neutralizing antibodies and antibody-dependent, cell-mediated cytotoxicity in human immunodeficiency virus infection. *AIDS Research and Human Retroviruses* 6, 341-356.

Scheid, J.F., Mouquet, H., Feldhahn, N., Seaman, M.S., Velinzon, K., Pietzsch, J., Ott, R.G., Anthony, R.M., Zebroski ,H., Hurley, A., Phogat, A., Chakrabarti, B., Li, Y., Connors, M., Pereyra ,F., Walker, B.D., Wardemann, H., Ho, D., Wyatt, R.T., Mascola, J.R., Ravetch, J.V., & Nussenzweig, M.C. (2009). Broad diversity of neutralizing antibodies isolated from memory B cells in HIV-infected individuals. *Nature* 458, 636-640.

Seaman, M.S., Janes, H., Hawkins, N., Grandpre, L.E., Devoy, C., Giri, A., Coffey, R.T., Harris, L., Wood, B., Daniels, M.G., Bhattacharya, T., Lapedes, A., Polonis, V.R., McCutchan, F.E., Gilbert, P.B., Self, S.G., Korber, B.T., Montefiori, D.C., & Mascola, J.R.. (2010). Tiered categorization of a diverse panel of HIV-1 Env pseudoviruses for assessment of neutralizing antibodies. *Journal of Virology* 84, 1439-1452.

Shattock, R.J., Griffin, G.E., & Gorodeski, G.I. (2000). In vitro models of mucosal HIV transmission. *Nature Medicine* 6,607-608.

Shen, X., & Tomaras, G.D. (2011). Alterations of the B-cell response by HIV-1 replication. *Current HIV/AIDS Reports* 8, 23-30.

Siegrist, C.A., Pihlgren, M., Tougne, C., Efler, S.M., Morris, M.L., AlAdhami, M.J., Cameron, D.W., Cooper, C.L., Heathcote, J., Davis, H.L., & Lambert, P.H. (2004). Co-administration of CpG oligonucleotides enhances the late affinity maturation process of human anti-hepatitis B vaccine response. *Vaccine* 23, 615-622.

Simek, M.D., Rida, W., Priddy, F.H., Pung, P., Carrow, E., Laufer, D.S., Lehrman, J.K., Boaz, M., Tarragona-Fiol, T., Miiro, G., Birungi, J., Pozniak, A., McPhee, D.A., Manigart, O., Karita, E., Inwoley, A., Jaoko, W., DeHovitz, J., Bekker, L-G., Pitisuttithum, P., Paris, R., Walker, L.M., Poignard, P., Wrin, T., Fast, P.E., Burton, D.R., & Koff, W.C. (2009). *Journal of Virology* 83, 7337-7348.

Stratov, I., Chung, A., & Kent, S.J. (2008). Robust NK cell-mediated human immunodeficiency virus (HIV)-specific antibody-dependent responses in HIV infected subjects. *Journal of Virology* 82, 5450–5459.

Titanji, K., De Milito, A., Cagigi, A., Thorstensson, R., Grutzmeier, S., Atlas, A., Hejdeman, B., Kroon, F.P., Lopalco, L., Nilsson, A., & Chiodi, F. (2006). Loss of memory B cells impairs maintenance of long-term serologic memory during HIV-1 infection. *Blood* 108, 1580-1587.

Titanji, K., Velu, V., Chennareddi, L., Vijay-Kumar, M., Gewirtz, A.T., Freeman, G.J., & Amara, R.R. (2010). Acute depletion of activated memory B cells involves the PD-1 pathway in rapidly progressing SIV-infected macaques. *Journal of Clinical Investigation* 120, 3878-3890.

Tomaras, G.D., Yates, N.L., Liu, P., Qin, L., Fouda, G.G., Chavez, L.L., Decamp, A.C., Parks, R.J., Ashley, V.C., Lucas, J.T., Cohen, M., Eron, J., Hicks, C.B., Liao, H-X., Self, S.G., Landucci, G., Forthal, D.N., Weinhold, K.J., Keele, B.F., Hahn, B.H., Greenberg, M.L., Morris, L., Abdool Karim, S.S., Blattner, W.A., Montefiori, D.C., Shaw, G.M., Perelson, A.S., & Haynes, B.F. (2008). Initial B-cell responses to transmitted human immunodeficiency virus type 1: Virion-binding immunoglobulin M (IgM) and IgG antibodies followed by plasma anti-gp41 antibodies with ineffective control of initial viremia. *Journal of Virology* 82, 12449-12463.

Trkola, A., Purtscher, M., Muster, T., Ballaun, C., Buchacher, A., Sullivan, N., Srinivasan, K., Sodroski, J. Moore, J.P., & Katinger, H. (1996). Human monoclonal antibody 2G12 defines a distinctive neutralization epitope on the gp120 glycoprotein of human immunodeficiency virus type 1. *Journal of Virology* 70, 1100-1108.

Vagenas, P., Williams, V.G., Piatak, M., Jr., Bess, J.W., Jr., Lifson, J.D., Blanchard, J.L., Gettie, A., & Robbiani, M. (2009). Tonsillar application of AT-2 SIV affords partial protection against rectal challenge with SIVmac239. *Journal of Acquired Immune Deficiency Syndromes* 52, 433-442.

Volgmann, T., Klein-Struckmeier, A., & Mohr, H. (1989). A fluorescence-based assay for quantitation of lymphokine-activated killer cell activity. *Journal of Immunological Methods* 119, 45-51.

Walker, L.M. & Burton, D.R. (2010). Rational antibody-based HIV-1 vaccine design: current approaches and future directions. *Current Opinion in Immunology* 22, 358-366.

Walker, L.M., Phogat, S.K., Chan-Hui, P-Y., Wagner, D., Phung, P., Goss, J.L., Wrin, T., Simek, M.D., Fling, S., Mitchan, J.L., Lehrman, J.K., Priddy, F.H., Olsen, O.A., Frey, S.M., Hammond, P.W., Protocol G Principal Investigators, Kaminsky, S., Zamb, T., Moyle, M., Koff, W.C., Poignard, P., & Burton, D.R. (2009). Broad and potent neutralizing antibodies from an African donor reveal a new HIV-1 vaccine target. *Science* 326, 285-289.

Wang, S., Bertley, F.M.N., Kozlowski, P.A., Herrmann, L., Manson, K., Mazzara, G., Piatak, M., Johnson, R.P., Carville, A., Mansfield, K., & Aldovini, A. (2004). An SHIV DNA/MVA rectal vaccination in macaques provides systemic and mucosal virus-specific responses and protection against AIDS. *AIDS Research and Human Retroviruses* 20, 846-859.

Weinhold, K.J. (1990). Nonrestricted forms of anti-HIV-1 cytotoxicity. In: *Techniques in HIV Research,* Aldovini, A & Walker, BD, pp. 187 - 199. Stockton Press, ISBN 0-935859-88-8, New York.

Wilkinson, R.W., Lee-MacAry, A.E., Davies, D., Snary, D., & Ross, E.L. (2001). Antibody-dependent cell-mediated cytotoxicity: a flow cytometry-based assay using fluorophores. *Journal of Immunological Methods* 258, 183-191.

Wu, X., Yang, Z., Li, Y., Hogerkorp, C-M., Schief, W.R., Seaman, M.S., Zhou, T., Schmidt, S.D., Wu, L., Xu, L., Longo, N.S., McKee, K., O'Dell, S., Louder, M.K., Wycuff, D.L., Feng, Y., Nason, M., Doria-Rose, N., Connors, M., Kwong, P.D., Roederer, M., Wyatt, R.T., Nabel, G.J., & Mascola, J.R. (2010). Rational design of envelope identifies broadly neutralizing human monoclonal antiobides to HIV-1. *Science* 329, 856-861.

Xiao, P., Zhao, J., Patterson, L.J., Brocca-Cofano, E., Venzon, D., Kozlowski, P.A., Hidajat, R., Demberg, T., & Robert-Guroff, M. (2010). Multiple vaccine-elicited nonneutralizing antienvelope antibody activities contribute to protective efficacy by reducing both acute and chronic viremia following simian/human immunodeficiency virus SHIV89.6P challenge in rhesus macaques. *Journal of Virology* 84, 7161-7173.

Yamada, T., Watanabe, N., Nakamura, T., & Iwamoto, A. (2004). Antibody-dependent cellular cytotoxicity via humoral immune epitope of Nef protein expressed on cell surface. *Journal of Immunology* 172 2401-2406.

Zhao, J., Lai, L., Amara, R.R., Montefiori, D.C., Villinger, F., Chennareddi, L., Wyatt, L.S., Moss, B., & Robinson, H.L. (2009). Preclinical studies of human immunodeficiency virus/AIDS vaccines: inverse correlation between avidity of anti-Env antibodies and peak postchallenge viremia. *Journal of Virology* 83, 4102-4111.

Zolla-Pazner, S. & Cardozo, T. (2010). Structure-function relationships of HIV-1 envelope sequence-variable regions refocus vaccine design. *Nature Reviews Immunology* 10, 527-535.

Zwick, M.B., Labrijn, A.F., Wang, M., Spenlehauer, C., Saphire, E.O., Binley, J.M., Moore, J.P., Stiegler, G., Katinger, H., Burton, D.R., & Parren, P.W.H.I. (2001). Broadly neutralizing antibodies targeted to the membrane-proximal external region of human immunodeficiency virus type 1 glycoprotein gp41. *Journal of Virology* 75, 10892-10905.

11

Role of Cytokines and Chemokines in HIV Infection

Vishwanath Venketaraman et al.*
College of Osteopathic Medicine of the Pacific, Western University of Health Sciences, USA

1. Introduction

Human immunodeficiency virus (HIV) is the cause of acquired immunodeficiency syndrome (AIDS). Blood monocytes and resident macrophages are important *in vivo* cell targets for HIV infection and their role in AIDS pathogenesis are well documented. These cells of innate immune defenses usually survive HIV infection, serve as a major virus reservoir, and function as immunoregulatory cells through secretion of several pro-inflammatory cytokines and chemokines in response to HIV infection, thereby recruiting and activating new target cells for the virus, including CD4+ T cells. This review describes the alterations in the synthesis of host cytokines and chemokines following HIV infection thereby favoring successful survival of the virus inside the host and enhancing the susceptibility of the host to opportunistic infections.

2. HIV and chemokine receptors

HIV infects immune cells of the macrophage and T-cell lineage. Entry into these cells requires CD4 as a receptor in addition to a co-receptor which most frequently is either chemokine receptor CCR5 or CXCR4 (Gorry & Ancuta, 2011). Binding and entry into human cells requires the two HIV envelope glycoproteins gp120 and gp41. Gp41 possesses a transmembrane domain and is associated with the viral envelope while Gp120 is present in association with Gp41 but does not insert into or contact the viral membrane (Tagliamonte *et al*; 2010). These two viral glycoproteins are present in HIV as tetramers. Therefore, three Gp41 molecules associate within the viral membrane, while three molecules of Gp120 associate with Gp41 (Tagliamonte *et al*; 2010). To facilitate HIV-1 entry into human cells, Gp120 binds to human cellular CD4 with high affinity. Binding causes a conformational change in Gp120 that reveals a co-receptor binding site. Binding to one of the chemokine

*Devin Morris[2], Clare Donohou[5], Andrea Sipin[4], Steven Kung[4], Hyoung Oh[2], Mesharee Franklin[2], John P. Murad[3], Fadi T. Khasawneh[3], Beatrice Saviola[1], Timothy Guilford[6] and Clare Donahue[6]
[1]*College of Osteopathic Medicine of the Pacific, Western University of Health Sciences, USA*
[2]*Graduate College of Biomedical Sciences, USA*
[3]*College of Pharmacy, Western University of Health Sciences, USA*
[4]*California State Polytechnic University, USA*
[5]*Pitzer College, USA*
[6]*Your Energy Systems, USA*

receptors is then facilitated which in turn induces a conformational change in the glycoprotein gp41 N-terminus (Tagliamonte *et al*; 2010). A fusion peptide portion of gp41 inserts into the host cell membrane and lowers energy that is required for fusion of the host and viral membranes (Tagliamonte *et al*; 2010). The viral core is then translocated into the cytoplasm of the host cell.

HIV-1 viral variants can in general use either the CCR5 or CXCR4 co-receptor for entry into human cells (Gorry & Ancuta, 2011). They may also at times use a variety of other chemokine receptors for entry (Gorry *et al*; 2007). The normal function of chemokine receptors is to bind chemokines that target immune cells to areas of inflammation within the human body. Certain HIV-1 viruses may have an increased ability to either bind the CCR5 receptor and are known as R5 viruses, bind to CXCR4 and are known as X4 viruses, or bind with mixed affinity to either receptor. This differential affinity lies within the specific alterations in amino acid sequence of the gp120 glycoprotein (Gorry & Ancuta, 2011). Although not correlating completely, macrophage tropic HIV-1 viruses generally are R5 and T-cell tropic viruses are X4 viruses (Gorry & Ancuta, 2011). Early during infection R5 viruses predominate, and it appears that there is some mechanism which selects these viruses during the transmission process (Grivel *et al*; 2010). For example, an HIV-1 naive individual may be exposed to both R5 and X4 virus particles from an infected individual, but only become infected with the R5 viral particles. There may be multiple factors which affect this process, including co-receptor availability and pH at the sites of infection. Acidic pH may act to disrupt the cationic charge present in gp120 proteins which bind to CXCR4 preferentially (Kwong *et al*; 2010, Edo-Matas *et al*; 2010). R5 viruses are also prominent during chronic infection. X4 viruses or R5X4 viruses which have mixed affinity can arise later during infection and often their presence precedes disease progression and immune cell depletion (Mariani, 2010).

Deletion of the CCR5 receptor can in many cases abrogate infection with HIV-1 completely. It has previously been identified that individuals homozygous for a 32 base pair deletion within the *CCR5* gene resulting in a nonfunctional CCR5 molecule are resistant to infection with the HIV-1 virus, though there have been some instances where homozygous *CCR5Δ32* individuals were infected with X4 HIV-1 (Samson, 1996). Additionally, people who carry one allele of *CCR5Δ32* have a slower progression of the disease. This knowledge has led to the development of treatments for HIV-1 infection. Transplantation of stem cells from individuals homozygous for *CCR5Δ32* into CCR5 HIV-1 positive individuals resulted in clearing of the virus from the infected patients (Hutter, 2009). Monoclonal antibodies against CCR5 to inhibit binding of HIV-1 to this co-receptor are a potential therapeutic to prevent viral entry and replication (Tenorio, 2011, Suleiman, 2010). In addition there are plans to use an individual's native stem cells as a target to disrupt the *CCR5* receptor gene which can then be transplanted back into the HIV infected patient to effect elimination of the HIV-1 virus from the body (Cannon and June, 2011). Pitfalls of these therapies include the problem that the CCR5 chemokine receptor has a native function within the body, and that disrupting this receptor may cause unforeseen deficits in the immune system. In fact, lack of the CCR5 receptor gene has been associated with increased risk of severe infection with other viruses such as the West Nile Virus, and certain flaviviruses (Lin *et al*; 2008, Kindberg *et al*; 2008). Notwithstanding the previously mentioned caveat, interference with the CCR5 receptor may indeed be a promising target to treat those infected with HIV-1 as well as prevent infection for those exposed to the virus via sexual activity, needle sharing, or accidental hospital transmission.

3. Chemokine ligand-2 (CCL2)

CCL2 or monocyte chemotactic protein-1 (MCP-1), of the C-C chemokine family, is a cytokine with the ability to influence both innate and adaptive immune responses (Daly *et al*; 2003). This chemokine is produced by a variety of different cell types including endothelial cells, fibroblasts, epithelial cells, smooth muscle cells, mesangial cells, astrocytic cells, and microglial cells. However, despite the wide range of cell types that have the ability to manufacture CCL2, the majority of CCL2 is produced by macrophages and monocytes (Deshmane *et al*; 2009).

Although technically a chemokine, CCL2 is often classified as an inflammatory cytokine due to its ability to attract various leukocytes (monocytes, memory T cells, basophils, natural killer (NK) cells etc.) to sites of trauma, bacterial and mycobacterial infection, toxin exposure, and ischemia (Daly *et al*; 2003, Deshmane *et al*; 2009, Mahad *et al*; 2003,, Charo *et al*; 2006). Besides attracting various leukocytes, CCL2 also specifically regulates the infiltration of monocytes, memory T lymphocytes, and NK cells (Deshmane *et al*; 2009). In addition, CCL2 has been found to have a profound effect on the differentiation of naïve helper T cells (Daly *et al*; 2003). Interestingly, studies have found that CCL2 expression tends to lead to the development of a Th2 immune response. Taking this tendency into account, it seems likely that CCL2 concentrations in HIV patients, which Weiss *et al.* (Weiss *et al*; 1997) found were correlated with viral load, can be linked to the Th1 to Th2 cytokine response switch often observed in HIV-1-infected patients (Deshmane *et al*; 2009).

CCL2 has also been found to play other roles in HIV pathogenesis. Eugenin *et al.* (Eugenin *et al*; 2006) noted that CCL2 in the central nervous system (CNS) attracts HIV-infected leukocytes into the brain thereby increasing the rate of HIV-1-infected cell-dispersal and causing the eventual impairment of the blood-brain-barrier. In fact, multiple studies indicate that CCL2 is largely responsible for the development of HIV encephalitis (HIVE), HIV-1-associated dementia (HAD), and NeuroAIDS (Deshmane *et al*; 2009, Eugenin *et al*; 2006).

4. HIV and the Th1 to Th2 Cytokine shift

Under normal conditions, the immune system utilizes a Th1 subset response to viral infections. Activated antigen presenting cells (APC) secrete interleukin-12 (IL-12) which causes Th cell differentiation into the Th1 subset of cells (Clerci et al; 1993). These Th1 cells then secrete a characteristic Th1 profile of cytokines consisting of interleukin-2 (IL-2), interferon-gamma (IFN-γ), and tumor necrosis factor-beta (TNF-β). IL-2 induces proliferation of naïve Th cells (T_0), amplifying the Th response. IFN-γ induces further IL-12 production in activated APCs, amplifying the Th1 response, and suppressing any Th2 response. IFN-γ also plays an important role in the activation of cytotoxic T_C cells which destroy virally infected cells.

In individuals infected with HIV, the normal Th1 response to viral infection is shifted to a Th2 response (Klein et al; 1997, Osakwe et al; 2010). Measurement of the serum cytokine levels of HIV infected patients has revealed an increase in Th2 cytokines as well as a decrease in Th1 cytokines (Klein et al; 1997, Osakwe et al; 2010). Assays have shown elevated serum IL-4 levels in HIV seropositive individuals (Clerci et al; 1993). IL-4 in the presence of proliferating T_0 cells leads to their differentiation into the Th2 subset. Th2 cells promote B-cell proliferation, class switching, and eosinophil activation (Clerci et al; 1993). This Th2 response is not appropriate for control of intracellular pathogens such as HIV, and so allows it to persist and spread in $CD4^+$ T-cells.

5. TNF-α and HIV infection

It has also been shown that HIV infection induces increased production of TNF-α by macrophages. TNF-α stimulates the production of free radicals. Moreover, enhanced levels of free radicals are likely to increase TNF-α in various cells. TNF-α consists of 233 amino acids and is expressed on all somatic cells, particularly on the cell membrane where it becomes hydrolyzed to its soluble form. TNF-α is considered as one of the most highly studied pro-inflammatory cytokines because it plays a critical role in the origin and progression of diseases such as HIV-1 (Bahia and Silakari, 2010). The immuno-regulatory response of the host influences the pathogenesis of HIV-1 infection, triggering monocytes, macrophages, and natural killer cells to produce TNF-α (Alfano and Poli, 2005). As a result, there is a positive correlation between HIV-1 viremia and TNF-α levels in serum of HIV-1 infected patients. This relationship suggests that reducing TNF-α levels may also reduce occurrence of HIV-1 viremia. In excess, TNF-α may cause severe inflammatory damage and toxicity, making control of its production and secretion highly important. Regulating its release serves as a potential means of therapy for HIV-1 and other diseases. TNF-α can also induce other pro-inflammatory cytokines such as IL-6 and IL-8, which aid in the upregulation of viral replication (Fernandez-Ortega et al; 2004). Studies have also shown the ability of TNF-α to stimulate production of anti-inflammatory cytokine IL-10, preventing further inflammation by causing TNF-α inhibition (Leghmari et al; 2008). TNF-α is secreted during the early phase of acute inflammatory diseases. Its pathogenic role in HIV-1 infection involves activation of nuclear factor kB (NF-κB), stimulating apoptosis of T lymphocytes. Tissue and plasma samples of hosts express high levels of TNF-α, contributing to fever, anorexia, and other symptoms of HIV/AIDS. TNF-α must be targeted at an appropriate time during production to prevent progression to the chronic stage. Local effect of the cytokine may be beneficial to the host, so monitoring its development is critical. Highly active antiretroviral therapy helps to reduce mortality rates, and development of potent antiretroviral drugs blocking HIV transcription continues to be successful. However, drug resistance and toxicity remains a challenge in this field of medicine (Fernandez-Ortega et al; 2004).

6. Interleukin 1 (IL-1) and HIV infection

HIV infection and its viral proteins can disturb the production of cytokines and disrupt their usual interactions resulting in disruption of the normal immune function. IL-1 and TNF-α are produced by activation of mononuclear phagocytes as well as microglia in the brain in response to normal immune stimuli such as immune complexes, lipopolysaccharides and phorbol esters (Burchett et al; 1998). It has been reported that IL-1 and TNF-α will be produced by either the binding of gp120 to the CD4 molecules on mononuclear phagocytes or infection with HIV (Merrill et al; 1989, Cheung et al; 2008).

IL-1 is the first discovered and most studied member of the cytokine family (Fantuzzi, 2003). IL-1 is a pro-inflammatory cytokine that plays a fundamental role in host defense by inducing acute and chronic inflammation through activation of the innate and acquired immune systems (Nambu and Nakae, 2010). IL-1 has been described as the prototypic pro-inflammatory cytokine as it was originally described as the first "endogenous" pyrogen due to its fever-inducing properties in both rabbits and humans (Dinarello, 1999). However, in spite of much research in the area of fever induction, the role of IL-1 in this area is still undefined (Fantuzzi, 2003). IL-1 consists of two distinct ligands (IL-1α and IL-1β) with two indistinguishable biological activities that signal through the IL-1 receptor (IL-1R1) (Bujak and Frangogiannis, 2009). Both IL-1α and IL-1β can also bind the IL-1 receptor accessory protein (IL-1RAcP). Once bound to the receptor, the complex transduces a signal that initiates a wide variety of inflammatory genes by activating the NF-κB system. The NF-κB transcribed genes can produce a variety of inflammatory products including chemokines, pro-inflammatory cytokines, such as TNF-α, IL-6 or IL-8 (Nambu and Nakae, 2010), adhesion molecules, such as vascular cell adhesion molecule-1 (VCAM-1) (Marui et al; 1993), colony-stimulating factors, and mesenchymal growth factor genes (Bujak and Frangogiannis, 2009). In addition, expression of inducible nitric oxide synthase, type 2 cyclooxygenase (COX)-2, and type 2 phospholipase A_2 is exquisitely sensitive to IL-1 (Bujak and Frangogiannis, 2009). IL-1 has also been associated with augmentation of the mast cell activation and Th2 cytokine secretion, suggesting involvement of IL-1 in allergic diseases such as allergic asthma (Dinarello, 1999).

Knockouts of IL-1 have been used to study acute and chronic neurodegenerative conditions, in which a role for IL-1 has been well established (Fantuzzi, 2003). For example, in rodent studies the presence of IL-1 after occlusion of the middle cerebral artery will increase the ischemic damage area. It has been shown that caspase-1 cleaves the inactive pre-form to the active mature form of IL-1β, which contributes to the damage from ischemia (Bujak and Frangogiannis, 2009). In resting cells, procaspase-1 is bound to an inhibitory molecule that prevents its activation. After damage to cells, conversion of procaspase-1 to caspase-1 is triggered by a molecular complex termed the "IL-1β inflammasome" (Martinon, 2002).

Macrophages and dendritic cells produce IL-1, IL-12 and other cytokines that permit CD4 cells to reach the level of maturation needed to produce IL-2, which is needed for self-replication of the CD4 cells and for the growth and function of CD8 cells (Levy, 2007). Thus IL-1 plays a role in maintaining normal immune function.

Elevation of IL-1 and TNF-α has been demonstrated in the serum of some patients with HIV-1 (Lepe-Zuniga et al; 1987). High levels of IL-1 (Lepe-Zuniga et al; 1987, Weiss et al; 1989, Molina et al; 1989, Roux-Lombard et al; 1989, Emilie et al; 1990) and TNF-α (Roux-Lombard et al; 1989) are produced in the supernatant of cultured peripheral blood monocyte early in the onset of HIV disease. The levels of TNF-α and IL-1 in the serum were positively correlated in symptomatic versus asymptomatic individuals (Lepe-Zuniga et al; 1987). HIV virus is present in mononuclear phagocytes and in the blood and brain of AIDS patients. Production of IL-1 and TNF-α from mononuclear phagocytes after stimulation with HIV-1 may contribute to some of the symptoms of AIDS such as fever, cachexia and aseptic meningitis (Merrill et al; 1989).

Chronic infection and viral latency are typical of HIV-1 infection. Stimulation with IL-1β as well as TNF-α can stimulate viral replication in chronically infected cells (Devadas et al; 2004). Monocytes are also major reservoirs for HIV-1 in infected tissue and vectors for virus transmission to target cells, as well as sources of potent cytokines that can affect cell function and virus replication (Devadas et al; 2004). It is thought that stimulation of viral replication in chronically infected cells is due to activation of NF-κB. In addition to IL-1 and TNF-α, contact with macrophages as well as a number of stressors can stimulate NF-κB, including phorbol esters, radical oxygen intermediates, and UV irradiation (Devadas et al; 2004).

Clinical manifestations of AIDS include both immunologic and neurologic disorders. In the brain it has been shown that IL-1 induces activation and proliferation of astrocytes, while TNF-α contributes to necrosis of cerebral blood vessels and possibly to demyelination

(Merrill et al; 1989). A feedback process has been described in which HIV-1 and TNF-α can each induce expression of the other. It has been proposed that IL-1 will participate in this feedback loop by inducing TNF-α or by direct T-cell activation, which is needed for HIV-1 replication (Merrill et al; 1989).

IL-1 has been implicated in the pathogenesis of HIV associated dementia (HAD) (Kaul et al; 2001). Both IL-1β and TNF-α are highly expressed in the central nervous system (CNS) of individuals with HAD, correlate with neuronal injury and are implicated in the pathogenesis of HAD (Epstein and Gendelman, 1993,, Brabers and Nottet, 2006). HIV-1, recombinant gp120, and viral transactivator Tat can activate astrocytes to secrete pro-inflammatory cytokines TNF-α, IL-6, and IL-1β (Corasaniti et al; 2001), which may contribute to the inflammatory environment in the brain (Herbein and Varin, 2010). Microglia and macrophages in the brain can release IL-1β after stimulation with HIV-1 envelope protein gp120 (Merrill et al; 1992, Wahl et al; 1989), which is elevated in brain during HIV (Tyor et al; 1992) and has been shown to be elevated in the cerebral spinal fluid during HIV infection (Gallo et al; 1989).

About 25% of subjects with HIV will develop dementia, particularly HIV encephalitis (HIVE), which can occur in spite of the use of HAART (Levy, 2007). Macrophage inflammatory products including IL-1β have been demonstrated in HIV related encephalitis in mouse and human brain tissue (Persidsky et al; 1997). It has been suggested that the release of neurotoxins, including L-cysteine, from macrophages in the brain is mediated by IL-1 following stimulation of the macrophages by the HIV membrane protein gp120.

L-Cysteine can be released from human monocyte derived macrophages stimulated by either gp120 (Lipton, 1998), or by IL-1 (Yeh et al; 2000). It has been suggested that cytokines including IL-1 may mediate the neurotoxic actions of gp120 (Yeh et al; 2000). Cysteine can act as an endogenous neurotoxin (Olney et al; 1990), which under both physiologic and pathophysiologic conditions stimulates *N*-methyl-D-aspartate subtype of glutamate receptor (NMDARs) and leads to neuronal apoptosis (Yeh et al; 2000). Thus, immune activation of macrophages in the brain without direct HIV infection may lead to neural damage (Yeh et al; 2000).

Autopsy evaluation of brain tissue from HIVE cases shows increased IL-1β in the frontal white matter of all 11 of the brains evaluated (67). Additionally, IL-1β, but not TNF-α expression was detected in HIVp24-positive cells in the HIVE patients, which indicates that IL-1β is induced by HIV-1 infection. The authors concluded that a macrophage/microglia lineage is the main cell type to release cytokines in HIVE, and IL-1β expression by HIV-1-infected cells may be one of the important factors for induction of HIVE (67).

7. Interleukin-6 (IL-6)

The family of IL-6-type cytokines comprises IL-6, IL-11, LIF (leukaemia inhibitory factor), OSM (oncostatin M), CNTF (ciliary neurotrophic factor), CT-1 (cardiotrophin-1) and CLC (cardiotrophin-like cytokine) (Heinrich et al; 2003). IL-6 is a pleiotropic cytokine that is commonly produced at local tissue sites and released into circulation in almost all situations of homeostatic perturbation typically including endotoxemia, endotoxic lung, trauma, and acute infections. In addition to its critical participation in the generation of immunity against chronic intracellular infections, circulating IL-6, together with other alarm cytokines TNF-α and IL-1, is known to be required for the induction of acute phase reactions composed of fever, corticosterone release, and hepatic production of acute phase proteins many of which are protease inhibitors (Xing et al; 1998). They activate target genes involved in differentiation, survival, apoptosis and proliferation. The members of this cytokine family have pro- as well as anti-inflammatory properties and are major players in haematopoiesis, as well as in acute-phase and immune responses of the organism. IL-6-type cytokines bind to plasma membrane receptor complexes containing the common signal transducing receptor chain gp 130 (glycoprotein 130). Signal transduction involves the activation of JAK (Janus kinase) tyrosine kinase family members, leading to the activation of transcription factors of the STAT (signal transducers and activators of transcription) family. Another major signaling pathway for IL-6-type cytokines is the MAPK (mitogen-activated protein kinase) cascade (Heinrich et al; 2003). IL-6 was originally identified as β2 (IFN-β2), IL-1-inducible 26kD protein and as a factor that induces the differentiation of B cells to antibody producing plasma cells (Hibi et al; 1996).

The induction of IL-6 by live HIV preparations occurred in the absence of T cells and could be neutralized by human anti-HIV serum indicating that HIV was responsible for this IL-6 inducing activity. It has been demonstrated that IL-6 can be produced by a variety of cells upon various kinds of stimulation: T cells infected with HTLV-1, fibroblasts stimulated with polyI:C, IL-1, platelet-derived growth factor, TNF-α, FCS, or LPS, and monocyte/macrophages stimulated with LPS. Monocyte/ macrophages, one of the target cells of HIV, produced IL-6 upon stimulation with both live and inactivated HIV (Nakajima et al; 1989). A study of women treated for cervical intraepithelial lesions showed that after treatment, there were increased levels of genital HIV, TNF-α, IL-6, and other activation markers in cervicovaginal lavage (Spear et al; 2008). In univariate analysis, genital tract HIV RNA was significantly associated with plasma HIV RNA and several of the cytokines, while in multivariate analysis, genital tract HIV RNA was significantly associated only with plasma HIV RNA and IL-6 (Spear et al; 2008). Another study was done to determine the effect of HIV on thymic stromal cells and the production of cytokines important in thymocyte development, three types of adherent thymic cultures were established and studied: thymic epithelial cells (TECs), macrophage-enriched, and mixed cultures of macrophages and TECs (M phi/TEC). M phi/TEC and macrophage-enriched cultures were infected by both HIV strains without cytopathic changes. The TECs grew well in culture exposed to HIV-1 strains HIV-1IIIB and HIV-1Ba-L for at least 6 weeks and showed no evidence of infection, cytopathology, or changes in cytokine production with HIV. Only cultures containing macrophages (M phi/TEC or macrophage enriched) showed changes in cytokine (IL-1 alpha, IL-1 beta, and IL-6) production with HIV. Unstimulated macrophage-enriched cultures produced small amounts of IL-6 that were increased by HIV 20-fold (Sandborg et al; 1994).

There are many studies showing the increase of IL-6 expression within HIV infected cells but not many studies suggesting what IL-6 does to HIV. In a study done by Miles in 1990, it was found that IL-6 might actually be a growth factor for the HIV virus (Miles et al; 1990). There was a proliferative response of the AIDS-Kaposi sarcoma (AIDS-KS) cells to high concentrations of hrIL-6 and the detection of IL-6-rRNA in the areas of the skin involved with Kaposi sarcoma. AIDS-KS cells synthesized, released, and responded to biologically active IL-6. AIDS-KS cells, in which IL-6 protein translation arrest was induced by an IL-6 anti sense oligodeoxynucleotide, did not proliferate optimally unless exogenous hrIL-6 was added (Miles et al; 1990).

8. Interleukin-17 (IL-17)

IL-17 is an inflammatory cytokine that is exclusively produced by a recently discovered subset of CD4+ T helper (Th) cells, referred to as Th17 cells (Crome et al; 2009). This cytokine has been found to help regulate the inflammatory response by activating fibroblasts, recruiting neutrophils, and acting on macrophages to promote both their recruitment and survival (Crome et al; 2009, Chang et al; 2007). In addition, IL-17 is thought to play a significant role in activating and inducing anti-microbial peptides and pro-inflammatory cytokines like IL-6, CCL2, and TNF-α (Crome et al; 2009, Chang et al; 2007). Furthermore, high levels of this cytokine have been linked to a number of inflammatory diseases including rheumatoid arthritis, multiple sclerosis (MS), and asthma. Low levels, on the other hand, are thought to cause both impaired host defense against mycobacterial infection and decreased antibacterial immunity (Crome et al; 2009, Brenchley et al; 2008).

Studies of the effects of HIV on IL-17 concentrations using flow cytometry have found that HIV-infected patients have significantly increased levels of IL-17 (Giorgio, 2003). Venketaraman *et al.* (unpublished data) was also able to show increased levels of IL-17 in HIV-infected blood plasma using ELISA assays. However, Brenchley *et al.*; 2008 noted that there were significantly fewer IL-17 producing Th17 cells in the gastrointestinal tract of HIV-infected patients. In fact, the study indicated that Th17 cells were preferentially targeted during HIV infection.

The decrease of IL-17 concentrations at the mucosal wall of the gastrointestinal tract could greatly increase the probability of bacterial infections, which could in turn have significant implications for the speed of HIV pathogenesis (Brenchley et al; 2008). As Levy et al; 2009 noted, chronic immune activation increases the production of pro-inflammatory cytokines (IL-6, IL-17, TNF-α, etc.). This up-regulation of pro-inflammatory cytokines often leads to the rapid loss of CD4+ T cells via apoptosis. Decreased IL-17 concentrations due to HIV infection can therefore ultimately lead to the general advancement of HIV by creating an environment favorable to opportunistic infection and chronic immune activation (Maek-A-Nantawat et al; 2007).

9. Interleukin-12 (IL-12)

IL-12 is a heterodimeric pro-inflammatory cytokine that is produced by dendritic cells and phagocytes during an infection (Giorgio, 2003). It is a cytokine identified as a master switch for leading the naïve CD4+ T cells towards the Th1 pathway and also activating NK cells (Villinger and Ansari, 2010). Not only does it directly induce T, NK, and NKT cell cytotoxicity, IL-12 also promotes macrophage activity via T- and NK-cell-produced IFN-γ (Giorgio, 2003, Egilmez et al; 2011). The pathway is antagonized in the presence of IL-10 (Villinger and Ansari, 2010).

IL-12 plays important roles in protecting the body from various microbial infections such as parasites, bacteria, and viruses (Yang et al; 2010). With mutations in genes of the IL-12, the cells are susceptible to intracellular pathogens such as tuberculosis, leprosy, HIV-1, hepatitis and malaria (Vannberg et al; 2011). One of the characteristics of HIV infection is the gradual deterioration of cellular effector responses. Studies has concluded that CD4+ and CD8+ T cell responses were enhanced *ex vivo* by the addition of IL-12, but that capacity to respond is decreased in patients with marked CD4 loss (Villinger and Ansari, 2010). Louis *et al;*. 2010, also added that IL-12 production required the presence of IFN-γ. Therefore, as HIV

progresses, decreased IFN-γ leads to decrease in IL-12 which leads to decreased CD4+ and CD8+ T cell response.
A decrease of IL-12 concentration increases the probability for opportunistic infections. Taoufik *et al*; 1997 and Mirani *et al*; 2002, showed IL-12 mRNA was diminished while IL-10 production was up-regulated in the presence of *Staphylococcus aureus* and HIV gp120, further inhibiting IL-12 cytokine production. Even though IL-12 is potent, Villinger and Ansari 2010, noted that when IL-12 therapy was administered in the late stages of HIV, it failed to restore normal levels of CD4 T cells and IFN-γ.

10. Additional effects of HIV on IFN-γ signaling

In addition to the Th1 subset response mediation mentioned earlier, IFN-γ normally acts on APCs to enhance their expression of major histocompatibility complex II (MHC-II), thereby enhancing their antigen presentation ability (Li et al; 2011). HIV transactivator protein (TAT) interferes with the intracellular signaling normally performed by the IFN-γ bound IFN-γ receptor (Cheng et al; 2009). In so doing, the TAT protein lowers the antigen presentation capacity of dendritic cells and macrophages, further limiting the immune response to the invading virus (Salgame et al; 2009).

11. The transforming growth factor β (TGF-β)

TGF-β cytokine family are closely related polypeptides which include tissue growth factors that have a diverse range of proteins that regulate many physiological processes including embryonic development, homeostasis, wound healing, chemotaxis, cell cycle control, cell proliferation, differentiation, apoptosis, adhesion, and migration (Leask and Abraham, 2004). TGF-β is one of the most immunosuppressive substances produced in the body and yet may inhibit or stimulate cell growth, depending on the cell type and culture conditions (Liu and Gaston Pravia, 2010). TGF-β is produced in many immune cells including lymphocytes, macrophages and dendritic cells (Liu and Gaston Pravia, 2010). Receptors for TGF-β have been found on all cell lines tested, allowing this cytokine to have effects on almost any tissue in the body (Leask and Abraham, 2004). It has also been shown to play a central role in tissue fibrosis (Leask and Abraham, 2004). Because of the multifunctional role played by TGF-β, it plays a central role in the pathogenesis of many diseases.(Leask and Abraham, 2004).
There are three forms of TGF-β (TGF-β1, TGF-β2, and TGF-β3) in mammalian cells. TGF-βs are synthesized using inactive precursors and cannot bind receptors until they are activated. After release of TGF-β from cells they associate with latency-associated protein and form a small inactive complex. In the extracellular matrix, this complex is bound by latent TGF-β-binding protein (LTBP), a component of the extracellular matrix that is necessary for the secretion and storage of TGF-β (Letterio and Roberts, 1998). Intracellular activity of TGF-β is mediated by the actions of Smad transcription factors as well as independent factors (Letterio and Roberts, 1998). Active Smad complexes bind to DNA weakly and high affinity binding is achieved by the association of Smad proteins with a large number of transcription factor partners (Massague, 1992). The variations of Smad proteins in transcriptional regulations and the diversity of Smad-independent pathways allow the pleiotropic actions of TGF-β (Letterio and Roberts, 1998).

HIV infection leads to a variety of disturbances in cytokine expression that can lead to a state of chronic activation of B cells and release of cytokines that may actually play an important role in the pathogenesis of HIV infection (Li and Flavell, 2008). Early HIV-1 infection is associated with a massive oligoclonal expansion of CD8 T cells (Massague and Gomis, 2006), however despite the high number of circulating CD8+ T cells the cytotoxic T lymphocyte (CTL) response is highly variable among HIV-1 infected individuals (Poli and Fauci, 1993). It has also been shown that the immune dysfunction in the initial phase of HIV infection exceeds CD4+ T cell infection and loss (Pantaleo et al; 1994). It appears that the immunosuppression effect occurs almost immediately upon infection (Garba et al; 2002). The result is diminished T cell response to antigen stimulation and persistence of HIV replication (Pantaleo and Fauci, 1995).

HIV-1 products such as TAT, induce the transcription of cytokines with immunosuppressive effects, including TGF-β (Cohen et al; 1999). It has been reported that extracellular TAT can be taken up by bystander cells and that it is possible that exogenous TAT, not associated with direct infection of a cell, can induce TGF-β transcription in immune competent cells (Pantaleo et al; 1993). Macrophages appear to be very sensitive to TAT and are affected by TAT concentrations 1,000-fold lower (500 pM) than those that affect T cells (Cohen et al; 1999). Macrophages stimulated by TAT either by infection or by the uptake of soluble TAT (sTat) induce Fas ligand (FasL), which in turn can trigger the apoptosis of antigen-reacting, Fas-expressing helper T cells. This mechanism would suppress T-cell dependent cellular and humoral immune responses to both HIV and other antigens (Cohen et al; 1999).

The transactivating effect of HIV-1 TAT is mediated by activator protein-1, which is the same multimolecular complex that is activated by TGF-β (Cohen et al; 1999). HIV-1 can induce both the transcription and secretion of TGF-β (Reinhold et al; 1999) and the induction of TGF-β can increase the apoptosis of NK cells (Poggi and Zocchi, 2006). TGF-β and Tat have been detected in the sera of early HIV-1 infected individuals at levels that were biologically active *in vitro* (Reinhold et al; 1999).

Some HIV-infected individuals have been shown to lose the ability of their cytotoxic T lymphocytes CTL ($CD8^+$) to control infection in cells that carry HIV as well as other infectious agents (Pantaleo et al; 1993). About 25% of HIV infected individuals have been shown to produce TGF-β1 in response to stimulation with HIV proteins or peptides (Garba et al; 2002). It has been shown that the loss of CTL activity is related to the production of TGF-β1 in sufficient amounts to significantly reduce the IFN-γ response of $CD8^+$ cells to both HIV and other viral proteins such as vaccinia virus (Garba et al; 2002).

It has been established that feline $CD4^+CD25^+$ T regulatory (T reg) cells share phenotypic and functional characteristics with human and murine T reg cells (Vahlenkamp et al; 2004). Early in the infection with feline immunodeficiency virus (FIV), $CD4^+CD25^+$ T reg cells exhibit increased expression of a membrane TGF- β (mTGF-β) (Mexas et al; 2008). The appearance of $TGF\text{-}\beta^+CD4^+CD25^+$ lymphocytes within the lymph node of FIV^+ cats occurs in both acute and chronic FIV, even though mTGF-β does not appear in the blood (Fogle et al; 2010). There is also evidence of increased expression of TGF-βRII, the receptor of TGF-β1, on $CD8^+$ lymphocytes in FIV^+ cats that would make the $CD8^+$ lymphocytes much more sensitive to TGF-β inhibition (Fogle et al; 2010). In FIV lentiviral infection, during both the acute and chronic stages of infection, $CD4^+CD25^+$ Tregs suppress $CD8^+$ responses and the $CD4^+CD25^+$ Tregs use mTGF-β to suppress IFN-γ expression resulting in suppression of $CD8^+$ lymphocyte function (Fogle et al; 2010). These findings help explain the paradox of chronic HIV-1 infection, in which $CD8^+$ T cells display an activated phenotype but exhibit reduced effector function (Fogle et al; 2010, Bucci et al; 1998, Tompkins and Tompkins 2008). IL-10 and TGF-β overlap with each other in many of their biological effects including inhibition of T cell proliferation and IFN-γ production (Othieno et al; 1999).

12. Interleukin-10 (IL-10)

IL-10 is an anti-inflammatory cytokine that essentially plays two regulatory roles in innate and adaptive immunity. It suppresses the up-regulation of various genes in macrophages and dendritic cells that are normally stimulated via toll-like receptors and promotes the proliferation of cytotoxic T cells, activates B cells, and induces the upregulation of specific genes in toll-like receptor activated phagocytic and dendritic cells (Trincheri, 2007). In addition, a critical function of IL-10 is its ability to inhibit pro-inflammatory cytokines such as TNF-α, IFN-γ, IL-1, IL-6, IL-2, and IL-12 (Trincheri, 2007). IL-10 decreases the production of pro-inflammatory cytokines by limiting the major histocompatibility class II and CD80/CD 86 expressed on monocytes and macrophage (Wang et al; 2005). IL-10 was believed to be produced by CD4+ Th2 cells; however, studies have shown that it is secreted by both Th1 and Th2 cells (Brockman et al; 2009). Also, cells from the myeloid lineage which include macrophages and dendritic cells also produce cytokine IL-10 (Hedrich and Bream, 2010). Furthermore, IL-10 is regulated both at the transcriptional and post-translational level and is involved in various signaling pathways (Couper et al; 2008).

There are several speculations of the role of IL-10 in HIV pathogenesis and the subject has been a popular interest in many studies. Ji *et al.*, 2005 reported that CD14+ monocytes are the main cells producing cytokine IL-10 in PBMCs after HIV-1 infection via interactions independent of CD4+ molecules, thus, concluding that IL-10 production is dependent on the presence of CD14+ monocytes. Moreover, as the patient progresses to advanced stages of HIV disease, the frequency of IL-10 producing cells increases significantly (118). On the other hand, Naicker *et al.*, 2009, stated that different stages of the HIV disease will govern what role IL-10 will play in infected individuals. For instance, in acute HIV-1 individuals, IL-10 may promote viral replication by inhibiting effector immune response from both arms of the innate and adaptive immunity (Naicker et al; 2009). Furthermore, it was proposed in a chronic phase, that IL-10 resembled a protective role by reducing immune activation, inhibiting virus replication in macrophages, and the increase in production of IL-10 levels lowered plasma viral load and increased CD4+ cell count (Naicker et al; 2009).

13. HIV and free radicals

It has been shown that HIV infection induces increased production of free radicals by macrophages. Free radical formation occurs as a byproduct of oxidative stress. Oxidative stress occurs when there is a disproportion between the reactive oxygen elements in the body versus the ability of the body to properly eliminate these reactive species. The presence of free radicals has been implicated in disturbing and damaging a number of biological processes (Karthikeyan et al; 2010). With regards to HIV infection the increase of oxidative stress has been seen to influence components in antioxidant defense in physiological antioxidants such as glutathione which are seen to decrease dramatically in HIV patients (Pace and Leaf, 1995). In addition to glutathione, vitamin A, C, and E at high doses as well as improving low levels of selenium were associated with assisting the prevention of HIV infection progression by working as antioxidants to remove free radicals

(Garland and Fawzi, 1999). The aforementioned studies may provide a low cost method for improving the prognosis of HIV infected patients in high risk, underprivileged areas of the world.

Chronic oxidative stress is often associated with HIV infection and research indicates a benefit for increased antioxidant vitamins and supplements in reduction of DNA base damage, which in turn can slow progression of infection (Jaruga et al; 2002). Neutrophils from asymptomatic HIV patients show increased oxygen radical production which can be modified by treating with N-acetyl cysteine, a compound used as an antioxidant (Smietana et al; 2008). The role of free radical oxidative stress on DNA damage is correlated with stimulated DNA repair mechanisms which activate enzymes associated with initiation of apoptosis such as poly ADP-ribose transferase and p53. Reduced NAD/NADH production would lower ATP synthesis that in turn correlates with a deficiency in glutathione; which as mentioned is an endogenous antioxidant important in resolving imbalance of free radicals (Dobmeyer et al; 1997).

The progression of HIV is correlated with a decreased immunity. One way in which this decreased immunity progresses is by free radical overload of monocytes and granulocytes which leads to deficiency of antioxidant mechanisms which may lead to the loss of CD4 cells often seen in the progression of HIV (Dobmeyer et al; 1997). The decreased immunity may also be related to the reactive oxygen species and free radical presence which is higher in HIV infected patients. With HIV infection progression there is an increased production of reactive oxygen species which leads to the theory of free radical mediated apoptosis of lymphocytes which reduces the ability for immune response to progressive HIV infections (Dobmeyer et al; 1997). With regards to CD4 cell counts the apoptosis of lymphocytes by free radicals leads to progression of immunodeficiency and makes for a quicker transition from HIV infection to AIDS (Bautisita, 2001). It has been published that during HIV-1 infection, hematopoietic cells are exposed to high amounts of free radicals. Subsequently there is a reduction of leukocytopoiesis and increase susceptibility to further infections (Masutani, 2000). Furthermore, there is a link to lipid peroxidation observed in patients with HIV or AIDS to a deficiency of antioxidants which leads to free radical proliferation (Favier et al; 1994).

Rate of viral replication is a key process to the proliferation of HIV infection. The conditions in which viruses such as HIV will proliferate seem to correlate with the presence of oxidative stress/free radicals *in vitro* (Fuchs et al; 1991). There tends to be an increase in nuclear transcription factor and inflammatory cytokine activation of the immune system (Brach et al; 1992). The progression of the virus/infection will then allow for opportunistic infections which then would also promote more oxidative stress due to increased free radical elements, again improving viral replication and weakening antioxidant defense (Knysz, 2007).

Damage or altering of the DNA repair machinery is an important aspect of the progression of HIV infection pathogenesis (Olinski et al; 2002). There is a slow and deliberate degradation of cellular components such as membrane blebbing, chromatin condensation, and DNA cleavage ability. Additionally, there is evidence that shows oxidative DNA damage will lead to the apoptotic cell death in HIV infected patients. There appears to be an increase in oxidatively modified DNA bases in HIV infected patients leading to what is known as pyrimidine and purine derived lesions. One specific lesion labeled, 8-OH-Gua was found in isolated lymphocytes of HIV patients. The presence of this lesion leads to transversions of DNA base pairs unless repaired before replication. The number of these lesions was seen to be reduced in response to antioxidant supplement and vitamin treatments, which correlates to free radical influence in DNA damage, and potential progression of HIV infection (Olinski et al; 2002).

14. Conclusion

Both HIV-1 and HIV-2 cause AIDS, but HIV-1 is found worldwide, whereas HIV-2 is found primarily in West Africa. Chemokine receptors, such as CXCR4 and CCR5 proteins, are required for the entry of HIV into CD4-positive cells. After establishing infection, HIV alters the synthesis of host cytokines and chemokines and kills CD4+ T lymphocytes thereby resulting in the loss of cell-mediated immunity and a high probability that the host will develop opportunistic infections.

15. References

Alfano, M and Poli, G. 2005. Role of cytokines and chemokines in the regulation of innate immunity and HIV infection. Molecular Immunology 42: 161-182.

Bahia, M.S and Silakari, O. 2010. Tumor Necrosis Factor Alpha Converting Enzyme: An Encouraging Target for Various Inflammatory Disorders. Chemical Biology & Drug Design. 75: 415-443.

Bautista AP. 2001 Free radicals, chemokines, and cell injury in HIV-1 and SIV infections and alcoholic hepatitis. Free Radical Biology and Medicine. 31(12):1527-1532.

Brabers NA and Nottet HS. 2006. Role of the pro-inflammatory cytokines TNF-alpha and IL-1beta in HIV-associated dementia. European journal of clinical investigation. 36(7):447-58.

Brach MA, de Vos S, Arnold C, Gruss HJ, Mertelsmann R and Herrmann F. 1992. Leukotriene B4 transcriptionally activates interleukin-6 expression involving NK-chi B and NF-IL6. Eur J Immunol. Oct 22(10):2705-2711.

Brenchley, Jason M., Paiardini, M., Knox, Kenneth S., Asher, Ava I., Cervasi, B., Asher, Tedi E., Scheinberg, P., Price, David A., Hage, Chadi A., Kholi, Lisa M., Khoruts, A., Frank, I., Else, J., Schacker, T., Silvestri, G and Daniel C. Douek. 2008. Differential Th17 CD4 T-cell depletion in pathogenic and nonpathogenic lentiviral infections. Blood 112(7): 2826-2835.

Brockman MA, Kwon DS, Tighe DP, Pavlik DF, Rosato PC, Sela J, Porichis F, Le Gall S, Waring MT, Moss K, Jessen H, Pereyra F, Kavanagh DG, Walker BD and Kaufmann DE. 2009. IL-10 is up-regulated in multiple cell types during viremic HIV infection and reversibly inhibits virus-specific T cells. Blood. 114(2):346-56.

Bucci JG, Gebhard DH, Childers TA, English RV, Tompkins MB and Tompkins WA. 1998. The CD8+ cell phenotype mediating antiviral activity in feline immunodeficiency virus-infected cats is characterized by reduced surface expression of the CD8 beta chain. The Journal of infectious diseases.178(4):968-77.

Bujak M and Frangogiannis NG. 2009. The role of IL-1 in the pathogenesis of heart disease. Arch Immunol Ther Exp (Warsz). 57(3):165-76.

Burchett SK, Weaver WM, Westall JA, Larsen A, Kronheim S and Wilson CB. 1998. Regulation of tumor necrosis factor/cachectin and IL-1 secretion in human mononuclear phagocytes. Journal of immunology. 140(10):3473-81.

Cannon, P and June, C. 2011. Chemokine receptor 5 knockout strategies. Current Opinion in HIV and AIDS. 6: 74-79.

Chang, Seon H., and Chen Dong. 2007. A novel heterodimeric cytokine consisting of IL-17 and IL-17F regulates inflammatory responses. *Cell Research* 17: 435-440.

Charo, Israel F. and Richard M. Ransohoff. 2006. The many roles of chemokines and chemokine receptors in inflammation. The New England Journal of Medicine. 345: 610-621.

Cheng SM, Li JCB, Lin SS, Lee DCW, Liu L, Chen Z, and Lau ASY. 2009. HIV-1 transactivator protein induction of suppressor cytokine signaling-2 contributes to dysregulation of IFN-g signaling. Blood. 13: 5192-5201.

Cheung R, Ravyn V, Wang L, Ptasznik A and Collman RG. 2008. Signaling mechanism of HIV-1 gp120 and virion-induced IL-1beta release in primary human macrophages. Journal of immunology. 180(10):6675-84.

Clerici M, Frances TH, Venzon D J, Blatt S, Hendrix CW, Wynn TA and Shearer GM. 1993. Changes in Interleukin-2 and Interleukin-4 Production in Asymptomatic Human Immunodeficiency Virus-seropositive Individuals. J Clin Invest. 91:759-765.

Cohen SS, Li C, Ding L, Cao Y, Pardee AB, Shevach EM, et al. 1999. Pronounced acute immunosuppression in vivo mediated by HIV Tat challenge. Proceedings of the National Academy of Sciences of the United States of America. 96(19):10842-7.

Corasaniti MT, Bilotta A, Strongoli MC, Navarra M, Bagetta G and Di Renzo G. 2001. HIV-1 coat protein gp120 stimulates interleukin-1beta secretion from human neuroblastoma cells: evidence for a role in the mechanism of cell death. British journal of pharmacology. 134(6):1344-50.

Couper, K. N., Blount, D. G and Riley, E. M. 2008. IL-10: the master regulator of immunity to infection. J Immunol. 180(9): 5771-5777.

Crome, S.Q., Wang, A.Y and M.K. Levings. 2009. Translational Mini-Review Series on Th17 Cells: Function and regulation of human T helper 17 cells in health and disease. The Journal of Translational Immunology. 159: 109-119.

Daly, Christine and Barrett J. Rollins. 2003. Monocyte Chemoattractant Protein-1 (CCL2) in Inflammatory Disease and Adaptive Immunity: Therapeutic opportunities and controversies. Microcirculation. 10: 247-257.

Deshmane, Satish L., Kremlev, S., Amini, S and Bassel E. Sawaya. 2009. Monocyte chemoattractant protein-1 (MCP-1): an overview. Journal of Interferon & Cytokine Research. 29(6): 313-326.

Devadas K, Hardegen NJ, Wahl LM, Hewlett IK, Clouse KA, Yamada KM, et al. 2004. Mechanisms for macrophage-mediated HIV-1 induction. Journal of immunology. 173(11):6735-44.

Dinarello CA. 1999. Cytokines as endogenous pyrogens. The Journal of infectious diseases.179 Suppl 2:S294-304.

Dobmeyer TS, Findhammer S, Dobmeyer JM, et al. 1997. Ex vivo induction of apoptosis in lymphocytes is mediated by oxidative stress: role for lymphocyte loss in HIV infection. Free Radic Biol Med. 22(5):775-785.

Edo-Matas D., van Dort KA, Setiawan LC, Schuitemaker H, Kootstra NA. 2011. Comparison of in vivo and in vitro evolution of CCR5 to CXCR4 co-receptor use of primary human Immunodeficiency type 1 variants. Virology. 412(2):269-77.

Egilmez NK, Harden JL, Virtuoso LP, Schwendener RA and Kilinc MO. 2011. Nitric oxide short-circuits interleukin-12-mediated tumor regression. Cancer Immunology, Immunotherapy 2011; 1-7.

Emilie D, Peuchmaur M, Maillot MC, Crevon MC, Brousse N, Delfraissy JF, et al. 1990. Production of interleukins in human immunodeficiency virus-1-replicating lymph nodes. The Journal of clinical investigation. 86(1):148-59.

Epstein LG and Gendelman HE. 1993. Human immunodeficiency virus type 1 infection of the nervous system: pathogenetic mechanisms. Annals of neurology. 33(5):429-36.

Eugenin, Eliseo A., Osiecki, K., Lopez, L., Goldstein, H., Calderon, Tina M and Joan W. Berman. 2006. CCL2/monocyte chemoattractant protein-1 mediates enhanced transmigration of human immunodeficiency virus (HIV)-infected leukocytes across the blood-brain-barrier: a potential mechanism of HIV-CNS invasion and NeuroAIDS. The Journal of Neuroscience. 26(4): 1098-1106.

Fantuzzi G. 2003. Cytokine knockouts. Totawa, NJ: Humana Press; p. 471.

Favier A, Sappey C, Leclerc P, Faure P and Micoud M. 1994. Antioxidant status and lipid peroxidation in patients infected with HIV. Chem Biol Interact. 91(2-3):165-180.

Fernandez-Ortega, C., Dubed, M., Ramos, T., Navea, L., Alvarez, G., Lobaina, L., Lopez, L., Casilla, D and Rodriguez, L. 2004. Non-induced leukocyte extract reduces HIV replication and TNF secretion. Biochemical and Biophysical Research Communications. 325: 1075-1081.

Fogle JE, Mexas AM, Tompkins WA and Tompkins MB. 2010. CD4(+)CD25(+) T regulatory cells inhibit CD8(+) IFN-gamma production during acute and chronic FIV infection utilizing a membrane TGF-beta-dependent mechanism. AIDS research and human retroviruses. 26(2):201-16.

Fuchs J, Ochsendorf F, Schofer H, Milbradt R and Rubsamen-Waigmann H. 1991. Oxidative imbalance in HIV infected patients. Med Hypotheses. 36(1):60-64.

Gallo P, Frei K, Rordorf C, Lazdins J, Tavolato B and Fontana A. 1989. Human immunodeficiency virus type 1 (HIV-1) infection of the central nervous system: an evaluation of cytokines in cerebrospinal fluid. J Neuroimmunol. 23(2):109-16.

Garba ML, Pilcher CD, Bingham AL, Eron J and Frelinger JA. 2002. HIV antigens can induce TGF-beta(1)-producing immunoregulatory CD8+ T cells. Journal of immunology. 168(5):2247-54.

Garland M and Fawzi WW. 1999. Antioxidants and progression of human immunodeficiency virus (HIV) disease. Nutrition Research.19(8):1259-1276.

Gorry, P.R. and Ancuta, P. 2011. Coreptors and HIV-1 Pathogenesis. Curr HIV/AIDS Rep. 8(1):45-53.

Gorry, P.R., et al. 2007. Changes in region of gp120 contribute to unusually broad co-receptor usage of an HIV-1 isolate from CCR5 Delta32 heterozygote. Virology. 362: 163-178.

Grivel, J., et al. 2010. Selective transmission of R5 HIV-1 variants: where is the gatekeeper? Journal of Transitional Medicine. 9 (Suppl 1): S6.

Hedrich, C. M., & Bream and J. H. 2010. Cell type-specific regulation of IL-10 expression in inflammation and disease. Immunol Res. 47(1-3): 185-206.

Heinrich, Peter C., Iris Behrmann, Serge Haan, Heike M. Hermanns, Gerhard Müller-Newen and Fred Schaper. 2003. Principles of Interleukin (IL)-6-type Cytokine Signalling and Its Regulation. Institut Für Biochemie. 374: 1-20.

Herbein G and Varin A. 2010. The macrophage in HIV-1 infection: from activation to deactivation? Retrovirology. 7:33.

Hibi M K. Nakajima and T. Hirano. 1996. IL-6 Cytokine Family and Signal Transduction: a Model of the Cytokine System. Journal of Molecular Medicine. 74.1: 1-12.

Hutter G. 2009. Long-term control of HIV by CCR5 Delta32/Delta32 stem-cell transplantation. N. Engl J Med. 360: 692-698.

Jaruga P, Jaruga B, Gackowski D, et al. 2002. Supplementation with antioxidant vitamins prevents oxidative modification of DNA in lymphocytes of HIV-infected patients. Free Radic Biol Med. 32(5):414-420.

Ji, J., Sahu, G. K., Braciale, V. L and Cloyd, M. W. 2005. HIV-1 induces IL-10 production in human monocytes via a CD4-independent pathway. Int Immunol. 17(6): 729-736.

Karthikeyan R, Manivasagam T, Anantharaman P, Balasubramanian T and Somasundaram S. 2010. Chemopreventive effect of Padina boergesenii extracts on ferric nitrilotriacetate (Fe-NTA)-induced oxidative damage in Wistar rats. Journal of Applied Phycology. 1-7

Kaul M, Garden GA and Lipton SA. 2001.Pathways to neuronal injury and apoptosis in HIV-associated dementia. Nature. 410(6831):988-94.

Kindberg, E., Mickiene A, Ax C, Akerlind B, Vene S, Lindquist L, Lundkvist A, Svensson L. 2008. A deletion in the chemokine receptor 5 (CCR5) gene is associated with tickborne encephalitis. J Infect Dis. 197:266-9.

Kwong P.D., Wyatt R, Sattentau QJ, Sodroski J, Hendrickson WA. 2000. Oligomeric modeling and electrostatic analysis of the gp120 envelope glycoprotein of human immunodeficiency virus. J Virol. 74:1961-1972.

Klein SA, Dobmeyer JM, Dobmeyer TS, Pape M, Ottmann OG, Helm EB, Hoelzer D and Rossol R, 1997. Demonstration of the Th1 to Th2 cytokine shift during the course of HIV-1 infection using cytoplasmic cytokine detection on single cell level by flow cytometry. AIDS. 11:1111-1118

Knysz B, Szetela B and Gladysz A. 2007. Pathogenesis of HIV-1 infection - chosen aspects. HIV & AIDS Review. 6(1):7-11.

Leask A and Abraham DJ. 2004. TGF-beta signaling and the fibrotic response. The FASEB journal : official publication of the Federation of American Societies for Experimental Biology. 18(7):816-27.

Leghmari, K., Bennasser, Y., Tkaczuk, J and Bahraoui, E. 2008. HIV-1 Tat protein induces IL-10 production by an alternative TNF-a-independent pathway in monocytes: Role of PKC-δ and p38 MAP kinase. Cellular Immunology. 253: 45-53.

Lepe-Zuniga JL, Mansell PW and Hersh EM. 1987. Idiopathic production of interleukin-1 in acquired immune deficiency syndrome. Journal of clinical microbiology. 25(9):1695-700.

Letterio JJ and Roberts AB. 1998. Regulation of immune responses by TGF-beta. Annual review of immunology. 16:137-61.

Levy J. 2007. HIV and the pathogenesis of AIDS. Washington, DC: ASM Press.

Levy and Jay A. 2009. HIV pathogenesis: 25 years of progress and persistent challenges. AIDS. 23:147-160.

Li JCB, Au K, Fang J, Yim HCH, Chow K, Ho P and Lau ASY. 2011. HIV-1 trans-activator protein dysregulates IFN-g signaling and contributes to the suppression of autophagy induction. AIDS. 25:15-25.

Li MO and Flavell RA. 2008. TGF-beta: a master of all T cell trades. Cell. 134(3):392-404.

Lim JK, Louie CY, Glaser C, Jean C, Johnson B, Johnson H, McDermott DH, Murphy PM. 2008. Genetic deficiency of chemokine receptor CCR5 is a strong risk factor for symptomatic West Nile virus infection: a meta-analysis of 4 cohorts in the US epidemic. J Infect Dis. 197:262-5.

Lipton SA. 1998. Neuronal injury associated with HIV-1: approaches to treatment. Annu Rev Pharmacol Toxicol. 38:159-77.

Liu RM and Gaston Pravia KA. 2010. Oxidative stress and glutathione in TGF-beta-mediated fibrogenesis. Free radical biology & medicine. 48(1):1-15.

Louis S., Dutertre CA., Vimeux L., Fery L., Henno L., Dioccous S., Kahi S., Deveau C., Meyer L., Goujard C and Hosmalin A. 2010. IL-23 and IL-12p70 production by monocytes and dendritic cells in primary HIV-1 infection. Journal of Leukocyte Biology. 87(4):645.

Maek-A-Nantawat, W, Buranapraditkun, S, Klaewsongkram, J and Kiat Ruxrungthum. 2007. Increased interleukin-17 production both in helper T cell subset Th17 and CD4-negative T cells in human immunodeficiency virus infection. Viral Immunology. 20(1): 66-75.

Mahad, Don J and Richard M. Ransohoff. 2003. The role of MCP-1 (CCL2) and CCR2 in multiple sclerosis and experimental autoimmune encephalomyelitis (EAE). Seminars in Immunology. 15: 23-32.

Marui N, Offermann MK, Swerlick R, Kunsch C, Rosen CA, Ahmad M, et al. 1993. Vascular cell adhesion molecule-1 (VCAM-1) gene transcription and expression are regulated through an antioxidant-sensitive mechanism in human vascular endothelial cells. The Journal of clinical investigation. 92(4):1866-74.

Martinon F, Burns K and Tschopp J. 2002. The inflammasome: a molecular platform triggering activation of inflammatory caspases and processing of proIL-beta. Molecular cell. 10(2):417-26.

Massague J. 1992.Receptors for the TGF-beta family. Cell. 69(7):1067-70.

Massague J and Gomis RR. 2006. The logic of TGF-beta signaling. FEBS letters. 580(12):2811-20.

Mariani, S.A. 2010. Asymmetric HIV-1 co-receptor use and replication in CD4+ T lymphocytes. Journal of Translational Medicine. 9 (Suppl 1):S8.

Masutani H. 2000. Oxidative stress response and signaling in hematological malignancies and HIV infection. Int J Hematol. 71(1):25-32.

Merrill JE, Koyanagi Y and Chen IS. 1989. Interleukin-1 and tumor necrosis factor alpha can be induced from mononuclear phagocytes by human immunodeficiency virus type 1 binding to the CD4 receptor. Journal of virology. 63(10):4404-8.

Merrill JE, Koyanagi Y, Zack J, Thomas L, Martin F and Chen IS. 1992. Induction of interleukin-1 and tumor necrosis factor alpha in brain cultures by human immunodeficiency virus type 1. Journal of virology. 66(4):2217-25.

Mexas AM, Fogle JE, Tompkins WA and Tompkins MB. 2008. CD4+CD25+ regulatory T cells are infected and activated during acute FIV infection. Vet Immunol Immunopathol. 126 (3-4):263-72.

Miles, Steven A., Ahmad R. Rezai, Jesus F. Salazar-Gonzalez, Meta Vander Meyden, Ronald H. Stevens, Diane M. Logan, Ronald T. Mitsuyasu, Tetsuya Taga, Toshio Hirano, Tadamitsu Kishimoto and Otoniel Matinez-Maza. 1990. AIDS Kaposi Sarcoma-

Derived Cells Produce and Respond to Interleukin 6. Proceedings of the National Academy of Sciences. 87.11: 4068-072.

Mirani M, Elenkov I, Volpi S, Hiroi N, Chrousos GP and Kino T. 2002. HIV-1 protein Vpr suppresses IL-12 production from human monocytes by enhancing glucocorticoid action: potential implications of Vpr coactivator activity for the innate and cellular immunity deficits observed in HIV-1 infection. Journal of Immunology.169:6361.

Molina JM, Scadden DT, Byrn R, Dinarello CA and Groopman JE. 1989. Production of tumor necrosis factor alpha and interleukin 1 beta by monocytic cells infected with human immunodeficiency virus. The Journal of clinical investigation. 84(3):733-7.

Naicker, D. D., Werner, L., Kormuth, E., Passmore, J. A., Mlisana, K., Karim, S. A., et al. 2009. Interleukin-10 promoter polymorphisms influence HIV-1 susceptibility and primary HIV-1 pathogenesis. J Infect Dis. 200(3): 448-452.

Nakajima K, Martínez-Maza O, Hirano T, Breen EC, Nishanian PG, Salazar-Gonzalez JF, Fahey JL and Kishimoto T. 1989. Induction of IL-6 (B cell stimulatory factor-2/IFN-beta 2) production by HIV. J Immunol.142(2):531-6

Nambu A and Nakae S. 2010. IL-1 and Allergy. Allergol Int. 59(2):125-35.

Olinski R, Gackowski D, Foksinski M, Rozalski R, Roszkowski K and Jaruga P. 2002. Oxidative DNA damage: assessment of the role in carcinogenesis, atherosclerosis, and acquired immunodeficiency syndrome. Free Radical Biology and Medicine. 33(2):192-200.

Olney JW, Zorumski C, Price MT and Labruyere J. 1990. L-cysteine, a bicarbonate-sensitive endogenous excitotoxin. Science (New York, NY. 248(4955):596-9.

Osakwe CE, Bleotu C, Chifiriuc MC, Crancea C, Otelea D, Paraschiv S, Petrea S, Dinu M, Baicus C, Streinu-Cercel A and Lazar V. 2010. TH1/TH2 Cytokine Levels as an Indicator for Disease Progression in Human Immunodeficiency Virus Type 1 Infection and Response to Antiretroviral Therapy. Roum Arch Microbiol Immunol. 69(1):24-34.

Othieno C, Hirsch CS, Hamilton BD, Wilkinson K, Ellner JJ and Toossi Z. 1999. Interaction of Mycobacterium tuberculosis-induced transforming growth factor beta1 and interleukin-10. Infect Immun. 67(11):5730-5.

Pace GW and Leaf CD. 1995. The role of oxidative stress in HIV disease. Free Radic Biol Med. 19(4):523-528.

Pantaleo G, Graziosi C, Demarest JF, Butini L, Montroni M, Fox CH, et al. 1993. HIV infection is active and progressive in lymphoid tissue during the clinically latent stage of disease. Nature. 362(6418):355-8.

Pantaleo G, Demarest JF, Soudeyns H, Graziosi C, Denis F, Adelsberger JW, et al. 1994. Major expansion of CD8+ T cells with a predominant V beta usage during the primary immune response to HIV. Nature. 370(6489):463-7.

Pantaleo G and Fauci AS. 1995. New concepts in the immunopathogenesis of HIV infection. Annual review of immunology. 13:487-512.

Persidsky Y, Buttini M, Limoges J, Bock P and Gendelman HE. 1997. An analysis of HIV-1-associated inflammatory products in brain tissue of humans and SCID mice with HIV-1 encephalitis. Journal of neurovirology. 3(6):401-16.

Poggi A and Zocchi MR. 2006. HIV-1 Tat triggers TGF-beta production and NK cell apoptosis that is prevented by pertussis toxin B. Clinical & developmental immunology. 13(2-4):369-72.

Poli G and Fauci AS. 1993. Cytokine modulation of HIV expression. Semin Immunol. 5(3):165-73.

Reinhold D, Wrenger S, Kahne T and Ansorge S. 1999. HIV-1 Tat: immunosuppression via TGF-beta1 induction. Immunology today. 20(8):384-5.

Salgame P, Guan MX, Agahtehrani A and Henderson EE. 1998. Infection of T Cell Subsets by HIV-1 and the Effects of Interleukin-12. J. Interferon and Cytokine Res. 18:521-528.

Samson, M. 1996. Resistance to HIV-1 infection in Caucasian individuals bearing mutant alleles of the CCR-5 chemokine receptor gene. Nature. 382: 722-725.

Sandborg, Christy I., Karen L. Imfeld, Frank Zaldivar and Monique A. Berman. 1994. HIV Type 1 Induction of Interleukin 1 and 6 Production by Human Thymic Cells. AIDS Research and Human Retroviruses. 10.10: 1221-229.

Smietana M, Clayette P, Mialocq P, Vasseur J-J and Oiry J. 2008. Synthesis of new N-isobutyryl-l-cysteine/MEA conjugates: Evaluation of their free radical-scavenging activities and anti-HIV properties in human macrophages. Bioorganic Chemistry. 36(3):133-140.

Spear, Gregory T., M. Reza Zariffard, Hua Y. Chen, Joshua J. Anzinger, Kathryn Anastos, John Rusine, John Gatabazi, Audrey L. French, Mardge Cohen and Alan L. Landay. 2008. Positive Association between HIV RNA and IL-6 in the Genital Tract of Rwandan Women. AIDS Research and Human Retroviruses. 24.7: 973-76.

Suleiman, J. 2010. Vicriviroc in combination therapy with an optimized regimen for treatment-experienced subjects: 48-week results of the VICTOR-E1 phase 2 trial. J Infect Dis. 201:590-9.

Tagliamonte, M, Tornesello ML, Buonaguro FM, Buonaguro L. 2011. Conformational HIV-1 envelope on particulate structures: a tool for chemokine coreceptor binding studies. Journal of Translational Medicine. 9 (Suppl 1):S1.

Taoufik Y, Lantz O, Wallon C, Charles A, Dussaix E and Delfraissy JF. 1997. Human immunodeficiency virus gp120 inhibits interleukin-12 secretion by human monocytes: an indirect interleukin-10-mediated effect. Blood. 89: 2842.

Tenorio, A. R. 2011. The monoclonal CCR5 antibody PRO-140: the promise of once-weekly HIV therapy. Curr HIV/AIDS Rep. 8(1):1-3.

Tompkins MB and Tompkins WA. 2008. Lentivirus-induced immune dysregulation. Vet Immunol Immunopathol. 123(1-2):45-55.

Trinchieri Giorgio. 2003. Interleukin-12 and the regulation of innate resistance and adaptive immunity. Nature Reviews Immunology. 3: 133.

Trinchieri, G. 2007. Interleukin-10 production by effector T cells: Th1 cells show self control. J Exp Med. 204(2): 239-243.

Tyor WR, Glass JD, Griffin JW, Becker PS, McArthur JC, Bezman L, et al. 1992.Cytokine expression in the brain during the acquired immunodeficiency syndrome. Annals of neurology. 31(4):349-60.

Vahlenkamp TW, Tompkins MB and Tompkins WA. 2004. Feline immunodeficiency virus infection phenotypically and functionally activates immunosuppressive CD4+CD25+ T regulatory cells. Journal of immunology. 172(8):4752-61.

Vannberg FO, Chapman SJ and Hill AVS. 2011. Human genetic susceptibility to intracellular pathogens. Immunological Reviews. 240:105.

Villinger F and Ansari AA. 2010. Role of IL-12 in HIV infection and vaccine. European Cytokine Network. 21:215.

Wahl LM, Corcoran ML, Pyle SW, Arthur LO, Harel-Bellan A and Farrar WL. 1989. Human immunodeficiency virus glycoprotein (gp120) induction of monocyte arachidonic acid metabolites and interleukin 1. Proceedings of the National Academy of Sciences of the United States of America. 86(2):621-5.

Wang, Z. Y., Sato, H., Kusam, S., Sehra, S., Toney, L. M and Dent, A. L. 2005. Regulation of IL-10 gene expression in Th2 cells by Jun proteins. J Immunol. 174(4): 2098-2105.

Weiss L, Haeffner-Cavaillon N, Laude M, Gilquin J and Kazatchkine MD. 1989. HIV infection is associated with the spontaneous production of interleukin-1 (IL-1) in vivo and with an abnormal release of IL-1 alpha in vitro. AIDS (London, England). 3(11):695-9.

Weiss L, Si-Mohamed A, Giral P, Castiel P, Ledur A, Blondin C, Kazatchkine MD and N Haeffner-Cavaillon. 1997. Plasma levels of monocyte chemoattractant protein-1 but not those of macrophage inhibitory protein-1α and RANTES correlate with virus load in human immunodeficiency virus infection. Journal of Infectious Diseases. 176: 1621-1624.

Xing HQ, Hayakawa H, Izumo K, Kubota R, Gelpi E, Budka H, et al. In vivo expression of proinflammatory cytokines in HIV encephalitis: an analysis of 11 autopsy cases.

Xing, Z., J. Gauldie, G. Cox, H. Baumann, M. Jordana, X. F. Lei and M. K. Achong. 1998. IL-6 Is an Anti-inflammatory Cytokine Required for Controlling Local or Systemic Acute Inflammatory Responses. Journal of Clinical Investigation. 101.2: 311-20.

Yang H, Wei J, Zhang H, Song W, Wei W, Zhang L, Qian K and He S. 2010.Upregulation of Toll-like Receptor (TLR) expression and release of cytokines from mast cells by IL-12. Cell Physiol Biochem. 26(3):337-46.

Yeh MW, Kaul M, Zheng J, Nottet HS, Thylin M and Gendelman HE, et al. 2000. Cytokine-stimulated, but not HIV-infected, human monocyte-derived macrophages produce neurotoxic levels of L-cysteine. Journal of immunology. 164(8):4265-70.

12

The Role of Genetic Polymorphisms in the Chemokine and Their Receptors and Cytokines in the Human Immunodeficiency Virus Type 1 (HIV-1) Infection

Edna Maria Vissoci Reiche, Marla Karine Amarante and
Maria Angelica Ehara Watanabe
State University of Londrina
Brazil

1. Introduction

The natural history and pathogenic processes of human immunodeficiency virus type 1 (HIV-1) infection are complex and variable, and depend on many viral and host factors and their interactions (Pantaleo et al., 1997). Individuals are not equal susceptible to the infection and have differences in their viral set points, rates of decline of $CD4^{+}$ T cells, levels of viremia, emergence of citotoxic T lymphocyte (CTL) escape mutants, and development of opportunistic infections resulting in varying incubation periods of the virus (Kaur & Mehra, 2009). HIV-1 infected individuals present different rates of disease progression; while a majority of individual progress to acquired immunodeficiency syndrome (AIDS) after the infection, most of them can be turned aviremic even the absence of antiretroviral therapy (ARV) up to ten years and are called typical progressors. Most importantly, ~5% to 10% of persistently infected individuals show no signs of disease progression for over 12 years and remain asymptomatic and aviremic and are classified as long term nonprogressors (LTNPs). On the other hand, rapid progressors are individuals that rapidly progress to AIDS within four years after primary HIV-1 infection and some individuals have been known to progress to AIDS and death within a year after primary infection (Fauci et al., 1996; Rosenberg & Fauci, 1991).

Genetic factors may be one of the host factors responsible for the susceptibility to infection and disease progression. However, no single gene or polymorphism is likely to be responsible for these effects. Brass et al. (2008) have reported that HIV-1 uses at least 250 host-derived dependency factors for gaining entry into target cells and completing its life cycle. Hence, multiple genetic factors are expected to be involved in susceptibility, disease pathogenesis, and progression following HIV-1 infection. Some of these genes that have been established with HIV/AIDS conclusively involve are: (1) genes influencing viral entry by altering the expression on cell surface the levels of chemokine receptors and their ligands as well cytokines (Seisdedos & Parmentier, 2006; Reiche et al., 2007); (2) genes involved in anti-HIV immune response including the antiviral Apolipoprotein B mRNA-editing enzyme, catalytic polypeptide-like 3G (APOBEC3G) gene family on chromosome 22q13 (An et al., 2009); the virus restriction factor Tripartite Interaction Motif 5 α (TRIM5α) on chromosome 11p15; (3) the human leukocyte antigens (HLA) polymorphic loci and their associated genes including HCP5, RNF39, and ZNRD1 on the short arm of human chromosome 6; (4) Dendritic Cell Specific Intracellular adhesion molecule-3-Grabbing Non-integrin (DC-SIGN) on chromosome 19q13; (5) interferon regulatory factor 1; (6) killer cell immunoglobulin-like receptor (KIR) KIR3DSI on chromosome 19q13; and (7) Ly6 family of G [glycosylphosphatidylinositol (GPI)-anchored proteins] (Kaur & Mehra, 2009).

This chapter reviews the most important genetic polymorphisms already described in the chemokine, cytokine and their receptors, and their role on the host susceptibility or resistance to HIV-1 infection, on the clinical course of the disease and on the response to the ARV. For this purpose, *in vitro* and *in vivo* studies for inclusion were identified by a systematic search through PubMed for English-language literature, included original and review articles published up to 2010. These data could contribute to identify some genetic biomarkers for infection, transmission, disease progression or ARV therapeutic failure.

2. Genetic polymorphisms in CC chemokines and their receptors

Chemokines are low-molecular-weight potent chemoattractants produced by a variety of cell types that include T cells, macrophages, natural killer (NK) cells, B cells, fibroblasts, and mast cells. These are involved in cell trafficking and immunomodulation of inflammation and immune responses. The chemokines are subdivided into CC, CXC, and CX_3C subfamilies, according to the number of cysteine residues in the molecule. Members of CC chemokines are CCL3 [macrophage inflammatory protein-1 (MIP-1α)], CCL4 [macrophage inflammatory protein 1β (MIP-1β)], and CCL5 [regulated upon activation normally T-expressed (RANTES)]. They are natural ligands for CC chemokine receptor R 5 (CCR5). One member of CXC chemokines is CXC ligand 12 (CXCL12), previously named stromal cell-derived factor 1 (SDF1), a natural ligand for CXC receptor 4 (CXCR4). In certain instances, the chemokine receptors serve as entry portals for pathogens to gain entry into target cells and establish infection. Based on cell tropism, HIV-1 isolates are classified into two main groups. The vast majority of primary HIV-1 isolates is, predominantly, tropic for CCR5 and gradually tends to become CXCR4 tropic during late infection. All non-syncytium-inducing (NSI) strains of HIV-1 require CCR5 to gain entry into target cells and are also named R5 strains, while the syncytium-inducing (SI) strains use CXCR4 to enter into host cells and are also named as X4 strains (Berger et al., 1999). Functional genetic polymorphisms are known to occur in these proteins that affect their levels of expression and therefore might modulate their molecular interactions.

2.1 CCL3, CCL4 and CCL18

The genes coding for CCL3 (MIP-1α), CCL4 (MIP-1β), and CCL18 [also referred to as small inducible cytokine subfamily A member 18 or pulmonary and activation-regulated chemokine (PARC)], are clustered together within a 47-kb region on chromosome 17q12. These are potent chemokines produced by macrophages, NK cells, fibroblasts, and T cells. Of these, CCL2, CCL3 and CCL4 are natural ligands for the primary HIV-1 coreceptor CCR5, and their genetic polymorphisms have been implicated in HIV-1 acquisition and disease progression, although these associations are complicated because of strong linkage disequilibrium between them (Modi et al., 2006).

2.2 CCL5

The CCL5 (RANTES) gene is located on chromosome 17 which encodes a chemokine ligand for CCR1, CCR3, and CCR5. It suppresses infection for R5 strains of HIV-1 by blocking CCR5 (Paxton et al., 1996; Arenzana-Seisdedos et al., 1996). Some polymorphisms in *CCL5* promoter region protect HIV-1 infected subjects against disease progression as a result of increased CCL5 synthesis (Liu et al., 1999; Wichukchinda et al., 2006). Three single nucleotide polymorphisms (SNPs) in this gene (-28C→G, -403G→A, and in 1.1C) were reported for their roles in progression to AIDS in HIV-1 infected individuals. The variant alleles -28G and -403A were found to be associated with delayed progression to AIDS in Japanese population by increasing levels of CCL5 transcription and by reducing rates of $CD4^+$ T-cell depletion (Liu et al., 1999). Other study also suggested that polymorphisms in the CCL5 promoter gene can influence the risks for HIV-1 infection and disease progression by increasing the CCL5 levels (McDermott et al., 2000; Koning et al., 2003). In the other hand, the SNP In 1.1C, nested within an intronic regulatory sequence element, accelerated the progression to AIDS in African Americans and European Americans by downregulating the CCL5 gene transcription (An et al., 2002). Study by Wichukchinda et al. (2006) demonstrated the mutation's protective effect by comparing disease progression in seroconverters carrying either the CCL5-*28G* or the CCL5 *In.1.1C* polymorphism. Individuals carrying the CCL5 *In.1.1C* allele progressed significantly faster to AIDS compared with those carrying the CCL5 - *28G* allele, along with those HIV-1-infected subjects without these mutations.

2.3 CCL3L1, CCL4L1

Human CC chemokine ligand 3 like 1 gene (CCL3L1) is a natural ligand of HIV-1 coreceptor CCR5 and a potent HIV-1 supressive chemokine that can physically block the entry of HIV-1. The CCL3L1 gene is located on human chromosome 17q11.2 and shares 96.0% amino acid homology with CCL3. The copy number of the CCL3L1 gene varies among different individuals and populations groups (Kaur & Mehra, 2009). CCL3L1 and CCL4L1 genes harbor several SNPs and hotspots for duplication, resulting in distinct haplotypes and copy number variations, respectively, in different individuals (Modi et al., 2006). The copy numbers are highest in Africans, followed by Asians, Amerindians Central and South Asians, Middle East individuals and Europeans. Variations in a copy numbers of CCL3L1 alter the expression of this potent CCR5 ligand and might influence the entry of HIV-1 into host cells. Copy number variations in CCL3L1 have been associated with susceptibility to HIV-1 infection (Gonzalez et al., 2005). However, the results are contradictory in different populations. A study carried out in the Japanese population (Nakajima et al., 2007) has shown that HIV-1 infected individuals have lower copy number than healthy controls. On the contrary, studies in North Indian population showed that the copy number variation in CCL3L1 gene has no effect on acquisition in HIV-1 infected individuals compared with healthy controls (Nakajima et al., 2008). Another study showed an association of CCR5-59029 A/G and CCL3L1 copy number polymorphism with HIV-1 transmission and progression among HIV-1 seropositive and repeatedly sexually exposed HIV-1 seronegative North Indians individuals, suggesting that these polymorphisms appeared to have synergistic or interactive effects and are expected to be involved in the host innate resistance to HIV-1 infection (Rathore et al., 2009).

2.4 CCR5

CCR5 is normally expressed at very low levels on the surface of naïve CD4+ T cells and at higher levels in activated CD4+ memory T cells as well as in monocytes and macrophages (Potter et al., 2007). Multiple polymorphic variations have been described in the *CCR5* gene that is located on chromosome 3p21. CCR5-Δ32 polymorphism is the first and most well characterized host restriction allele associated with AIDS. This natural knockout deletion of 32 base-pair creates a premature stop codon resulting in truncated protein product, a shortened protein which remains intracellular and fails to reach the cell surface in individuals homozygous for the variant. The first study described a frequency of approximately 0.100 for the null-mutant allele of the *CCR5* gene in the Caucasian population. Heterozygotes for the allele have reduced levels of quantifiable CCR5 receptors in the cell surface and were present at similar frequencies among infected and uninfected cohort controls. Among HIV-1 infected homosexual cohorts, heterozygosity correlated well with decreased disease progression. However, no correlation was apparent among the haemophilic population (Dean et al., 1996).

A second study identified the same mutant allele of CCR5 in two homozygous individuals who had been repeatedly exposed to the HIV-1 but remained uninfected (Liu et al., 1997). The results also showed that the mutation makes the CCR5 protein incapable of mediating infection by HIV-1 *in vitro*. A third study suggested that heterozygosity also provides some protection from HIV-1 infection (Samson et al., 1996) and the discrepancy regarding the protection from HIV-1 infection was most likely due to the difference between the populations evaluated. The first study (Dean et al., 1996) compared large and matched cohorts of individuals, whereas the third (Samson et al., 1996) examined only non-cohort population matched by geographical location and the use of a French surname.

Even though homozygosity for the CCR5-Δ32 results in near-total protection for the HIV-1 infection, subjects can still be infected with T-tropic or SI strains of the virus, which use the CXCR4 coreceptor for cell entry (Dean et al., 1996; Samson et al., 1996; Zimmerman et al., 1997; O'Brien et al., 1997; Theodorou et al., 1997). Studies of HIV-1 infected homozygous for the CCR5-Δ32 mutation have been reported, but are rare (O'Brien et al., 1997; Theodorou et al., 1997; Balotta et al., 1997; Biti et al., 1997), probably due to a T-tropic virus, strain which only uses CXCR4 as coreceptor for cell entry.

Heterozygosity for the CCR5-Δ32 is significantly higher in cohorts of HIV-1 infected LTNPs compared to HIV-1 infected typical progressors (Cohen et al., 1997; Zimmerman et al., 1997; Eugen-Olsen et al., 1997). Although the heterozygosity was not related to the complete protection against HIV-1 infection (Dean et al., 1996; Samson et al., 1996), it may confer partial protection against disease progression or death in HIV-1 infected individuals (Zimmerman et al., 1997; Smith et al., 1997; Martin et al., 1998; de Roda et al., 1997; Meyer et al., 1999; Ionnadis et al., 1998). Presumably, heterozygosity limits the number of coreceptors available for HIV-1 binding. Indeed, CCR5 density of the surface of the CD4+ T cell has been correlated with viral load in persons with untreated HIV-1 infection (Reynes et al., 2000). Studies incorporating viral phenotype have suggested that the protective effect of CCR5-Δ32 heterozygosity against disease progression is lost when the infection virus is T-tropic (Michael et al., 1997).

An international meta-analysis showed that HIV-1 infected subjects heterozygous for the CCR5-Δ32 displayed lower HIV-1 RNA level than wild type patients. This result appears to be supported by the simple explanation that the fewer available CCR5 portals on cells of

CCR5-Δ32 delay HIV-1 replication and the virus-mediated destruction of the CD4+/ CCR5+ T-cell lymphocyte population (Ioannidis et al., 2001). The observation that this naturally-occurring genetic mutation can slow or delay the onset of AIDS in patient populations was the basis of therapeutic interventions targeting the interaction between the virus and the coreceptor CCR5.

Several other mutations in the coding region of the *CCR5* gene have been identified (Carrington et al., 1997). Ten common SNPs within the 1,000 base-pairs region upstream of CCR5-coding exons that exhibit promoter and regulatory activity have been described, possibly affecting the levels of CCR5 expression (Carrington et al., 1999; Martin et al., 1998; Kostrikis et al., 1998; Quillent et al., 1998; Piacentini et al., 2009). These polymorphisms are identified as CCR5P1 to CCR5P10 and the most common of them are CCR5P1 and CCR5P4 (Chatterjee, 2010).

The CCR5P1/P1 promoter allele was the first genetic variant in the CCR5 promoter to be associated with rapid progression of AIDS, although variants of other genes have been described more recently to be AIDS-accelerating (Carrington et al., 1997; Faure et al., 2000). The hypothesis that the genetic effect is mediated by an increase in available CCR5 portals is also supported by the epidemiologic pattern. The strongest acceleration mediated by the CCR5P1/P1 genotype occurs in the first five years of infection, a period when R5 (NSI) virus strains predominate in 90.0-95.0% of patients (Schuitemaker et al., 1992).

The A/G polymorphism at base-pair 59029 in the CCR5 promoter was identified and appears to affect the rate of progression to AIDS in HIV-1 infected homosexuals. The CCR5 59029 G/G genotype appears to be more protective than CCR5 59029 A/A, and this effect may be the result of a reduced CCR5 mRNA production. The A allele exhibits a 50.0% higher expression of CCR5 *in vitro* and confers faster disease progression than the G allele (Passam et al., 1999). These results indicated that this site in the CCR5 promoter is important and may be a useful target for treatment of the HIV-1 infection (McDermott et al., 1998).

It is estimated that homozygozity for the CCR5P1/P1 promoter allele was responsible for the development of the disease in 10.0% to 17.0% of the patients who developed AIDS within 3.5 years of HIV-1 infection, irrespective of the CCR5-Δ32 and CCR2-64I (defined in this chapter in the next sections) genotypes. The frequency of this susceptible genotype in the general population is only 7.0% to 13.0% (Martin et al., 1998).

Homozygosity for CCR5-59356-T, a polymorphism more frequent in the African-American rather than in Caucasian or Hispanic populations, has been strongly associated with an increased rate of perinatal HIV-1 transmission (Kostrikis et al., 1999). Additionally, the *59353C* allele is found in higher frequency in some progressors compared with LTNPs (Jang et al., 2008).

Complete linkage disequilibrium between CCR5P1 and CCR5-2459A sites and the CCR5P1 haplotype was shown to be associated with rapid progression to AIDS endpoints in both African-American and Caucasians cohorts. This effect was recessive in Caucasians and dominant in African-Americans, probably due to the presence of modulating genes or as yet unidentified polymorphisms with different frequencies among the racial groups (An et al., 2000). This same study described that both CCR5P1 homozygous and heterozygous African-Americans showed a trend towards more rapid progression to AIDS endpoints. Similar to the recessive effect of the CCR5P1 allele in Caucasians, which was strongest in the first 4-6 years following seroconversion, the dominant effect of the CCR5P1 allele in African-Americans was also evident in the first 4 years. This result is consistent with both the function of CCR5 as the coreceptor for early transmissible M-tropic HIV-1 strains and also with the studies of CCR5-Δ32 showing an early effect (Dean et al., 1996).

Unlikely the CCR5-Δ32 mutation which is found only in people of Northern European descent, the CCR5P1 allele has a frequency larger than 40.0% both in Caucasians, Asians and populations of African descent, suggesting that the CCR5P1 allele may have a more general effect on AIDS pathogenesis worldwide (An et al., 2000).

Another SNP in *CCR5* gene is a T→A substitution (named CCR5-m303A polymorphism) and results in a Threonine to Alanine transition at position 303. It encodes a truncated protein and abolishes the coreceptor activity of CCR5. This polymorphism shows a weak association with delayed progression to AIDS. When is present in heterozygous state with CCR5-Δ32, produces a phenotype of resistance to HIV-1 in primary isolates *in vitro* (Quillent et al., 1998).

Based on a unique constellation of additional multisite polymorphisms in CCR5 regulatory 5′ region, a number of CCR5 haplotypes have been identified (Gonzalez et al.,1999; Martin et al., 1998). They have been designed based on the nucleotide position in the 5′ untranslated region (UTR) and are referred to as human haplogroups A to G. Of these, HHE has been associated with accelerated disease progression in Caucasians (Gonzalez et al., 1999) and Thais (Nguyen et al., 2004) but not in African Americans. The HHC and HHD haplotypes showed positive association with fast progression to AIDS in African Americans (Kostrikis et al., 1999; Nguyen et al., 2004). In the Indian population, HHE has been implicated with susceptibility to infection and development of AIDS (Kaur et al., 2007). Whether this haplotype also influences disease progression is not clear because long-term follow-up is desirable to reach such a conclusion (Kaur & Mehra, 2009).

2.5 CCR2

Although the HIV-1 virus does not directly use CCR2 for host cell entry, and CCR2 is considered a minor coreceptor for HIV-1 infection, a Valine to Isoleucine substitution at position 64 in the first transmembrane domain of CCR2 (named CCR2-64I, V64I or G190A) has been associated with delayed progression to AIDS (Smith et al., 1997). HIV-1 infected individuals heterozygous or homozygous for this mutation appear to progress to AIDS or death more slowly. However, this mutation results in normal levels of expression of the CCR2 receptor and has not been shown to affect the susceptibility to HIV-1 infection (Smith et al., 1997; Martin et al., 1998; de Roda et al., 1997; Kostrikis et al., 1998; Mummidi et al., 1998; Mulherin et al., 2003).

Even though the change of the Valine to Isoleucine in a position buried in one of the seven transmembrane segments of this receptor could be considered innocuous, the epidemiological effect on AIDS progression was surprising. It has been shown that the CCR2-64I protein product can preferentially dimerizes with the CXCR4 polypeptide, sequestering it in the endoplasmic reticulum, while the CCR2 peptides cannot. Such differential intracellular kinetics between CCR2 allele products and primary HIV-1 coreceptors *in vivo* could reduce the rate of disease progression by limiting the number of available CXCR4 coreceptors, therefore also reducing indirectly the rate of viral replication (O'Brien and Moore, 2000). However, this effect on disease progression has not confirmed (Michael et al., 1997; Eugen-Olsen et al., 1998).

The distribution of CCR2-64I varies among different ethnic groups. Unlike the CCR5-Δ32 mutation, which is found primarily in Caucasians, the frequency of the CCR2-64I allele varies from 10.0% to 25.0% in both African-Americans and Caucasians, and in all other ethnic groups studied. The protective allele A occurs at a population frequency of 15.0%-17.0% in Chinese, ~12.0% in the North Indians (Kaur et al., 2007), and 3.0%-15.0% in the South Indian populations (Ramana et al., 2001). Studies of HIV-1 infected commercial sex workers in Nairobi and Kenya, suggested that the presence of the mutation helped to explain slow progression in 21.0% to 46.0% of slow progressors (Anzala et al., 1998). The effect of the CCR5-Δ32 allele on HIV-1 disease progression was also different from the effect of the CCR2 allele. The protection against AIDS provided by CCR5-Δ32 was continuous during the course of infection, while the protection provided by CCR2-64I was the greatest early in the course of infection (Mulherin et al., 2003).

A meta-analysis study found that in the absence of highly active antiretroviral therapy (HAART), both CCR5-Δ32 and CCR2-64I carriers progressed to AIDS at a 25.0% slower rate than individuals who lacked either of these protective alleles. They also progressed more slowly to death, approximately 35.0% and 25.0% slower, respectively (Ioannidis et al., 2001). Mabuka et al. (2009) verified that the presence of the CCR2-64I allele was associated with reduced viral load and with protection against early HIV-1 transmission among pregnant women who received short course zidovudine. In Kenya and other African countries, where approximately one quarter of individuals carry the variant allele, understanding this genetic mutation may help explain disparities in transmission risk and rates of disease progression and could contribute to vaccine development and other prevention interventions.

Because the genetic loci for *CCR5* and *CCR2* are in strong linkage disequilibrium, their combined analysis is greatly helpful to define CCR2-CCR5 extended haplotypes for disease association purposes (Kaur & Mehra, 2009).

3. Genetic polymorphisms in CXC chemokines and their receptors

3.1 CXCL12 (SDF1)

CXCL12 (SDF1) is a highly potent α chemokine, the natural ligand for the CXCR4, and a potent entry inhibitor for T-tropic (X4 or SI) HIV-1 strains that generally emerge during the late-stage of HIV-1 infection (Bleul et al., 1996). The CXCL12-CXCR4 interactions are essential for the homing and retention of hematopoietic progenitor cells in the bone marrow and have been shown to control the navigation of progenitor cells between the bone marrow and the blood. The gene for CXCL12 (SDF1) is ~10kb long and located on human chromosome 10q11.1. It exists in two isoforms, α and β, obtained as a consequence of alterative splicing. A common G to A transition, initially referred to as SDF1-3′A and currently named CXCL12-3′A, was described at an evolutionarily conserved sequence of the 3′UTR of the β transcript gene. The polymorphism at the 801 position (G801A or CXCL12′A) has been shown to have a recessive protective effect against HIV-1 infection. Homozygotes for the CXCL12-3′A variant showed a remarkable level of protection against AIDS, supporting the hypothesis that the CXCL12-3′A variant restricts the emergency of X4 HIV-1 strains, with overproduction of CXCL12 in local compartments, which binds to and blocks the CXCR4 receptors required for X4 viruses to emerge and multiply (Winkler et al., 1998). However, direct evidence for an effect of CXCL12-3′A on the synthesis, quantity or half life of the ligand has not been obtained *in vitro* (Arya et al., 1999). Because CXCL12 expression is limited to stromal cells and other tissues that are not easy to quantify, this hypothesis is difficult to test *in vivo* (Bleul et al., 1996).

Global, regional, and ethnic distributions of frequencies of CXCL12 genotypes and of the CXCL12-3'A allele vary significantly, ranging from 0.029-0.091 in Africans, 0.056-0.150 in American Indians, 0.149-0.217 in Europeans, 0.09- 0.380 in North Asians, 0.06-0.43 in South Asians, and 0.536- 0.7145 in Oceanian population (Su et al., 1999). In other ethnic cohorts, the allelic frequency of CXCL12-3'A ranged from 0.100 to 0.332 (Passam et al., 2005; Williamson et al., 2000; Wang et al., 2003). The frequency of the CXCL12 polymorphisms was also investigated in various cohorts of HIV-1 exposed but uninfected and among HIV-1 infected individuals. The results showed that the CXCL12-3'A allele delayed progression to AIDS but not decreased the susceptibility to HIV-1 infection (Winkler et al., 1998). Another study showed that the CXCL12-3'A homozygous mutation did not influence the clinical course of asymptomatic patients. However, the lower number of deaths during the follow-up period among symptomatic patients who were homozygotes and heterozygotes for the CXCL12-3'A allele, suggested that both genotypes could have a possible late-stage protective effect on the clinical outcome of HIV-1 patients after the AIDS diagnosis (Reiche et al., 2006). However, the disease-retarding role of homozygosity for the CXCL12-3'A allele has not been confirmed in other cohorts (Mummidi et al., 1998; Wang et al., 2003; van Rij et al., 1998; Magierowska et al., 1999; Rousset et al., 1999; Brambilla et al., 2000; Soriano et al., 2002).

Verma et al. (2007) observed a low frequency of CCR5-Δ32 (1.5%) and of CCR2-64I (9.1%) in healthy Northern Indians, suggesting high vulnerability of North Indians to HIV-1 infection. However, the allelic frequency of the CXCL12 3'A was high (20.4%) in the healthy HIV-1 seronegative Northern Indians included in their study, which was similar to that observed in South Indians (17.0%-35.0%) and South European populations (14.0%-33.0%) (Ramana et al., 2001).

Chaudhary et al. (2008) examined the SNP of CXCL12 3'A by polymerase chain reaction-restriction fragment length polymorphism (PCR-RFLP), cloning and sequencing in individuals from Northen India and showed that the genotypic frequency of CXCL12 3'A/CXCL12 3'A in the 100 HIV-1 seronegative healthy individuals, in 150 HIV-1 seronegative individuals with high risk for sexually transmitted disease (STD), and in 100 HIV-1 seropositive patients were 4.0%, 18.0% and 7.0%, respectively. A significantly higher frequency of CXCL12 3'A/CXCL12 3'A was observed in high risk STD individuals as compared to HIV-1 seropositive (p = 0.014) and healthy HIV-1 seronegative tested individuals (p = 0.001), suggesting a protective role of CXCL12 3'A allele in HIV-1 infection. In this study it was observed a significant increase in the homozygous genotype for the mutant allele CXCL12 3'A in the high risk STD individuals as compared to both the healthy seronegative and HIV-1 seropositive individuals, suggesting a possible protective role of this allele in the homozygous state against HIV-1 infection.

The frequencies of CXCL12 3'A, CCR5-Δ32, CCR5-m3030, and CCR2-64I allelic variants were investigated in unrelated healthy Bahraini individuals without any known history of HIV-1 infection or AIDS symptoms. The results showed that CCR2-64I allele (8.9%) and especially the CXCL12 3'A allele (26.5%) were predominant and may be associated with resistance to fast HIV-1 infection in this population, and thus their genotyping could be used for prognosis in HIV-1 infected individuals. No mutant alleles were detected for CCR5-m303A mutation and the frequency of 2.8% for CCR5-Δ32 allele may be attributed to the admixture with people of European descent (Salem et al., 2009).

The epidemiological interaction of CCR5/CCR2 and CXCL12-3'A suggests that a functional interaction might explain the enhanced protection. One hypothesis is that CCR2 and CCR5 variants slow AIDS by limiting the number of CCR5 coreceptors that mediate the replication and spread of primary, early stage R5 HIV-1 strains, while the CXCL12-3'A variant restricts the emergence of X4 HIV-1 strains and the ensuing AIDS-accelerating process (O'Brien and Moore, 2000).

However, several studies show a lack of relationship between CXCL12 3'A and HIV-1 disease non-progression (Vidal et al., 2005a; Ioannidis et al., 2001; Tresoldi et al., 2002). For instance, in their international meta-analysis, Ioannidis et al. (2001) measured the effects of subjects homozygous for the CXCL12 3'A polymorphism by reviewing studies that prospectively followed HIV-1 infected patients from seroconversion to AIDS diagnosis and death. Results showed that being homozygous for the polymorphism had no effect on disease progression and there was no significant difference in HIV-1 RNA levels among persons with and without the polymorphism.

Recently, Tan et al. (2010) showed that the allelic frequency of CCR5-Δ32, CCR5m303A, CCR2-64I and CXCL12-3'A in HIV-1 infected and uninfected high-risk Uighurs individuals, the largest population of minority in China, was 4.4%, 2.7%, 25.7% and 57.4%, respectively. While there was no significant difference in the frequency of CCR5-Δ32, CCR2-64I and CXCL12-3'A between HIV-1 seropositive and seronegative group, the frequency of CCR5m3030A in HIV-1 seropositive group was significantly higher than that in seronegative group. Furthermore, a woman who carried homozygous CCR5-Δ32 was positive for HIV-1 infection. Therefore, these data suggest that the CCR5-Δ32 CCR2-64I and CXCL1´3'A alleles may have limited effect on protecting from HIV-1 infection and CCR5m303A variant may be associated with the risk for HIV-1 infection in high-risk Uighurs individuals.

The distribution of CCR5-Δ32, CCR2-64I, and CXCL12 3'A alleles was evaluated in Guangxi Province Zhuang population, the largest minority ethnic population with over 15 million people, mainly located in Guangxi Province, China. The CCR5-Δ32 was absent, and CCR2-64I and CXCL12 3'A alleles were relatively common and seem not to confer protection against HIV-1 infection in this population. The results suggest that the Zhuang people may have a similar genetic susceptibility to HIV-1 infection with most other Chinese ethnic groups (Qijian et al., 2010).

3.2 CXCR1, CXCR2

CXCR1 (IL-8RA) and CXCR2 (IL-8RB) are receptors for IL-8, a proinflammatory cytokine involved in chemoattraction and activation of neutrophils. CXCR1 and CXCR2 genes are located o chromosome 2q35 and several polymorphisms have been described including SNPs T92G (CXCR1 -300) and C1003T (CXCR1-142) that result in a CXCR1 haplotype Ha. A genetic study on French cohort composing of rapid and slow progressors HIV-1 infected individual identified a strong association of CXCR1 haplotype Ha with protection against rapid progression to AIDS (Vasilescu et al., 2007). It was suggested that the inhibitory effect of CXCR1 Ha could be mediated by suppressing $CD4^+$ and CXCR4 expression (Kaur & Mehra, 2009).

3.3 CXCR4

The highly conserved *CXCR4* gene is an obvious target as CXCR4 serves a coreceptor for X4 (SI) strains of HIV-1 to gain entry into cells. This gene is located on chromosome 2 and the screening of entire transcription unit resulted in the detection of two rare polymorphisms.

One of these CXCR4 mutations was silent, and each was unique to two nonprogressors. However, no association with progression to AIDS was found (Cohen et al., 1998).

3.4 CXCR6

The CXCR6 is a chemokine receptor that is known as a minor coreceptor in HIV-1 infection but could participate in disease progression through its role as a mediator of inflammation. Petit et al. (2008) described the effects of mutation of acidic extracellular CXCR6 residues on receptor function. Although most CXCR6 mutants examined were expressed at levels similar to wild-type CXCR6, the N-terminal E3Q mutant was poorly expressed, which may explain previously reported protective effects of a similar SNP, with respect to late-stage HIV-1 infection. In contrast to several other chemokine receptors, mutation of the CXCR6 N-terminal and inhibition of post-translational modifications of this region were without effect on receptor function. This data suggests a novel paradigm for the CXCR6:CXCL16 interaction, a finding which may impact the discovery of small-molecule antagonists of CXCR6.

Study by Limou et al. (2010) verified that the rs2234358 polymorphism in the CXCR6 gene was the strongest signal obtained for the genomewide association study comparing the 186 Genomics of Resistance to Immunodeficiency Virus (GRIV) LTNPs who were not elite controlls with 697 uninfected control subjects. This association was replicated in 3 additional independent European studies, reaching genomewide significance. This association with LTNPs is independent of the CCR2-CCR5 loci and the HCP5 polymorphisms. The statistical significance, the replication, and the magnitude of the association demonstrate that CXCR6 is likely involved in the molecular etiology of AIDS and, in particular, in LTNPs, emphasizing the power of extreme-phenotype cohorts.

4. Genetic polymorphisms in CX_3C Chemokine Receptor (CX_3CR)

4.1 CX_3CR1

CX_3CR1, a leukocyte chemotactic and adhesion receptor for the human chemokine fractalkine, has also been defined as a minor HIV-1 coreceptor, particularly expressed on brain. Mutations on the CX_3CR1 gene, located at chromosome 3, have been described, such as V249I (substitution changed Valine to Isoleucine) and T280M (substitution changed Threonine to Methionine) (Faure et al., 2000), with frequency of 26.0% and 13.0%, respectively. The impact of CX_3CR1 polymorphisms on HIV-1 pathogenesis is controversial, with conflicting reports of their role in disease progression in HIV-1 infected patients. Individuals homozygous for the 280M allele exhibited accelerated disease progression (Faure et al., 2000, 2003), with a small but statistically significant correlation with slightly earlier immunological and virologic failure (Brumme et al., 2003). However, further studies did not confirm this observation (McDermott et al., 2000; Kwa et al., 2003).

Polymorphisms in CCR2 and CX_3CR1, which HIV-1 sometimes uses as coreceptors, have also been associated with slowing HIV-1 disease progression. For example, the *CCR2-64I* mutation has been shown to reduce CXCR4 expression on $CD4^+$ T cells, thereby interfering with X4-tropic virus infection (Kalinkovich et al., 1999). In one study's cohort of HIV-1 positive Kenyan sex workers (Anzala et al., 1998), the frequency of being positive for *CCR2-64I* was highest in LTNPs, which was three times greater than that for progressors. In a separate study, Vidal et al. (2005b) found that the *CX_3CR1 V249I* polymorphism is significantly more frequent in LTNPs than progressors, but not than healthy controls. It has been observed that there was a large discrepancy between these alleles among populations of the north and south. Populations in the same language-speaking family or with the same origin shared similar allele distributions.

Puissant et al. (2006) observed that some genetic polymorphisms had an impact on the evolution of plasma virus load and peripheral T lymphocyte counts in HIV-1 infected patients under HAART. After 1 year of HAART, patients with a virological response (undetectable plasma HIV-1 RNA) have a higher frequency of the homozygous CXCL12 3'A genotype than patients with other polymorphisms such as CCR5-Δ32, CCR2-64I, CX_3CR1-249I, and CX_3CR1-280M. Similarly, patients with a $CD4^+$ T cell increase of over 200/mm^3 from baseline after 1 year of HAART display higher frequencies of homozygous CXCL12 3'A and homozygous CX_3CR1-280M genotypes than other patients. Moreover, the authors showed that CX_3CR1-280M allele was associated with high peripheral $CD4^+$ T cell counts not only in HIV-1 soropositive patients but also in healthy controls.

Qian et al. (2008) showed that the frequencies of CX_3CR1-249I and 280M alleles varied substantially among different population and were independent risk factors for accelerating the progression to AIDS. Further, Parczewski et al. (2009) studied the influence of genetic variants for CCR5-Δ32, CCR5 -G2459A, CCR2- G190A, CX_3CR1- G744A, and CX_3CR1-C838T in a cohort of 168 HIV-1 seropositive adults and 151 healthy newborns from northwestern Poland. The results showed that haplotypes containing CCR5-Δ32, CCR2-G190A, and CX_3CR1- G744A were significantly more common in the healthy newborns suggesting an association between these haplotypes and resistance to HIV-1 infection in this population.

5. Genetic polymorphism in cytokines and their receptors

Like chemokines, the role of cytokines in the modulation of HIV-1 infection and the rate of disease progression remains to be fully understood. Evidence of strong epidemiological associations between cytokines and HIV-1 disease progression has been limited and, in some cases, inconsistent across studies. Studies have shown that cytokines can have inhibitory, stimulatory or both effects on HIV-1 replication (Han et al., 1996; Naif et al., 1997).

5.1 Interleukin-4 (IL-4) and IL-4 Receptor (IL-4R)

IL-4 is an important cytokine that induces differentiation of $CD4^+$ Th cells. It also regulates the expression of the HIV-1 coreceptors CCR5 and CXCR4. IL-4 decreases the levels of CCR5 on the surfaces of CD4-bearing cells and increases CXCR4 levels on the same or other cells. *IL-4* gene is located on chromosome 11 and a SNP in the regulatory region of IL-4 gene (IL4-589 C/T), initially identified among HIV-1 seropositive Japanese individuals, has been reported to have a protective effect against transmission of HIV-1 through heterosexual contact. The IL4-R alpha I50V polymorphism in exon 5 of IL-4R gene affects the functional responsiveness of the gene (Risma et al., 2002). The SNP I50V was found to be associated with slow progression to AIDS in HIV-1 infected individuals (Soriano et al., 2005). However, another study suggested an association of IL-4R alpha I50V allele with increased likelihood of HIV-1 infection in North Indian population (Chatterjee et al., 2009).

5.2 Interleukin 10 (IL-10)

The interleukin-10 (IL-10) is known to inhibit HIV-1 replication in macrophages *in vivo* (Kollmann et al., 1996). The gene encoding IL-10 is situated on chromosome 1 and a polymorphism with C→A transition in the promoter region at position -592, named IL10-C592A, has been associated with diminished IL-10 production and accelerated progression to AIDS with a dominant effect (Winkler et al., 1998). This SNP is carried by 23.6% of the Caucasians, 40.0% of the African Americans, 33.0% of Hispanics, and 60.0% of the Asians. The molecular mechanism behind this SNP is not well understood but is has been predicted that IL-10 may control proliferation of HIV-1 by limiting the number of activated macrophages available for HIV-1 replication (Chatterjee, 2010).

5.3 Tumor Necrosis Factor Alpha (TNF-α)

TNF-α is a pro-inflammatory cytokine and is known to be involved in the various immunogenetic events that influence HIV-1 infection. The gene encoding TNF-α is located on chromosome 6 and four polymorphisms in the TNF-α promoter have been identified, all with G→A transitions; however, the information available of how TNF-α genetic variants affect vulnerability to HIV-1 infection is inconsistent (reviewed by Chatterjee, 2010). Veloso et al. (2010) determined whether carriage of the TNF- α-238G/A, -308G/A, and -863 C/A gene promoter SNPs influence the risk of HIV-1 infection and disease progression in Caucasian Spaniards. For this purpose, 239 heavily exposed but uninfected individuals (EU), 203 healthy controls (HC), 109 HIV-1 infected typical progressors (TP) and 75 HIV-1 infected LTNPs were evaluated. The results showed that the distribution of TNF-α variants did not differ among HIV-1 infected compared with EU and among TP and LTNPs. The analysis in LTNPs subset indicated that TNF-α-238A variant allele was significantly overrepresented in patients who spontaneously controlled plasma viremia compared with those who had a detectable plasma viral load. Taken together, the results suggested that TNF-α genetic variants were unrelated to disease progression in infected subjects but the -238 G/A SNP may modulate the control of viremia in LTNPs.

5.4 Interferon alpha receptor 1 (IFNAR1)

Interferon alpha (IFN-α) elicits a pleotropic antiviral response and form the first line of defense against HIV-1 infection. This cytokine acts through the IFN-α receptor (IFNAR) that is composed of two subunits, IFNAR1 and IFNAR2, encoded by the gene located at chromosome 21q (Kim et al., 1997). Two SNPs in the *IFNAR1* gene, IFNAR1-18339G→C (Valine to Leucine change in exon) and IFNAR1-30127C→T (in intron), found in tight linkage disequilibrium were associated with susceptibility to HIV-1 infection (Diop et al., 2006).

6. Genetic polymorphism and the response to antiretroviral therapy

The observations that genetic markers influence the natural history of HIV-1 and that the infection and the immunological and virologic responses to HAART is neither universal nor homogeneous (DeHovitz et al., 2000), lead to the thought that the response to treatment may also be genetically determined. Polymorphisms in the chemokine and chemokine receptor genes may affect response to HAART, in addition to other host factors governing poor immune response to HAART, such as increasing age (Viard et al., 2001), injection drug use

(Dronda et al., 2002), hepatitis C virus coinfection (Greub et al., 2000), and lower baseline CD4+ T cell count (Vaamonde et al., 2006).

Genetic polymorphisms could also explain the heterogeneity in sustaining viral suppression observed among patients receiving HAART (O'Brien et al., 2000). Approximately 10.0% of HIV-1 infected patients do not respond to HAART with a reduction of viral load, even if there is good compliance and no evidence of viral resistance (Lederberger et al., 1999).

However, studies investigating the association between genetic polymorphisms and response to HAART have provided conflicting data. An improvement in the immunological and the virological responses in association with the CCR5-Δ32, CCR2-64I, CXCL12-3'A, and CCR5-59029G/A polymorphisms has been reported (O'Brien et al., 2000; Guerin et al., 2000; Kasten et al., 2000; Yamashita et al., 2001). HIV-1 infected patients with wild type genotypes for the CCR5, CCR2, and 59029A alleles treated with HAART had the poorest response to therapy compared with patients with other genotypes combined with the CCR5-Δ32, CCR-64I or 59029G alleles (O'Brien et al., 2000). Polymorphism within the *CX₃CR1* gene was associated with accelerated virological and immunological therapy failure (Brumme et al., 2003). One report (Puissant et al., 2006) showed that, after one year of HAART, patients with undetectable plasma HIV-1 RNA levels have a higher frequency of the homozygous CXCL12-3'A genotype than other patients. Similarly, patients with a CD4+T cell count increase of over 200/mm^3 from baseline after one year of HAART display higher frequencies of homozygous CXCL12-3'A and CX_3CR1-280M genotypes than other patients.

Another study that evaluated a subgroup of patients with baseline CD4+ T cell count of 201-500 cells/mm^3, showed that both the CXCL12-3'A and CCR2-64I alleles displayed a positive influence on clinical progression after HAART initiation. The CXCL12-3'A allele showed this effect through a more rapid CD4+ T lymphocyte restoration counts above the level of 500 cells/mm^3, while CCR2-64I was associated with stronger viral suppression. Regarding the CCR5-Δ32 and CCR5-59029G/A alleles, they had no effects on the response to HAART initiation (Passam et al., 2005). In contrast, other studies did not find such correlation (Brumme et al., 2001; Bratt et al., 1998; Wit et al., 2002). However, one of these studies (Bratt et al., 1998) did not exclude nonadherent patients, and analyzed their data on an intent-to-treat basis, thus reducing the likelihood of finding a difference. In addition, 69.0% of their CCR5/Δ32 heterozygous patients had SI virus isolates, and therefore, tended to have lower CD4+ T cell counts, higher plasma HIV-1 RNA levels, and a greater proportion of azidothymidine resistance mutations.

Another study evaluated the CCR5-Δ32, CXCL12-3'A, and CCR2-64I genetic polymorphisms in HIV-1 infected patients receiving HAART and the results showed that successful treatment was associated with heterozygosity for the CCR5-Δ32, underscoring that the chemokine receptor polymorphisms have a modifying effect on the virological response to HAART. The course of mean viral load was significantly worse for patients without the CCR5-Δ32 allele and the multivariate analysis demonstrated that heterozygosity for the CCR5-Δ32 variant is an independent prognostic factor for treatment outcome (Bogner et al., 2004).

The frequency of the CXCL12- 3'A, CCR2-64I, CCR5-Δ32, and CCR5-Promoter-59029-A/G polymorphisms was also evaluated in 155 Brazilian HIV-1 infected on pre and post-HAART and their influence on CD4+ T cell counts. The results showed that the CD4+ T cell gain was influenced by carriage of one or more of these polymorphisms, highlighting the possibility that these genetic traits can be useful to identify patients at risk for faster progression to AIDS or therapeutic failure (Rigatto et al., 2008).

The chemokine polymorphisms CXCR6-3E/K, In1.1T/C, H7 haplotype, CX_3CR1-V249I, and CX_3CR1-T280M have been shown to affect the course of HIV-1 infection. The influence on immunologic and virologic response to HAART in a group of 143 HIV-1 patients was studied by Passam et al. (2007). The results revealed an improved immunologic response to HAART in patients with the CX_3CR1-249I or CX3CR1-280M allele. On the contrary, patients with initial viral load suppression due to HAART showed a faster virologic failure in the presence of the CXCR6-3K allele. The In1.1T/C polymorphism and H7 haplotype did not reveal any specific effect on HAART response.

7. Conclusion

So far, the CCR5-Δ32 allele remains the most important host factor known to be associated to the resistance to the HIV-1 infection. However, high frequencies of CCR5-Δ32, CCR2-64I, and CXCL12-3′A alleles could be all the aftermath or adaptive episodes in which a pathogen exerted selective pressure favoring the survival of persons with these beneficial alleles.

Taken together, the reviewed studies suggest that the existence of genetic polymorphisms must be taken into account in the virological and immunological follow-up of HIV-1 infected patients under treatment with HAART, and that pharmacogenetics is very likely to influence the future individualization of HAART. The individual genetic conditions could be of interest not only in terms of disease progression, but also on the drug metabolism, and therapy response. The identification of genetic polymorphisms in the HIV-1 infected individuals could be useful to identify a possible genotype or genotype associations that could serve as a marker of either the disease progression in HIV-1 infected individuals or of a higher probability of HAART failure.

Genetic markers could also be useful to better characterize the genetic epidemiology of HIV-1 infection and to detect individuals at high risk of a faster disease progression. This information could lead to the use of different or more aggressive therapeutic strategies, the monitoring in shorter interval of time, or both procedures. Most of the studies reviewed here signaled that the chemokine receptor antagonists are important new antiviral drugs to combat the HIV-1 infection. HIV-1 infected patients in the advanced stages of the disease and/or with multiresistance to the antiretroviral agents currently available could benefit from these new therapeutic strategies.

It is possible that a multifaceted approach to antiretroviral therapy, which takes into account the genetic host factors and the use of combinations of inhibitors that target different steps of the viral life cycle, has the best potential for long-term control of HIV-1 infection. Such approach could lead to the optimal therapeutic effects of reducing viral loads and some immune restoration response, and also to an increase in the span of life of infected individuals. In this post-genomic era, the study of host factors and their genetic contribution to HIV-1 infection, addresses fundamental issues in our understanding of the pathogenesis of the infection and opens new opportunities for therapeutic intervention to be developed.

8. References

An, P.; Johnson, R.; Phair, J.; Kirk, G.D.; Yu, X-F.; Donfield, S.; Buchbinder, S.; Goedert, J.J. & Winkler, C.A. (2009). *APOBEC3B* deletion and risk of HIV-1 acquisition. *The Journal of Infectious Diseases*, v.200, pp.1054-1058, ISSN 0022-1899.

An, P.; Martin, M.P.; Nelson, G.W.; Carrington, M.; Smith, M.W.; Gong, K.; Vlahov, D.; O'Brien, S.J. & Winkler, C.A. (2000). Influence of CCR5 promoter haplotypes on AIDS progression in African-Americans. *AIDS*, v. 14, n. 14, pp. 2117-2122, ISSN 0269-9370.

An, P.; Nelson, G.W.; Wang, L.; Donfield, S.; Goedert, J.J.; Phair, J.; Vlahov, D.; Buchbinder, S.; Farrar, W.L.; Modi, W.; O'Brien, S.J. & Winkler, C.A. (2002). Modulating influence on HIV/AIDS by interacting RANTES gene variants. *Proceedings National Academy of Sciences U S A*, v. 99, pp. 10002-10007, ISSN 0027-8424.

Anzala, A.O.; Ball, T.B.; Rostron, T.; O'Brien, S. J.; Plummer, F.A. & Rowland-Jones, S.L. (1998). CCR2-64I allele and genotype association with delayed AIDS progression in African women. University of Nairobi Collaboration for HIV Research. *The Lancet*, v. 351, pp. 1632–1633, ISSN 0099-5355.

Arenzana-Seisdedos, F. & Parmentier, M. (2006). Genetics of resistance to HIV infection: role of co-receptors and co-receptor ligands. *Seminars in Immunology*, v. 18, pp. 387-403, ISSN 1044-5323.

Arenzana-Seisdedos, F.; Virelizier, J-L.; Rousset, D.; Clark-Lewis, I.; Loetscher, P.; Moser, B. & Baggiolini, M. (1996). HIV blocked by chemokine antagonist. *Nature*, v. 383, n. 6599, pp.400, ISSN 0028-0836.

Arya, S.K.; Ginsberg, C.C.; Davis-Warren, A. & D'Costa, J. (1998). In vitro phenotype of SDF1 gene mutant that delay the onset of human immunodeficiency virus disease in vivo. *Journal of Human Virology*, v.2, p. 133-138, ISSN 1090-9508.

Balotta, C.; Bagnarelli, P.; Violin, M.; Ridolfo, A.L.; Zhou, D.; Berlusconi, A.; Corvasce, S.; Corbellino, M.; Clementi, M.; Clerici, M.; Moroni, M. & Galli, M. (1997). Homozygous delta 32 deletion of the CCR5-chemokine receptor gene in an HIV-1-infected patient. *AIDS*, v. *11*, n.10, pp. F67-F71, ISSN 0269-9370.

Biti, R.; Ffrench, R.; Young, J.; Bennets, B.; Steward, G. & Liang, T. (1997). HIV-1 infection in an individual homozygous for the CCR5 deletion allele. *Nature Medicine.*, v. 3, n.3, pp. 252-253, ISSN 1078-8956.

Bleul, C.C.; Farzan, M.; Choe, H.; Parolin, C.; Clark-Lewis, I.; Sodoski, J.; Springer, T.A. (1996). The lymphocyte chemoattractant SDF-1 is a ligand for LESTR/fusin and blocks HIV-1 entry. *Nature*, v. 382, n. 6594, p. 829-833, ISSN 0028-0836.

Bogner, J.; Lutz, B.; Klein, H.G.; Pollerer, C.; Troendle, U. & Goebel, F.D. (2004). Association of highly active antiretroviral therapy failure with chemokine receptor 5 wild type. *HIV Medicine*, v. 5, n. 4, pp. 264-272, ISSN 1464-2662.

Brambilla, A.; Villa, C.; Rizzardi, G.; Veglia, F.; Ghezzi, S.; Lazzarin, A.; Cusini, M.; Muratori, S.; Santagostino, E.; Gringeri, A.; Louie, L.G.; Sheppard, H.W.; Poli, G.; Michael, N.L.; Pantaleo, G. & Vicenzi, E. (2000). Shorter survival of SDF1-3'A homozygotes linked to CD4+ T cell decrease in advanced human immunodeficiency virus type 1 infection. *The Journal of Infectious Diseases*, v. 182, n. 1, p. 311-315, ISSN 0022-1899.

Brass, A.L.; Dykxhoom, D.M.; Benita, Y.; Yan, N.; Engelman, A.; Xavier, R.J.; Lieberman, J. & Elledge, S.J. (2008) Identification of host proteins required for HIV infection through a functional genomic screen. *Science*, v. 319, n.5868, pp.921-926, ISSN 0036-8075.

Bratt, G.; Karlsson, A.; Leandersson, A.C.; Albert, J.; Wahren, B. & Sandstrom, E. (1998). Treatment history and baseline viral load, but not viral tropism or CCR-5 genotype, influence prolonged antiviral efficacy of highly active antiretroviral treatment. *AIDS*, v. *12*, n.16, pp. 2193-2202, ISSN 0269-9370.

Brumme, Z.L.; Chan, K.J.; Dong, W.; Hogg, R.; O'Shaughnessy, M.V.; Montaner, J.S. & Harrigan, P.R. (2001). CCR5Delta32 and promoter polymorphisms are not correlated with initial virological or immunological treatment response. *AIDS*, v. 15, n.17, pp. 2259-2266, ISSN 0269-9370.

Brumme, Z.L.; Dong, W.W.Y.; Chan, K.J.; Hogg, R.S.; Montaner, J.S.C.; O'Shaughnessy, M.V. & Harrigan, P.R. (2003). Influence of polymorphisms within the CX3CR1 and MDR-1 genes on initial antiretroviral therapy response. *AIDS*, v. 17, n.2, pp. 201-208, ISSN 0269-9370.

Carrington, M.; Kissner, T.; Gerrard, B.; Ivaniv, S.; O'Brien, S.J.; Dean, M.A. (1997). Novel alleles of the chemokine-receptor gene CCR5. *Journal of Human Genetics*, v. 61, n. 6, pp. 1261-1267, ISSN 1434-5161.

Carrington, M.; Nelson, G.W.; Martin, M.P.; Kissner, T.; Vlahov, D.; Goedert, J.J.; Kaslow, R.; Buchbinder, S.; Hoots, K. & O'Brien, S.J. (1999). HLA and HIV-1: heterozygosity advantage and B*35-Cw*04 disadvantage. *Science*, v. 283, p. 1748-1752, ISSN 0036-8075.

Chatterjee, A.; Rathone, A. & Dhole, T.N. (2009). Association of IL-4 589 C/T promoter and Il-4RalphaI50V receptor polymorphism with susceptibility to HIV-1 infection in North Indians. *Journal of Medical Virology*, v.81, n.6, pp.959-956, ISSN 0146-6615.

Chatterjee, K. (2010). Host genetic factors in susceptibility to HIV-1 infection and progression to AIDS. *Journal of Genetics*, v.89, n.1, pp.109-116, ISSN 0022-1333.

Chaudhary, O.; Rajsekar, K.; Ahmed, I.; Verma, R.; Bala, M.; Bhasinc, R. & Luthra, K. (2008). Polymorphic variants in DC-SIGN, DC-SIGNR and SDF-1 in high risk seronegative and HIV-1 patients in Northern Asian Indians. *Journal of Clinical Virology*, n. 43, pp. 196–201, ISSN 1386-6532.

Cohen, O.J.; Kinter, A. & Fauci, A.S. (1997). Host factors in the pathogenesis of HIV disease. *Immunological Reviews*, v. 159, pp. 31-48, ISSN 0105-2896.

Cohen, O.J.; Paolucci, S.; Bende, S. M.; Daucher, M.; Moriuchi, H.; Moriuchi, M.; Cicala, C.; Davey, R.T. Jr.; Baird. B. & Fauci, A.S. (1998). CXCR4 and CCR5 genetic polymorphisms in long-term nonprogressive human immunodeficiency virus infection: lack of association with mutations other than CCR5-Delta32. *Journal of Virology*, v.72, n. 7, pp. 6215-6217, ISSN 0022-538X.

Cohen, O.J.; Vaccarezza, M.; Lam, G.K.; Baird, B.; Wildt, K.; Murphy, P.M.; Zimmerman, P.A.; Nutman, T.B.; Fox, C.H.; Hoover, S.; Adelsberger, K.J.; Baseler, M.; Arthos, J.; Davey, R.T.; Dewar, R.L.; Metcalf, J.; Schwartzentruber, D.J.; Orenstein, J.M.; Buchbinder, S.; Saah, A.J.; Detels, R.; Phair, J.; Rinaldo, C.; Margolick, J.B.; Pantaleo, G. & Fauci, A.S. (1997). Heterozygosity for a defective gene for CC chemokine receptor 5 is not the sole determinant for the immunologic and virologic phenotype of HIV-infected long-term nonprogressors. *The Journal of Clinical Investigation*, v. 100, n. 6, pp. 1581-1589, ISSN 0021-9738.

de Roda Husman, A.M.; Koot, M.; Cornelissen, M.; Keet, I.P.M.; Brouwer, M.; Broersen, S.M.; Bakker, M.; Roos, M.T.; Prins, M.; de Wolf, F.; Coutinho, R.A.; Miedema, F.; Goudsmit, J. & Schuitemaker, H. (1997). Association between CCR5 genotype and the clinical course of HIV-1 infection. *Annals of Internal Medicine*, v. 127, n. 10, pp. 882-890, ISSN 0003-4819.

Dean, M.; Carrington, M.; Winkler, C.; Huttley, G.A.; Smith, M.W.; Allikmets, R.; Goedert, J.J.; Buchbinder, S.P.; Vittinghoff, E.; Gomperts, E.; Donfield, S.; Vlahov, D.; Kaslow, R.; Saah, A.; Rinaldo, C.; Detels, R. & O'Brien, S.J. (1996). Hemophilia growth and development study, Multicenter AIDS Cohort Study, Multicenter Hemophilia Cohort Study, San Francisco City Cohort, Alive Study, O'Brien, S.J†. Genetic restriction of HIV-1 infection and progression to AIDS by a deletion allele of the CKR5 structural gene. *Science*, v. 273, n.5823, pp. 1856-1862, ISSN 0036-8075.

DeHovitz, J.A.; Kovacs, A.; Feldman, J.G.; Anastos, K.; Young, M.; Cohen, M.; Gange, S.J.; Melnick, S. & Greenblatt, R.M. (2000). The relationship between virus load response to highly active antiretroviral therapy and change in CD4 cell counts: A report from the Women's interagency HIV study. *The Journal of Infectious Diseases*, v. 182, n. 5, pp. 1527-1530, ISSN 0022-1899.

Diop, G.; Hirtzig, T.; Do, H.; Coulonges, C.; Vasilescu, A.; Labib, T.; Spadoni, J.L.; Therwath, A.; Lathrop, M.; Matsuda, F. & Zagury, J.F. (2006). Exhaustive genotyping of the interferon alpha receptor 1 (IFNAR1) gene and association of an IFNAR1 protein variant with AIDS progression or susceptibility to HV-1 infection in a French AIDS cohort. *Biomedicine and Pharmacotherapy*, v.60, n.9, pp. 569-577, ISSN 0753-3322.

Dronda, F.; Moreno, S.; Moreno, A.; Casado, J.L.; Perez-Elias, M.J. & Antela, A. (2002). Long-term outcomes among antiretroviral-naive human immunodeficiency virus-infected patients with small increases in CD4+ cell counts after successful virologic suppression. *Clinical Infectious Diseases*, v. 35, n. 8, pp. 1005-1009, ISSN 1058-4838.

Eugen-Olsen, J.; Iversen, A.K.; Benfield, T.L.; Koppelhus, U. & Garred, P. (1998). Chemokine receptor CCR2b 64I polymorphism and its relation to CD4 T-cell counts and disease progression in a Danish cohort of HIV-infected individuals. Copenhagen AIDS cohort. *Journal of Acquired Immune Deficiency Syndrome and Human Retrovirology*, v. 18, n. 2, pp. 110-116, ISSN 1077-9450.

Eugen-Olsen, J.; Iversen, A.K.; Garred, P.; Koppelhus, U.; Pedersen, C.; Benfield, T.L.; Sorensen, A.M.; Katzenstein, T.; Dickmeiss, E.; Gerstoft, J.; Skinhoj, P.; Svejgaard, A.; Nielsen, J.O. & Hofmann, B. (1997). Heterozygosity for a deletion in the CKR-5 gene leads to prolonged AIDS-free survival and slower CD4 T-cell decline in a cohort of HIV-seropositive individuals. *AIDS* v. 11, n.3, pp. 305–310, ISSN 0269-9370.

Fauci, A.S.; Pantaleo, G.; Stanley, S. & Weissman, D. (1996). Immunopathogenic mechanisms of HIV infection. *Annals of Internal Medicine*, v. 124, pp. 654-663, ISSN 0003-4819.

Faure, S.; Meyer, L.; Costagliola, D.; Vaneensberghe, C.; Genin, E.; Autran, B.; Delfraissy, J.F.; McDermott, D.H.; Murphy, P.M.; Debré, P.; Théodorou, I. & Combadière, C. (2000). Rapid progression to AIDS in HIV+ individuals with a structural variant of the chemokine receptor CX3CR1. *Science*, v. 287, n. 5461, pp. 2274-2277, ISSN 0036-8075.

Faure, S.; Meyer, L.; Genin, E.J.; Pellet, P.; Debre, P.; Theodorou, I. & Combadiere, C. SEROCO Study Group. (2003). Deleterious genetic influence of CX3CR1 genotypes on HIV-1 disease progression. *Journal of Acquired Immune Deficiency Syndrome*, v. 32, n.3, pp. 335-337, ISSN 1525-4135.

Gonzalez, E.; Bamshad, M.; Sato, N.; Mummidi, S.; Dhanda, R.; Catano, G.; Cabrera, S.; McBride, M.; Cao, X.H.; Merrill, G.; O'Connell, P.; Bowden, D.W.; Freedman, B.I.;

Anderson, S.A.; Walter, E.A.; Evans, J.S.; Stephan, K.T.; Clark, R.A.; Tyagi, S.; Ahuja, S.S.; Dolan, M.J. & Ahuja, S.K. Race-specific HIV-1 disease-modifying effects associated with CCR5 haplotypes. *Proceedings of the National Academy of Sciences USA*, v.96, pp12004-12009, ISSN 0027-8424.

Gonzalez, E.; Kulkarni, H.; Bolivar, H.; Mangano, A.; Sanchez, R.; Catano, G.; Invs., R.J.; Freedman, B.I.; Quinones, M.P.; Bamshad, M.J.; Murthy, K.K.; Rovin, B.H.; Bradley, W.; Clark, R.A.; Anderson, S.A.; O'Connell, R.J.; Agan B.K.; Ahuja, S.S.; Bologna, R.; Sen, L.; Dolan, M.J & Ahuja, S.K. (2005). The influence of CCL3L1 gene-containing segmental duplications on HIV-1/AIDS susceptibility. *Science*, v. 307, n. 5714, pp. 1434-1440, ISSN 0036-8075.

Greub, G.; Ledergerber, B.; Battegay, M.; Grob, P.; Perrin, L.; Furrer, H.; Burgisser, P.; Erb, P.; Boggian, K.; Piffaretti, J.C.; Hirschel, B.; Janin, P.; Francioli, P.; Flepp, M. & Telenti, A. (2000). Clinical progression, survival, and immune recovery during antiretroviral therapy in patients with HIV-1 and hepatitis C virus coinfection: the Swiss HIV Cohort Study. *The Lancet*, v. *356*, n.9244, pp. 1800-1805, ISSN 0099-5355.

Guerin, S.; Meyer, L.; Theodorou, I.; Boufassa, F.; Magierowska, M.; Goujard, C.; Rouzious, C.; Debre, P.; Delfraissy, J.F.; SEROCO/HEMOCO Study Group. (2000). CCR5 delta32 deletion and response to highly active antiretroviral therapy in HIV-1-infected patients. *AIDS*, v. 14, n. 17, pp. 2788-2790, ISSN 0269-9370.

Han, X.; Becker, K.; Degen, H.J. Jablonowski, H. & Strohmeyer, G. (1996). Synergistic stimulatory effects of tumor necrosis factor alpha and interferon gamma on replication of human immunodeficiency virus type 1 and on apoptosis of HIV-1-infected host cells. *European Journal of Clinical Investigation*, v.26, n.4, pp. 286-292, ISSN 0014-2972.

Ioannidis, J.P.; O'Brien, T.R.; Rosenberg, P.S.; Contopoulos-Ioannidis, D.G. & Goedert, J.J. (1998). Genetic effects on HIV disease progression. *Nature Medicine*, v. *4*, n.5, pp. 536, ISSN 1078-8956.

Ioannidis, J.P.A.; Rosenberg, P.S.; Goedert, J.J.; Ashton, L.J.; Benfield, T.L.; Buchbinder, S.P.; Coutinho, R.A.; Eugen-Olsen, J.; Gallart, T.; Katzenstein, T.L.; Kostrikis, L.G.; Kuipers, H.; Louie, L.G.; Mallal, S.A.; Margolick, J.B.; Martinez, O.P.; Meyer, L.; Michael, N.L.; Operskalski, E.; Pantaleo, G.; Rizzardi, G.P.; Schuitemaker, H.; Sheppard, H.; Stewart, G.J.; Theodorou, I.D.; Henrik, U.; Vicenzi, E.; Vlahov, D.; Wilkinson, D.; Workman, C.; Zagury, J-F. & O'Brien, T.R. (2001). Effects of CCR5-Delta32, CCR2-64I, and SDF-1 3'A alleles on HIV-1 disease progression: an international meta-analysis of individual-patient data. *Annals of Internal Medicine*, v. 135, pp. 782–795, ISSN 0003-4819.

Jang, D. H.; Choi, B.S. & Kim, S.S. (2008). The effects of RANTES/CCR5 promoter polymorphisms on HIV disease progression in HIV-infected Koreans. *International Journal of Immunogenetics*, v. 35, pp. 101–105, ISSN 1744-3121.

Kalinkovich, A.; Weisman, Z. & Bentwich, Z. (1999). Chemokines and chemokine receptors: role in HIV infection. *Immunological Letters*, v. 68, pp. 281–287.

Kasten, S.; Goldwich, A.; Schmitt, M.; Rascu, A.; Grunke, M.; Dechant, C.; Kalden, J.R. & Harrer. T. (2000). Positive influence of the Delta32CCR5 allele on response to highly active antiretroviral therapy (HAART) in HIV-1 infected patients. *European Journal of Medical Research*, v. *5*, n. 8, pp. 323-328, ISSN: 0949-2321.

Kaur, G. & Mehra, N. (2009). Genetic determinants of HIV-1 infection and progression to AIDS: susceptibility to HIV infection. *Tissue Antigens*, v.73, pp.289-301, ISSN 0001-2815.

Kaur, G.; Singh, P.; Kumar, N.; Rapthap, C.C.; Sharma, G.; Vajpayee, M.; Wig, N.; Sharma, S.K. & Mehra, N.K. (2007). Distribution of CCR2 polymorphism in HIV-1 infected and healthy subjects in North India. *International Journal of Immunogenetics,* v. 34, n.3, pp. 153-156, ISSN 1744-3121.

Kaur, G.; Singh, P.; Rapthap, C.C.; Kumar, N.; Vajpayee, M.; Sharma, S.K.; Wanchu, A. & Mehra, N.K. (2007). Polymorphism in the CCR5 gene promoter and HIV-1 infection in North Indians. *Human Immunology*, v. 68, n.5, pp. 454-461, ISSN 0198-8859.

Kim, S.H.; Cohen, B.; Novick, D. & Rubinstein, M. (1997). Mamalian type I interferon receptors consits of two subunits: IFNaR1 and IFNaR2. *Gene*, v. 196, n.1-2, pp.279-286, ISSN 0378-1119.

Kolmann, T.R.; Pettoello-Mantovani, M.; Katopodis, N.F.; Hachamovitch, M.; Rubistein, A.; Kim, A. & Goldstein, H. (1996). Inhibition of acute in vivo human immunodeficiency virus infection by human interleukin 10 treatment of SCID mice implanted with human fetal thymus and liver. *Proceedings of the National Academy of Sciences USA*, v.93, n.7, pp. 3126-3131, ISSN 0027-8424.

Koning, F.A.; Kwa, D.; Boeser-Nunnink, B.; Dekker, J.; Vingerhoed, J.; Hiemstra, H. & Schuitemaker, H. (2003). Decreasing sensitivity to RANTES (regulated on activation, normally T cell-expressed and -secreted) neutralization of CC chemokine receptor 5-using, non-syncytium-inducing virus variants in the course of human immunodeficiency virus type 1 infection. *The Journal of Infectious Diseases*, v. 188, pp. 864–872, ISSN 0022-1899.

Kostrikis, L.G. ; Neumann, A.U. ; Thomson, B. ; Korber, B.T. ; McHardy, P. ; Karanicolas, R. ; Deustch, L. ; Lew, J.F. ; McIntoch, K. ; Pollack, H. ; Borkowsky, W. ; Spiegel, H.M. ; Palumbo, P. ; Oleske, J. ; Bardeguez, A. ; Luzuriaga, K. ; Sullivan, J. ; Wolinsky, S.M. ; Koup, R.A.; Ho, D.D. & Moore, J.P. (1999). A polymorphism in the regulatory region of the CC-chemokine receptor 5 gene influences perinatal transmission of human immunodeficiency virus type 1 to African-American infants *Journal of Virology*, v. 73, n. 12, pp. 10264-10271, ISSN 0022-538X.

Kostrikis, L.G.; Huang, Y.; Moore, J.P.; Wolinsky, S.M.; Zhang, L.; Guo, Y.; Deutsch, L.; Phair, J.; Neumann, A.U.; Ho, D.D. (1998). A chemokine receptor CCR2 allele delays HIV-1 disease progression and is associated with a CCR5 promoter mutation. *Nature Medicine*, v. 4, n. 3, pp. 350-353, ISSN 1078-8956.

Kwa, D.; Boeser-Nunnink, B. & Schuitemaker, H. (2003). Lack of evidence for an association between a polymorphism in CX3CR1 and the clinical course of HIV infection or virus phenotype evolution. *AIDS*, v. 17, n. 5, pp. 759-761, ISSN 0269-9370.

Ledergerber, B.; Egger, M.; Opravil, M.; Telenti, A.; Hirschel, B.; Battegay, M.; Vernazza, P.; Sudre, P.; Flepp, M.; Furrer, H.; Francioli, P. & Weber, R. (1999). Clinical progression and virological failure on highly active antiretroviral therapy in HIV-1 patients: a prospective cohort study. Swiss HIV Cohort Study. *The Lancet*, v. 353, n.9156, pp. 863-868, ISSN 0099-5355.

Limou, S.; Coulonges, C.; Herbeck, J.T.; van Manen, D.; An, P.; Le Clerc, S.; Delaneau, O.; Diop, G.; Taing, L.; Montes, M.; van't Wout, A.B., Gottlieb, G.S.; Therwath, A.; Rouzioux, C.; Delfraissy, J.F.; Lelièvre, J.D.; LévyM Y,L HercbergM S,L DinaM C,L.;

Phair, J.; Donfield, S.; Goedert, J.J.; Buchbinder, S.; EstaquierM J,L; Schächter, F.; Gut, I.; Froguel, P.; Mullins, J.I.; Schuitemaker, H.; Winkler, C. & Zagury, J.F. (2010). Multiple-cohort genetic association study reveals CXCR6 as a new chemokine receptor involved in long-term nonprogression to AIDS. *The Journal of Infectious Diseases*, v. 202, n. 6, pp. 908-915, ISSN 0022-1899.

Liu, H.; Chao, D.; Nakayama, E.E.; Taguchi, H.; Goto, M.; Xin, X.; Takamatsu, J.K.; Saito, H.; Ishikawa, Y.; Akaza, T.; Juji, T.; Takebe, Y.; Ohishi, T.; Fukutake, K.; Maruyama, Y.; Yashiki, S.; Sonoda, S.; Nakamura, T.; Nagai, Y.; Iwamoto, A. & Shioda, T. (1999). Polymorphism in RANTES chemokine promoter affects HIV-1 disease progression. *Proceedings National Academy of Sciences USA*, v. 96, n. 8, pp. 4581–4585, ISSN 0027-8424.

Liu, S-L.; Schacker, T.; Musey, L.; Shriner, D.; McElrath, M.J.; Corey, L. & Mullins, J.I. (1997). Divergent patterns of progression to AIDS after infection from the same source: human immunodeficiency virus type 1 evolution and antiviral responses. *Journal of Virology*, v. 71, n. 6, pp. 4284-4295, ISSN 0022-538X.

Mabuka, J.M.; Mackelprang, R.D.; Lohman-Payne, B.; Majiwa, M.; Bosire, R.; John-Stewart, G.; Rowland-Jones, S.; Overbaugh, J. & Farquhar, C. (2009). CCR2-64I polymorphism is associated with lower maternal HIV-1 viral load and reduced vertical HIV-1 transmission. *Journal of Acquired Immune Deficiency Syndrome*, v. 51, n. 2, pp. 235-237, ISSN 1525-4135.

Magierowska, M.; Theodorou, I.; Debré, P.; Sanson, F.; Autran, B.; Rivière, Y.; Charron, D.; French ALT and IMMUNOCO Study Groups & Costagliola, D. (1999). Combined genotypes of CCR5, CCR2, SDF1, and HLA genes can predict the long-term nonprogressor status in human immunodeficiency virus-1-infected individuals. *Blood*, v. 93, n. 3, p. 936-941, ISSN 0006-4971.

Martin, M.P.; Dean, M.; Smith, M.W.; Winkler, C.; Gerrard, B.; Michael, N.L.; Lee, B.; Doms, R.W.; Margolick, J.; Buchbinder, S.; Goedert, J.J.; O'Brien, T.R.; Hilgartner, M.W.; Vlahov, D.; O'Brien, S.J. & Carrington, M. (1998). Genetic acceleration of AIDS progression by a promoter variant of CCR5. *Science*, v. 282, n. 5395, pp. 1907-1911, ISSN 0036-8075.

McDermott, D.H.; Beecroft, M.J.; Kleeberger, C.A.; Al-Sharif, F.M.; Ollier, W.E.; Zimmerman, P.A.; Boatin, B.A.; Leitman, S.F.; Detels, R.; Hajeer, A.H. & Murphy, P.M. (2000). Chemokine RANTES promoter polymorphism affects risk of both HIV infection and disease progression in the Multicenter AIDS Cohort Study. *AIDS*, v. 14, n. 17, pp. 2671–2678, ISSN 0269-9370.

McDermott, D.H.; Colla, J.S.; Kleeberger, C.A.; Plankey, M.; Rosenberg, P.S.; Smith, E.D.; Zimmerman, P.A.; Combadiere, C.; Leitman, S.F.; Kaslow, R.A.; Goedert, J.J.; Berger, E.A.; O'Brien, T.R. & Murphy, P.M. (2000). Genetic polymorphism in CX3CR1 and risk of HIV disease. *Science*, v. *290*, n.5499, pp. 2031, ISSN 0036-8075.

McDermott, D.H.; Zimmernan, P.A.; Guignard, F.; Kleeberger, C.A.; Leitman, S.F. & Murphy, P.M. (1998). CCR5 promoter polymorphism and HIV-1 disease progression. Multicenter AIDS Cohort Study (MACS). *The Lancet*, v. 352, n.9131, pp.866-870, ISSN 0099-5355.

Meyer, L.; Magierowska, M.; Hubert, J-B.; Theodorou, I.; van Rij, R.; Prins, M.; de Roda, H.; Coutinho, R. & Schuitemaker, H. (1999). CC-chemokine receptor variants, SDF-1 polymorphism, and disease progression in 720 HIV-infected patients. *AIDS*, v. 13, n. 5, p. 624-626, ISSN 0269-9370.

Michael, N.L.; Louie, L.G.; Rohrbaugh, A.L.; Schultz, K.A.; Dayhoff, D.E.; Wang, C.E. & Sheppard, H.W. (1997). The role of CCR5 and CCR2 polymorphisms in HIV-1 transmission and disease progression. *Nature Medicine,* v.3, n.10, pp.1160-1162, ISSN 1078-8956.

Modi, W.S.; Lautenberger, J.; An, P.; Scott, K.; Goedert, J.J.; Kirk, G.D.; Buchbinder, S.; Phair, J.; Donfield, S.; O'Brien, S.J. & Winkler, C. (2006). Genetic variation in the CCL18-CCL3-CCL4 chemokine gene cluster influences HIV type transmission and AIDS disease progression. *American Journal of Human Genetics*, v. 79, n.1, pp; 120-128, ISSN 1434-5161.

Mulherin, S.A.; O'Brien, T.R.; Ioannidis, J.P.A.; Goedert, J.J.; , Buchbinder, S.P.; Coutinho, R.A.; Jamieson, B.D.; Meyers, L.; Michael, N.L.; Pantaleo, G.; Rizzardi, G.P.; Schuitemaker, H.; Shepaard, H.W.; Theodorou, I.D.; Vlahov, D. & Rosenberg, P.S. (2003). Effects of CCR5-Delta32 and CCR2-64I alleles on HIV-1 disease progression: the protection varies with duration of infection. *AIDS,* v. 17, n. 3, pp. 377-387, ISSN 0269-9370.

Mummidi, S.; Ahuja, S.S.; Gonzalez, E.; Anderson, S.A.; Santiago, E.N.; Stephan, K.T.; Craig, F.E.; O'Connell, P.; Tryon, V.; Clark, R.A.; Dolan, M.J. & Ahuja, S.K. (1998). Genealogy of the CCR5 locus and chemokine system gene variants associated with altered rate if HIV-1 disease progression. *Nature Medicine*, v. 4, n.7, pp. 786-793, ISSN 1078-8956.

Naif, H.M.; Li, S.; Ho-Shon, M.; Mathijs, J.M.; Williamson, P. & Cunningham, A.L. (1997). The state of maturation of monocytes into macrophages determines the effects of IL-4 and IL-13 on HIV replication. *Journal of Immunology*, v. 158, n. 1, pp. 501-511, ISSN 0016-5751.

Nakajima, T.; Kaur, G.; Mehra, N. & Kimura, A. (2008). HIV-1/AIDS susceptibility and copy number variations in CCL3L1, a gene enconding a natural ligand for HIV-1 coreceptor CCR5. *Cytogenetic and Genome Research,* v.123, n.1-4, pp. 156-160, ISSN 1424-8581.

Nakajima, T.; Ohtani, H.; Naruse, T.; Shibata, H.; Mimaya, J.I.; Terunuma, H. & Kimura, A. (2007). Copy number variations of CCL3L1 and long-term prognosis of HIV-1 infection in asymptomatic HIV-infected Japanese with hemophilia. *Immunogenetics*, v.59, n.10, pp. 793-798, ISSN 0093-7711.

Nguyen, L.; Li, M.; Chaowanachan, T.; Hu, D.J.; Vanichseni, S.; Mock, P.A.; van Griensven, F.; Martin, M.; Sangkum, U.; Choopanya, K.; Tappero, J.W.; Lal, R.B. & Yang, C. (2004). CCR5 promoter haplotypes associated with HIV-1 discordant progression in Thai injection drug users. *AIDS*, v.18, n.9, pp.1327-1333, ISSN 0269-9370.

O' Brien, S.J.& Moore, J.P. (2000). The effect of genetic variation in chemokines and their receptors on HIV transmission and progression to AIDS. *Immunological Reviews*, v. 177, pp. 99-111, ISSN 0105-2896.

O' Brien, T.R.; McDermott, D.H.; Ioannidis, J.P.A.; Carrington, M.; Murphy, P.M.; Havlir, D.V. & Richman, D.D. (2000). Effect of chemokine receptor gene polymorphisms on the response to potent antiretroviral therapy. *AIDS*, v. 14, n. 7, p. 821-826, ISSN 0269-9370.

O'Brien, W.A.; Hartigan, P.M.; Daar, E.S.; Simberkoff, M.S. Hamilton, J.D. (1997). Changes in plasma HIV RNA levels and CD4+ lymphocyte counts predict both response to antiretroviral therapy and therapeutic failure. VA Cooperative Study Group on AIDS. *Annals of Internal Medicine,* v. 126, n.12, pp. 939-945, ISSN 0003-4819.

Pantaleo, G.; Demarest, J.F.; Schacker, T.; Vaccarezza, M.; Cohen, O.J.; Daucher, M.; Graziosi, C.; Schnittman, S.S.; Quinn, T.C.; Shaw, G.M.; Perrin, L.; Tambussi, G.; Lazzarin, A.; Sekaly, R.P.; Soudeyns, H.; Corey, L. & Fauci, A.S. (1997). The qualitative nature of the primary immune response to HIV infection is a prognosticator of disease progression independent of the initial level of plasma viremia. *Proceedings National Academy of Sciences USA,* v. 94, n.1, pp. 254-258, ISSN 0027-8424.

Parczewski, M.; Leszczyszyn-Pynka, M.; Kaczmarczyk, M.; Adler, G.; Binczak-Kuleta, A.; Loniewska, B.; Boron-Kaczmarska, A. & Ciechanowicz, A. (2009). Sequence variants of chemokine receptor genes and susceptibility to HIV-1 infection. *Journal of Applied Genetics,* v. 50, n. 2, pp. 159-166, ISSN 1234-1983.

Passam, A.M.; Sourvinos, G.; Krambovitis, E.; Miyakis, S.; Stavrianeas, N.; Zagoreos, I. & Spandidos, D.A. (2007). Polymorphisms of CX(3)CR1 and CXCR6 receptors in relation to HAART therapy of HIV type 1 patients. *AIDS Research and Human Retroviruses,* v. 23, n. 8, pp.1026-1032, ISSN 0889-2229.

Passam, A.M.; Zafiropoulos, A.; Miyakis, S.; Zagoreos, I.; Stavrianeas, N.G.; Krambovitis, E. & Spandidos, D.A. (2005). CCR2-64I and CXCL12 3'A alleles confer a favorable prognosis to AIDS patients undergoing HAART therapy. *Journal of Clinical Virology,* v. 34, pp. 302-309, ISSN 1386-6532.

Paxton, W.A.; Martin, S.R.; Tse, D.; O'Brien, T.R.; Skurnick, J.; VanDevanter, N.; Padian, N.; Braun, J.F.; Kotler, D.P.; Wolinsky, S.M. & Koup RA. (1996). Relative resistance to HIV-1 infection of CD4 lymphocytes from persons who remain uninfected despite multiple high-risk sexual exposure. *Nature Medicine,* v.2, n.4, pp. 412-417, ISSN 1078-8956.

Petit, S.J.; Chayen, N.E. & Pease, J.E.(2008). Site-directed mutagenesis of the chemokine receptor CXCR6 suggests a novel paradigm for interactions with the ligand CXCL16. *European Journal of Immunology,* v. 38, n. 8, pp. 2337-2350.

Piacentini, L., Biasin, M., Fenizia, C. & Clerici, M. (2009). Genetic correlates of protection against HIV infection: the ally within. *Journal of Internal Medicine,* v. 265, pp. 110–124, ISSN 0954-6820.

Potter, S. J., Lacabaratz, C., Lambotte, O., Perez-Patrigeon, S., Vingert, B., Sinet, M., Colle, J. H., Urrutia, A., Scott-Algara, D.; Boufassa, F.; Delfraissy, J.F.; Thèze, J.; Venet, A. & Chakrabarti, L.A. (2007). Preserved central memory and activated effector memory $CD4^+$ T-cell subsets in human immunodeficiency virus controllers: an ANRS EP36 study. *Journal of Virology,* v. 81, n.24, pp. 13904–13915, ISSN 0022-538X

Puissant, B.; Roubinet, F.; Massip, P.; Sandres-Saune, K.; Apoil, P-A.; Abbal, M.; Pasquier, C.; Izopet, J. & Blancher, A. (2006). Analysis of CCR5, CCR2, CX3CR1, and SDF1 polymorphisms in HIV-positive treated patients: impact on response to HAART and o peripheral T lymphocyte counts. *AIDS Research and Human Retroviruses,* v. 22, n. 2, pp. 153-162, ISSN 0889-2229.

Qian, Y.; Sun, H.; Lin, K.; Shi, L.; Shi, L. & Chu, J. (2008). Distribution of CCR5-Delta32, CCR2-64I, SDF1-3'A, CX3CR1-249I, and CX3CR1-280M in Chinese populations. *AIDS Research Human Retroviruses,* v. 24, n. 11, pp. 1391-1397.

Quillent, C.; Oberlin, E.; Braun, J.; Rousset, D.; Gonzales-Canali, G.; Métais, P.; Montagnier, L.; Virelizier, J-L.; Arenzana-Seisdedos, F. & Beretta, A. (1998). HIV-1 resistance phenotype conferred by combination of two separate inherited mutations of CCR5 gene. *The Lancet*, v. 351, pp. 14-18, ISSN 0099-5355.

Ramana, G.V.; Vasanthi, A.; Khaja, M.; Su, B.; Govindaiah, V.; Jin, L.; Singh, L. & Chakraborty, R. (2001). Distribution of HIV-1 resistance-conferring polymorphic alleles SDF-1-3'A, CCR2-64I and CCR5-Delta32 in diverse populations of Andhra Pradesh, South India. *Journal of Genetics*, v. 80, n.3, pp. 137–140.

Rathore, A.; Chatterjee, A.; Sivarama, P.; Yamamoto, N.; Singhal, P.K. & Dhole, T.N. (2009). Association of CCR5-59020 A/G and CCL3L1 copy number polymorphism with HIV type 1 transmission/progression among HIV type 1-seropositive and repeatedly sexually exposed HIV type 1-seronegative North Indians. *AIDS Research and Human Retroviruses*, v.25, n.11, pp.1149-1156, ISSN 0889-2229.

Reiche, E. M.; Ehara Watanabe, M.A.; Bonametti, A. M.; Kaminami Morimoto, H.; Akira Morimoto, A.; Wiechmann, S.L.; Breganó, J.W.; Matsuo, T.; Vissoci Reiche, F.; Miranda, H.C.; Brajão Oliveira, K.; Vogler, I.H.; Siscar, A.R. (2006). The effect of stromal cell-derived factor 1 (SDF1/CXCL12) genetic polymorphism on HIV-1 disease progression. *International Journal of Molecular Medicine*, v. 18, n.4, pp. 785-793, ISSN 1107-3756.

Reiche, E.M.V.; Bonametti, A.M.; Voltarelli, J.C.; Morimoto, H.K. & Watanabe, M.A.E. (2007). Genetic polymorphisms in the chemokine and chemokine receptors: impact on clinical course and therapy of the human immunodeficiency virus type 1 infection (HIV-1). *Current Medicinal Chemistry*, v.14, n. 12, pp. 1325-1334, ISSN 0929-8673.

Reynes, J.; Portales, P.; Segondy, M.; Baillat, V.; André, P.; Réant, B.; Avinens, O.; Couderc, G.; Benkirane, M.; Clot, J.; Eliaou, J.F. & Corbeau, P. (2000). CD4+ T cell surface CCR5 density as a determining factor of virus load in persons infected with human immunodeficiency virus type 1. *The Journal of Infectious Diseases*, v. 181, n.3, pp. 927-932, ISSN 0022-1899.

Rigato, P.O.; Hong, M.A.; Casseb, J.; Ueda, M.; de Castro, I.; Benard, G. & Duarte, A.J. (2008). Better CD4+ T cell recovery in Brazilian HIV-infected individuals under HAART due to cumulative carriage of SDF-1-3'A, CCR2-V64I, CCR5-Δ32 and CCR5-promoter 59029A/G polymorphisms. *Current HIV Research*, v. 6, n. 5, pp. 466-473, ISSN 1570-162X.

Risma, K.A.; Wang, N.; Andrews, R.P.; Cunningham, C.M.; Ericksen, M.B.; Bernstein, J.A.; Chakraborty, R & Hershey, G.K. (2002). V75R567 Il-4 receptor alpha is associated with allergic asthma and enhanced IL-4 receptor function. *Journal of Immunology*, v.169, n.3, pp. 1604-1610, ISSN 0016-5751.

Rosenberg, Z.F. & Fauci, A.S. (1991). Immunopathogenesis of HIV infection. *FASEB Journal*, v. 5, pp. 2382-2390.

Salem, A.H.; Farid, E.; Fadel, R.; Abu-Hijleh, M.; Almawi, W.; Han, K.; Batzer, M.A. (2009). Distribution of four HIV type 1-resistance polymorphisms (CCR5-Delta32, CCR5-m303, CCR2-64I, and SDF1-3'A) in the Bahraini population. *AIDS Res Hum Retroviruses*, v. 25, n.10, pp 973-977.

Samsom, M.; Libert, F.; Doranz, B.J.; Rucker, J.; Liesnard, C.; Farber, C.M.; Saragosti, S.; Lapoumeroulie, C.; Cognaux, J.; Forceille, C.; Muyldermans, G.; Verhofstede, C.; Burtonboy, G.; Georges, M.; Imai, T.; Rana, S.; Yi, Y.; Smyth, R.J.; Collman, R.G.;

Doms, R.W.; Vassart, G. & Parmentier, M. (1996). Resistance to HIV-1 infection in Caucasian individuals bearing mutant alleles of the CCR-5 chemokine receptor gene. *Nature*, v. 382, n. 6593, pp. 722-726, ISSN 0028-0836.

Schuitemaker, H.; Koot, M.; Kootstra, N.A.; Dercksen, M.W.; de Goede, R.E.Y.; van Steenwijk, R.P.; Lange, J.M.; Schattenkerk, J.K.M.; Miedema, F. & Tersmette, M. (1992). Biological phenotype of human immunodeficiency virus type 1 clones at different stages of infection: progression of disease is associated with a shift from monocytotropic to T-cell-tropic virus populations. *Journal of Virology*, n. 66, n.3, pp. 1354-1360, ISSN 0022-538X.

Smith, M.W.; Carrington, M.; Winkler, C.; Lomb, D.; Dean, M.; Huttley, G. & O'Brien, S.J. (1997). CCR2 chemokine receptor and AIDS progression. *Nature Medicine*, v.3, pp. 1052-1053, ISSN 1078-8956.

Smith, M.W.; Dean, M.; Carrington, M.; Winkler, C.; Huttley, G.A.; Lomb, D.A.; Goedert, J.J.; O'Brien, T.R.; Jacobson, L.P.; Kaslow, R.; Buchbinder, S.; Vittinghoff, E.; Vlahov, D.; Hoots, K.; Hilgartner, M.W. & O'Brien, S.J. (1997). Contrasting genetic influence of CCR2 and CCR5 variants on HIV-1 infection and disease progression. Hemophilia Growth and Development Study (HGDS), Multicenter AIDS Cohort Study (MACS), Multicenter Hemophilia Cohort Study (MHCS), San Francisco City Cohort (SFCC), ALIVE Study. *Science*, v. *277*, pp. 959–965, ISSN 0036-8075.

Soriano, A.; Lozano, F.; Oliva, H.; Garcia, F.; Nomdedeu, M.; De Lazzari, E.; Rodríguez, C.; Barrasa, A.; Lorenzo, J.I.; Del Romero, J.; Plana, M.; Miró, J.M.; Gatell, J.M.; Vives, J. & Gallart, T. (2005). Polymorphisms in the interleukin-4 receptor alpha chain gene influence susceptibility to HIV-1 infection and its progression to AIDS. *Immunogenetics*, v.57, n.9, pp.644-654, ISSN 0093-7711.

Soriano, A.; Martínez, C.; García, F.; Plana, M.; Palou, E.; Lejeune, M.; Aróstegui, J.I.; De Lazzari, E.; Rodriguez, C.; Barrasa, A.; Lorenzo, J.I.; Alcamí, J.; Romero, J.D.; Miró, J.M.; Gatell, J.M. & Gallart, T. (2002). Plasma stromal cell-derived factor (SDF)-1 levels, SDF1-3'A genotype, and expression of CXCR4 on T lymphocytes: their impact on resistance to in human immunodeficiency virus type 1 infection and its progression. *The Journal of Infectious Diseases*, v. 186, n. 7, pp. 922-931, ISSN 0022-1899.

Su, B.; Jin, L.; Hu, F.; Xiao, J.; Luo, J.; Lu, D.; Zhang, W.; Chu, J.; Du, R.; Geng, Z.; Qiu, X.; Xue, J.; Tan, J.; O'Brien, S.J. & Chakraborty, R. (1999). Distribution of two HIV-1 resistant polymorphisms (SDF1-3'A and CCR2-64I) in East Asia and world populations and its implication in AIDS epidemiology. *American Journal of Human Genetics*, v. 65, n. 4, pp. 1047-1053, ISSN 1434-5161.

Su, Q.; Mai, Z.; Zang, N.; Wu, S.; Xiao, X. & Liang, H. (2010). Distribution of CCR5-delta-32, CCR2-64I, and SDF1-3'A in Guangxi Zhuang population. *Journal of the International Association of Physicians in AIDS Care*, v. 9, n. 3, pp. 145-149.

Tan, X.H.; Zhang, J.Y.; Di, C.H.; Hu, A.R.; Yang, L.; Qu, S.; Zhao, R.L.; Yang, P.R. & Guo, S.X. (2009). Distribution of CCR5-Delta32, CCR5m303A, CCR2-64I and SDF1-3'A in HIV-1 infected and uninfected high-risk Uighurs in Xinjiang, China. *Infection, Genetics and Evolution*, v. 10, n. 2, pp. 268-272.

Theodorou, I.; Meyer, L.; Magierowska, M.; Katlama, C. & Rouzioux, C. (1997). HIV-1 infection in an individual homozygous for CCR5 delta 32. Seroco Study Group. *The Lancet*, v. 349, n.9060, pp. 1219-1220, ISSN 0099-5355.

Tresoldi, E.; Romiti, M.L.; Boniotto, M.; Crovella, S.; Salvatori, F.; Palomba, E.; Pastore, A.; Cancrini, C.; Martino, M.; Plebani, A.; Castelli, G.; Rossi, P.; Tovo, P.A.; Amoroso, A.; & Scarlatti, G. in Cooperation with the European Shared Cost Project Group and the Italian Register for GIV Infection in Children. (2002). Prognostic value of the stromal cell-derived factor 1 3'A mutation in pediatric human immunodeficiency virus type 1 infection. *The Journal of Infectious Diseases,* v. 185, pp. 696–700, ISSN 0022-1899.

Vaamonde, C.M.; Hoover, D.R.; Anastos, K.; Tan, T.; Shi, Q.; Gao, W.; Kovacs, A.; Cohen, M.; De Hovitz J. & Glesby, M.J. (2006). Factors associated with poor immunologic response to virologic suppression by highly active antiretroviral therapy in HIV-infected women. *AIDS Research and Human Retroviruses,* v. 22, n.3, pp. 222-231, ISSN 0889-2229.

van Rij, R.P.; Broersen, S.; Goudsmit, J.; Coutinho, R.A. & Schuitemaker, H. (1998). The role of a stromal cell-derived factor-1 chemokine gene variant in the clinical course of HIV-1 infection. *AIDS,* v. 12, n. 9, pp. F-85-F90, ISSN 0269-9370.

Vasilescu, A.; Terashima, Y.; Enbomoto, M.; Heath, S.; Poonpiriya, V.; Gatanaga, H.; Do, H.; Diop, G.; Hirtzig, T.; Auewarakul, P.; Lauhakirti, D.; Sura, T.; Charneau, P.; Marullo, S.; Therwath, A.; Oka, S.; Kanegasaki, S.; Lathrop, M.; Matsushima, K.; Zagury, J.F. & Matsuda, F. (2007). A haplotype of the human CXCR1 gene protective against rapid disease progression in HIV-1+ patients. *Proceedings of the National Academy of Sciences USA,* v. 104, n.9, pp. 3354-3359, ISSN 0027-8424.

Veloso, S.; Olona, M.; García, F.; Domingo, P.; Alonso-Villaverde, C.; Broch, M.; Peraire, J.; Viladés, C.; Plana, M.; Pedrol, E.; López-Dupla, M.; Aguilar, C.; Gutiérrez, M.; Leon, A.; Tasias, M.; Gatell, J.M.; Richart, C. & Vidal, F. (2010). Effect of *TNF-α* genetic variants and *CCR5-Δ32* on the vulnerability to HIV-1 infections and disease progression in Caucasian Spaniards. *BMC Medical Genetics,* v.11, pp.63, ISSN 1471-2350.

Verma, R.; Guptya, R.B.; Singh, K.; Bhasin, R.; Shukla, A.A.; Chauhan, S.S. & Luthra, K. (2007). Distribution of CR5Δ32, CCR2-64I and SDF1-3'A and plasma levels of SDF-1 in HIV-1 seronegative North Indians. *Journal of Clinical Virology,* v. 38, pp. 198–203, ISSN 1386-6532.

Viard, J.P.; Mocroft, A.; Chiesi, A.; Kirk, O.; Roge, B.; Panos, G.; Vetter, N.; Bruun , J.N.; Jonson, M. & Lundgren, J.D.(2001) Influence of age on CD4 cell recovery in human immunodeficiency virus-infected patients receiving highly active antiretroviral therapy: evidence from the Euro SIDA study. *The Journal of Infectious Diseases,* v. 183 n.8, pp. 1290-1294, ISSN 0022-1899.

Vidal, F., Peraire, J., Domingo, P., Broch, M., Knobel, H., Pedrol, E., Dalmau, D., Vilades, C. & Sambeat, MA. (2005a). Lack of association of SDF-1 3'A variant allele with long-term nonprogressive HIV-1 infection is extended beyond 16 years. *Journal of Acquired Immune Deficiency Syndrome,* v. 40, pp. 276–279, ISSN 1525-4135.

Vidal, F., Vilades, C., Domingo, P., Broch, M., Pedrol, E., Dalmau, D., Knobel, H., Peraire, J., Gutierrez, C.; Sambeat, M.A.; Fontanet, A.; Deig, E.; Cairó, M.; Montero, M.; Richart, C.; Mallal, S. & Chemokines LTNP Study Group. (2005b). Spanish HIV-1-infected long-term nonprogressors of more than 15 years have an increased frequency of the CX3CR1 249I variant allele. *Journal of Acquired Immune Deficiency Syndrome,* v. 40, n.5, pp. 527–531, ISSN 1525-4135.

Wang, F-S.; Hong, W-G.; Cao, Y.; Liu, M-X.; Jin, L.; Hu, L-P.; Wang, Z.; Feng, T-J.; Hou, J.; Zhang, B.; Shi, M.; Xu, D-P.; Lei, Z-Y.; Wang, B.; Liu, Z-D.; Ye, J-J.; Peng, L.; Qiu, Y. & Winkler, C. (2003). Population survey of CCR5-Δ32, CCR m3030, CCR2b 64I, and SDF1 3'A allele frequencies in indigenous Chinese healthy individuals, and HIV-1 infected and HIV-1-unifected individuals in HIV-1 risk groups. *Journal of Acquired Immune Deficiency Syndrome*, v. 32, n. 2, pp. 124-130, ISSN 1525-4135.

Wichukchinda, N., Nakayama, E. E., Rojanawiwat, A., Pathipvanich, P., Auwanit, W., Vongsheree, S., Ariyoshi, K., Sawanpanyalert, P. & Shioda, T. (2006). Protective effects of IL4–589T and RANTES-28G on HIV-1 disease progression in infected Thai females. *AIDS*, v. 20, pp.189–196, ISSN 0269-9370.

Williamson, C.; Loubser, S.A.; Brice, B.; Joubert, G.; Smit, T.; Thomas, R.; Visagie , M.; Cooper M, Ryst E van der. (2000). Allelic frequencies of host genetic variants influencing susceptibility to HIV-1 infection and disease in South African populations. *AIDS*, v. 14, n. 4, p. 449-451, ISSN 0269-9370.

Winkler, C.; Modi, W.; Smith, M.W.; Nelson, G.W.; Wu, X.; Carrington, M.; Dean, M.; Honjo, T.; Tashiro, K.; Yabe, D.; Buchbinder, S.; Vittinghoff, E.; Goedert, J.J.; O'Brien, T.R.; Jacobson, L.P.; Detels, R. Donfield, S.; Willoughby, A.; Gomperts, E.; Vlahov, D.; Phair, J. & O'Brien, S.J. (1998). Genetic restriction of AIDS pathogenesis by an SDF-1 chemokine gene variant. ALIVE study, Hemophilia Growth and Development Study (HGDS), Multicenter AIDS Cohort Study (MACS), Multicenter Hemophilia Cohort Study (MHCS), San Francisco City Cohort (SFCS). *Science*, v. 279, n. 5349, pp. 389-393, ISSN 0036-8075.

Wit, F.W.; van Rij. R.P.; Weverling, G.J.; Jange, J.M. & Schuitemaker, H. (2002). CC chemokine receptor 5 delta32 and CC chemokine receptor 2 64I polymorphisms do not influence the virologic and immunologic response to antiretroviral combination therapy in human immunodeficiency virus type 1-infected patients. *The Journal of Infectious Diseases*, v. 186, n.12, pp. 1726-1732, ISSN 0022-1899.

Yamashita, T.E.;, Phair, J.P.; Muñoz, A.; Margolick, J.B.; Detels, R.; O'Brien, S.J.; Mellors, J.W.; Wolinsky, S.M. & Jacobson, L.P. (2001). Immunologic and virologic response to highly active antiretroviral therapy in the Multicenter AIDS Cohort Study. *AIDS*, v. 15, p. 735-746, ISSN 0269-9370.

Zimmerman, P.; Buckler-White, A.; Alkhatib, G.; Spalding, T.; Kubofcik, J.; Combadiere, C.; Weissman, D.; Cohen, O.; Rubbert, A.; Lam, G.; Vaccarezza, M.; Kennedy, P.E.; Kumaraswami, V.; Giorgi, J.V.; Detels, R.; Hunter, J.; Choper, M.; Berger, E.A.; Fauci, A.S.; Nutman, T.B. & Murphy, P.M. (1997). Inherited resistance to HIV-1 conferred by an inactivating mutation in CC chemokine receptor 5: studies in populations with contrasting clinical phenotypes, defined racial background, and quantified risk. *Molecular Medicine*, v. *3*, n. 1, pp. 23-26, ISSN 1077-1551.

13

CXCL8 Regulation and Function in HIV Infections and Potential Treatment Strategies

Per-Erik Olsson, Hazem Khalaf and Jana Jass
Örebro Life Science Center, School of Science and Technology, Örebro University
Sweden

1. Introduction

Interleukin-8 (CXCL8) is a chemokine that was originally identified as a key factor in neutrophil recruitment and activation. Numerous cell types produce CXCL8, including immune cells, mucosal epithelial cells, endothelial cells and smooth muscle cells (Garcia-Vicuna et al., 2004). CXCL8 is one of the important inflammatory mediators responsible for the recruitment of neutrophils and T-cells to the site of infection, therefore it is an attractive target for therapy against diseases that affect immune cells such as HIV. HIV directly targets the host's immune system and thus reduces the ability of the innate and adaptive immune system to fight disease. As a chemokine, CXCL8 is a potential target for controling HIV infection by reducing the migration of T-cells to the site of infection. It is therefore necessary to identify the signaling pathways involved in CXCL8 regulation in order to develop viable CXCL8 based treatment strategies. In line with this, we have recent shown that CXCL8 activation in Jurkat T-cells is not primarily under the control of NFκB, but that the AP-1 signaling pathway appears to be central for the regulation of CXCL8 (Khalaf et al., 2010). An understanding of the regulation and function of cytokines and chemokines, while complex, remains important for the development of new strategies in the development of HIV treatments. It is interesting to note that several lactobacilli strains are able to modulate CXCL8 expression and release (Anukam et al., 2009; Zhang et al., 2005). Disturbance of the lactobacilli flora in the vaginal tract has been shown to increase the risk of infections and acquisition of HIV type 1 (Taha et al., 1998). Several studies have shown that treatment with certain *Lactobacillus* species and strains have positive effects on women with HIV infections and have been successful in trials to counteract vaginal infections (Hummelen et al., 2010; Spear et al., 2007).

In the present chapter we give a background to CXCL8 regulation and function as well as its involvement in HIV etiology. We also provide an overview of the available information on the possible uses of *Lactobacillus* species in treatment of infections with special emphasis on HIV. In addition, the effects obtained by using lactobacilli treatment together with expression of adhesion inhibitors will be discussed. The aim is to give the reader an overview of the role of CXCL8 in HIV infections and combine this with information on how lactobacilli treatment influences the chemokine levels and evaluate these systems potential in the treatment of HIV patients.

1.1 Inflammatory responses

Pro-inflammatory cytokines, such as TNF, IL-1 and IL-6, as well as the chemokine CXCL8 promote inflammation, whereas anti-inflammatory cytokines, including IL-4, IL-10 and IL-13, suppress the activity of pro-inflammatory cytokines (Dinarello, 2000). Gene-expression and release of cytokines, such as TNF, IL-1 and IL-6, and cell adhesion molecules, including ICAM-1, P selectin, and E selectin, are indicators of induced inflammatory responses (Pearson et al., 2003). NF-κB has been proposed as the main transcriptional regulator of cytokine expression, adhesion factors and anti-apoptotic factors (McKay & Cidlowski, 1999). It has been suggested that inflammatory cytokines, such as TNF, are involved in the induction of reactive oxygen intermediates (O_2^-) that cause DNA damage (Shoji et al., 1995). Recent observations have shown that elevated levels of IL-6 and C-reactive protein are associated with the development of atherosclerosis and type II diabetes (Libby et al., 2002). Elevated cytokine levels are also associated with cellular senescence and may be involved in telomere shortening and continuous cell divisions (Itahana et al., 2001).

1.2 T-cell derived inflammatory responses

Optimal T-cell activation is achieved following antigen binding to the T-cell receptor (TCR), together with co-stimulatory signals followed by cytokine expression (Gonzalo et al., 2001). T-cells produce a broad range of pro- and anti-inflammatory cytokines, including IL-2, IL-6, IL-10 and TNF, in response to infections (Opal & DePalo, 2000). IL-10 is another important anti-inflammatory cytokine expressed by activated T-cells, providing control of intestinal inflammatory responses, but is also important for normal T-cell function (Asseman et al., 1999). Chemokine expression (CXCL8) by $CD8^+$ T-cells is crucial in immune responses by inducing cytokines, such as TNF and IFN-γ by $CD4^+$ cells, and antibody secretion by B-cells (Kim et al., 1998). Recent findings provide evidence indicating expression of several types of Toll-like receptors (TLRs), including TLR4, on T-cells (Caramalho et al., 2003). These results demonstrate a specific role of T-cells in the induction of inflammatory responses by direct recognition of antigens, independent of antigen-presenting cells.

1.3 Epithelial cell derived inflammatory responses

Wounds, chemical irritation or infection may cause inflammation of the epithelial surface. Acute inflammation induces expression of pro-inflammatory cytokines and chemokines that attract immune cells, such as neutrophils, followed by the production of anti-inflammatory cytokines thereby initiating the healing process (Philip et al., 2004). The balance between pro- and anti-inflammatory cytokines determines the severity of an infection. However, prolonged inflammatory responses are prevented by the expression of IL-1ra, glucocorticoids and IL-10, which also improves cell survival (Berg et al., 1995; van der Poll et al., 1997; Walley et al., 1996). Lipopolysaccharides (LPS) are well-known bacterial toxins and potent inducers of inflammatory responses. It has been suggested that epithelial cells are refractory to LPS since they do not express surface CD14, an important signaling protein that functions by docking the LPS/LBP (Lipid binding protein)- complex with TLR4 to initiate intracellular signaling cascades (Svanborg et al., 1999). However, in the presence of serum cells, epithelial cells respond to LPS, demonstrating the presence of a second soluble form of CD14 (sCD14) (Noel et al., 1995; Riedel et al., 2006). Furthermore, CD14-independent pathways are also present in epithelial cells that can be triggered by substances such as peptidoglycan and result in the release of pro-inflammatory cytokines (Sato et al.,

2003). While inflammatory responses are mainly induced through signals transduced via TLRs on epithelial cell surface, there is evidence indicating involvement of other membrane receptors, including Dectin-1, in the enhancement of inflammatory responses (Gantner et al., 2003).

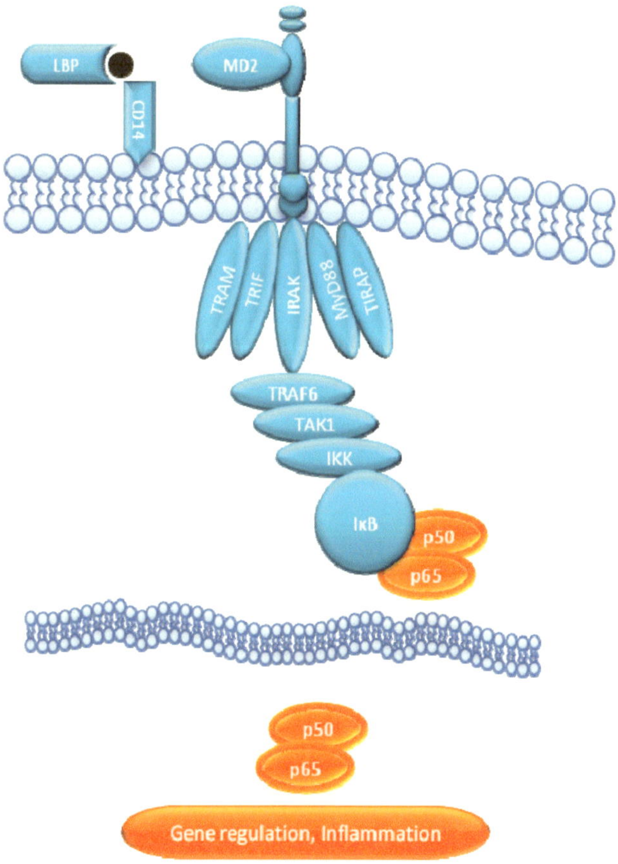

Fig. 1. Inflammation induced by LPS, which binds to TLR4 and signals for MyD88 activation that in turn starts a phosphorylation cascade leading to NF-κB activation and nuclear translocation.

1.4 NF-κB and MAPK signaling pathways

Recognition of toxins by epithelial- and immune cells occurs via TLRs that activate specific intracellular signaling pathways and result in the transcription of essential proteins for survival. Currently, more than 10 TLRs have been identified and recognize; among others, zymosan (TLR1/TLR2), LPS-LTA (TLR4-TLR2/TLR6) and dsRNA (TLR3) (Xu et al., 2001). NF-κB has a central role in the induction of inflammatory responses by regulating a wide range of genes. Several stress factors can activate NF-κB, including bacterial toxins, cytokines, reactive oxygen species and UV light. Bacterial toxins, such as LPS and peptidoglycan, activate NF-κB via TLRs whereas cytokines, TNF, IL-1, signal via TNF-R1 and IL-1R on the membrane surface (Dinarello, 2000). LPS activates NF-κB following binding to a LPS-binding protein, which facilitates LPS binding to CD14. Once bound to CD14, the LPS-binding protein dissociates, and the LPS-CD14 complex associates with TLR4 with the help of the extracellular protein MD2. The binding of LPS-CD14 complex leads to the activation and binding of a cytoplasmic signaling molecule called myeloid differentiation factor 88 (MyD88). Binding of MyD88 leads to the activation of interleukin-1-receptor-associated kinase (IRAK), which phosphorylates TNF-receptor-associated factor (TRAF) 6. TRAF6 leads to the activation of TGF-beta activated kinase (TAK) 1, which activates NF-κB-inducible kinase (NIK). IκB kinase (IKK), activated by NIK, phosphorylates the inhibitory protein IκB followed by subsequent degradation in the proteasome. This leads to NF-κB activation, which translocates into the nucleus and initiates transcription of a wide range of inflammatory genes (Fig. 1) (Ali & Mann, 2004).

An additional important signaling pathway involved in the induction of cytokines and inflammation is the mitogen-activated protein kinase (MAPK) pathway. Several stress factors can induce the activation of MAPK pathway, however only pro-inflammatory cytokines and growth factors can induce inflammation, apoptosis or differentiation through either p38 MAPK or c-Jun NH_2-terminal kinase (JNK). There are three major groups of MAPKs; p38 Map kinase family, extracellular signal-regulated kinase (Erk) family and JNK family (McCarroll et al., 2003). A series of phosphorylation steps are the key events leading to MAPK activation and gene-expression (Faure et al., 1994). Furthermore, activation of the Raf/MAPK pathway has been shown to stimulate transcription of, among others, cytokines through AP-1, NF-IL6 and NF-κB (Bruder & Kovesdi, 1997).

Since T-cells lack TLRs, antigens are recognized by the TCR with the help of co-stimulatory receptors, such as CD28. This results in the activation of resting T-cells and a signaling cascade that activates phospholipase C (PLC) and cleavage of phosphatidylinositol bis-phosphate (PIP2) to inositol (1,4,5)-trisphosphate (IP3) and diacylglycerol (DAG) (Teixeira et al., 2003). IP3 mobilize Ca^{2+} from intracellular stores and together with DAG activates PKC (Gajewski et al., 1994; Werlen et al., 1998). In addition, Ca^{2+} also activates calcineurin/calmodulin and RasGRP, which is a Ras activator and is directly connected to the MAPK pathway (Dower et al., 2000). Recent reports have revealed the importance of three additional intracellular proteins, namely CARMA1, Bcl10 and MALT1 (CBM) in the induction of NF-κB (Scharschmidt et al., 2004). Down regulation of Bcl10 was shown to result in inhibition of NF-κB, transduced via TCR/CD28 and PKC. It was suggested that Bcl10 is initially activated by TCR/PKC but further activation (>1h) promotes its degradation. Furthermore, deletion of any component of the CBM complex impairs antigen receptor activation of NF-κB (Gaide et al., 2002; Narayan et al., 2006). CARMA1 has been shown to be required for NF-κB activation through Akt signaling, in cooperation with PKC following short-term exposure (30min) of Jurkat T-cells with PMA (Narayan et al., 2006). These studies indicate that PKC is crucial for NF-κB activation, following short-term exposure; from signals transduced via TCR and co-stimulatory receptors, such as CD28, and that the CBM complex proteins play a key role in these signaling processes (Fig. 2).

NF-κB is an important transcription factor complex involved in almost every aspect of cell regulation including apoptosis, differentiation, proliferation and initiation of immune responses (Barnes & Adcock, 1997; Makarov, 2000; Tergaonkar, 2006). NF-κB is an attractive therapeutic target since it is constitutively active in many human malignancies (Dolcet et al., 2005).

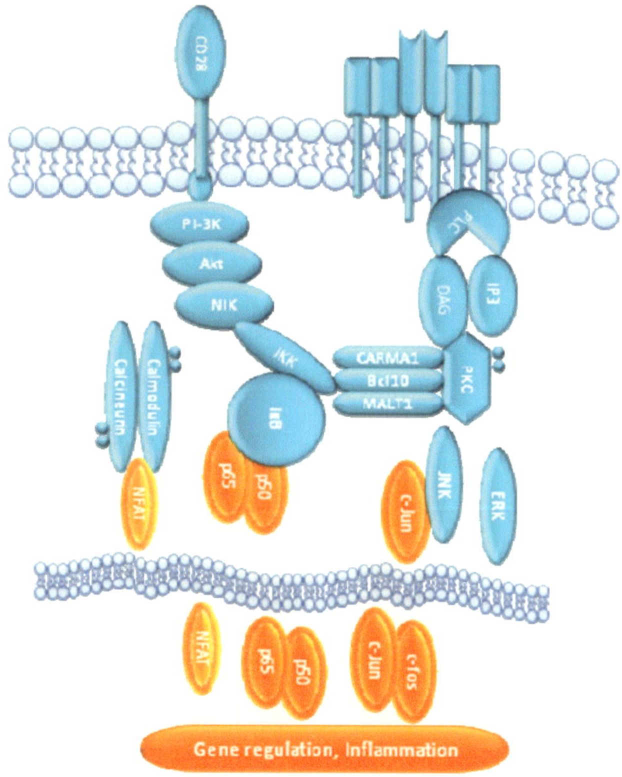

Fig. 2. T-cells recognize antigens via TCR and co-stimulatory receptors (CD28), leading to a downstream signaling cascade involving PKC activation and several transcription factors including NF-κB, AP-1 and NFAT.

2. CXCL8 regulation and signal transduction

In order to understand how CXCL8 contributes to the etiology of HIV, it is important to characterize the cellular signal transduction pathways regulating CXCL8. There are over 50 chemokines identified and almost 18 chemokine receptors have been characterized (Alfano & Poli, 2005). Chemokines are divided into four categories according to the location of two cysteine residues at the N-terminal region. These include C, CC, CXC and CX_3C chemokines (Zlotnik & Yoshie, 2000). Chemokine receptors have been designated the same nomenclature as for their respective chemokine. Besides several immune cells, many other cell types have been described to express chemokine receptors, including endothelial cells, fibroblasts and smooth muscle cells (Garcia-Vicuna et al., 2004). This indicates that chemokines are not only implicated in the regulation of cell trafficking but also in cell proliferation and gene regulation (Wong & Fish, 2003).

Several chemokines share the same receptor but possess different binding affinities to each one. We have previously shown an association between IL-6 release and NF-κB activity while CXCL8 release was more closely correlated with activator protein (AP)-1 activity (Khalaf et al., 2010). Blocking NF-κB activation resulted in a complete inhibition of IL-6 while the CXCL8 levels remained elevated as shown both at the protein and mRNA levels.

Our results indicate that in Jurkat T-cells, IL-6 is regulated through NF-κB while CXCL8 regulation is independent of NF-κB and is closely associated with AP-1 activation. The interplay between immune cells and the expression levels of different cytokines/chemokines is an important factor for consideration.

The gram-negative derived endotoxin, LPS, is a known factor reported to induce CXCL8 expression and release. However, pre-treatment with anti-inflammatory cytokines, including IL-4, IL-10 and TGF-β1, resulted in a significant reduction in CXCL8 expression (Ehrlich et al., 1998). Thus, the balance between pro- and anti-inflammatory cytokines is a determinant factor for immune cell activation as well as the expression levels of cytokines and chemokines released by different cells. Maintaining this balance is therefore of great importance, however there is a need to improve our understanding about the regulatory mechanisms controlling the expression of inflammatory mediators and their effect(s) on different immune cells.

The main regulators of *cxcl8* gene expression are NF-κB and the MAP kinases JNK, ERK and p38 leading to the assembly and activation of the transcription factor AP-1. NF-κB is required for CXCL8 release in most cell types, while optimal induction is achieved following binding of additional transcription factor including MAP kinases and C/EBP (Hoffmann et al., 2002). However, the ratio of activation between NF-κB to MAPK and other transcription factors in this regulatory mechanism seems to differ depending on the pressure caused by a specific stress factor and cell type. In airway epithelial cells NF-κB, ERK and JNK were found to be essential for TNF-induced CXCL8 expression, while p38 acted as a posttranscriptional regulator (Li et al., 2002). Even though p38 is not required for *cxcl8* gene expression, it plays a major role in CXCL8 release by stabilizing its mRNA through protein kinase-2 (Hoffmann et al., 2002). A simplified representation of the signaling pathways involved in CXCL8 expression and regulation is shown in figure 3. Furthermore, reactive oxygen intermediates (ROI) are important regulators of cytokine and chemokine expression and has been shown to mediate a dose-dependent CXCL8 expression (DeForge et al., 1993). They further demonstrated that the effect of these potent immune regulators could be almost completely abolished by applying the OH-radical scavenger DMSO, which reduced CXCL8 expression by 90%.

There are two well-characterized receptors for CXCL8, namely CXC chemokine receptor (CXCR)-1 and -2. CXCL8 binds to these receptors with high affinity (Bertini et al., 2004), while CXCR1 is specific for CXCL8, (NAP)-2 and granulocyte chemotactic protein (GCP)-2, CXCR2 can bind additional chemokines, including CXCL1, 2, 3, 5, 6 and 7 (Acosta et al., 2008). Despite their structural similarities, these receptors possess different biological effects through distinct signaling pathways (Gabellini et al., 2009).

Signals transduced through CXCR1 stimulate neutrophil migration through epithelial layers, while CXCR2 signaling promotes angiogenesis (Sturm et al., 2005). The intracellular protein Bcl-10 has been proposed to play a critical role in the signaling pathway leading to CXCL8 expression and its enhancement of angiogenesis through CXCR2 (Karl et al., 2005). Both NF-κB and C/EBP have been reported to be downstream targets of activation in the CXCR2 signaling cascade, ultimately leading to CXCL8 expression, creating a positive feedback loop (Acosta & Gil, 2009). This positive feedback loop leading to neutrophil activation and migration is regulated by internalization of CXCR1 and CXCR2 upon ligand binding. Furthermore, a second regulatory mechanism of CXCL8 receptor expression involves metalloproteinases as important regulatory factors (Khandaker et al., 1999). They demonstrated a significant reduction of CXCR1 and CXCR2 following exposure of neutrophils with LPS or TNF that was shown to act through activation of serine proteinases. This may indicate that a mechanism used by microorganisms to evade the immune system is by reducing neutrophil migration towards the infected site. CXCR1 was further shown to be expressed on cytotoxic CD8+ effector T-cells, indicating the vital physiological role of CXCL8 in recruiting lymphocytes and therefore acting as an important link between innate and adaptive immunity (Takata et al., 2004).

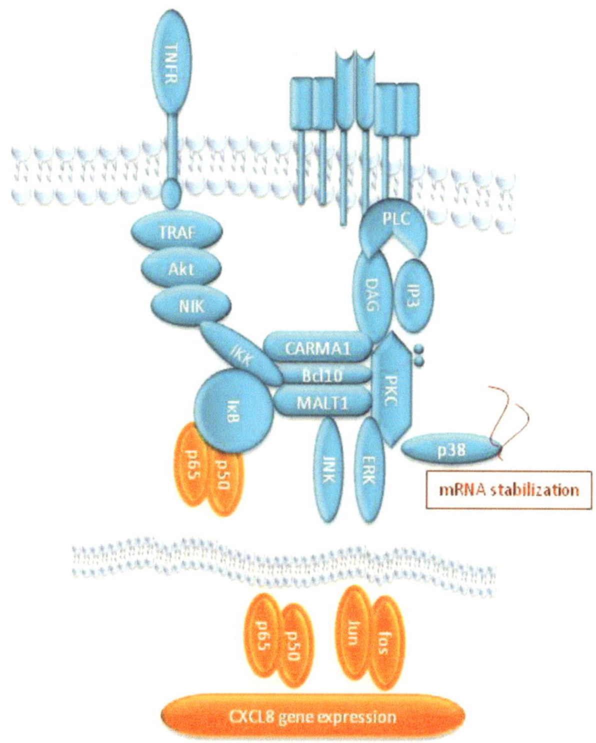

Fig. 3. Intracellular signaling cascade leading to *cxcl8* gene expression. NF-κB (p50, p65) and AP-1 (jun, fos) are the main regulators at the transcriptional level, while p38 serves to stabilize the mRNA molecules.

3. Targeting CXCL8 in HIV treatment strategies

CXCL8 has been implicated in many cellular responses, such as HIV pathogenesis, angiogenesis and cell growth and survival. HIV-infected individuals have elevated CXCL8 levels that, due to the potent chemo-attractant characteristics of CXCL8, can result in the recruitment of target cells, leading to a progressive infection and HIV-1 replication (Ott et al., 1998). However, it has also been suggested that CXCL8 is involved in decreased replication of HIV-1 during the early stages of infection (Rollenhagen & Asin, 2010). In addition, CXCL8 can act as a potent anti-apoptotic agent, inducing the expression of pro-survival proteins, including Bcl-2 and Bcl-x_L (Li et al., 2003). While the role of CXCL8 remains complex it remains an interesting candidate as a suitable therapeutic target in HIV treatment.

Cellular HIV infection involves interactions between glycoprotein gp120, CD4 and CC/CXC receptors (Suresh & Wanchu, 2006). It is therefore possible that an HIV infection can be interrupted and the progression of an established infection can be delayed by targeting CC and/or CXC chemokine receptors. There are two well characterized chemokine receptors by which HIV can bind, enter and infect monocytes, microglia and T-lymphocytes, namely CCR5 and CXCR4 (Ghafouri et al., 2006). CXCL8 dependent activation of CXCR1 has also been suggested to result in inhibited HIV infection and entry into cells (Richardson et al., 2003). Richardson and colleagues showed that CXCR1 activation and internalization resulted in a cross-phosphorylation and internalization of CCR5. Furthermore, C-terminal mutation of CXCR1 internalized both CCR5 and CXCR4 and thus inhibited HIV-1 infection and entry. Furthermore, since HIV-1 competes with CCL5 and CXCL8 for the chemokine receptor DARC (duffy antigen receptor for chemokines) the serum levels of these chemokines may affect the progression of HIV by binding to their respective receptors (He et al., 2008). HIV-1 binding to DARC was also shown to affect chemokine-induced inflammation.

Even though CXCL8 expression is impaired in HIV-infected cells, pro-inflammatory cytokines such as TNF can induce CXCL8 production and expression from other immune cells. It was recently demonstrated that HIV-infected macrophages secrete TNF and IL-1β that in turn act on astrocytes to induce CXCL8 production (Zheng et al., 2008). CXCL8 production was mediated through the MAPK-associated pathways, including p38, c-Jun N-terminal kinase (JNK) and extracellular signal-regulated kinases (ERK1/2). This inflammatory process plays an important role in the pathogenesis of HIV-associated dementia. Reduction of CXCL8 production can therefore be used to control immune cell migration into the central nervous system, which will reduce the overall inflammatory responses at this site. In addition, CXCL8 is co-localize with CD68/CD40 cells, and CD40 receptor expression on microglial cells act as potent inducers of CXCL8 expression, through AP-1 and NF-κB, following ligation of its ligand CD40L, which is expressed on monocytes and T-lymphocytes (D'Aversa et al., 2008). Taken together, these studies show the importance of understanding the regulatory mechanisms leading to chemokine expression in T-cells and other immune cells in order to find a suitable target to control HIV replication and progression.

Antiretroviral drugs that target different structural properties in HIV have failed to eradicate the virus but rather suppressed its spreading and pathogenesis. These difficulties have been due to the variability and ability of HIV to internalize without being detected, followed by reactivation (Archer et al., 2009). These drugs are therefore applied in a combination to inhibit several steps of the viral life cycle, including proteases to inhibit maturation, reverse transcription inhibitors and inhibitors for HIV integration into the genome (Arhel & Kirchhoff, 2010). Other difficulties include drug-drug interactions and long-term toxicities (Tilton & Doms, 2010). However, as chemokine levels are severely altered in HIV infected individuals and are involved in HIV replication this has led to an interest in applying this knowledge to controling HIV infections (Llano & Esté, 2005). Alternative treatment methods have been developed, targeting host proteins/receptors that are used by the virus to enter and infect a cell, such as maraviroc, which is a CCR5 antagonist (Swenson et al., 2011). As viruses are divided into CCR5- and CXCR4-dependent (Pilcher et al., 2004), it is important to accurately determine this mechanism before applying a specific treatment to successfully reduce/inhibit HIV spread and pathogenesis. However, although an initial virus infection is CCR5-dependent, a large subset will switch to using CXCR4 as a co-receptor. This is a major concern since maraviroc has little or no effect on CXCR4-dependent viruses (Kuritzkes, 2011). The interplay between different immune cells during an established HIV infection remains important to understand. Determination of cytokine expression by specific cells and the effect that these inflammatory mediators have on other cells to produce chemokines is also important. Further investigations are needed to evaluate the patterns of immune cell activation and cytokine/chemokine regulation in order to find suitable therapeutic targets.

4. Probiotic *Lactobacillus* as an alternative HIV treatment strategy

Lactobacillus spp are part of the healthy human microbiota, found primarily in the gastrointestinal and vaginal tracts. Certain *Lactobacillus* spp have been identified as health promoting probiotic bacteria by inhibiting pathogen colonization and modulating the immune response in the host (reviewed in Reid et al., 2003). Evidence of immune modulating properties exhibited by certain lactobacilli strains has been shown through their ability to alter cytokine expression in tissue cells infected by pathogens, *in vitro* and *in vivo*, and thus helping maintain homeostasis (Anukam et al., 2009; Frick et al., 2007; Moorthy et al., 2010; Nandakumar et al., 2009; van Hemert et al., 2010; Zhang et al., 2005). Altered cytokine responses, including TNF, NF-κB, IL-6, IL-1β, CXCL8, IL-10 and IL-12, are dependent on cell type (human mucosal epithelial cells, human mononuclear cells, T-cells, dendritic cells etc) and *Lactobacillus* species and strain (Nandakumar et al., 2009; van Hemert et al., 2010). From these reports, probiotic lactobacilli demonstrate a clear potential for both development of new strategies to reduce the risk of HIV infection and combat AIDS progression through their anti-infective and immune-modulating properties.

Vaginal infections such as bacterial vaginosis (BV) and candidiasis have been correlated with an increased risk of HIV infection (Sha et al., 2005; St John et al., 2007). BV and candidiasis are characterized by microbiota that is comprised of a range of anaerobic bacteria or *Candida albicans*, respectively, while deficient in lactobacilli (Sha et al., 2005). Furthermore, women already infected with HIV that lacked vaginal lactobacilli and had BV or candidiasis had higher levels of HIV shedding in the genital tract (Coleman et al., 2007; Spinillo et al., 2005). Increased HIV transcripts in vaginal cells and viral shedding increases the risk of HIV transmission. Furthermore, vaginal secretions from women with BV increased HIV expression in chronically infected monocyte cell line *in vitro*, while secretions from women without BV had no effect on HIV expression (Spear et al., 2007). This is believed to be due to the higher levels of proinflammatory cytokines primarily those that function through NF-κB (Al-Harthi et al., 1998). *C. albicans* infections increase vaginal CXCL8 levels and neutrophil presence while higher levels of vaginal lactobacilli reduced CXCL8 levels and other pro-inflammatory cytokines (Spear et al., 2008). CXCL8 is a potent chemokine that recruits neutrophils to the site of infections, thus by reducing chemokine levels, the target cells for HIV infection are limited. Using lactobacilli to modulate the CXCL8 levels and other pro-inflammatory signals may thus reduce the risk of HIV infection and reduce viral replication.

Certain *Lactobacillus* spp have been shown to reduce pro-inflammatory cytokine release from stimulated cells. The probiotic *Lactobacillus rhamnosus* GG reduced the *cxcl8* expression and CXCL8 and CCL11 secretion in TNF or IL-1β - stimulated human intestinal epithelial cells

(Caco-2bbe) by blocking NF-κB activation and nuclear translocation (Donato et al., 2010). In the same study, related bacteria *Lactobacillus farciminis* and *Lactobacillus plantarum* RO403 did not alter the CXCL8 or CCL11 levels in the stimulated cells. Others reported that *L. plantarum* 299v showed differential influence on expression and secretion of CXCL8 in HT-29 colonic epithelial cells that were treated with TNF. *L. plantarum* 299v enhanced the *cxcl8* mRNA above that of TNF treatment alone while decreasing CXCL8 secretion from HT-29 cells (McCracken et al., 2002). The *L. plantarum* 299v alone did not induce CXCL8. This is especially interesting since CXCL8 has been shown to decreases transcription of RS-Tropic HIV-1 in peripheral blood lymphocytes and decreases replication in ectocervical tissue explants (Rollenhagen & Asin, 2010; Tiemessen et al., 2000). However, another study had reported that increased levels of CXCL8 stimulated HIV-1 replication in T lymphocytes and macrophages, and this could be significantly inhibited using CXCL8 antibodies or blocking CXCR1 and CXCR2 receptors (Lane et al., 2001). High levels of secreted CXCL8 have been associated with chronic infections in HIV infected persons, thus recruiting and exposing the target cells for HIV infection. Modulation of CXCL8 suggests a potential role for certain strains of lactobacilli in reducing the risk for HIV infection and disease progression.

5. Genetically modified lactobacilli for HIV treatment

Commensal *Lactobacillus* spp from the gastrointestinal and vaginal tract have been considered safe and thus have been used to develop genetically engineered lactobacilli as potential live antiviral-fusion delivery systems. Several investigators have genetically engineered a human isolate of *Lactobacillus jensenii* to secrete fusion inhibitors that target necessary receptors for HIV infection with the aim of being used as a vaginal topical treatment. Chang and colleagues have genetically engineered *L. jensenii* to produce a two-domain CD4 protein that bound the HIV-1 gp120 moderately inhibiting HIV binding and entry into Hela cells expressing CD4-CXCR4 *in vitro* (Chang et al., 2003). Similarly, other fusion inhibitors have been successfully expressed from *L. jensenii* such as the anti-HIV-1 chemokine RANTES and a mutated CCR5 antagonist that showed inhibition of infecting T-cells and macrophages in a concentration dependent manner (Vangelista et al., 2010). A recent patent has been filed for genetically engineered *L. reuteri* RC-14 to be used in treatment of HIV and AIDS after infection by secreting fusion inhibitors in the gastrointestinal tract to reduce or slow the progression of AIDS (Lemke 2010; Patent #US 2010/0143305 A1). One report showed that *L. rhamnosus* GR-1 and *L reuteri* RC-14 did not naturally have the ability to alter RANTES in yeast-infected epithelial cells and *L. rhamnosus* GG did not induce the expression of CCL5 (Martinez et al., 2009; Nandakumar et al., 2009). However, to the authors' knowledge, there has been no systematic evaluation of lactobacilli for inducing HIV-1 fusion inhibitors in cell. The combination of genetically engineered lactobacilli strains to express fusion inhibitor molecules, including CXCR1 and 2 and CXCL8 modulation may further reduce HIV infection and AIDS progression.

6. Conclusions

It is clear that cytokines and chemokines are important factors in HIV infection and disease progression, making them plausible targets for anti-HIV therapy and to slow the progression to AIDS. CXCL8 is an important factor to consider in HIV therapy, as it is responsible for the recruitment of neutorphils and T-cells to the site of infection. As HIV

targets immune cells and thereby interferes with the innate immune systems, it is of interest to develop methods to block or reduce the ability of HIV to infect immune cells. Therefore, in order to develop viable CXCL8 based treatment strategies it is important to identify the signaling pathways involved in CXCL8 regulation as well as to determine the function of CXCL8 and its receptors in different physiological responses.
Certain lactobacilli have been shown to have immune modulating abilities. There is a clear potential for using probiotic lactobacilli to counter infections, including HIV, as they have both anti-infective and immune-modulating properties. From this aspect, the ideal probiotic *Lactobacillus* species/strain for therapeutic use is one that increases intracellular CXCL8, while maintains a low level of secreted pro-inflammatory cytokines, such as NF-kB, TNF, CXCL8 and IL-6, that promote HIV replication and recruit HIV-target cells. Combining the health promoting properties of lactobacilli with modulation of *cxcl8* expression and release can be of great importance in fighting HIV infections.

7. Acknowledgement

The present study was made possible by grants from The Knowledge Foundation, Sweden, Sparbanksstiftelsen Nya, Sweden and funding from the Faculty of Business, Science and Engineering, Örebro University, Sweden.

8. References

Acosta, J.C., O'Loghlen, A., Banito, A., Guijarro, M.V., Augert, A., Raguz, S., Fumagalli, M., Da Costa, M., Brown, C., Popov, N., Takatsu, Y., Melamed, J., d'Adda di Fagagna, F., Bernard, D., Hernando, E. & Gil, J. (2008). Chemokine signaling via the CXCR2 receptor reinforces senescence. *Cell*, Vol. 133 (No. 6): 1006-1018.

Acosta, J.C. & Gil, J. (2009). A role for CXCR2 in senescence, but what about in cancer? *Cancer Res*, Vol. 69 (No. 6): 2167-2170.

Al-Harthi, L., Spear, G.T., Hashemi, F.B., Landay, A., Sha, B.E. & Roebuck, K.A. (1998). A human immunodeficiency virus (HIV)-inducing factor from the female genital tract activates HIV-1 gene expression through the kappaB enhancer. *The Journal of Infectious Diseases*, Vol. 178 (No. 5): 1343-1351.

Alfano, M. & Poli, G. (2005). Role of cytokines and chemokines in the regulation of innate immunity and HIV infection. *Mol Immunol*, Vol. 42 (No. 2): 161-182.

Ali, S. & Mann, D.A. (2004). Signal transduction via the NF-kappaB pathway: a targeted treatment modality for infection, inflammation and repair. *Cell Biochem Funct*, Vol. 22 (No. 2): 67-79.

Anukam, K.C., Hayes, K., Summers, K. & Reid, G. (2009). Probiotic Lactobacillus rhamnosus GR-1 and Lactobacillus reuteri RC-14 may help downregulate TNF-Alpha, IL-6, IL-8, IL-10 and IL-12 (p70) in the neurogenic bladder of spinal cord injured patient with urinary tract infections: a two-case study. *Advances in urology*: 680363.

Archer, J., Braverman, M.S., Taillon, B.E., Desany, B., James, I., Harrigan, P.R., Lewis, M. & Robertson, D.L. (2009). Detection of low-frequency pretherapy chemokine (CXC motif) receptor 4 (CXCR4)-using HIV-1 with ultra-deep pyrosequencing. *AIDS*, Vol. 23 (No. 10): 1209-1218.

Arhel, N. & Kirchhoff, F. (2010). Host proteins involved in HIV infection: new therapeutic targets. *Biochim Biophys Acta*, Vol. 1802 (No. 3): 313-321.

Asseman, C., Mauze, S., Leach, M.W., Coffman, R.L. & Powrie, F. (1999). An essential role for interleukin 10 in the function of regulatory T cells that inhibit intestinal inflammation. *J Exp Med*, Vol. 190 (No. 7): 995-1004.

Barnes, P.J. & Adcock, I.M. (1997). NF-kappa B: a pivotal role in asthma and a new target for therapy. *Trends Pharmacol Sci*, Vol. 18 (No. 2): 46-50.

Berg, D.J., Leach, M.W., Kuhn, R., Rajewsky, K., Muller, W., Davidson, N.J. & Rennick, D. (1995). Interleukin 10 but not interleukin 4 is a natural suppressant of cutaneous inflammatory responses. *J Exp Med*, Vol. 182 (No. 1): 99-108.

Bertini, R., Allegretti, M., Bizzarri, C., Moriconi, A., Locati, M., Zampella, G., Cervellera, M.N., Di Cioccio, V., Cesta, M.C., Galliera, E., Martinez, F.O., Di Bitondo, R., Troiani, G., Sabbatini, V., D'Anniballe, G., Anacardio, R., Cutrin, J.C., Cavalieri, B., Mainiero, F., Strippoli, R., Villa, P., Di Girolamo, M., Martin, F., Gentile, M., Santoni, A., Corda, D., Poli, G., Mantovani, A., Ghezzi, P. & Colotta, F. (2004). Noncompetitive allosteric inhibitors of the inflammatory chemokine receptors CXCR1 and CXCR2: prevention of reperfusion injury. *Proc Natl Acad Sci U S A*, Vol. 101 (No. 32): 11791-11796.

Bruder, J.T. & Kovesdi, I. (1997). Adenovirus infection stimulates the Raf/MAPK signaling pathway and induces interleukin-8 expression. *J Virol*, Vol. 71 (No. 1): 398-404.

Caramalho, I., Lopes-Carvalho, T., Ostler, D., Zelenay, S., Haury, M. & Demengeot, J. (2003). Regulatory T cells selectively express toll-like receptors and are activated by lipopolysaccharide. *J Exp Med*, Vol. 197 (No. 4): 403-411.

Chang, T.L., Chang, C.H., Simpson, D.A., Xu, Q., Martin, P.K., Lagenaur, L.A., Schoolnik, G.K., Ho, D.D., Hillier, S.L., Holodniy, M., Lewicki, J.A. & Lee, P.P. (2003). Inhibition of HIV infectivity by a natural human isolate of Lactobacillus jensenii engineered to express functional two-domain CD4. *Proc Natl Acad Sci U S A*, Vol. 100 (No. 20): 11672-11677.

Coleman, J.S., Hitti, J., Bukusi, E.A., Mwachari, C., Muliro, A., Nguti, R., Gausman, R., Jensen, S., Patton, D., Lockhart, D., Coombs, R. & Cohen, C.R. (2007). Infectious correlates of HIV-1 shedding in the female upper and lower genital tracts. *AIDS*, Vol. 21 (No. 6): 755-759.

D'Aversa, T.G., Eugenin, E.A. & Berman, J.W. (2008). CD40-CD40 ligand interactions in human microglia induce CXCL8 (interleukin-8) secretion by a mechanism dependent on activation of ERK1/2 and nuclear translocation of nuclear factor-kappaB (NFkappaB) and activator protein-1 (AP-1). *J Neurosci Res*, Vol. 86 (No. 3): 630-639.

DeForge, L.E., Preston, A.M., Takeuchi, E., Kenney, J., Boxer, L.A. & Remick, D.G. (1993). Regulation of interleukin 8 gene expression by oxidant stress. *J Biol Chem*, Vol. 268 (No. 34): 25568-25576.

Dinarello, C.A. (2000). Proinflammatory cytokines. *Chest*, Vol. 118 (No. 2): 503-508.

Dolcet, X., Llobet, D., Pallares, J. & Matias-Guiu, X. (2005). NF-kB in development and progression of human cancer. *Virchows Arch*, Vol. 446 (No. 5): 475-482.

Donato, K.A., Gareau, M.G., Wang, Y.J. & Sherman, P.M. (2010). Lactobacillus rhamnosus GG attenuates interferon-{gamma} and tumour necrosis factor-alpha-induced barrier dysfunction and pro-inflammatory signalling. *Microbiology*, Vol. 156 (No. Pt 11): 3288-3297.

Dower, N.A., Stang, S.L., Bottorff, D.A., Ebinu, J.O., Dickie, P., Ostergaard, H.L. & Stone, J.C. (2000). RasGRP is essential for mouse thymocyte differentiation and TCR signaling. *Nat Immunol*, Vol. 1 (No. 4): 317-321.

Ehrlich, L.C., Hu, S., Sheng, W.S., Sutton, R.L., Rockswold, G.L., Peterson, P.K. & Chao, C.C. (1998). Cytokine regulation of human microglial cell IL-8 production. *J Immunol*, Vol. 160 (No. 4): 1944-1948.

Faure, M., Voyno-Yasenetskaya, T.A. & Bourne, H.R. (1994). cAMP and beta gamma subunits of heterotrimeric G proteins stimulate the mitogen-activated protein kinase pathway in COS-7 cells. *J Biol Chem*, Vol. 269 (No. 11): 7851-7854.

Frick, J.S., Schenk, K., Quitadamo, M., Kahl, F., Koberle, M., Bohn, E., Aepfelbacher, M. & Autenrieth, I.B. (2007). Lactobacillus fermentum attenuates the proinflammatory effect of Yersinia enterocolitica on human epithelial cells. *Inflammatory bowel diseases*, Vol. 13 (No. 1): 83-90.

Gabellini, C., Trisciuoglio, D., Desideri, M., Candiloro, A., Ragazzoni, Y., Orlandi, A., Zupi, G. & Del Bufalo, D. (2009). Functional activity of CXCL8 receptors, CXCR1 and CXCR2, on human malignant melanoma progression. *Eur J Cancer*, Vol. 45 (No. 14): 2618-2627.

Gaide, O., Favier, B., Legler, D.F., Bonnet, D., Brissoni, B., Valitutti, S., Bron, C., Tschopp, J. & Thome, M. (2002). CARMA1 is a critical lipid raft-associated regulator of TCR-induced NF-kappa B activation. *Nat Immunol*, Vol. 3 (No. 9): 836-843.

Gajewski, T.F., Qian, D., Fields, P. & Fitch, F.W. (1994). Anergic T-lymphocyte clones have altered inositol phosphate, calcium, and tyrosine kinase signaling pathways. *Proc Natl Acad Sci U S A*, Vol. 91 (No. 1): 38-42.

Gantner, B.N., Simmons, R.M., Canavera, S.J., Akira, S. & Underhill, D.M. (2003). Collaborative induction of inflammatory responses by dectin-1 and Toll-like receptor 2. *J Exp Med*, Vol. 197 (No. 9): 1107-1117.

Garcia-Vicuna, R., Gomez-Gaviro, M.V., Dominguez-Luis, M.J., Pec, M.K., Gonzalez-Alvaro, I., Alvaro-Gracia, J.M. & Diaz-Gonzalez, F. (2004). CC and CXC chemokine receptors mediate migration, proliferation, and matrix metalloproteinase production by fibroblast-like synoviocytes from rheumatoid arthritis patients. *Arthritis Rheum*, Vol. 50 (No. 12): 3866-3877.

Ghafouri, M., Amini, S., Khalili, K. & Sawaya, B.E. (2006). HIV-1 associated dementia: symptoms and causes. *Retrovirology*, Vol. 3: 28.

Gonzalo, J.A., Tian, J., Delaney, T., Corcoran, J., Rottman, J.B., Lora, J., Al-garawi, A., Kroczek, R., Gutierrez-Ramos, J.C. & Coyle, A.J. (2001). ICOS is critical for T helper cell-mediated lung mucosal inflammatory responses. *Nat Immunol*, Vol. 2 (No. 7): 597-604.

He, W., Neil, S., Kulkarni, H., Wright, E., Agan, B.K., Marconi, V.C., Dolan, M.J., Weiss, R.A. & Ahuja, S.K. (2008). Duffy antigen receptor for chemokines mediates trans-infection of HIV-1 from red blood cells to target cells and affects HIV-AIDS susceptibility. *Cell Host Microbe*, Vol. 4 (No. 1): 52-62.

Hoffmann, E., Dittrich-Breiholz, O., Holtmann, H. & Kracht, M. (2002). Multiple control of interleukin-8 gene expression. *J Leukoc Biol*, Vol. 72 (No. 5): 847-855.

Hummelen, R., Changalucha, J., Butamanya, N.L., Cook, A., Habbema, J.D. & Reid, G. (2010). Lactobacillus rhamnosus GR-1 and L. reuteri RC-14 to prevent or cure bacterial vaginosis among women with HIV. *Int J Gynaecol Obstet*, Vol. 111 (No. 3): 245-248.

Itahana, K., Dimri, G. & Campisi, J. (2001). Regulation of cellular senescence by p53. *Eur J Biochem*, Vol. 268 (No. 10): 2784-2791.

Karl, E., Warner, K., Zeitlin, B., Kaneko, T., Wurtzel, L., Jin, T., Chang, J., Wang, S., Wang, C.Y., Strieter, R.M., Nunez, G., Polverini, P.J. & Nor, J.E. (2005). Bcl-2 acts in a proangiogenic signaling pathway through nuclear factor-kappaB and CXC chemokines. *Cancer Res*, Vol. 65 (No. 12): 5063-5069.

Khalaf, H., Jass, J. & Olsson, P.E. (2010). Differential cytokine regulation by NF-kappaB and AP-1 in Jurkat T-cells. *BMC Immunol*, Vol. 11: 26.

Khandaker, M.H., Mitchell, G., Xu, L., Andrews, J.D., Singh, R., Leung, H., Madrenas, J., Ferguson, S.S., Feldman, R.D. & Kelvin, D.J. (1999). Metalloproteinases are involved in lipopolysaccharide- and tumor necrosis factor-alpha-mediated regulation of CXCR1 and CXCR2 chemokine receptor expression. *Blood*, Vol. 93 (No. 7): 2173-2185.

Kim, J.J., Nottingham, L.K., Sin, J.I., Tsai, A., Morrison, L., Oh, J., Dang, K., Hu, Y., Kazahaya, K., Bennett, M., Dentchev, T., Wilson, D.M., Chalian, A.A., Boyer, J.D., Agadjanyan, M.G. & Weiner, D.B. (1998). CD8 positive T cells influence antigen-specific immune responses through the expression of chemokines. *J Clin Invest*, Vol. 102 (No. 6): 1112-1124.

Kuritzkes, D.R. (2011). Genotypic tests for determining coreceptor usage of HIV-1. *J Infect Dis*, Vol. 203 (No. 2): 146-148.

Lane, B.R., Lore, K., Bock, P.J., Andersson, J., Coffey, M.J., Strieter, R.M. & Markovitz, D.M. (2001). Interleukin-8 stimulates human immunodeficiency virus type 1 replication and is a potential new target for antiretroviral therapy. *Journal of virology*, Vol. 75 (No. 17): 8195-8202.

Li, A., Dubey, S., Varney, M.L., Dave, B.J. & Singh, R.K. (2003). IL-8 directly enhanced endothelial cell survival, proliferation, and matrix metalloproteinases production and regulated angiogenesis. *J Immunol*, Vol. 170 (No. 6): 3369-3376.

Li, J., Kartha, S., Iasvovskaia, S., Tan, A., Bhat, R.K., Manaligod, J.M., Page, K., Brasier, A.R. & Hershenson, M.B. (2002). Regulation of human airway epithelial cell IL-8 expression by MAP kinases. *Am J Physiol Lung Cell Mol Physiol*, Vol. 283 (No. 4): L690-699.

Libby, P., Ridker, P.M. & Maseri, A. (2002). Inflammation and atherosclerosis. *Circulation*, Vol. 105 (No. 9): 1135-1143.

Llano, A. & Esté, J.A. (2005). Chemokines and other cytokines in human immunodeficiency virus type 1 (HIV-1) infection. *Inmunología*, Vol. 24: 246-260.

Makarov, S.S. (2000). NF-kappaB as a therapeutic target in chronic inflammation: recent advances. *Mol Med Today*, Vol. 6 (No. 11): 441-448.

Martinez, R.C., Seney, S.L., Summers, K.L., Nomizo, A., De Martinis, E.C. & Reid, G. (2009). Effect of Lactobacillus rhamnosus GR-1 and Lactobacillus reuteri RC-14 on the ability of Candida albicans to infect cells and induce inflammation. *Microbiology and immunology*, Vol. 53 (No. 9): 487-495.

McCarroll, J.A., Phillips, P.A., Park, S., Doherty, E., Pirola, R.C., Wilson, J.S. & Apte, M.V. (2003). Pancreatic stellate cell activation by ethanol and acetaldehyde: is it mediated by the mitogen-activated protein kinase signaling pathway? *Pancreas*, Vol. 27 (No. 2): 150-160.

McCracken, V.J., Chun, T., Baldeon, M.E., Ahrne, S., Molin, G., Mackie, R.I. & Gaskins, H.R. (2002). TNF-alpha sensitizes HT-29 colonic epithelial cells to intestinal lactobacilli. *Experimental biology and medicine*, Vol. 227 (No. 8): 665-670.

McKay, L.I. & Cidlowski, J.A. (1999). Molecular control of immune/inflammatory responses: interactions between nuclear factor-kappa B and steroid receptor-signaling pathways. *Endocr Rev*, Vol. 20 (No. 4): 435-459.

Moorthy, G., Murali, M.R. & Niranjali Devaraj, S. (2010). Lactobacilli inhibit Shigella dysenteriae 1 induced pro-inflammatory response and cytotoxicity in host cells via impediment of Shigella-host interactions. *Digestive and liver disease : official journal of the Italian Society of Gastroenterology and the Italian Association for the Study of the Liver*, Vol. 42 (No. 1): 33-39.

Nandakumar, N.S., Pugazhendhi, S. & Ramakrishna, B.S. (2009). Effects of enteropathogenic bacteria & lactobacilli on chemokine secretion & Toll like receptor gene expression in two human colonic epithelial cell lines. *The Indian journal of medical research*, Vol. 130 (No. 2): 170-178.

Narayan, P., Holt, B., Tosti, R. & Kane, L.P. (2006). CARMA1 is required for Akt-mediated NF-kappaB activation in T cells. *Mol Cell Biol*, Vol. 26 (No. 6): 2327-2336.

Noel, R.F., Jr., Sato, T.T., Mendez, C., Johnson, M.C. & Pohlman, T.H. (1995). Activation of human endothelial cells by viable or heat-killed gram-negative bacteria requires soluble CD14. *Infect Immun*, Vol. 63 (No. 10): 4046-4053.

Opal, S.M. & DePalo, V.A. (2000). Anti-inflammatory cytokines. *Chest*, Vol. 117 (No. 4): 1162-1172.

Ott, M., Lovett, J.L., Mueller, L. & Verdin, E. (1998). Superinduction of IL-8 in T cells by HIV-1 Tat protein is mediated through NF-kappaB factors. *J Immunol*, Vol. 160 (No. 6): 2872-2880.

Pearson, T.A., Mensah, G.A., Alexander, R.W., Anderson, J.L., Cannon, R.O., 3rd, Criqui, M., Fadl, Y.Y., Fortmann, S.P., Hong, Y., Myers, G.L., Rifai, N., Smith, S.C., Jr., Taubert, K., Tracy, R.P. & Vinicor, F. (2003). Markers of inflammation and cardiovascular disease: application to clinical and public health practice: A statement for healthcare professionals from the Centers for Disease Control and Prevention and the American Heart Association. *Circulation*, Vol. 107 (No. 3): 499-511.

Philip, M., Rowley, D.A. & Schreiber, H. (2004). Inflammation as a tumor promoter in cancer induction. *Semin Cancer Biol*, Vol. 14 (No. 6): 433-439.

Pilcher, C.D., Eron, J.J., Jr., Galvin, S., Gay, C. & Cohen, M.S. (2004). Acute HIV revisited: new opportunities for treatment and prevention. *J Clin Invest*, Vol. 113 (No. 7): 937-945.

Reid, G., Jass, J., Sebulsky, M.T. & McCormick, J.K. (2003). Potential uses of probiotics in clinical practice. *Clinical microbiology reviews*, Vol. 16 (No. 4): 658-672.

Richardson, R.M., Tokunaga, K., Marjoram, R., Sata, T. & Snyderman, R. (2003). Interleukin-8-mediated heterologous receptor internalization provides resistance to HIV-1 infectivity. Role of signal strength and receptor desensitization. *J Biol Chem*, Vol. 278 (No. 18): 15867-15873.

Riedel, C.U., Foata, F., Philippe, D., Adolfsson, O., Eikmanns, B.J. & Blum, S. (2006). Anti-inflammatory effects of bifidobacteria by inhibition of LPS-induced NF-kappaB activation. *World J Gastroenterol*, Vol. 12 (No. 23): 3729-3735.

Rollenhagen, C. & Asin, S.N. (2010). IL-8 decreases HIV-1 transcription in peripheral blood lymphocytes and ectocervical tissue explants. *J Acquir Immune Defic Syndr*, Vol. 54 (No. 5): 463-469.

Sato, M., Sano, H., Iwaki, D., Kudo, K., Konishi, M., Takahashi, H., Takahashi, T., Imaizumi, H., Asai, Y. & Kuroki, Y. (2003). Direct binding of Toll-like receptor 2 to zymosan, and zymosan-induced NF-kappa B activation and TNF-alpha secretion are down-regulated by lung collectin surfactant protein A. *J Immunol*, Vol. 171 (No. 1): 417-425.

Scharschmidt, E., Wegener, E., Heissmeyer, V., Rao, A. & Krappmann, D. (2004). Degradation of Bcl10 induced by T-cell activation negatively regulates NF-kappa B signaling. *Mol Cell Biol*, Vol. 24 (No. 9): 3860-3873.

Sha, B.E., Zariffard, M.R., Wang, Q.J., Chen, H.Y., Bremer, J., Cohen, M.H. & Spear, G.T. (2005). Female genital-tract HIV load correlates inversely with Lactobacillus species but positively with bacterial vaginosis and Mycoplasma hominis. *The Journal of infectious diseases*, Vol. 191 (No. 1): 25-32.

Shoji, Y., Uedono, Y., Ishikura, H., Takeyama, N. & Tanaka, T. (1995). DNA damage induced by tumour necrosis factor-alpha in L929 cells is mediated by mitochondrial oxygen radical formation. *Immunology*, Vol. 84 (No. 4): 543-548.

Spear, G.T., St John, E. & Zariffard, M.R. (2007). Bacterial vaginosis and human immunodeficiency virus infection. *AIDS Res Ther*, Vol. 4: 25.

Spear, G.T., Zariffard, M.R., Cohen, M.H. & Sha, B.E. (2008). Vaginal IL-8 levels are positively associated with Candida albicans and inversely with lactobacilli in HIV-infected women. *Journal of reproductive immunology*, Vol. 78 (No. 1): 76-79.

Spinillo, A., Zara, F., Gardella, B., Preti, E., Mainini, R. & Maserati, R. (2005). The effect of vaginal candidiasis on the shedding of human immunodeficiency virus in cervicovaginal secretions. *American journal of obstetrics and gynecology*, Vol. 192 (No. 3): 774-779.

St John, E., Mares, D. & Spear, G.T. (2007). Bacterial vaginosis and host immunity. *Current HIV/AIDS reports*, Vol. 4 (No. 1): 22-28.

Sturm, A., Baumgart, D.C., d'Heureuse, J.H., Hotz, A., Wiedenmann, B. & Dignass, A.U. (2005). CXCL8 modulates human intestinal epithelial cells through a CXCR1 dependent pathway. *Cytokine*, Vol. 29 (No. 1): 42-48.

Suresh, P. & Wanchu, A. (2006). Chemokines and chemokine receptors in HIV infection: role in pathogenesis and therapeutics. *J Postgrad Med*, Vol. 52 (No. 3): 210-217.

Svanborg, C., Godaly, G. & Hedlund, M. (1999). Cytokine responses during mucosal infections: role in disease pathogenesis and host defence. *Curr Opin Microbiol*, Vol. 2 (No. 1): 99-105.

Swenson, L.C., Mo, T., Dong, W.W., Zhong, X., Woods, C.K., Jensen, M.A., Thielen, A., Chapman, D., Lewis, M., James, I., Heera, J., Valdez, H. & Harrigan, P.R. (2011). Deep sequencing to infer HIV-1 co-receptor usage: application to three clinical trials of maraviroc in treatment-experienced patients. *J Infect Dis*, Vol. 203 (No. 2): 237-245.

Taha, T.E., Hoover, D.R., Dallabetta, G.A., Kumwenda, N.I., Mtimavalye, L.A., Yang, L.P., Liomba, G.N., Broadhead, R.L., Chiphangwi, J.D. & Miotti, P.G. (1998). Bacterial vaginosis and disturbances of vaginal flora: association with increased acquisition of HIV. *AIDS*, Vol. 12 (No. 13): 1699-1706.

Takata, H., Tomiyama, H., Fujiwara, M., Kobayashi, N. & Takiguchi, M. (2004). Cutting edge: expression of chemokine receptor CXCR1 on human effector CD8+ T cells. *J Immunol*, Vol. 173 (No. 4): 2231-2235.

Teixeira, C., Stang, S.L., Zheng, Y., Beswick, N.S. & Stone, J.C. (2003). Integration of DAG signaling systems mediated by PKC-dependent phosphorylation of RasGRP3. *Blood*, Vol. 102 (No. 4): 1414-1420.

Tergaonkar, V. (2006). NFkappaB pathway: a good signaling paradigm and therapeutic target. *Int J Biochem Cell Biol*, Vol. 38 (No. 10): 1647-1653.

Tiemessen, C.T., Kilroe, B. & Martin, D.J. (2000). Interleukin-8 fails to induce human immunodeficiency virus-1 expression in chronically infected promonocytic U1 cells but differentially modulates induction by proinflammatory cytokines. *Immunology*, Vol. 101 (No. 1): 140-146.

Tilton, J.C. & Doms, R.W. (2010). Entry inhibitors in the treatment of HIV-1 infection. *Antiviral Res*, Vol. 85 (No. 1): 91-100.

van der Poll, T., Jansen, P.M., Montegut, W.J., Braxton, C.C., Calvano, S.E., Stackpole, S.A., Smith, S.R., Swanson, S.W., Hack, C.E., Lowry, S.F. & Moldawer, L.L. (1997). Effects of IL-10 on systemic inflammatory responses during sublethal primate endotoxemia. *J Immunol*, Vol. 158 (No. 4): 1971-1975.

van Hemert, S., Meijerink, M., Molenaar, D., Bron, P.A., de Vos, P., Kleerebezem, M., Wells, J.M. & Marco, M.L. (2010). Identification of Lactobacillus plantarum genes modulating the cytokine response of human peripheral blood mononuclear cells. *BMC microbiology*, Vol. 10: 293.

Vangelista, L., Secchi, M., Liu, X., Bachi, A., Jia, L., Xu, Q. & Lusso, P. (2010). Engineering of Lactobacillus jensenii to secrete RANTES and a CCR5 antagonist analogue as live HIV-1 blockers. *Antimicrobial agents and chemotherapy*, Vol. 54 (No. 7): 2994-3001.

Walley, K.R., Lukacs, N.W., Standiford, T.J., Strieter, R.M. & Kunkel, S.L. (1996). Balance of inflammatory cytokines related to severity and mortality of murine sepsis. *Infect Immun*, Vol. 64 (No. 11): 4733-4738.

Werlen, G., Jacinto, E., Xia, Y. & Karin, M. (1998). Calcineurin preferentially synergizes with PKC-theta to activate JNK and IL-2 promoter in T lymphocytes. *Embo J*, Vol. 17 (No. 11): 3101-3111.

Wong, M.M. & Fish, E.N. (2003). Chemokines: attractive mediators of the immune response. *Semin Immunol*, Vol. 15 (No. 1): 5-14.

Xu, X.H., Shah, P.K., Faure, E., Equils, O., Thomas, L., Fishbein, M.C., Luthringer, D., Xu, X.P., Rajavashisth, T.B., Yano, J., Kaul, S. & Arditi, M. (2001). Toll-like receptor-4 is expressed by macrophages in murine and human lipid-rich atherosclerotic plaques and upregulated by oxidized LDL. *Circulation*, Vol. 104 (No. 25): 3103-3108.

Zhang, L., Li, N., Caicedo, R. & Neu, J. (2005). Alive and dead Lactobacillus rhamnosus GG decrease tumor necrosis factor-alpha-induced interleukin-8 production in Caco-2 cells. *The Journal of nutrition*, Vol. 135 (No. 7): 1752-1756.

Zheng, J.C., Huang, Y., Tang, K., Cui, M., Niemann, D., Lopez, A., Morgello, S. & Chen, S. (2008). HIV-1-infected and/or immune-activated macrophages regulate astrocyte CXCL8 production through IL-1beta and TNF-alpha: involvement of mitogen-activated protein kinases and protein kinase R. *J Neuroimmunol*, Vol. 200 (No. 1-2): 100-110.

Zlotnik, A. & Yoshie, O. (2000). Chemokines: a new classification system and their role in immunity. *Immunity*, Vol. 12 (No. 2): 121-127.

14

Emerging Roles of Prostaglandins in HIV-1 Transcription

Nancy Dumais, Sandra C. Côté and Anne-Marie Ducharme
Université de Sherbrooke
Canada

1. Introduction

Prostaglandins (PG), generated by cyclooxygenase (COX), are a group of lipid mediators formed in response to various stimuli. They include PGD_2, PGE_2, PGF_{2alpha}, and PGI_2. Immediately after synthesis, they are released outside the cell and exert their actions by binding to a G-protein-coupled rhodopsin-type receptor on the surface of target cells. There are seven types of prostaglandin receptors: the PGD receptor, four subtypes of PGE receptor, the PGF receptor, and the PGI receptor. Prostaglandins are involved in host defense against various pathogens. Along with mediating inflammatory symptoms, PGs might suppress some innate immune factors, including nitric oxide (NO) production. These immunomodulatory molecules have been shown to participate in the regulation of virus replication and the modulation of inflammatory responses following infection. Moreover, virus infection also stimulates the expression of a number of proinflammatory gene products, including COX-2, inducible nitric oxide synthase (iNOS) as well as proinflammatory cytokines.

An overproduction of PGE_2 (as high as 10^{-4}M) is seen in a number of disorders (e.g. allergy, hyper-IgE syndrome, Hodgkin lymphoma, trauma, sepsis, and transplantation), most of which are characterized by elevated Th2 and IgE responses. Elevated levels of PGE_2 have also been reported in individuals infected with HIV-1 and it has been postulated that this may contribute to the immunosuppressive state seen in such virally infected patients. The mechanism(s) responsible for the enhanced prostaglandin formation is still undefined. The initial contact between the virus particle and its target cell might represent the crucial step leading to the production of PGE_2 by macrophages. This concept is supported by the finding that a significant production of endogenous PGE_2 is induced (20- to 40-fold increase) following incubation of primary human monocytes with the HIV-1 external envelope glycoprotein gp120. Given that pro-inflammatory molecules such as PGE_2 are up-regulated during HIV-1 infection, an imbalance in PGJ_2 production is observed in HIV+ individuals.

This book chapter will focus on roles of prostaglandins in HIV-1 replication and their potential therapeutic implications. We propose to review mechanisms by which the pro-inflammatory prostaglandin PGE_2 and the anti-inflammatory prostaglandin PGJ_2 regulate HIV-1 transcription and replication. Specific attention will be placed on how prostaglandins affect the nuclear translocation of NF-κB (nuclear factor kappa B), an essential transcription factor for HIV-1 transcription. In addition, signaling pathways as well as other transcription factors that are activated or repressed by prostaglandins that regulate HIV-1 gene expression will be reviewed.

2. Prostaglandins: Their synthesis and roles in the regulation of inflammation

2.1 Prostaglandins synthesis

The initial reaction in prostaglandin production is phospholipase A_2 (PLA_2)-mediated liberation of a 20-carbon essential fatty acid, arachidonic acid, from membrane phospholipids. Cyclooxygenase (COX) is the rate-limiting enzymes catalysing oxidation of arachidonic acid to the hydroperoxyendoperoxide, prostaglandin G_2 (PGG_2). Subsequently, PGG_2 is reduced to form the hydroxylendoperoxide, prostaglandin H_2 (PGH_2). Then, prostanoids including prostaglandin D_2 (PGD_2), prostaglandin E_2 (PGE_2), prostaglandin F_{2alpha} ($PGF_2\alpha$), prostacyclin (PGI_2), and thromboxane A_2 (TXA_2) are formed by the action of discrete prostaglandins synthases (reviewed in Coleman et al., 1994). Figure 1 reviews the arachidonic cascade.

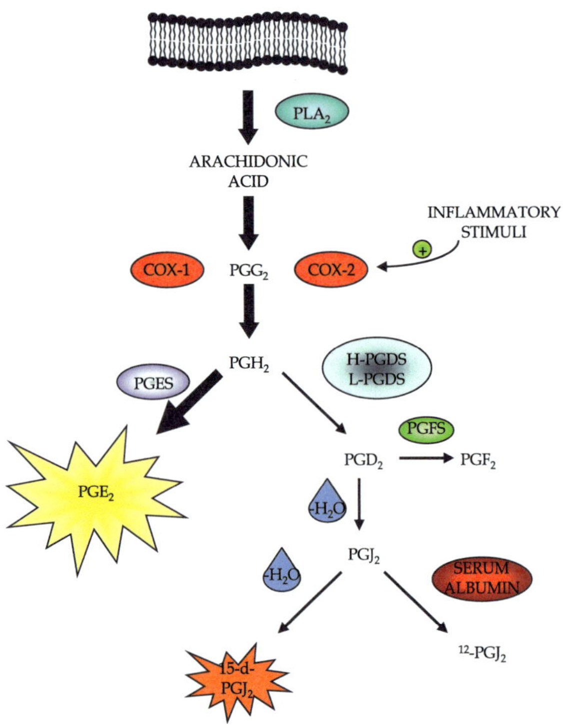

Fig. 1. A model for prostaglandins synthesis.

Prostaglandin E_2 (PGE_2), an oxygenated polyunsaturated fatty acid that contains a cyclopentane ring structure, is present in high concentrations in individuals infected with numerous pathogens (Abel et al., 1992; Ben-Hur et al., 1996; Farrell & Kirkpatrick, 1987; Foley et al., 1992; Griffin et al., 1994a; Henke et al., 1992; Kernacki & Berk, 1994; Midulla et al., 1989; Onta et al., 1993; Ramis et al., 1992; Rastogi et al., 1992; Reiner & Malemud, 1984; Sorrell et al., 1989; Wang & Chadee, 1992, 1995). PGE_2 are molecules that have been shown to modulate the immune response both *in vitro* and *in vivo* (Goodwin & Webb, 1980). Macrophages, follicular dendritic cells, fibroblasts, and vascular endothelial cells synthesize

PGE_2, while lymphocytes do not secrete this major product of arachidonic acid metabolism (Frey et al., 1986; Heinen et al., 1986; Kurland & Bockman, 1978; Phipps et al., 1988). A marked increase in PGE_2 production is generated in response to a variety of immunological stimuli including interleukin (IL)-1, tumor necrosis factor-α (TNF-α), antigen-antibody complexes, and lipopolysaccharide (Roper & Phipps, 1994) in addition to exposition to microorganisms. PGE_2 has been implicated in decreasing T-cell proliferation, IL-2 production, and IL-2 receptor expression (Goodwin et al., 1977; Goodwin & Ceuppens, 1983; Rincon et al., 1988; Roper & Phipps, 1994; Walker et al., 1983). PGE_2 shifts the balance of the cellular immune response away from T-helper type 1 (Th1) favouring a Th2 response which drives humoral responses toward the production of IgE (Fedyk & Phipps, 1996). However, other findings have depicted PGE_2 as a pleiotropic molecule that can act both negatively or positively on the immune system (Phipps et al., 1991). Depending on the cell type, binding of PGE_2 to one of its six described receptors (EP_1, EP_2, EP_{3I}, EP_{3II}, EP_{3III}, and EP_4) can lead to phospholipase C activation, phosphatidylinositol turnover increase, activation of adenylate cyclase through cholera toxin-sensitive $G_{\alpha s}$ proteins and mobilization of intracellular Ca^{2+} concentration (Coleman et al., 1994). PGE_2 facilitates expansion of the Th17 subset of T helper cells of both human and mouse through elevation of cAMP via PGE_2 receptors EP_2 and EP_4 (Sakata et al., 2010).

The balance of opposing prostaglandins produced in tissues profoundly influences inflammatory responses (Harris et al., 2002). The J series of prostaglandins are the end product metabolites of PGD_2 and are abundantly produced by mast cells, platelets, as well as alveolar macrophages (Ito et al., 1989; Straus & Glass, 2001). One of these molecules, 15-d-PGJ_2, is a natural activator of the peroxisome proliferators-activated receptor-γ (PPAR-γ), a nuclear receptor family member that elicits anti-inflammatory activities in macrophages (Hinz et al., 2003; Hortelano et al., 2000; Jiang et al., 1998; Ricote et al., 1998), lymphocytes (Clark et al., 2000; Padilla et al., 2000; Yang et al., 2000), dendritic cells (Faveeuw et al., 2000), and endothelial cells (Imaizumi et al., 2003). Currently, the mechanisms regulating the anti-inflammatory effects of 15-d-PGJ_2 and other PPAR-γ agonists are poorly understood, but it has been suggested to involve the inhibition of the nuclear factor κB (NF-κB) signaling pathway (Daynes & Jones, 2002; Rossi et al., 2000). PPAR-γ is also expressed at high levels both in the colonic epithelium and intestinal epithelial cells (Lefebvre et al., 1998; Saez et al., 2004; Saez et al., 1998; Sarraf et al., 1998; Sarraf et al., 1999), where, depending on the model system studied, it can result in either an increase or a decrease in proliferation (Brockman et al., 1998; Lefebvre et al., 1998).

2.2 Prostaglandins and HIV infection

An overproduction of PGE_2 as high as 10^{-4}M is seen in a number of disorders (e.g.allergy, hyper-IgE syndrome, Hodgkin lymphoma, trauma, sepsis, and transplantation), most of which are characterized by elevated Th2 and IgE responses (Fedyk & Phipps, 1996; Haraguchi et al., 1995a; Phipps et al., 1991; Roper & Phipps, 1994). Elevated levels of PGE_2 have also been reported in individuals infected with HIV-1 (Abel et al., 1992; Foley et al., 1992; Griffin et al., 1994a; Ramis et al., 1992) and it has been postulated that this may contribute to the immunosuppressive state seen in such virally-infected patients (Hui et al., 1995). *In vitro*, peripheral blood monocytes and macrophages from AIDS patients exhibit abnormal production of cyclooxygenase products (Coffey et al., 1999; Fernandez-Cruz et al., 1989; Foley et al., 1992; Mastino et al., 1993; Ramis et al., 1991). The mechanism(s) responsible for the enhanced prostaglandin formation is still undefined. The initial contact between the virus particle and its target cell might represent the crucial step leading to the production of PGE_2 by macrophages. Significant production of endogenous PGE_2 is induced (20- to 40-fold increase) following incubation of primary human monocytes with the HIV-1 external envelope glycoprotein gp120 (Wahl et al., 1989). However, in sharp contrast with this report, a previous study has demonstrated that interaction between gp120 and THP-1, a human monocytoid cell line, does not increase exogenous production of PGE_2 (Hui et al., 1995). It is important to specify that, unlike monocyte/macrophages, promonocytoid THP-1 cells are not at a terminal stage of differentiation. In addition, a monomer form of gp120 was used in this study which might not parallel physiological conditions where gp120 is under a multimeric form (Pinter et al., 1989).

3. PGE_2 and HIV transcription

3.1 Importance of NF-κB in HIV-1 gene transcription

HIV-1 gene expression is regulated in a cell type- and differentiation-dependent manner by the binding of both host and viral proteins to the long terminal repeat (LTR), which serves as the viral promoter. Host transcription factors such as the Sp family, NF-κB family, activator protein 1 (AP-1) proteins, nuclear factor of activated T cells (NFAT), and CCAAT enhancer binding protein (C/EBP) family members play essential roles in the regulation of HIV-1 transcription by binding sites in the LTR that display different levels of sequence conservation (Fig 2). Viral proteins such as HIV Vpr and Tat also bind to the LTR to regulate transcription (Kilareski et al., 2009). Many of these host and viral proteins engage in extensive protein-protein interactions, leading to a complex system of transcriptional regulation.

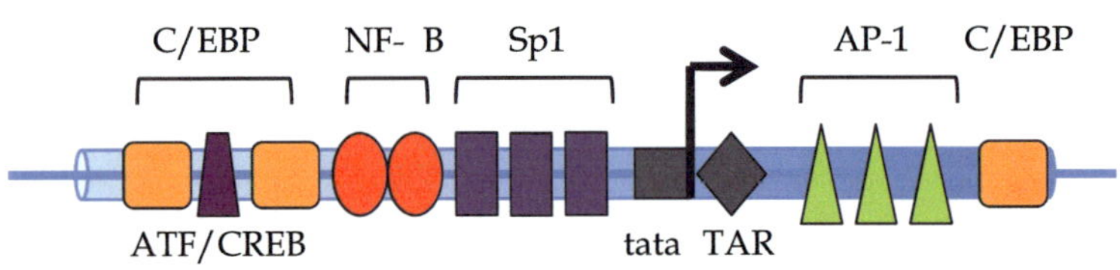

Fig. 2. A schematic representation of a typical HIV-1 LTR.

The transcription factor NF-κB is known to play a central role in the activation of HIV-1 gene expression. The enhancer in the U3 region of LTR contains two NF-κB binding sites (Siebenlist et al., 1994) that are critical for LTR promoter activity and important for optimal HIV-1 replication (Santoro et al., 2003; Siebenlist et al., 1994). NF-κB is an inducible transcription factor that plays an important role in cellular gene expression associated with immune responses, inflammation and cell survival (Ghosh et al., 1998; Viatour et al., 2005). In the host cytoplasm, NF-κB is a heterodimeric molecule (p50/p65) that forms an inactive complex with its inhibitor IκB. Stimulation with inflammatory cytokines, such as TNF-α and IL-1β, viral and bacterial antigens, and stress-inducing agents leads to immediate phosphorylation and subsequent degradation of IκB by the proteasome, resulting in the translocation of NF-κB from the cytoplasm to nucleus.

3.2 Activation of HIV-1 LTR activity by PGE_2

Immune and inflammatory responses are triggered by microorganisms such as bacteria, viruses, and protozoan, all known to be potential opportunistic pathogens in HIV-1-positive patients. The formation and production of elevated levels of inflammatory mediators such as PGE_2 is a hallmark of the HIV-1 infection (Foley et al., 1992; Griffin et al., 1994a; Ramis et al., 1992). Prostaglandins play a role in disease exacerbation by directly altering T-cell functions or macrophage activation. Although it was thought that PGE_2 is primarily an immunosuppressive molecule that acts as a down-regulator of many aspects of B- and T-cell function and proliferation, other findings support a role for PGE_2 as a potentiator of immunoglobulin class switching and cytokines and cytokine receptors synthesis (Phipps et al., 1991). Moreover, knowing that PGE_2 is a good inducer of cAMP and that a 4-fold increase in intracellular levels of cAMP is seen in asymptomatic HIV-1-seropositive subjects as compared with uninfected controls (Hofmann et al., 1993), it is thus of prime importance to study the putative effect of PGE_2 on the regulatory elements of HIV-1 in T cells considered to be the major cellular reservoir for HIV-1 in the human peripheral blood. As shown in Fig 3, exogenous PGE_2 could further increase the overall positive effect mediated by various HIV-1 LTR-activating agents confirming that PGE_2 could be considered by itself as a potent inducer of HIV-1 LTR transcription in T cells.

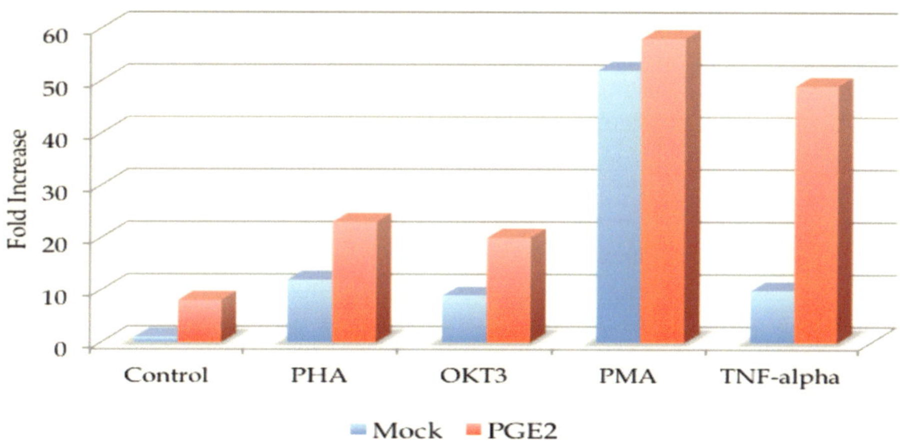

Fig. 3. Activation of HIV-1 LTR by several stimuli in the absence or presence of PGE_2. 1G5 cells, a clonal cell line derived from Jurkat E6.1 cells which has been with stably transfected with a luciferase gene driven by the HIV-1 LTR (Aguilar-Cordova et al., 1994), were either left untreated (control) or treated with PHA (3 µg/ml), OKT3 (1 µg/ml), PMA (20 ng/ml), or TNF-α (2 ng/ml) in the absence or presence of 100 nM PGE_2 for 8 h. Cell lysates were evaluated for luciferase activity and are expressed as fold induction relative to basal luciferase activity in untreated control cells (considered as 1).

Northern blot assays, flow cytometric analyses, and pharmacological studies showed that the EP_4 gene is expressed on T lymphoid cells such as Molt-4, KM-3, IG5 and Jurkat E6.1 (Blaschke et al., 1996; De Vries et al., 1995; Dumais et al., 1998; Mori et al., 1996). It has been demonstrated that EP_4 receptors are coupled to adenylate cyclase via a stimulatory G protein ($G_{\alpha s}$) and that such activation results in an enhancement of intracellular cAMP levels (Coleman et al., 1995; Nishigaki et al., 1995). Interestingly, PGE_2 has been shown to lead to an increase in intracellular cAMP levels partly via the EP_4 receptor (Rodbell, 1980), a finding which lend credence to the potential implication of the EP_4 receptor in the PGE_2-induced up-regulation of HIV-1 LTR activity.

3.2.1 NF-κB-dependent signaling pathways involved in activation of HIV-1 LTR by PGE_2 in T cells

The involvement of specific intracellular second messengers in PGE_2-mediated up-regulation of HIV-1 LTR activity has been dissected using several signal transduction inhibitors. Only exogeneous PGE_2 plays a role in the activation of HIV-1 LTR-driven gene expression as shown with experiments using indomethacin, a potent inhibitor of the cyclooxygenase pathway (Dumais et al., 1998). Moreover, it was demonstrated that T cells had a limited capacity to metabolize arachidonic acid to prostaglandins (Auberger et al., 1989; Fu et al., 1990; Goldyne & Rea, 1987). Interaction between PGE_2 and an adenylate cyclase-coupled stimulatory receptor leads to activation of adenylate cyclase, hydrolysis of ATP, enhanced turnover of intracellular cAMP and binding to PKA (Kammer, 1988). In T cells, PGE_2-induced enhancement of HIV-1 LTR dependent activity requires the participation of adenylate cyclase, cAMP as well as protein kinase A (Dumais et al., 1998) and elevation of cAMP levels resulted in HIV-1 replication (Nokta & Pollard, 1992). It is also well known that cAMP-dependent pathways regulate the immune effector functions of lymphocytes and macrophages. For example, during immune response, cAMP exhibits positive regulatory effects at low concentrations whereas inhibitory effects are seen at high concentrations (Koh et al., 1995). Many of the earlier studies have shown that PGE_2 interaction with T cells *in vitro* resulted in an elevation of the cAMP level (Rincon et al., 1988) and that such elevated intracellular cAMP levels were responsible for the proliferative disturbances in T cells (Baker et al., 1981; Lingk et al., 1990; Munoz et al., 1990). In T cells, experiments with the calcium chelator BAPTA/AM and the calcium inhibitor CAI are suggestive of the importance of Ca^{2+} in the PGE_2-induced activation of HIV-1 transcription (Dumais et al., 1998). However, given that there is no published report indicating Ca^{2+} influx through the EP_4 receptor, our results with BAPTA/AM and carboxyamido-triazole (CAI), two inhibitors of intracellular calcium mobilization, lead us to postulate that PGE_2 could generate calcium release from intracellular storage organelles. Up-regulation of HIV-1 LTR requires the implication of cAMP and calcium, as well as the participation of the NF-κB transcription factor.

Several agents known as potent activators of HIV-1 transcription (e.g. PMA, PHA, TNF-α, and anti-CD3 antibody) are all acting through a common mechanism, namely via the nuclear translocation of the transcription factor NF-κB which binds to the enhancer region of the HIV-1 LTR (Nabel, 1991). This transcription factor is sequestered in the cytoplasm due to its physical association with the inhibitor named IκB. NF-κB is a pleiotropic transcription factor that controls the expression of a wide variety of genes, including cytokines such as IL-1, IL-2, IL-6, IL-8, interferon-β, and TNF-α, as well as known genes for some cell adhesion molecules including ICAM-1 and VCAM-1. Its importance in the regulation of HIV-1 gene expression has been stated in numerous studies (Siebenlist et al., 1994). Results from mobility shift assays suggest that the PGE_2-mediated effect on HIV-1 LTR activity is due to activation of the transcription factor NF-κB. This is in agreement with the previous demonstration that PGE_2 activates NF-κB in the macrophage-like cell line J774 (Muroi & Suzuki, 1993). The fact that we have noticed that both NF-κB and Ca^{2+} are key elements in the PGE_2 effect on HIV-1 transcription is of interest considering that calcineurin, a Ca^{2+}/calmodulin-dependent serine/threonine protein phosphatase, has been reported to activate NF–κB through the inactivation of IκB (Frantz et al., 1994). Moreover, researchers had earlier found that cAMP-mediated enhancement of PKA might be involved in the dissociation of IκB from NF-κB (Nabel and Baltimore, 1987). Recent studies have revealed that NF-κB is regulated through phosphorylation of the p65 subunit by PKA which is directly regulated by intracellular levels of cAMP (Zhong et al., 1997). Experiments in Jurkat E6.1 T cells performed with κB-driven reporter gene constructs (pκB-TATA-LUC and pNF-κB-LUC) and HIV-1 LTR-based vectors (pLTR-LUC and pmκBLTR-LUC), suggest that NF-κB-binding regions and another element(s) in the HIV-1 LTR are involved in the activation of HIV-1 LTR-dependent transcription induced by PGE_2 (fig 4). These results hence support the notion that PGE_2 might be activating the transcription factor NF-κB via cAMP/PKA and calcium signaling pathways in human T lymphoid cells.

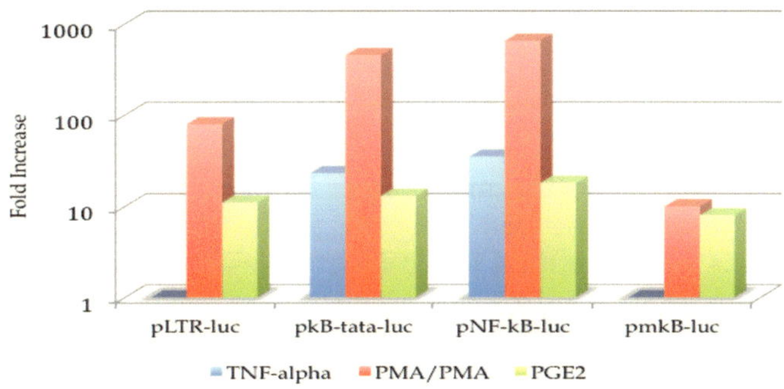

Fig. 4. NF-κB-dependent and -independent activation of HIV-1 LTR by PGE_2. Jurkat E6.1 cells were transiently transfected with pLTR-LUC, pmκBLTR-LUC, pNF-κB-LUC or pκB-TATA-LUC and were either left untreated or were treated for 8 h with TNF-α (2 ng/ml), PHA/PMA (3 μg/ml and 20 ng/ml, respectively), or PGE_2 (100 nM). Results shown are expressed as fold induction relative to basal luciferase activity in untreated control cells (considered as 1).

3.2.2 Other transcription factors implicated in the PGE_2-induced HIV-1 gene transcription

PGE_2 could have the capacity to modulate several signal transduction pathways through its effect on transcription factors regulated by cAMP such as the cAMP response-element binding factor, the activating protein-1 (Haraguchi et al., 1995b) and Sp1 (Rohlff et al., 1997). The involvement of these three transcription factors in the observed NF-κB-independent activation of HIV-1 LTR mediated by PGE_2 was further investigated. We have previously discussed that interaction of PGE_2 with EP_4 receptor subtype in human T cells can up-regulate HIV-1 replication via both NF-κB-dependent and -independent pathways (Dumais et al., 1998). In this section, we will address the functional role played by other transcription factors in the PGE_2-induced HIV-1 LTR activation.

Several signal transduction pathways have been shown to regulate the expression of target genes by inducing the phosphorylation of specific transcription factors (Hunter & Karin, 1992). The second messenger cAMP mediates the transcriptional induction of numerous genes through protein kinase A (PKA)-dependent phosphorylation of the CREB at Ser^{133} (Gonzalez et al., 1989). CREB is a stimulus-induced 43-kDa basic leucine zipper (b-ZIP) transcription factor that binds to an octanucleotide cAMP-responsive element (CRE) (i.e., TGANNTCA) both as a homodimer and as a heterodimer in conjunction with other members of the activation transcription factor (ATF)/CREB superfamily of transcription factors (Gonzalez & Montminy, 1989; Habener, 1990; Hoeffler et al., 1988). It is now believed that the transcriptional regulation of genes containing either CCAAT/enhancer binding protein (C/EBP) or ATF/CREB recognition sites may involve the heterodimerization between different members of the b-ZIP family. This is clearly illustrated by the demonstration that transcription of HIV-1 in monocytic cells is regulated by a synergistic interaction between ATF/CREB and C/EBP protein families (Ross et al., 2001). The C/EBP-related family of nuclear transcription factors constitutes a class of proteins characterized by their ability to bind the CCAAT consensus sequence, inducing either transcriptional activation or repression of target genes (Cao et al., 1991; Chodosh et al., 1988; Johnson & McKnight, 1989; Williams et al., 1991). Members of this family include C/EBPα, C/EBPβ (also termed LAP, NF-IL6α, IL-6DBP, AGP/EBP), C/EBPγ, C/EBPδ (NF-IL6) and C/EBPε (Mueller et al., 1990). Interestingly, regulatory sequences of HIV-1, which are located within the LTR, harbor three C/EBP sites that bind C/EBPβ (Tesmer et al., 1993) (Fig 2) and these sites are essential to initiate virus replication in cells of the monocyte/macrophage lineage (Henderson et al., 1995) and in endothelial cells as recently described (Lee et al., 2001). PKA and transcription factors of the ATF/CREB family may be critical for HIV-1 expression and regulation. In this regard, HIV-1 infection has been associated with sustained elevation of cAMP in T cell lines and in normal peripheral blood mononuclear lymphocytes (Nokta & Pollard, 1992). Moreover, HIV-1 replication has been shown to be modulated by intracellular levels of cAMP (Dumais et al., 1998; Nokta & Pollard, 1992). For example, activation of the cAMP/PKA pathway by cholera toxin enhances HIV-1 transcription in latently infected monocytoid U1 cells (Chowdhury et al., 1993). It is still unknown whether the HIV-1 genome, especially the LTR, possesses CRE sequences. However, the downstream sequence elements located in the U5 domain of HIV-1 LTR has been proposed to act as 12-O-tetradecanoylphorbol-13-acetate/phorbol ester responsive element (TRE)-like CRE that bind both AP-1 and CREB/ATF, allowing the induction of HIV-1 LTR activity through both protein kinase C and PKA activation signals (Rabbi et al., 1998).

PGE_2 can act as a potent activator of HIV-1 LTR-driven transcription through effects on both NF-κB-dependent and -independent signaling events (Dumais et al., 1998). More recently, calcium and the CREB transcription factor were also found to be essential second messengers in the PGE_2-mediated up-regulation of LTR activity in T cells (our unpublished observation). Although the binding of a member of the CREB family to the HIV-1 LTR via the CRE consensus sequence has not yet been described, it has been postulated that CREB can act indirectly on the regulatory elements of this retrovirus. For example, it has been shown that CREB interacts with HIV-1 LTR through an association with transcription factors such as TFIID and TFIIB (Ferreri et al., 1994; Rohr et al., 1999; Xing et al., 1995) or with the adapter CBP; the latter is known to interact with the general transcription machinery (Nordheim, 1994). Recently, a recognition sequence for members of the ATF/CREB family was identified within the untranslated leader region of HIV-1 as a novel TRE-like CRE capable of binding both AP-1 and ATF/CREB (Rabbi et al., 1997). However, the U5 region of the HIV-1 LTR is absent from our molecular constructs, rejecting the possible implication of TRE-like CRE in the noticed PGE_2-induced viral activation. A recent report has shown that dopamine treatment of HIV-1-infected T cells leads to the binding of CREB to the COUP-TF sequence that is located at the 5' end of the HIV-1 LTR in a region called the NRE (Rohr et al., 1999). The various LTR constructs used in our study do not bear the NRE, suggesting that the COUP-TF binding domain is not participating in PGE_2-mediated effect.

The C/EBP family of nuclear proteins is a member of a larger superfamily of transcription factors characterized by the b-ZIP motif that also includes the ATF/CREB family (Johnson, 1993). In a number of cell types, C/EBPβ has been shown to function as a cAMP-activated transcription factor (Metz & Ziff, 1991; Roesler et al., 1988; Tae et al., 1995). Treatment of Jurkat cells with PGE_2 resulted in a noticeable induction of nuclear translocation and activation of C/EBPβ. Indeed, DNA mobility shift assays provided clear evidence that PGE_2 and forskolin treatment of human T cells increases the level of specific protein-DNA complexes when the consensus C/EBP binding site is used as a molecular probe. Although treatment of Jurkat cells with PGE_2 did not alter the protein level of C/EBPβ in whole cell extracts, there was a redistribution of this protein from the cytoplasm to the nucleus upon exposure to PGE_2 (Dumais et al., 2002).

It has been previously demonstrated that individual C/EBP proteins can homodimerize or heterodimerize with other members of the C/EBP family of b-ZIP domain proteins to elicit specific cAMP-mediated transcriptional stimulation or repression (Metz & Ziff, 1991; Vinson et al., 1989; Williams et al., 1991). Moreover, it is now believed that transcriptional regulation of genes containing the recognition sites of either C/EBP or ATF/CREB may result from heterodimeric formation between different members in each of the C/EBP and ATF/CREB families (Vallejo, 1994). This mechanism may be used to respond to complex signals and transcriptional cues through single sequence elements including a response to cAMP, despite the absence of active CRE, AP1, and AP2 consensus nucleotide sequences (Kagawa & Waterman, 1990; Lund et al., 1990; Pittman et al., 1995). The best example is provided by the CFTR gene promoter that is controlled by interactions between C/EBP and ATF/CREB family members with CREB1 and ATF1 binding to the inverted CCAAT element of this gene to finely regulate its transcription (Pittman et al., 1995). Although the absence of CRE certainly may not preclude ATF or CREB protein from targeting promoters devoid of such cis-acting elements, it is interesting to note that regulation of the somatostatin gene requires protein-protein interaction between C/EBP and ATF/CREB transcription factors to elicit a cAMP-dependent response through the CRE element (Vallejo, 1994). Inversely, C/EBP proteins have been shown to bind specifically to the phosphoenolpyruvate carboxykinase gene CRE with high affinity to promote cAMP-mediated transcriptional activation (Park et al., 1993). In addition, previous studies identified C/EBP as an effector of cAMP-mediated transcription of the phosphoenolpyruvate carboxykinase gene through combined interactions with liver-specific transcription factors (Roesler, 2000; Roesler et al., 1995). Experiments conducted with a vector coding for LIP suggested that C/EBP was playing a crucial role in activation of HIV-1 LTR-driven gene expression that is seen following treatment of human T cells with PGE_2 (Dumais et al., 2002). It should be noted that the β-isoform of C/EBP has been intimately linked with the cAMP signaling system, as exemplified by the reported capacity of cAMP to stimulate C/EBPβ gene expression (Park et al., 1993) and translocation of C/EBPβ from the cytosol to the nucleus (1991). Thus, we propose that the PGE_2-dependent increase in HIV-1 LTR transcriptional activity is mediated in part by C/EBPβ. The dominant negative form of C/EBP, i.e., LIP, has less impact on PGE_2-mediated induction of HIV-1 LTR-driven activity than mutating the C/EBP binding sites, suggesting that factors in addition to C/EBP may be binding to C/EBP sites.

We have identified C/EBPβ as a PGE_2-activated transcriptional regulator of HIV-1 LTR in Jurkat cells and demonstrated that C/EBP binding sites are functionally important for virus transcription. We also suggest that functional and physical association between members of two important transcription factor families, i.e., C/EBPβ and CREB, are required for activation of HIV-1 transcription by PGE_2 (Dumais et al., 2002). Our findings represent a further indication of the high complexity of the molecular mechanisms that regulate HIV-1 gene expression following treatment of human T cells with PGE_2. Fig 5 reviews the effect of PGE_2 on HIV-1 LTR transcription.

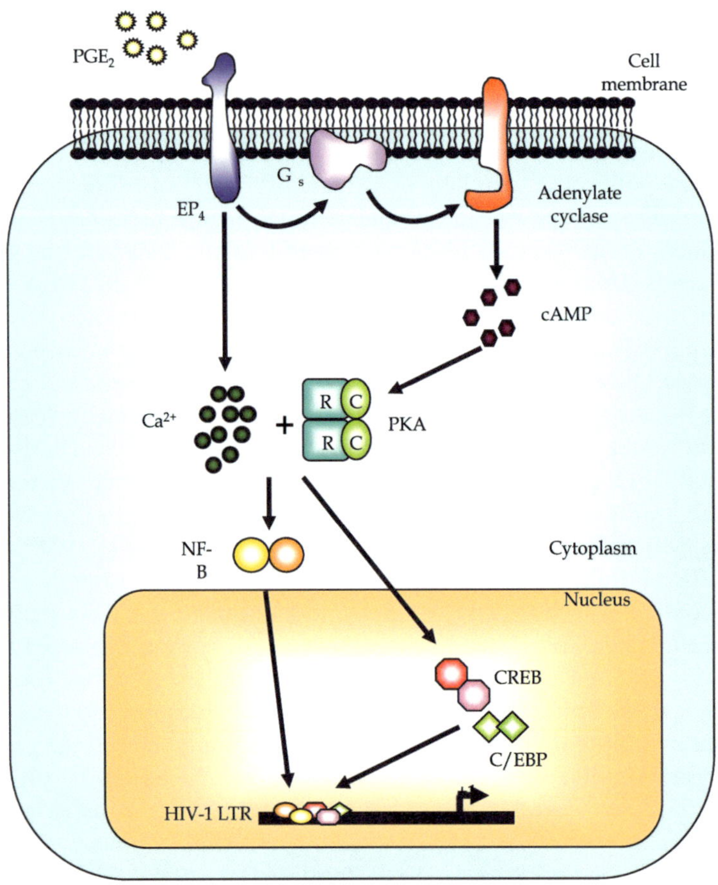

Fig. 5. A model of PGE_2-induced HIV-1 LTR activation in T cells.

3.2.3 Significance

Results from several studies showed that PGE_2 have a major impact in HIV-1 pathogenesis exacerbation. Knowing that HIV-infected individuals have a deficiency in the production of anti-inflammatory molecules, more knowledge are required to fully understand the potential benefit of the resolution of inflammation for people on HAART. Because they are clinically important molecules, a further understanding of the roles that prostaglandins played in host defense and HIV pathogenesis will have great impact on therapeutic research. Detailed characterization of prostaglandins interactions with cells infected with

HIV-1 will help us to understand their mechanism of action and establish their therapeutic potential in the resolution of inflammation in HIV+ individuals.

3.3 15-d-PGJ_2 and HIV-1 replication/production in intestinal epithelial cells

Sexual transmission is the predominant mode for epidemic spread of HIV-1 infection worldwide. Because semen contains both free HIV-1 virions and HIV-1-infected cells (Bouhlal et al., 2002; Royce et al., 1997; Shepard et al., 2000), it can lead to both free and cell-associated viral transmission. The intestinal mucosa of the rectum, which serves as a site for virus entry, is known to play a fundamental role in early HIV-1 infection (Belyakov & Berzofsky, 2004; Kozlowski & Neutra, 2003; Neutra et al., 1996). In contrast, the mechanism of HIV-1 transmission across the epithelium is not well understood. While it is known that the penetration of HIV-1 may occur through lesions in the epithelium (Dickerson et al., 1996; Kozak et al., 1997), the existence of lesions is not required (Miller et al., 1990; Spira et al., 1996). Some studies suggest that HIV-1 can be carried to lymphocytes by dendritic cells (Geijtenbeek et al., 2000; Pohlmann et al., 2001). It has been proposed that HIV-1 can cross the epithelium barrier via epithelial cell infection. A quantitative analysis of enhanced green fluorescent protein-tagged HIV infection of cells derived from the female reproductive tract, brain and colon demonstrated that gp120-independent HIV infection occurs in intestinal epithelial cells (Zheng et al., 2006). These results clearly illustrate the importance of such cells in viral latency and transmission during mucosal HIV-1 infection. Earlier *in vitro* studies showed that HIV can infect human intestinal cell lines lacking CD4 (Fantini et al., 1991; Fantini et al., 1993). These studies also demonstrated that galactosylceramide (GalCer), which binds with high-affinity to gp120, can act as a CD4 surrogate HIV-1 receptor (Meng et al., 2002). In fact, Caco-2 cells, a human intestinal cell line, can be infected by HIV-1 via GalCer and CXCR4, one of the two known HIV chemokine coreceptors (Delezay et al., 1997; Fantini et al., 1993). Also, primary human intestinal cells are capable of selectively transferring R5 HIV-1 to CCR5+ cells (cells that express both GalCer and CCR5 on their cell surface) (Meng et al., 2002). Thus, they proposed that infection of epithelial cells might facilitate HIV-1 penetration into the epithelium barrier (Zheng et al., 2006). Following viral replication in the infected epithelial cells, newly formed HIV virions may be discharged into the basolateral side of the epithelium and exposed to immune cells present in the mucosal milieu. This process may ultimately lead to the dissemination of the virus throughout the body. Therefore, it is essential to understand the mechanisms by which HIV replication in epithelial cells can be modulated by the immune system molecules present in the mucosal milieu. Prostaglandins play key roles in inflammation. During the time course of inflammation, the prostaglandins profile shifts from the predominantly pro-inflammatory PGE_2 to the anti-inflammatory PGJ_2, which is the end product metabolite of PGD_2 (Gilroy et al., 1999; Ianaro et al., 2001; Kapoor et al., 2005a; Kapoor et al., 2005b). Pro-inflammatory molecules such as PGE_2 are up-regulated during HIV-1 infection (Griffin et al., 1994b; Ramis et al., 1991) leading to an imbalance in PGJ_2 production. Given that the cyclopentone prostaglandin PGJ_2 has potent anti-inflammatory properties, it is important to determine whether the addition of PGJ_2 could inhibit HIV-1 transcription in intestinal epithelial cells.

Cyclopentone prostaglandins such as PGA_1 possess potent antiviral activity against a wide variety of viruses such as herpesviruses (Hughes-Fulford et al., 1992; Yamamoto et al., 1987), poxviruses (Santoro et al., 1982), paramyxoviruses (Amici et al., 1992; Santoro et al., 1980), orthomyxoviruses (Santoro et al., 1988), picornaviruses (Ankel et al., 1985), togaviruses

(Mastromarino et al., 1993), rhabdoviruses (Ankel et al., 1985; Santoro et al., 1983) and retroviruses (Hayes et al., 2002; Rozera et al., 1996; Skolnik et al., 2002). In macrophages, rosiglitazone, troglitazone, and PGJ_2 as well as fenofibrate (a PPAR-α agonist) can inhibit HIV-1 replication in U1 cells (Skolnik et al., 2002), while PGA_1 and PGA_2 can inhibit HIV-1 replication in U937 cells and human monocyte-derived macrophages (Hayes et al., 2002). During acute HIV-1 infection in the well-characterized T cell line CEM-SS, treatment with cyclopentone prostaglandins such as PGA_1 and PGJ_2 profoundly alters viral replication (Rozera et al., 1996). Moreover, this antiviral effect does not seem to be mediated by alterations in the expression of α-, β-, or γ-interferon, TNF-α, TNF-β, IL-6 or IL-10 in HIV-infected CEM-SS but rather by a direct, as yet unidentified, mechanism (Rozera et al., 1996).

3.3.1 15-d-PGJ_2 inhibition of HIV-1 transcription and viral production

The potent anti-inflammatory molecule 15-d-PGJ_2 strongly suppresses HIV-1 replication and particle production in Caco-2 cells, a human intestinal cell line that mimics rectal epithelium susceptible to HIV-1 (Delezay et al., 1997; Fantini et al., 1991; Fantini et al., 1992; Fantini et al., 1993; Zheng et al., 2006). Prophylactic or co-treatment with 15-d-PGJ_2 of intestinal epithelial cells significantly reduces HIV replication as well as p24 core antigen production (Boisvert et al., 2008). The 15-d-PGJ_2-mediated suppression of HIV-1 replication is a result of the inhibition of promoter activity as shown by the utilization of a pLTR-luc reporter plasmid (Fig 6). This suppression of HIV-1 LTR activity is dose-dependant and is optimal 24h post-treatment. Moreover, 15-d-PGJ_2 inhibition of sodium butyrate (NaBut)-induced LTR activity is not specific to Caco-2 cells but can be observed in other intestinal epithelial cell lines such as HT-29 and SW620. Sodium butyrate plays major roles in HIV infection. Indeed, urinary butyrate levels were increased in the AIDS patients with weight loss (2.83±0.67 µmol/l) relative to the controls (1.31±0.13 µmol/l, $P<0.05$), with the HIV+ patients (1.65±0.18 µmol/l) and AIDS patients without weight loss (1.90±0.22 µmol/l) falling in between (Stein et al., 1997). NaBut is a deacetylase inhibitor that has been shown to activate HIV-1 replication in cells of T-lymphoid and monocytoid origin (Golub et al., 1991). Thus, 15-d-PGJ_2, without significantly changing cell viability or the cell cycle by blocking them in G1 phase or altering apoptosis, profoundly affects HIV-1 replication and gene expression in intestinal epithelial cell lines (Boisvert et al., 2008).

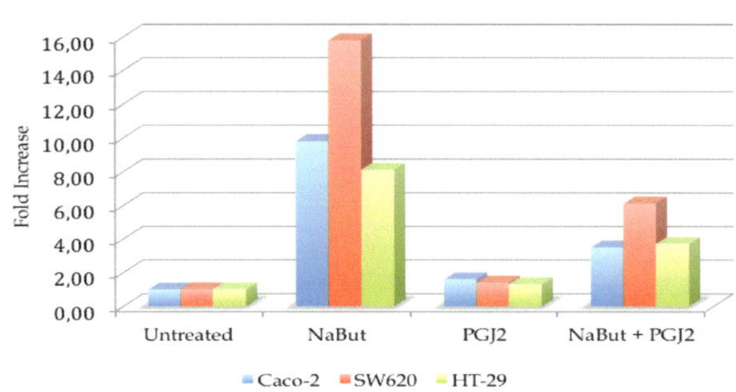

Fig. 6. 15-d-PGJ_2-mediated negative effect on HIV-1 LTR activity. Caco-2, SW620 and HT-29 cells were transiently transfected with pLTR-luc and treated with 15-d- PGJ_2 (20 µM) used in combination with 2 mM NaBut in a 24 h incubation period. Results shown are expressed as fold induction relative to basal luciferase activity in untreated control cells (considered as 1).

3.3.2 15-d-PGJ_2-inhibition of HIV-1 LTR activation is linked to modification to NF-kB signaling pathway

It has been shown previously that 15-d-PGJ_2 exerts its effect(s) on cells by activating the PPAR-γ transcription factor via PPAR-γ, the natural ligand of PGJ_2 (Schoonjans et al., 1996; Spiegelman, 1998). However, several studies have reported PPAR-γ independent effects of PGJ_2 on transcriptional regulation via the modulation of NF-κB (Rossi et al., 2000; Straus et al., 2000). In Caco-2, ciglitazone, a PPAR-γ agonist, failed to mimic the PGJ_2-induced suppression of LTR activity, a result that suggests a PPAR-γ-independent mechanism, such as the NF-κB pathway, may play a role in this effect in intestinal epithelial cells (Boisvert et al., 2008). This result is in contrast to those of Skolnik et al. in 2002 (Skolnik et al., 2002) that showed that ciglitazone was able to reduce the HIV-1 promoter activity in monocytes and in peripheral blood mononuclear cells (PBMCs). In contrast, ciglitazone induces luciferase activity in this experimental model. The induction of NF-κB activity in colon cancer cells via p65 phosphorylation has been previously reported (Chen & Harrison, 2005), and this phenomenon may explain why we observed an increase in luciferase expression following the ciglitazone treatment of Caco-2 cells. The blockade of PPAR-γ receptor activation by using a specific human PPAR-γ antagonist (GW9662) confirms that 15-d-PGJ_2 repress LTR activity by a mechanism independent of PPAR-γ (Boisvert et al., 2008). Similarly, expression of IL-1β in human chondrocytes is inhibited by 15-d-PGJ_2 by a PPAR-γ-independent mechanism (Boyault et al., 2001) as well as IL-8 expression in endothelial cells (Jozkowicz et al., 2001).

The PPAR-γ-independent mechanism by which 15-d-PGJ_2 mediates its anti-inflammatory effect can be dependent upon the inhibition of the NF-κB signaling pathway (Daynes & Jones, 2002; Rossi et al., 2000). The NF-κB binding sites within the HIV-1 promoter confer a high level of viral transcription in many cell types (Rabson & Lin, 2000). Previous studies have shown that cyclopentone prostaglandins via their ability to modulate NF-κB activity, significantly alter HIV-1 replication in T cells, monocytes/macrophages and intestinal epithelial cells (Boisvert et al., 2008; Hayes et al., 2002; Rozera et al., 1996; Skolnik et al., 2002). In Caco-2 cells, the functional role of NF-κB was determined using pκB-TATA-luc or pNFκB-luc expression plasmids (Fig 7). The results demonstrated that the NaBut-induced

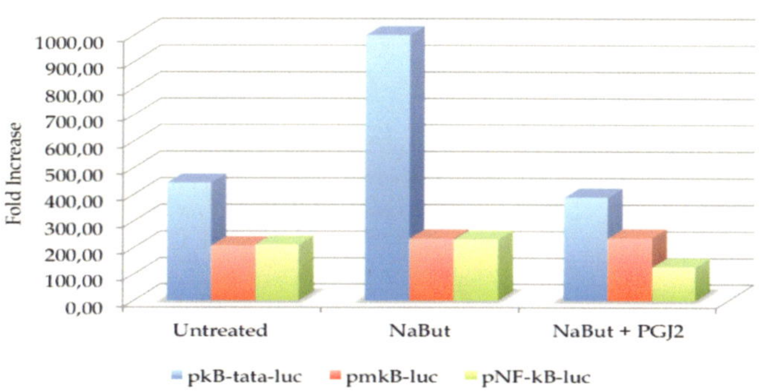

Fig. 7. NF-κB-dependent inhibition of HIV-1 LTR by 15-d-PGJ_2. Caco-2 cells were transiently transfected with pκB-TATA-luc, pmκB-luc and pNF-κB-luc. Then, cells were treated with 20 μM 15-d-PGJ_2 used in combination with 2 mM NaBut in a 24 h incubation period. Caco-2 cells were lysed and luciferase activity was monitored. Results shown are expressed as fold induction relative to basal luciferase activity in untreated control cells (considered as 1).

luciferase activity of the pκB-TATA-luc construct, which contains the HIV-1 enhancer, is abrogated by 15-d-PGJ_2 in a dose-dependent manner. A control construct containing the HIV-1 enhancer with inactivated NF-κB binding sites, pmκB-luc, was used to show that NF-κB is necessary for the NaBut activation of the HIV-1 LTR in Caco-2. Similar results to pκB-TATA-luc were found using the pNFκB-luc construct, which contains five consensus NF-κB binding sites. Together, these data suggest that NF-κB is involved in the 15-d-PGJ_2-mediated suppression of HIV-1 LTR activation in Caco-2 cells.

15-d-PGJ_2 alters the stability of IκBα proteins thereby altering NF-κB activation. Moreover in human bronchial epithelium, cyclopentone prostaglandin such has PGA_1, has been shown to enhance the expression of IκBα, a primary inhibitor of the pro-inflammatory transcription factor NF-κB (Thomas et al., 1998). In intestinal epithelial cells, IKK activity was lower in Caco-2 cells treated with 15-d-PGJ_2 and the inhibition of IKK activity was direct without increasing IκBα mRNA expression. Another group (Scher & Pillinger, 2005) reported an inhibitory effect of 15-d-PGJ_2 on NF-κB activation and expression of pro-inflammatory genes such as COX-2, IL-1β and TNF-α. Interestingly in human chondrocytes, 15d-PGJ_2, but not troglitazone, modulates IL-1β expression by inhibiting NF-κB and AP-1 activation pathways, a mechanism independent of PPAR-γ as observed with 15-d-PGJ_2 and NaBut-induced LTR activation. Moreover, it was shown by electrophoretic mobility shift assays that 15-d-PGJ_2 represses the nuclear translocation of the ubiquitous transcription factor NF-κB, which also results in the repression of HIV-1 transcription (Boisvert et al., 2008). Taken together results showed that the cyclopentone PGJ_2 inhibits NaBut-induced NF-κB binding activity in Caco-2 cells. This effect is caused by a reduction in the activity of IKK which results in reduced NF-κB nuclear translocation but not alterations in IκBα gene expression (Fig 8).

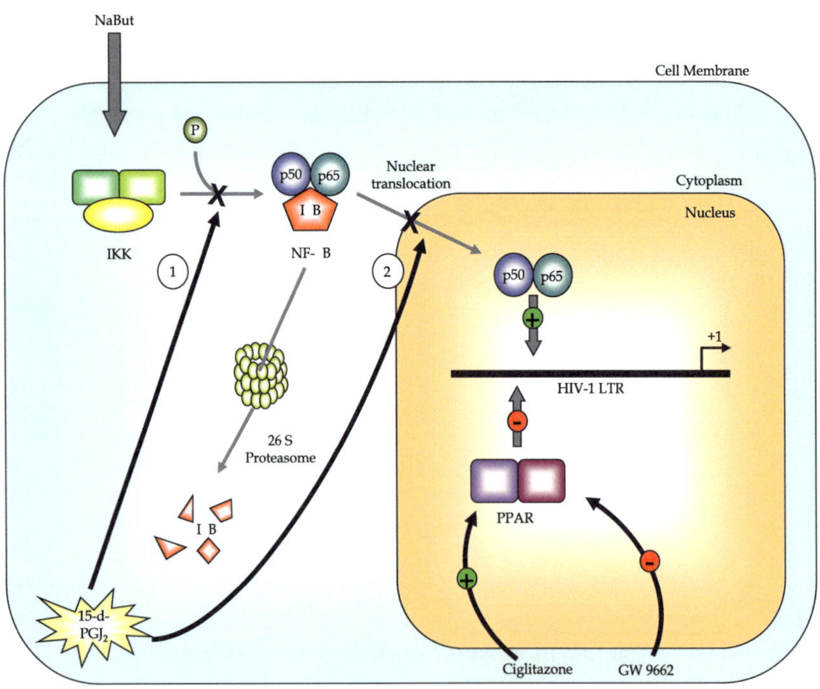

Fig. 8. Effect of 15-d-PGJ_2 on NF-κB and impact on HIV-1 transcription.

4. Conclusion

AIDS patients exhibit abnormal production of cyclooxygenase products. Prostaglandins are complex immunomodulatory molecules that shape, on one hand, the immune system and, on the other hand, have an influence on gene transcription by inducing or repressing several transcription factors in cells. Recent studies have led to a better understanding of the unique characteristics and importance of prostaglandins on HIV-1 transcription and replication (Fig 9).

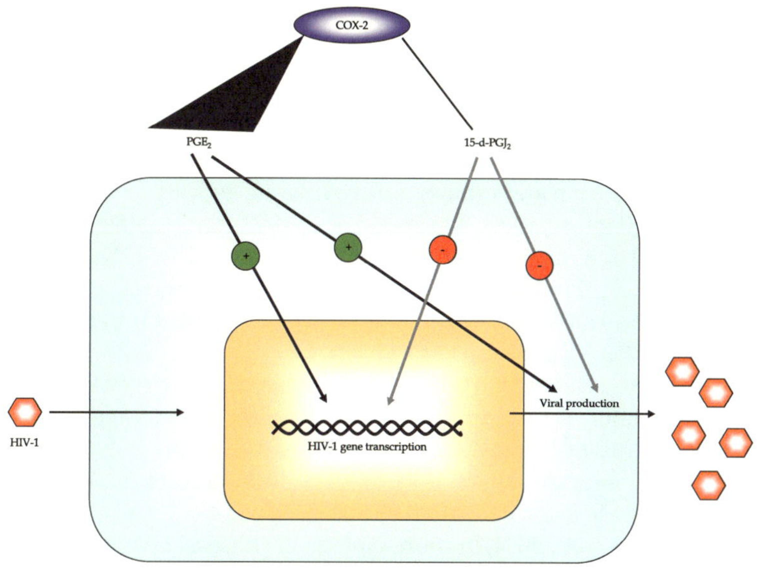

Fig. 9. A model for prostaglandins actions on HIV-1 pathogenesis.

Because of their intrinsic intracellular obligatory parasitic form of life, viruses depend heavily on cell metabolic machinery for their replication. Thus, changes in cellular metabolism might influence the viral life cycle. The data reported in this chapter highlight the positive action of PGE_2, a powerful cAMP-inducing agent, on the regulatory elements of HIV-1. PGE_2 has now emerged as an immuno-activator that acts on the EP_4 receptor that facilitates HIV-1 LTR activation. Elevated levels of PGE_2 detected in HIV-1-infected persons or induced by opportunistic pathogens might actively participate to immunological disturbances associated with AIDS and modify the pathogenesis of this retroviral disease by inducing a higher viral load. High concentrations of PGE_2 (up to 100 μM) found in seminal fluids of HIV-1-infected persons might directly enhance virus replication and facilitate viral transmission during sexual activities. Thus, analysis of the role of the PGE_2 signaling may provide deeper insight into the pathological mechanisms underlying HIV/AIDS exacerbation, which should be fully taken into account in developing an EP_4 antagonist as a therapeutic agent and its clinical application.

Accumulating data from several studies suggest that PGJ_2 has intracellular effects that may suppress inflammation. They include inhibition of NF-κB by multiple mechanisms such as IκB kinase inhibition, blockade of NF-κB nuclear binding and activation of PPAR-γ. The consequences of these activities are complex, but are likely to play a role in the prevention and/or resolution of inflammation. In this chapter, we showed the potentiality of the anti-inflammatory molecule, PGJ_2, to modulate the NaBut effect on HIV-1 LTR in intestinal epithelial cells by a PPAR-γ-independent mechanism via the inhibition of NF-κB translocation to the nucleus. These results suggest that such prostaglandins may have therapeutic value in the treatment of HIV-1 infected individuals where inhibition of NF-κB activity may be required.

5. References

Abel, P.M., McSharry, C., Galloway, E., Ross, C., Severn, A., Toner, G., Gruer, L., Wilkinson, P.C., 1992. Heterogeneity of peripheral blood monocyte populations in human immunodeficiency virus-1 seropositive patients. FEMS Microbiol Immunol 5, 317-323.

Aguilar-Cordova, E., Chinen, J., Donehower, L., Lewis, D.E., Belmont, J.W., 1994. A sensitive reporter cell line for HIV-1 tat activity, HIV-1 inhibitors, and T cell activation effects. AIDS research and human retroviruses 10, 295-301.

Amici, C., Sistonen, L., Santoro, M.G., Morimoto, R.I., 1992. Antiproliferative prostaglandins activate heat shock transcription factor. Proc Natl Acad Sci U S A 89, 6227-6231.

Ankel, H., Mittnacht, S., Jacobsen, H., 1985. Antiviral activity of prostaglandin A on encephalomyocarditis virus-infected cells: a unique effect unrelated to interferon. J Gen Virol 66 (Pt 11), 2355-2364.

Auberger, P., Didier, M., Didier, J., Aussel, C., Fehlmann, M., 1989. A chymotryptic-type protease inhibitor decreases interleukin 2 synthesis and induces prostaglandin production in Jurkat T cells. Cellular signalling 1, 289-294.

Baker, P.E., Fahey, J.V., Munck, A., 1981. Prostaglandin inhibition of T-cell proliferation is mediated at two levels. Cellular immunology 61, 52-61.

Belyakov, I.M., Berzofsky, J.A., 2004. Immunobiology of mucosal HIV infection and the basis for development of a new generation of mucosal AIDS vaccines. Immunity 20, 247-253.

Ben-Hur, T., Rosenthal, J., Itzik, A., Weidenfeld, J., 1996. Rescue of HSV-1 neurovirulence is associated with induction of brain interleukin-1 expression, prostaglandin synthesis and neuroendocrine responses. Journal of neurovirology 2, 279-288.

Blaschke, V., Jungermann, K., Puschel, G.P., 1996. Exclusive expression of the Gs-linked prostaglandin E2 receptor subtype 4 mRNA in mononuclear Jurkat and KM-3 cells and coexpression of subtype 4 and 2 mRNA in U-937 cells. FEBS letters 394, 39-43.

Boisvert, M., Cote, S., Vargas, A., Pasvanis, S., Bounou, S., Barbeau, B., Dumais, N., 2008. PGJ2 antagonizes NF-kappaB-induced HIV-1 LTR activation in colonic epithelial cells. Virology 380, 1-11.

Bouhlal, H., Chomont, N., Haeffner-Cavaillon, N., Kazatchkine, M.D., Belec, L., Hocini, H., 2002. Opsonization of HIV-1 by semen complement enhances infection of human epithelial cells. J Immunol 169, 3301-3306.

Boyault, S., Simonin, M.A., Bianchi, A., Compe, E., Liagre, B., Mainard, D., Becuwe, P., Dauca, M., Netter, P., Terlain, B., Bordji, K., 2001. 15-Deoxy-delta12,14-PGJ2, but not troglitazone, modulates IL-1beta effects in human chondrocytes by inhibiting NF-kappaB and AP-1 activation pathways. FEBS Lett 501, 24-30.

Brockman, J.A., Gupta, R.A., Dubois, R.N., 1998. Activation of PPARgamma leads to inhibition of anchorage-independent growth of human colorectal cancer cells. Gastroenterology 115, 1049-1055.

Cao, Z., Umek, R.M., McKnight, S.L., 1991. Regulated expression of three C/EBP isoforms during adipose conversion of 3T3-L1 cells. Genes & development 5, 1538-1552.

Chen, F., Harrison, L.E., 2005. Ciglitazone induces early cellular proliferation and NF-kappaB transcriptional activity in colon cancer cells through p65 phosphorylation. Int J Biochem Cell Biol 37, 645-654.

Chodosh, L.A., Baldwin, A.S., Carthew, R.W., Sharp, P.A., 1988. Human CCAAT-binding proteins have heterologous subunits. Cell 53, 11-24.

Chowdhury, M.I., Koyanagi, Y., Horiuchi, S., Hazeki, O., Ui, M., Kitano, K., Golde, D.W., Takada, K., Yamamoto, N., 1993. cAMP stimulates human immunodeficiency virus (HIV-1) from latently infected cells of monocyte-macrophage lineage: synergism with TNF-alpha. Virology 194, 345-349.

Clark, R.B., Bishop-Bailey, D., Estrada-Hernandez, T., Hla, T., Puddington, L., Padula, S.J., 2000. The nuclear receptor PPAR gamma and immunoregulation: PPAR gamma mediates inhibition of helper T cell responses. Journal of immunology 164, 1364-1371.

Coffey, M.J., Phare, S.M., Cinti, S., Peters-Golden, M., Kazanjian, P.H., 1999. Granulocyte-macrophage colony-stimulating factor upregulates reduced 5-lipoxygenase metabolism in peripheral blood monocytes and neutrophils in acquired immunodeficiency syndrome. Blood 94, 3897-3905.

Coleman, R.A., Eglen, R.M., Jones, R.L., Narumiya, S., Shimizu, T., Smith, W.L., Dahlen, S.E., Drazen, J.M., Gardiner, P.J., Jackson, W.T., et al., 1995. Prostanoid and leukotriene receptors: a progress report from the IUPHAR working parties on classification and nomenclature. Advances in prostaglandin, thromboxane, and leukotriene research 23, 283-285.

Coleman, R.A., Smith, W.L., Narumiya, S., 1994. International Union of Pharmacology classification of prostanoid receptors: properties, distribution, and structure of the receptors and their subtypes. Pharmacol Rev 46, 205-229.

Daynes, R.A., Jones, D.C., 2002. Emerging roles of PPARs in inflammation and immunity. Nat Rev Immunol 2, 748-759.

De Vries, G.W., Guarino, P., McLaughlin, A., Chen, J., Andrews, S., Woodward, D.F., 1995. An EP receptor with a novel pharmacological profile in the T-cell line Jurkat. British journal of pharmacology 115, 1231-1234.

Delezay, O., Koch, N., Yahi, N., Hammache, D., Tourres, C., Tamalet, C., Fantini, J., 1997. Co-expression of CXCR4/fusin and galactosylceramide in the human intestinal epithelial cell line HT-29. AIDS 11, 1311-1318.

Dickerson, M.C., Johnston, J., Delea, T.E., White, A., Andrews, E., 1996. The causal role for genital ulcer disease as a risk factor for transmission of human immunodeficiency virus. An application of the Bradford Hill criteria. Sex Transm Dis 23, 429-440.

Dumais, N., Barbeau, B., Olivier, M., Tremblay, M.J., 1998. Prostaglandin E2 Up-regulates HIV-1 long terminal repeat-driven gene activity in T cells via NF-kappaB-dependent and -independent signaling pathways. J Biol Chem 273, 27306-27314.

Dumais, N., Bounou, S., Olivier, M., Tremblay, M.J., 2002. Prostaglandin E(2)-mediated activation of HIV-1 long terminal repeat transcription in human T cells necessitates CCAAT/enhancer binding protein (C/EBP) binding sites in addition to cooperative interactions between C/EBPbeta and cyclic adenosine 5'-monophosphate response element binding protein. J Immunol 168, 274-282.

Fantini, J., Baghdiguian, S., Yahi, N., Chermann, J.C., 1991. Selected human immunodeficiency virus replicates preferentially through the basolateral surface of differentiated human colon epithelial cells. Virology 185, 904-907.
Fantini, J., Bolmont, C., Yahi, N., 1992. Tumor necrosis factor-alpha stimulates both apical and basal production of HIV in polarized human intestinal HT29 cells. Immunology letters 34, 85-90.
Fantini, J., Cook, D.G., Nathanson, N., Spitalnik, S.L., Gonzalez-Scarano, F., 1993. Infection of colonic epithelial cell lines by type 1 human immunodeficiency virus is associated with cell surface expression of galactosylceramide, a potential alternative gp120 receptor. Proc Natl Acad Sci U S A 90, 2700-2704.
Farrell, J.P., Kirkpatrick, C.E., 1987. Experimental cutaneous leishmaniasis. II. A possible role for prostaglandins in exacerbation of disease in Leishmania major-infected BALB/c mice. Journal of immunology 138, 902-907.
Faveeuw, C., Fougeray, S., Angeli, V., Fontaine, J., Chinetti, G., Gosset, P., Delerive, P., Maliszewski, C., Capron, M., Staels, B., Moser, M., Trottein, F., 2000. Peroxisome proliferator-activated receptor gamma activators inhibit interleukin-12 production in murine dendritic cells. FEBS letters 486, 261-266.
Fedyk, E.R., Phipps, R.P., 1996. Prostaglandin E2 receptors of the EP2 and EP4 subtypes regulate activation and differentiation of mouse B lymphocytes to IgE-secreting cells. Proceedings of the National Academy of Sciences of the United States of America 93, 10978-10983.
Fernandez-Cruz, E., Gelpi, E., Longo, N., Gonzalez, B., de la Morena, M.T., Montes, M.G., Rosello, J., Ramis, I., Suarez, A., Fernandez, A., et al., 1989. Increased synthesis and production of prostaglandin E2 by monocytes from drug addicts with AIDS. AIDS 3, 91-96.
Ferreri, K., Gill, G., Montminy, M., 1994. The cAMP-regulated transcription factor CREB interacts with a component of the TFIID complex. Proceedings of the National Academy of Sciences of the United States of America 91, 1210-1213.
Foley, P., Kazazi, F., Biti, R., Sorrell, T.C., Cunningham, A.L., 1992. HIV infection of monocytes inhibits the T-lymphocyte proliferative response to recall antigens, via production of eicosanoids. Immunology 75, 391-397.
Frantz, B., Nordby, E.C., Bren, G., Steffan, N., Paya, C.V., Kincaid, R.L., Tocci, M.J., O'Keefe, S.J., O'Neill, E.A., 1994. Calcineurin acts in synergy with PMA to inactivate I kappa B/MAD3, an inhibitor of NF-kappa B. The EMBO journal 13, 861-870.
Frey, J., Janes, M., Engelhardt, W., Afting, E.G., Geerds, C., Moller, B., 1986. Fc gamma-receptor-mediated changes in the plasma membrane potential induce prostaglandin release from human fibroblasts. European journal of biochemistry / FEBS 158, 85-89.
Fu, J.Y., Masferrer, J.L., Seibert, K., Raz, A., Needleman, P., 1990. The induction and suppression of prostaglandin H2 synthase (cyclooxygenase) in human monocytes. The Journal of biological chemistry 265, 16737-16740.
Geijtenbeek, T.B., Kwon, D.S., Torensma, R., van Vliet, S.J., van Duijnhoven, G.C., Middel, J., Cornelissen, I.L., Nottet, H.S., KewalRamani, V.N., Littman, D.R., Figdor, C.G., van Kooyk, Y., 2000. DC-SIGN, a dendritic cell-specific HIV-1-binding protein that enhances trans-infection of T cells. Cell 100, 587-597.

Ghosh, S., May, M.J., Kopp, E.B., 1998. NF-kappa B and Rel proteins: evolutionarily conserved mediators of immune responses. Annual review of immunology 16, 225-260.

Gilroy, D.W., Colville-Nash, P.R., Willis, D., Chivers, J., Paul-Clark, M.J., Willoughby, D.A., 1999. Inducible cyclooxygenase may have anti-inflammatory properties. Nat Med 5, 698-701.

Goldyne, M.E., Rea, L., 1987. Stimulated T cell and natural killer (NK) cell lines fail to synthesize leukotriene B4. Prostaglandins 34, 783-795.

Golub, E.I., Li, G.R., Volsky, D.J., 1991. Induction of dormant HIV-1 by sodium butyrate: involvement of the TATA box in the activation of the HIV-1 promoter. AIDS 5, 663-668.

Gonzalez, G.A., Montminy, M.R., 1989. Cyclic AMP stimulates somatostatin gene transcription by phosphorylation of CREB at serine 133. Cell 59, 675-680.

Gonzalez, G.A., Yamamoto, K.K., Fischer, W.H., Karr, D., Menzel, P., Biggs, W., 3rd, Vale, W.W., Montminy, M.R., 1989. A cluster of phosphorylation sites on the cyclic AMP-regulated nuclear factor CREB predicted by its sequence. Nature 337, 749-752.

Goodwin, J.S., Bankhurst, A.D., Messner, R.P., 1977. Suppression of human T-cell mitogenesis by prostaglandin. Existence of a prostaglandin-producing suppressor cell. The Journal of experimental medicine 146, 1719-1734.

Goodwin, J.S., Ceuppens, J., 1983. Regulation of the immune response by prostaglandins. Journal of clinical immunology 3, 295-315.

Goodwin, J.S., Webb, D.R., 1980. Regulation of the immune response by prostaglandins. Clinical immunology and immunopathology 15, 106-122.

Griffin, D.E., Wesselingh, S.L., McArthur, J.C., 1994a. Elevated central nervous system prostaglandins in human immunodeficiency virus-associated dementia. Ann Neurol 35, 592-597.

Griffin, J.W., Wesselingh, S.L., Griffin, D.E., Glass, J.D., McArthur, J.C., 1994b. Peripheral nerve disorders in HIV infection. Similarities and contrasts with CNS disorders. Res Publ Assoc Res Nerv Ment Dis 72, 159-182.

Habener, J.F., 1990. Cyclic AMP response element binding proteins: a cornucopia of transcription factors. Mol Endocrinol 4, 1087-1094.

Haraguchi, S., Good, R.A., Day, N.K., 1995a. Immunosuppressive retroviral peptides: cAMP and cytokine patterns. Immunology today 16, 595-603.

Haraguchi, S., Good, R.A., James-Yarish, M., Cianciolo, G.J., Day, N.K., 1995b. Induction of intracellular cAMP by a synthetic retroviral envelope peptide: a possible mechanism of immunopathogenesis in retroviral infections. Proceedings of the National Academy of Sciences of the United States of America 92, 5568-5571.

Harris, S.G., Padilla, J., Koumas, L., Ray, D., Phipps, R.P., 2002. Prostaglandins as modulators of immunity. Trends in immunology 23, 144-150.

Hayes, M.M., Lane, B.R., King, S.R., Markovitz, D.M., Coffey, M.J., 2002. Peroxisome proliferator-activated receptor gamma agonists inhibit HIV-1 replication in macrophages by transcriptional and post-transcriptional effects. J Biol Chem 277, 16913-16919.

Heinen, E., Cormann, N., Braun, M., Kinet-Denoel, C., Vanderschelden, J., Simar, L.J., 1986. Isolation of follicular dendritic cells from human tonsils and adenoids. VI. Analysis of prostaglandin secretion. Ann Inst Pasteur Immunol 137D, 369-382.

Henderson, A.J., Zou, X., Calame, K.L., 1995. C/EBP proteins activate transcription from the human immunodeficiency virus type 1 long terminal repeat in macrophages/monocytes. Journal of virology 69, 5337-5344.

Henke, A., Spengler, H.P., Stelzner, A., Nain, M., Gemsa, D., 1992. Lipopolysaccharide suppresses cytokine release from coxsackie virus-infected human monocytes. Res Immunol 143, 65-70.

Hinz, B., Brune, K., Pahl, A., 2003. 15-Deoxy-Delta(12,14)-prostaglandin J2 inhibits the expression of proinflammatory genes in human blood monocytes via a PPAR-gamma-independent mechanism. Biochemical and biophysical research communications 302, 415-420.

Hoeffler, J.P., Meyer, T.E., Yun, Y., Jameson, J.L., Habener, J.F., 1988. Cyclic AMP-responsive DNA-binding protein: structure based on a cloned placental cDNA. Science 242, 1430-1433.

Hofmann, B., Nishanian, P., Nguyen, T., Liu, M., Fahey, J.L., 1993. Restoration of T-cell function in HIV infection by reduction of intracellular cAMP levels with adenosine analogues. AIDS 7, 659-664.

Hortelano, S., Castrillo, A., Alvarez, A.M., Bosca, L., 2000. Contribution of cyclopentenone prostaglandins to the resolution of inflammation through the potentiation of apoptosis in activated macrophages. Journal of immunology 165, 6525-6531.

Hughes-Fulford, M., McGrath, M.S., Hanks, D., Erickson, S., Pulliam, L., 1992. Effects of dimethyl prostaglandin A1 on herpes simplex virus and human immunodeficiency virus replication. Antimicrob Agents Chemother 36, 2253-2258.

Hui, R., Curtis, J.F., Sumner, M.T., Shears, S.B., Glasgow, W.C., Eling, T.E., 1995. Human immunodeficiency virus type 1 envelope protein does not stimulate either prostaglandin formation or the expression of prostaglandin H synthase in THP-1 human monocytes/macrophages. Journal of virology 69, 8020-8026.

Hunter, T., Karin, M., 1992. The regulation of transcription by phosphorylation. Cell 70, 375-387.

Ianaro, A., Ialenti, A., Maffia, P., Pisano, B., Di Rosa, M., 2001. Role of cyclopentenone prostaglandins in rat carrageenin pleurisy. FEBS Lett 508, 61-66.

Imaizumi, T., Kumagai, M., Hatakeyama, M., Tamo, W., Yamashita, K., Tanji, K., Yoshida, H., Satoh, K., 2003. 15-Deoxy-delta 12,14-prostaglandin J2 inhibits the expression of granulocyte-macrophage colony-stimulating factor in endothelial cells stimulated with lipopolysaccharide. Prostaglandins & other lipid mediators 71, 293-299.

Ito, S., Narumiya, S., Hayaishi, O., 1989. Prostaglandin D2: a biochemical perspective. Prostaglandins, leukotrienes, and essential fatty acids 37, 219-234.

Jiang, C., Ting, A.T., Seed, B., 1998. PPAR-gamma agonists inhibit production of monocyte inflammatory cytokines. Nature 391, 82-86.

Johnson, P.F., 1993. Identification of C/EBP basic region residues involved in DNA sequence recognition and half-site spacing preference. Molecular and cellular biology 13, 6919-6930.

Johnson, P.F., McKnight, S.L., 1989. Eukaryotic transcriptional regulatory proteins. Annu Rev Biochem 58, 799-839.

Jozkowicz, A., Dulak, J., Prager, M., Nanobashvili, J., Nigisch, A., Winter, B., Weigel, G., Huk, I., 2001. Prostaglandin-J2 induces synthesis of interleukin-8 by endothelial cells in a PPAR-gamma-independent manner. Prostaglandins Other Lipid Mediat 66, 165-177.

Kagawa, N., Waterman, M.R., 1990. cAMP-dependent transcription of the human CYP21B (P-450C21) gene requires a cis-regulatory element distinct from the consensus cAMP-regulatory element. The Journal of biological chemistry 265, 11299-11305.

Kammer, G.M., 1988. The adenylate cyclase-cAMP-protein kinase A pathway and regulation of the immune response. Immunology today 9, 222-229.

Kapoor, M., Clarkson, A.N., Sutherland, B.A., Appleton, I., 2005a. The role of antioxidants in models of inflammation: emphasis on L-arginine and arachidonic acid metabolism. Inflammopharmacology 12, 505-519.

Kapoor, M., Shaw, O., Appleton, I., 2005b. Possible anti-inflammatory role of COX-2-derived prostaglandins: implications for inflammation research. Curr Opin Investig Drugs 6, 461-466.

Kernacki, K.A., Berk, R.S., 1994. Characterization of the inflammatory response induced by corneal infection with Pseudomonas aeruginosa. J Ocul Pharmacol 10, 281-288.

Kilareski, E.M., Shah, S., Nonnemacher, M.R., Wigdahl, B., 2009. Regulation of HIV-1 transcription in cells of the monocyte-macrophage lineage. Retrovirology 6, 118.

Koh, W.S., Yang, K.H., Kaminski, N.E., 1995. Cyclic AMP is an essential factor in immune responses. Biochemical and biophysical research communications 206, 703-709.

Kozak, S.L., Platt, E.J., Madani, N., Ferro, F.E., Jr., Peden, K., Kabat, D., 1997. CD4, CXCR-4, and CCR-5 dependencies for infections by primary patient and laboratory-adapted isolates of human immunodeficiency virus type 1. J Virol 71, 873-882.

Kozlowski, P.A., Neutra, M.R., 2003. The role of mucosal immunity in prevention of HIV transmission. Curr Mol Med 3, 217-228.

Kurland, J.I., Bockman, R., 1978. Prostaglandin E production by human blood monocytes and mouse peritoneal macrophages. The Journal of experimental medicine 147, 952-957.

Lee, E.S., Zhou, H., Henderson, A.J., 2001. Endothelial cells enhance human immunodeficiency virus type 1 replication in macrophages through a C/EBP-dependent mechanism. Journal of virology 75, 9703-9712.

Lefebvre, A.M., Chen, I., Desreumaux, P., Najib, J., Fruchart, J.C., Geboes, K., Briggs, M., Heyman, R., Auwerx, J., 1998. Activation of the peroxisome proliferator-activated receptor gamma promotes the development of colon tumors in C57BL/6J-APCMin/+ mice. Nature medicine 4, 1053-1057.

Lingk, D.S., Chan, M.A., Gelfand, E.W., 1990. Increased cyclic adenosine monophosphate levels block progression but not initiation of human T cell proliferation. Journal of immunology 145, 449-455.

Lund, J., Ahlgren, R., Wu, D.H., Kagimoto, M., Simpson, E.R., Waterman, M.R., 1990. Transcriptional regulation of the bovine CYP17 (P-450(17)alpha) gene. Identification of two cAMP regulatory regions lacking the consensus cAMP-responsive element (CRE). The Journal of biological chemistry 265, 3304-3312.

Mastino, A., Grelli, S., Piacentini, M., Oliverio, S., Favalli, C., Perno, C.F., Garci, E., 1993. Correlation between induction of lymphocyte apoptosis and prostaglandin E2 production by macrophages infected with HIV. Cell Immunol 152, 120-130.

Mastromarino, P., Conti, C., Petruzziello, R., De Marco, A., Pica, F., Santoro, M.G., 1993. Inhibition of Sindbis virus replication by cyclopentenone prostaglandins: a cell-mediated event associated with heat-shock protein synthesis. Antiviral Res 20, 209-222.

Meng, G., Wei, X., Wu, X., Sellers, M.T., Decker, J.M., Moldoveanu, Z., Orenstein, J.M., Graham, M.F., Kappes, J.C., Mestecky, J., Shaw, G.M., Smith, P.D., 2002. Primary intestinal epithelial cells selectively transfer R5 HIV-1 to CCR5+ cells. Nat Med 8, 150-156.

Metz, R., Ziff, E., 1991. cAMP stimulates the C/EBP-related transcription factor rNFIL-6 to trans-locate to the nucleus and induce c-fos transcription. Genes & development 5, 1754-1766.

Midulla, F., Huang, Y.T., Gilbert, I.A., Cirino, N.M., McFadden, E.R., Jr., Panuska, J.R., 1989. Respiratory syncytial virus infection of human cord and adult blood monocytes and alveolar macrophages. Am Rev Respir Dis 140, 771-777.

Miller, C.J., Alexander, N.J., Sutjipto, S., Joye, S.M., Hendrickx, A.G., Jennings, M., Marx, P.A., 1990. Effect of virus dose and nonoxynol-9 on the genital transmission of SIV in rhesus macaques. J Med Primatol 19, 401-409.

Mori, K., Tanaka, I., Kotani, M., Miyaoka, F., Sando, T., Muro, S., Sasaki, Y., Nakagawa, O., Ogawa, Y., Usui, T., Ozaki, S., Ichikawa, A., Narumiya, S., Nakao, K., 1996. Gene expression of the human prostaglandin E receptor EP4 subtype: differential regulation in monocytoid and lymphoid lineage cells by phorbol ester. Journal of molecular medicine 74, 333-336.

Mueller, C.R., Maire, P., Schibler, U., 1990. DBP, a liver-enriched transcriptional activator, is expressed late in ontogeny and its tissue specificity is determined posttranscriptionally. Cell 61, 279-291.

Munoz, E., Zubiaga, A.M., Merrow, M., Sauter, N.P., Huber, B.T., 1990. Cholera toxin discriminates between T helper 1 and 2 cells in T cell receptor-mediated activation: role of cAMP in T cell proliferation. The Journal of experimental medicine 172, 95-103.

Muroi, M., Suzuki, T., 1993. Role of protein kinase A in LPS-induced activation of NF-kappa B proteins of a mouse macrophage-like cell line, J774. Cellular signalling 5, 289-298.

Nabel, G., Baltimore, D., 1987. An inducible transcription factor activates expression of human immunodeficiency virus in T cells. Nature 326, 711-713.

Nabel, G.J., 1991. HIV. Tampering with transcription. Nature 350, 658.

Neutra, M.R., Frey, A., Kraehenbuhl, J.P., 1996. Epithelial M cells: gateways for mucosal infection and immunization. Cell 86, 345-348.

Nishigaki, N., Negishi, M., Honda, A., Sugimoto, Y., Namba, T., Narumiya, S., Ichikawa, A., 1995. Identification of prostaglandin E receptor 'EP2' cloned from mastocytoma cells EP4 subtype. FEBS letters 364, 339-341.

Nokta, M.A., Pollard, R.B., 1992. Human immunodeficiency virus replication: modulation by cellular levels of cAMP. AIDS research and human retroviruses 8, 1255-1261.

Nordheim, A., 1994. Transcription factors. CREB takes CBP to tango. Nature 370, 177-178.

Onta, T., Sashida, M., Fujii, N., Sugawara, S., Rikiishi, H., Kumagai, K., 1993. Induction of acute arthritis in mice by peptidoglycan derived from gram-positive bacteria and its possible role in cytokine production. Microbiology and immunology 37, 573-582.

Padilla, J., Kaur, K., Cao, H.J., Smith, T.J., Phipps, R.P., 2000. Peroxisome proliferator activator receptor-gamma agonists and 15-deoxy-Delta(12,14)(12,14)-PGJ(2) induce apoptosis in normal and malignant B-lineage cells. J Immunol 165, 6941-6948.

Park, E.A., Gurney, A.L., Nizielski, S.E., Hakimi, P., Cao, Z., Moorman, A., Hanson, R.W., 1993. Relative roles of CCAAT/enhancer-binding protein beta and cAMP regulatory element-binding protein in controlling transcription of the gene for

phosphoenolpyruvate carboxykinase (GTP). The Journal of biological chemistry 268, 613-619.
Phipps, R.P., Illig, K., Schad, V., Bhimani, K., 1988. Differential presentation of tolerogenic immunoglobulin in vivo by macrophages and by a lymphoid dendritic cell-like tumor line. Journal of leukocyte biology 43, 271-278.
Phipps, R.P., Stein, S.H., Roper, R.L., 1991. A new view of prostaglandin E regulation of the immune response. Immunology today 12, 349-352.
Pinter, A., Honnen, W.J., Tilley, S.A., Bona, C., Zaghouani, H., Gorny, M.K., Zolla-Pazner, S., 1989. Oligomeric structure of gp41, the transmembrane protein of human immunodeficiency virus type 1. Journal of virology 63, 2674-2679.
Pittman, N., Shue, G., LeLeiko, N.S., Walsh, M.J., 1995. Transcription of cystic fibrosis transmembrane conductance regulator requires a CCAAT-like element for both basal and cAMP-mediated regulation. The Journal of biological chemistry 270, 28848-28857.
Pohlmann, S., Baribaud, F., Doms, R.W., 2001. DC-SIGN and DC-SIGNR: helping hands for HIV. Trends Immunol 22, 643-646.
Rabbi, M.F., al-Harthi, L., Saifuddin, M., Roebuck, K.A., 1998. The cAMP-dependent protein kinase A and protein kinase C-beta pathways synergistically interact to activate HIV-1 transcription in latently infected cells of monocyte/macrophage lineage. Virology 245, 257-269.
Rabbi, M.F., Saifuddin, M., Gu, D.S., Kagnoff, M.F., Roebuck, K.A., 1997. U5 region of the human immunodeficiency virus type 1 long terminal repeat contains TRE-like cAMP-responsive elements that bind both AP-1 and CREB/ATF proteins. Virology 233, 235-245.
Rabson, A.B., Lin, H.C., 2000. NF-kappa B and HIV: linking viral and immune activation. Adv Pharmacol 48, 161-207.
Ramis, I., Rosello-Catafau, J., Gelpi, E., 1992. In vivo transformation of arachidonic acid into 12-hydroxy-5,8,10,14-eicosatetraenoic acid by human nasal mucosa. Journal of chromatography 575, 143-146.
Ramis, I., Rosello-Catafau, J., Gomez, G., Zabay, J.M., Fernandez Cruz, E., Gelpi, E., 1991. Cyclooxygenase and lipoxygenase arachidonic acid metabolism by monocytes from human immune deficiency virus-infected drug users. J Chromatogr 557, 507-513.
Rastogi, N., Bachelet, M., Carvalho de Sousa, J.P., 1992. Intracellular growth of Mycobacterium avium in human macrophages is linked to the increased synthesis of prostaglandin E2 and inhibition of the phagosome-lysosome fusions. FEMS Microbiol Immunol 4, 273-279.
Reiner, N.E., Malemud, C.J., 1984. Arachidonic acid metabolism in murine leishmaniasis (Donovani): ex-vivo evidence for increased cyclooxygenase and 5-lipoxygenase activity in spleen cells. Cellular immunology 88, 501-510.
Ricote, M., Li, A.C., Willson, T.M., Kelly, C.J., Glass, C.K., 1998. The peroxisome proliferator-activated receptor-gamma is a negative regulator of macrophage activation. Nature 391, 79-82.
Rincon, M., Tugores, A., Lopez-Rivas, A., Silva, A., Alonso, M., De Landazuri, M.O., Lopez-Botet, M., 1988. Prostaglandin E2 and the increase of intracellular cAMP inhibit the expression of interleukin 2 receptors in human T cells. European journal of immunology 18, 1791-1796.

Rodbell, M., 1980. The role of hormone receptors and GTP-regulatory proteins in membrane transduction. Nature 284, 17-22.
Roesler, W.J., 2000. What is a cAMP response unit? Mol Cell Endocrinol 162, 1-7.
Roesler, W.J., Graham, J.G., Kolen, R., Klemm, D.J., McFie, P.J., 1995. The cAMP response element binding protein synergizes with other transcription factors to mediate cAMP responsiveness. The Journal of biological chemistry 270, 8225-8232.
Roesler, W.J., Vandenbark, G.R., Hanson, R.W., 1988. Cyclic AMP and the induction of eukaryotic gene transcription. The Journal of biological chemistry 263, 9063-9066.
Rohlff, C., Ahmad, S., Borellini, F., Lei, J., Glazer, R.I., 1997. Modulation of transcription factor Sp1 by cAMP-dependent protein kinase. The Journal of biological chemistry 272, 21137-21141.
Rohr, O., Schwartz, C., Aunis, D., Schaeffer, E., 1999. CREB and COUP-TF mediate transcriptional activation of the human immunodeficiency virus type 1 genome in Jurkat T cells in response to cyclic AMP and dopamine. Journal of cellular biochemistry 75, 404-413.
Roper, R.L., Phipps, R.P., 1994. Prostaglandin E2 regulation of the immune response. Advances in prostaglandin, thromboxane, and leukotriene research 22, 101-111.
Ross, H.L., Nonnemacher, M.R., Hogan, T.H., Quiterio, S.J., Henderson, A., McAllister, J.J., Krebs, F.C., Wigdahl, B., 2001. Interaction between CCAAT/enhancer binding protein and cyclic AMP response element binding protein 1 regulates human immunodeficiency virus type 1 transcription in cells of the monocyte/macrophage lineage. Journal of virology 75, 1842-1856.
Rossi, A., Kapahi, P., Natoli, G., Takahashi, T., Chen, Y., Karin, M., Santoro, M.G., 2000. Anti-inflammatory cyclopentenone prostaglandins are direct inhibitors of IkappaB kinase. Nature 403, 103-108.
Royce, R.A., Sena, A., Cates, W., Jr., Cohen, M.S., 1997. Sexual transmission of HIV. N Engl J Med 336, 1072-1078.
Rozera, C., Carattoli, A., De Marco, A., Amici, C., Giorgi, C., Santoro, M.G., 1996. Inhibition of HIV-1 replication by cyclopentenone prostaglandins in acutely infected human cells. Evidence for a transcriptional block. J Clin Invest 97, 1795-1803.
Saez, E., Rosenfeld, J., Livolsi, A., Olson, P., Lombardo, E., Nelson, M., Banayo, E., Cardiff, R.D., Izpisua-Belmonte, J.C., Evans, R.M., 2004. PPAR gamma signaling exacerbates mammary gland tumor development. Genes & development 18, 528-540.
Saez, E., Tontonoz, P., Nelson, M.C., Alvarez, J.G., Ming, U.T., Baird, S.M., Thomazy, V.A., Evans, R.M., 1998. Activators of the nuclear receptor PPARgamma enhance colon polyp formation. Nature medicine 4, 1058-1061.
Sakata, D., Yao, C., Narumiya, S., 2010. Prostaglandin E2, an immunoactivator. J Pharmacol Sci 112, 1-5.
Santoro, M.G., Benedetto, A., Carruba, G., Garaci, E., Jaffe, B.M., 1980. Prostaglandin A compounds as antiviral agents. Science 209, 1032-1034.
Santoro, M.G., Benedetto, A., Zaniratti, S., Garaci, E., Jaffe, B.M., 1983. The relationship between prostaglandins and virus replication: endogenous prostaglandin synthesis during infection and the effect of exogenous PGA on virus production in different cell lines and in persistently infected cells. Prostaglandins 25, 353-364.
Santoro, M.G., Favalli, C., Mastino, A., Jaffe, B.M., Esteban, M., Garaci, E., 1988. Antiviral activity of a synthetic analog of prostaglandin A in mice infected with influenza A virus. Arch Virol 99, 89-100.

Santoro, M.G., Jaffe, B.M., Garaci, E., Esteban, M., 1982. Antiviral effect of prostaglandins of the A series: inhibition of vaccinia virus replication in cultured cells. The Journal of general virology 63, 435-440.

Santoro, M.G., Rossi, A., Amici, C., 2003. NF-kappaB and virus infection: who controls whom. The EMBO journal 22, 2552-2560.

Sarraf, P., Mueller, E., Jones, D., King, F.J., DeAngelo, D.J., Partridge, J.B., Holden, S.A., Chen, L.B., Singer, S., Fletcher, C., Spiegelman, B.M., 1998. Differentiation and reversal of malignant changes in colon cancer through PPARgamma. Nature medicine 4, 1046-1052.

Sarraf, P., Mueller, E., Smith, W.M., Wright, H.M., Kum, J.B., Aaltonen, L.A., de la Chapelle, A., Spiegelman, B.M., Eng, C., 1999. Loss-of-function mutations in PPAR gamma associated with human colon cancer. Mol Cell 3, 799-804.

Scher, J.U., Pillinger, M.H., 2005. 15d-PGJ2: the anti-inflammatory prostaglandin? Clin Immunol 114, 100-109.

Schoonjans, K., Staels, B., Auwerx, J., 1996. Role of the peroxisome proliferator-activated receptor (PPAR) in mediating the effects of fibrates and fatty acids on gene expression. J Lipid Res 37, 907-925.

Shepard, R.N., Schock, J., Robertson, K., Shugars, D.C., Dyer, J., Vernazza, P., Hall, C., Cohen, M.S., Fiscus, S.A., 2000. Quantitation of human immunodeficiency virus type 1 RNA in different biological compartments. J Clin Microbiol 38, 1414-1418.

Siebenlist, U., Franzoso, G., Brown, K., 1994. Structure, regulation and function of NF-kappa B. Annu Rev Cell Biol 10, 405-455.

Skolnik, P.R., Rabbi, M.F., Mathys, J.M., Greenberg, A.S., 2002. Stimulation of peroxisome proliferator-activated receptors alpha and gamma blocks HIV-1 replication and TNFalpha production in acutely infected primary blood cells, chronically infected U1 cells, and alveolar macrophages from HIV-infected subjects. J Acquir Immune Defic Syndr 31, 1-10.

Sorrell, T.C., Rochester, C.P., Breen, F.N., Muller, M., 1989. Eicosanoids produced during interactions between Pseudomonas aeruginosa and alveolar macrophages are species-dependent. Immunol Cell Biol 67 (Pt 3), 169-176.

Spiegelman, B.M., 1998. PPAR-gamma: adipogenic regulator and thiazolidinedione receptor. Diabetes 47, 507-514.

Spira, A.I., Marx, P.A., Patterson, B.K., Mahoney, J., Koup, R.A., Wolinsky, S.M., Ho, D.D., 1996. Cellular targets of infection and route of viral dissemination after an intravaginal inoculation of simian immunodeficiency virus into rhesus macaques. J Exp Med 183, 215-225.

Straus, D.S., Glass, C.K., 2001. Cyclopentenone prostaglandins: new insights on biological activities and cellular targets. Med Res Rev 21, 185-210.

Straus, D.S., Pascual, G., Li, M., Welch, J.S., Ricote, M., Hsiang, C.H., Sengchanthalangsy, L.L., Ghosh, G., Glass, C.K., 2000. 15-deoxy-delta 12,14-prostaglandin J2 inhibits multiple steps in the NF-kappa B signaling pathway. Proc Natl Acad Sci U S A 97, 4844-4849.

Tae, H.J., Zhang, S., Kim, K.H., 1995. cAMP activation of CAAT enhancer-binding protein-beta gene expression and promoter I of acetyl-CoA carboxylase. The Journal of biological chemistry 270, 21487-21494.

Tesmer, V.M., Rajadhyaksha, A., Babin, J., Bina, M., 1993. NF-IL6-mediated transcriptional activation of the long terminal repeat of the human immunodeficiency virus type 1.

Proceedings of the National Academy of Sciences of the United States of America 90, 7298-7302.

Thomas, S.C., Ryan, M.A., Shanley, T.P., Wong, H.R., 1998. Induction of the stress response with prostaglandin A1 increases I-kappaBalpha gene expression. FASEB J 12, 1371-1378.

Vallejo, M., 1994. Transcriptional control of gene expression by cAMP-response element binding proteins. J Neuroendocrinol 6, 587-596.

Viatour, P., Merville, M.P., Bours, V., Chariot, A., 2005. Phosphorylation of NF-kappaB and IkappaB proteins: implications in cancer and inflammation. Trends Biochem Sci 30, 43-52.

Vinson, C.R., Sigler, P.B., McKnight, S.L., 1989. Scissors-grip model for DNA recognition by a family of leucine zipper proteins. Science 246, 911-916.

Wahl, L.M., Corcoran, M.L., Pyle, S.W., Arthur, L.O., Harel-Bellan, A., Farrar, W.L., 1989. Human immunodeficiency virus glycoprotein (gp120) induction of monocyte arachidonic acid metabolites and interleukin 1. Proceedings of the National Academy of Sciences of the United States of America 86, 621-625.

Walker, C., Kristensen, F., Bettens, F., deWeck, A.L., 1983. Lymphokine regulation of activated (G1) lymphocytes. I. Prostaglandin E2-induced inhibition of interleukin 2 production. Journal of immunology 130, 1770-1773.

Wang, W., Chadee, K., 1992. Entamoeba histolytica alters arachidonic acid metabolism in macrophages in vitro and in vivo. Immunology 76, 242-250.

Wang, W., Chadee, K., 1995. Entamoeba histolytica suppresses gamma interferon-induced macrophage class II major histocompatibility complex Ia molecule and I-A beta mRNA expression by a prostaglandin E2-dependent mechanism. Infection and immunity 63, 1089-1094.

Williams, S.C., Cantwell, C.A., Johnson, P.F., 1991. A family of C/EBP-related proteins capable of forming covalently linked leucine zipper dimers in vitro. Genes & development 5, 1553-1567.

Xing, L., Gopal, V.K., Quinn, P.G., 1995. cAMP response element-binding protein (CREB) interacts with transcription factors IIB and IID. The Journal of biological chemistry 270, 17488-17493.

Yamamoto, N., Fukushima, M., Tsurumi, T., Maeno, K., Nishiyama, Y., 1987. Mechanism of inhibition of herpes simplex virus replication by delta 7-prostaglandin A1 and delta 12-prostaglandin J2. Biochem Biophys Res Commun 146, 1425-1431.

Yang, X.Y., Wang, L.H., Chen, T., Hodge, D.R., Resau, J.H., DaSilva, L., Farrar, W.L., 2000. Activation of human T lymphocytes is inhibited by peroxisome proliferator-activated receptor gamma (PPARgamma) agonists. PPARgamma co-association with transcription factor NFAT. The Journal of biological chemistry 275, 4541-4544.

Zheng, J., Xie, Y., Campbell, R., Song, J., Wang, R.Q., Chiu, R., Berenson, J., Razi, M., Massachi, S., Yang, O.O., Chen, I.S., Pang, S., 2006. gp120-independent HIV infection of cells derived from the female reproductive tract, brain, and colon. J Acquir Immune Defic Syndr 43, 127-136.

Zhong, H., SuYang, H., Erdjument-Bromage, H., Tempst, P., Ghosh, S., 1997. The transcriptional activity of NF-kappaB is regulated by the IkappaB-associated PKAc subunit through a cyclic AMP-independent mechanism. Cell 89, 413-424.

Part 3

From the Clinic to the Patients: HIV and Clinical Manifestations

15

Pathology of HIV/AIDS: Lessons from Autopsy Series

Andrey Bychkov[1,2], Shunichi Yamashita[1] and Alexander Dorosevich[2]
[1]*Nagasaki University Graduate School of Biomedical Sciences*
[2]*Smolensk Regional Institute of Pathology*
[1]*Japan*
[2]*Russia*

1. Introduction

HIV infection is a global disease and despite considerable efforts of the international community it is a main cause of human mortality (UNAIDS, 2009). Morphological insights into HIV/AIDS are based on the study of clinical cases by means of biopsy and autopsy. Morphological changes during development of HIV infection and, especially, through AIDS progression are variable and specified mainly by characteristics of widespread secondary infections and tumors. Opportunistic infections account for approximately 80% of deaths in patients with AIDS and their spectrum is constantly changing, as a result of improvements in treatment options and prophylaxis along with the increasing life span of HIV-infected individuals. Postmortem examinations provide important diagnostic and epidemiological data and represent a most reliable source for estimation of the full spectrum of diseases in individual patients and the general population.

2. Pathomorphology of HIV/AIDS

Morphology of HIV/AIDS is manifested by wide range of indicative (secondary) diseases while specific changes caused by HIV are mainly detected in immune system at the early stages of infection and in central nervous system.

Lymphadenopathy is the marked feature of acute HIV infection defined as generalized enlargement of lymph nodes. Histologically, this process passes through a series of changes: hyperplasia, involution, depletion, and sclerosis (Baroni & Uccini, 1993). In the stage of hyperplasia, the lymph nodes are characterized by disorderly grouped multiple follicles with 'starry sky' pattern due to arrangement of macrophages. Formation of multinuclear cells resembling symplasts is result of merging of lymphocytes infected by virus. With the progression of disease, lymphoid depletion becomes extensive and a fibrovascular carcass appears more evident along with increasing vascularity (angiomatosis). Finally, lymph nodes harbor 'burnt-out' appearance. Although profound depletion of lymphoid tissues is driven by cytotoxic effect of HIV but there is no histologic picture diagnostic of this condition (O'Murchadha et al., 1987).

Large proportion of patients at different stages of disease has morphological proofs of HIV-induced brain damage (Kibayashi et al., 1996). HIV neuropathology is comprised of following patterns (in order of appearance): lymphocyte infiltration of the leptomeninges, microglial nodules formation and HIV encephalitis. The latter lesion consists of numerous foci with mononuclear cells typical of small macrophages, microglia, and multinucleated giant cells. The giant cells are the hallmark of HIV infection since viral antigens can be detected in their cytoplasm (Gyorkey et al., 1987).

Development of indicative diseases which include opportunistic infections and secondary neoplasms which reflects severe deficiency of immune system and in most of cases determines progression of the disease to full-blown AIDS. Morphological descriptions given below represent our common findings of infectious and neoplastic diseases in AIDS.

2.1 Morphology of mycobacterial Infections in HIV patients

Tuberculosis in HIV-patients is characterized by a prevalence of its generalized form with extensive dissemination and acute progression of specific processes. Notable histological features are loss of granuloma formation and abundance of necrotic changes. Generally, all the forms of tuberculosis seen in the terminal stages are actively progressive. The main forms of tuberculosis are generalized, pulmonary (often disseminated) and extrapulmonary. Thus, various organs are affected, most often the lungs, lymph nodes, liver, kidneys, spleen, intestine, and central nervous system (Smith et al., 2000). Tissue reaction in the terminal stage shows typical tuberculous granulomas with giant and epithelioid cells in only 20% of lesions, whereas the remaining 80% demonstrates numerous foci of nonreactive caseous necrosis abundant of acid-fast bacilli (Parkhomenko et al., 2003).

Pulmonary tuberculosis is manifested as a bilateral disseminated type or polycavernous variant. In disseminated tuberculosis, foci of specific lesions (granulomas) comprise large central zones of caseous necrosis surrounded by a few inflammatory cells. Giant cells are uncommon. Ziehl-Neelsen staining shows numerous acid-fast bacteria in the foci of caseous necrosis. All these histological signs characterize tuberculosis as progressive and highly active. Macroscopic study of the lungs often reveals miliary disseminated tuberculosis, while macrofocal dissemination and caseous pneumonia are rare. The pattern of dissemination is bilateral, with a predominance of micronodular, miliary and submiliary types. Tubercles evenly spread to the whole organ or localized to one of the lobes. In a large proportion of cases, macroscopic detection of tuberculous changes in lungs is difficult, but histological examination reveals miliary and submiliary necrotic foci (Berdnikov et al., 2011). The characteristic microscopic picture is a predominance of alterative and exudative changes with the lack of a productive component of inflammation or its minimal manifestation (Fig. 1a). The latter is marked by the absence of signs of encapsulation and organization of inflammatory foci. Classic granulomas are infrequent and only few of them contain giant cells of Langhans (Fig. 1b). Initially, there is formation of colonies of *Mycobacteria* in the pulmonary parenchyma, which is accompanied by cellular infiltration with a significant predominance of polymorphonuclear leucocytes. The cells phagocytose the bacteria and this step is marked by karyorrhexis. Later, this process is associated with massive breakdown of leucocytes resulting in necrosis and microabscesses. Tissue sections stained by Ziehl–Neelsen showed numerous acid-fast bacteria in the foci of caseous necrosis. An exudative reaction in the form of serous-fibrinous pneumonia or fibrinous-purulent pneumonia with predominance of neutrophilic leucocytes is detected at the periphery of caseous foci. Such exudation may extent from lobular up to sub-lobar area. Some alveoli contain accumulations of foamy macrophages that are characteristic for typical tuberculous inflammation. There is an increase in the thickness of the pleura caused by extensive hyperemia and edema. The intrathoracic lymph nodes are also affected, enlarged (3–4 cm in diameter), and aggregated. Partial or total caseous lymphadenitis is detected with the spread of inflammatory processes to the surrounding soft tissues. Evident reduction of follicular structures and lymphoid depletion is a characteristic feature of these lymph nodes.

Extrapulmonary tuberculosis is detected as a component of a generalized type of tuberculosis. Monomorphic miliary foci of caseous necrosis are found in various internal organs, more often in the spleen, kidneys, liver, and rarely in the meninges, peritoneum, exo- and endocrine glands (pancreas, adrenals, prostate, thyroid, ovaries). As a whole, in cases of generalized tuberculosis, *Mycobacteria* cause alterative and exudative reactions simultaneously in several organs with the mean number of organs involved is 5.4 (own data). Most of the foci are suspected to be spread via hematogenous dissemination from lungs. Histopathology of the parenchymatous organs reveals monomorphic miliary nodules of caseous necrosis with rare giant cells, as in the lungs. In many cases, tubercles are not visible by visual inspection. In the spleen, the foci of caseous necrosis have a tendency to fuse and may cover up to 50% of the cut surface.

Tuberculous meningitis is characterized grossly by typical basilar localization with poorly detected gray-white exudates and tubercles in the subarachnoid space. Microscopic examination of the meninges reveals evident hyperemia and edema accompanied by alterative reactions. The latter is manifested as areas of caseous necrosis extensively infiltrated by polymorphs, lymphocytes, and macrophages. Various types of vasculitis such as endovasculitis, panvasculitis, thrombovasculitis, and perivasculitis are evident. Perivasculitis is more often present with edema and excessive mononuclear, neutrophilic, eosinophilic, and plasma cell infiltration in all layers of the vessel wall (Fig. 1c). Destructive process may extent into brain tissue with formation of localized abscesses.

Mycobacterium avium-intracellulare (MAI) infection leads to massive necrotic destruction of lymph nodes with minor involvement of the lungs. Mostly granulomas are difficult to detect throughout the inner organs by naked eye. The only exception is spleen which is filled with miliary granulomas in roughly half of cases. Different groups of visceral lymph nodes are enlarged and show characteristic yellow tone of cut surface. Microscopically, proliferation of large round to elliptical striated pale blue macrophages is noted. Cytoplasm of these cells is packed with huge number of acid-fast bacilli. Well-formed granulomas with fibrosis, necrosis, and epithelioid histiocytes are present in less than one third of cases (Klatt et al., 1987).

2.2 Morphology of bacterial infections

Bacterial Pneumonia

There is a broad spectrum of causative agents of pneumonia revealed by microbiology. Besides typical microflora, bacterial pneumonia can be caused by opportunistic agents, which are activated under immunodeficiency. The most common causative agents of pneumonia are *Staphylococcus aureus, Pseudomonas aeruginosa, Klebsiella pneumoniae, Streptococcus pneumoniae, Haemophilus influenzae* and *Escherichia coli* (Afessa et al., 1998).

Hematoxylin and eosin together with Gram staining of sections of lungs helps in revealing nonspecific microflora. At autopsy, staining of smears of lung sections using Romanovskii-Giemsa and Gram stains is also useful in establishing the nonspecific character of microflora in cases of bacterial pneumonia. Bacteriological culture of lung tissue helps in revealing the nature of the causative agents of pneumonia most accurately. Grossly, patchy areas of red or grey consolidation involve more often the lower zones of the lungs. On cut surface, these patchy consolidated lesions are dry, granular, firm, red or grey in color, slightly elevated over the surface and are often located around a bronchiole. Histologically, suppurative exudate, consisting of neutrophils with admixture of fibrin, fills alveoli and alveolar septa are dilated by congested capillaries and leucocytic infiltration. Often, the course of pneumonia in HIV-infected patients has a tendency to form microabscesses, and in such cases, the microscopic changes resembles to microfocal dissemination in pulmonary tuberculosis. In microabscesses, purulent necrotic foci are found with expressed perifocal exudative reaction, which strengthened their resemblance to pulmonary tuberculosis in HIV-infected patients.

Sepsis

Pneumonia and primary bloodstream infections are the main sites of infections for almost all patients with sepsis, followed by angiogenic-related bacteremia originated from thrombophlebitis in intravenous drug users or from venous catheter in bedridden patients and urinary tract infections. Nosocomial infections compose the major part of etiology of severe sepsis. Microbiology of infections is comprised of different species, mostly *Pseudomonas aeruginosa, Klebsiella pneumoniae* and *Staphylococcus spp.,* while *Streptococcus spp., Escherichia coli* and *Salmonella spp.* are detected with lower frequency (Japiassú et al., 2010). Microorganisms impact small vessels in the primary site and cause local injury both by obstructing the vessels and by releasing toxins. Subsequently a combination of necrosis, hemorrhage and suppuration occurs, with further formation of pyemic abscesses in the various organs and their distribution depends on the site of the original septic thrombosis. Microscopically, pyemic abscesses are typically surrounded by a zone of hemorrhage and an early lesion may show a central zone of necrosis often containing huge numbers of bacteria. This is surrounded by a zone of suppuration and an outermost zone of acutely inflamed and often hemorrhagic tissue. In septic thrombosis of major veins, larger fragments may be released into the circulation, and by impacting in arteries give rise to correspondingly larger foci of necrosis and suppuration (septic infarcts). In case if it involves heart, pyogenic bacteria may produce endocarditis and severely damage cardiac valves. The vegetations on valve are tend to break down and the valve cusps are largely covered by crumbling masses, which consist of layers of fibrin containing clumps of bacteria enclosed by a zone of leukocytes, macrophages and granulation tissue. The substance of the cusps may be extensively destroyed by suppuration.

2.3 Invasive fungal infections

Pneumocystis jirovecii (former *Pneumocystis carinii*) typically produces pneumonia that is widespread throughout the lungs with a chronic course of disease and rapid progression. Pulmonary pneumocystosis is a disease caused by intense multiplication of relatively pathogenic single-celled saprophyte *Pneumocystis jirovecii* in the human respiratory tract.

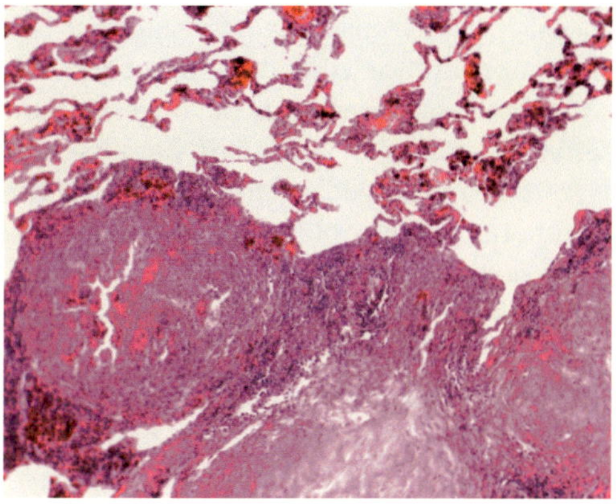

(a) Pulmonary tuberculosis,
foci of caseous necrosis. H&E, × 100

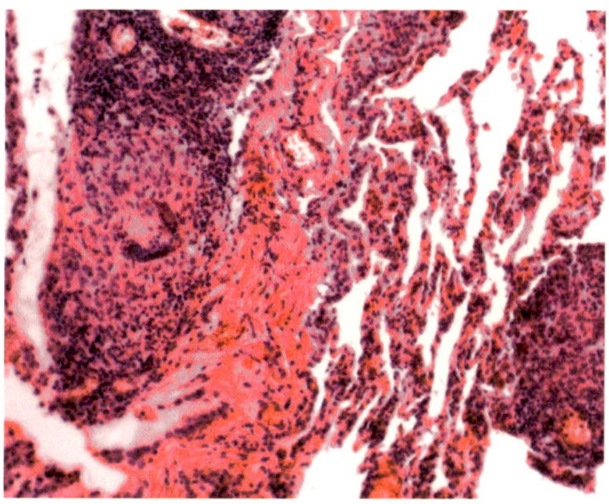

(b) Pulmonary tuberculosis,
granuloma with giant cell. H&E, × 140

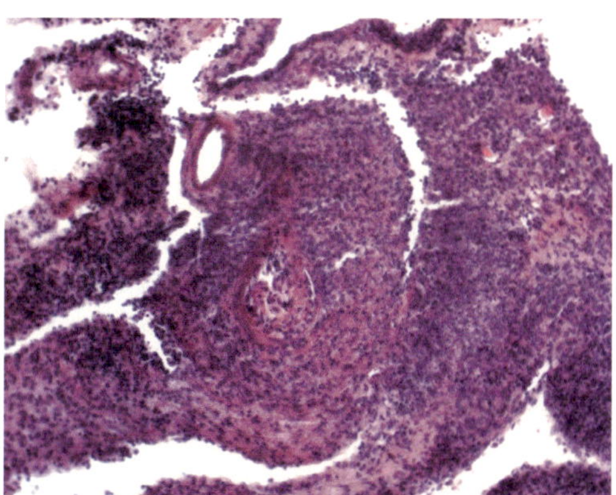

(c) Tuberculous meningitis,
panvasculitis with alteration. H&E, × 140

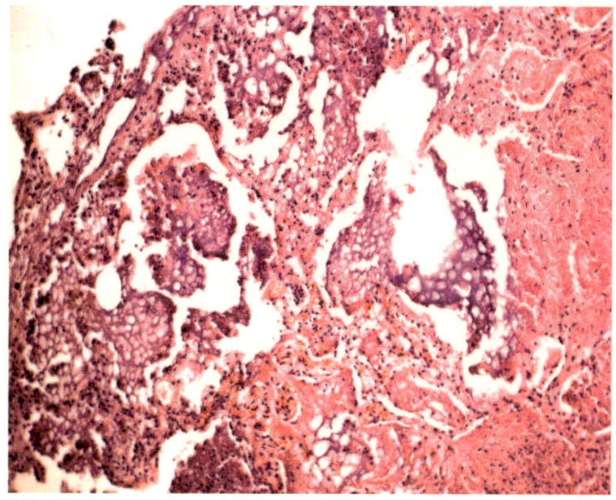

(d) Pneumocystic pneumonia,
foamy exudate. H&E, × 100

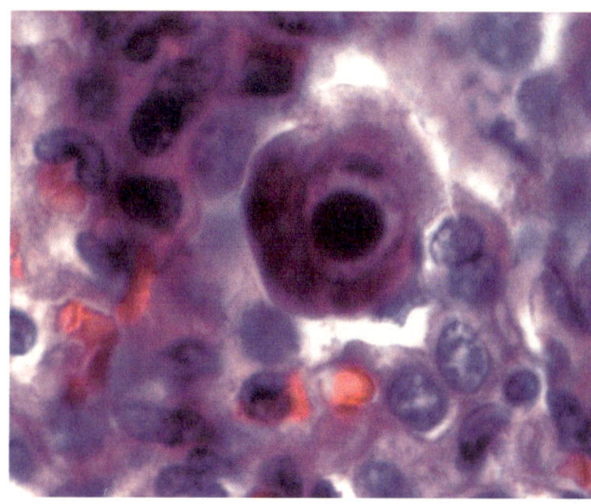

(e) Cytomegalovirus infection of lung,
cell with 'owl-eye' appearance. H&E, × 1200

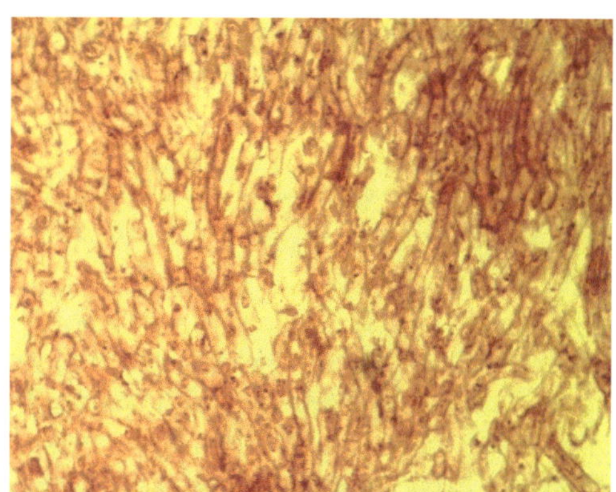

(f) Pulmonary aspergillosis,
branching hyphae of fungus. PAS, × 600

Fig. 1. Microscopic patterns of opportunistic infections in AIDS

The terminal period of pneumocystosis is pneumonia, manifested in the later stages of HIV infection, which often leads to death. The gross appearance resembles to pneumonic consolidation. The cut surface of the lung is pale pink with scattered areas of congestion and rarely hemorrhages. Microscopically, in the edematous stage, characteristic homogenous, foamy protein-containing eosinophilic exudate is found in the alveolar lumen (Fig. 1d). This is a pathognomonic sign of pneumocystic pneumonia. Neutrophils, macrophages and plasma cells are detected around the collections of *Pneumocystis jirovecii.*

Cryptococcus neoformans in immunocompromised hosts may spread from lungs, which is the site of primary infection, to distant organs anh most frequently affecting the central nervous system and causes meningitis. Pulmonary manifestations exhibit pneumonitis, pulmonary nodules or less commonly pleural effusions. Sometimes variably sized pale soft granulomas are grossly visible in the lungs. If fungi with capsules are numerous, a grossly apparent mucoid exudate may be seen in the cerebral ventricles or on the meninges. Microscopically, the yeast cells appear pale blue and ovoid while the capsule is round and clear. Inflammatory reaction is weak and represented by a few scattered lymphocytes or macrophages with phagocytized organisms. PAS stain is effective for detection of the capsule and nucleus of the organisms.

Candida albicans infection is one of the most prevalent in patients with AIDS, ranging from localized skin and mucosa lesions to widely disseminated disease. Characteristic gross findings of candidiasis are prominent in the pharynx, larynx, and trachea with invasion into principle bronchi, which includes a pseudomembranous form with white, elevated mucosal plaques. Bronchopulmonary aspergillosis and candidiasis are characterized by the collection of fungal mycelia in the lumen of small bronchi and invasion of fungus into the acini. *Candida* microabscesses are common and they had a typical polymorphonuclear leucocytes infiltration. Histologically, *Candida* organisms could be identified by their size, budding property, and pseudohyphae. The pseudohyphae could be distinguished from *Aspergillus* hyphae by the lack of branching, the smaller size, and frequent absence of true septations in the former. Histological diagnosis may be confirmed using the Romanovskii staining technique, which is helpful in differentiation between *Candida* and *Aspergillus.* Bronchopulmonary aspergillosis is characterized by the collection of branching mycelia of *Aspergillus* in the bronchial lumen with involvement of the bronchial wall and further invasion of the fungus into the acini (Fig. 1f).

2.4 Viral and parasitic infections

Cytomegalovirus (CMV) *infection* is one the most prevalent secondary diseases in AIDS. It is featured by multiple organs involvement, including lungs, digestive system, brain and eyes. CMV infection proceeds diversely from latent infection to severe acute generalization in the later stages of HIV infection. Microscopically, CMV lesions appear as characteristic metamorphosis of alveolar and bronchial epithelium (Fig. 1e). The persistence of viruses in the epithelial cells leads to cytomegalic giant cell formation. Alveolar cells increase in size up to 25–40 μm. About 1–2 nuclear inclusions are detected containing viral particles in the chromatin in each cell and there is a thin perinuclear clear halo. The nucleus of each affected cell is usually eccentrically positioned and the cell border is not prominent. Additionally, the cytoplasm of affected cells may contain coarse dark basophilic bodies. Characteristic infiltrative changes and CMV transformations are numerous. Moderate cytomegalic transformation of alveolar and bronchial epithelial cells (2–3 typical cells in the form of an 'owl-eye' in the field of view) is accompanied with focal accumulations of serous fluid and protein masses in the alveolar cavities along with admixtures of macrophages and weak infiltration of interstitial tissue. If the lung changes consist of diffuse persisting alveolitis with CMV transformation (up to 20 cells per field of view), then this process is accompanied by extensive fibrosis, but uncommonly leads to the formation of a 'honeycomb-like' appearance of the lungs. The outcome of CMV infection of the lungs is peribronchial and widespread interstitial fibrosis with thickening and vast deformation of the interalveolar septa. Thus, heterogeneous patterns of CMV infection of the lung represent continuous progression of disease and include the following events as virus-induced transformation of the cells, pneumonias with cavity formation, productive granulomatous alveolitis and eventually pulmonary fibrosis (Parkhomenko et al., 2004).

Toxoplasma gondii is a protozoan parasite which is highly prevalent among humans and animals throughout the world. Immunocompromised patients are especially prone to develop disseminated toxoplasmosis, either from acute exposure to the organisms or from reactivation of latent infection. Multiple organ systems are often involved, including the CNS, heart, lungs and skeletal muscle. Damage to the CNS by *Toxoplasma gondii* is characterized by numerous foci of enlarging necrosis and microglia nodules. The former are often resolved with cyst formation or calcification. Presence of many brain abscesses with almost universal involvement of the cerebral hemispheres is the most characteristic feature of toxoplasmic encephalitis in AIDS patients. The diagnosis of toxoplasmosis is readily made from histologic analysis of tissue specimens by observing any of the three infectious stages of *T. gondii*: tachyzoites in groups, bradyzoites (parasitic tissue cysts) or sporozoites within oocysts. Tachyzoites and cysts are seen in and adjacent to necrotic foci near or in glial nodules, perivascular regions, and even in uninvolved cerebral tissue. Reactive inflammatory reaction is comprised of mixed infiltrate distributed in patchy pattern.

2.5 HIV-associated neoplasia

Kaposi's sarcoma is a low-grade mesenchymal tumor which arises initially as an angioproliferative disorder caused by *Kaposi's sarcoma-associated herpes virus* (Du et al., 2007). Skin involvement is common and manifested by the presence of red to red-purple lesions ranging from flat patches to slightly raised plaques and nodules. Visceral involvement frequently includes the lung, lymph nodes, and gastrointestinal tract. Microscopically, Kaposi's sarcoma features clusters of tiny apparent capillaries budding off normal blood vessels. It grows as massed bundles of spindle cells, with red blood cells in slits between them. Hemosiderin pigmentation and hyaline globules usually accompany the spindle cell proliferation. Tumor has an ability to infiltrate around large vascular structures, near epithelial or mesothelial surfaces, or near the capsules of organs.

Non-Hodgkin lymphomas (NHL) risk in AIDS patients is increased more than 70 times comparing with general population (Frisch et al., 2001). Malignant non-Hodgkin's lymphomas (mostly intermediate- to high-grade tumors) exhibit two major patterns which include systemic and CNS lymphomas. These lymphomas often show evidence of *Epstein-Barr virus* as etiologic agent (Fassone et al., 2002). AIDS-related lymphomas consistently determine a B-cell phenotype and are histogenetically related to germinal center or postgerminal center B-cells in the vast majority of cases. About 80% of NHL's in AIDS arise systemically, either nodally or extranodally, while 20% arise in the central nervous system. Almost any extranodal site can be involved with predominance of bone marrow, gastrointestinal tract and liver. NHLs appear as small infiltrates, focal nodular lesions, or larger tumor masses with accompanying necrosis and hemorrhage. Microscopically, tumors generally referred to diffuse large B-cell lymphomas or high-grade B-cell (small non-cleaved) Burkitt-like lymphomas, according to REAL classification. Immunohistochemistry is a routine diagnostic tool in typing of these lesions.

3. Autopsy series

AIDS was recognized in 1981 for the first time, resulting in the deaths of more than 25 million people. Since the late 1990s approximately 2 million HIV-infected persons are reported to have died annually (UNAIDS, 2009). Distribution of the regions with the highest death tolls is determined by the prevalence of HIV infection. Countries of Sub-Saharan Africa are the worst-affected, followed by South and South-East Asia. Most countries with high rates of AIDS prevalence have published reports on autopsy series to date (Fig. 2). Currently, there is a global decline of autopsy rates as a consequence of improved patient management, introduction of etiologic therapy and preventive measures. However such advances are available only in developed countries, where postmortem examination has lost the status of routine diagnostic procedure. Concurrently only few recent reports from Sub-Saharan Africa are available while the pace of HIV epidemics is still very high. Moreover, some countries with high AIDS burden (more than 500,000 infected) including Thailand, China and Ukraine are yet to present large autopsy series.

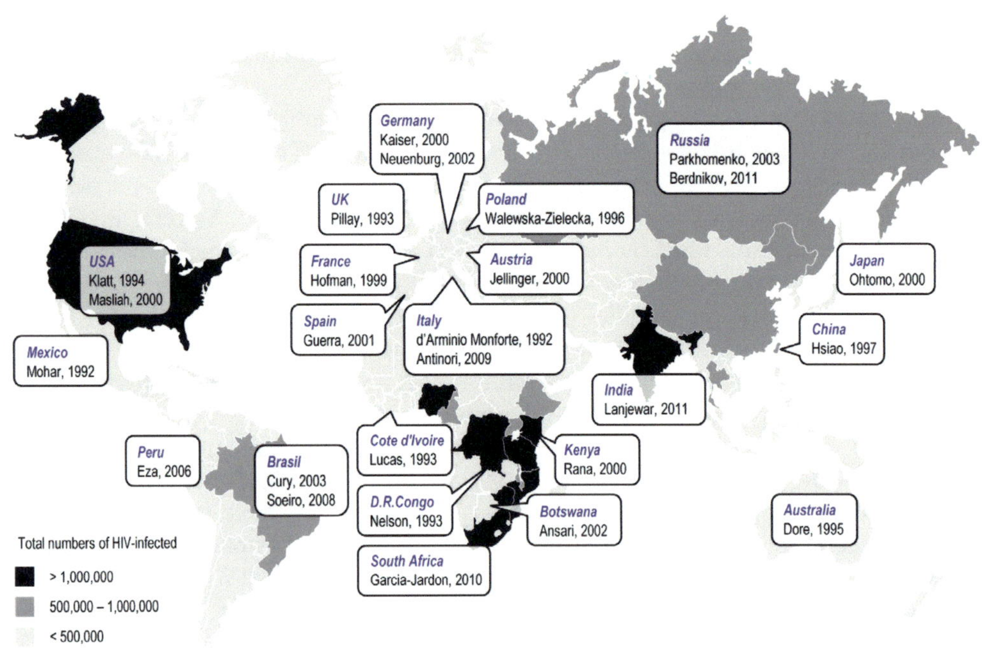

Fig. 2. Worldwide representative autopsy series

3.1 Value of autopsy

Since the first years of HIV/AIDS pathology has contributed significantly to study of new disease. Before mid-1990s various changes of organs and systems studied with different pathological techniques were described in numerous publications. The data taken from the study of autopsy series have shown that postmortem examination is extremely valuable for determining wide range of AIDS-related diseases. Diagnostic role of the autopsy is enhanced considerably by employment of histological examination of the organs. Such specimens can be further proceeded to staining with special techniques useful in detection of microorganisms or immunohistochemistry and even to molecular biological techniques. Thus, complete postmortem study allows determining the cause of death and contributed pathologies, it may identify diseases and etiological agents that were clinically unsuspected or undiagnosed. By providing these types of data, the autopsy serves as an important measure in monitoring the quality of care, basically comparing antemortem with postmortem findings. Autopsy remains established tool for obtaining epidemiological information about diseases and producing vital statistics, since systematic postmortem examination provides representative data on the main pathologies in distinct communities and permits evaluation of changes that may occur over time (Lanjewar, 2011; Lyon et al., 1996). Postmortem surveillance is vital for monitoring the course of HIV-infection and promotes clinicians awareness (Sehonanda et al., 1996).

However, over the past decades, autopsy rates have markedly declined all over the world due to various reasons (Table 1). Advances in laboratory and radiological diagnostics contribute in recognizing different AIDS-related diseases and diminish diagnostic value of autopsy.

Benefits	Limitations
Diagnostic value: - gross findings, - histological analysis, - correlations with antemortem diagnosis *Epidemiological needs:* - death records, - trends over time periods *Educational goals:* - for students, - for professionals (clinical conferences) *Scientific potential:* - case reports, - series reports, - sample collection/further reevaluation	*Difficulties in obtaining consent* *High efficiency of clinical diagnostic tools:* - laboratory diagnostics, - diagnostic radiology, - endoscopy *Risk of infection for staff* *Choice of 'alternative autopsy' techniques:* - needle autopsy, - virtual autopsy, - verbal autopsy *High costs*

Table 1. The AIDS autopsies today: *Pros & Cons*

Health care systems of developed countries offer high-quality diagnostic opportunities for HIV patients, while in developing countries such options have limited availability. Another one concern is that most relatives of died patients are not willing to provide consent for an autopsy because of cultural, traditional and other beliefs (Garcia-Jardon et al., 2010). It is important for clinicians to approach families for autopsy consent. From the other hand, some pathologists and technicians avoid to carry out autopsies on HIV infected cases, because of risk to be infected (Lanjewar, 2011). A major challenge in applying autopsy for AIDS cases is the rising trend of so-called 'alternative autopsy' techniques. Whereas incomplete autopsies such as examination of selected organs or needle autopsy may be accepted partially as being equivalent to a full autopsy, non-invasive procedures like virtual autopsy and echopsy cannot substitute for conventional necropsy techniques (Burton & Underwood, 2007). Verbal autopsy which appears to be gaining acceptance in developing countries (Bhattacharya & Neogi, 2008) is in no way an objective diagnostic technique. Postmortem examination should include collection of organs specimens for histological study; any exception to this rule will markedly decrease the value of autopsy.

3.2 Results

We have analyzed the largest autopsy series from different continents that covered the time period from 1982 to 2011 (Table 2). The main focus was on the prevalence of AIDS-indicative diseases and their distribution according to time periods and geography. Opportunistic infections were the most common autopsy findings, followed by less frequent secondary neoplasms.

Mycobacterial infections were detected in all the series with the lowest frequency around 20% (Afessa et al., 1998; Guerra et al., 2001; Soeiro et al., 2008). In developed countries such as Italy, Germany and Japan, the prevalence of tuberculosis in autopsies of patients with HIV/AIDS is 5-7%, whereas these rates were found to be 38-59% mostly in developing countries (Ansari et al., 2002; d'Arminio Monforte et al., 1992; Hsiao et al., 1997; Kaiser et al., 2000; Lucas et al., 1993; Ohtomo et al., 2000). Pulmonary lesions tend to hematogenous spread, thus the disseminated variant was described in 60-90% cases (Ansari et al., 2002; Cury et al., 2003; Parkhomenko et al., 2003; Rana et al., 2000; Soeiro et al., 2008). Extremely high rates of tuberculosis were reported in recent studies from Russia and India, 82% and 68%, respectively (Berdnikov et al., 2011; Lanjewar, 2011). Emergence of tuberculosis became obvious only in the last decade, when dramatic increase of this infection was implicated as a prime cause of death in AIDS patients. The main reason for such burden in Russia is the overlapping of prior independent epidemics of HIV and tuberculosis with subsequent merging and fast spread through neglected population groups like intravenous drug users, prisoners, alcoholics, homeless persons. Modern HIV-associated tuberculosis is a highly aggressive destructive process in the lungs caused by multidrug resistant strains of *Mycobacteria* and characterized by widespread dissemination and extrapulmonary involvement (Berdnikov et al., 2011).

Currently MAI infections are not of major significance, but they featured notably in the early series from USA and Europe (Guerra et al., 2001; Jellinger et al., 2000; Klatt et al., 1994; Masliah et al., 2000).

Country	USA	USA	USA	USA	USA	Austria	Spain	Botswana	Brasil	Russia	Brasil	SouthAfrica	Russia	India	Russia
Source	Klatt, *1994*	Lyon, *1993*	Sehonanda, *1996*	Afessa, *1998*	Masliah, *2000*	Jellinger, *2000*	Guerra, *2001*	Ansari, *2002*	Cury *2003*	Parkhomenko, *2003*	Sceiro, *2008*	Garcia-Jardon, *2010*	Berdnikov, *2011*	Lanjewar, *2011*	*own data (unpublished)*
Period	1982-1993	1984-1993	1982-1993	1985-1996	1982-1998	1993-1999	1987-1997	1997-1998	1993-2000	1991-2001	1990-2000	2000-2008	2003-2010	1988-2007	2000-2011
Cases	**565**	**279**	**168**	**233**	**390**	**260**	**150**	**104**	**92**	**321**	**250**	**86**	**264**	**223**	**155**
Opportunistic Infections															
MycoBact		**64** 23%							**25** 27%						
TB	**76** 13%		**45** 27%	**13** 5%		**15** 6%	**12** 8%	**42** 40%		**99** 31%	**36** 14%	**25** 32%	**216** 82%	**152** 68%	**72** 46%
MAI	**104** 18%		**26** 15%	**31** 13%	**85** 21%	**36** 14%	**17** 11%	**2** 2%			**15** 6%		**7** 3%		**1** 1%
Bacterial		**81** 29%			**149** 41%	**138** 53%									
Pneum	**52** 9%			**98** 42%			**14** 9%	**24** 23%		**48** 15%	**91** 36%	**17** 22%	**26** 10%	**48** 21%	**40** 26%
Sepsis	**32** 6%						**1** 1%	**4** 4%	**13** 14%	**23** 8%	**36** 14%	**4** 5%	**10** 4%		**6** 4%
Meningitis								**2** 2%	**5** 5%	**5** 2%	**4** 2%	**8** 10%			**1** 1%
Viral															
CMV	**286** 51%	**128** 46%	**36** 21%	**40** 17%	**196** 50%	**127** 49%	**19** 13%	**16** 15%	**16** 17%	**59** 19%	**33** 13%		**3** 1%	**35** 16%	**10** 7%
HSV	**92** 16%	**20** 7%				**11** 4%	**1** 1%								**1** 1%
Fungal															
PCP	**308** 55%	**80** 29%	**55** 33%	**56** 24%	**100** 26%	**30** 12%	**21** 14%	**11** 11%	**15** 16%	**6** 2%	**68** 27%	**7** 9%	**6** 2%	**11** 5%	**17** 11%
Asperg	**6** 1%	**3** 1%	**9** 5%	**2** 1%		**12** 5%	**3** 2%				**1** 1%		**1** 1%		**1** 1%
Cryptoc	**78** 14%	**25** 9%	**9** 5%	**23** 10%	**119** 30%	**25** 10%	**3** 2%	**7** 7%	**4** 4%	**3** 1%	**9** 3%	**6** 7%	**9** 3%	**18** 8%	**5** 3%
Cand	**240** 42%	**30** 11%	**23** 14%	**6** 2%		**46** 18%	**1** 1%		**6** 6%	**3** 1%			**44** 17%	**6** 3%	**9** 6%
Histoplasm	**13** 2%	**29** 10%	**3** 2%	**2** 1%		**2** 1%			**5** 5%		**3** 1%	**1** 1%	**3** 1%		
Parasitic															
Toxo	**51** 9%	**9** 3%	**5** 3%		**11** 3%	**18** 7%	**1** 1%	**1** 1%	**9** 10%	**22** 7%	**18** 7%	**1** 1%		**15** 6%	
Cryptosp	**5** 1%	**7** 3%												**6** 3%	
Helminthes											**5** 2%	**1** 1%		**3** 1%	
Secondary Neoplasms															
KS		**138** 24%		**19** 8%	**41** 10%	**41** 16%	**1** 1%	**11** 11%		**33** 10%	**11** 4%	**1** 1%	**2** 1%	**2** 1%	
NHL		**81** 14%		**3** 1%	**20** 5%	**17** 7%	**13** 9%	**3** 3%	**2** 2%	**3** 1%	**5** 2%		**6** 2%	**8** 3%	**2** 2%
Frequency hierarchy	CMV PCP-Bact	PCP-CMV	PCP TB-CMV	Pneum PCP-CMV	CMV-Bact PCP	Bact-CMV	PCP-CMV	TB Pneum-CMV	TB Bact-CMV	TB CMV-Pneum	Pneum-PCP	TB Pneum	TB	TB Pneum	TB Pneum

Abbreviations: MycoBact, mycobacterial infections; TB, tuberculosis; MAI, *Mycobacterium avium-intracellulare* infection; Pneum, pneumonia; CMV, *Cytomegalovirus* infection; HSV, *Herpes Simplex Virus* infection; PCP, pneumocystic pneumonia; Asperg, aspergillosis; Cryptoc, cryptococcosis; Cand, candidiasis; Histoplasm, histoplasmosis; Toxo, toxoplasmosis; Cryptosp, cryptosporidiosis; KS, Kaposi's sarcoma; NHL, non-Hodgkin's lymphoma; Bact, bacterial infections

Table 2. Autopsy findings from the largest autopsy series.

Similarly, bacterial infections in the same way as tuberculosis showed a marked rise in the last decades and represent an important cause of mortality in AIDS patients. Bacterial pneumonias were identified in 21-36% of cases from low- and middle-income countries (Ansari et al., 2002; Garcia-Jardon et al., 2010; Lanjewar, 2011; Soeiro et al., 2008). Early American sets often not mentioned pneumonias apart from pyogenic infections like sepsis, because they were included in the list of AIDS criteria subsequently. HIV patients are prone to nosocomial pneumonias caused by bacterial associations which demonstrate relapsing course with complications such as abscess formation and pleural effusion (Parkhomenko et al., 2003).

The prevalence of *Cytomegalovirus* infection ranges from 13-19% in African, Indian and Brasilian series to 46-69% cases from USA and Europe (Jellinger et al., 2000; Klatt et al., 1994; Lyon et al., 1996; Masliah et al., 2000; Pillay et al. 1993; Walewska-Zielecka et al., 1996). The highest rates of 74-76% were described in Japan and Australia (Dore et al., 1995; Ohtomo et al., 2000). Among invasive fungal infections pneumocystosis exhibits most significant decline due to effective prophylaxis and introduction of highly active anti-retroviral therapy (HAART). Early reports described high prevalence of pneumocystic pneumonias in more than half of all patients (Klatt et al., 1994), however recent studies could reveal *Pneumocystis jirovecii* pneumonia in less than 10% cases (Parkhomenko et al., 2003). Low levels of pneumocystosis are also specific for African countries regardless time period (Garcia-Jardon et al., 2010; Lucas et al., 1993; Nelson et al., 1993). A large retrospective study of an Italian cohort showed that the prevalence of opportunistic mycoses decreased over time, owing mainly to a significant decrease in pneumocystosis and cryptococcosis, whereas the prevalence of aspergillosis and histoplasmosis remained relatively stable while that of candidiasis tended to increase in the last years (Antinori et al., 2009). Rates of toxoplasmosis showed no significant variation for decades and comprise 1-10% of cases (Cury et al., 2003; Guerra et al., 2001; Sehonanda et al., 1996). The levels of HIV-related neoplasms seem to be decreasing over time, which was demonstrated for both non-Hodgkin's lymphomas and Kaposi's sarcomas in reviewed series (Jones et al., 1999; Launay & Guillevin, 2003).

The main patterns of organ/system involvement in AIDS are pulmonary, generalized or system isolated (CNS, digestive system). In most autopsy series of HIV-infected patients, pulmonary pattern was the most common with an incidence of 60–88%, followed by the CNS (60–80%), and the gastrointestinal tract (Concepcion et al., 1996; Cox et al., 2010; Hofman et al., 1999; Jellinger et al., 2000; Mohar et al., 1992; Sehonanda et al., 1996). Opportunistic monoinfection was observed on the highest level only in 40% cases, while most postmortem studies detected several microbial agents (Rana et al., 2000; Soeiro et al., 2008).

Cases with advanced CNS alterations have a high frequency of opportunistic infections and neoplasms (Masliah et al., 2000). A generalized pattern may be caused by virtually all opportunistic agents, but the most disseminating microorganism today is *Mycobacterium tuberculosis* (Parkhomenko et al., 2003).

Not all deaths of AIDS patients are related to HIV. The percentage of deaths from AIDS-related diseases has decreased, especially in those countries where highly active antiretroviral therapy is widely available. Non-AIDS causes in high-income countries account for at least a third of deaths, and include non-natural causes such as drug overdose, suicide, and violence along with various somatic diseases (Kohli et al., 2005; Krentz et al., 2005). Important non-HIV-related complications contributing to mortality of AIDS patients are chronic liver diseases, cardiovascular pathology and malignancies (d'Arminio Monforte, 2009; Friis-Møller et al., 2010; Lucas et al., 2008; Sackoff et al., 2006). Cases of hepatic involvement are extremely common in HIV-infected cohort of intravenous drug users with HCV co-infection which may die from liver cirrhosis or necrotizing liver failure (Guerra et al., 2001).

One of the important utilities of autopsy is the correlation between antemortem and postmortem diagnosis. A recent review from the UK spanning 23 years showed that the autopsy findings altered the primary diagnosis in 70% of cases, and that 36% of opportunistic infections were not diagnosed prior to death (Beadsworth et al., 2009). An Indian series showed discordance between antemortem and postmortem diagnosis in 42% cases (Lanjewar, 2011). Russian authors reported that in 7% of cases HIV infection (!) was detected only postmortem (Berdnikov et al., 2011). Both false positive as well as false negative antemortem diagnoses are described (Martinson et al., 2007). Infections such tuberculosis, *Cytomegalovirus* and invasive mycoses are missed with the highest rate (Antinori et al., 2009; Beadsworth et al., 2009; Eza et al., 2006; Tang et al., 2006; Wilkes et al., 1988).

3.3 Current trends

The most notable changes described in reviewed series are the rise of tuberculosis infection and bacterial pneumonias for last 10 years (Fig. 3). Tuberculosis is often represented by generalized and disseminated forms. Bacterial infections still occur more frequently than other opportunistic infections in patients with HIV. Multiple infections with involvement of several organs are common.

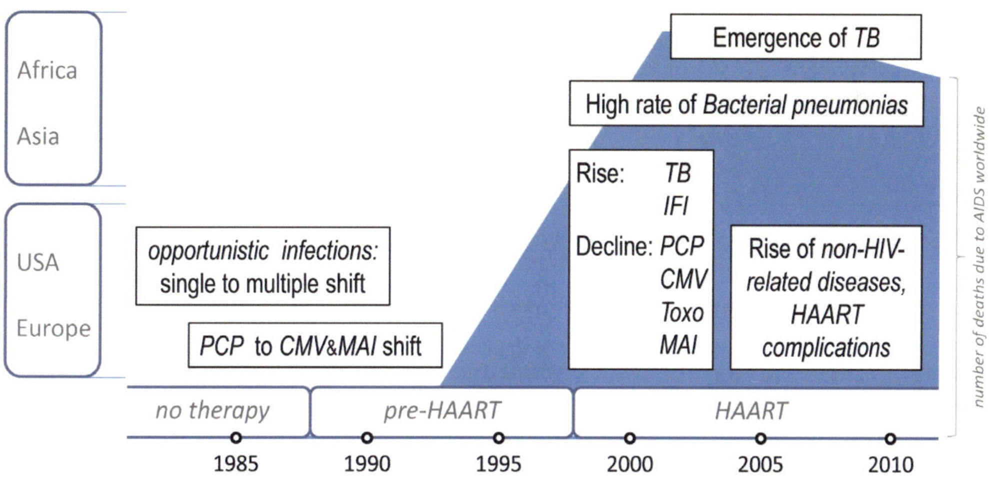

Abbreviations: PCP, pneumocystic pneumonia; CMV, *Cytomegalovirus* infection; MAI, *Mycobacterium avium-intracellulare* infection; TB, tuberculosis; IFI, invasive fungal infections; Toxo, toxoplasmosis

Fig. 3. Major changing patterns of AIDS reported in retrospective studies.

Lungs and central nervous system are the most common targets for pathological processes. The incidence of pneumocystic pneumonia has declined significantly as a result of antiretroviral therapy and chemoprophylaxis. Rates of CMV infection also had been decreased, but not so markedly as pneumocystosis.

The possible concern of described results is that early autopsy series from our set represent high-income developed countries and the most recent series are from low- and middle-income countries. Therefore, it is more correct to report about emergence of HIV-related tuberculosis in developing countries than all over the world. Actually, in Western world (high-income model) tuberculosis spreads through HIV-infected cohort, while in Russia and India social conditions drives tuberculosis in neglected population (alcoholics, imprisons, homeless), that is superimposed by HIV. Contribution of non-HIV-related pathology in AIDS mortality depends on availability of HAART and, consequently, economical development of the country.

Finally, we may suppose that current trends in AIDS mortality for low- and high-income countries are different. Emergence of tuberculosis and high prevalence of bacterial infections are typical for Sub-Saharan Africa, South-East Asia and Eastern Europe. Growth of non-AIDS-related diseases is observed in USA and Western Europe.

4. Conclusion

Through the whole timeline of HIV epidemics significant differences in epidemiology contributed to evolution of disease. Thus, changing patterns of geographic distribution, modes of infection, spectrum of secondary diseases were widely described and explained. Since the first reports on AIDS autopsy has playing an important role in study of HIV infection. Autopsy series and case reports provided abundance of data on various aspects of AIDS. Soon after introduction of HAART large retrospective autopsy studies covering several thousand cases were published (Jellinger et al., 2000; Morgello et al., 2002; Neuenburg et al., 2002; Vago et al., 2002). Results of comprehensive post-mortem examinations were in concordance with data from numerous clinical studies declaring efficacy of therapy and marked reduction of mortality from AIDS (de Martino et al., 2000; Mocroft et al., 1998; Palella et al., 1998). HAART contributed the most important shift in the history of HIV epidemics. However, currently only 10% (roughly) of HIV patients globally are receiving ART (Brown et al., 2010). Moreover, rates of non-adherence to antiretroviral therapy has been shown to range from 33% to 88% (Mills et al., 2006). Access to antiretroviral therapy in developing high-burden countries is restricted and number of AIDS-related deaths in only Sub-Saharan Africa for the last 10 years has exceeded 10 million (UNAIDS, 2009).

The total number of HIV autopsies declined worldwide after the advent of combination therapy. It is thought, that recruiting of such sophisticated studies like autopsy series to analysis of morbidity and mortality trends is not reasonable. Instead of that new methods are established to assess mortality statistics in developing countries (Bhattacharaya & Neogi, 2008). Currently, the popularity of studies evaluating AIDS-related mortality by means of verbal autopsy is increasing (Bundhamcharoen et al., 2011; Lopman et al., 2010; Negin et al., 2010).

We believe that autopsy series represent most reliable sources in estimation of mortality trends. While in the early years of HIV epidemics autopsy function was largely scientific (e.g. recognizing and describing), nowadays the epidemiological data are of main value. Systematic retrospective study of autopsy series worldwide is a valuable tool that should contribute to the study of AIDS epidemics evolution.

5. Acknowledgment

Authors would like to thank Dr. Jimson W. D'Souza (Smolensk State Medical Academy), Dr. Florence Orim (Nagasaki University Graduate School of Biomedical Sciences), Dr. Jitender Singh (Sir Ganga Ram Hospital, New Delhi) and Dr. Larisa Skrobut (Smolensk Regional Institute of Pathology) for their help in preparation of manuscript.

This work was supported by Grant-in-Aid for Scientific Research by Ministry of Health, Labor and Welfare of Japan #H22-AIDS-nominated type-G009, "Patients' participated clinical research on long term therapy of HIV/HCV co-infected hemophiliacs".

6. References

Afessa, B., Green, W., Chiao, J. & Frederick, W. (1998). Pulmonary Complications of HIV Infection: Autopsy Findings. *Chest*, Vol. 113, No. 5, pp. 1225-1229.

AIDS Epidemic Update: November 2009, UNAIDS, ISBN 978 92 9173 832 8, Geneva.

Ansari, N., Kombe, A., Kenyon, T., Hone, N., Tappero, J., Nyirenda, S., Binkin, N. & Lucas, S. (2002). Pathology and Causes of Death in a Group of 128 Predominantly HIV-Positive Patients in Botswana, 1997-1998. *The International Journal of Tuberculosis and Lung Disease*, Vol. 6, No. 1, pp. 55-63.

Antinori, S., Nebuloni, M., Magni, C., Fasan, M., Adorni, F., Viola, A., Corbellino, M., Galli, M., Vago, G., Parravicini, C. & Ridolfo, A. (2009). Trends in the Postmortem Diagnosis of Opportunistic Invasive Fungal Infections in Patients with AIDS: a Retrospective Study of 1,630 Autopsies Performed Between 1984 and 2002. *American Journal of Clinical Pathology*, Vol. 132, No. 2, pp. 221-227.

Baroni, C. & Uccini, S. (1993). The Lymphadenopathy of HIV Infection. *American Journal of Clinical Pathology*, Vol. 99, No. 4, pp. 397-401.

Beadsworth, M., Cohen, D., Ratcliffe, L., Jenkins, N., Taylor, W., Campbell, F., Beeching, N. & Azadeh, B. (2009). Autopsies in HIV: Still Identifying Missed Diagnoses. *International Journal of STD & AIDS*, Vol. 20, No. 2, pp. 84-86.

Berdnikov, R., Grinberg, L., Sorokina, N., Zhidkova, O. & Nevolin, A. (2011). HIV and Tuberculosis by Data Gained from Pathologic Anatomy Autopsy. *Ural'skiĭ Meditsinskiĭ Zhurnal*, Vol. 79, No. 1, pp. 67-71.

Bhattacharya, M. & Neogi, S. (2008). Estimation of Mortality Due to AIDS – A Review. *Indian Journal of Public Health*, Vol. 52, No. 1, pp. 21-27.

Brown, T., Bao, L., Raftery, A., Salomon J., Baggaley, R., Stover, J. & Gerland P. (2010). Modelling HIV Epidemics in the Antiretroviral Era: the UNAIDS Estimation and Projection Package 2009. *Sexually Transmitted Infections*, Vol. 86, ii3-ii10.

Bundhamcharoen, K., Odton, P., Phulkerd, S. & Tangcharoensathien, V. (2011). Burden of Disease in Thailand: Changes in Health Gap between 1999 and 2004. *BMC Public Health*, Vol.11:53.

Burton, J. & Underwood, J. (2007). Clinical, educational, and epidemiological value of autopsy. *Lancet*, Vol. 369, No. 9571, pp. 1471-1480.

Concepcion, L., Markowitz, G., Borczuk, A. & Factor, S. (1996). Comparison of Changing Autopsy Trends in the Bronx Population with Acquired Immunodeficiency Syndrome. *Modern Pathology*, Vol. 9, No. 10, pp. 1001-1006.

Cox, J., Lukande, R., Lucas, S., Nelson, A., Van Marck, E. & Colebunders, R. (2010). Autopsy Causes of Death in HIV-Positive Individuals in sub-Saharan Africa and Correlation with Clinical Diagnoses. *AIDS Reviews*, Vol. 12, No. 4, pp. 183-194.

Cury, P., Pulido, C., Furtado, V. & da Palma, F. (2003). Autopsy Findings in AIDS Patients from a Reference Hospital in Brazil: Analysis of 92 Cases. *Pathology, Research & Practice*, Vol. 199, No. 12, pp. 811-814.

d'Arminio Monforte, A., Vago, L., Lazzarin, A., Boldorini, R., Bini, T., Guzzetti, S., Antinori, S., Moroni, M. & Costanzi, G. (1992). AIDS-Defining Diseases in 250 HIV-Infected Patients; a Comparative Study of Clinical and Autopsy Diagnoses. *AIDS*, Vol. 6, No. 10, pp. 1159-1164.

d'Arminio Monforte, A. (2009). Malignancy-Related Deaths Among HIV-infected Patients. *Clinical Infectious Diseases*, Vol. 48, No. 5, pp. 640-641.

de Martino, M., Tovo, P., Balducci, M., Galli, L., Gabiano, C., Rezza, G. & Pezzotti, P. (2000). Reduction in Mortality with Availability of Antiretroviral Therapy for Children with Perinatal HIV-1 Infection. Italian Register for HIV Infection in Children and the Italian National AIDS Registry. *Journal of American Medical Association*, Vol. 284, No. 2, pp. 190-197.

Dore, G., Marriott, D. & Duflou, J. (1995). Clinico-Pathological Study of Cytomegalovirus (CMV) in AIDS Autopsies: Under-Recognition of CMV Pneumonitis and CMV Adrenalitis. *Australian and New Zealand Journal of Medicine*, Vol. 25, No. 5, pp. 503-506.

Du, M., Bacon, C. & Isaacson, P. (2007). Kaposi Sarcoma-Associated Herpesvirus/Human Herpesvirus 8 and Lymphoproliferative Disorders. *Journal of Clinical Pathology*, Vol. 60, No. 12, pp. 1350-1357.

Eza, D., Cerrillo, G., Moore, D., Castro, C., Ticona, E., Morales, D., Cabanillas, J., Barrantes, F., Alfaro, A., Benavides, A., Rafael, A., Valladares, G., Arevalo, F., Evans, C. & Gilman, R. (2006). Postmortem Findings and Opportunistic Infections in HIV-Positive Patients from a Public Hospital in Peru. *Pathology, Research & Practice*, Vol. 202, No. 11, pp. 767-775.

Fassone, L., Cingolani, A., Martini, M., Migliaretti, G., Oreste, P., Capello, D., Gloghini, A., Vivenza, D., Dolcetti, R., Carbone, A., Antinori, A., Gaidano, G. & Larocca L. (2002). Characterization of Epstein-Barr Virus Genotype in AIDS-Related Non-Hodgkin's Lymphoma. *AIDS Research and Human Retroviruses*, Vol. 18, No. 1, pp. 19-26.

Friis-Møller, N., Thiébaut, R., Reiss, P., Weber, R., Monforte, A., De Wit, S., El-Sadr, W., Fontas, E., Worm, S., Kirk, O., Phillips, A., Sabin, C., Lundgren, J. & Law, M. (2010). Predicting the Risk of Cardiovascular Disease in HIV-Infected Patients: the Data Collection on Adverse Effects of Anti-HIV Drugs Study. *European Journal of Cardiovascular Prevention and Rehabilitation*, Vol. 17, No. 5, pp. 491-501.

Frisch, M., Biggar, R., Engels, E. & Goedert J. (2001). Association of Cancer with AIDS-related Immunosuppression in Adults. *Journal of American Medical Association*, Vol. 285, No. 13, pp. 1736-1745.

Garcia-Jardon, M., Bhat, V., Blanco-Blanco, E. & Stepian, A. (2010). Postmortem Findings in HIV/AIDS Patients in a Tertiary Care Hospital in Rural South Africa. *Tropical Doctor*, Vol. 40, No. 2, pp. 81-84.

Guerra, I., Ortiz, E., Portu, J., Atarés, B., Aldamiz-Etxebarría, M. & De Pablos, M. (2001). Value of Limited Necropsy in HIV-Positive Patients. *Pathology, Research & Practice*, Vol. 197, No. 3, pp. 165-168.

Gyorkey, F., Melnick, J. & Gyorkey, P. (1987). Human Immunodeficiency Virus in Brain Biopsies of Patients with AIDS and Progressive Encephalopathy. *Journal of Infectious Diseases*, Vol. 155, No. 5, pp. 870-876.

Hofman, P., Saint-Paul, M., Battaglione, V., Michiels, J. & Loubière, R. (1999). Autopsy Findings in the Acquired Immunodeficiency Syndrome (AIDS). A Report of 395 Cases from the South of France. *Pathology, Research & Practice*, Vol. 195, No. 4, pp. 209-217.

Hsiao, C., Huang, S., Huang, S., Song, C., Su, I., Chuang, C., Yao, Y., Lin, C. & Hsu, H. (1997). Autopsy Findings on Patients with AIDS in Taiwan. *Zhonghua Min Guo Wei Sheng Wu Ji Mian Yi Xue Za Zhi*, Vol. 30, No. 3, pp. 145-159.

Japiassú, A., Amâncio, R., Mesquita, E., Medeiros, D., Bernal, H., Nunes, E., Luz, P., Grinsztejn, B. & Bozza, F. (2010). Sepsis is a Major Determinant of Outcome in Critically Ill HIV/AIDS Patients. *Critical Care*, Vol. 14, No. 4, R152, 8 pages.

Jellinger, K., Setinek, U., Drlicek, M., Böhm, G., Steurer, A. & Lintner, F. (2000). Neuropathology and General Autopsy Findings in AIDS During the Last 15 Years. *Acta Neuropathologica*, Vol. 100, No. 2, pp. 213-220.

Jones, J., Hanson, D., Dworkin, M., Ward, J. & Jaffe, H. (1999). Effect of Antiretroviral Therapy on Recent Trends in Selected Cancers among HIV-Infected Persons. Adult/Adolescent Spectrum of HIV Disease Project Group. *Journal of Acquired Immune Deficiency Syndromes*, Vol. 1, No. 21, Suppl. 1, pp. S11-S17.

Kaiser, A., Weng, L., Brockhaus, W. & Wünsch, P. (2000). Opportunistic Infections and HIV-Associated Malignancies. An Evaluation of 58 autopsy Cases Within 10 Years. *Medizinische Klinik*, Vol. 95, No. 9, pp. 482-486.

Kibayashi, K., Mastri, A. & Hirsch C. (1996). Neuropathology of Human Immunodeficiency Virus Infection at Different Disease Stages. *Human Pathology*, Vol. 27, No. 7, pp. 637-642.

Klatt, E., Jensen, D. & Meyer, P. (1987). Pathology of Mycobacterium Avium-Intracellulare Infection in Acquired Immunodeficiency Syndrome. *Human Pathology*, Vol. 18, No. 7, pp. 709-714.

Klatt, E., Nichols, L. & Noguchi, T. (1994). Evolving Trends Revealed by Autopsies of Patients with the Acquired Immunodeficiency Syndrome. 565 Autopsies in Adults with the Acquired Immunodeficiency Syndrome, Los Angeles, California, 1982-1993. *Archives of Pathology & Laboratory Medicine*, Vol. 118, No. 9, pp. 884-890.

Kohli, R., Lo, Y., Howard, A., Buono, D., Floris-Moore, M., Klein, R. & Schoenbaum, E. (2005). Mortality in an Urban Cohort of HIV-Infected and at-Risk Drug Users in the Era of Highly Active Antiretroviral Therapy. *Clinical Infectious Diseases*, Vol. 41, No. 6, pp. 864-872.

Krentz, H., Kliewer, G. & Gill, M. (2005). Changing Mortality Rates and Causes of Death for HIV-Infected Individuals Living in Southern Alberta, Canada from 1984 to 2003. *HIV Medicine*, Vol. 6, No. 2, pp. 99-106.

Lanjewar, D. (2011). The Spectrum of Clinical and Pathological Manifestations of AIDS in a Consecutive Series of 236 Autopsied Cases in Mumbai, India. *Pathology Research International*, Vol. 2011, Article ID 547618, 12 pages

Launay, O. & Guillevin, L. (2003). Epidemiology of HIV-Associated Malignancies. *Bulletin du Cancer*, Vol. 90, No. 5, pp. 387-392.

Lopman, B., Cook, A., Smith, J., Chawira, G., Urassa, M., Kumogola, Y., Isingo, R., Ihekweazu, C., Ruwende, J., Ndege, M., Gregson, S., Zaba, B. & Boerma, T. (2010). Verbal Autopsy Can Consistently Measure AIDS Mortality: a Validation Study in Tanzania and Zimbabwe. *Journal of Epidemiology and Community Health*, Vol. 64, No. 4, pp. 330-334.

Lucas, S., Hounnou, A., Peacock, C., Beaumel, A., Djomand, G., N'Gbichi, J., Yeboue, K., Hondé, M., Diomande, M., Giordano, C., Doorly, R., Brattegaard, K., Kestens, L., Smithwick, R., Kadio, A., Ezani, N., Yapi, A. & De Cock, K. (1993). The Mortality and Pathology of HIV Infection in a West African City. *AIDS*, Vol. 7, No. 12, pp. 1569-1579.

Lucas, S., Curtis, H. & Johnson, M. (2008). National Review of Deaths Among HIV-Infected Adults. *Clinical Medicine*, Vol. 8, No. 3, pp. 250-252.

Lyon, R., Haque, A., Asmuth, D. & Woods, G. (1996). Changing Patterns of Infections in Patients with AIDS: a Study of 279 Autopsies of Prison Inmates and Nonincarcerated Patients at a University Hospital in Eastern Texas, 1984-1993. *Clinical Infectious Diseases*, Vol. 23, No. 2, pp. 241-247.

Martinson, N., Karstaedt, A., Venter, W., Omar, T., King, P., Mbengo, T. Marais, E., McIntyre, J, Chaisson, R. & Hale, M. (2007). Causes of Death in Hospitalized Adults with a Premortem Diagnosis of Tuberculosis: an Autopsy Study. *AIDS*, Vol. 21, No. 15, pp. 2043-2050.

Masliah, E., DeTeresa, R., Mallory, M. & Hansen, L. (2000). Changes in Pathological Findings at Autopsy in AIDS Cases for the Last 15 Years. *AIDS*, Vol. 14, No. 1, pp. 69-74.

Mills, E., Nachega, J., Bangsberg, D., Singh, S., Rachlis, B., Wu, P., Wilson, K., Buchan, I., Gill, C. & Cooper, C. (2006). Adherence to HAART: a Systematic Review of Developed and Developing Nation Patient-Reported Barriers and Facilitators. *PLoS Medicine*, Vol. 3, No. 11, e438.

Mocroft, A., Vella, S., Benfield, T., Chiesi, A., Miller, V., Gargalianos, P., d'Arminio Monforte, A., Yust, I., Bruun, J., Phillips, A. & Lundgren, J. (1998). Changing Patterns of Mortality Across Europe in Patients Infected with HIV-1. EuroSIDA Study Group. *Lancet*, Vol. 352, No. 9142, pp. 1725-1730.

Mohar, A., Romo, J., Salido, F., Jessurun, J., Ponce de León, S., Reyes, E., Volkow, P., Larraza, O., Peredo, M., Cano, C., Gomez, G., Sepulveda, J. & Mueller, N. (1992). The Spectrum of Clinical and Pathological Manifestations of AIDS in a Consecutive Series of Autopsied Patients in Mexico. *AIDS*, Vol. 6, No. 5, pp. 467-473.

Morgello, S., Mahboob, R., Yakoushina, T., Khan, S. & Hague, K. (2002). Autopsy Findings in a Human Immunodeficiency Virus-Infected Population Over 2 Decades: Influences of Gender, Ethnicity, Risk Factors, and Time. *Archives of Pathology & Laboratory Medicine*, Vol. 126, No. 2, pp. 182-190.

Negin, J., Wariero, J., Cumming, R., Mutuo, P. & Pronyk, P. (2010). High Rates of AIDS-Related Mortality among Older Adults in Rural Kenya. *Journal of Acquired Immune Deficiency Syndromes*, Vol. 55, No. 2, pp. 239-244.

Nelson, A., Perriëns, J., Kapita, B., Okonda, L., Lusamuno, N., Kalengayi, M., Angritt, P., Quinn, T. & Mullick, F. (1993). A Clinical and Pathological Comparison of the

WHO and CDC Case Definitions for AIDS in Kinshasa, Zaïre: is Passive Surveillance Valid? *AIDS*, Vol. 7, No. 9, pp. 1241-1245.

Neuenburg, J., Brodt, H., Herndier, B., Bickel, M., Bacchetti, P., Price, R., Grant, R. & Schlote, W. (2002). HIV-Related Neuropathology, 1985 to 1999: Rising Prevalence of HIV Encephalopathy in the Era of Highly Active Antiretroviral Therapy. *Journal of Acquired Immune Deficiency Syndromes*, Vol. 31, No. 2, pp. 171-177.

Ohtomo, K., Wang, S., Masunaga, A., Iwamoto, A. & Sugawara I. (2000). Secondary Infections of AIDS Autopsy Cases in Japan with Special Emphasis on Mycobacterium Avium-Intracellulare Complex Infection. *The Tohoku Journal of Experimental Medicine*, Vol. 192, No. 2, pp. 99-109.

O'Murchadha, M., Wolf, B. & Neiman, R. (1987). The Histologic Features of Hyperplastic Lymphadenopathy in AIDS-Related Complex are Nonspecific. *American Journal of Surgical Pathology*, Vol. 11, No. 2, pp. 94-99.

Palella, F., Delaney, K., Moorman, A., Loveless, M., Fuhrer, J., Satten, G., Aschman, D. & Holmberg, S. (1998). Declining Morbidity and Mortality among Patients with Advanced Human Immunodeficiency Virus Infection. HIV Outpatient Study Investigators. *New England Journal of Medicine.*, Vol. 338, No. 13, pp. 853-860.

Parkhomenko, I., Tishkevich, O., Shagil'dian, V., Solnyshkova, T. & Nikonova, E. (2004). Pathomorphogenesis of Cytomegalovirus Lungs Lesions in HIV Infection. *Arkhiv Patologii*, Vol. 66, No. 4, pp. 20-23.

Parkhomenko, I., Tishkevich, O. & Shakhgil'dian, V. (2003). Analysis of Autopsies in HIV Infection. *Arkhiv Patologii*, Vol. 65, No. 3, pp. 24-29.

Pillay, D., Lipman, M., Lee, C., Johnson, M., Griffiths, P. & McLaughlin, J. (1993). A Clinico-Pathological Audit of Opportunistic Viral Infections in HIV-Infected Patients. *AIDS*, Vol. 7, No. 7, pp. 969-974.

Rana, F., Hawken, M., Mwachari, C., Bhatt, S., Abdullah, F., Ng'ang'a, L., Power, C., Githui W., Porter, J. & Lucas, S. (2000). Autopsy Study of HIV-1-Positive and HIV-1-Negative Adult Medical Patients in Nairobi, Kenya. *Journal of Acquired Immune Deficiency Syndromes*, Vol. 24, No. 1, pp. 23-29.

Sackoff, J., Hanna, D., Pfeiffer, M. & Torian, L. (2006). Causes of Death among Persons with AIDS in the Era of Highly Active Antiretroviral Therapy: New York City. *Annals of Internal Medicine*, Vol. 145, No. 6, pp. 397-406.

Sehonanda, A., Choi, Y. & Blum, S. (1996). Changing Patterns of Autopsy Findings Among Persons with Acquired Immunodeficiency Syndrome in an Inner-City Population. A 12-Year Retrospective Study. *Archives of Pathology & Laboratory Medicine*, Vol. 120, No. 5, pp. 459-464.

Smith, M., Boyars, M., Veasey, S. & Woods, G. (2000). Generalized Tuberculosis in the Acquired Immune Deficiency Syndrome. *Archives of Pathology & Laboratory Medicine*, Vol. 124, No. 9, pp. 1267-1274.

Soeiro, A., Hovnanian, A., Parra, E., Canzian, M. & Capelozzi, V. (2008). Post-mortem Histological Pulmonary Analysis in Patients with HIV/AIDS. *Clinics*, Vol. 63, No. 4, pp. 497-502.

Tang, H., Liu, Y., Yen, M., Chen, Y., Wann, S., Lin, H., Lee, S., Lin, W., Huang, C., Su, B., Chang, P., Li, C. & Tseng, H. (2006). Opportunistic Infections in Adults with Acquired Immunodeficiency Syndrome: a Comparison of Clinical and Autopsy Findings. *Journal of Microbiology, Immunology, and Infection*, Vol. 39, No. 4, pp. 310-315.

Vago, L., Bonetto, S., Nebuloni, M., Duca, P., Carsana, L., Zerbi, P. & D'Arminio-Monforte, A. (2002). Pathological Findings in the Central Nervous System of AIDS Patients on Assumed Antiretroviral Therapeutic Regimens: Retrospective Study of 1597 Autopsies. *AIDS*, Vol. 16, No. 14, pp. 1925-1928.
Walewska-Zielecka, B., Kamiński, Z. & Nowosławski, A. (1996). AIDS Pathology: Infections and Neoplasms in 55 Fatal AIDS Cases. A Postmortem Study. *Polish Journal of Pathology*, Vol. 47, No. 4, pp. 163-170.

16

HIV and Lung Cancer

Yusuke Okuma, Naoki Yanagisawa, Yukio Hosomi,
Atsushi Ajisawa and Masahiko Shibuya
Tokyo Metropolitan Cancer and Infectious diseases Center, Komagome Hospital
Japan

1. Introduction

Lung cancer patients with HIV infection are expected to become an emerging issue with respect to morbidity and mortality, as the number of such patients is rapidly increasing. However, few reports or textbooks dealing with this issue have documented the details of these cases. Thus, in clinical settings, infectious disease physicians or medical oncologists occasionally hesitate to treat HIV-infected patients with lung cancer. Since 1996, the outcome of HIV-infected patients has improved, because CD4 cell counts and viral load are generally well controlled with the advent of highly active antiretroviral therapy (HAART), which strongly inhibits HIV viral proliferation and restores the patient's immunological status. Furthermore, the prognosis in the HIV population has improved significantly due to the prevention and treatment of opportunistic infections (OIs). As a result, HIV infection is chronically manageable. In the pre-HAART era, the median survival time in the HIV population was 10 years, while, at present, 85% of patients survive more than 10 years.(Sepkowitz, 2001)

In the pre-HAART era, most HIV-infected patients died of acquired immunodeficiency syndrome (AIDS). Recently, however, one-third of all such patients die of malignant tumor,(Bonnet *et al.*, 2009) and deaths due to AIDS-defining cancers (ADCs), such as Kaposi's sarcoma (KS), primary central nervous system lymphoma (PCNSL) and non-Hodgkin's lymphoma (NHL), and invasive cervical carcinoma, which were defined by the Centers for Disease Control and Prevention (CDC), are decreasing. On the other hand, the number of deaths due to non-AIDS-defining cancers (NADCs) is increasing.(Engels *et al.*, 2008, Silverberg *et al.*, 2009) At present, in the population with HIV infection, lung cancer accounts for 5% of all deaths and 15% of all deaths by malignant tumors.(Bonnet *et al.*, 2009) Of all of the NADCs, lung cancer is the most common,(Engels *et al.*, 2006, Lavole *et al.*, 2006, Patel *et al.*, 2008) followed by breast cancer, soft tissue sarcoma, Hodgkin's lymphoma (HL), penile cancer, lip cancer, and testicular seminoma.(Frisch *et al.*, 2001) In 1984, Irwin *et al.* reported the first case with simultaneous HIV infection and lung cancer,(Irwin *et al.*, 1984) and several dozen patients have since been reported in the United States and Europe. (Table. 1) The clinical demographics of lung cancer with HIV infection differ slightly from the general population and are characterized by younger age, advanced stage at diagnosis, and aggressive tumor extension. Thus, the prognosis of lung cancer in the HIV population is poorer than that of lung cancer in the general population.(Lavole *et al.*, 2006) Moreover, patient fragility to treatment needs to be considered.

In the general population, lung cancer is the most common cause of cancer death worldwide. Furthermore, in the last decade, there has been progress in lung cancer treatment modalities. The development of novel antitumor agents and molecular targeted drugs has increased the lines of chemotherapy, and new treatment strategies, such as maintenance therapy and biomarker-based therapy (personalized therapy), provide diverse options. At present, in front-line chemotherapy for lung cancer patients, platinum-doublet chemotherapy with the third-generation antitumor agent has been shown to prolong survival and contribute to symptom palliation. Before the 1990s, the median survival time with the best supportive care was 4-5 months, and the 1-year survival rate was 10% in Stage IV non-small cell lung cancer (NSCLC). In 1995, the benefits of chemotherapy for Stage IV NSCLC were confirmed, and the median survival time was prolonged to 8 months.(Non-small Cell Lung Cancer Collaborative Group, 1995) At present, median survival time is 12 months, and the 1-year survival rate has improved to 50-60% from 30-35% in 2002.(Azzoli *et al.*, 2009) Thus, the reported data dealing with lung cancer in HIV patients are not comparable. In addition, drug interactions between antiviralagents and antitumor agents

Author	Nº of patients	Years	Median age (y)	Male (%)	Smoking (%)	Median pack-years	IVDU (%)	Homosexual (%)	NSCLC (%)	Adenocarcinoma	Squamous cell carcinoma	SCLC (%)	Median CD4 (cells/µL)	CD4 < 200 cells/µL	Latency (y)	PS > 2 (%)	Stage III/IV	Median Survival (mo)
Sridhar et al.	19	86-91	47	100	94	60	21	32	95	42	31	5	121	53	-	37	79	3
Trielli et al.	36	86-98	38	89	94	40	69	17	86	36	33	14	150	44	-	43	84	5
Brock et al.	92	86-04	46	67	99	30	58	-	91	48	17	9	305	-	5.5	-	87	6.3
Vyzula et al.	16	88-95	45	94	100	30	63	38	88	50	19	12	184	54	-	69	81	5.4
Alshafie et al.	11	90-94	50	82	90	-	81	0	100	46	36	0	329	30	-	-	90	3
Spano et al.	22	93-02	45	86	95	40	23	45	95	36	50	5	364	30	-	-	90	3
Pakkala et al.	80	95-08	52	80	100	37	25	33	91	41	32	9	304	-	-	-	-	-
Lavole et al.	49	96-07	46	67	99	33	17	18	100	67	17	0	350	-	8.6	71	84	8.1
D'Jaen et al.	75	96-08	50	83	99	41	30	47	81	46	35	19	340	-	11	-	77	9
Bertolaccini et al.	26	03-07	39	85	85	30	58	23	81	-	-	19	143	-	-	-	76	23

IVDU: intravenous drug user; NSCLC: non-small cell lung cancer; SCLC: small cell lung cancer; PS: performance status

Table 1. Documented clinical demographics of lung cancer patients with HIV.

must be considered, as they may increase or decrease efficacy by inhibiting cytochrome P450 (CYP450) induction, and the actual efficacy of and tolerance to therapy in such patients are uncertain.

In this chapter, we discuss the epidemiology, frequency, risk factors, clinical management, and treatment of HIV-infected lung cancer patients.

2. Incidence

Between 2001 and 2006, 71% of deaths were due to malignant tumors, as compared to only 20% in the pre-HAART era.(Crum-Cianflone *et al.*, 2009) It is evident that the HIV-infected population has a higher risk for lung cancer. In many studies comparing the incidence of lung cancer in patients with HIV to that in the general population, the standardized incidence ratio (SIR), adjusted for age and sex, has been calculated. SIR is an estimate of the ratio of the incidence of cancer in a given patient subset compared with the projected cancer incidence in the population at large. For instance, an SIR > 1 would indicate that lung cancer occurs more frequently in HIV-infected patients than in the general population; in fact, the SIR was 1.4-4.5. In the period before the advent of HAART, the SIR was 6.5 (95% confidential interval (CI) 4.5-8.9),(Frisch & Hjalgrim, 1999, Parker *et al.*, 1998) from 1978-1996, the SIR was 4.5 with 808 patients,(Frisch *et al.*, 2001) and in most European studies, the SIR did not exceed 1.13.(Bower *et al.*, 2003, Herida *et al.*, 2003, Powles *et al.*, 2009) In the HAART era, the SIR was 2.27-3.3.(Powles *et al.*, 2009, Patel *et al.*, 2008) In a meta-analysis with seven observational studies of NADCs (n=1016), the SIR was 2.72 (95% CI 1.91-3.87).(Grulich *et al.*, 2007) In many studies, the number of lung cancer patients with HIV infection has been shown to increase from the HAART era to the post-HAART era. The incidence, however, has not changed. On the other hand, there are few data from Asian countries. The TAHOD study, a retrospective study of 617 patients between 2000 and 2008 in 10 Asian countries, reported that the number of patients with simultaneous HIV infection and NADCs is increasing, even in developing countries. Infection-unrelated NADCs (NADC-IURs), including lung cancer, account for 22%, with lung cancer being the most common (1.9%, 12 patients). In this study, the authors concluded that the Asian patient demographic differs from the Western demographic.(Petoumenos *et al.*, 2010)

3. Pathogenesis & risk factors

The risk factors for lung cancer in the HIV population are strongly associated with immunity and cigarette smoking. The higher risk for carcinogenesis in immune-compromised patients and the increased risk for lung cancer occurrence are particularly well known; kidney transplant patients have a significantly higher incidence of lung cancer than hemodialysis patients.(Vajdic *et al.*, 2006) Carcinogenesis in lung cancer is not directly associated with viral load and CD4 cell counts, and the mechanism of the increased risk for lung cancer is not fully understood. The reasons for the increased incidence of lung cancer in HIV-infected patients therefore remain uncertain.

3.1 Smoking exposure & other traditional risk factors

Cigarette smoking in the HIV population is a major contributing factor for carcinogenesis, as in the general population. The American Lung Association has reported that 87% of all lung cancer is caused by smoking, and smoking cessation decreases the annual risk.(Samet *et al.*, 1988) The rate of smoking in the HIV population is 57%, higher than in the general population (33%),(Saves *et al.*, 2003) and a smoking history of 30-40 pack-years is seen in the HIV population.(Benard *et al.*, 2007, Friis-Moller *et al.*, 2003) In particular, in the Women's Interagency HIV Study (WIHS) cohort study in the HIV population in the United States, female lung cancer patients with HIV infection were significantly more common than in the general population, showing the increased risk for lung cancer.(Levine *et al.*, 2010) Thus, smoking cessation programs need to be directed to the HIV population when infection is diagnosed. On the other hand, smoking is reported to be an independent risk factor for carcinogenesis in lung cancer.(Kirk *et al.*, 2007)

Recently, the National Cancer Institute reported that an annual low-dose computed tomography (CT) scan in the general population decreased lung cancer death by 80% by detecting the early stages of lung cancer.(Aberle *et al.*, 2010) In a study at Johns Hopkins University and associated hospitals, most of the 92 lung cancer patients with HIV infection died of lung cancer. Overall, 60% of the 32 patients who underwent chest radiography were not diagnosed as having lung cancer within a year. With regard to CT, 1 out of 28 patients was not diagnosed.(James, 2006) Smoking cessation and low-dose CT scans to detect the early stages of lung cancer would therefore be beneficial for HIV population.

Among other behavioral risk factors, intravenous drug users had been considered as a higher risk for developing lung cancer. However, the higher rate of smoking among intravenous drug users may be a confounding factor in some studies.

3.2 Immunosuppression as a risk factor

Immunodeficiency is a significant risk factor for carcinogenesis in some types of cancer. However, there is no evidence that decreased CD4 cell counts are associated with carcinogenesis in NADCs.(Clifford & Franceschi, 2007) In many case-control studies, the incidence of NADCs was not associated with the CDC classification (Table 2).

CD4 Cell Categories	Clinical Categories		
	A Asymptomatic, Acute HIV, or PGL	**B** Symptomatic Conditions, not A or C	**C** AIDS-Indicator Conditions
>500/μL	A1	B1	C1
200-500/μL	A2	B2	C2
< 200/μL	A3	B3	C3

CDC = U.S. Centers for Disease Control and Prevention; PGL = persistent generalized lymphadenopathy.

Table 2. CDC Classification System for HIV-Infected Adults and Adolescents

However, the incidence in HL, anal cancer, or hepatocellular carcinoma is affected by decreased CD4 cell counts. CD4 cell counts less than 200 cells/μL were associated with the incidence of NADCs (hazard ratio (HR), 1.67).(Powles *et al.*, 2009) CD4 cell counts increased by 100 cells/μL with the introduction of HAART, and the risk for NADCs decreased by 19%.(Bruyand *et al.*, 2009) However, carcinogenesis in lung cancer is not considered to be associated with immunological status (CD4 cell counts and viral load).(Kirk *et al.*, 2007, Spano *et al.*, 2004)

3.3 HIV as a risk factor

Many cases of carcinogenesis in HIV-related carcinomas are related to viruses such as Epstein Barr virus or Human Herpes virus-8. The International Agency for Research on Cancer (IARC), an agency of the World Health Organization (WHO), is examining the relationship between viruses and carcinogenesis, including: Epstein Barr virus for HL, NHL, nasopharyngeal carcinoma, and Burkitt's lymphoma; human herpes virus-8 for KS and primary effusion lymphoma; human papilloma virus for cervical, vulvar, and vaginal carcinoma, penile carcinoma, anal carcinoma, oral cavity carcinoma, and oropharyngeal and tonsillar carcinoma; hepatitis C virus for hepatocellular carcinoma and NHL; hepatitis B virus for hepatocellular carcinoma; and HIV for cervical and conjunctival squamous cell carcinoma, NHL, PCNSL, KS, and HL (particularly mixed cellularity and lymphocyte depleted subtypes). Of these, HIV is not organ-specific and is unique in that carcinogenesis occurs indirectly through immune suppression. Considering immunological status and infection, carcinomas accompanying HIV infection are classified into three categories: first, KS, NHL, and head and neck cancer, including AIDS-defining disease; second, NADC-IRs (infection-related), related to infection, hepatocellular carcinoma, HL, leiomyosarcoma, anal cancer, bladder cancer, laryngeal cancer, oral cavity cancer, penile cancer, gastric cancer, tongue cancer, and tonsillar cancer; and lastly, NADC-IURs (infection-unrelated), not related to infection, such as lung cancer and breast cancer.

Currently, carcinogenesis in lung cancer is considered not to be associated with HIV infection itself. On the other hand, microsatellite alternation resulting in genetic instability is seen in lung cancer patients with HIV infection.(Wistuba *et al.*, 1998) In another study, HIV-infected patients easily developed pulmonary disease because of decreased glutathione and antioxidant levels, as well as increased lysosome and chemokine ligand 5 (CCL5) levels in broncho-alveolar lavage fluid.(Agostini *et al.*, 1995, Allard *et al.*, 1998, Buhl *et al.*, 1989, Gordon *et al.*, 2005) Chronic inflammation is associated with carcinogenesis in lung cancer.(Buhl *et al.*, 1989) (Fig. 1) Furthermore, downregulation of HIV Tat-interacting protein

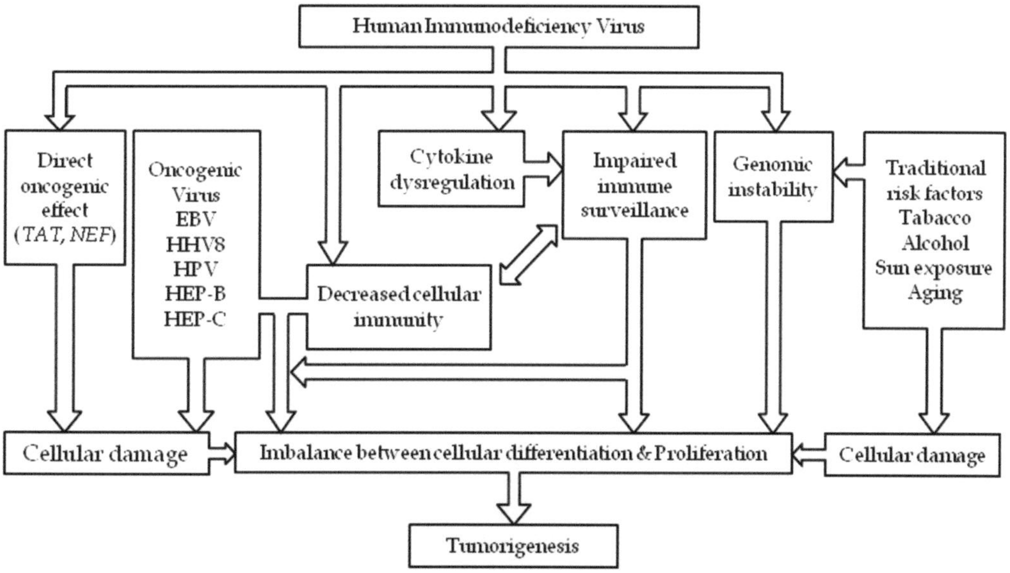

Fig. 1. Potential mechanisms for carcinogenesis in non-AIDS-defining cancer(Nguyen *et al.*)

30 (TIP30) has been verified to promote metastasis of lung cancer *in vitro* and in nude mice.(Baker *et al.*, 2000, Tong *et al.*, 2009) Thus, lung cancer in the HIV population tends to be aggressive with poor prognosis. Inhibiting HIV appears to inhibit carcinogenesis in lung cancer; however, there is no clear evidence of decreased incidence of lung cancer with the use of HAART. HAART reconstitutes immunity and decreases the risk of OIs.

4. Clinical manifestations

When compared to lung cancer in the general population, lung cancer in HIV-infected patients affects younger patients and is more aggressive. The median age of HIV-infected lung cancer patients is 45-50 years, while it is 62 years in the general population.(Spano *et al.*, 2004) With regard to the clinical stage of the lung cancer, 75-90% of all HIV-infected patients are advanced, 18-29% are in a locally advanced stage, and 50-68% are in the metastatic stage.(Lavole *et al.*, 2006) Adenocarcinoma is the most common (31-52%), followed by squamous cell carcinoma (17-39%), large cell carcinoma (3-16%), small cell carcinoma (SCLC) (1-14%), and bronchial alveolar carcinoma (less than 2%).(Tirelli *et al.*, 2000, Vyzula & Remick, 1996, Sridhar *et al.*, 1992, Alshafie *et al.*, 1997, D'Jaen *et al.*, 2010) This is similar to the distribution seen in the general population, as NSCLC accounts for 85% of all lung cancer patients in the general population. Comparing the pre-HAART era and the HAART era, the rate of adenocarcinoma was unchanged (48%), but the rate of squamous cell carcinoma was 21% in the pre-HAART era, as compared to 10% in the HAART era.(Brock *et al.*, 2006) Epidermal growth factor receptor (EGFR) mutation is a predictive factor for EGFR-tyrosine kinase inhibitors (EGFR-TKIs), and the incidence of harboring EGFR mutation among Asians is 30-35%, while it is ~10% among Caucasians.(Maemondo *et al.*, 2010, Mitsudomi *et al.*, 2009, Rosell *et al.*, 2009) A lung cancer patient harboring EGFR mutations with HIV infection has been reported.(Erickson *et al.*, 2008) CD4 cell counts at diagnosis range between 120 and 360 cells/µL,(Spano *et al.*, 2004, Tirelli *et al.*, 2000, Vyzula & Remick, 1996, Sridhar *et al.*, 1992, Brock *et al.*, 2006, Bedimo *et al.*, 2009, Tenholder & Jackson, 1993) while median CD4 cell counts in the HAART era are more than 300 cells/µL.

Overall, 25-50% of lung cancer patients with HIV infection had AIDS,(Alshafie *et al.*, 1997, Lavole *et al.*, 2006, Spano *et al.*, 2004, Sridhar *et al.*, 1992, Tirelli *et al.*, 2000, Vyzula & Remick, 1996) and 55% underwent HAART. The latency from diagnosis of HIV infection to the diagnosis of lung cancer differs by sex, being 4.1 years in women and 7.7 years in men ($p=0.02$). However, the gender-based difference has not been discussed.(Pakkala *et al.*, 2010) The frequency of metastatic organ involvement is uncertain. Release of interleukin-1 by intracerebral gp-120 components with HIV promotes brain metastasis *in vivo*.(Hodgson *et al.*, 1998) In the clinical setting, a patient with two intracerebral hemorrhages has been reported (the incidence of intratumoral hemorrhage in NSCLC is 0.52%).(Okuma *et al.*, 2010) Of note, HIV-infected patients have a higher risk of intracranial events(d'Arminio Monforte *et al.*, 2004); thus, careful follow-up is required for HIV-infected patients in clinical settings.

5. Multidisciplinary treatments & management

The fundamental modalities of treatment for lung cancer are surgery, radiotherapy, and chemotherapy.

SCLC is sensitive to both chemotherapy and radiotherapy; thus, radical concurrent chemoradiotherapy is indicated for limited-disease SCLC. When compared to NSCLC,

SCLC is characterized by higher grade, rapid progression with proliferation, and ease of metastasis to lymph nodes/distant organs in the early stage. Untreated, the median survival time is between 2 and 4 months. The response rate and median survival time in limited-disease SCLC are 70% and between 14 and 20 months, respectively. In extended-disease SCLC, chemotherapy is basic, and palliative radiotherapy is added according to the symptoms. The response rate in extended disease is 45-95%, and the median survival time is 7-10 months.(El Maalouf *et al.*, 2007)

In NSCLC, radiotherapy or chemotherapy is less sensitive than SCLC. Radical surgery is limited in Stage I-III NSCLC, and palliative chemotherapy is indicated in Stage IV NSCLC, while surgery alone is for Stage IA, and surgery-based multidisciplinary treatment is required in Stage IB-III. A decision on the treatment strategy should take into account histology, age, performance status (PS), and co-morbidities. In Stage IV patients with poor PS (≥ 3) best supportive care is recommended. The 5-year survival is 50% in Stage IA, 43% in Stage IB, 36% in Stage IIA, 25% in Stage IIB, 19% in Stage IIIA, 7% in Stage IIIB, and 2% in Stage IV. The median survival time is 14 months in Stage III and 10 months in Stage IV.(Goldstraw *et al.*, 2007)

In the period before the advent of HAART, HIV-infected patients were considered to have decreased immune competence of lymphocytes or CD4 cell counts because of accompanying complications or fragility to treatment. Toxicity and tolerance data in the treatment of other cancers are available. No fewer than 25% of advanced cancer patients with HIV infection were not treated,(Achenbach *et al.*) and among NSCLC patients with HIV infection, initial treatment consisted of chemotherapy in 31%, radiotherapy in 23%, and both in 15%.(D'Jaen *et al.*, 2010)

5.1 Surgery

Surgery is a promising modality of treatment for Stage I and II NSCLC, and is the first-line choice of treatment for all operable patients. In previous reports, patients with CD4 cell counts of more than 500 cells/μL were considered operable, while in those with lower CD4 cell counts, the indication for surgery needed careful consideration. The treatment of HIV-infected lung cancer patients at present, however, should follow the standard of care for safety and efficacy, as their prognosis depends on their lung cancer, not their HIV status. Moreover, complications, such as cardiovascular diseases and interstitial pneumonia associated with cigarette smoking, need to be taken into account, because more of these patients have a history of smoking.(Aberg, 2009)

With surgery, a reported case series did not demonstrate an increased risk of postoperative complications because of CD4 cell counts or immunological status.(Massera *et al.*, 2000) Thus, the indication for surgery in HIV-infected lung cancer patients should be determined based on pulmonary function, PS, and staging, as in the general population. Furthermore, the prognosis of such patients is good.(Spano *et al.*, 2004) In addition, the clinician should consider the medical staff's perioperative risk for blood-borne infection and ensure that standard precautions are taken. The reported blood-borne infection rate associated with surgery ranges from 0.2-0.5%.(Bell, 1997)

In determining the clinical stage, ^{18}F-fluorodeoxyglucose-positoron emission tomography-computed tomography (PET-CT) scan is a highly sensitive and specific examination. However, prudent assessment with regard to lymph nodal diagnosis is needed in the HIV population because of potential false positive to lymph nodes and upstaging in anal cancer.(Cotter *et al.*, 2006)

With respect to adjuvant chemotherapy (postoperative chemotherapy) for patients with NSCLC, a 13% decrease in the risk of death was demonstrated with chemotherapy (HR 0.87, 95%CI 0.74-1.02, p=0.08) in 1995.(Non-small Cell Lung Cancer Collaborative Group, 1995) This rate is equivalent to a 5% improvement in the 5-year survival rate. In later studies, a 5-15% improvement in the 5-year survival rate was demonstrated (HR 0.89, 95%CI 0.82-0.96, p=0.005) in NSCLC patients with Stage II-IIIA with cisplatin-based chemotherapy.(Pignon *et al.*, 2008) However, as described later, toxicity, efficacy and prognostic factors for HIV-infected lung cancer patients are uncertain.

5.2 Radiotherapy

The role of radiotherapy in HIV-infected lung cancer patients is uncertain. In general, radiation therapy for ether ADCs or NADCs leads to severe mucosal toxicity in acute phase and late-phase disturbances, even when low-dose radiation is used. In KS patients who undergo thoracic irradiation, esophagitis occurs frequently and is often severe.(Chak *et al.*, 1988, Cooper *et al.*, 1984) The mechanism of the more severe mucositis is considered to be related to decreased mucosal restoration due to a shortage of glutathione antioxidant(Buhl *et al.*, 1989, Vallis, 1991) or to be related to OIs (Fungi, Candida species, herpes, cytomegalovirus, and Cryptococcus infections).(Boal *et al.*, 1979, Rodriguez *et al.*, 1989)

In the patient with good PS or without weight loss, unresectable locoregionally advanced NSCLC or limited-disease SCLC, the standard of care is concurrent chemoradiotherapy. The 3-year survival rate in unresectable locoregionally advanced NSCLC is around 10% with radiotherapy alone, and at present, the 3-year survival rate improves by more than 25% with concurrent platinum-based chemoradiotherapy.(Blackstock & Govindan, 2007) Concurrent chemoradiotherapy is more effective but more toxic than sequential chemoradiotherapy. At present, it is recommended that HIV-infected lung cancer patients be treated with the same standard care as the general population. However, aggressive treatment requires consideration of the risk of interactions between antiretroviral agents and antitumor agents, and fragility to treatment and safety of chemoradiotherapy are uncertain. A reported case having locally advanced squamous cell lung cancer, concurrently treated with nelfinavir and 5 species of HAART and intensity modulated radiotherapy, died of massive hemoptysis because of bronchial perforation, whereas pathological complete response (CR) was achieved with intensity modulated radiotherapy at a dose of 20 Gy.(Chapman *et al.*, 2009) In a phase I study involving pancreatic cancer patients with HIV infection, a radiosensitizing effect with nelfinavir was reported.(Brunner *et al.*, 2008)

Conformal radiotherapy is appropriate, as in the general population, because of narrowing of the irradiation fields. Palliative radiotherapy is indicated according to symptoms in Stage IV.

5.3 Chemotherapy

With regard to chemotherapy, adjuvant chemotherapy is used for Stage IB-IIIA NSCLC, concomitant chemoradiotherapy is given in locoregionally advanced NSCLC, and palliative chemotherapy is given in Stage IV.(Azzoli *et al.*, 2009) In the meta-analysis of Stage IV NSCLC, which accounts for 40% of all lung cancer, platinum doublet chemotherapy prolonged the median survival to 1.5-2.8 months and improved the 1-year survival rate to 10%.(Non-small Cell Lung Cancer Collaborative Group, 2008, Grilli *et al.*, 1993, Marino *et al.*, 1994, Souquet *et al.*, 1993) Chemotherapy significantly improved survival, with a HR of 0.73 (p<0.0001) in 1995.(Kivisto *et al.*, 1995) In 2008, the same group reported the results of a meta-analysis of 16 randomized studies, and chemotherapy showed a survival benefit with an HR of 0.73 (95% CI 0.71-0.83, $p < 0.0001$) again. On the other hand, the survival benefit is no different between 1995 and later studies ($p = 0.77$) (Non-small Cell Lung Cancer Collaborative Group, 2008). However, the survival time has gradually improved because of trials with novel antitumor drugs that were excluded from this meta-analysis and diversification of treatment strategies. As the population with HIV infection is excluded from clinical trials, information regarding the efficacy and safety of chemotherapy in these patients is limited to retrospective reports.

5.3.1 Chemotherapy for metastatic stage in patients with HIV infection

5.3.1.1 Front-line setting

Chemotherapy is more frequently used for advanced lung cancer in HIV-infected patients because 75-90% of lung cancer patients with HIV infection have advanced disease.(Lavole *et al.*, 2006, Lavole *et al.*, 2009, Cadranel *et al.*, 2006) However, the benefit of chemotherapy is questionable, as the prospective clinical benefits and toxicities have not been realistically evaluated. In a phase II prospective study with carboplatin and gemcitabine combination chemotherapy followed by paclitaxel maintenance therapy involving 47 patients consisting mainly of lung cancer patients with poor PS (2 or 3) and immunologically fragile patients, including HIV infection and post-bone marrow transplantation, tolerance and efficacy were demonstrated to be adequate.(Bridges *et al.*, 2008) Previous reports have concluded that the benefit of chemotherapy was controversial, but the prognosis of NSCLC patients with HIV infection treated with chemotherapy was reported to be the same as the prognosis of the general population with NSCLC. D'Jean *et al.* reported that, among HIV-infected lung cancer patients, 81% (taxanes 45%, gemcitabine 26%, vinca alkaloid 10%) were treated with platinum-doublet chemotherapy in the front-line setting. Patients treated with singlet chemotherapy or oral antitumor agents outside of standard regimens were 3% each.(Previous study, 2010) Elderly lung cancer patients and lung cancer patients with poor PS in the general population have a poorer prognosis with chemotherapy and singlet chemotherapy, not platinum-doublet chemotherapy, is generally recommended.(D'Addario *et al.*, 2009) Among lung cancer patients with HIV infection, PS is poor (before 1996, 37~57% of patients had PS of more than 2; after 1996, this decreased to less than 30% of patients)(Spano *et al.*, 2004) Thus, for treatment of fragile patients, chemotherapy would be applied to lung cancer patients with HIV infection.

Current standard chemotherapy for advanced NSCLC is based on platinum doublet (cisplatin or carboplatin) plus third-generation antitumor drugs (irinotecan, docetaxel, gemcitabine, vinorelbine, paclitaxel,(Schiller *et al.*, 2002, Kelly *et al.*, 2001, Ohe *et al.*, 2007) and pemetrexed(Scagliotti *et al.*, 2008)) or EGFR-TKIs; gefitinib(Maemondo *et al.*, 2010, Mitsudomi *et al.*, 2009) and erlotinib(Rosell *et al.*, 2009), and an antiangiogenic inhibitor (bevacizumab).(Sandler *et al.*, 2006) Maintenance therapy with pemetrexed(Ciuleanu *et al.*, 2009) and erlotinib(Cappuzzo *et al.*, 2010) is known to prolong survival. In SCLC, platinum and etoposide or irinotecan combination therapy is used.(Murray & Turrisi, 2006) For relapsed SCLC, amrubicin or topotecan is given. In locally advanced NSCLC and limited disease (LD) SCLC, thoracic irradiation is added. D'Jean *et al.* reported that, among HIV-infected lung cancer patients, the agents combined with platinum agents were topoisomerase in 67%, vinca alkaloid in 22%, and taxanes in 11%. The response rate to front-line chemotherapy was 39% in 41 patients. Of the treated patients, 63% had adverse events, and 34% were Grade 3/4. Treatment-related deaths were seen in 2 patients (0.05%); 1 with pneumonitis, and 1 from an unknown cause.(Previous study, 2010)

5.3.1.2 Second-line setting

Overall, 60% of lung cancer patients treated with front-line chemotherapy proceed to second-line chemotherapy. In NSCLC patients with good PS, the standard of care is docetaxel (Shepherd *et al.*, 2001, Fossella *et al.*, 2000), pemetrexed(Hanna *et al.*, 2004) and erlotinib.(Shepherd *et al.*, 2005) Docetaxel is indicated for all histological types of NSCLC. Pemetrexed is expected to be active for non-squamous cell histology.(Scagliotti *et al.*, 2009) Erlotinib is effective for both patients harboring EGFR mutation and EGFR wild-type,(Ciuleanu *et al.*, 2010) although the response rate and survival time differ between them. Platinum doublet chemotherapy or non-platinum doublet chemotherapy is not anticipated to have efficacy in the second-line setting.(Azzoli *et al.*, 2009) For SCLC, intravenous or oral topotecan,(Eckardt *et al.*, 2007, von Pawel *et al.*, 1999) amrubicin,(Inoue *et al.*, 2008, Onoda *et al.*, 2006) and carboplatin and paclitaxel, re-treatment for sensitive-relapse cases are considered.(Giaccone *et al.*, 1987, Postmus *et al.*, 1987, Groen *et al.*, 1999) In the HIV population, details concerning second-line chemotherapy in Stage IV are uncertain. The rates of HIV-infected lung cancer patients treated with second-line chemotherapy in HIV population were 32% (17/53) in NSCLC and 10% (1/9) in SCLC. The response rate in this study was 11%, as in the general population.(D'Jaen *et al.*, 2010)

5.3.1.3 Molecular targeted agents

The understanding of cancer at the molecular level is profound, and proteins playing significant roles in tumor proliferation, invasion, and metastasis have been identified. As a result, molecular targeted inhibitors or antibodies for these proteins have recently been developed. Of these, drugs targeting EGFR, vascular endothelial growth factor (VEGF), and echinoderm microtubule-associated protein-like 4-anaplastic lymphoma kinase translocation (EML4-ALK)(Kwak *et al.*, 2010) have been shown to be efficacious. EGFR-targeted drugs have particularly strong evidence supporting their use. In NSCLC harboring EGFR mutation in the general population, use of EGFR-TKIs doubles survival.(Mitsudomi *et al.*, 2009, Maemondo *et al.*, 2010, Rosell *et al.*, 2009) Thus, despite the potential for drug interactions, use of EGFR-TKIs is indicated in HIV-infected patients. Though no drug interactions are expected, prudence is required from the perspective of cost and safety.

5.3.2 Pharmacodynamic interactions between HAART & cytotoxic antitumor agents

HAART reconstructs immunity and decreases risk of OIs to inhibit HIV viral load and increase CD4 cell counts for patients infected with HIV. The goal for HAART is to continuously suppress the viral load to undetectable and maintain CD4 cell counts above 500 cells/μL.(Silverberg *et al.*, 2007) However, decreases in antiretroviral agent concentrations can exacerbate clinical status, and increased/decreased concentrations of antitumor agents lead to severe toxicity or reduced antitumor effects. Both increases and decreases in serum concentrations can occur for either/both antiretroviral agents and/or cytotoxic antitumor agents.(Kivisto *et al.*, 1995) Therefore, decreased effectiveness and increased toxicity of chemotherapy must be considered. In addition, failure of virological treatment may occur. Interactions between antiretroviral agents and chemotherapeutic agents must always be considered and are a cause for concern for oncologists in clinical settings.

	Expected chemotherapeutic concentration modifications based on antiretroviral drugs used						Expected interactions between HAART and chemotherapy
	NRTI	NNRTI	PI	INSTI	FI	MVC	
Platinum	→	→	→	→	→	→	Hematological toxicity with ZDV, Neuropathy, Nephropathy with TDF
Taxanes	→	↓	↑	→	→	→	Hematological toxicity with ZDV Neuropathy with d4T and DDI
Etoposide	→	↓	↑	→	→	→	Hematological toxicity with ZDV
Gemcitabine	→	→	→	→	→	→	Hematological toxicity with ZDV Nephropathy with TDF
Pemetrexed	→	→	→	→	→	→	Hematological toxicity with ZDV
Topotecan	→	→	→	→	→	→	Hematological toxicity with ZDV
Irinotecan	→	↓	↑	→	→	→	Hematological toxicity with ZDV
Gefitinib Erlotinib	→	↓	↑	→	→	→	None
Bevacizumab	→	→	→	→	→	→	None

INSTI: integrase strand transfar inhibitor; FI: fusion inhibitor; MVC: maraviroc; ZDV: zidovudine; TDF: tenofovir; ddI: didanosine

Table 3. Expected drug interactions between antiretroviral agents and antitumor agents commonly used in NSCLC and SCLC.(Makinson *et al.*, 2010)

However, the available pharmacokinetic data for antiretroviral drugs and antitumor agents are not predictive: 1. available pharmacokinetic data are limited to case reports, and limited individual data cannot be generalized; 2. antitumor agents of a similar class can have variable pharmacokinetics; and 3. unexpected drug interactions can occur because metabolism by CYP450 is associated with single nucleotide polymorphisms (SNPs).

Antiretroviral agents are classified into six categories: nucleoside reverse transcriptase inhibitors (NRTIs); non-nucleoside reverse transcriptase inhibitors (NNRTIs); protease inhibitors (PIs); integrase inhibitors; fusion inhibitor enfuvirtide; and C-C chemokine receptor type 5 (CCR5) coreceptor antagonists. Interactions among these during treatment for ADCs, such as PCNSL or KS, enhance adverse toxicities. For instance, KS patients with CD4 cell counts greater than 200 cells/μL are reported to have a good response to paclitaxel treatment, with the same prognosis as patients with a normal immunological status.

Drug interaction between antiretroviral agents and antitumor agents is assumed when the drug is metabolized by CYP450 pathway. Many PIs and NNRTIs are metabolized by this pathway, and competitive metabolism between antitumor drugs must be considered. (Table 3) Increases in toxicity between antiretroviral agents and antitumor agents have been reported. Among NNRTIs, efavirenz increases toxicity with concomitant use of vinka alkaloids and taxanes.(Makinson *et al.*, 2010) All NRTIs and most PIs have increased drug sensitivities *in vitro*, and this leads to increased toxicity. The NRTIs efavirenz, delavirdine, and nevirapine are primarily metabolized by CYP450.(Gulick, 1998, Flexner, 1998) In a study of patients with NHL undergoing treatment with concomitant antiretroviral agents and cyclophosphamide, doxorubicin, and etoposide, significantly lower nadir neutrophil counts were seen. As compared to the group with/without PIs, the group with PIs had greater toxicity (48% vs. 27%; p=0.0025). Drug interactions have also been confirmed *in vitro*; cultured cells that expressed P-glycoprotein (P-gp) accumulated increased concentrations of paclitaxel or vinblastine concomitant with PIs.(Washington *et al.*, 1998) PIs such as ritonavir and indinavir have a strong affinity for CYP450 and also strongly inhibit CYP3A4. These enzymes are used in metabolic pathways with ifosfamide, docetaxel, paclitaxel, irinotecan, vinca alkaloids, and etoposide.(Rowinsky & Donehower, 1997, Stebbing & Bower, 2006) Severe myelosuppression with atazanavir(Richman *et al.*, 1987, Tan & Ratner, 1997) and peripheral neuropathy with didanosine, stavudine, and zalcitabine occur.(Rowinsky & Donehower, 1997) Thus, their combined use with platinum or paclitaxel leads to increased toxicities. Combination treatment with irinotecan and atazanavir is also contraindicated. Cisplatin, the key drug in lung cancer chemotherapy,(Azzoli *et al.*, 2009, Barlesi & Pujol, 2005) is not metabolized by the CYP450 enzyme pathway. Thus, drug interactions with HAART do not occur, but accumulating toxicity, such as nephrotoxicity and neurotoxicity, must be considered. In addition, patients on antiretroviral agents having nephrotoxicity such as tenofovir disoproxil require careful follow-up.

Of the molecular targeted agents, EGFR-TKIs have been poorly evaluated, but they are known to be metabolized by CYP3A4, and ritonavir should be avoided. Raltegravir is metabolized by UGT1A1 (uridine diphosphate glucuronosyl transferase isoform 1) and does not induce or inhibit hepatic enzymes; thus, drug interactions appear to be absent. Maraviroc, a CCR5 antagonist, also does not interact with CYP3A4. As for PIs, indinavir and sequinavir inhibit cell proliferation or invasion by acting through matrix metalloprotease.(Toschi *et al.*, 2011) Due to the increased toxicity of such drug interactions, the drugs that are better to apply in HAART regimens with antiretroviral drug are those not associated with CYP450, such as NRTI, raltegravir, or enfuvirtide.

In the future, dose adjustments will be used to investigate Pharmacokinetic data via a prospective study; however, the prognosis of lung cancer patients with HIV infection is anticipated to be similar to that in the general population. Thus, conventional doses and regimens are adequate.

5.3.3 Prevention of opportunistic infections & potential complications

An increased risk of OIs is considered to be a complication of chemotherapy because of the associated decrease in CD4 cell counts. In lung cancer patients, changes in CD4 cell counts with chemotherapy are unclear. However, previous reports on treatment for ADCs provide information about changes in CD4 cell counts. CD4 cell counts in NHL on chemotherapy decreased to 50% of baseline at the nadir and recovered within a month. CD4 cell counts and viral load do not change with chemotherapeutic treatment.(Powles *et al.*, 2002) In addition, in ADCs, CD4 cell counts in patients receiving concomitant HAART or HIV viral load-negative patients are considered to recover sooner.(Powles *et al.*, 2002, Hakim *et al.*, 1997) OIs on chemotherapy occurred in 8 of 25 patients (32%), and their CD4 cell counts were less than 150 cells/µL. These patients also had poor PS, and half of the patients developed Grade 3 or 4 hematological toxicity.(Tirelli *et al.*, 2000) Recent few reports have discussed the occurrence of OIs during chemotherapy. Primary prevention of OIs is adequate; no specific preventive therapies are necessary in patients with a well-controlled viral load. Generally, in patients with less than 200 cells/µL, trimethoprim-sulfamethoxazole or pentamidine inhalation is used for pneumocystis pneumonia prevention, and in patients with less than 50 cells/µL, a macrolide is used for Mycobacteriaum avium complex (MAC) prevention. Thus, a monthly CD4 cell count check is preferred during chemotherapy and one month after treatment.

5.4 Supportive care

In supportive care, drug interactions between antiretroviral agents and other agents must be considered (Table 4). However, in clinical settings, physicians must administer palliative therapy. Interactions between morphine and some HAART drugs have been shown, but the benefit of morphine for palliation remains. In Stage IV NSCLC, early induction of palliative therapy after diagnosis significantly improves quality of life and mood, and prolongs survival by 2 months.(Temel *et al.*, 2010) As in patients from the general population, early palliative therapy is indicated for HIV-infected patients, as well as psychological support at the end-stage. As for the lung cancer patients with bone metastasis, zoledronic acid, a new bisphosphonate, is an appropriate palliative treatment for skeletal-related events (SREs) and symptoms associated with bone metastases.(Rosen *et al.*, 2003a, Rosen *et al.*, 2003b) The efficacy and safety of zoledronic acid given concomitantly with HAART for the osteoporosis that is associated with long-term HAART administration have been evaluated in a clinical trial and found to be advantageous.(Bolland *et al.*, 2008, Bolland *et al.*, 2007, Huang *et al.*, 2009) When SREs occur, they are associated with decreased activities of daily living and shorter survival.(Tsuya *et al.*, 2007) Thus, zoledronic acid should be given to patients with bone metastases of lung cancer, even asymptomatic.

	Expected concentration modifications in drugs used supportive care based on antiretroviral drugs used					
	NRTI	NNRTI	PI	INSTI	FI	MVC
Dexamethasone	→	↓	↓	→	→	→
Lorazepam	→	↓	↑	→	→	→
Tricyclic antidepressants	→	→	↑	→	→	→
Fentanyl	→	→	↑	→	→	→
Carbamazepine	→	↓	↓	→	→	→

Table 4. Expected drug interactions between antiretroviral agents and frequently used supportive agents for chemotherapy.

6. Prognosis

Lung cancer patients with HIV infections are considered to have a poorer prognosis than the general population because of their younger age, immunodeficiency, aggressive extension, and more advanced stage at diagnosis. In a meta-analysis, the median survival time was 5-9 months.(Powles *et al.*, 2003, Karp *et al.*, 1993, Sridhar *et al.*, 1992, Tirelli *et al.*, 2000, Spano *et al.*, 2004, Alshafie *et al.*, 1997) The 1-year survival of HIV-infected lung cancer patients was 10% (0-15%), as compared to 40% (20-50%) in the general population.(Cadranel *et al.*, 2006, Cinti *et al.*, 2008, Grubb *et al.*, 2006, Vyzula & Remick, 1996) Over the last 20 years, survival by histology was about 7 months in SCLC and 5 months in NSCLC.(Hakimian *et al.*, 2007) Favorable prognostic factors are reported to be good PS and early stage at diagnosis. The concomitant use of HAART is controversial as a prognostic factor. The reason for these patients' poor prognosis is considered to be their more advanced stage at diagnosis.(Lavole *et al.*, 2009)

CD4 cell count is sometimes considered to be a prognostic factor for chemotherapy. The prognosis for patients with a CD4 cell count greater than 200 cells/μL is 11.5 months, while that for patients with a CD4 cell count less than 200 cells/μL is 3.4 months.(Hakimian *et al.*, 2007) At present, patients with CD4 cell counts greater than 200 cells/μL can be given chemotherapy, and they have been demonstrated to have the comparable survival to non-HIV patients. (Hakimian *et al.*, 2007)

7. Future directions

Lung cancer has become common in HIV-infected patients and appears to be increasing in clinical settings, and NADCs have become the main cause of death. Thus, lung cancer has significant clinical meaning in the management of HIV-infected patients. Knowledge about its epidemiology, screening, risk factors, and intervention will reduce the incidence of lung cancer. In particular, aggressively promoting smoking cessation programs and screening for lung cancer for earlier detection will play important roles as strategies in preventing lung cancer.

HIV-infected patients should receive standard care for lung cancer, and it is anticipated that they will have the same prognosis as the general population. However, for these patients, we need to consider previously reported toxicities and fragility to treatment. In addition, increased intensity of treatment due to drug interactions and increased radiosensitization with HAART must be considered. As the clinical details of such patients have not been well reported, infectious disease physicians and oncologists must collaborate when treating HIV-infected lung cancer patients.

8. References

Aberg, J.A. (2009). Cardiovascular complications in HIV management: past, present, and future. *J Acquir Immune Defic Syndr,* Vol.50, No.1, pp. 54-64

Aberle, D.R., Berg, C.D., Black, W.C. et al. (2010). The National Lung Screening Trial: overview and study design. *Radiology,* Vol.258, No.1, pp. 243-253

Achenbach, C.J., Cole, S.R., Kitahata, M.M. et al. Mortality after cancer diagnosis in HIV-infected individuals treated with antiretroviral therapy. *AIDS*, pp.

Agostini, C., Sancetta, R., Cerutti, A. et al. (1995). Alveolar macrophages as a cell source of cytokine hyperproduction in HIV-related interstitial lung disease. *J Leukoc Biol,* Vol.58, No.5, pp. 495-500

Allard, J.P., Aghdassi, E., Chau, J. et al. (1998). Oxidative stress and plasma antioxidant micronutrients in humans with HIV infection. *Am J Clin Nutr,* Vol.67, No.1, pp. 143-147

Alshafie, M.T., Donaldson, B. & Oluwole, S.F. (1997). Human immunodeficiency virus and lung cancer. *Br J Surg,* Vol.84, No.8, pp. 1068-1071

Azzoli, C.G., Baker, S., Jr., Temin, S. et al. (2009). American Society of Clinical Oncology Clinical Practice Guideline update on chemotherapy for stage IV non-small-cell lung cancer. *J Clin Oncol,* Vol.27, No.36, pp. 6251-6266

Baker, M.E., Yan, L. & Pear, M.R. (2000). Three-dimensional model of human TIP30, a coactivator for HIV-1 Tat-activated transcription, and CC3, a protein associated with metastasis suppression. *Cell Mol Life Sci,* Vol.57, No.5, pp. 851-858

Barlesi, F. & Pujol, J.L. (2005). Combination of chemotherapy without platinum compounds in the treatment of advanced non-small cell lung cancer: a systematic review of phase III trials. *Lung Cancer,* Vol.49, No.3, pp. 289-298

Bedimo, R.J., Mcginnis, K.A., Dunlap, M. et al. (2009). Incidence of non-AIDS-defining malignancies in HIV-infected versus noninfected patients in the HAART era: impact of immunosuppression. *J Acquir Immune Defic Syndr,* Vol.52, No.2, pp. 203-208

Bell, D.M. (1997). Occupational risk of human immunodeficiency virus infection in healthcare workers: an overview. *Am J Med,* Vol.102, No.5B, pp. 9-15

Benard, A., Bonnet, F., Tessier, J.F. et al. (2007). Tobacco addiction and HIV infection: toward the implementation of cessation programs. ANRS CO3 Aquitaine Cohort. *AIDS Patient Care STDS,* Vol.21, No.7, pp. 458-468

Bertolaccini, L., Lybéris, P., Soncini, S. et al. (2008). Clinical characteristic lung cancer in HIV-infected patients. *Cancer Therapy,* Vol.6, pp. 903-906

Blackstock, A.W. & Govindan, R. (2007). Definitive chemoradiation for the treatment of locally advanced non small-cell lung cancer. *J Clin Oncol,* Vol.25, No.26, pp. 4146-4152

Boal, D.K., Newburger, P.E. & Teele, R.L. (1979). Esophagitis induced by combined radiation and adriamycin. *AJR Am J Roentgenol,* Vol.132, No.4, pp. 567-570

Bolland, M.J., Grey, A.B., Horne, A.M. et al. (2008). Effects of intravenous zoledronate on bone turnover and BMD persist for at least 24 months. *J Bone Miner Res,* Vol.23, No.8, pp. 1304-1308

Bolland, M.J., Grey, A.B., Horne, A.M. et al. (2007). Annual zoledronate increases bone density in highly active antiretroviral therapy-treated human immunodeficiency virus-infected men: a randomized controlled trial. *J Clin Endocrinol Metab,* Vol.92, No.4, pp. 1283-1288

Bonnet, F., Burty, C., Lewden, C. et al. (2009). Changes in cancer mortality among HIV-infected patients: the Mortalite 2005 Survey. *Clin Infect Dis,* Vol.48, No.5, pp. 633-639

Bower, M., Powles, T., Nelson, M. et al. (2003). HIV-related lung cancer in the era of highly active antiretroviral therapy. *AIDS,* Vol.17, No.3, pp. 371-375

Bridges, B.B., Thomas, L., Hausner, P.F. et al. (2008). Phase II trial of gemcitabine/carboplatin followed by paclitaxel in patients with performance status=2,3 or other significant co-morbidity (HIV infection or s/p organ transplantation) in advanced non-small cell lung cancer. *Lung Cancer,* Vol.61, No.1, pp. 61-66

Brock, M.V., Hooker, C.M., Engels, E.A. et al. (2006). Delayed diagnosis and elevated mortality in an urban population with HIV and lung cancer: implications for patient care. *J Acquir Immune Defic Syndr,* Vol.43, No.1, pp. 47-55

Brunner, T.B., Geiger, M., Grabenbauer, G.G. et al. (2008). Phase I trial of the human immunodeficiency virus protease inhibitor nelfinavir and chemoradiation for locally advanced pancreatic cancer. *J Clin Oncol,* Vol.26, No.16, pp. 2699-2706

Bruyand, M., Thiebaut, R., Lawson-Ayayi, S. et al. (2009). Role of uncontrolled HIV RNA level and immunodeficiency in the occurrence of malignancy in HIV-infected patients during the combination antiretroviral therapy era: Agence Nationale de Recherche sur le Sida (ANRS) CO3 Aquitaine Cohort. *Clin Infect Dis,* Vol.49, No.7, pp. 1109-1116

Buhl, R., Jaffe, H.A., Holroyd, K.J. et al. (1989). Systemic glutathione deficiency in symptom-free HIV-seropositive individuals. *Lancet,* Vol.2, No.8675, pp. 1294-1298

Cadranel, J., Garfield, D., Lavole, A. et al. (2006). Lung cancer in HIV infected patients: facts, questions and challenges. *Thorax,* Vol.61, No.11, pp. 1000-1008

Cappuzzo, F., Ciuleanu, T., Stelmakh, L. et al. (2010). Erlotinib as maintenance treatment in advanced non-small-cell lung cancer: a multicentre, randomised, placebo-controlled phase 3 study. *Lancet Oncol,* Vol.11, No.6, pp. 521-529

Chak, L.Y., Gill, P.S., Levine, A.M. et al. (1988). Radiation therapy for acquired immunodeficiency syndrome-related Kaposi's sarcoma. *J Clin Oncol,* Vol.6, No.5, pp. 863-867

Chapman, C.H., Shen, J., Filion, E.J. et al. (2009). Marked tumor response and fatal hemoptysis during radiation for lung cancer in a human immunodeficiency virus-positive patient taking nelfinavir. *J Thorac Oncol,* Vol.4, No.12, pp. 1587-1589

Cinti, S.K., Gandhi, T. & Riddell, J.T. (2008). Non-AIDS-defining cancers: should antiretroviral therapy be initiated earlier? *AIDS Read,* Vol.18, No.1, pp. 18-20, 26-32

Ciuleanu, T., Brodowicz, T., Zielinski, C. et al. (2009). Maintenance pemetrexed plus best supportive care versus placebo plus best supportive care for non-small-cell lung cancer: a randomised, double-blind, phase 3 study. *Lancet,* Vol.374, No.9699, pp. 1432-1440

Ciuleanu, T., Stelmakh, L., Cicenas, S. et al. (2010). LBOA5 - Erlotinib versus docetaxel or pemetrexed as second-line therapy in patients with advanced non-small-cell lung cancer (NSCLC) and poor prognosis: efficacy and safety results from the phase III TITAN study. *2010 Chicago Multidisciplinary Symposium in Thoracic Oncology,* Vol.*Abstract*, pp.

Clifford, G. & Franceschi, S. (2007). Immunity, infection, and cancer. *Lancet,* Vol.370, No.9581, pp. 6-7

Cooper, J.S., Fried, P.R. & Laubenstein, L.J. (1984). Initial observations of the effect of radiotherapy on epidemic Kaposi's sarcoma. *JAMA,* Vol.252, No.7, pp. 934-935

Cotter, S.E., Grigsby, P.W., Siegel, B.A. et al. (2006). FDG-PET/CT in the evaluation of anal carcinoma. *Int J Radiat Oncol Biol Phys,* Vol.65, No.3, pp. 720-725

Crum-Cianflone, N., Hullsiek, K.H., Marconi, V. et al. (2009). Trends in the incidence of cancers among HIV-infected persons and the impact of antiretroviral therapy: a 20-year cohort study. *AIDS,* Vol.23, No.1, pp. 41-50

D'addario, G., Fruh, M., Reck, M. et al. Metastatic non-small-cell lung cancer: ESMO Clinical Practice Guidelines for diagnosis, treatment and follow-up. *Ann Oncol,* Vol.21 Suppl 5, pp. v116-119

D'arminio Monforte, A., Cinque, P., Mocroft, A. et al. (2004). Changing incidence of central nervous system diseases in the EuroSIDA cohort. *Ann Neurol,* Vol.55, No.3, pp. 320-328

D'jaen, G.A., Pantanowitz, L., Bower, M. et al. (2010). Human immunodeficiency virus-associated primary lung cancer in the era of highly active antiretroviral therapy: a multi-institutional collaboration. *Clin Lung Cancer,* Vol.11, No.6, pp. 396-404

Eckardt, J.R., Von Pawel, J., Pujol, J.L. et al. (2007). Phase III study of oral compared with intravenous topotecan as second-line therapy in small-cell lung cancer. *J Clin Oncol,* Vol.25, No.15, pp. 2086-2092

El Maalouf, G., Rodier, J.M., Faivre, S. et al. (2007). Could we expect to improve survival in small cell lung cancer? *Lung Cancer,* Vol.57 Suppl 2, pp. S30-34

Engels, E.A., Biggar, R.J., Hall, H.I. et al. (2008). Cancer risk in people infected with human immunodeficiency virus in the United States. *Int J Cancer,* Vol.123, No.1, pp. 187-194

Engels, E.A., Brock, M.V., Chen, J. et al. (2006). Elevated incidence of lung cancer among HIV-infected individuals. *J Clin Oncol,* Vol.24, No.9, pp. 1383-1388

Erickson, T.M., Koeppe, J.R., Miller, Y.E. et al. (2008). Bronchioloalveolar carcinoma presenting as chronic progressive pulmonary infiltrates in a woman with HIV: a diagnosis worth making. *J Thorac Oncol,* Vol.3, No.11, pp. 1353-1355

Flexner, C. (1998). HIV-protease inhibitors. *N Engl J Med,* Vol.338, No.18, pp. 1281-1292

Fossella, F.V., Devore, R., Kerr, R.N. et al. (2000). Randomized phase III trial of docetaxel versus vinorelbine or ifosfamide in patients with advanced non-small-cell lung cancer previously treated with platinum-containing chemotherapy regimens. The TAX 320 Non-Small Cell Lung Cancer Study Group. *J Clin Oncol,* Vol.18, No.12, pp. 2354-2362

Friis-Moller, N., Weber, R., Reiss, P. et al. (2003). Cardiovascular disease risk factors in HIV patients--association with antiretroviral therapy. Results from the DAD study. *AIDS,* Vol.17, No.8, pp. 1179-1193

Frisch, M., Biggar, R.J., Engels, E.A. et al. (2001). Association of cancer with AIDS-related immunosuppression in adults. *JAMA,* Vol.285, No.13, pp. 1736-1745

Frisch, M. & Hjalgrim, H. (1999). Re: Nonmelanomatous skin cancer following cervical, vaginal, and vulvar neoplasms: etiologic association. *J Natl Cancer Inst,* Vol.91, No.6, pp. 565-566

Giaccone, G., Ferrati, P., Donadio, M. et al. (1987). Reinduction chemotherapy in small cell lung cancer. *Eur J Cancer Clin Oncol,* Vol.23, No.11, pp. 1697-1699

Goldstraw, P., Crowley, J., Chansky, K. et al. (2007). The IASLC Lung Cancer Staging Project: proposals for the revision of the TNM stage groupings in the forthcoming (seventh) edition of the TNM Classification of malignant tumours. *J Thorac Oncol,* Vol.2, No.8, pp. 706-714

Gordon, S.B., Janoff, E.N., Sloper, D. et al. (2005). HIV-1 infection is associated with altered innate pulmonary immunity. *J Infect Dis,* Vol.192, No.8, pp. 1412-1416

Grilli, R., Oxman, A.D. & Julian, J.A. (1993). Chemotherapy for advanced non-small-cell lung cancer: how much benefit is enough? *J Clin Oncol,* Vol.11, No.10, pp. 1866-1872

Groen, H.J., Fokkema, E., Biesma, B. et al. (1999). Paclitaxel and carboplatin in the treatment of small-cell lung cancer patients resistant to cyclophosphamide, doxorubicin, and etoposide: a non-cross-resistant schedule. *J Clin Oncol,* Vol.17, No.3, pp. 927-932

Grubb, J.R., Moorman, A.C., Baker, R.K. et al. (2006). The changing spectrum of pulmonary disease in patients with HIV infection on antiretroviral therapy. *AIDS,* Vol.20, No.8, pp. 1095-1107

Grulich, A.E., Van Leeuwen, M.T., Falster, M.O. et al. (2007). Incidence of cancers in people with HIV/AIDS compared with immunosuppressed transplant recipients: a meta-analysis. *Lancet,* Vol.370, No.9581, pp. 59-67

Gulick, R. (1998). Combination therapy for patients with HIV-1 infection: the use of dual nucleoside analogues with protease inhibitors and other agents. *AIDS,* Vol.12 Suppl 3, pp. S17-22

Hakim, F.T., Cepeda, R., Kaimei, S. et al. (1997). Constraints on CD4 recovery postchemotherapy in adults: thymic insufficiency and apoptotic decline of expanded peripheral CD4 cells. *Blood,* Vol.90, No.9, pp. 3789-3798

Hakimian, R., Fang, H., Thomas, L. et al. (2007). Lung cancer in HIV-infected patients in the era of highly active antiretroviral therapy. *J Thorac Oncol,* Vol.2, No.4, pp. 268-272

Hanna, N., Shepherd, F.A., Fossella, F.V. et al. (2004). Randomized phase III trial of pemetrexed versus docetaxel in patients with non-small-cell lung cancer previously treated with chemotherapy. *J Clin Oncol,* Vol.22, No.9, pp. 1589-1597

Herida, M., Mary-Krause, M., Kaphan, R. et al. (2003). Incidence of non-AIDS-defining cancers before and during the highly active antiretroviral therapy era in a cohort of human immunodeficiency virus-infected patients. *J Clin Oncol,* Vol.21, No.18, pp. 3447-3453

Hodgson, D.M., Yirmiya, R., Chiappelli, F. et al. (1998). Intracerebral HIV glycoprotein (gp120) enhances tumor metastasis via centrally released interleukin-1. *Brain Res,* Vol.781, No.1-2, pp. 244-251

Huang, J., Meixner, L., Fernandez, S. et al. (2009). A double-blinded, randomized controlled trial of zoledronate therapy for HIV-associated osteopenia and osteoporosis. *AIDS,* Vol.23, No.1, pp. 51-57

Inoue, A., Sugawara, S., Yamazaki, K. et al. (2008). Randomized phase II trial comparing amrubicin with topotecan in patients with previously treated small-cell lung cancer: North Japan Lung Cancer Study Group Trial 0402. *J Clin Oncol,* Vol.26, No.33, pp. 5401-5406

Irwin, L.E., Begandy, M.K. & Moore, T.M. (1984). Adenosquamous carcinoma of the lung and the acquired immunodeficiency syndrome. *Ann Intern Med,* Vol.100, No.1, pp. 158

James, J.S. (2006). Lung cancer: very high death rate with HIV, huge reduction possible with CT screening for early diagnosis. *AIDS Treat News*, No.420, pp. 5-6

Karp, J., Profeta, G., Marantz, P.R. et al. (1993). Lung cancer in patients with immunodeficiency syndrome. *Chest,* Vol.103, No.2, pp. 410-413

Kelly, K., Crowley, J., Bunn, P.A., Jr. et al. (2001). Randomized phase III trial of paclitaxel plus carboplatin versus vinorelbine plus cisplatin in the treatment of patients with advanced non--small-cell lung cancer: a Southwest Oncology Group trial. *J Clin Oncol,* Vol.19, No.13, pp. 3210-3218

Kirk, G.D., Merlo, C., P, O.D. et al. (2007). HIV infection is associated with an increased risk for lung cancer, independent of smoking. *Clin Infect Dis,* Vol.45, No.1, pp. 103-110

Kivisto, K.T., Kroemer, H.K. & Eichelbaum, M. (1995). The role of human cytochrome P450 enzymes in the metabolism of anticancer agents: implications for drug interactions. *Br J Clin Pharmacol,* Vol.40, No.6, pp. 523-530

Kwak, E.L., Bang, Y.J., Camidge, D.R. et al. (2010). Anaplastic lymphoma kinase inhibition in non-small-cell lung cancer. *N Engl J Med,* Vol.363, No.18, pp. 1693-1703

Lavole, A., Chouaid, C., Baudrin, L. et al. (2009). Effect of highly active antiretroviral therapy on survival of HIV infected patients with non-small-cell lung cancer. *Lung Cancer,* Vol.65, No.3, pp. 345-350

Lavole, A., Wislez, M., Antoine, M. et al. (2006). Lung cancer, a new challenge in the HIV-infected population. *Lung Cancer,* Vol.51, No.1, pp. 1-11

Levine, A.M., Seaberg, E.C., Hessol, N.A. et al. (2010). HIV as a risk factor for lung cancer in women: data from the Women's Interagency HIV Study. *J Clin Oncol,* Vol.28, No.9, pp. 1514-1519

Maemondo, M., Inoue, A., Kobayashi, K. et al. (2010). Gefitinib or chemotherapy for non-small-cell lung cancer with mutated EGFR. *N Engl J Med,* Vol.362, No.25, pp. 2380-2388

Makinson, A., Pujol, J.L., Le Moing, V. et al. (2010). Interactions between cytotoxic chemotherapy and antiretroviral treatment in human immunodeficiency virus-infected patients with lung cancer. *J Thorac Oncol,* Vol.5, No.4, pp. 562-571

Marino, P., Pampallona, S., Preatoni, A. et al. (1994). Chemotherapy vs supportive care in advanced non-small-cell lung cancer. Results of a meta-analysis of the literature. *Chest,* Vol.106, No.3, pp. 861-865

Massera, F., Rocco, G., Rossi, G. et al. (2000). Pulmonary resection for lung cancer in HIV-positive patients with low (<200 lymphocytes/mm(3)) CD4(+) count. *Lung Cancer,* Vol.29, No.2, pp. 147-149

Mitsudomi, T., Morita, S., Yatabe, Y. et al. (2009). Gefitinib versus cisplatin plus docetaxel in patients with non-small-cell lung cancer harbouring mutations of the epidermal growth factor receptor (WJTOG3405): an open label, randomised phase 3 trial. *Lancet Oncol,* Vol.11, No.2, pp. 121-128

Murray, N. & Turrisi, A.T., 3rd (2006). A review of first-line treatment for small-cell lung cancer. *J Thorac Oncol,* Vol.1, No.3, pp. 270-278

Nguyen, M.L., Farrell, K.J. & Gunthel, C.J. Non-AIDS-Defining Malignancies in Patients with HIV in the HAART Era. *Curr Infect Dis Rep,* Vol.12, No.1, pp. 46-55

Non-small Cell Lung Cancer Collaborative Group (1995). Chemotherapy in non-small cell lung cancer: a meta-analysis using updated data on individual patients from 52 randomised clinical trials. Non-small Cell Lung Cancer Collaborative Group. BMJ, Vol.311, No.7010, pp. 899-909

Non-small Cell Lung Cancer Collaborative Group (2008). Chemotherapy in addition to supportive care improves survival in advanced non-small-cell lung cancer: a systematic review and meta-analysis of individual patient data from 16 randomized controlled trials. J Clin Oncol, Vol.26, No.28, pp. 4617-4625

Ohe, Y., Ohashi, Y., Kubota, K. et al. (2007). Randomized phase III study of cisplatin plus irinotecan versus carboplatin plus paclitaxel, cisplatin plus gemcitabine, and cisplatin plus vinorelbine for advanced non-small-cell lung cancer: Four-Arm Cooperative Study in Japan. *Ann Oncol,* Vol.18, No.2, pp. 317-323

Okuma, Y., Hosomi, Y., Takagi, Y. et al. (2010). Long-term survival following metachronous intratumoral hemorrhage in an HIV-infected patient with lung cancer. *Int J Clin Oncol,* Vol.15, No.5, pp. 515-518

Onoda, S., Masuda, N., Seto, T. et al. (2006). Phase II trial of amrubicin for treatment of refractory or relapsed small-cell lung cancer: Thoracic Oncology Research Group Study 0301. *J Clin Oncol,* Vol.24, No.34, pp. 5448-5453

Pakkala, S., Chen, Z., Rimland, D. et al. (2010). HIV-associated lung cancer in the era of highly active antiretroviral therapy (HAART): Correlation between CD4 count and outcome. *J Clin Oncol,* Vol.28, No.15s, pp. suppl; abstr 7632

Parker, M.S., Leveno, D.M., Campbell, T.J. et al. (1998). AIDS-related bronchogenic carcinoma: fact or fiction? *Chest,* Vol.113, No.1, pp. 154-161

Patel, P., Hanson, D.L., Sullivan, P.S. et al. (2008). Incidence of types of cancer among HIV-infected persons compared with the general population in the United States, 1992-2003. *Ann Intern Med,* Vol.148, No.10, pp. 728-736

Petoumenos, K., Hui, E., Kumarasamy, N. et al. (2010). Cancers in the TREAT Asia HIV Observational Database (TAHOD): a retrospective analysis of risk factors. *J Int AIDS Soc,* Vol.13, No.1, pp. 51

Pignon, J.P., Tribodet, H., Scagliotti, G.V. et al. (2008). Lung adjuvant cisplatin evaluation: a pooled analysis by the LACE Collaborative Group. *J Clin Oncol,* Vol.26, No.21, pp. 3552-3559

Postmus, P.E., Berendsen, H.H., Van Zandwijk, N. et al. (1987). Retreatment with the induction regimen in small cell lung cancer relapsing after an initial response to short term chemotherapy. *Eur J Cancer Clin Oncol,* Vol.23, No.9, pp. 1409-1411

Powles, T., Imami, N., Nelson, M. et al. (2002). Effects of combination chemotherapy and highly active antiretroviral therapy on immune parameters in HIV-1 associated lymphoma. *AIDS,* Vol.16, No.4, pp. 531-536

Powles, T., Robinson, D., Stebbing, J. et al. (2009). Highly active antiretroviral therapy and the incidence of non-AIDS-defining cancers in people with HIV infection. *J Clin Oncol,* Vol.27, No.6, pp. 884-890

Powles, T., Thirwell, C., Newsom-Davis, T. et al. (2003). Does HIV adversely influence the outcome in advanced non-small-cell lung cancer in the era of HAART? *Br J Cancer,* Vol.89, No.3, pp. 457-459

Richman, D.D., Fischl, M.A., Grieco, M.H. et al. (1987). The toxicity of azidothymidine (AZT) in the treatment of patients with AIDS and AIDS-related complex. A double-blind, placebo-controlled trial. *N Engl J Med,* Vol.317, No.4, pp. 192-197

Rodriguez, R., Fontanesi, J., Meyer, J.L. et al. (1989). Normal-tissue effects of irradiation for Kaposi's sarcoma/AIDS. *Front Radiat Ther Oncol,* Vol.23, pp. 150-159

Rosell, R., Moran, T., Queralt, C. et al. (2009). Screening for epidermal growth factor receptor mutations in lung cancer. *N Engl J Med,* Vol.361, No.10, pp. 958-967

Rosen, L.S., Gordon, D., Kaminski, M. et al. (2003a). Long-term efficacy and safety of zoledronic acid compared with pamidronate disodium in the treatment of skeletal complications in patients with advanced multiple myeloma or breast carcinoma: a randomized, double-blind, multicenter, comparative trial. *Cancer,* Vol.98, No.8, pp. 1735-1744

Rosen, L.S., Gordon, D., Tchekmedyian, S. et al. (2003b). Zoledronic acid versus placebo in the treatment of skeletal metastases in patients with lung cancer and other solid tumors: a phase III, double-blind, randomized trial--the Zoledronic Acid Lung Cancer and Other Solid Tumors Study Group. *J Clin Oncol,* Vol.21, No.16, pp. 3150-3157

Rowinsky, E. & Donehower, R. 1997. Pharmacology of cancer chemotherapy-antimicrotubule agents. In *Cancer principles and practice of oncology, 5th ed.* (Ed. De Vitavt, H., Rosembersa, Editors), pp. 467-483. Lippincott-Raven Publishers, Philadelphia

Samet, J.M., Wiggins, C.L., Humble, C.G. et al. (1988). Cigarette smoking and lung cancer in New Mexico. *Am Rev Respir Dis,* Vol.137, No.5, pp. 1110-1113

Sandler, A., Gray, R., Perry, M.C. et al. (2006). Paclitaxel-carboplatin alone or with bevacizumab for non-small-cell lung cancer. *N Engl J Med,* Vol.355, No.24, pp. 2542-2550

Saves, M., Chene, G., Ducimetiere, P. et al. (2003). Risk factors for coronary heart disease in patients treated for human immunodeficiency virus infection compared with the general population. *Clin Infect Dis,* Vol.37, No.2, pp. 292-298

Scagliotti, G., Hanna, N., Fossella, F. et al. (2009). The differential efficacy of pemetrexed according to NSCLC histology: a review of two Phase III studies. *Oncologist,* Vol.14, No.3, pp. 253-263

Scagliotti, G.V., Parikh, P., Von Pawel, J. et al. (2008). Phase III study comparing cisplatin plus gemcitabine with cisplatin plus pemetrexed in chemotherapy-naive patients with advanced-stage non-small-cell lung cancer. *J Clin Oncol,* Vol.26, No.21, pp. 3543-3551

Schiller, J.H., Harrington, D., Belani, C.P. et al. (2002). Comparison of four chemotherapy regimens for advanced non-small-cell lung cancer. *N Engl J Med,* Vol.346, No.2, pp. 92-98

Sepkowitz, K.A. (2001). AIDS--the first 20 years. *N Engl J Med,* Vol.344, No.23, pp. 1764-1772

Shepherd, F.A., Fossella, F.V., Lynch, T. et al. (2001). Docetaxel (Taxotere) shows survival and quality-of-life benefits in the second-line treatment of non-small cell lung cancer: a review of two phase III trials. *Semin Oncol,* Vol.28, No.1 Suppl 2, pp. 4-9

Shepherd, F.A., Rodrigues Pereira, J., Ciuleanu, T. et al. (2005). Erlotinib in previously treated non-small-cell lung cancer. *N Engl J Med,* Vol.353, No.2, pp. 123-132

Silverberg, M.J., Chao, C., Leyden, W.A. et al. (2009). HIV infection and the risk of cancers with and without a known infectious cause. *AIDS,* Vol.23, No.17, pp. 2337-2345

Silverberg, M.J., Neuhaus, J., Bower, M. et al. (2007). Risk of cancers during interrupted antiretroviral therapy in the SMART study. *AIDS,* Vol.21, No.14, pp. 1957-1963

Souquet, P.J., Chauvin, F., Boissel, J.P. et al. (1993). Polychemotherapy in advanced non small cell lung cancer: a meta-analysis. *Lancet,* Vol.342, No.8862, pp. 19-21

Spano, J.P., Massiani, M.A., Bentata, M. et al. (2004). Lung cancer in patients with HIV Infection and review of the literature. *Med Oncol,* Vol.21, No.2, pp. 109-115

Sridhar, K.S., Flores, M.R., Raub, W.A., Jr. et al. (1992). Lung cancer in patients with human immunodeficiency virus infection compared with historic control subjects. *Chest,* Vol.102, No.6, pp. 1704-1708

Stebbing, J. & Bower, M. (2006). Comparative pharmacogenomics of antiretroviral and cytotoxic treatments. *Lancet Oncol,* Vol.7, No.1, pp. 61-68

Tan, B. & Ratner, L. (1997). The use of new antiretroviral therapy in combination with chemotherapy. *Curr Opin Oncol,* Vol.9, No.5, pp. 455-464

Temel, J.S., Greer, J.A., Muzikansky, A. et al. (2010). Early palliative care for patients with metastatic non-small-cell lung cancer. *N Engl J Med,* Vol.363, No.8, pp. 733-742

Tenholder, M.F. & Jackson, H.D. (1993). Bronchogenic carcinoma in patients seropositive for human immunodeficiency virus. *Chest,* Vol.104, No.4, pp. 1049-1053

Tirelli, U., Spina, M., Sandri, S. et al. (2000). Lung carcinoma in 36 patients with human immunodeficiency virus infection. The Italian Cooperative Group on AIDS and Tumors. *Cancer,* Vol.88, No.3, pp. 563-569

Tong, X., Li, K., Luo, Z. et al. (2009). Decreased TIP30 expression promotes tumor metastasis in lung cancer. *Am J Pathol,* Vol.174, No.5, pp. 1931-1939

Toschi, E., Sgadari, C., Malavasi, L. et al. (2011). Human immunodeficiency virus protease inhibitors reduce the growth of human tumors via a proteasome-independent block of angiogenesis and matrix metalloproteinases. *Int J Cancer,* Vol.128, No.1, pp. 82-93

Tsuya, A., Kurata, T., Tamura, K. et al. (2007). Skeletal metastases in non-small cell lung cancer: a retrospective study. *Lung Cancer,* Vol.57, No.2, pp. 229-232

Vajdic, C.M., Mcdonald, S.P., Mccredie, M.R. et al. (2006). Cancer incidence before and after kidney transplantation. *JAMA,* Vol.296, No.23, pp. 2823-2831

Vallis, K.A. (1991). Glutathione deficiency and radiosensitivity in AIDS patients. *Lancet,* Vol.337, No.8746, pp. 918-919

Von Pawel, J., Schiller, J.H., Shepherd, F.A. et al. (1999). Topotecan versus cyclophosphamide, doxorubicin, and vincristine for the treatment of recurrent small-cell lung cancer. *J Clin Oncol,* Vol.17, No.2, pp. 658-667

Vyzula, R. & Remick, S.C. (1996). Lung cancer in patients with HIV-infection. *Lung Cancer,* Vol.15, No.3, pp. 325-339

Washington, C.B., Duran, G.E., Man, M.C. et al. (1998). Interaction of anti-HIV protease inhibitors with the multidrug transporter P-glycoprotein (P-gp) in human cultured cells. *J Acquir Immune Defic Syndr Hum Retrovirol,* Vol.19, No.3, pp. 203-209

Wistuba, Ii, Behrens, C., Milchgrub, S. et al. (1998). Comparison of molecular changes in lung cancers in HIV-positive and HIV-indeterminate subjects. *JAMA,* Vol.279, No.19, pp. 1554-1559

17

Neuropsychiatric Manifestations of HIV Infection and AIDS

Victor Obiajulu Olisah
Department of Psychiatry, Ahmadu Bello University Teaching Hospital, Zaria, Nigeria

1. Introduction

Acquired Immune Deficiency Syndrome (AIDS) was first reported in the United States in 1981 and has since become a major worldwide epidemic. AIDS is caused by the human immunodeficiency virus (HIV). By killing or damaging cells of the body's immune system, HIV progressively destroys the body's ability to fight infections and certain cancers. The term AIDS applies to the most advanced stages of HIV infection.

Statistics on the world epidemic of HIV/AIDS indicates that 39.5 million people are living with HIV/AIDS worldwide. Of these, 24.7 million (63%) live in Sub-Saharan Africa, a region that is home to just 10% of the world's population (UNAIDS/WHO report, 2006).

HIV is a retrovirus, which is immunosuppressive, predisposing the individual to opportunistic infections and certain neoplasm (Wiley, 1994). In addition to impairment in immune functions, evidence has suggested that HIV is neurotropic. It should therefore be anticipated that neuropsychiatric complication might be common in HIV positive individuals during all phases of HIV related illness.

Over the years, researchers have developed antiretroviral drugs to fight both HIV infection and its associated infections and cancers. Currently available drugs do not cure people with HIV infection or AIDS, and they all have side effects that can be severe. Because no vaccine for HIV is available, the only way to prevent infection is to avoid behaviours that put a person at risk of infection, such as sharing needles and unprotected sex.

It is believed that neuropsychiatric disorders account for over 15% of the world's disease burden. Due to the recent advances in antiretroviral therapy, the life expectancy of people living with HIV has increased, and thus clinicians are more likely to encounter the neuropsychiatric manifestations of the disease. In as many as 20% of HIV infected individuals, neurologic or neuropsychiatric symptoms may be the presenting features, prior to other medical symptoms of AIDS. Despite improvement in and combination of antiretroviral therapy, neuropsychiatric complications still occur in as many as 50% of people living with HIV and are mostly undiagnosed and untreated. Assessment and management of mental disorders is integral to an effective HIV/AIDS intervention program. Mental health professionals will increasingly be called upon to assist in the management of people living with HIV/AIDS. Thus psychiatrists will need to be familiar with disorders that are prevalent in HIV infection. It is now estimated that 40-70% of patients with AIDS develop clinical neurologic abnormalities. The most common neurologic manifestations are minor cognitive motor disorder (MCMD) and HIV-associated dementia (HAD). On the other hand, depression is the most common psychiatric condition in people living with

HIV/AIDS with estimated life time prevalence in the range of between 21% and 61% (Elliot et al, 1998). This category of psychiatric disorders presents diagnostic challenges because of the many neurovegetative confounding factors that are present in association with HIV illness. In both cases, the impact of these syndromes on seropositive patients is significant and appropriate intervention is required, the key to optimal treatment resting with early diagnosis and aggressive treatment.

Initially, the neuropsychiatric manifestations of HIV/AIDS were attributed to psychological reactions to a systemic illness, the effects of psychosocial stressors associated with the disease, or the consequences of opportunistic infections or neoplasms within the central nervous system (CNS). It is now recognized that the psychiatric sequelae of HIV infection and AIDS are numerous and have etiologies that involve neurobiological and psychosocial factors. These include the direct or primary effects of HIV on nervous tissue, the consequences of secondary viral and nonviral opportunistic infections, tumors, cerebrovascular disease, and the complications of systemic therapies for AIDS and associated disorders.

Some previous studies have indicated that Neuropsychiatric disorders in people living with HIV/AIDS are associated with disease progression, poor adherence to antiretroviral drugs, increased incidence of high risk sexual behavior with the potential for further HIV transmission, and deterioration in their quality of life.

Mental and neurological disorders have an intertwined relationship with HIV and AIDS, yet sadly are often overlooked when HIV interventions are planned and implemented. Several important aspects of HIV care and treatment place psychiatrists at the forefront of this epidemic, these include:

- psychiatric disorders (including substance use) can increase an individual's risk of acquiring sexually transmitted diseases, including HIV;
- pre-existing mental disorders (including substance use) can predate and/or complicate HIV-related illness;
- neuropsychiatric complications and psychiatric illness can affect adherence to antiretroviral therapy regimens;
- new antiretroviral treatments and combination therapies can affect the CNS and/or contribute to the development of psychiatric side effects/symptoms;
- individuals with waning immunity and high viral loads may be at particular risk for the HIV-related CNS complications that can cause acute mental status changes;
- the proportion of mental health and/or substance abuse disorders among people living with HIV/AIDS is nearly 5 times greater than the proportion found in the general population;
- persons living with a severe mental illness are disproportionately vulnerable (as high as 23%) to infection with HIV and other sexually transmitted diseases;
- psychiatric syndromes can be especially challenging to recognize and accurately diagnose in the medically ill; and
- as HIV/AIDS becomes increasingly a chronic disorder with the improvement of treatments and longer survival times, the need for comprehensive psychiatric care and services is expected to rise.

2. Biology and pathophysiology of HIV infection

HIV is a lentivirus, a subgroup of retroviruses. As with other retroviruses, HIV has rapid rate of genetic mutation. This family of viruses is known for latency, persistent viremia, infection of the nervous system and weakening of the host immune responses. HIV-1 is the form of the virus that causes disease in most part of the world. HIV-2 discovered in 1986, causes a relatively small proportion of cases clustered in West Africa. HIV has high affinity for CD4 T lymphocytes and monocytes. When HIV binds to CD4 cells, it becomes internalized. The virus replicates itself by generating a DNA copy using reverse transcriptase enzyme. Viral DNA becomes incorporated into the host DNA, enabling further replication (Green, 1991, Stebbing et al, 2004). HIV causes the lysis of CD4 lymphocytes. These cells are critical in cell-mediated immunity. The course of HIV infection is characterized by latency. Unfortunately, profound immune deficiency eventually develops, as CD4 cell count drops below 200cells per mm3. At this point, the patient becomes vulnerable to opportunistic infections and malignancies (Centers for Disease Control, 1982). Progression from HIV to AIDS occurs at a median of 11years after infection. In the recent past, most patients would not survive more than 1 to 2 years after diagnosis of AIDS. However, since the introduction of antiretroviral drugs and prophylaxis against opportunistic pathogens, death rates from AIDS have begun to decline significantly.

3. Treatment of HIV infection

Treatment is accomplished through numerous combinations of antiretroviral agents belonging to the following groups: Nucleoside analogue reverse transcriptase inhibitors, nonnucleoside reverse transcriptase inhibitors, protease inhibitors and nucleoside analogues. In the mid-1990s, several investigators studied combination therapies of two reverse transcriptase inhibitors and a protease inhibitor. This therapy was later referred to as Highly Active Antiretroviral Therapy (HAART). HAART dramatically reduced viral load and often resulted in an increase in CD4 cell count. The current goal of treatment is to reduce viral load to undetectable levels and maintain such remission without interruption. Evidence suggests that the therapies suppress replication but do not eradicate HIV from all parts of the body, particularly lymphoid tissue and the brain. Not all patients who initiate antiretroviral therapy respond. The lack of clinical response is likely explained by problems with adherence, suboptimal antiretroviral treatment potency, and genetic mutation of HIV strains (Descamps et al, 2000). Many patients experience substantial side effects, and it is not uncommon for changes to be made in antiretroviral regimens because of such side effects. Adverse effects include lipodystrophy, hyperlipidemia, nephrotoxicity, bone marrow suppression, neuropathy and elevation of blood glucose to possibly diabetes mellitus levels (Deeks et al, 1997). Patients often experience nausea, vomiting, diarrhea, sleep disturbances and rashes.

Adherence is of utmost concern with antiretroviral treatment because even minor deviations from the prescribed regimen can result in viral resistance and permanent loss of efficacy for existing medications (Practice guidelines for HIV treatment, 2000). Studies of antiretroviral treatment continue to indicate that a near-perfect adherence is needed to adequately repress viral replication (Demasi et al, 2001).

As the world HIV epidemic spreads increasingly among disadvantaged persons with limited resources who have multiple comorbid disorders, significantly more psychosocial stressors, and less access to ongoing primary or mental health care, these individuals are at risk of not receiving the recommended treatment for HIV infection. Services for HIV patients must balance medical interventions with the emotional, economic, and social supports required for good quality of life and prevention of further transmission (Practice guidelines for HIV treatment, 2000).

4. Etiology of the neuropsychiatric manifestations of HIV/AIDS

4.1 Impact of HIV on the Central Nervous System (CNS)

Clinical evidence for direct infection of the CNS by HIV emerged in the mid- 1980s, when patients began to survive their presenting opportunistic infections but went on to develop neuropsychiatric syndromes that could not be attributed to CNS opportunistic infections and neoplasm. Additional evidence included signs of neuro-cognitive impairment in adults, loss or arrest of developmental milestones in children, ability to culture HIV from the cerebrospinal fluid, neuropathological lesions of the brain at autopsy, and abnormalities observed through brain imaging techniques, including cerebral atrophy (Deeks et al, 1997).

HIV invades the CNS early in the course of infection entering by way of macrophages, which along with microgial cells are largely responsible for HIV replication within the CNS. While HIV does not infect neurons in the CNS, it causes neuronal death by causing the elaboration of neurotoxins which in turn induce a variety of inflammatory factors that cause apoptosis, or programmed cell death of neurons (Swindells et al, 1999).

The pathogenesis of HIV infection within the brain and its relationship to neurologic and psychiatric complications remains obscure, but there is evidence that cellular and molecular components of the immune system are involved (Bloom & Rausch, 1997).

Several different mechanisms may explain the effects of HIV on the CNS. Researchers have hypothesized that pathogenesis begins with viral penetration of the CNS and associated loss of integrity of the blood-brain barrier. This may allow cellular and non-cellular inflammatory components of the immune system to enter the CNS, resulting in damage to neurons and non-neuronal support cells (Rabkin & Ferrando, 1997).

Some studies have examined viral load and CD4 cell counts, measures typically used to monitor immunologic function in patients with HIV infection, as potential markers of CNS injury and vulnerability to CNS complications. A study that followed viral loads and CD4 cell counts in a large cohort of HIV-infected men without AIDS found that relatively high plasma HIV RNA (> 3000 copies/ml) and low CD4 T-lymphocyte counts (< 500 x 106 cells/l) were predictive of both dementia and neuropathy (Childs et al., 1999).The authors suggested that effective suppression of HIV may reduce the risk of developing these neurological complications.

Based on evidence of basal ganglia dysfunction in HIV-associated dementia (Berger & Nath, 1997), some researchers proposed that microvascular abnormalities would be found in the basal ganglia of patients with this condition (Berger, 2000).Using time-course magnetic resonance imaging, these investigators observed increased enhancement, both immediate and late, in the basal ganglia of individuals with HIV infection and moderate-to-severe dementia, relative to HIV patients without dementia. These data suggested that increases in regional cerebral blood volume and disruption of the blood-brain barrier have an etiologic role in the development of HIV-associated dementia.

Most HIV DNA in the brain has been found in macrophages/microglia, often near apoptotic neurons, suggesting that cytokines produced by the infected cells might contribute to neuronal destruction (Shapshak et al., 1995). Macrophages may infiltrate the CNS by interacting with the endothelial cells that form the blood-brain barrier, causing endothelial cell damage and disrupting the barrier (Nottet, 1999). Chemokines (cytokines that act as macrophage attractants) and their receptors on neurons and glial cells appear to play a central role in HIV entry into the CNS and eventual cellular destruction (Gabuzda &Wang, 2000; Zheng, 1999).Synaptic damage, without neuronal loss, has been observed in patients with mild HIV-associated cognitive disorders. Using synaptic density as an indicator of damage in post-mortem brain samples from HIV-infected patients, Everall and colleagues found that reduced synaptic density correlated significantly with ante-mortem neuropsychological functioning, and stressed that early diagnosis and treatment could potentially reverse synaptic damage and prevent cognitive decline(Everall et al., 1999). Loss of subcortical neurons in the brain of people infected with HIV may be associated with the experience of depression.

Evidence is accumulating to suggest roles for several HIV proteins, including glycoprotein 120 (gp120), HIV-1 negative factor (Nef), and transactivating protein (Tat), in HIV-induced neuropathogenesis. For example, the viral envelope protein gp120 appears to bind to rat dorsal root ganglia and human neuroblastoma cells (Apostolski et al., 1993), and in rats exposure to gp120 has been shown to cause swelling and increase tumor necrosis factor in the sciatic nerve trunk, induce astrocyte and microglial infiltration into the spinal cord, and cause neuropathic pain behaviours (Herzberg & Sagen, 2001). *In vitro*, studies have shown that Nef induces macrophage chemotaxis (Koedel et al., 1999) and acts as a potent neurotoxin (Trillo-Pazos et al., 2000). Astrocytes treated with Tat *in vitro* produced pro-inflammatory cytokines and chemokines that may contribute to neuronal injury (Galey et al., 2001). Tat also stimulates macrophage production of metalloproteinases, enzymes that are expressed at increased levels in certain neurologic diseases and in the brain tissues of patients with AIDS (Johnston et al.2000). Although the significance of these laboratory findings for patients with HIV or AIDS remains to be clarified, it is probable that many of these mechanisms combine to produce the neurologic and psychiatric changes seen with HIV infection and AIDS. Identifying and characterizing the mechanisms involved may open new avenues for prevention and treatment.

4.2 Psychosocial factors

The psychosocial stress associated with a socially stigmatizing terminal illness and frequent infections carries with it tremendous emotional upheaval in vulnerable individuals. There is usually a sense or loss of health, financial security, independence and relationships in HIV infected persons. This is made worse when relevant social support is missing (Katalan et al, 1989).

Specific crisis points and psychosocial factors can precipitate psychiatric disorders especially anxiety and depression in HIV-infected persons. These crisis points includes- learning of HIV positive status, disclosure of HIV status to family and friends, introduction of medication, occurrence of any physical illness, recognition of new symptoms/ progression of disease, necessity for hospitalization, death of a partner, diagnosis of AIDS, changes in major aspects of lifestyle, necessity for making end of life and permanency decisions (HIV clinical guidelines, 2000).

5. Neurologic manifestations of HIV

HIV is classified among the lentiviruses, a family of viruses characterized in part by their tendency to cause chronic neurologic disease in their animal hosts. It is not surprising, then, that neurologic complications of HIV infection are common and not confined to opportunistic infections. All levels of the neuraxis can be involved, including the brain, meninges, spinal cord, nerve, and muscle. Neurologic disease is the first manifestation of symptomatic HIV infection in roughly 10-20% of persons, while about 60% of patients with advanced HIV disease will have clinically evident neurologic dysfunction during the course

of their illness (Koppel et al., 1985). The incidence of subclinical neurologic disease is even higher: autopsy studies of patients with advanced HIV disease have demonstrated pathologic abnormalities of the nervous system in 75-90% of cases (De la Monte et al., 1987).
HIV has been cultured from brain, nerve, and cerebrospinal fluid (CSF) from persons at all stages of the disease, including those without neurologic signs or symptoms. Positive HIV cultures in CSF do not predict the presence or development of neurologic signs or symptoms later on. The development of neurologic manifestations of AIDS depends on a number of factors, such as antiretroviral treatment history, degree of immunosuppression, and the molecular biology of the viral strain, particularly its neurovirulence(McGuire & Greene, 1996) Host factors, including genetic makeup, undoubtedly play a role in selective vulnerability to neurologic manifestations.
The initial infection of the nervous system by HIV is usually asymptomatic, although acute aseptic meningitis, encephalitis, and inflammatory polyneuropathy have all occurred in this setting. Despite its potential to cause disease at all levels of the nervous system, HIV does not directly infect central or peripheral neurons, astrocytes, or oligodendroglial cells. Latent or low level HIV infection in the CNS is maintained by virus-infected cells of the monocyte/macrophage lineage. "Indirect effects" of macrophage activation--such as dysregulation of cytokines and chemokines, free-radical (oxidative stress) injury, and secretion of soluble factors that are potently neurotoxic, have been implicated as effectors of nervous Minor Cognitive system injury in HIV.

5.1 Minor cognitive impairment

Despite evidence of early infection of the CNS, symptoms of cognitive impairment typically occur late in symptomatic HIV disease, usually in the setting of severe immunosuppression (Miller et al., 1990).
Cognitive impairment has long been recognized as part of manifestation of human immune deficiency virus infection. These changes include loss of cognitive flexibility, difficulty in problem solving, mental slowness and difficulty in concentration. There are also difficulties in memory which manifest as delayed recall. Despite the wide spread use of highly active antiretroviral therapy (HAART), at least in developed nations and some developing nations, cognitive impairment and other neurological complications of HIV infection persist with devastating personal and socioeconomic consequences. Even though neurons are rarely infected by human immunodeficiency virus especially at early stage of the infection, neuronal loss is quite common in patient with HIV infection.
Although as many as 40% of patients with HIV/AIDS will have some form of cognitive impairment even before the development of full dementia, only a small percentage (5-10%) may go on to develop dementia itself. Various type of cognitive impairment in HIV infection has been documented and the American academy of Neurology (AAN) published a diagnostic criteria for HIV associated dementia (HAD) and minor cognitive motor disorder (MCMD); which include motor, affective and behavioural abnormalities, consistent with the early description of AIDS dementia complex.

5.2 AIDS Dementia Complex (ADC)

Some investigators hold that increased HIV proliferation in the brain is necessary for the development of ADC. Others propose that a macrophage-initiated cascade of events can lead to brain dysfunction and clinical dementia, even in the absence of high viral load in the brain. Activated macrophages, whether infected with HIV or not, are capable of secreting potent neurotoxins, inducing pro-inflammatory cytokines, and generating oxygen free radicals that can damage cells and lead to neuronal dysfunction or death (Glass et al., 1995). A particular subtype of monocyte/macrophages derived from the peripheral blood was found to be greatly increased among patients with AIDS dementia compared with both HIV infected and uninfected controls. Soluble factors from these macrophages were found to be highly neurotoxic--that is, they killed human brain cells in culture (Pulliam et al., 1997).

Although the incidence of nearly all nervous system opportunistic infections has declined dramatically in the era of potent antiretroviral therapy, the impact on the incidence and prevalence of HIV-associated cognitive impairment including frank ADC--has been low. The prevalence of ADC in HIV-infected individuals with higher CD4 counts (200-350 cells/μL) actually appears to have increased since 1996. Pathologically, the prevalence of HIV-associated brain disease, or encephalopathy, is rising despite suppressive antiretroviral therapy (Neuenburg et al., 2002). Poor penetration of the blood-brain barrier by many of the antiretroviral drugs, particularly the protease inhibitors, has been suggested as a reason for the persistence of ADC.

There is some evidence that, despite the poor CNS penetration of most antiretrovirals, effective antiretroviral therapy may attenuate the neurotoxicity of circulating monocytes/macrophages. Among individuals with ADC receiving effective antiretroviral regimens, macrophage-derived soluble factors were found to be less neurotoxic than observed prior to the availability of combination antiretroviral therapy (Pulliam et al., 1997).

The major difference between "HIV associated dementia complex" and "HIV associated minor cognitive/ motor disorder" is the severity of impairment in activities of daily living. That is, by definition, dementia must have cognitive impairment severe enough to interfere with occupational or social functioning. In "HIV associated minor cognitive/motor disorder," activities of daily living are generally intact with the possible exception of mild difficulties in the most demanding activities.

The initial features of HIV associated dementia include an overall slowing in cognition (i.e., bradyphrenia) and movement (i.e., bradykinesia) as well as difficulties in motor dexterity and coordination, forgetfulness, poor concentration, and marked apathy. Although dysphoric mood is not a common feature, the pronounced slowing and apathy may appear as if the patient is depressed. Furthermore, assessing other aspects of depression (e.g., weight loss, cognitive disturbance and insomnia) is difficult for patients with this disorder due to shared symptomatology that may be indistinguishable from the psychiatric symptoms.

Later in the course of HIV associated dementia, the patient may exhibit myoclonus, bowel and bladder incontinence, and, eventually, mutism and a vegetative state. Once these advanced features are present, death is typically imminent.

Because the above initial symptoms are similar to those seen in other patient groups with subcortical impairment (e.g., Parkinson's disease, progressive supranuclear palsy, multiple sclerosis) and because of the neuroimaging findings of subcortical neuropathology, HIV associated dementia was originally described as a subcortical dementia. However, in light of the more recent findings of cortical atrophy and higher cortical function deficits in AIDS patients, this characterization may not fully describe the spectrum of neuropsychiatric deficits associated with HIV infection and AIDS.

Antiretroviral therapy may be helpful in treating Minor Cognitive /Motor Disorder and HIV associated dementia and should be recommended for all patients, unless there are contraindications. The ability of particular antiretroviral drugs to penetrate the blood-brain barrier may be less important to treatment success than the overall potency of the regimen and the ability of the patient to adhere to it.

Studies from the 1980s showed that zidovudine monotherapy was beneficial in patients with HAD, so some clinicians include it in the ART regimen for anyone with neurocognitive impairment. Others suggest using at least 2 drugs that cross the blood-brain barrier (eg, zidovudine, stavudine, abacavir, lamivudine, and nevirapine). Efavirenz, didanosine, and lamivudine cross to a lesser degree. As a class, protease inhibitors (PIs) have poor blood-brain barrier penetration. Nevertheless, patients have shown neurocognitive improvement while taking PI-containing regimens, perhaps because of indirect effects on HIV activity in the CNS.

When present, depressive symptoms should be treated with low dosages of selective serotonin reuptake inhibitors (SSRIs).

Antipsychotic medications may be useful in treating agitation and hallucinations, but patients with these conditions are often extremely sensitive to anticholinergic adverse effects and extrapyramidal symptoms. Newer neuroleptic or antipsychotic agents, such as olanzapine and risperidone, have lower rates of significant side effects compared with older drugs. The starting dosage of olanzapine is 2.5 mg orally at bedtime; that for risperidone is 0.5-1 mg orally at bedtime. Note that these drugs may interact with antiretroviral medications, especially ritonavir, and can cause weight gain and other metabolic adverse effects. Avoid benzodiazepines, which tend to increase confusion and decrease concentration.

Psychostimulants such as methylphenidate (Ritalin) and dextroamphetamine (Dexedrine) have been used to improve attention, concentration, and psychomotor function. Dosages of methylphenidate start at 5 mg for a test dose, then 2.5-5.0 mg twice daily, increasing by doses of 5 mg every other day until the desired effect is achieved. Usual dosages are in the range of 20-30 mg per day. Monitor blood pressure, heart rate, and symptoms of restlessness, agitation, nausea, and psychosis.

For a patient who is knowledgeable about HIV, a dementia workup or diagnosis often precipitates a crisis, with an increased risk of suicide. Carefully screen for depression and suicidality, and treat these if they develop.

Behavioral management strategies may assist the patient with early manifestations of dementia to continue living with some degree of independence and safety in the home. Memory aids such as posted notes, calendars, alarmed pill-boxes, and other environmental cues may help.

It is critical to enlist the support of family members and significant others at an early stage of the illness. Because the disease is frightening and may be progressive, the patient and members of the support system need assistance in anticipating and planning for the future. Plans for assisted living or other in-home custodial care should be made early. Severe or late dementia causes fear, misunderstanding, and frustration for both the patient and care givers. All involved will require help from visiting nurses, social workers, hospice workers, and physicians. Recommend the preparation of an advance directive for the patient with early manifestations of dementia.

5.3 Overview of clinical neurologic disease

5.3.1 Cerebral symptoms and signs

Apart from dementia, HIV-infected patients are at risk for a wide range of neurologic diseases. Cerebral signs and symptoms are the most common. Global cerebral disease can present with altered mental status or generalized seizures, whereas focal disease often produces hemiparesis, hemisensory loss, visual field cuts, or disturbances in language use. Fungal, viral, and mycobacterial meningoencephalitides are the most common causes of global cerebral dysfunction, and progressive multifocal leukoencephalopathy (PML), primary CNS lymphoma, and toxoplasmosis account for the majority of focal presentations. As the epidemic has progressed, the epidemiology of CNS complications has changed. In general, availability of effective antiretroviral regimens has been associated with a dramatic decline in incidence and severity of opportunistic infections of the CNS. Even before the availability of these regimens, the incidence of CNS toxoplasmosis had declined among patients receiving trimethoprim-sulfamethoxazole prophylaxis against Pneumocystis. Unfortunately, antiretroviral regimens have not demonstrably decreased the prevalence of PML, and the incidence among individuals with higher CD4 counts may be increasing. However, the prognosis of this once uniformly fatal disease has improved dramatically, with long-term remissions now fairly common among patients receiving antiretroviral therapy (Berger et al., 1998).

5.3.2 Syndromes affecting cord, nerve roots, and muscle

Viral and, rarely, fungal and parasitic opportunistic infections can affect the spinal cord. Systemic lymphoma can infiltrate nerve roots and meninges, occasionally causing a mass lesion within the cord. In addition, HIV itself is associated with a spastic paraparesis similar to that seen with vitamin B12 deficiency. Peripheral nerve injury is very common, particularly a painful distal neuropathy seen late in HIV infection. About 35% of hospitalized patients with advanced HIV disease have peripheral neuropathy (Hall et al., 1991).

Although myalgias or muscle pains are a frequent complaint, frank muscle disease is less common. Both inflammatory myopathies and a toxic myopathy secondary to zidovudine have been observed. More recently, a syndrome of acute neuromuscular weakness, often associated with lactic acidosis, has been described in association with several nucleoside analogue reverse transcriptase inhibitors, including zidovudine (AZT), stavudine (d4T), didanosine (ddI), and lamivudine (3TC), either alone or in combination. Any patient on antiretroviral therapy presenting with a "Guillain-Barré-type" picture of ascending neuromuscular weakness should be tested for lactic acidosis and evaluated with electromyography and nerve conduction studies.

Among patients infected with HIV, serious neurologic disease may present with relatively trivial symptoms and signs. Therefore, a high index of suspicion must be maintained to detect disease early in these patients. A careful neurologic examination to attempt anatomic localization is necessary to guide further laboratory and imaging studies. Because multiple neurologic diseases often coexist in patients, close follow-up is needed even if a presumptive diagnosis has been made. A change in clinical condition often necessitates a thorough reevaluation.

5.3.3 Pain

There is growing awareness that pain from a variety of etiologies commonly complicates HIV disease. In general, patients with AIDS have pain comparable in prevalence and intensity to

pain in patients with cancer, with similar mixtures of neuropathic and visceral-somatic etiologies. However, although efforts to improve malignant pain management have benefited many patients with cancer, pain in patients with AIDS is dramatically undertreated.
Aggressive pain treatment can be the single most important and most challenging intervention in the care of patients with HIV disease. In a recent U.S. study, only 15% of ambulatory AIDS patients with severe pain received adequate pain management. The principles of pain assessment and treatment in the patient with HIV/AIDS are not fundamentally different from those in the patient with cancer and should be followed.
These principles are described in the WHO analgesic ladder (WHO clinical guidelines, 1994), a well-validated, stepwise approach to pain management related to pain severity. Therapy ranges from nonopioid analgesics and adjuvants to systemic weak and strong opioids to intraspinal drug delivery for refractory severe pain. Opioids, except in quite high doses, can be ineffective in neuropathic pain; adjuvants (namely, tricyclics, anticonvulsants) are often more successful. Where neuropathic pain is refractory to such therapies, pain management specialists should be consulted.

5.4 Specific neurologic conditions

5.4.1 Neuromuscular disorders

A wide range of peripheral nervous system disorders develop in patients with HIV infection, leading to pain, sensory symptoms, and muscle weakness. Both "primary" HIV associated nerve disorders, and those secondary to opportunistic processes are well described. In addition, certain antiretroviral drugs may cause or exacerbate peripheral neuropathies.
Classification of Neuromuscular Disorders
Four types of neuropathy are important to recognize in clinical practice, either because of their high prevalence or their therapeutic implications, or both. They are:

1. Distal symmetric polyneuropathy (DSPN)
2. Mononeuropathy multiplex
3. Chronic inflammatory demyelinating polyneuropathy
4. Progressive lumbosacral polyradiculopathy

The incidence of neuropathy increases with declining CD4 cell count and advancing systemic HIV disease. Familiar causes of neuropathy, such as nutritional deficiency and diabetes mellitus, account for only a small percentage of the neuropathy in these patients. Toxicity of therapeutic drugs, notably zalcitabine (ddC) is responsible for some cases of neuropathy, or for progression; however, antiretroviral toxicity is probably overdiagnosed as a primary cause of HIV-associated neuropathy.
Proper recognition of the different types of peripheral nerve dysfunction is essential for patient management. Except for the few neuropathies with known causes, most of these disorders are characterized on the basis of clinical features alone. The rate of symptom progression, the degree of weakness relative to sensory loss, and the severity of immunosuppression guide the differential diagnosis. The electrophysiologic features of nerve conduction and electromyographic studies remain the gold standard for diagnosis, and may lead to different therapeutic options.

5.4.2 Myopathy

Symptomatic primary muscle disease is uncommon in patients with HIV infection. A polymyositislike syndrome occurs rarely, with few cases encountered even in large referral centers. A secondary myopathy attributable to the muscle toxicity of AZT emerged in the latter half of the 1980s with widespread use of the drug. The hallmark of myopathy is diffuse, symmetric weakness of "proximal" muscles, hip or shoulder girdle muscles, with a sparing of sensory and autonomic functions. Difficulty with squatting, rising from a chair, or walking upstairs is often the presenting symptom of myopathy. Some patients have myalgia and muscle tenderness, but these complaints are also common in patients without myopathy. In patients receiving AZT, discontinuation of the drug may result in clinical improvement of myopathy. Muscle pain and serum creatine kinase levels decrease first, followed by a more delayed improvement in strength. Some patients may tolerate rechallenging with lower doses of AZT, although the use of other antiretroviral therapy is probably preferable (Dalakas et al., 1990).

5.4.3 Spinal cord disorders

Clinically significant spinal cord disorders are less common in HIV disease than are peripheral nervous system diseases. The neurologic signs of myelopathy such as increased tone and hyperreflexia in the legs and Babinski signs (extensor plantar responses) may be elicited even in the absence of subjective complaints. In most cases, such asymptomatic signs reflect mild HIV-associated spinal cord disease that may or may not progress. Patients with symptomatic myelopathy usually complain first of clumsy gait and urinary hesitancy. The clinical course is typically one of slow progression, and most patients remain ambulatory. A more fulminant course may be seen with wheelchair dependence within a few months. Upper extremities are affected very late, if at all. Baclofen (10-30 mg three times daily) or tizanidine (4 mg three times daily) may attenuate leg spasticity and reduce leg cramps. Painful dysesthesias may be treated with "neuropathic pain" adjuvants, such as lamotrigine or desipramine.

5.4.4 Intracranial disorders

The CNS disorders in the setting of HIV disease can be divided into four general categories: a) primary infection of the brain by HIV; b) opportunistic infections by parasitic, fungal, viral, and bacterial organisms; b) CNS neoplasms; and d) complications of systemic disorders.

Primary HIV Infection of the Brain: HIV Associated Dementia Complex has already been discussed above.

5.4.5 Intracranial opportunistic infections

CNS toxoplasmosis has been the most common cause of intracerebral mass lesion in HIV-infected patients. Its incidence has declined dramatically among patients receiving PCP prophylaxis, and further declined among patients treated with effective antiretroviral therapy. Earlier reports described frequencies of 3-40%, reflecting the considerable regional variation in exposure to the parasite. CT scan of the brain usually shows multiple ring-enhancing lesions with predilection for cortex and deep gray-matter structures such as the basal ganglia. The cerebellum and brain stem are less commonly involved. Radiologic appearance can vary markedly; single lesions and lesions with diffuse enhancement, as well as nonenhancing lesions can appear.

5.4.6 Aseptic meningitis

Patients with aseptic meningitis often present initially with headache and occasionally with altered mental status or cranial neuropathies. Many patients with this syndrome probably have primary HIV meningoencephalitis. In investigating symptoms such as headache, altered mental status, and cranial neuropathy, aseptic meningitis must be a diagnosis of exclusion.

5.4.7 Viral encephalitis

Among the opportunistic viral infections of the CNS, the most important are the herpes viruses: herpes simplex types 1 and 2 (HSV-1 and -2), herpes varicella-zoster (VZV), and CMV. Each can cause a meningoencephalitis with mental status changes and focal neurologic findings. Diagnosis is complicated by the low yield of CSF viral cultures in herpesvirus encephalitis in general. In general, the onset of headache, fever, and seizures should, in the absence of other clear etiologies, prompt empiric treatment for herpes simplex encephalitis with acyclovir (10.0 to 12.5 mg/kg intravenously every 8 hours).

5.4.8 Fungal encephalitis

Candida Albicans, which commonly infects the oral mucosa of patients with HIV disease, can cause a meningoencephalitis, usually in the setting of fungemia. Microabscesses are the usual pathologic findings in the brain. Mucormycosis, especially among injection drug users, and aspergillosis have been reported causes of meningoencephalitis in patients with advanced HIV disease.

5.4.9 Systemic neoplasms

Although Kaposi sarcoma (KS) is the most common systemic neoplasm in HIV disease, it rarely spreads to the CNS. Among the systemic cancers, non-Hodgkin lymphoma is the most important cause of neurologic dysfunction in HIV disease and invades the CNS by spreading along the leptomeninges. Common signs and symptoms include cranial nerve palsies and polyradiculopathy and less commonly, myelopathy due to epidural metastasis with spinal cord compression.

5.4.10 Central nervous system lymphoma

Primary CNS lymphoma (PCNSL) is a fairly common cause of cerebral mass lesions in patients with advanced HIV disease. The most common signs and symptoms are confusion, lethargy, and personality changes, usually with focal deficits, such as hemiparesis, hemisensory loss, ataxia, and aphasia. Seizures are less common, but not rare.

5.4.11 Metabolic encephalopathy

Metabolic encephalopathy occurs frequently in patients with advanced HIV disease. Adverse reactions to therapeutic drugs, hypoxia, electrolyte imbalance, and multiorgan failure are common etiologies. Efavirenz can cause a transient encephalopathy for a few weeks after initiation of therapy. In the cachectic patient or in patients with significant liver disease or history of protracted vomiting, Wernicke encephalopathy due to thiamine deficiency should be considered.

5.4.12 Stroke

Cerebral infarction and transient ischaemic attacks are seen infrequently in HIV infected patients, with a reported incidence ranging from 0.5% to 8.0%. Based on a case control study, this incidence is less than that among age-matched young adults with other terminal illnesses. Among patients with advanced HIV disease, cerebral ischemic disease is more common than hemorrhagic stroke.

6. Psychiatric manifestations of HIV infection

Recognizing the psychiatric manifestations of HIV disease can be complicated by the complex biologic, psychologic and social circumstances associated with this illness, and psychiatric symptoms often go unrecognized and untreated(Evans et al., 1999). The significance of these findings is magnified by emerging evidence that certain symptoms, such as depression, may be associated with an increase in mortality rate among HIV-seropositive women and with disease progression in HIV-seropositive men.

The psychiatric sequelae of HIV infection and AIDS are numerous and have etiologies that involve neurobiological and psychosocial factors. These include the natural and expected grief response to being diagnosed with a terminal illness, later reactions to disability and illness, exacerbation of preexisting psychiatric illness, development of new primary psychiatric symptoms and syndromes, and the neuropsychiatric manifestations of HIV associated neurological illness.

It is understandable that individuals who receive notification of positive HIV test results will be emotionally distressed as they adjust to the knowledge of their HIV serostatus. The severity of the acute distress will vary from individual to individual. Whereas some individuals may react with little distress, others may be at increased risk of suicide. Thus, it appears that although individuals are often distraught after receiving positive HIV test results, after an adjustment period lasting weeks to a few months, most will cope well and will show a reduction in anxiety and depressive symptoms. Consequently, it appears that symptoms of depression and anxiety should not be considered "normal" in asymptomatic HIV infection. Rather, significant symptoms should warrant careful clinical evaluation.

6.1 Depressive disorder in patients with HIV/AIDS

Depressive symptoms are the commonest psychiatric complication of chronic medical illnesses (Practice guidelines for HIV treatment, 2000). Studies have shown that the prevalence of depression in people living with HIV/AIDS is 2 to 3 times higher than that in the general population (Bing et al, 2001). Depressive disorder is the most common psychiatric condition in people living with HIV/AIDS with estimated life time prevalence in the range of between 21% and 61% (Elliot et al, 1998). A recent meta-analysis of data from ten studies examining the prevalence of depression among HIV-infected individuals reveal a two-fold increase in rates of depression compared with HIV-negative individuals (Ciesla et al, 2001).The current estimates may represent an underestimation as there is evidence that depression may be under diagnosed in the context of HIV medical care (Steven et al, 2003). Previous research has also shown that depression in patients with HIV/AIDS may be associated with disease progression (Cook et al, 2004), reduced compliance with antiretroviral treatment (Rabkin et al, 2002), and as a result of additional illness burden, lead to a reduction in the quality of life (Sherbourne et al, 2000). Depressed individuals with HIV use significantly more health care and related services (Williams et al, 2005). Despite all of these important evidences, depression remains underrecognized, underdiagnosed and undertreated in medical clinics. Thus, recognizing and treating depression is important

because of its association with poor self-care and worse health outcomes in those with HIV (Paterson et al, 2000).
The relationship between depression and HIV/AIDS may be complex. Firstly, populations at risk for HIV infection have elevated rates of major depression. High rates of major depression have been found in homosexual men (Sittirai et al, 1993) and patients with substance use disorders (Mc Kinon et al, 1996). Secondly, major depression is a risk factor for HIV infection by virtue of its impact on behavior, intensification of substance abuse, exacerbation of self-destructive behaviors, and promotion of poor partner choice in relationships. In this way, depression can be seen as a vector of HIV transmission. Patients with depression have also been shown to be at increased risk for disease progression and mortality. Thirdly, HIV increases the risk of developing major depression through a variety of mechanisms, including direct injury to subcortical areas of the brain, chronic stress, stigma, worsening social isolation, bereavement, debilitation and intense demoralization (Zisook et al, 1998). Although direct evidence for a relationship between worsening HIV disease and the development of depression is limited, there are several studies that support this link, particularly the study based on the Multicenter AIDS Cohort Study showing that there is a two and half fold increase in rates of depression as patients CD4 cell count falls below 200cells per mm[3.]
Symptoms of depression include persistent sadness, loss of interest, decreased energy and appetite, low concentration, sleep problems, guilt/worthlessness feelings, psychomotor retardation or agitation, and suicidal ideations. In addition to significant distress, symptoms of depression can also cause other health-related functional and quality of life impairments.

6.2 Mania

Higher rates of mania have also been noted with progression of HIV infection. In early HIV infection, 1%-2% of patients experience manic episodes (Lyketsos &Treisman, 2001), which is only slightly higher than the rate in the general population. However, after the onset of AIDS, 4%-8% of patients appear to experience mania (Lyketsos et al., 1993). This increased frequency of mania around the time of onset of AIDS has been closely associated with cognitive changes or dementia and is thought to be a secondary manic syndrome due to HIV infection of the CNS. In a 17-month chart review, among the 8% of patients with manic episodes, counts of helper/inducer lymphocyte (CD3+/CD4+) cells were significantly higher in those with a history of mood disorder, suggesting that mania may be a direct effect of HIV on the CNS (Lyketsos et al., 1993).In a case-control study of 19 patients with HIV-associated mania and 57 HIV-seropositive controls, AIDS dementia was significantly more common in patients with mania, which suggests a strong association between HIV neuropathology and manic symptoms(Mijch et al., 1999). Sometimes referred to as "AIDS mania," this condition is phenomenologically different from the typical manic syndrome of bipolar disorder in both its symptom profile and severity, and it is often characterized by irritability rather than euphoria.

6.3 Anxiety

Anxiety is common in patients with HIV seropositivity. Individuals with pre-existing disorder may be at increased risk for exacerbation of symptoms, due to the numerous stresses of HIV positivity. Concern over possible progression of HIV disease, the impact of illness on social status, friends, family and work, as well as existential concerns all may result in significant anxiety.

6.4 Psychosis

Psychosis is a recognized, but relative to the mood disorders, an uncommon psychiatric manifestation of AIDS. Even less commonly, antiretroviral therapy may precipitate psychosis. For example, there have been anecdotal reports of psychosis associated with ganciclovir and efavirenz. Paranoid delusions, and auditory hallucination have been reported most frequently and manic symptoms and catatonia have also been described. Psychosis has been found more frequently in patients with AIDS-related neurocognitive impairments and can be a manifestation of psychiatric conditions such as delirium, affective disorders, or schizophrenia, but it also may occur in the absence of these conditions. Estimates of the prevalence of new-onset psychosis in patients with HIV range from 0.5 to 15% (which is considerably higher than would be expected in the general population).

6.5 Delirium

Delirium is a frequent consequence of the severe medical illnesses or treatment that occurs over the course of AIDS. Behavioural manifestations include agitation, psychosis, aggressive behaviour, mutism and marked withdrawal. The delirium in AIDS is usually indistinguishable from the delirium resulting from any other serious acute medical illness.

6.6 Substance abuse

Abuse of variety of substances, including alcohol, and other illicit drugs may be common in groups at high risk of HIV infection. Continued abuse of substances may have many adverse consequences, including interference with patients adherence to needed medical treatment, increased risk of behaviour that could result in further transmission of HIV (such as unsafe sex while intoxicated, sharing needles etc.), as well as morbidity related directly to the use of the substance. It is therefore necessary to do a careful assessment for an existing substance use disorder in HIV positive patients.

6.7 Suicide

Several epidemiological studies suggest that AIDS patients are at increased risk of death by suicide. The relative prevalence is estimated to range from 7 to 36 times the rate in demographically similar control populations. Other studies, however, have not found patients with AIDS to have higher suicidal ideation, especially when comparing persons with AIDS to other medically or neuropsychiatrically ill patients.

HIV infection may exacerbate psychiatric conditions, including major depression, bipolar disorder, and schizophrenia. One study of patients who had schizophrenia before they were diagnosed with HIV infection found that the patients had more severe depressive episodes and reduced tolerance to psychopharmacologic medications (including benzodiazepines and neuroleptics) after infection than before. Although methodological issues make such studies difficult, more research is needed to understand better the role of HIV infection in worsening pre-existing psychiatric disorders.

Various complications of HIV infection including opportunistic infections of the CNS, tumors, systemic disease, and adverse effects of medications may mimic psychiatric illnesses, producing symptoms that resemble mania, depression, psychosis, or drug intoxication. In all cases, any underlying medical problem should be addressed. The acute onset of psychiatric symptoms in a patient with no such prior history should prompt a complete neuropsychiatric evaluation, toxicology and laboratory screens, and when appropriate, neuroimaging studies and lumbar puncture to help identify possible causes.

7. Assessment and treatment of psychiatric disorders in people living with HIV/AIDS

A comprehensive history from the patient and/or caregiver is needed. There should be special focus on the history of the current complaint, past psychiatric history, past and present substance abuse history, full medical history and sexual risk history and the patient's adherence to previous treatment regimens. Of equal importance is identification of social support systems.

A mental status examination (MSE) of the patient's level of cognitive (knowledge-related) ability, appearance, emotional mood, and thought patterns at the time of evaluation should be conducted. In the psychotic patient one needs to focus specifically on the behaviour and appearance of the patient. His or her speech and speed of thoughts should be assessed, and mood symptoms, affect, suicidality and neuro-vegetative symptoms evaluated. Perceptual disturbances, thought form, thought content and finally insight and judgment also need to be assessed.

A comprehensive and meticulous physical and neurological examination should be performed to exclude any organic causes for the presenting psychiatric symptoms. One should first examine for signs of delirium and rule out HIV-associated cognitive disorders. Medical diagnoses should first be considered and only after that should a psychiatric diagnosis be entertained.

Differential diagnosis needs to consider the presence of a pre-existing psychiatric illness, use of illicit substances and the presence of cognitive impairment.

Assessment and treatment of psychotic disorders in people living with HIV/AIDS (PLWHA) can be very challenging. A useful delineation may be to divide psychosis in the PLWHA into: (i) psychiatric disorders predating HIV infection; (ii) new-onset psychotic disorders; and (iii) disorders associated with medical conditions (delirium) or substance intoxication or withdrawal, and those that are likely to be complications of treatment (i.e. antiretrovirals or antituberculosis drugs). A good history, mental state and physical examination is usually important in making this delineation. Laboratory investigations are crucial in the assessment of delirium and substance intoxication.

The choice of antipsychotic drugs depends largely on the patient, presenting symptoms, past response, potential side-effect profile, possible drug interactions, cost, and pill burden of the chronically ill patient. Many patients with new-onset psychosis or psychosis associated with various medical conditions may only require short-term treatment with antipsychotic medication. However, some patients may require long-term maintenance treatment with antipsychotic agents, and here special attention must be paid to the following factors. The typical antipsychotics are commonly used in resource-constrained settings. Here low doses of haloperidol or chlorpromazine can be used. Vigilance is required with regard to extrapyramidal side effects. Newer atypical antipsychotics such as Risperidone or Olanzepine are now widely used in the treatment of psychotic disorders in HIV/AIDS. They have lower propensity to cause extrapyramidal side effects.

The impact of depression on the course of HIV has initiated the application of specific psychosocial and pharmacologic treatments targeting individuals with HIV and comorbid depression. Pharmacotherapy is the mainstay of treatment of moderate to severe depression. Several studies have demonstrated efficacy of various antidepressant agents in HIV patients, but no single antidepressant has been found superior in treating HIV-infected patients as a group (Olatunji et al, 2006).

Aside from how well the pharmacology of the antidepressant matches a patient's disease, the engine that drives effectiveness is patient adherence. The general rule is to start at low doses of any medication and titrate up to a therapeutic dose slowly, so as to minimize early side effects that may act as obstacles to adherence. Patients who show partial response to antidepressant after adequate dosage and duration should be offered an augmentation strategy. The choice of an antidepressant is largely based on their side effect profile. Some of the antidepressant drugs that are useful in treatment of depression in patients with HIV/AIDS include Amitriptyline, Imipramine, Clomipramine, Fluoxetine, Paroxetine, Sertraline, Fluvoxamine and Venlafaxine (Elliot et al, 1998). The use of psychostimulants such as Methylphenidate and Dextroamphetamine has also been found effective (Wagner et al, 2000).

Some clinicians often wonder about the interaction of antidepressants and HAART. Some interactions may occur but two points deserve emphasis. Firstly, because depression is associated with reduction in adherence to HAART, untreated depression may be equally or more detrimental to disease progression than any medication interaction. Secondly, experience in working with comorbid HIV and depression has not shown clinical significance to antidepressant-HAART interaction.

Psychosocial intervention is an integral part of treatment for depression in patients with HIV/AIDS. A combination of psychosocial intervention and medication was shown to be more effective for patients than either modality alone. Among the individual psychotherapies, interpersonal psychotherapy, cognitive-behavioral psychotherapy and supportive psychotherapy are effective in treatment of depression in patients with HIV/AIDS (Markowitz et al, 1995). A social intervention such as social support group therapy is also effective (Kelly et al, 1993).

Identifying and treating depression in patients with HIV/AIDS could result in substantial improvement in quality of life and potentially increase medication adherence, which would in turn affect illness severity and progression.

Treatment of anxiety disorders in HIV/AIDS also requires a combination of psychosocial intervention and medication. Adequate counseling and relaxation techniques are sufficient to treat mild anxiety associated with the various crisis points in the course of HIV/AIDS. For the more severe anxiety disorders, antidepressants and cognitive behavioural techniques are useful.

Every patient with HIV/AIDS presenting with psychiatric disorder must also be assessed for suicidal risk and cases where risk is high, patients should be hospitalized for detailed evaluation and appropriate treatment.

Substance abuse is a common problem in patients with HIV/AIDS. Physicians should have a high index of suspicion while assessing patients. When present, motivational interviews are important. Patients with severe problems who are motivated should be hospitalized for detoxification and appropriate pharmacological and psychosocial treatment.

8. Neurologic and psychiatric complications of antiretroviral drugs

Much progress has been made in treating HIV infection in the last several years and people infected with HIV are now living longer, healthier lives. What was once considered a progressive, ultimately fatal disease has become, in developed countries, a chronic condition that often can be managed long term.

In large part, this change has resulted from the introduction of protease inhibitors (PI), nucleoside reverse transcriptase inhibitors (NRTI), and non-nucleoside reverse transcriptase inhibitors (NNRTI) in highly active antiretroviral treatment (HAART) regimen. Now, carefully selected combinations of these agents can bring viral loads below detectable levels, increase CD4 T-lymphocyte counts, and improve immune function.

Investigators have realized that HIV cannot be completely eradicated with the treatments that are currently available and that long-term HAART may have side-effects that are severe or health- complicating enough to require modification or temporary cessation of treatment. Even when the virus is virtually undetectable in the blood, it appears to remain sequestered in host reservoirs that are inaccessible to HAART and may provide a source for viral rebound if therapy is withdrawn. With the treatments currently available, HAART will probably need to continue for the patient's lifetime, and clinicians need a thorough understanding of the health implications associated with long-term HAART, the potential complications of HIV infection even in the absence of overt illness, and the strategies for maintaining treatment adherence and minimizing treatment side-effects.

Unfortunately, complications of HAART and complications of HIV infection, particularly in patients with advanced disease and AIDS, overlap significantly. Among health risks that may be associated with HIV or HAART are neurologic complications (such as myelopathy, neuropathy and neuropathic pain, changes in cognition, and dementia), and psychiatric complications (such as mania, depression, schizophrenia, and substance abuse and dependence). CNS complications in patients with HIV, including psychiatric syndromes, delirium, seizures, and cognitive impairment, may in some cases reflect consequences of treatment with antiretroviral drugs that penetrate the CNS. For example, zidovudine and efavirenz, both considered attractive choices for patients with CNS complications because they have good CNS penetration, are themselves associated with potentially significant neuropsychiatric complications. Peripheral neurologic complications including neuropathic pain, neuropathic weakness, and denervation syndromes have been attributed to various toxic and metabolic factors in association with antiretroviral treatment. In managing neurologic complications, it is important to distinguish, when possible, between symptoms related to the HIV disease process and side-effects of HAART. To make such distinctions, clinicians need to understand which antiretroviral agents may cause neurologic and psychiatric symptoms.

Zidovudine, a nucleoside analogue that inhibits replication of HIV by interfering with viral reverse transcriptase, was the first agent to significantly reduce mortality and opportunistic infections in HIV-infected patients. Zidovudine has been found effective at high doses in slowing the progression of AIDS dementia, and can penetrate the blood-brain barrier. Zidovudine is therefore an attractive choice in HAART regimens targeting dementia and other CNS complications of HIV. However, its CNS penetration may also explain the confusion, agitation, and insomnia in up to 5% of people who took zidovudine for one year. In addition, there are anecdotal reports of psychiatric symptoms, including mania and depression, in patients treated with zidovudine. Several case reports document manic episodes in association with zidovudine treatment, even in patients with no previous psychiatric history. In some patients, mania was severe enough to necessitate hospitalization. In recent years, fewer problems have been reported, in part because zidovudine is now used in lower doses‹approximately of 600 mg/day (or 300 mg twice a day) versus the up to 2000 mg/day doses used in the pre-HAART era.

The mechanisms involved in zidovudine-associated psychiatric effects are unknown. For some patients, dose reduction is beneficial, but for others, discontinuation may be necessary. Discontinuing zidovudine treatment has been shown to rapidly reduce manic symptoms (and symptoms returned upon reintroduction of the drug, suggesting a causal relationship). However, patients have been able to resume zidovudine treatment if they also received treatment for mania.

Other adverse neurologic effects of zidovudine treatment are insomnia, myalgia, and severe headaches. Zidovudine also has been associated with seizures, particularly in cases of overdose, which have on rare occasions been fatal. Because HIV infection is associated with similar neurological problems, it is important to exclude other causes before attributing them to zidovudine treatment. However, the severity of these side-effects suggests the need to closely monitor patients taking this drug.

Neurologic symptoms associated with other NRTI may include headache, malaise, and fatigue; for most patients, these symptoms are not severe enough to discontinue HAART. A more serious side-effect is peripheral neuropathy and may be seen with didanosine, zalcitabine, or stavudine treatment but not with zidovudine treatment. The mechanism is unknown, but in vitro studies have shown that zalcitabine, stavudine, and didanosine but not zidovudine - inhibit nerve growth factor (NGF)-stimulated differentiation of a neuronal cell line.

For patients with peripheral neuropathy, symptomatic treatment with ibuprofen or topical analgesic creams can sometimes be effective. Tricyclic antidepressants have been used to manage pain in patients with HIV-associated peripheral neuropathy. In clinical practice, we have found that Tricyclic antidepressants can be partially effective, but for many patients, the pain of neuropathy can be severe, irreversible, and debilitating. Therefore, patients with HIV who develop neuropathy require careful evaluation to determine the risks and benefits of continuing NRTI treatment. In some cases, decreasing dosage may help, but in others, the contributing drug must be discontinued.

Three NNRTIs - efavirenz, delavirdine, and nevirapine - are currently available for the treatment of HIV infection. They are usually prescribed in combination with NRTI. Clinical trials of delavirdine and nevirapine revealed few adverse events affecting the CNS; therefore, the relatively more substantial CNS side-effects seen in clinical trials of efavirenz were unexpected.

CNS side-effects observed with efavirenz include dizziness, headache, confusion, stupor, impaired concentration, agitation, amnesia, depersonalization, hallucinations, insomnia, and abnormal or vivid dreams. For most patients, these side-effects resolve within 6-10 weeks of starting treatment, but for some patients, symptoms seem to wax and wane over a long term. For most patients, these disturbances diminished or resolved within 2 months. Neither dose reduction nor dose splitting shortened or reduced the intensity of symptoms.

Psychiatric effects also have been noted with efavirenz, though they occur less frequently than neurologic effects.When efavirenz-associated psychiatric effects occur, they may be serious and may include anxiety, depression, and suicidal ideation.

Clinicians should advise patients of possible CNS effects of efavirenz, and should watch for changes in behavior, cognition, or mood. If side-effects persist or patients find them intolerable, a switch in HAART regimen may be appropriate. Although efavirenz is often a first-line treatment, many patients receive it after experiencing treatment failure on earlier HAART regimens. Therefore, patients who switch to efavirenz and then experience neurologic or psychiatric side-effects may have limited options for future antiretroviral treatment. It is important to carefully consider risks and treatment alternatives for these patients.

The combination of HIV Protease Inhibitor with the older antiretroviral agents brought about substantial decreases in viral loads and opportunistic infections with concomitant increases in CD4 T-cell counts. As a result, HIV-associated morbidity and mortality has declined dramatically in recent years.

Although PI may have neurologic side-effects, they tend to be variable and less prominent than those seen with NRTI or NNRTI. Neurologic symptoms may occur more often with ritonavir or ritonavir/saquinavir combination treatments than with indinavir treatment.

9. Consequences of neuropsychiatric problems in patients with HIV/AIDS

Some previous studies have indicated that Neuropsychiatric disorders in people living with HIV/AIDS are associated with disease progression, poor adherence to antiretroviral drugs, increased incidence of high risk sexual behavior with the potential for further HIV transmission, and deterioration in their quality of life. Thus, the place of psychiatrists in the treatment and care of patients with HIV/AIDS is crucial.

There is a consistently strong evidence from high income countries that adherence to Highly Active Antiretroviral Therapy is lowered by depression, cognitive impairment, alcohol use and substance use disorders. A study in Ethiopia showed that depression was associated with less than 95% self reported adherence (Ambebir et al., 2008). Previous research has also shown that depression in patients with HIV/AIDS may be associated with reduced adherence with antiretroviral treatment (Byakika-Tusuiime et al., 2009; Dimatteo et al., 2000; Mugavero et al., 2000; Phyllips et al., 2002; Rabkin & Goetz 2002)and disease progression(Cook 2004; Paterson 2000).They concluded that identifying and treating depression in these patients may improve medication adherence.

In a study of women who were medically eligible to receive Highly Active Antiretroviral Therapy (HAART), its non receipt was associated with substance use. Furthermore, other epidemiological studies indicate that the presence of drug use disorder can complicate the management of HIV illness and compromise adherence to HIV medication and secondary preventive efforts (HIV clinical resource 2009).

HIV-infected subjects in several studies reported "forgetting" as one of the most common reasons for poor adherence to antiretroviral drugs. It is also possible that HIV-associated neurocognitive disturbances, which are common and more prominent as the disease advances, might be responsible for some of the cases of poor medication adherence. Other studies have reported a significantly greater risk of poor adherence to HAART in HIV-infected persons with neurocognitive impairment (Hinkin et al. 2002).

Depression has been associated with immune suppression and other health outcomes in studies of individual with and without chronic disease (; Herbert & Cohen 1993; Rover et al., 1991). Studies have documented association between depression and HIV progression (Lesserman et al., 1997; Lesserman et al, 1999), HIV-related symptoms (Leketsos et al., 1993) and mortality (Lesserman et al., 1997). Some studies found that HIV-sero-positive gay men who reported depressive symptoms demonstrated immunological changes associated with HIV activity and progression, for example CD4, CD8 cell count proliferate.

Some studies have compared pattern of neuropsychiatric disorder especially the neurocognitive impairment at various level of CD4 cell counts namely 200, 250, 300, 350 and 400 cells /ml and found that there is generally worsening trend of neurocognitive impairment as the CD4 cell count decreases and therefore recommended the serial determination of CD4 cell count in HIV infected patient and screening for neuropsychiatric syndromes in those with CD4 count values of less than 350 cell/ml(Bornstein et al., 1992; Heaton et al., 1995; Miller et al., 1990).

Research has shown that neuropsychiatric disorders in patients with HIV/AIDS complicates help seeking, diagnosis, quality of care provided, treatment and its outcome and adherence(World Health Organization report, 2008). Regardless of aetiology, the co morbidity of mental illness and HIV poses special challenge for HIV care. Individual with these co morbidity face even greater barriers to care than those with HIV alone. Once in care, their treatment is more complex (Francine et al., 2009). Mental and substance use disorders in HIV/AIDS affects help seeking behaviour or uptake of diagnostic and treatment services for HIV and AIDS.

People with alcohol use disorders are more likely than the general population to contract HIV. Similarly, rates of alcohol problems are high among HIV/AIDS patients (Petry, 1999). Lifetime prevalence rates of alcohol use disorders ranging from 29% to 60% have been found among HIV positive populations (Bryant, 1998). This is 2 to 4 times higher than in the general population. Alcohol use is associated with high-risk sexual behaviors and intravenous drug use which are two major modes of HIV transmission.

In persons already infected, the combination of heavy drinking and HIV has been associated with increased medical and psychiatric complications, delays in seeking treatment (Samet et al., 1998), difficulties with HIV medication adherence (Cook et al., 2001; Wagner et al., 2001), and poorer HIV treatment outcomes (Lucas et al., 2002). Decreasing alcohol use in people who have HIV or who are at risk for becoming infected reduces the spread of HIV and the diseases associated with it.

People who abuse alcohol are more likely to engage in behaviors that place them at risk for contracting or transmitting HIV. A history alcohol use has been correlated with a lifetime tendency toward high-risk sexual behaviors, including multiple sex partners, unprotected intercourse, sex with high-risk partners (e.g., injection drug users, prostitutes), and the exchange of sex for money or drugs (Avins et al., 1994; Boscarino et al., 1995; Malow et al., 2001; Windle, 1997).There may be many reasons for this association. For example, alcohol can act directly on the brain to reduce inhibitions and diminish risk perception (Cooper, 2002; Fromme et al., 1999; MacDonald et al., 2000).

Decreasing alcohol use among HIV patients not only reduces the medical and psychiatric consequences associated with alcohol consumption but also decreases other drug use and risky sexual behavior and hence reduces HIV transmission (Lucas et al., 2002). Thus, alcohol and other drug abuse treatment can be considered primary HIV prevention as well (Metzger et al., 1998).

With improved treatments and longer survival times for persons with HIV infection, the maintenance and improvement of their functioning and well-being (collectively referred to as "health-related quality of life") have become major goals of treatment. The World Health

Organization (WHO) defined quality of life (QOL) as an individual's perception of their position in life in the context of the culture and value systems in which they live and in relation to their goals, expectations, standards and concerns. It is a broad-ranging concept affected in a complex way by the person's physical health, psychological state, level of independence, social relationships and their relationship to salient features of their environment (WHOQOL Group, 1995).

We know from studies of patients and general populations that mood disorders, particularly depression, have a substantial negative impact on a person's health-related quality of life (Jia et al, 2004). In fact, for most domains of functioning and well-being, depression is more debilitating than most medical conditions (Sherbourne et al, 2000). In a study conducted by Sherbourne et al (2000) to assess the impact of psychiatric conditions on health related quality of life, they recruited a national probability sample of persons with HIV, receiving medical care in the United States. Subjects were screened for psychiatric conditions and their health-related quality of life was assessed. They found that 36% of subjects screened positive for a current depressive disorder and 26% for dysthymia. Subjects with a probable diagnosis of any mood disorder had significantly worse functioning and well-being than those without a mood disorder diagnosis on all health-related quality of life measures, including the physical and mental health composites. These findings substantiate the considerable additional illness burden associated with mood disorders in HIV infected people.

This chapter is intended to help create awareness about mental health problems and its consequences in patients with HIV/AIDS, so as to facilitate routine screening of mental disorders and mental health integration in the comprehensive care
of people living with HIV/AIDS.

10. References

Ambebir A, Woldemicheal K, Getachew S, Girma B & Deribe K.(2008). Predictors of adherence to antiretroviral therapy among HIV infected persons: a prospective study in Southwest Ethiopia. *BMC Public Health*, 30(8): 265.

Apostolski S,McAlarney T,Quattrini A, Steven WL, Rosoklija G, Lugaressi A, Cobo M, Sadiq SA, Lederman S, Hays AP & Latov N. (1993). The gp120 glycoprotein of human immunodeficiency virus type 1 binds to sensory ganglion neurons. *Annals of Neurology*, 34:855-863.

Avins, A.L., Woods, W.J., Lindan, C.P., Hudes, E.S., Clark, W., & Hulley, S.B. (1994). HIV infection and risk behaviors among heterosexuals in alcohol treatment programs. *Journal of the American Medical Association*, 271(7), 515–518.

Berger JR & Nath A.(1997). HIV dementia and the basal ganglia. *Intervirology*, 40:122-131.

Berger JR, Levy RM, Flomenhoft D & Dobbs M. (1998). Predictive factors for prolonged survival in acquired immunodeficiency syndrome-associated progressive multifocal leukoencephalopathy. *Annals of Neurology*. 44(3):341-9.

Berger JR,Nath A, Greenberg RN, Anderson AH, Greene RA, Bognar A & Avison MJ. (2000). Cerebrovascular changes in the basal ganglia with HIV dementia. *Neurology*, 54:921-926.

Bing EG, Burnam MA, Longshore D, Fleishman JA, Sherbourne CD, London SA, Turner BJ, Eggan F, Beckman R, Vitiello B, Morton SC, Orlando M, Bozzette SA, Ortiz-Borron L & Shapiro M. (2001). The estimated prevalence of psychiatric disorders, drug use and dependence among people with HIV disease in the United States. *Archives of General Psychiatry*, 58 : 721-28.

Bloom FE & Rausch DM.(1997). HIV in the brain: pathology and neurobehavioral consequences. *Journal of Neurovirology*, 3:102-109.

Bornstein RA, Nasrallah HA & Para MF. (1992). Neuropsychological performance in asymptomatic HIV infection. *Journal of Neuropsychiatry and clinical Neuroscience*, 4:386-394.

Boscarino, J.A., Avins, A.L., Woods, W.J., Lindan, C.P., Hudes, E.S. & Clark, W. (1995). Alcohol-related risk factors associated with HIV infection among patients entering alcoholism treatment: Implications for prevention. *Journal of Studies on Alcohol*, 56(6), 642–653.

Bryant, K. (1998).Alcohol and AIDS: A Guide to Research Issues and Opportunities: *National Institute on Alcohol Abuse and Alcoholism.*

Byakika-Tusuiime J, Crane J, Oyugi JH, Ragland K, Kayume A, & Musoke P.(March, 2009). Longitudinal antiretroviral adherence in HIV +ve Ugandan parents and their children initiating HAART in the MTCT-Plus family treatment model: role of depression in declining adherence over time. *AIDS Behaviour.* (Epub ahead of print) Pubmed PMID: 19301113

Centers for Disease Control (1982): Undifferentiated non-Hodgkins Lymphoma among homosexual males in United States. *MMWR* 31: 227 - 30.

Childs EA,Lyles RH,Selnes OA, Chen B, Miller EN, Cohen BA, Becker JT, Mettors J & Mc Arthur JC. (1999). Plasma viral load and CD4 lymphocytes predict HIV-associated dementia and sensory neuropathy.*Neurology*,52:607-613.

Ciesla MA & Robert JE.(2001). Meta-analysis of the relationship between HIV infection and risk for depressive disorders. *American Journal of Psychiatry*, 158, 5 : 725-30.

Cook, R.L., Sereika, S.M., Hunt, S.C., Woodward, W.C., Erlen, J.A. & Conigliaro, J. (2001). Problem drinking and medication adherence among patients with HIV infection. *Journal of General Internal Medicine*, 16(2), 83–88.

Cook J. (2004). Depressive symptoms increase AIDS-related death. *American Journal of Public Health*, 150 {10}: 85-94.

Cooper, M.L. (2002). Alcohol use and risky sexual behavior among college students and youth: Evaluating the evidence. *Journal of Studies on Alcohol*, 14,101–117.

Dalakas MC, Illa I, Pezeshkpour GH, Laukaitis JP, Cohen B & Griffin JL.(1990). Mitochondrial myopathy caused by long-term zidovudine therapy. *New England Journal of Medicine*, 322(16):1098-105.

Deeks SG, Smith M, Holodniy M & Kahn JO.(1997). HIV-1 Protease inhibitor: A review of clinicians. *JAMA*, 277: 145 - 53.

de la Monte SM, Ho DD, Schooley RT, Hirsch MS & Richardson EP. (1987). Subacute encephalomyelitis of AIDS and its relation to HTLV-III infection. *Neurology*, 37(4):562-9.

Demasi RA, Graham MN, Tolson JM, Pham SV, Capuano GA, Fisher RL, Shaefer MS, Pakes GE, Sawyerr GA & Eron JJ. (2001). Correlation between self reported adherence to highly active antiretroviral therapy and virologic outcome. *Advances in Therapy*, 18(4): 163 - 73.

Descamps D, Flandre P, Calvez V, Pentavin G, Meiffredy V, Collin G, Delangerre C, Robert-Delmas S, Bazin B, Aboulker JP, Pialoux G, Raffi F & Brun-Vezinet F. (2000). Mechanisms of virologic failure in previously untreated HIV-infected patients from a trial of Induction-Maintenance Therapy. *JAMA*, 283: 205 - 19.

Dimatteo MR, Lepper HS, & Croghan TW.(2000). Meta-analysis of the effects of anxiety and depression on patient adherence. *Archives of Internal Medicine*, 160:2101-07.

Elliot AJ & Roy-Byrne PP.(1998). Major depressive disorder and HIV-1 infection. *Seminars in Clinical Neuropsychiatry*, 3:137-50.

Evans DL, Staab JP, Petitto JM, Morrison MF, Szuba MP, Ward HE, Wingate B, Luber MP, & O'Reardon JP. (1999). Depression in the medical setting: biopsychological interactions and treatment considerations. *Journal of Clinical Psychiatry*, 60(Suppl 4):40-55.

Everall IP,Heaton RK,Marcotte TD, Ellis RJ, McCutchan JA, Atkinson JH, Grant I, Mallory M & Mastiah E. (19999). Cortical synaptic density is reduced in mild to moderate human immunodeficiency virus neurocognitive disorder.HNRC Group. HIV Neurobehavioral Research Center.*Brain Pathology*, 9:209-217.

Francine C, Karen M & Milton W. (2005). Official journal of the world psychiatry association. Pmcid: pmci414758 [online] 2005 Oct [cited 2009 Nov 16]; Available from: URL:http://www.unaids.org/en/default.asp

Fromme, K., D'Amico, E. & Katz, E.C. (1999).Intoxicated sexual risk taking: An expectancy or cognitive impairment explanation? *Journal of Studies on Alcohol*, 60(1), 54–63.

Gabuzda D & Wang J.(2000). Chemokine receptors and mechanisms of cell death in HIV neuropathogenesis. *Journal of Neurovirology*, 6(Suppl 1):S24-S32.

Galey D, Woodward J & Nath A.(2001). Regulation of cytokines and chemokines by HIV, Tat, and gp120 in astrocytes. *Eighth Conference on Retroviruses and Opportunistic Infections*. Chicago, February 2001 [abstract 70].

Glass JD, Fedor H, Wesselingh SL & McArthur JC.(1995). Immunocytochemical quantitation of human immunodeficiency virus in the brain: correlations with dementia. *Annals of Neurology*, 38(5):755-62.

Green WC. (1991). The molecular biology of HIV-1 infection. *New England Journal of Medicine*, 324: 308 - 16.

Hall CD, Snyder CR, Messenheimer JA, Wilkins JW, Robertson WT, Whaley RA & Robertson KR.(1991). Peripheral neuropathy in a cohort of human immunodeficiency virus-infected patients. Incidence and relationship to other nervous system dysfunction. *Archives of Neurology*, 48(12):1273-4.

Heaton RK, Grant I & Butters N.(1995). The HNRC 500-Neuropsychology of HIV in function at different disease stages. *Journal of international neuropsychological Society*, 1:231-251.

Herbert TB & Cohen S.(1993). Depression and immunity: a meta-analytical review. *Psychology Bulletin*, 113:472-486.

Herzberg U & Sagen J.(2001). Peripheral nerve exposure to HIV viral envelope protein gp120 induces neuropathic pain and spinal gliosis. *Journal of Neuroimmunology*,116:29-39.

Hinkin CH, Castellon SA, Durvasula RS, Hardy DJ, Lam MN, Mason KI, Thrasher D, Goetz MB & Stefaniak M.(2002). Medication adherence among HIV+ adults: effects of cognitive dysfunction and regimen complexity. *Neurology*, 59:1944–1950.

HIV clinical guidelines for the primary care practitioner. Mental health care for people with HIV infection. Published by the AIDS Institute, New York State department of health, 2000. Pg. 2.

HIV clinical resource. Depression and mania in patient with HIV/AIDS. [online] 2008 Jun [cited 2009 Nov16]; Available from: URL:http://www.hivguidelines.org/guideline.aspx?guidelineid=13

Jia H, Uphold CR, Wu S, Reid K, Findley K & Duncan PW. (2004). Health-related quality of life among men with HIV infection: effects of social support, coping and depression. *AIDS Patient Care STDS*, 18: 594 - 603.

Johnston J, Zhang K & Silva C. (2000). HIV-1 Tat induction of matrix metalloproteinases causes neuronal damage. Seventh Conference on Retroviruses and Opportunistic Infections. San Francisco, [abstract 439].

Katalan J. (1989). HIV disease and Psychiatry practice. *Psychiatric Bulletin*, 13: 316 - 22.

Koedel U,Kohleisen B,Sporer B, Lahrtz F, Ovod V, Fontana A, Erfle V & Pfister H. (1999). HIV type 1 Nef protein is a viral factor for leukocyte recruitment into the central nervous system. *Journal of Immunology*, 163:1237-1245.

Koppel BS, Wormser GP, Tuchman AJ, Maayan S, Hewlett D Jr & Daras M.(1985). Central nervous system involvement in patients with acquired immune deficiency syndrome (AIDS). Acta Neurology Scandinavica, 71(5):337-53.

Lesserman J, Petitton JM, Perkins DO, Folds TD, Golden RN & Evans DL.(1997). Severe stress, depressive symptoms and changes in lymphocytes subsets in HIV- infected men: a 2-year follow -up study. *Archives of General Psychiatry*, 54:279-285.

Lyketsos CG, Hoover DR & Guccione MS.(1993). Depressive symptoms as predictors of medical outcomes in HIV infection. *JAMA*, 270:2563-2567.

Lyketsos CG, Hanson AL, Fishman M, Rosenblatt A, McHugh PR & Treisman GJ. (1993). Manic syndrome early and late in the course of HIV. *American Journal of Psychiatry*, 150:326-7.

Lyketsos CG & Treisman GJ.(2001). Mood disorders in HIV infection. *Psychiatry Annals*, 31:45-50.

MacDonald, T.K., MacDonald, G., Zanna, M.P. & Fong, G.T. (2000).Alcohol, sexual arousal, and intentions to use condoms in young men: Applying alcohol myopia theory to risky sexual behavior. *Health Psychology*, 19(3), 290–298.

Malow, R.M., Dévieux, J.G., Jennings, T.E., Lucenko, B.A. & Kalichman, S.C. (2001). Substance-abusing adolescents at varying levels of HIV risk: Psychosocial characteristics, drug use, and sexual behavior. *Journal of Substance Abuse*, 13,103-117.

Markowitz JC, Klerman GL, Clougherty KF, Spielman LA, Jocobsberg LB, Fishman B, Frances AJ, Kocsis JH & Perry SW. (1995). Individual Psychotherapies for depressed HIV-positive patients. *American Journal of Psychiatry*, 152: 1504 - 9.

McGuire D & Greene WC.(1996). Neurological damage in HIV infection: the Molecular Biology of HIV/AIDS. *New York: John Wiley & Sons*,127-142.

Mc Kinon K, Cournos F, Sugden R, Guido JR & Herman R.(1998). The relative contributions of psychiatric symptoms and AIDS knowledge to HIV risk behaviours among people with severe mental illness. *Journal of Clinical Psychiatry*, 57(11): 506 - 13.

Metzger, D.S., Navaline, H. & Woody, G.E. (1998). Drug abuse treatment as HIV prevention. *Public Health Reports,* 113(1), 97–106.

Miller EN, Selnes OA & McArthar JC.(1990). Neuropsychological performance in HIV-1 infected homosexual men; the multicenter AIDS cohort study. *Neurology,* 40 197-203.

Mijch AM, Judd FK, Lyketsos CG, Ellen S & Cockram A.(1999). Secondary mania in patients with HIV infection: Are antiretrovirals protective? *Journal of Neuropsychiatry Clinical Neuroscience*, 11:475-80.

Mugavero M, Ostermann J, Whetten K, Leserman J, Swartz M, Stangl D & Thielman. (2006). Barriers to antiretroviral adherence: the importance of depression, abuse, and other traumatic events. *AIDS Patient Care STDS*, 20(6):418-28.

Neuenburg JK, Brodt HR, Herndier BG, Bickel M, Bacchetti P, Price RW, Grant RM & Schlote W.(2002). HIV-related neuropathology, 1985 to 1999: rising prevalence of HIV encephalopathy in the era of highly active antiretroviral therapy. *Journal of Acquired Immune Deficiency Syndrome*, 31(2):171-7.

Nottet HS. (1999). Interactions between macrophages and brain microvascular endothelial cells: role in pathogenesis of HIV-1 infection and blood - brain barrier function. *Journal of Neurovirology,5:659*-669.

Olatunji BO, Mimiaga MJ, O'cleirigh C & Safren SA.(2006). Review of treatment studies of depression in HIV. *Top HIV Medicine* , 14(3): 112 - 24.

Paterson DL, Swindells S, Mohr J, Brester M, Vergis EM, Squier C, Wagener MM & Singh N. (2000). Adherence to protease inhibitor therapy and outcomes in patients with HIV infection. *Annals of Internal Medicine*, 133: 21 - 30.

Petry, N.M. (1999). Alcohol use in HIV patients. *International Journal of STD and AIDS,* 10(9), 561–570.

Phyllips KD, Moneyham L, Murdaugh C, Boyd MR, Tavakoli A, Jackson K & Vyavaharkar M. (2005). Sleep disturbance and depression as barriers to adherence. *Clinical Nursing Research,* 14:273-293.

Practice guidelines for the treatment of patients with HIV/AIDS. American Psychiatric Association 2000. www.psych.org

Pulliam L, Gascon R, Stubblebine M, McGuire D & McGrath MS.(1997). Unique monocyte subset in patients with AIDS dementia. *Lancet*, 349(9053):692-5.

Rabkin JG & Ferrando S.(1997). A 'second life' agenda. Psychiatric research issues raised by protease inhibitor treatments for people with the human immunodeficiency virus or the acquired immunodeficiency syndrome. *Archives of General Psychiatry, 54:1049-1053.*

Rabkin JG & Goetz RR.(2002). Effects of depressive symptoms and mental health quality of life on use of highly active antiretroviral therapy among HIV sero-positive women. *AIDS Journal*, 30: 401-9.

Rover BW German PS, Brant LJ, dark R, Burton L & Folstein MF. (1991). Depression and mortality in nursing homes. *JAMA*, 265:993-996.

Samet, J.H., Freedberg, K.A., Stein, M.D., Lewis, R., Savetsky, J., Sullivan, L, Levenson SM & Hingson R. (1998). Trillion virion delay: Time from testing positive for HIV to presentation for primary care. *Archives of Internal Medicine,* 158(7), 734–740.

Shapshak P,Nagano I,Xin K, Bradley W, McCoy CB, Sun NC, Stewart RV, Yoshioka M, Petito C & Goodkin K. (1995). HIV-1 heterogeneity and cytokines. Neuropathogenesis.*Advances in Experimental Medicine & Biology,* 373:225-238.

Sherbourne CD, Hays RD, Fleishman JA, Vitiello B, Magruder KM, Bing EG, McCaffrey D, Burnam A, Longshore D, Eggon F, Bozzette SA & Shapiro MF. (2000). Impact of psychiatric conditions on health related quality of life in persons with HIV infection. *American Journal of Psychiatry,* 157 {2} 248-54.

Sittirai W, Brown T & Sakondhavat C.(1993). Level of HIV risk behavior and AIDS knowledge in Thai men having sex with men. *AIDS Care,* 5(3): 261 - 71.

Stebbing J, Gazzard B & Douck DC.(2004). Where does HIV live? New England Journal of Medicine, 350 (24) 2487 - 98.

Steven MA, Kilbourne AM, Gifford AL, Burnam MA, Turner B et al. (2003). Underdiagnosis of depression in HIV. *Journal of General Internal Medicine,* 18(6): 450-60.

Swindells S, Zheng J & Gendelman HE.(1999). HIV associated dementia: new insight into disease pathogenesis and therapeutic interventions. *AIDS Patient Care STDS* , 3: 153 - 63.

Trillo-Pazos G,McFarlane-Abdulla E,Campbell IC,Pilkington GJ & Everall IP.(2000). Recombinant nef HIV-IIIB protein is toxic to human neurons in culture.*Brain Research,* 864:315-326.

UNAIDS/WHO report on Global HIV/AIDS statistics. November 2006.

Wagner GJ & Rabkin R.(2000). Effects of Dextroamphetamine on depression and fatigue in men with HIV: a double-blind, placebo-controlled trial. *Journal of Clinical Psychiatry,* 61: 436 - 40.

Wagner, J.H., Justice, A.C., Chesney, M., Sinclair, G., Weissman, S. & Rodriguez-Barradas, M. (2001). Patient and provider-reported adherence: Toward a clinically useful approach to measuring antiretroviral adherence. *Journal of Clinical Epidemiology,* 54(1), 91–98.

Wiley AC. (1994). Pathology of neurologic diseases in AIDS. *Psychiatric Clinics of North America,* 17: 1 - 15.

Williams P, Narciso L, Browne G, Roberts J, Weir R & Gafni A. (2005). The prevalence, correlates, and cost of depression in people living with HIV/AIDS in Ontario: Implications for service directions. *AIDS Education and Prevention,* 17: 119 - 30.

World Health Organization. Clinical practice guidelines. Washington DC: U.S. Department of Health and Human Services AHCPR Pub. #94-0592. 1994;14.

World Health Organization. HIV/AIDS and mental health. [online] 2008 Nov [cited 2009 Nov]; 24th session.

WHOQOL Group.(1995). *Social Science Medicine,* 41(10): 1403 - 9.

Zheng J,Ghorpade A,Niemann D, Shapiron MF & Bozzette SA. (1999). Lymphotropic virions affect chemokine receptor-mediated neural signaling and apoptosis: implications for human immunodeficiency virus type 1-associated dementia. *Journal of Virology*, 73:8256-8267.

Zisook S, Peterkin J, Goggin KJ, Sledge P, Atkinson JH, Cotter RL, Thylin MR, Epstein L, Swartz JM, Shepard RB, Liu X, Nukuna A & Gendelman HE. (1998). Treatment of major depression in HIV positive men. *Journal of Clinical Psychiatry*, 59: 217 - 24.

18

AIDS and Trauma

Erik Vakil, Caroline Zabiegaj-Zwick and AB (Sebastian) van As
University of Cape Town
South Africa

1. Introduction

Trauma is a significant cause of mortality (10%) worldwide and is responsible for 15% of all disability-adjusted life years (DALYs) (Murray & Lopez, 1997). Seven of the top 30 contributors to the global burden of disease are due to injury, including motor vehicle accidents, falls, war injuries, self-inflicted injuries, violence, drowning and burns. All of these injuries are seen in the trauma setting and places trauma workers at risk of exposure to blood and other body fluids. The relevance of HIV and trauma is increasing as the global prevalence of HIV continues to rise. Sixty million have been infected with HIV since the beginning of the epidemic and 25 million have died of HIV-related causes (UNAIDS, 2009). Of those newly infected, 40% were young people - the group most likely to be involved in trauma.

2. Universal precaution

In general, the risk of transmission of any infectious disease may be minimised in the trauma setting by implementing universal precautions. The World Health Organization (WHO) has developed universal precaution guidelines which are summarised below (WHO, 2007).

- Hand wash after any direct contact with patients
- Safe collection and disposal of sharps
- Gloves for contact with body fluids, non intact skin and mucous membranes
- Wearing a mask, eye protection and a gown if blood or other body fluids might splash
- Covering cuts and abrasions
- Cleaning of spills of blood and other bodily fluids
- Safe system for hospital waste management and disposal

In addition, the WHO advocates Hepatitis B virus (HBV) vaccination of healthcare workers, development of post exposure protocols for those at risk of contact with infected body fluids, adequate provision of personal protective equipment (PPE) with appropriate means of disposal, and monitoring of staff training and use of PPE.

Historically, trauma workers have generally had poor compliance with universal precaution guidelines. In a Jamaican study, where health care workers were interviewed to determine the reason for not adhering to universal precautions, numerous reason were provided including: (1) increase in workload made adherence difficult, (2) a perceived reduction in dexterity when wearing gloves, (3) insufficient supply of PPE and (4) lack of penalties for not adhering to universal precautions (Vaz et al., 2010). Other studies in the United States have reached similar conclusions and also highlighted that trauma workers have a poor knowledge of infection risk (Kelen et al. 1990; Kim et al., 1999)

3. Post-exposure prophylaxis

Post-exposure prophylaxis (PEP) is the collection of measures taken after exposure to a pathogen in order to prevent or reduce the risk of transmission. In the case of HIV, such measures should include, but are not limited to, first-aid, appropriate HIV testing, counselling, anti-retroviral (ARV) chemotherapy, and follow-up. The risk of occupational exposure to healthcare workers in the trauma setting depends on the relative prevalence of HIV in the trauma population and the level of exposure. The use of PEP in patients attending the trauma service should also be considered in cases of sexual assault and other forms of acute non-occupational exposure. It is strongly recommended that all trauma services have well established PEP protocols, sufficient resources and necessary training for effective implementation.

The only direct evidence supporting the prophylactic use of ARV chemotherapy (zidovudine) for healthcare associated HIV exposure comes from a single case-control study involving patients from the United States, United Kingdom, France and Italy (Cardo et al., 1997). Healthcare workers were 81% less likely to seroconvert if they received zidovudine after a needlestick injury and the risk of seroconversion was linked to the volume of blood transmitted and the HIV blood titre level. Indirect evidence supporting the prophylactic use of ARVs include reduced rates of vertical transmission in HIV positive mothers who received zidovudine and the success of ARVs in raising $CD4^+$ counts, reducing viral titres, and decreasing morbidity and mortality in HIV positive patients (Connor et al., 1996).

3.1 Occupational exposure

The risk of HIV transmission through needlestick injury is 0.3%. The risk of transmission from contact of contaminated fluids with mucous membranes or damaged skin is approximately 0.09%. However, the risk of occupational exposure in trauma may be higher than in other hospital settings. This is because the HIV status of patients is usually unknown, the prevalence of HIV in the trauma population is generally greater than the community, the mechanism of injury is often violent and may increase the level of exposure, and the emergent nature of trauma increases the situational stress and may lead to riskier practice.

PEP is only indicated in cases where there is a risk of transmission (Table 1) and contra-indicated in cases where there is no appreciable benefit (Table 2). For occupational exposure, this includes contact between body fluids at risk of HIV contamination and non-intact skin or mucous membranes. Indirect evidence from animal studies suggest that initiation of PEP after 72 hours following exposure is not effective at reducing rates of seroconversion. PEP should therefore not be offered in such cases and strategies should exist to offer PEP as soon as possible after exposure (Martin et al., 1993). Starter packs are well-suited to the emergency department as they offer quick access to ARVs, may result in less wasted medication if PEP is not continued, requires the patient to attend follow-up to obtain additional ARVs ensuring appropriate testing and counselling, and can easily be placed in small or under-serviced departments. Theoretical risk of HIV resistance may develop if starter packs are inappropriately used or ARV courses are not routinely completed.

Exposure between body fluids suspected of, or confirmed to be, HIV positive and:
• Non-intact skin (needlestick, sharp injury, skin abrasion)
• Mucous membranes (oral cavity, nasal cavity, eyes)
• Sexual contact in cases where a condom was not used, broke or fell off during intercourse
• Oral sex with ejaculation[1]

Table 1. Indications for PEP[2]

• Patient is already HIV positive from previous exposure
• Exposure has been chronic[3]
• Exposure through intact skin
• Sexual contact with condom use that remains intact
• Exposure to non-infectious body fluids such as saliva, faeces, urine, and sweat
• Exposure to HIV negative body fluids
• Greater than 72 hours have elapsed since exposure

Table 2. Contraindications to PEP[2]

3.2 Exposure as a result of sexual assault

The risk of non-occupational exposure depends on the nature of contact with contaminated fluids. In cases of sexual assault, the method of assault, the condition of genital or oral mucosa, the circumcision status, and the level of HIV virulence all play a role. Risk is increased in cases of rape, where there is decreased lubrication and may be associate with violent penetration. Children, especially small children, are also at an increased risk for anatomical reasons. Generalised risk from a single sexual contact depends on the method of exposure. Published estimates of HIV transmission for receptive anal intercourse are 1-30%, insertive anal intercourse 0.1-10%, receptive vaginal intercourse 0.1-10%, and insertive vaginal intercourse 0.1-1% (Boily et al., 2009). Case studies have also reported transmission from oral sex with ejaculation (Lifson et al., 1990; Rozenbaum et al., 1988).

PEP should be offered to all victims of sexual assault attending the trauma service where the act occurred within 72 hours. In many cases, particularly with children, the assault may be on a background of chronic abuse, in which case PEP is not indicated. However, special care should be taken to distinguish between cases of chronic abuse and cases of acute-on-chronic abuse where a different perpetrator is responsible for the most recent assault. In such cases, PEP should be offered.

---

[1] The risk for oral transmission is considered very low but PEP may be offered in cases where the exposure is in association with significat oral disease such as ulceration or dysplasia

[2] Adapted from: WHO. Post-exposure prophylaxis to prevent HIV infection: Joint WHO/ILO guidelines on post-exposure prophylaxis (PEP) to prevent HIV infection. *HIV/AIDS Programme: Strengthening health services to fight HIV/AIDS.* 2007

[3] Chronic exposure should be distinguished from episodic exposure where PEP may still be effective. This distinction may be challenging.

3.3 Other types of exposure

Routine PEP after community-acquired needlestick injury is controversial and administration should be based on risk assessment. At risk populations include children, security workers and cleaners (Celenza et al., 2011). Children from communities with low prevalence of HIV may not warrant PEP (Makwana & Riordan, 2005). Care should also be taken to ensure exposure was within 72 hours as presentation to the emergency department may be delayed (Johnston & O'Conor, 2005).

The risk associated with needle-sharing is approximately 0.67%. PEP for needle-sharing may also be offered if presented within 72 hours and where exposure is likely to be acute rather than chronic.

3.4 PEP regimens

When indicated, the ARV regimen used depends on various factors including national policy, institutional policy, level of resources, toxicity and side-effects, daily pill burden, drug contra-indications and compliance. Although a single drug regimen using zidovudine has shown to be effective, multi-drug regimens are now more commonly used in order to cover drug-resistant HIV clones. The use of two drugs must be weighed against cost, toxicity and availability. A third drug may be considered in cases where the background prevalence of ARV resistance is greater than 15%.

Two drug regimens include fixed-dose dual nucleoside reverse transcriptase inhibitor (NRTI) therapy with combination zidovudine-lamivudine or combination tenofovir-emtricitabine. A protease inhibitor (PI), usually in combination with ritonavir, which increases PI plasma levels, are usually added if a third drug is necessary. Combination ritonavir-lopinavir, -atazanavir, -darunavir have all been used. All PEP regimens are given for 28 days post exposure.

3.5 Testing, follow-up and counselling

Testing of the source patient, in cases where HIV status is unknown, should include rapid-ELISA testing for HIV as well as testing for HBV (surface antigen - HBsAg) and Hepatitis C virus (HCV). In cases where HIV or HCV infection has occurred within the last 2-4 weeks, HIV or HCV RNA PCR may be indicated.

Testing of the exposed patient should be carried out as soon as possible to establish a baseline for follow-up testing. Tests should include a rapid-ELISA for HIV, HBV immunity status (anti-HB antibodies), HBsAg and HCV antibodies. Baseline full blood count, liver enzymes and creatinine should also be obtained to monitor for PEP side-effects and sequelae from hepatitis infection. Screening for other sexually transmitted infections may be warranted in cases of sexual assault or in patients with high risk behaviour.

At the minimum, follow-up testing at 6 months should be performed to document HIV negative status. Seroconversion after 6 months in those receiving PEP has been reported but is extremely rare (Ippolito et al., 1999). More intensive follow-up can include HIV and HCV antibody testing at 4-6 weeks, 3 months, and 6 months. Relevant additional testing should be offered in patients who become symptomatic or experience drug toxicity.

Post-exposure counselling should form an integral part of the PEP protocol. Services should be available to address HIV testing, follow-up testing, ARV treatment, legal issues and compensation claims should they arise. In the event that HIV is contracted, services should be available to address relevant needs. Counselling to address special needs of certain population sub-groups such as children and victims of sexual assault should also be made available.

4. Management and outcome of HIV positive patients in trauma

The function of a trauma unit is to stabilise and treat life threatening injuries. It has been shown that HIV alone is not responsible for mortality in trauma but rather the patient's ability to mount an immune response (Allard & Meintjies, 2005). It is also unethical to not treat life-threatening conditions based on a patient's HIV status (Smit 2010). In fact, a number of studies have suggested that HIV positive patients have the same mortality rate as non-infected patients, especially if they are in the early stages of the disease (Smit, 2010).

With regard to surgical outcomes, early views were often pessimistic. It was felt that HIV positive patients were prone to poor wound healing, high post-operative complication rates, a prolonged post-operative period and higher mortality rates. This helped trigger a number of studies investigating the morbidity and complication rates among HIV positive patients both in general and orthopaedic surgery.

Many such studies have produced conflicting results. Duane et al conducted a retrospective study comparing outcomes of HIV positive and HIV negative patients over a 5-year period in the trauma unit. They found no difference in infection rates or overall complications based on $CD4^+$ count alone (Duane et al., 2008). Conversely, Karpelowsky et al showed that in children who were HIV positive or exposed to HIV had increased rates of poor wound healing and breakdown of reconstruction sites (Karpelowsky et al., 2009). Other post-operative complications cited in the study were likely due to non-HIV related factors. For example, a large proportion of the children studied underwent emergency surgery, which is known to have higher rates of post-operative complications since the children tend to be sicker at presentation. This is true for both HIV positive and HIV negative patients. It was also found that up to 79% of children included in the study were undernourished and 36% had other co-morbid diseases including major respiratory and nutritional problems prior to undergoing surgery.

Stawicki et al found that HIV positive patients had both longer length of hospital stay as well as longer length of stay in ICU (Stawicki et al., 2005). They noted however, that HIV positive patients had more pulmonary, infectious and renal complications than the control group and suggested that the mortality of HIV positive patients was likely linked to these co-morbid processes. They also found that HIV positive patients needed greater numbers of surgical procedures but failed to state what the indication for these procedures were. Studies by Morrison et al and Horberg et al found similar findings to Stawicki et al, stating that HIV positive patients had higher post-operative complication rates, especially respiratory complications (Horberg et al., 2006; Morrison et al., 2010).

Studies comparing complication rates in orthopaedic surgeries have been small and only tentative conclusions can be drawn. It has been shown that HIV positive patients with an open fracture (depending on the contamination of the wound) have a higher rate of infection, especially deep infection. There is also a higher rate of late sepsis with procedures that need internal instrumentation, but sepsis may have been avoided with improved medical management including prophylactic antibiotic use before invasive procedures as well as early evaluation and treatment of possible infections (Luck Jr, 1994; Van Aardt, 2010).

The overwhelming conclusion in all these studies however, has been that there is not enough evidence to properly evaluate the relationship between HIV and outcomes after trauma. There is a significant deficiency in research in this particular area and often available data is extrapolated from studies determining the effect of HIV on patients undergoing surgical procedures, either emergency or elective. Unfortunately, researchers face an ethical challenge when testing for HIV in the trauma setting and it is unlikely that sufficiently powered studies with adequate controls are possible in the current medical climate.

5. Drug interference between ARVs and commonly used trauma drugs

Currently available ARVs inhibit the reverse transcriptase and protease enzymes of the human immunodeficiency virus. These drugs are associated with many side-effects and close monitoring is mandatory. It is also important in the trauma setting to recognise a patient's HIV status and the possible concurrent use of ARVs since administration of drugs with potential for interaction may to lead to adverse outcomes.

First-line treatment of HIV involves the use of 2 NRTIs and a non-nucleoside transcriptase inhibitor (NNRTI). Protease inhibitors are used as second line therapies (Town, 2003). Common side effects of NRTIs include lactic acidosis, hypersensitivity reactions, pancreatitis, peripheral neuropathy and hepatic dysfunction (as most are metabolised in the liver). NNRTIs are known inducers or inhibitors of other drugs due to their effect on the hepatic cytochrome systems, and hypersensitivity reactions are common. Protease inhibitors undergo hepatic cytochrome P450 (CYP450) metabolism and many in this class are potent hepatic inhibitors.

Table 3 outlines the drug interactions between NNRTIs or protease inhibitors and other drugs that are dependent on CYP450 metabolism. Many potential interactions of other commonly used drugs remain unknown and have not been included. It is important to take a drug history to ensure that potential side effects can be avoided or closely monitored. In cases where drugs must be administratered, dose adjustment may limit side-effects.

	Drugs	ARV interaction	Clinical Effects	Management
A	Aminophylline	Protease inhibitors	Decreased theophylline effects	Monitor and adjust theophylline levels as indicated
	Amiodarone	NNRTI Protease inhibitors	Increased amiodarone effects (hypotension, bradycardia, cardiac arrhythmias	Monitor and adjust amiodarone as indicated, with reduction of amiodarone dose as needed Should not be co-administered with PIs

	Drugs	ARV interaction	Clinical Effects	Management
B	Bactrim	Lamivudine	Increased Lamivudine levels?	Unknown at present but no dose adjustment necessary for either drug
	Beta- Blockers	Protease inhibitors	Increased effects of Beta-blockers	Use with caution
D	Diazepam	Zidovudine, Protease inhibitors, Efavirenz	Increased diazepam levels (increased sedation, respire-atory depression)	Do not co-administer Alternative agents: Lorazepam, oxazepam, temazepam
	Digoxin	Protease inhibitor	Increased digoxin levels	Monitor digoxin levels closely
	Dilitiazem	Efavirenz	Decreased dilitiazem effects	Titrate dilitiazem to clinical effect
F	Fentanyl	NNRTI Protease inhibitors	Increased effects of Fentanyl	Close monitoring necessary
	Flagyl	Protease Inhibitors	Disulfiram-like reaction	Do not co-administer
	Furosemide	NNRTI Protease inhibitors Lamivudine	Increased effects of ARVS?	Use with caution
H	Haloperidol	NNRTIs PIs	Increased haloperidol effects	Monitor and adjust dosage as indicated
I	Ipecac	All	Decreased effects of ARVs if recently ingested due to induced vomiting	Avoid concurrent use
K	Ketamine	NNRTIs	Reduced effects of ketamine	Monitor and adjust dose as necessary
L	Lidocaine	Protease Inhibitors	Increased lidocaine levels	Monitor and adjust lidocaine dose
M	Methyl-prednisone	NNRTIs Protease Inhibitors	Possibly increased methylprednisone effects	Monitor while using
	Midazolam	NNRTI Protease inhibitors	Increased midazolam effects (increased sedation, confusion, respire-atory depression)	Single dose IV midazolam may be used; chronic midazolam administration should be avoided

	Drugs	ARV interaction	Clinical Effects	Management
	Morphine	Protease inhibitors	Increased morphine levels (increased sedation and respir-atory depression)	Monitor closely when using together
N	Nitroglycerine	Protease inhibitors	Possible increase in effects of nitro-glycerine	Not known- but monitor for hypotension
P	Phenergan	NNRTIs Protease inhibitors	Unknown	Monitor closely in used concurrently for side effects
	Phenobarbitol	NNRTIs, Protease inhibitors	Decreased NNRTI and PI levels	Avoid combination if possible
	Phenytoin	NNRTIs Protease inhibitors	Decreased NNRTI and PI levels	Avoid combination if possible
	Prednisone	NNRTIs Protease Inhibitors	Possibly increased prednisone effects	Close monitoring
S	Succinylcholine	NNRTI Protease inhibitors	Possible prolongation of effects of succinylcholine	Use with caution

Table 3. Commonly used drugs in the trauma unit and possible complications (McNicholl 2011; University of Cape Town 2003; University of Liverpool 2010)

6. Conclusion

It is likely that trauma units will see an increasing number of HIV positive patients in the years to come. In an area still lacking adequate research, trauma workers need to be diligent to approach the HIV positive patient in the context of their presentation. They must also stay vigilant to protect themselves against transmission. It is hoped that as HIV prevention and treatment improve, HIV patients will no longer represent a unique cohort and their management, and most importantly, their outcomes, will be as good as those without HIV.

7. References

Allard, D. & Meintjies, G. (2005). HIV and Trauma, In: *Handbook of Trauma for Southern Africa*, A. Nicol, (Ed.), pp. 374-380, Oxford University Press, ISBN 978-019-5780-80-2, Cape Town, South Africa

Boily, M.; Baggaley R. F.; Wang L.; Masse, B.; White, R. G.; Hayes, R. J. & Alary M. (2009). Heterosexual Risk of HIV-1 Infection Per Sexual Act: Systematic Review and Meta-Analysis of Observational Studies. *The Lancet Infectious Diseases*, Vol.9, No.2, (February 2009), pp. 118-129, ISSN 1473-3099

Cardo, D. M.; Culver, D. H.; Ciesielski, C. A.; Srivastava, P. U.; Marcus, R.; Abiteboul, D.; Heptonstall, J.; Ippolito, G.; Lot, F.; McKibben, P. S. & Bell, D. M. (1997). A Case-

Control Study of HIV Seroconversion in Health Care Workers after Percutaneous Exposure. *New England Journal of Medicine*, Vol.337, No.21, (November 1997), pp. 1485-1490, ISSN 0028-4793

Celenza, A.; D'Orsogna, L. J.; Tosif, S. H.; Bateman, S. M.; O'Brien, D.; French, M. A. & Martinez O. P. (2011). Audit of Emergency Department Assessment and Management of Patients Presenting with Community-Acquired Needle Stick Injuries. *Australian Health Review*, Vol.35. No.1, (February 2011), pp. 57-62, ISSN 0156-5788

Connor, E. M.; Sperling, R. S.; Gelber, R.; Kiselev, P.; Scott, G.; O'Sullivan, M. J.; VanDyke, R.; Bey, M.; Shearer, W.; Jacobson, R. L.; Jimenez, E.; O'Neill, E.; Bazin, B.; Delfraissy, J. F.; Culnane, M.; Coombs, R.; Elkins, M.; Moye, J.; Stratton, P. & Balsley, J. (1994). Reduction of Maternal-Infant Transmission of Human Immunodeficiency Virus Type 1 with Zidovudine Treatment. *New England Journal of Medicine*, Vol.331, No.18, (November 1994), pp. 1173-1180, ISSN 0028-4793

Duane, T. M.; Sekel, S.; Wolfe, L. G.; Malhotra, A. K.; Aboutanos, M. B. & Ivatury, R. R. (2008). Does HIV Infection Influence Outcomes After Trauma. *The Journal of Trauma*, Vol.65, No.1 (July 2008), pp. 63-65, ISSN 1529-8809

Horberg, M. A.; Hurley, L. B.; Klein, D. B.; Follansbee, S. E.; Quesenberry, C.; Flamm, J. A.; Green, G. M. & Luu, T. (2006). Surgical Outcomes in Human Immunodeficiency Virus-Infected Patients in the Era of Highly Active Antiretroviral Therapy. *Archives of Surgery*, Vol.141, No.12. (December 2006), pp. 1238-1245, ISSN 0004-0010

Ippolito, G.; Puro, V.; Heptonstall, J.; Jagger, J.; De Carli, G. & Petrosillo, N. (1999). Occupational Human Immunodeficiency Virus Infection in Health Care Workers: Worldwide Cases Through September 1997. *Clinical Infectious Diseases*, Vol.28, No.2, (February 1999), pp. 365-383, ISSN 1058-4838

Johnston, J.J. & O'Conor, E. (2005). Neddlestick Injuries, Management and Education: A Role for Emergency Medicine?. *European Journal of Emergency Medicine*, Vol. 12, No.1, (February 2005), pp. 10-12, ISSN 0969-9546

Karpelowsky, J. S.; Leva, S. E.; Kelley, B.; Numanoglu, A.; Rode, H. & Millar, A. J. W. (2009). Outcomes of Human Immunodeficiency Virus-Infected and -Exposed Children Undergoing Surgery—A Prospective Study. *Journal of pediatric surgery*, Vol.44, No.4, (April 2009), pp. 681-687, ISSN 1531-5037

Kelen, G.D.; DiGiovanna, T.A.; Celentano, D.D.; Kalainov, D.; Bisson, L.; Junkins, E.; Stein, A.; Lofy, L.; Scott, C. R. J.; Sivertson, K.T. & Quinn, T. C. (1990). Adherence to Universal (Barrier) Precautions During Interventions on Critically Ill and Injured Emergency Department Patients. *Journal of Acquired Immune Deficiency Syndromes*, Vol.3, No.10, (October 1990), pp. 987-994, ISSN 0894-9255

Kim, L. E.; Evanoff, B. A.; Parks, R. L.; Jeffe, D. B.; Mutha, S.; Haase, C. & Fraser, V. J. (1999). Compliance with Universal Precautions Among Emergency Department Personnel: Implications for Prevention Programs. *American Journal of Infection Control*, Vol.27, No.5, (October 1999), pp. 453-455, ISSN 0196-6553

Lifson, A. R.; O'Malley, P. M.; Hessol, N.A.; Buchbinder, S.P.; Cannon, L. & Rutherford, G. W. (1990). HIV Seroconversion in Two Homosexual Men After Receptive Oral Intercourse with Ejaculation: Implications for Counseling Concerning Safe Sexual Practices. *American Journal of Public Health*, Vol.80, No.12, (December 1990), pp. 1509-1511, ISSN 0090-0036

Luck Jr., J.V. (1994). Orthopaedic Surgery on the HIV-Positive Patient: Complications and Outcomes. *Instructional Course Lectures*, Vol.43, pp. 543-549, ISSN 0065-6895

Makwana, N. & Riordan, F. A. (2005). Prospective Study of Community Needlestick Injuries. *Archives of Disease in* Childhood, Vol.90, No.5, (May 2005), pp. 523-524, ISSN 1468-2044

Martin, L. N.; Murphy-Corb, M.; Soike, K. F.; Davison-Fairburn, B. & Baskin, G. B. (1993). Effects of Initiation of 3'-Azido,3'-Deoxythymidine (Zidovudine) Treatment at Different Times after Infection of Rhesus Monkeys with Simian Immunodeficiency Virus. *Journal of Infectious Diseases*, Vol.168, No.4, (October 1993), pp. 825-835, ISSN 0022-1899

McNicholl, I. R. (Ed.) (2011). Database of Antiretroviral Drug Interaction, In: *HIV InSite, University of California San Francisco,* 06.05.2011, Available from http://hivinsite.ucsf.edu/insite?page=ar-00-02

Morrison, C. A.; Wyatt, M. M. & Carrick, M. M. (2010). Effects of Human Immunodeficiency Virus Status on Trauma Outcomes: A Review of the National Trauma Database. *Surgical Infections*, Vol.11, No.1, (February 2010) pp. 41-47, ISSN 1557-8674

Murray, C. J. L. & Lopez, A. D. (1997). Global Mortality, Disability, and the Contribution of Risk Factors: Global Burden of Disease Study. *The Lancet*, Vol.349, No.9063 (May 1997), pp. 1436-1442, ISSN 0140-6736

Rozenbaum, W.; Gharakhanian, S.; Duval, C. E. & Coulard, J. P. (1988). HIV Transmission By Oral Sex. *The Lancet*, Vol.331, No.8599, (June 1988), pp. 1395-1395, ISSN 0140-6736

Smit, S. (2010). Guidelines For Surgery in the HIV Patient. *CME*, Vol.28, No.8, (August 2010) pp. 356-358

Sperling, R. S.; Shapiro, D.; Coombs, R. W.; Todd, J. A.; Herman, S. A.; McSherry, G. D.; O'Sullivan, M. J.; VanDyke, R. B.; Jimenez, E.; Rouzioux, C.; Flynn, P. M.; Sullivan, J. L.; Spector, S. A.; Diaz, C.; Rooney, J.; Balsley, J.; Gelber, R. D. & Connor, E. M. (1996). Maternal Viral Load, Zidovudine Treatment, and the Risk of Transmission of Human Immunodeficiency Virus Type 1 from Mother to Infant. *New England Journal of Medicine*, Vol.335, No.22, (November 1996), pp. 1621-1629, ISSN 0028-4793

Stawicki, S. P.; Hoff, W. S.; Hoey, B. A.; Grossman, M. D.; Scoll, B. & Reed 3rd, J. F. (2005). Human Immunodeficiency Virus Infection in Trauma Patients: Where Do We Stand?" *The Journal of Trauma*, Vol.58, No.1, (January 2005), pp. 88-93, ISSN 0022-5282

University of Cape Town. (2003). *South African Medical Formulary*, South African Medical Association: Health and Medical Publishing Group, ISBN 1-875098-39-9 , Cape Town, South Africa.

UNAIDS. (2009). Global Facts and Figures, In: *Data and Analysis*, 06.05.2011, Available from http://data.unaids.org/pub/GlobalReport/2006/200605-fs_globalfactsfigures_en.pdf.

University of Liverpool. (July 2010). HIV Drug Interactions, In: *HIV Drug Interactions*, 06.05.2011, Available from http://www.hiv-druginteractions.org/PrintableCharts.aspx

Van Aardt, P. (2010). The Impact of HIV/AIDS on Orthopedic Surgery. *CME* Vol.28, (August 2010), pp. 384

Vaz, K.; McGrowder, D.; Alexander-Lindo, R.; Gordon, L.; Brown, P. & Irving, R. (2010). Knowledge, Awareness and Compliance with Universal Precautions Among Health Care Workers at the University Hospital of the West Indies, Jamaica. *The International Journal of Occupational and Environmental Medicine*, Vol.1, No.1, (October 2010), pp. 171-181, ISSN 2008-6814

WHO. (2007). Standard Precautions in Healthcare, In: *Global Alert and Response*. 06.05.2011, Available from http://www.who.int/csr/resources/publications/standardprecautions/en/index.html

19

Cutaneous Manifestations of HIV/AIDS in Sub-Sahara African

Innocent Ocheyana George[1] and Dasetima Dandison Altraide[2]
[1]*Department of Paediatrics, University of Port Harcourt Teaching Hospital,Port Harcourt,*
[2]*Department of Medicine, University of Port Harcourt Teaching Hospital, Port Harcourt, Nigeria*

1. Introduction

The burden of skin disease is high in developing countries particularly the sub-Saharan Africa. The HIV/AIDS epidemic does not make it any better. More than 90% of HIV positive patients may develop mucocutaneous problems at one stage of the disease or the other with significant morbidity and mortality.
The aim is to highlight common cutaneous manifestations of HIV/AIDS in sub-Sahara Africa. A good knowledge of these cutaneous lesions may aid in early diagnosis and appropriate treatment of HIV infection.

2. Cutaneous manifestations of HIV/AIDS

Cutaneous manifestations are common in patients with HIV infection in the sub-Saharan Africa and can be broadly classified into infection/infestation, malignancy, and cutaneous hypersensitivity. It may be the sentinel event that brings the patient to the physician. Majority of HIV-infected patients will have dermatologic problem at some time during their illness. This may provide a more accurate measure of the disease progression than other organs because the skin is much accessible (Johnson, 1999).
Skin disorders are mostly attributable to the alterations in immune function. Some of the skin diseases are unique to HIV infection, while some are really not new diseases (Aftergut and Cockerell , 1999; Olumide, 2002). The later diseases may be more widespread, have an unusual character or a more prolonged course and may be resistant to therapy. The affected individuals have a significantly increased incidence of skin complaints which rises as HIV infection progresses (Wiwanitkit, 2004). In the asymptomatic stage of HIV infection, cutaneous manifestations are non-specific. Common cutaneous disorders present with atypical features for instance, shingles (VZV) may be severe, recurrent, haemorrhagic or affect more than one dermatome; warts may be multiple and large. Seborrhoeic dermatitis, pityrosorum folliculitis, eosinophilic pustulosis and bacilliary angiomatosis are all well recognized. In the later symptomatic stages, in addition to those infections mentioned above, the following should also be remembered: mycobacterium tuberculosis and atypical mycobacteria, candida species; *Trichophyton rubrum, Malassezia furfur,* chronic herpes simplex, florid molluscum contagiosum. Neoplastic processes, especially Kaposi's sarcoma make their appearance at this time.

2.1 Mycobacteria

These organisms are important causes of systemic infection in HIV disease, but cutaneous lesions have also been recognized, both direct infection and papulonecrotic tuberculide. Cutaneous lesions of mycobacterium avium complex (MAC) include nodules (Fig 1), ulcerations, pustules abscesses, folliculitis and lymph adenitis. Cutaneous lesions of mycobacterium tuberculosis (TB) include scrofuloderma, papules, vesicles, necrotic ulcerations, subcutaneous nodules and pustules. Bacillus calmette - Guerin (BCG) vaccine may cause local and systemic infection in HIV patients especially after signs of defective immunity have appeared, it is regarded as contra-indicated except for children as yet asymptomatic in areas of high risk for tuberculosis.

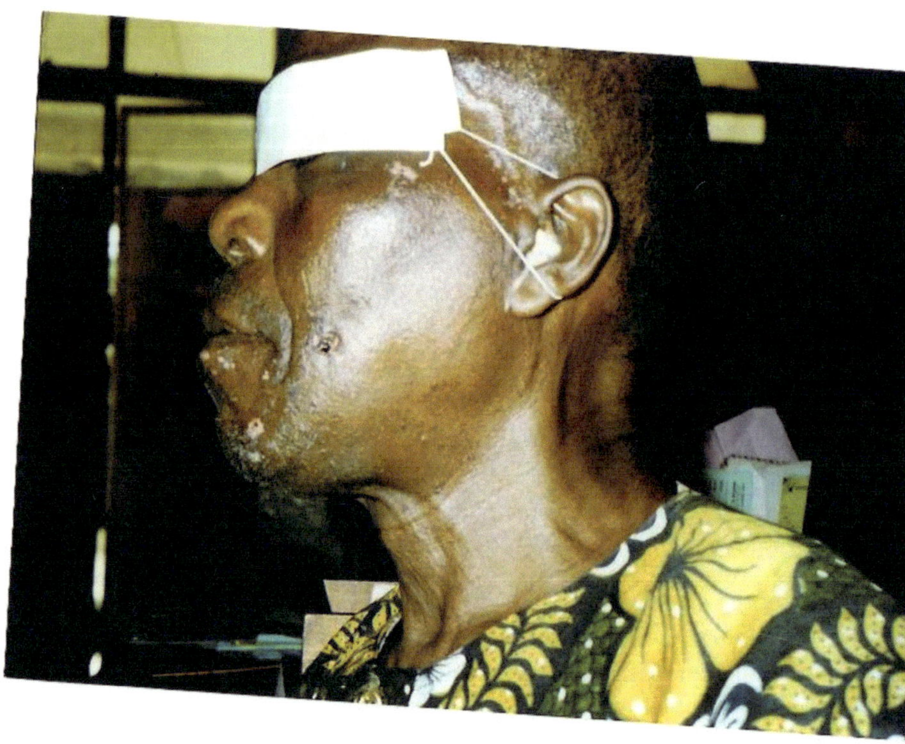

Fig. 1. Cutaneous nodule of Tuberculosis in HIV

The treatment of mycobacterium tuberculosis is the conventional DOTS using rifampicin, isonazid, ethambutol and pyrazinamide. It is recommended that for MAC treatment regimen should include at least 2 agents, with ethambutol being one of the agents.

2.2 Syphilis

Syphilis is a sexually transmitted disease due to infection with *Treponema pallidum*. Both syphilis and HIV infection are sexually transmitted diseases and so could occur concurrently (Olumide; 2002).

Unusual courses of syphilis have been reported in HIV infections. Not only may the serological response to *T. pallidum* be impaired but also syphilis may progress much more rapidly to advanced stages than in individuals without HIV. Moreover syphilis in patients with HIV infection may not respond to conventional treatment. Skin signs of syphilis in HIV infected patients are usually similar to that of HIV - negative patients but are often extensive and atypical.

A severe form of secondary syphilis or lues, 'syphilis maligna' can occur in HIV patients with papular, papulovesicular, pustular and necrotizing lesions which may form thick crusts and painful ulcers accompanying severe systemic symptoms . Tertiary gummata and neurosyphilis also appear more common.

Recommended treatment is benzathine penicilin 2.4 million units intramuscularly in a single dose given as 1.2 million units in each buttock. The treatment is repeated in a week. If there is central nervous system involvement 2.4 million units of aqueous penicillin is given intravenously every 4 hours for 10 - 14 days. This is because intramuscular benzathine penicillin does not give therapeutic levels in the CSF.

2.3 Staphylococcus aureus

Skin infections with *Staph aureus* are quite common in HIV infected patients and the frequency increases with progression of immune-deficiency. Not only is *Staph aureus* the most common bacterial pathogen in HIV infected patients but also a large percentage of patients become chronic carriers. Apart from the types of skin lesions commonly associated with *Staph aureus* in patients without HIV such as folliculitis, impetigo, ecthyma, abscesses and cellulitis, more unusual manifestations such as atypical plaque - like folliculitis, pyomyositis or botryomycosis are frequently encountered during HIV diseases.

Botryomycosis is characterized by chronic, Suppurating, granulomatous lesions which may present as inflammatory nodules, discharging ulcers, sinuses and fistulae. The lesions usually solitary can occur in the skin, liver, bones, etc, and on gross examination of the pus, pinhead - sized whitish yellow granules are evident. The granules simply contain a central mass of bacteria surrounded by a capsule and can be demonstrated on biopsy or smear of the purulent focus. The capsule is usually periodic - Acid - Schiff (PAS) positive. Botryomycosis is caused by bacteria with *Staph aureus* usually the major causal agent and *Pseudomonas aeruginosa* ranking second in frequency. The therapy of choice is surgical excision in conjunction with antibiotics.

2.4 Bacillary angiomatosis

These angioma-like lesions may affect skin, mucosal surfaces and internal organs, Cutaneous lesions typically begin as tiny pinpoint papules, resembling Campbel de Morgan sports, often in large numbers and very widespread. They enlarge rapidly both outwards and inwards, looking like pyogenic granulomas and subcutaneous nodules. They may resemble some forms of AIDS-related Kaposi's sarcoma (and indeed the two may coexist but can generally be distinguished by their faster growth, bright red color and rounder shape, with no elongation along skin crease). If injured, lesions bleed profusely. Visceral lesions may occur and deaths from laryngeal obstruction and disseminated intravascular obstruction are recorded. Bacillary angiomatosis has been seen mainly in HIV disease, but also in other immunodeficient patients and rarely in the otherwise healthy. It is caused by *Bartonella henselae* or occassional *B. quintana*, argyrophilic bacilli. Confirmation of diagnosis is by recognition of histological features or by PCR amplification of the organism's nucleic acid obtained from biopsy tissue.

Treatment - the recommended treatment for bacillary angiomatosis is erythromycin 500mg qds. If the patient has severe disease or can not tolerate orally, intravenous erythromycin can be given. Alternative to erythromycin include doxycline 100mg bid; minocycline 100mg bid or tetracycline 50mg qid, treatment should continue for 8-12 weeks and in case of systematic disease 3-4 months.

2.5 Demodicidosis

Folliculitis due to *Demodex folliculorum* may cause an itchy papular eruption in HIV patients. Affected areas include head and neck, and trunk and arms Microscopy of smears or scrapings, or histology confirms the presence of numerous mites. There is a rapid response to topical treatment with insecticides such as y-benzene hexachloride.

2.6 Viral infection

Viruses other than HIV-1 are common pathogens in HIV-1 disease and are probably important infectious co-factors for disease progression (Sterling and Kurtz, 1998). These opportunistic infections range from relatively benign disorder such as cosmetically disfiguring molluscum contagiosum to severe infections of the skin and mucus membranes such as ulcerating herpes simplex and oral hairy leukoplakia, which is attributed to Epstein Barr virus infection.

2.7 Herpes simplex

Chronic painful, non-healing ulcers found in herpes simplex virus (HDV) infections are commonly located at the junction between skin and mucous membranes, mainly in the perioral and perianal areas. Chronic ulcerating herpes simplex must first be differentiated from conventional recurrent HSV infection. Whereas the latter can occur at any stage of HIV-1 disease and is clinically and morphologically indistinguishable from the blistering eruptions commonly seen in patients without HIV-1 infection, the former heralds profound immunodeficiency. Chronic ulcerating herpes simplex is one of the AIDS-defining opportunistic infection according to Centers for Disease Control and Prevention. Systemic antiviral treatment is essential since these lesions show no tendency to resolve spontaneously. The differential diagnosis, which depends on the location of the lesions, includes pyoderma gangrenosum, bacterial and fungal infection, and cutaneous manifestation of lymphomas.

The recommended treatment for primary or recurrent HSV injection is oral acyclovir. In severe infections, intravenous acyclovir can be used. Other alternatives include famciclovir and fascarnet.

2.8 Varicella-zoster

Clinical manifestation of infection with the varicella-zoster virus (VZV), another member of the herpes virus family, depends largely on the age of the patient. Primary VZV infection in HIV-1 infected children is often severe, with dissemination and pneumoina, encephalitis, or pancreatitis. As with adult patients, epidemiological studies indicate that the frequency of reactivation of latent VZV, leading to herpes zoster, is greatly increased, with a relative risk in one study of 16.9 for HIV-1 infected person over non-infected persons. 8-13% of patients with AIDS have experienced at least one episode of herpes zoster and recurrent herpes zoster is observed more frequently in HIV-1 seropositive patients than in sero-negative individuals. However, herpes zoster is not a reliable sign of profound immunodeficiency because it can occur at any state of HIV infection. Clinical manifestations range from an uneventful vesicular eruption in a dermatomal pattern, similar to that in non-HIV-1 infected individuals, to severe haemorrhagic and necrotic lesions that may extend over several dermatomes, followed by cutaneous dissemination. In contrast to the high frequency of systemic dissemination associated with primary VZV infection, dissemination is infrequent in conventional herpes zoster. Nevertheless, chronic verrucous or ecthymatous VZV infections may persist for months.

2.9 Molluscum contagiosum

Poxvirus infection causing Molluscum contagiosum is ordinarily self-limited in immunocompetent individuals, occurring mainly in children. However, during HIV-1 disease molluscum contagiosum is seen in up to 20% of patients, and is usually associated with established immunodeficiency.

Characteristics lesions, which appear commonly on the face and in the genital regions, include skin-coloured umbilicated papules with one or more central hyperkeratotic pores. Individual lesions can grow to more than 1 cm in size and, if located on the face, may be disfiguring. If multiple nodular lesions become confluent they are difficult to treat, commonly recurring after conventional local destruction. The differential diagnosis includes basal-cell carcinoma, common warts, keratacanthoma, atypical mycobacterial infections, and, especially, cutaneous manifestations of systemic infections with *Cyptococcus neoformans*, *Histoplasma capsulatum*, or *Penicillium marneffei*. Since differentiation of molluscum contagiosum from these important fungal infections is often uncertain clinically, histopathological confirmation should always be sought.

Human Papilloma virus- Common warts may occur in unusual locations, with unusual severity, and with high frequency in HIV-1 infected patients but they are seldom serious. With respect to genital involvement in women (Fig2), both frequency of human papilloma virus (HPV) infection and the progression of HPV-associated cervical lesions correlate with the level of immune suppression. Moderate to severe cervical dysplasia and carcinoma-in-situ are part of category B symptomatic conditions in the revised classification system for HIV infection. In men, the rate of anogenital HPV infection is high in HIV-1 sero-positive and sero-negative homosexuals. However, as for women, HPV prevalence and symptoms tend to increase with disease progression.

3. Fungal infections

3.1 Dematophyte Infection

Tinea infections of varying sites do occur and may be chronic and widespread in HIV positive patient (Fig 3). The overall frequency is higher in non-infected control population. Nail involvement is common and can cause diffuse whitening. Proximal nail whitening or proximal subungual onychomycosis, unusual in immunocompetent individuals is regarded by some as characteristic of HIV-associated nail infection.

Treatment is standard with the use of topical and systemic anti-fungal agents.

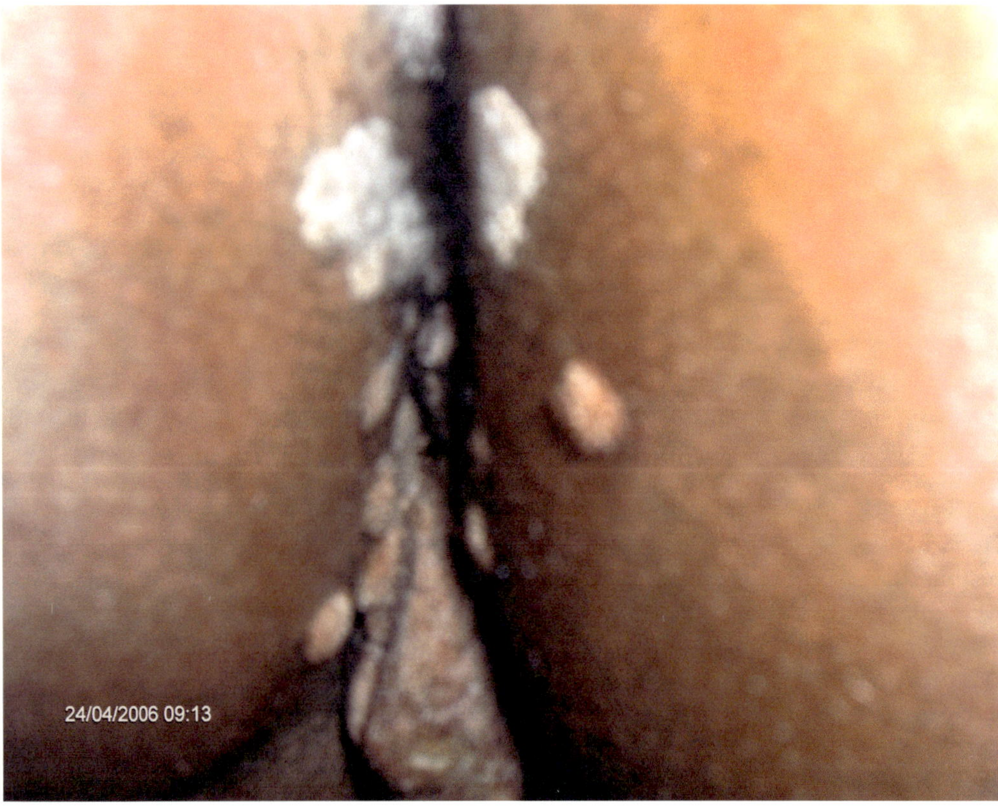

Fig. 2. Genital warts in HIV

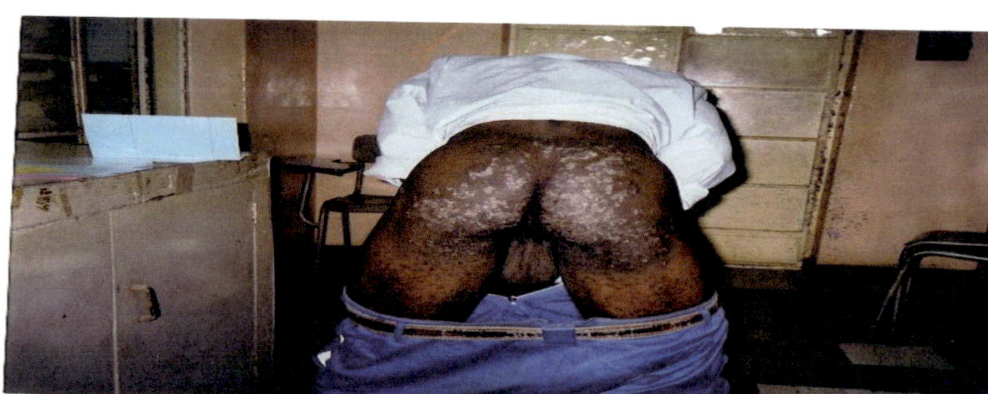

Fig. 3. Extensive tinea cruris and corporis

3.2 Candidiasis

This is common in all stages of HIV infection affecting the skin, nail, genitals and oral mucosa.Cutaneous lesions are often located in the intertriginous areas/ skin folds as highly pruritic inflamed areas with satellite lesions and/or follicular pustules. In addition to HIV, other risk factors are diabetes mellitus, obesity, malignancy, use of immunosuppressive therapy and cytotoxic drugs, use of systemic and topical corticosteroids and antibiotic therapy, hot humid environment, occlusion e.g. diapers, casts and dressings, blood malignancies and neutropenia and skin disease which disturb the cutaneous barrier e.g. psoriasis and contact dermatitis.

Nail lesions affect the proximal nail fold and nail plate. Nail fold lesions (paronychia) present as painful, erythematous swellings which may discharge purulent material. Genital lesions present as pruritic vulvo-vaginitis with discharge of a creamy white material. There may be involvement of the perineum with erythematous and satellite lesions. In severe cases, the oral mucosa may show extensive white plagues or widespread erythema, and esophageal involvement may give rise to dysphagia and retrosternal pain.

Standard topical therapy will suffice but in severe cases and nail involvement systemic therapy may be needed. Fluconazole (50mg daily) has a higher cure rate than ketoconazole (20mg daily) and intermittent administration of fluconazole (150mg) also proved effective.

3.3 Cutaneous malignancies

Persons infected with Human Immunodeficiency Virus (HIV) are at higher risk for the development of certain types of cancers. The AIDS was first reported in the summer of 1981 in Los Angeles among young homosexuals who were observed to have had a disseminated type of Kaposi's sarcoma and pneumocystis carini infection.

3.4 Kaposi's sarcoma

Kaposi's sarcoma (KS), the most common tumor in patients with AIDS, is strongly associated with immunosuppression (Schwartz et al., 2008). KS is a vascular neoplasm affecting the endothelial cell and that affects the skin, and the mucosa, less commonly involves other organs like the gastrointestinal tracts, lungs and lymph nodes. KS can occur in HIV-negative patients where it typically has a chronic indolent course. In HIV infected patients KS has a more aggressive course and may have systemic involvement.

Epidemiological data suggest that the cause is a sexually transmitted infectious agent and this has recently been supported by the finding of herpes virus nucleic acid in Kaposi's sarcoma lesions (Schwartz et al., 2008) .However, this virus called Kaposi's sarcoma associated herpes virus (or human herpes virus type 8) has also been detected in classical KS; Gut lymphomas and other skin lesions of AIDS patients. The role of HHV-8 in the pathogenesis of Kaposi's sarcoma is yet to be clearly defined.

The mucocutaneous lesions of KS are usually asymptomatic vary from the earliest pink macules to the thickened papules and plaques which later develop to nodules. Diffuse lesions may manifest mainly as oedema. The lesions initially may appear benign-looking and may be misdiagnosed as pigmented naevi, Spitz naevi, dermatofibroma, bruises, pyogenic granulomas, malignant melanoma, ecchymosis, molluscum contagiosum or lichen planus. The lesions may appear any where on the skin but the tip of the nose and the hard palate are common sites. Lesions in the feet may occasionally become warty. Lesions may develop at the site of trauma (Kobner Phenomenon).

Unlike the metastatic behavior of other malignant tumors, KS is a multifocal neoplasm in which each lesion seems to develop de novo from endothelial cells that line lymphatic or blood vessels into skin or visceral.

Progression of lesions depends upon the immune status. If the $CD4^{+}$ cell count rises, either with or without treatment lesion may regress at least temporary.

Treatment: This is not curative. Palliative therapy is indicated for lesions that are disfiguring, causing pains or with systemic symptoms.

Local therapy would include:

a. Surgery for large lesions. This would include the use of excision and laser.
b. Cryosurgery
c. Intralesional chemotherapy using vinblastine
d. The tumor is sensitive to radiotherapy.

Systemic therapy would include the following:

a. Chemotherapy including vinblastine, bleomycin, Doxorubicin
b. Biology response modifiers which include IFN-a, interleukin-2 and intravenous immunoglobulin
c. Antiretroviral therapy
d. Photodynamic therapy.

3.5 Other malignancies

AIDS-related lymphomas are not uncommon and are usually high grade of the immunoblastic or small-cell type.

3.6 Cutaneous hypersensitivity

This is a group of eruptions in patients with HIV disease. The pathophysiology of some of them is not well defined and therapeutic responses have been disappointing. However, some explanations have been advised based on some immunologic findings. Monocytes, macrophages, epidermal langerhans cells and dendritic cells of the dermis have CD4 antigen and are potential targets for infection by HIV. The decrease in langerhans cells as in AIDS may lead to altered cell mediated immunity.

3.7 Xeroderma

Dry skin is common in HIV/AIDS especially if chronic diarrhea is a masked feature and may be related to malabsorption. There is associated prutitus. In more severe cases with changes you have acquired ichthyosis. Icythuosis is a disorder of keratinization characterized clinically by dry scaly skin. It should be noted that acquired ichthyosis can also be found in lymphomas, lepromatous leprosy and sarcoidosis which are conditions with reduced immunity. Treatment is the use of emollients.

3.8 Pruritic Papular Eruption (PPE) of HIV

PPE of HIV is a unique manifestation of HIV which has not been seen in seronegative patients (Eisman, 2006, Machtinger et al., 2004). Clinically, the lesions are red or skin coloured papules that are symmetrically disseminated in the trunk, buttocks and extremities (Fig 4). The lesions are extremely pruritic. The lesions heal with post inflammatory hypopigmentation with new hyperpigmented lesions. The eruptions wax and wane during

the course of the illness. The cause of the lesion is not known but most people think that it is a hypersensitivity reaction to antigens or a direct effect of the HIV.
Treatment with antihistamines, phototherapy and photochemotherapy may be used but of limited success.Patient education as to the cause of the illness is important.

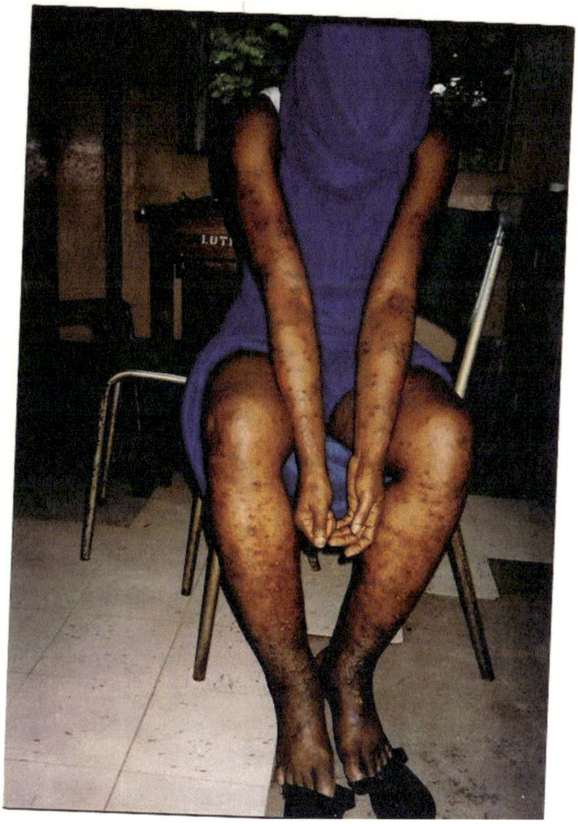

Fig. 4. Pruritic papular of HIV infection

3.9 Seborrheic Dermatitis

Seborrheic dermatitis (SD) is a chronic papulosquamous disorder characterized by distinctive morphology (red, sharply marginated lesion covered with greasy looking scales and hypopigmentation which is usually seen in dark skinned people) and a distinctive distribution in areas with a rich supply of sebaceous glands namely the scalp, forehead, eyebrows, lashline, nasolabial folds, beard and post auricular skin. Other areas include presternal region, inter scapular area, axillae, groin and gluteal crease.
The prevalence of seborrheic dermatitis is around 1-3% in the general population and 40-83% in HIV/AIDS patients.
The aetiology of SD is unclear. It has been suggested that the yeast *Pityrosporum ovale* is important in the aetiology of SD. Clinically, a wide spectrum of lesions exist but characteristic distribution; hypopigmented nummular patches which may coalesce to form polycyclic lesion on the back and presternal area; diffuse erythematous hypopigmented macules involving the scalp margins and butterfly areas of the face and trunk; scalp and

facial involvement presenting as dandruff and blepharitis; flexural, petaloid and pityrosporum folliculitis.
In Africa, hypopigmentation is a prominent feature which has been explained as a result of dicarboxylic acids produced by malassezia causing competitive inhibition of tyrosinase and perhaps a direct cytotoxic effect on hyperactive melanocytes (Altraide et al., 2010).
Seborrheic dermatitis in HIV/AIDS patients occur in varying severity (Altraide et al; 2010). It is usually characterized by thick micaceous scales and usually hyperkeratotic and inflammatory and more widespread and generalized.
Conclusion: Skin disorders are common in sub-Saharan African and may present with early, severe, unusual and atypical manifestations in the course of HIV infection. Awareness of the varied pattern of these manifestations would help in the early diagnosis and management of HIV infection, which would in turn decrease the morbidity and improve the quality of life of HIV-infected patients.

4. References

Aftergut K., Cockerell CJ (1999). Update on the cutaneous manifestations of HIV infection. Clinical and pathologic features. Dermatol. Clin. Vol.17, No.3, pp. 445-71.

Altraide DD, Olumide YM, Mohammed TT (2010). Predictive value of seborrheic dermatitis for HIV infection in Lagos Nigeria. Port Harcourt Medical Journal. 5(1): 30-36.

Eisman S (2006). Pruritic papular eruption in HIV. *Dermatol. Clin.* Vol.24, pp.449-457.

Johnson RA (1999). Cutaneous manifestations of human immunodeficiency virus disease.In: Friedberg IM, Eisen AZ, Wolf K, *et al.*, eds . *Fitzpatrick's Dermatology.* McGraw- Hill, pp. 2138-2150.

Machtinger EL, Van Beek M, Furmanski L, et al(2004).Etiology of pruritic papular eruption with HIV infection in Uganda. *JAMA.* ; vol292, pp.2614-2621.

Olumide YM (2002). A self-instructed textbook of acquired immune deficiency syndrome (HIV/AIDS) for medical students, resident doctors and medical practioners. Longman Nigeria PLC pp.22-80.

Schwartz RA, Micali G, Nasca MR, Scuderi L (2008). Kaposi sarcoma: a continuing conundrum. J Am Acad Dermatol. Vol.59, No. 2, pp. 179-206.

Sterling JC, Kurtz JB. Viral infections: In. Champion RH, Burton JL, Burns DA, Breathnach SM eds Rookwdkinson/Ebling, Textbook of dermatology 6th edition. London 1998: Blackwell science LTD 2: 1057-1079.

Tschachler E, Bergstresser PR, Stingl G (1996) . HIV-related skin diseases. *Lancet* Vol. 348, pp. 659-63.

Wiwanitkit V. Prevalence of dermatological disorders in Thai HIV-infected patients correlated with different CD4 lymphocyte count statuses: a note on 120 cases. *Int JDermatol* 2004; 43 (4): 265-8.

20

Benign and Malignant Lymphoproliferative Disorders in HIV/AIDS

Etienne Mahe and Monalisa Sur
McMaster University, Hamilton, Ontario
Canada

1. Introduction

Owing to the striking lymphotropsism exhibited by the human immunodeficiency virus, HIV/AIDS patients demonstrate a wide breadth of both benign and malignant lymphoproliferative disorders. These disorders span the spectrum from viral lymphadenopathy to lymphocentric opportunistic infections to proliferations of uncertain and frankly malignant potential. This chapter explores a number of the many possible HIV/AIDS associated disorders from the perspective of the lymphoid system. Notably, some of these disorders are themselves AIDS defining illnesses while others are entities known to occur frequently in the HIV/AIDS population but not directly influenced by HIV infection. In most cases, HIV-associated lymphoproliferative disorders are thought to result from an aberrant host immune response in the context of chronic inflammatory stimulation rather than as a direct consequence of HIV infection.

1.1 Pathogenesis

The human immunodeficiency virus is a member of the lentivirus genus (lenti- , *latin* "slow"), a group of viruses in the retrovirus family characterized by tropism for immune cells (Norkin, 2010). HIV demonstrates strong affinity for a specific cohort of human T-cells, the CD4 "Helper" T-cell; this is accomplished by means of the viral gp120 protein's strong affinity for the CD4 molecule (Wain-Hobson, 1996). HIV infects cells with CD4 cell-surface receptor molecules, using them to gain entry into the cell (Verani, et al., 2005). In early infection, HIV is widely disseminated by way of its interaction with antigen presenting cells (e.g. Langerhans and dendritic cells) which direct antigen obtained from mucous membranes toward the tissues of the adaptive immune system (namely the lymph nodes); HIV can accomplish this both by means of CD4 receptor binding but also by exploiting the immune response itself by allowing phagocytosis into these antigen presenting cells through either interations with complement or Fc receptors (Verani, et al., 2005). The result is a systemic dissemination of HIV infection to lymphoid tissues (Pantaleo, et al., 1993). Once gained access to the lymphoid tissues of the body, HIV may engage in a latent infection of T-cells by way of viral integration into resting or memory T-cells; these cells may then serve another reservoir of infection (Sierra, et al., 2005).
A number of studies have explored the biological influences that HIV may have on lymphomagenesis. The primary role of the CD4 T-cell is played out in the adaptive immune

response. More specifically, non-infected CD4 T-cells function as immune system modulators through interactions with a multitude of other cells of both the adaptive immune system (i.e. B-cells) as well as the innate immune system (e.g. macrophages and monocytes)(Robbins, et al., 2010). HIV infected CD4 cells cannot execute these normal immunomodulatory functions: HIV replication within CD4 cells is directly cytopathic (Hazenberg, et al., 2000); non-infected CD4 cells will be reduced in number due to activation-induced cell death under the influence of both HIV infection as well as other concomitant infections (McCune, 2001); HIV tropism for CD4 cells will result in colonization and persistent immunostimulation in lymphoid tissues; HIV will also infect immature CD4 positive precursor T-cells thereby further reducing the effective CD4 T-cell pool (Robbins, et al., 2010).

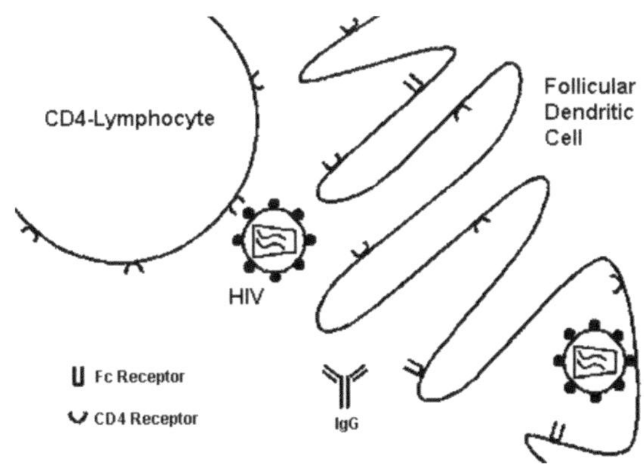

Fig. 1. HIV receptor-specific pathogenesis

In contrast to other viruses associated with neoplasms, HIV is not regarded as a directly transforming virus (i.e. its effect on the host cell genome does not directly initiate neoplastic transformation). This is evidenced by a number of observations regarding HIV-associated lymphomas: there is a wide etiologic range of possible HIV-associated lymphomas; there is frequent association of HIV-associated lymphomas with "super-infecting" known oncogenic pathogens (e.g. Kaposi-sarcoma virus and Epstein-Barr virus); and most HIV-associated lymphomas are lymphomas of B-cells (and not of T-cells, which one would expect if HIV were a uniformly transformative virus). Molecular studies have also noted a propensity for viral genomic integration at random active gene sites; while this may theoretically lead to an insertion at a transformative locus, HIV does not show consistent insertion at a transformative site (Mitchell, et al., 2004).

EBV has been shown to contribute to lymphomagenesis in a number of ways; the latent membrane proteins, in particular, have garnered much research interest in this vein. In the 1980s it was recognized that EBV latent membrane protein-1 gene was able to transform mouse cell models (Wang, et al., 1985). EBV-LMP has also been shown to activate the tumor necrosis factor and p38 mitogenic pathways (Mosialos, et al., 1995; Eliopoulos, et al., 1999); activation of these pathways may contribute to the ability of EBV-infected (and potentially transformed) cells to evade host defense mechanisms. Another EBV encoded protein, latent membrane protein A2 has been shown to stimulate lymphocyte development and proliferation in mouse models outside of the normal immunologic milieu (Caldwell, et al., 1998). Finally, Vockerodt and colleague recently demonstrated that latent membrane

protein-1 was capable of inducing a Hodgkin-like state in non-previously transformed germinal centre B-cells (Vockerodt, et al., 2008).
Less commonly, HIV-associated lymphomas demonstrate co-infection with the Kaposi sarcoma herpes virus, HHV-8. A number of HHV-8 viral proteins have been implicated in lymphomagenesis: the HHV-8 latency-associated nuclear antigen has been shown to interfere with normal p53 and Rb gene protein functions; the K13 viral protein interferes with host cell Fas-mediated apoptosis pathways; and the Kaposin B viral protein has been shown to prevent the normal degeneration of stimulatory cytokines (Wen & Damania, 2010). The combined influence of these and other HHV-8 encoded proteins, especially within the context of an already abnormal immunomodulation from HIV infection, places infected B-cells at high risk of malignant transformation.

2. Non-neoplastic lymphoid disorders in HIV/AIDS

2.1 HIV-associated lymphadenopathy

Lymphadenopathy is a characteristic (though certainly not specific) finding in HIV/AIDS patients. Variable definitions of lymphadenopathy exist in the medical literature, typically making reference to enlarged, swollen or painful lymph nodes as definitive. Size cut-offs have been proposed in some definitions and many clinicians will investigate lymph nodes exceeding 1 cm in size. Ioachim notes that lymph nodes larger than 3 cm should raise suspicion of neoplasia (Ioachim & Medeiros, 2009b). Often lymphadenopathy will come to clinical attention as rapidly enlarging lymph nodes; unfortunately, there is little data to suggest how the rapidity of lymph node enlargement pertains to the presence of absence of a neoplastic proliferation. Other features of clinical concern include matting or adherence of multiple nodes to one another, as well as enlargement of several nodes in a given nodal chain (Ioachim & Medeiros, 2009b). Most frequently, due to the frequent clinical concern that an enlarged lymph node may admonish, biopsy and pathological examination of lymph nodes is necessary, especially in the at risk HIV/AIDS community. For our purposes, HIV-associated lymphadenopathy refers to enlarged lymph nodes attributable strictly to a non-neoplastic viral process excluding other opportunistic pathogens (discussed later).
Lymphadenopathy was identified as one of the earliest clinical signs in early epidemiologic studies of patients with AIDS; the closely studied 1982 Vancouver cohort of at risk homosexual men demonstrated a prevalence of 50% of post-seroconversion lymphadenopathy (Boyko, et al., 1987). Similar values were noted in other cohorts, including heterosexual males and females, such as the Zimbabwean cohort of Latif, et al. (Latif, et al., 1989). Lymphadenopathy is also more commonly identified in HIV positive children than in non-HIV infected children (Bakaki, et al., 2001; Nielsen, et al., 1997). HIV-associated lymphadenopathy demonstrates preponderance for the head and neck area, often presenting as cervical lymphadenopathy (Prasad, et al., 2006). Other radiologic studies have also demonstrated frequent (typically occult) intra-abdominal lymphadenopathy in HIV positive patients, most commonly as a result of opportunistic infection but also due to lymphomas (Jasmer, et al., 2002). Concern over the latter not infrequently results in invasive abdominal lymph node biopsies for diagnostic purposes.
HIV-associated lymphadenopathy follows a consistent histological pattern of progression (see Figure 2). Lymphadenopathy typically begins with the onset of HIV viremia; this acute phase of HIV infection (the acute retroviral syndrome) is typically described as a

mononucleosis-like cluster of symptoms. Acute retroviral syndrome typically begins 2-6 weeks post-infection and may last for several weeks. Typical symptoms include fever, headache, malaise, pharyngitis and lymphadenopathy (Carpenter, et al., 2004). The lymphadenopathy, however, often persists beyond this acute phase. The histological features of early HIV-associated lymphadenopathy typically demonstrate exuberant hyperplastic changes: large lymphoid follicles with irregular serpiginous shapes are characteristic; irregular enlargement of germinal centres is noted; these large germinal centres typically demonstrate prominent apoptotic bodies and tingible body macrophages; and there may be expansion of the interfollicular zones by numerous transformed B lymphocytes (these have a monocytoid appearance and correspond to antigenically stimulated B-cells). These features are typical of the so-called Grade 1 HIV-associated lymphadenopathy.

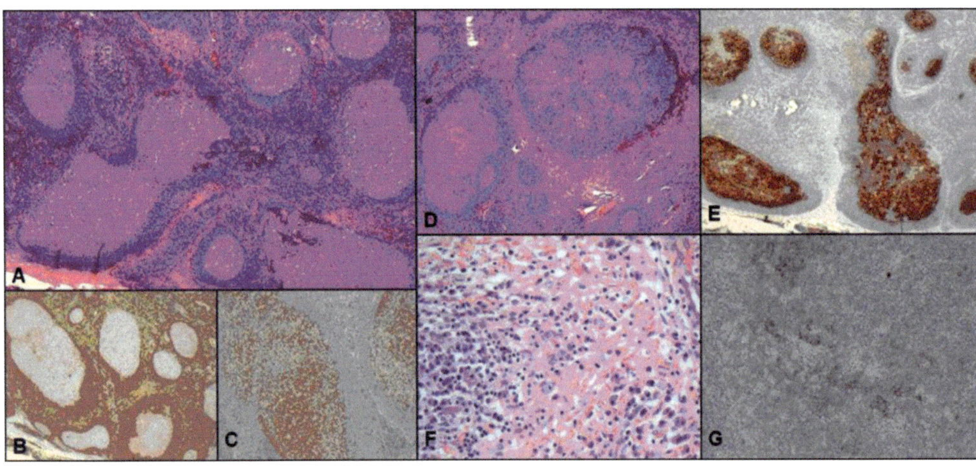

Fig. 2. HIV Lymphadenopathy: A: Early HIV Lymphadenopathy (Grade 1); B: BCL2 stain demonstrating benign follicle staining pattern (negative in follicles and positive in interfollicular zones); C: Ki67 demonstrating benign follicle staining pattern (high index nuclear staining in follicles with low index in interfollicular zones); D: Grade 2 HIV Lymphadenopathy demonstrating early follicular-lysis; E: Corresponding CD21 stain demonstrating hyperplastic moth-eaten follicular dendritic cell meshwork (replaced by fibrosis); F: Grade 3 HIV Lymphadenopathy demonstrating marked fibrosis and loss of follicles; G: Corresponding CD21 stain demonstrating near absence of follicular dendritic meshwork

As HIV infection progresses, the antigenic stimulation within the lymph node begins to wane. This leads to a Grade 2 pattern of HIV-associated lymphadenopathy characterized by a reduction in the number of lymphoid follicles, an increase in the number of plasma cells and a proliferation of perifollicular blood vessels. At the extreme of HIV-associated lymphadenopathy is the Grade 3 pattern in which the residual follicles begin to display sclerosis of their germinal centres.

Although consistent, none of the histologic features noted above are specific to HIV. The Grade 1 pattern, for example, is frequently observed in non-HIV viral lymphadenitides. The Grade 2 and 3 patterns show a significant overlap with those of Castleman's disease (see later). In such cases, a clinical history of known or suspected HIV infection is essential in order that the correct diagnosis be made and that the correct treatment regimen be instituted. The vascular proliferation noted in Grade 2 and 3 may also be misconstrued for Kaposi's sarcoma (see later for the lymph node features of Kaposi's sarcoma); immunohistochemistry for the Kaposi's sarcoma virus is now a commonplace tool to avoid this diagnostic confusion. Other more aggressive lymphoproliferative disorders need to be ruled out in lymph nodes sampled in the context of HIV; the key feature in HIV-associated lymphadenopathy of any Grade is the relative preservation of lymph node architecture which is often lost in lymphoid malignancies.

EBV seropositivity is widespread in HIV positive patients and in the context of lymphadenopathy EBV infection can confuse the histopathologic diagnosis (see Figure 3). More specifically, EBV infection may produce reactive cells demonstrating a striking resemblance to the Reed-Sternberg cells of Hodgkin's lymphoma. In such cases, immunohistochemistry is essential. In order to rule out Hodgkin's lymphoma, the atypical Reed-Sternberg like cells seen in lymphadenitis will typically stain positive for CD20, CD45, and may stain positive for CD30 (an activation marker); these cells, unlike true Reed-Sternberg cells, should not stain for CD15.

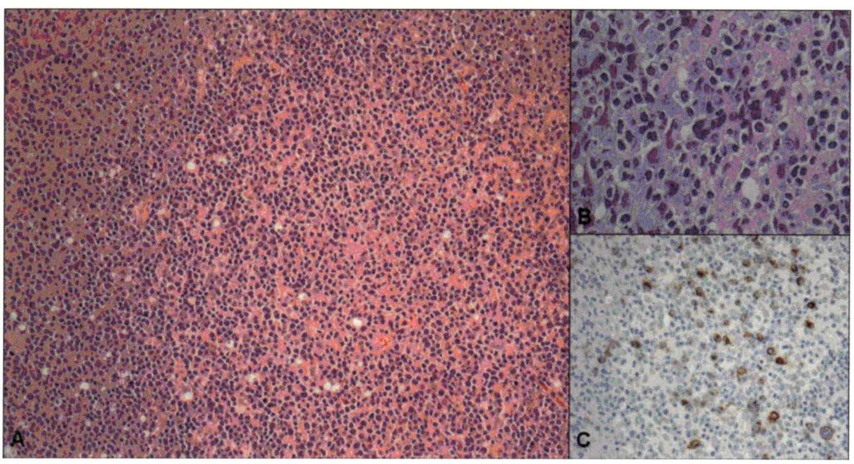

Fig. 3. HIV Lymphadenopathy with EBV related changes: A: Loss of normal lymph node architecture; B: Reed-sternberg-like cells present in EBV-related HIV Lymphadenopathy; C: Corresponding EBV Stain

Treatment for HIV-associated lymphadenopathy is focused around optimizing antiretroviral therapy, treated other concomitant infections as needed and clinical follow-up. The latter point is emphasized in order that lymphoid neoplasia not be missed. Studies have explored the outcomes of patients diagnosed with HIV-associated lymphadenopathy and graded according to the above scheme. In their cohort of HIV patients with lymphadenopathy, Ioachim and colleagues noted that most cases of HIV-associated lymphadenopathy began as Grade 1; many cases subsequently progressed from Grade 1 to 2 and from Grade 2 to 3; most cases with Grade 3 lymphadenopathy subsequently developed AIDS defining illnesses (Ioachim & Medeiros, 2009; Ioachim, et al., 1990). Ioachim et al also noted a distinct survival difference between the various grades of HIV-associated lymphadenopathy (Ioachim & Medeiros, 2009; Ioachim, et al., 1990). Grade 3 HIV-associated lymphadenopathy is also strongly associated with development of Kaposi's sarcoma (Ioachim & Medeiros, 2009c).

2.2 Bacillary angiomatosis

Bacillary Angiomatosis is a lesion of proliferating endothelial cells caused by *Bartonella* species occuring in immunocompromised patients, almost exclusively in patients with AIDS. The first documented case of HIV/AIDS associated bacillary angiomatosis was reported by Stoler and colleagues in 1983 (Cotell & Noskin, 1994; Stoler, et al., 1983); they reported a peculiar case of a young AIDS patient with multiple cutaneous nodules found to consist of proliferating endothelial cells forming lobular networks of small caliber blood vessels. Interspersed within this network were small gram-negative bacillary forms visible only on Warthin-Starry staining. For many years, efforts to speciate the organism observed histologically were unsuccessful; initial attempts at culturing the organism with a range of media produced no results (Cotell & Noskin, 1994; Stoler, et al., 1983). Finally, with the dawning of PCR based techniques, the organism believed to be the causal agent in bacillary angiomatosis was found to be genomically comparable to the species known to cause Cat Scratch Disease, the organism known today as *Bartonella henselae* (Relman, et al., 1990).

It is now known that bacillary angiomatosis may be associated with a number of *Bartonella* species, most common *B. henselae* and *B. quintana* (Maguina, et al., 2009). Interestingly, studies have shown high seroprevalence for *Bartonella* species in the population overall (Lamas, et al., 2010). Furthermore, clinically silent *Bartonella* seroprevalence has been observed in the HIV population, rarely with very high titres (Pape, et al., 2005; Yousif, et al., 1996). These laboratory data mirror the clinically evident divergence of *Bartonella* infection observed in the immunocompromised and immunocompetent populations. In immunocompetent individuals, *Bartonella* infection, if clinically evident, typically manifests as the so-called "cat-scratch disease," characterized by lymphadenopathy demonstrating caseating granuloma formation. In immunocompromised patients, on the other hand, the infection manifests as vascular lesions, sometimes progressing to a potentially fatal systemic infection. This stark contrast has spawned a number of studies demonstrating the importance of an intact adaptive immune system.

Bartonella infection is transmitted either by means of an insect vector (e.g. mites, lice) or by means of trauma by an animal vector (the namesake "cat-scratch" is evident) (Minnick, et al., 2003; Ioachim & Medeiros, 2009a; Wolff, et al., 2005). Studies exploring the comparative genomics of *Bartonella* infections in HIV patients and their pet cats have confirmed this long suspected epidemiologic link (Chang, et al., 2002). After inoculation, *Bartonella* species home to erythrocytes and endothelial cells, thereby allowing it access to multiple sites in the body (Minnick, et al., 2003). *Bartonella* then exploits a number of molecular pathways to evade its host's immune system (Minnick, et al., 2003); this evasion may explain the clinically observed propensity of *Bartonella* to produce granulomatous lymphadenitis. In immunocompromised patients, exploiting an already weakened immune system, *Bartonella* stimulates angiogenesis; *Bartonella* infection stimulates the production of hypoxia-induced factor and other cytokines, thereby upregulating angiogenesis (Minnick, et al., 2003).

Bacillary angiomatosis typically occurs in AIDS patients with low CD4 counts (typically less than $100/mm^3$) (Maguina, et al., 2009). Most patients present with skin lesions, characteristically as multiple violaceous or red papules; these lesions may be painful, typically progress over days to weeks and may resemble cherry hemangiomas or pyogenic granulomas (Wolff, 2005). In most cases a combination of clinical history, known HIV/AIDS status and clinical assessment will result in the correct diagnosis; the differential diagnosis, however, may include Kaposi's sarcoma thereby mandating histopathological assessment

(Maguina, et al., 2009). In a notable number of cases of BA, lymphadenopathy may be identified as the inciting event (Gasquet, et al., 1998). *B. henselae* BA, in particular, tends to demonstrate lymphadenoapthy, both with and without skin lesions (Ioachim & Medeiros, 2009a). Aggressive cases of bacillary angiomatosis may demonstrate splenic or hepatic involvement as bacillary peliosis, often with fatal outcomes.

The histologic features of bacillary angiomatosis in lymph nodes are similar to those seen in skin lesions and elsewhere (see Figure 4). Bacillary angiomatosis typically forms richly vascular nodules. Proliferating endothelial cells are evident, forming variably sized blood-filled vascular spaces into which their nuclei protrude. There may be notable anisonucleosis, multiple nucleoli and numerous mitoses; these features may suggest a malignant entity. Ancillary staining with Warthin-Starry silver stain invariably demonstrates numerous bacilli, 0.2-0.3 μm in size, often noted in clumps (Maguina, et al., 2009; Ioachim & Medeiros, 2009a). Electron microscopy will demonstrate a trilaminar bacillus in association with an obvious proliferation of endothelial cells with characteristic Weibel-Palade bodies (Kostianovsky & Greco, 1994). Modern attempts at developing reliable immunohistochemical markers to aid in the diagnosis of bacillary angiomatosis have been as yet unsuccessful; PCR techniques may be relied upon to confirm the presence of *Bartonella* infection in cases that may be diagnostically equivocal (Caponetti, et al., 2009).

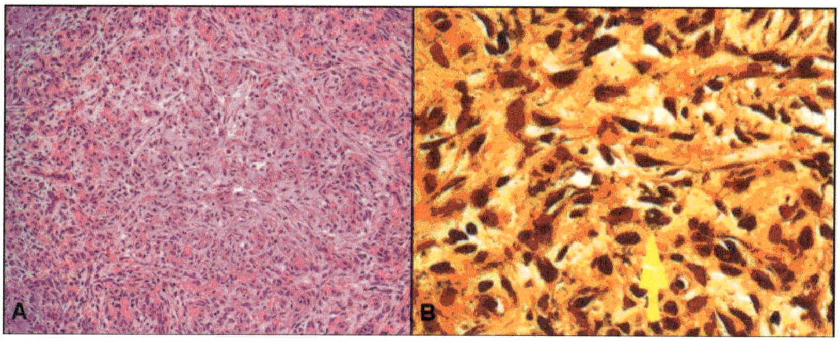

Fig. 4. Bacillary Angiomatosis: A: Low-power view demonstrating proliferating venules; B: Warthin-starry stain demonstrating extracellular clump of bacteria (arrow)

The differential diagnosis of bacillary angiomatosis may include a number of entities, especially if the HIV/AIDS status of the patient is unknown. On hematoxylin & eosin staining alone, bacillary angiomatosis may resemble a hemangioma. Gram staining may help distinguish bacillary angiomatosis from pyogenic granuloma (the former being invariably negative). Bacillary angiomatosis may sometimes be difficult to discern from Kaposi's sarcoma. Histologically, Kaposi's cells are more characteristically spindled and there is a predominance of slit-like vascular spaces. Nonetheless, most authories recommend using an immunohistochemical stain against HHV-8, the causal virus of Kaposi's sarcoma, in order to rule out this more serious condition. Another malignant condition that may be mimicked by bacillary angiomatosis is typical angiosarcoma; this entity is highly aggressive and demonstrates an infiltrative architecture.

Although the clinical course of bacillary angiomatosis is variable, the treatment of choice is antibiotics (typically a course of erythromycin or doxycycline); some cases may also resolve spontaneously even without treatment, however (Wolff, et al., 2005). Care should be taken in HIV/AIDS patients with very low CD4 counts; these patients not only require quick accurate diagnosis to define the appropriate treatment regimen, but further preventative action may also be beneficial, such as prevention of exposure to animals.

2.3 Other common infectious lymphadenitides in HIV/AIDS

While a complete review of the opportunistic and co-infectious agents encountered in HIV/AIDS is beyond the scope of this book, any discussion of the lymph node based disease entities encountered in HIV/AIDS would be remiss if not for a discussion of the commonest node-based co-infections. The following is a brief discussion of the most common opportunistic infections encountered in HIV/AIDS patients from the perspective of lymph node disease.

2.3.1 Pneumocystis

Pneumocystis jiroveci is a ubiquitous organism in nature manifesting as a disease-causing organism only in the immunocompromised. This fungus first came to broad clinical attention in the early 1980s when it was noted in 70-80%of AIDS patients, most commonly manifest as pneumonia. Rarely, however, pneumocystosis does involve the lymph nodes. Anderson and Barrie were probably the first to report pneumocystis in a lymph node, two decades prior to the first identified cases of HIV/AIDS (ANDERSON & BARRIE, 1960). Of the reported extra-pulmonary cases of pneumocystis, the lymphoreticular system is probably the most common (Grimes, et al., 1987; Ioachim & Medeiros, 2009d). When involving lymph nodes, pneumocystis most commonly involves the mediastinum and retroperitoneal lymph nodes (Ioachim & Medeiros, 2009d). The gross features typically reflect the presence of necrotizing granuloma: lymph nodes are typically enlarged with central areas of purulent material. Microscopically, granulomata with central necrotic eosinophilic material will be noted (see Figure 5). The causal microorganisms are generally not overtly evident on routine histologic stains but can be readily identified on fungal silver stains as helmet-shaped organisms within the necrotic foci. Immunohistochemical stains for *Pneumocystis jiroveci* are available, though a combination of clinical history of HIV infection and morphologic features identified on silver staining are often sufficient. The current treatment of choice is trimethoprim-sulfamethoxazole antibiotics; the US centres for disease control also recommend that all HIV-positive patients diagnosed with pneumocystosis be maintained on indefinite prophylactic anti-fungal agents provided that CD4 count remains below 200 cells/μL (Kaplan, et al., 2009).

2.3.2 Mycobacteria

Globally the risk of co-infection with *Mycobacteria tuberculosis* is 20-37 times higher in patients with HIV than those without (WHO Department of HIV/AIDS Stop TB Department, 2010). The WHO also estimates that 25% of HIV-positive patients will die due to concomitant tuberculosis (WHO Department of HIV/AIDS Stop TB Department, 2010). Other non-tuberculous infections are also frequent in (and many are characteristic of) HIV infection. In addition to their primary involvement of the lungs, mycobacteria are also frequently encountered in lymph nodes, especially in the context of HIV infection. Mycobacterial lymphadenitis, regardless of the underlying species, will characteristically produce lymph node enlargement with foci of necrosis. The histologic features are often characteristic, namely central eosinophilic necrosis surrounded by a rim of pallisading histiocytes and giant cells (see Figure 5). In this peripheral rim of histiocytes, mycobacteria may be identified, often few and far between, on acid fast staining (pathologists often use a Ziehl-Neelsen stain for this purpose). Positivity on acid-fast staining does not equate to tuberculosis, however, and in many cases distinguishing between *Mycobacteria tuberculosis*, atypical mycobacteria or the *Mycobacterium avium complex* can be challenging, often requiring molecular testing for speciation (which can fortunately be performed off formalin-fixed and paraffin-embedded tissues). The presence of the so-called Langhans giant cells (with peripherally rimmed nuclei) may hint at the presence of *Mycobacteria tuberculosis* but is by no means specific. Another advantage to molecular testing when acid-fast bacteria are encountered is the ability to test for antimicrobial resistant strains by PCR; this may be an invaluable aid given the burgeoning cohort of multidrug resistant TB cases encountered in HIV/AIDS.

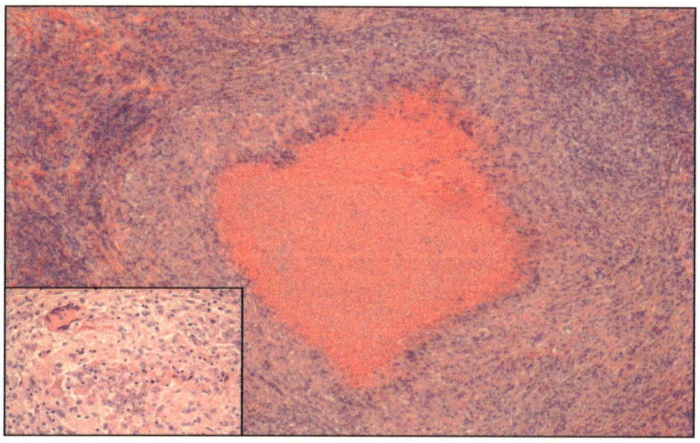

Fig. 5. Tuberculous Lymphadenitis: Granuloma with eosinophilic necrotic centre; inset: characteristics Langhans giant cell (top left) with adjacent necrosis (bottom right)

2.3.3 Toxoplasmosis

Toxoplasma gondii is the causative agent of toxoplasmosis, a parasitic infection believed to be one of the worlds most prevalent. *Toxoplasma gondii* seropositivity in the at-large population has previously been reported as high as 70-90%, though modern estimates in the range of 10-40% seem reasonable (Shin, et al., 2009; Kamani, et al., 2009; Fromont, et al., 2009). Not unexpectedly, the overall seroprevalence of *Toxoplasma gondii* is also high; while the estimates may be lower in North American and Europe, one recent Nigerian cohort demonstrated a seroprevalence of over 50% with active parasitism in the blood detected in over 20% (Lindstrom, et al., 2006). *Toxoplasma gondii* demonstrates parasitism of a number of animal hosts, most commonly of felines (the definitive host). Humans are typically infected by way of consumption of contaminated foods or exposure to contaminated soil or animal droppings. Vertical transmission is also possible, producing a dangerous congenital toxoplasmosis. One of the most frequent presentations of toxoplasmosis in the HIV population is toxoplasma encephalitis (Ioachim & Medeiros, 2009e); a histologically characteristic infection of lymph nodes is also common, however. Toxoplasmosis lymphadenopathy typically affects the lymph nodes of the head and neck; these are typically slightly enlarged and tender to palpation. The most frequently encountered histologic features are nodal follicular hyperplasia with interspersed aggregates and sheets of monocytoid lymphocytes and scattered clusters of epithelioid cells (see Figure 6). The monocytoid cells are immunoglobin producing B-cells (which will stain positive for B-cell markers) and can most typically be found in the subcapsular and paratrabecular locations while the epithelioid cells are histiocytes and are characteristically seen to encroach upon follicles but do not form true granulomas. Many HIV positive cases of toxoplasma lymphadenopathy will demonstrate free or engulfed trophozoites (which may be seen staining hook-like organisms H&E, either free floating or within macrophages); they are rarely observed in immunocompetent patients, however. The giemsa special stain can be used to highlight the organisms and some labs use immunohistochemistry with *Toxoplasma gondii* antibodies; PCR testing is the gold-standard, however. The histologic differential diagnosis is long—as would be expected in most cases with prominent collections of histiocytes. For this reason, it is advisable to use ancillary testing or special stains when examining lymph nodes with prominent collections of histiocytes. In addition to antibiotics for treatment of acute toxoplasmosis (such as pyrimethamine, sulfadiazine or clindamycin), the centres for disease control and prevention also currently recommend antibiotic prophylaxis for HIV patients with low CD4 counts (less than 200 cells/µL) (Kaplan, et al., 2009). Routine serologic testing of HIV positive patients is also recommended (Kaplan, et al., 2009).

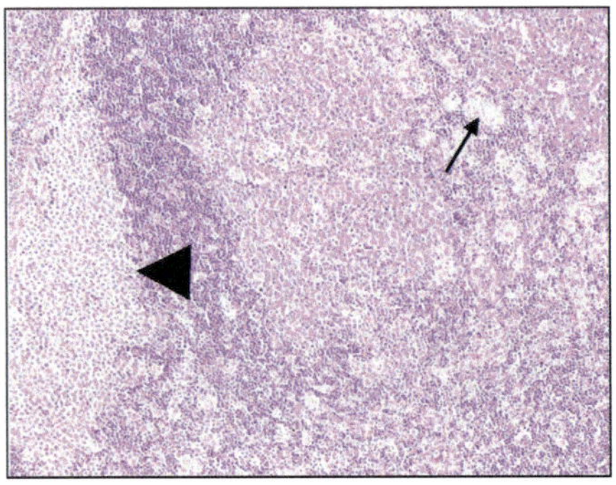

Fig. 6. Toxoplasma Lymphadenitis: Hyperplastic follicle with moth-eaten appearance infiltrated by epithelioid histiocytes (arrow) with adjacent collection of monocytoid B-cells (arrowhead)

2.4 Castleman's disease

Castleman's disease, also known as angiofollicular lymphadenopathy, was first described by Castleman and colleagues in the 1950's. The first studies of Castleman's disease predated the recongnition of HIV and it was not until decades later that its connection to HIV and HHV-8 was recognized. We now recognize two distinct histological forms, the hyaline-vascular and plasma variants. The plasma cell variant may further be categorized into unicentric and multicentric forms, the latter characteristically HIV-associated and of poorer prognosis.

The pathogenetic mechanisms leading to the development of Castleman's disease remain debated. Evidence supports HHV-8 as the etiologic agent in at least some cases; in one study, 50% of the unicentric plasma cell variant cases and nearly all cases of the mulcentric form were noted to be positive for HHV-8 (Soulier, et al., 1995). Further evidence in support of HIV and HHV-8 viral pathogens as etiologic agents stems from studies indicating a response of HIV associated multicentric Castleman's disease to antiviral agents (Casper, et al., 2004). Other studies have identified the lymphokine interleukin-6 (IL-6) as a potential contributor to the development of the plasma cell variant (Oksenhendler, et al., 2002). Interleukin-6 is a chemokine with a number of roles: it acts as an activator of T and B-cells; it also acts to downregulate pro-inflammatory cytokines by inhibiting interleukin-1 and tumour necrosis factor α (Jones, et al., 2001). Another study demonstrated that HHV-8 produces an interleukin-6 homologue (Osborne, et al., 1999). These factors together may account for the pathogenesis of the plasma cell variant, especially the multicentric form. The hyaline vascular variant, however, does not demonstrate as strong an association with HHV-8 and is most common in non-HIV patients, some with no evident immune dysregulation; in these cases, the pathogenesis has yet to be elucidated.

The hyaline vascular variant is the most common variant of the unicentric form, representing 80-90% of cases (Ioachim & Medeiros, 2009f). This variant typically presents as enlargement of a lymph node or lymph node group, often in the mediastinal region. This variant is also is more common than the plasma cell variant to affect younger patients. Few systemic symptoms are present in the hyaline vascular variant and most symptoms are related to mass effect. The classical histological features demonstrate preservation of overall lymph node architecture with an abundance of follicles (see Figure 7). In these follicles are one or two (sometime conjoined) germinal centres demonstrating prominent sclerosis and paucicellularity. The mantle/marginal cells of these follicles can be seen to form concentric layers (termed "onion-skinning") around the sclerosed germinal centres. The classic form also demonstrates a hyalinized penetrating vessel passing into the sclerotic germinal centre from the exterior of the follicle (forming so called "lollipop" lesions). Other interfollicular zone changes may be noted including extensive proliferation of small vascular channels (termed "high endothelial venules"). Sclerosis of the lymph node capsule is also a common finding. As noted previously, similar features may also be noted in cases of high-grade HIV-associated lymphadenopathy. The latter usually lack the classical lollipop lesions and the mantle/marginal zone onion-skinning is usually far less prominent. Ancillary tests for HHV-8 may be helpful but typically the diagnosis is made histologically.

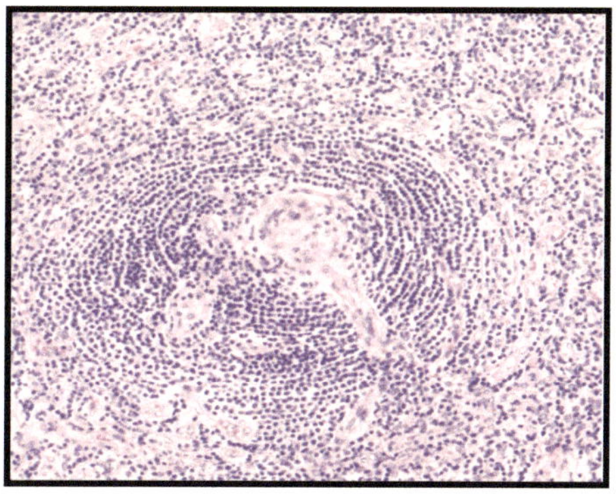

Fig. 7. Hyaline Vascular Variant of Castleman's Disease

The plasma cell variant is the less common of the unicentric forms (Ioachim & Medeiros, 2009f). As in the hyaline vascular variant, the unicentric plasma cell variant may present as an enlarging mass. Patients with this histological variant, however, are more prone to systemic clinical symptoms than those patients with the hyaline vascular variant. Typical symptoms include fevers, night sweats, malaise, and weight loss (these symptoms, in conjunction with enlarged lymph nodes often arouse suspicions of a lymphoproliferative disorder; biopsy for diagnosis is generally recommended). The plasma cell variant demonstrates the similar features of onion skinning and lollipop lesions, though the degree of hyalinization of the germinal centres is markedly reduced relative to the hyaline vascular variant; this may sometimes make the recognition of the lollipop lesions difficult (see Figure 8). Examination of the interfollicular zones is generally very helpful since it demonstrates numerous sheets of mature plasma cells (these generally stand out prominently since prominent plasma cells are rare in lymph nodes). The prominent vascularity noted in the interfollicular zones of the hyaline vascular variant is typically absent. Some cases may have foci demonstrating features of the hyaline vascular variant; when the histologic features of the plasma cell variant dominate, however, the latter diagnosis is appropriate. A number of studies have demonstrated a histological difference between plasma cell variant affected lymph nodes positive and negative for HHV-8 infection. In HHV-8 negative cases, residual hyperplastic follicles are usually notable; in contrast in HHV-8 positive cases, fewer residual follicles are noted and a more prominent interfollicular space vascular proliferation is present. Also, HHV-8 positive immunoblastic cells are also more prominent in the HHV-8 positive cases.

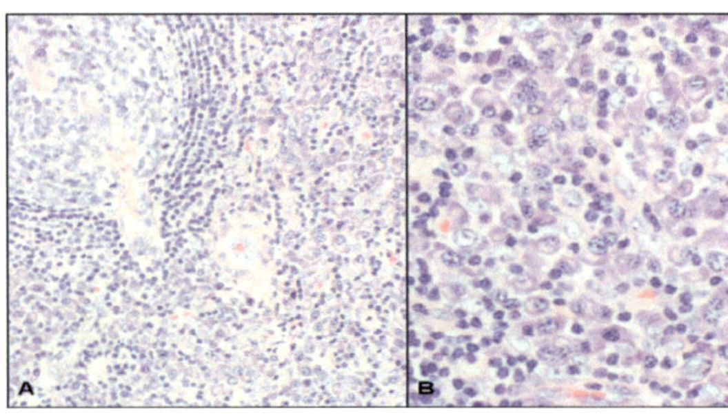

Fig. 8. Plasma Cell Variant of Castleman's Disease: A: Non-hyalinized "lollipop" lesion; B: High-power view demonstrating prominent interfollicular plasma cell infiltrates

Multicentric castleman's disease almost invariably involves multiple lymph nodes most typically demonstrating the histology seen in the unicentric plasma cell variant. The multicentric form has been traditionally under-recognized since its diagnosis requires positive detection of Castleman's disease in multiple locations. This form is also most often present in the context of HIV infection. Patients are nearly always symptomatic, usually presenting with fever, malaise, night sweats and weight loss (the so called B-symptoms) and may also present with hepatosplenomegaly, skin rash, edema and neurologic changes (Ioachim & Medeiros, 2009f). Other laboratory findings include cytopenias, elevated erythrocyte sedimentation rate and elevated C-reactive protein (Ioachim & Medeiros, 2009f). Diagnosis may be confused when a number of the latter clinical signs and symptoms are present, since these are suggestive of the so-called POEMS syndrome (this is a syndrome characterized by the presence of peripheral neuropathy, organomegaly, edema, monoclonal serum paraprotein, and skin changes). POEMS syndrome demonstrates significant diagnostic overlap Castleman's disease, especially the multicentric form. It is felt to be a para-neoplastic syndrome resulting from plasma cell disorders and is felt to have a common pathogenetic link with the plasma cell variant of Castleman's disease via interleukin-6 (Dispenzieri, 2007). The differential diagnosis can be further confused when HIV is considered; the latter, or rather the anti-retroviral drugs used to treat it, can cause peripheral neuropathies, skin changes, edema and other symptoms. In order to avoid diagnostic confusion, specific POEMS criteria have been set forth (Dispenzieri, 2007) and lymphadenopathy should be investigated histopathologically for features of Castleman's disease.

The treatment and prognosis of Castleman's disease depends greatly on both the histologic type as well as the presence of absence of multicentric disease. The hyaline vascular variant is often treated only with excision but adjuvant radiation therapy has been used in cases not amenable to complete resection (Roca, 2009). Some cases of both the hyaline vascular and plasma cell variants may be complicated by recurrence (chiefly the latter more than the former) (Roca, 2009). Cases of unicentric disease with persistent symptoms may also require steroids or chemotherapy (Roca, 2009). The multicentric form often requires aggressive treatment, frequently with chemotherapy (using regimens similar to those used in aggressive lymphomas, often combined with the anti-CD20 antibody rituximab) (Mylona, et al., 2008). There is controversy as to the actual benefit of anti-retroviral therapy; in their systematic review of Multicentric Castleman's disease in HIV, Mylona and colleagues determined that the survival outcomes from Multicentric Castleman's disease with and without antiretroviral therapies were comparable (Mylona, et al., 2008). The caveat to this latter observation is the reduction in incidence of Kaposi's sarcoma in patients on antiretrovirals (Mylona, et al., 2008).

2.5 Polymorphous post-transplant lymphoproliferative disease-like B-cell lymproliferative disorder

With the development of immunosuppressive medications permitting greatly improved successes of allogeneic transplant, it was noted that chronically immunosuppressed patients had a uniquely increased risk of a variety of lymphoproliferative disorders. These proliferations, 80% of B-cell lineage (Jacobson & LaCasce, 2010), were termed post-transplant lymphoproliferative disorders to reflect their unique clinicopathologic characteristics. For our purposes, it is interesting to note that, many decades after the concept of iatrogenic immunosuppression was introduced for the purposes of ameliorating transplant outcomes, the HIV/AIDS epidemic revealed an equally dangerous wave of immunosuppression in which many other cases clinically and histologically similar to post-transplant lymphoproliferative disorder were encountered.

The first series of HIV-associated post-transplant lymphoproliferative disorders was reported in 1987. Four infant autopsy cases from patients with HIV (at that time, the human T-lymphocyte virus-III) and a clinical picture compatible with AIDS were included in the report. At autopsy, splenic and liver infiltrates were noted. These infiltrates, as well as other microscopic infiltrates in the lungs, were noted to consist of a polymorphous collection of inflammatory cells with a preponderance of lymphocytes. These lymphocytes were noted to be polyclonal by kappa and lamda immunohistochemistry. Currently, this entity is known as HIV-associated polymorphous lymphoproliferative disorder (Raphaël, et al., 2008).

Though few cases have been reported, some small series have explored the clinical and pathologic characteristic of this entity. HIV-associated polymorphous lymphoproliferative disorder typically presents in adults with low CD4 counts (typically less than 200 cells/μL) (Nador, et al., 2003). This entity is identified both within and without lymph nodes and tends most often to present unifocally. In contrast to most HIV-associated lymphomas, HIV-associated polymorphous lymphoproliferative disorder tends to lack a monotonous morphology, often demonstrating a mixture of lymphocytes, plasma cells, immunoblasts and histiocytes (see Figure 9). Of particular interest is the tendency for the majority of cells to bear plasmacytoid morphology. A variable degree of cytologic atypia and even necrosis may also be observed.

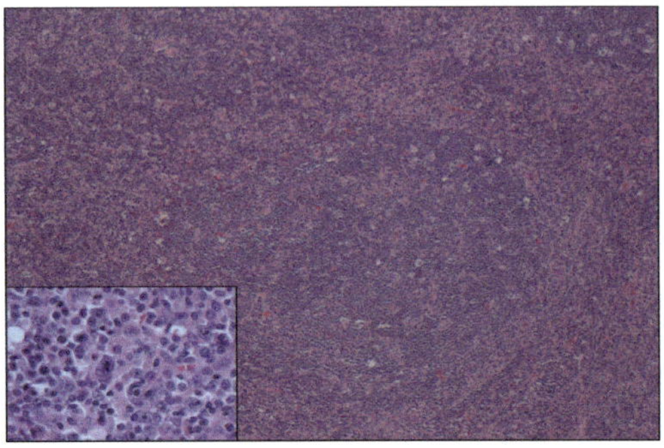

Fig. 9. HIV-associated Polymorphous post-transplant lymphoproliferative disease-like B-cell lymphoproliferative disorder: low-power view demonstrating follicular-lysis; inset: high-power view demonstrating polymorphous infiltrate

The immunophenotypic features of HIV-associated polymorphous lymphoproliferative disorder are also unique. Most cases will demonstrate some form of B-cell phenotype, either in the form of CD20 expression or by prevue of immunoglobulin expression (Nador, et al., 2003). Most, but certainly not all, will demonstrate kappa or lambda light-chain restriction and molecular evidence of clonal immunoglobulin gene rearrangement (Nador, et al., 2003). Some will even demonstrate co-expression of CD20 and CD43, considered an aberrant quality most often observed in B-cell lymphomas (Nador, et al., 2003). The largest series to our knowledge failed to demonstrate any cases demonstrating non-germline T-cell receptor rearrangements (Nador, et al., 2003). Most cases also demonstrate EBV co-infection with few also demonstrating HHV-8 co-infection (Nador, et al., 2003).

HIV-associated polymorphous lymphoproliferative disorders also tend to have a relatively better prognosis than other HIV-associated lymphomas, further reinforcing the debatable malignity of this entity. As noted by Nador and colleagues, many patients will do well, even in the absence of chemotherapy (Nador, et al., 2003). This observation was echoed in one such patient from our institution who responded well by way of optimization of his anti-retroviral therapy. Minimal data is available for the development of optimal treatment regimens, however.

3. HIV-associated lymphomas

HIV patients have a 60-110 fold increased risk of developing a lymphoma relative to the HIV negative population at large (Raphaël, et al., 2008; Lewden, et al., 2005; Whelan & Scadden, 2006). The incidence of HIV-associated lymphomas also increases with duration of disease (Besson, et al., 2001); this is a notable concern in the modern era of antiretrovirals in which the latency period from HIV infection to the development of AIDS is increasing. In recent studies exploring causes of death among HIV/AIDS patients treated with potent antiviral medications, lymphomas were reported as the most common malignancy (Lewden, et al., 2005; Besson, et al., 2001); this is in contrast to the evident predominance of Kaposi's sarcoma in the pre-anti-retroviral era (Carpenter, et al., 2004). Lymphomas in HIV also demonstrate unique preponderances for extra-nodal sites. Characteristic sites of extra-nodal primary involvement include the gastrointestinal tract and the central nervous system (Thirlwell, et al., 2003).

Epidemiological data suggests that the overall incidence of many lymphomas has fallen since the introduction of anti-retroviral treatment. In particular, Besson et al noted a significant reduction in AIDS-related lymphomas in a retrospective review of lymphoma rates before and after the introduction of anti-retroviral treatment (Besson, et al., 2001). The particularly devastating primary central nervous system lymphoma characteristic of AIDS in the pre-antiretroviral era was found to virtually disappear in Besson et al.'s post-antiretroviral cohort (Besson, et al., 2001). Similar observations were made in other studies, noting both improved survival for HIV-associated lymphoma patients and also an overall decrease in incidence (Wolf, et al., 2005; Biggar, et al., 2005; Sacktor, et al., 2001). (One notable exception is Hodgkin's lymphoma in HIV/AIDS patients which, in pre- and post-antiretroviral cohorts has shown an increased incidence; this phenomenon will be explored in the later section "Hodgkin's Lymphoma.")

3.1 Burkitt's lymphoma

Burkitt's lymphoma is a highly aggressive lymphoma eponimized for Denis Burkitt, a British surgeon working in Africa in the 1950s. In his seminal paper, Burkitt described a peculiar "sarcoma" demonstrating a predilection for the jaws of African children. This lesion, Burkitt noted, was first described in 1938 by Christiansen; it was Burkitt's attention to the geographic preponderance of this lesion in Africa, in addition to his detailed clinicopathologic description of 38 cases, which led the disease to be named after him however (BURKITT, 1958). In the 1960s, by way of the work of O'Conor and Wright, the pathologic nature of Burkitt's lymphoma was further detailed: in particular, O'Conor identified the lesion as a lymphoma and Wright demonstrated that the lesion could be accurately histologically distinguished from other lymphomas (O'CONOR & DAVIES, 1960; WRIGHT, 1963). Later, in the 1970s, the association of EBV infection and Burkitt's lymphoma was elucidated with the first publication of EBV viral culture from lymphoblasts obtained from Burkitt's lymphoma samples (EPSTEIN, et al., 1964).

The WHO currently acknowledges three major classes of Burkitt's lymphoma: the endemic form (referring to the entity described by Burkitt with a predilection for the jaws of African children); the sporadic form (more common to adults than children and without a specific geographical or anatomical predilection); and Burkitt's lymphoma arising in the context of immunocompromise (Leoncini, et al., 2008). The latter category was only recently added in order to highlight the unique clinical and pathogenetic features of this entity relative to the other two. Of note, all three entities share the common morphologic, immunophenotypic and molecular features which have come to define Burkitt's lymphoma; they are chiefly distinguished from one another, therefore, on the basis of clinical features.

The first few cases of HIV/AIDS associated Burkitt's lymphoma were reported in the early 1980s; likely the first case was reported by Doll and List (Doll & List, 1982) with a subsequent small case series reported by Ziegler and colleagues (Ziegler, et al., 1982). These cases all presented in homosexual men with AIDS-like clinical features (though these cases were documented prior to the definition of AIDS and before the discovery of HIV) and involved both nodal and extra-nodal sites. Interestingly, these cases were etiologically associated with immunosuppression, despite a lack of awareness of HIV; the immunocompromised in these cases was originally thought to be associated with CMV infection or drug use.

More than two decades later, Burkitt's lymphoma has become one of the most common malignancies in patients with HIV/AIDS. According to the WHO, Burkitt's lymphoma accounts for 30% of all HIV-associated lymphomas (Raphaël, et al., 2008); this number has been noted to reach as high as 40% in some series (Spina, et al., 1998). The WHO also notes that in patients with HIV, Burkitt's lymphoma is 1000 times more likely than in patients without concomitant HIV infection (Raphaël, et al., 2008). An HIV positive patient can furthermore expect a 10-20% lifetime risk of Burkitt's lymphoma (Noy, 2010). In contrast to other HIV/AIDS associated lymphomas, Burkitt's lymphoma often presents relatively early on in the course of infection, often before the severe immunocompromise that precedes most HIV-associated lymphomas (Gaidano, et al., 1998). A recent large study also noted an intriguing decrease in the incidence of Burkitt's lymphoma in cases of profoundly low CD4 counts relative to less immunocompromised AIDS patients (Guech-Ongey, et al., 2010). Despite the distinct classification status afforded to HIV-associated Burkitt's lymphoma relative to other non-immunocompromised Burkitt's cases, controversies persist regarding the need for the distinction. In their cohort of African children with Burkitt's lymphoma, Orem and colleagues noted more similarity than difference between HIV positive and negative patients, with the caveat that HIV-positive Burkitt's patients tended to present with less lymphadenopathy and at higher stage than the others (Orem, et al., 2009). This was in keeping with the previous observations of Spina and colleagues noting similar clinicopathologic features amongst their cohort of HIV-positive and negative Burkitt's patients, including comparable disease free survival rates in HIV patients receiving antiretroviral therapy (Spina, et al., 1998). In contrast, epidemiologic data have suggested that Burkitt's lymphoma age-adjusted incidence may be influenced by HIV status (Mbulaiteye, et al., 2010).

HIV-associated Burkitt's lymphoma demonstrates identical classic histologic features to the other classes of Burkitt's lymphomas (see Figure 10). Whether nodal or extra-nodal, the classic Burkitt's histomorphology is a diffuse effacement of normal tissue architecture by sheets of cohesive intermediately sized (~12 μm) cells with minimal basophilic cytoplasm and central round to oval nuclei usually with multiple distinct nucleoli. These cells are interspersed by larger macrophages (bearing characteristic reniform or kidney-bean shaped nuclei) with enlarged pale cytoplasm often containing engulfed cellular debris; these interspersed "tangible-body" macrophages produced the characteristic "starry-sky" appearance. The macroscopic corollary to this histomorphology is the typical fish-flesh tan white irregular tumour mass. As in most lymphomas, however, there are no macroscopic features characteristic of given specific entity. One unique histopathological feature observed more frequently in HIV-associated Burkitt's lymphomas is Burkitt's lymphoma with a lymphoblastic morphology. In these cases, the tumour cells are notable for their eccentric nuclei, prominent central large nucleoli, and often contain cytoplasmic eosinophilic globules representing immunoglobulin deposits (Leoncini, et al., 2008). These features are observed in up to two-thirds of cases according to the WHO (Leoncini, et al., 2008).

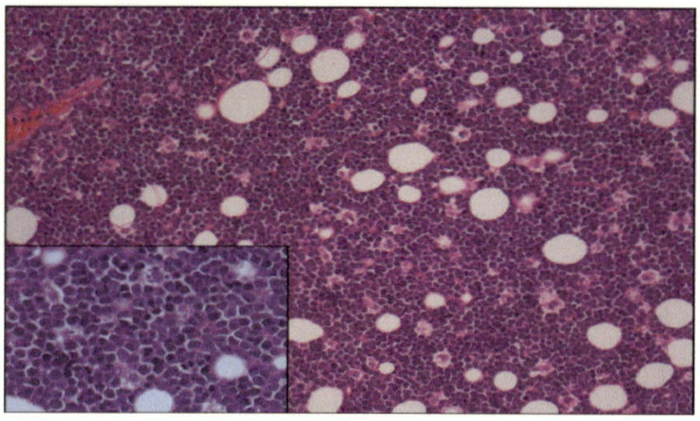

Fig. 10. HIV-associated Burkitt's lymphoma: diffuse "starry-sky" appearance of intermediate-sized cells; inset: high-power of Burkitt cells with scattered macrophages (containing tingible bodies or engulfed debris). The optically clear spaces are fat droplets (this biopsy was taken from a mesenteric lymph node).

Similar immunophenotypic features to the endemic and sporadic Burkitt's forms are observed in HIV-associated Burkitt's lymphoma. The tumour cells are B-cells, demonstrating a variety of possible B-cell antigens including CD19, CD20 and CD22. Burkitt's lymphomas of all types demonstrate characteristic positivity for BCL-6 and CD10 (both immunomarkers of germinal centre phenotype). Unlike diffuse large B-cell lymphomas of germinal centre origin, furthermore, Burkitt's cells are only weakly positive (and often completely negative) for BCL2-. The Ki-67 proliferation immunostain is also characteristically positive nearly in 100%of Burkitt's cells (indicating an extremely high cell proliferation index). To aid in distinguishing Burkitt's lymphomas from precursor B-cell neoplasms (such as pre-B ALL and others, which may have overlapping morphologic features with Burkitt's lymphoma), the TdT stain (a stain indicating a primitive phenotype) is characteristically negative in Burkitt's lymphoma.

The molecular and cytogenetic features in Burkitt's lymphomas (while not entirely specific) are also characteristic. Translocation of the proto-oncogenic MYC region (which encodes a highly conserved cellular transcription factor) to the transcriptionally active IG heavy chain gene, t(8:14), is the most frequently encountered cytogenetic mutation in Burkitt's lymphoma. As previously noted, this translocation is not specific; MYC:IGH translocations have been observed in many diffuse large B-cell lymphomas (often themselves demonstrating high cellular proliferation indices) as well as other malignancies. Using sensitive molecular techniques, EBV virus sequences are observed in 50-70% of HIV-associated Burkitt's lymphomas. This is in contrast to the endemic form, which are virtually all found to contain EBV sequences, as well as the sporadic form which only rarely are found to harbor EBV co-infection.

Chemotherapy for HIV-associated Burkitt's lymphoma is has evolved as the HIV/AIDS epidemic has progressed. Early on, when most HIV-associated Burkitt's patients presented having previously been diagnosed with AIDS, the chemotherapy treatment regimen applied to Burkitt's lymphomas focused on minimizing iatrogenic immunodeficiency. In these cases, the rapid progression characteristic of Burkitt's lymphoma was unfortunately allowed to sway the balance in favor of early mortality from lymphoma (Levine, et al., 2000). Later, with the introduction of anti-retrovirals and the accompanying benefit of improved immunostatus, chemotherapy has evolved toward similar regimens used in the endemic and sporadic Burkitt's lymphomas. Modern HIV-associated Burkitt's lymphomas seem to be treated most commonly with combinations of cyclophosphamide, vincristine, doxorubicin, cytarabine, methotrexate with or without rituximab. Use of the latter anti-CD20 antibody (used frequently to augment the chemotherapeutic response in numerous B-cell lymphomas) remains controversial, in particular relative to the potential immunocompromise that the latter may induce (Levine, et al., 2000); studies exploring optimal treatment regimens in HIV-associated Burkitt's lymphoma are limited given the relative rarity of cases (Noy, 2010).

3.2 Diffuse large B-cell lymphoma

Diffuse large B-cell lymphoma is a heterogeneous category of lymphomas typified by an aggressive clinical aspect, a large cell histomorphology (i.e. neoplastic cells greater than two-times the normal lymphocyte) and B-cell immunophenotype. This category has been the subject of a multitude of classifications over the course of the previous half-century. Currently, the most commonly used WHO classification acknowledges a number of possible "large B-cell" entities, of which diffuse large B-cell lymphoma not otherwise specified is probably the most common. Other diffuse large B-cell lymphoma subtypes (other than the NOS subtype) include rare entities such as primary diffuse large B-cell lymphoma of the central nervous system (an entity characteristically found in HIV/AIDS patients). The current WHO classification schema also allows for molecular and immunohistochemical subgroups in addition to morphologic classes; some of these subgroups have gained notoriety for their distinct therapeutic responses. While a complete description of diffuse large B-cell lymphoma is beyond the scope of this chapter, we will focus heretofore on the specific distinguishing features of HIV/AIDS related diffuse large B-cell lymphomas.

While the most recent edition of the WHO Classification of Hematolymphoid tumours suggests that diffuse large B-cell lymphoma in HIV is second to Burkitt's lymphoma as the most common lymphoma encountered in HIV/AIDS, newer studies have suggested that diffuse large B-cell lymphoma may in fact be more common (Raphaël, et al., 2008; Mantina, et al., 2010; Gucalp & Noy, 2010). There also appear to have been changes in the incidence of diffuse large B-cell lymphoma over the course of the HIV/AIDS epidemic: at the outset in the early to mid 1980s, diffuse large cell lymphoma was very infrequently diagnosed; a marked increase in this diagnosis was seen toward the mid to late 1990s, however (Levine, et al., 2000). These latter results may relate to the observation that diffuse large B-cell lymphoma in HIV/AIDS appears to afflict patients in the setting of long-standing infection with concomitantly low CD4 counts, in contrast to other HIV-associated lymphomas (Raphaël, et al., 2008). As with most HIV-associated lymphomas, diffuse large B-cell lymphoma can often be found in extra-nodal sites; this entity, furthermore, is commonly associated with central nervous system involvement (Agarwal, et al., 2009); furthermore, while overall numbers of central nervous system lymphomas in HIV/AIDS have dropped since the onset of the antiretroviral era, diffuse large-B-cell lymphoma currently seems to be the most frequent offender in the central nervous system (Agarwal, et al., 2009). Important clinical prognostic factors have been noted as pertaining to HIV-associated diffuse large B-cell lymphoma: Vaccher and colleagues noted the importance of CD4 counts, in addition to the other factors incorporated into the international prognostic index (namely age, advanced stage disease, elevated levels of serum lactate dehydrogenase as an indicator of rapid neoplastic cell turnover, extranodal spread and functional performance status) (Vaccher, et al., 1996).

The macroscopic and microscopic features of diffuse large B-cell lymphoma in HIV/AIDS are comparable to those seen in the non-HIV population. Diffuse large B-cell lymphoma generally causes uniform enlargement of a node or group of nodes, often with a characteristic "fish flesh" macroscopic cut surface. On microscopic exam, sheets of large cells typically efface the normal lymph node architecture (these cells are often greater than 12 μm in maximal dimension) (see Figure 11). These neoplastic cells will demonstrate variable cytoplasm, variably sized nuclei, often with clumping or vesciculated chromatin and variable nucleoli. Areas of necrosis may be present, either as individual cells or clusters of cells. Mitotic figures are common and markedly atypical mitoses may be frequent. Often, however, it is difficult to ascribe any specific morphologic features other than diffuse architecture and large cell size to diffuse large B-cell lymphomas. When involving extra-nodal sites, the same diffuse pattern of effaced normal tissue architecture can also be seen, sometimes producing an obvious mass suspicious for a metastatic lesion. The predominant cell type will be the large neoplastic B-cell with variable numbers of intervening fibroblasts and inflammatory cells, sometimes producing a desmoplastic response. In these circumstances, it may be necessary to exclude a malignancy of origin other than the hematolymphoid system such as a carcinoma; these differential diagnoses are usually quickly excluded using a panel of immunohistochemical stains.

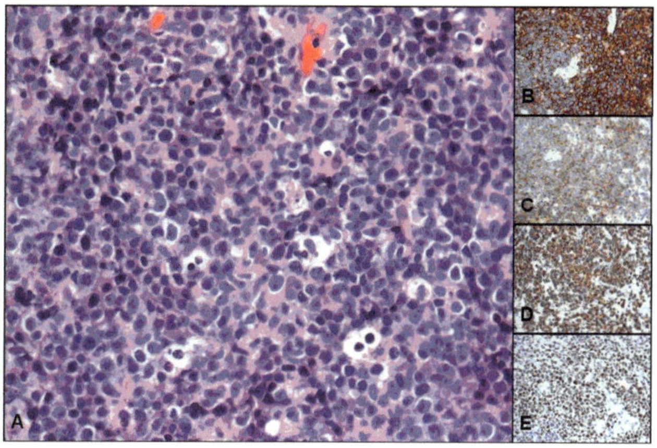

Fig. 11. Diffuse Large B-cell Lymphoma: A: Diffuse pattern of infiltration by pleomorphic large cells; B: CD20 immunostain confirming B-cell lineage; C: CD10 immunostain suggesting germinal centre phenotype; D: BCL2 immunostain strongly and diffusely positive, as is consistent with a B-cell neoplasm; E: BCL6 immunostain suggesting germinal centre phenotype

Immunophenotyping, either by immunohistochemistry or flow cytometry (or ideally both) is required. Diffuse large B-cell lymphomas must, by definition, express one or more of the B-cell markers (e.g. CD19, CD20, CD79a, PAX5, etc.). Diffuse large B-cell lymphomas will frequently be positive for BCL2, though poorly differentiated forms may show only focal or patchy staining. Subsequent stratification of the lesion into "germinal centre" or "non-germinal centre" types is then recommended; the former will generally demonstrate expression of either BCL6 or CD10 (both germinal centre markers) whereas the latter are typically both BCL6 and CD10 negative and may also be MUM-1 positive. This form of stratification can be helpful in directing treatment. More specifically, it has been

demonstrated by means of both gene expression profiling (and the surrogate use of immunophenotyping) that diffuse large B-cell lymphomas with a germinal centre phenotype/gene expression profile have a better prognosis (Chang, et al., 2004). Additional staining with Ki67 to demonstrate neoplastic cell proliferation index is also recommended. Diffuse large B-cell lymphomas typically demonstrate a Ki67 proliferation index less than 60-70%; higher indices may suggest a more aggressive entity. High Ki67 index in combination with BCL6 positivity and weak BCL2 staining raises the possibility of a lymphoma intermediate between a diffuse large B-cell and Burkitt's lymphoma. Staining with CD38 or CD138 is also helpful in ruling out a potentially highly aggressive plasmablastic phenotype. Studies have also demonstrated a negative association between HIV-associated diffuse large B-cell lymphoma progression free-survival as well as overall survival and co-infection with EBV (Park, et al., 2007). In our experience however studies exploring the contribution of EBV to the specific pathogenesis of HIV-associated diffuse large B-cell lymphoma are lacking.
The treatment of HIV-associated diffuse large B-cell lymphoma has traditionally been the same as those cases in the HIV-negative population, namely with a combination of cyclophosphamide, doxorubicin, vincristine, and prednisone. This approach has been met with controversy however as a variety of studies using more traditionally "aggressive" chemotherapy regimens, regimens with concomitant rituximab therapy and even regimens incorporating a reduction in antiretroviral therapy have shown promising results in their own rights. Navaro and colleagues demonstrated that patients with HIV-associated diffuse large B-cell lymphoma treated with routine chemotherapy but with additional antiretrovirals demonstrated no significant differences in clinical and laboratory parameters relative to HIV-negative cases of diffuse large B-cell lymphoma (with the caveat that HIV cases were more likely to present with B-symptoms) (Navarro, et al., 2005) Ezzat and colleagues recently indicated that a combination of rituximab with standard chemotherapy and antiretrovirals improved the survival of HIV patients with diffuse large B-cell lymphoma; this study also incorporated epidemiologic data from before and after the antiretroviral era to elucidate a difference in survivability (Ezzat, et al., 2007). In a recent study, Dunleavy and colleagues performed a trial of chemotherapy using short-course etoposide, prednisone, vincristine, cyclophosphamide, doxorubicin and rituximab after having halted antiretroviral therapy for the duration of the chemotherapy (with subsequent restart after completion) (Dunleavy, et al., 2010). In their cohort of 33 authors reported a progression free survival and overall survival of 84% and 68% respectively after a median follow-up of 5 years; 10 deaths were reported with 5 attributed to HIV (3 due to purported previous persistent mycobacterial infection) (Dunleavy, et al., 2010). Head-to-head outcome comparisons, with and without antiretroviral therapy (with particular attention to the long-term effects of short-term iatrogenic HIV-related immunosuppression) have yet to be reported.

3.3 Hodgkin's lymphoma

Thomas Hodgkin, a British physician, first described this strange disease in 1832. Over the course of his work as a pathologist working in Guy's Hospital's anatomical library in London, he noted a number of patients at autopsy with bizarre lymphadenopathy (Mukherhee, 2010). These patients were frequently young and male and died rapidly after a brief fever-stricken illness (Mukherhee, 2010). Having received a less than stellar response to his newly reported disease, he abandoned any further academic exploration of this peculiar lymphadenopathy (and, furthermore, abandoned his life's work soon after) (Mukherhee, 2010). The disease was later further characterized by Samuel Wilks, who coined the eponym "Hodgkin disease" (Stone, 2010). It was not until decades after the first descriptions of Hodgkin's lymphoma that the microscopic feature of the disease—the Reed-Sternberg cell—was discovered by Carl Sternberg of Germany (followed by Dorothy Reed Mendenhall) (Mukherhee, 2010). The current state of the art suggests that the Reed-Sternberg cell is a germinal centre B-cells, as evidenced by the detection of immunoglobulin gene re-arrangements; these cells, it is thought, demonstrate abortive differentiation and therefore do not proceed to produce immunoglobulin (Ioachim & Medeiros, 2009g). Reed-Sternberg cells have also been found to produce a number of pro-inflammatory cytokines; these, it is believed, contribute to the spectrum of "by-stander" non-neoplastic inflammatory cells which make up the majority of the cellular constituents in Hodgkin's lymphomas (Ioachim & Medeiros, 2009g).

One of the earliest series of Hodgkin's lymphomas in a cohort of probable AIDS patients was reported by Ioachim and colleagues (Ioachim, et al., 1985). In this series, only 3 of 21 patients in this study were diagnosed with Hodgkin's lymphoma (Ioachim, et al., 1985). Since these first cases were diagnosed, many more cases of Hodgkin's lymphoma in HIV/AIDS patients have been identified and modern epidemiologic data suggests that HIV-positive patients have at least a 2-10-fold increased risk of developing Hodgkin's lymphoma relative to the HIV-negative population (Carbone, et al., 2009; Sissolak, et al., 2010). Despite this increase, Hodgkin's lymphoma is infrequent relative to diffuse large B-cell lymphoma and Burkitt's lymphoma (the latter two accounting for at least 60% of HIV-associated lymphomas) (Raphaël, et al., 2008).

The pathobiology of HIV-associated Hodgkin's lymphoma serves to demonstrate the unique environment of immunocompromise that HIV infection causes, even in patients with relatively high CD4 counts or on antiretroviral regimens. More specifically, epidemiologists have observed not only an increased incidence of Hodgkin's lymphoma with severe AIDS related immunocompromise but also a paradoxical increased incidence of Hodgkin's lymphoma in HIV-positive patients without AIDS after the introduction of antiretrovirals. In their large cohort study for instance, Biggar and colleagues noted that there was an increased risk of development of Hodgkin's lymphoma in HIV-positive patients with only moderate immunosuppression (Biggar, et al., 2006). Experts have offered hypotheses to explain these unique observations. It is thought that the Reed-Sternberg cell of Hodgkin's lymphoma relies upon intact immunomodulatory signals from T-cells. With T-cell numbers sufficiently stabilized in HIV-infection treated with antiretrovirals—but in an immunologically active environment caused by chronic HIV infection with upregulated inflammatory cytokine production—Reed-Sternberg cells may be inadvertently stimulated and Hodgkin's lymphoma may develop (Sissolak, et al., 2010). Despite the relatively low risk of Hodgkin's lymphoma in HIV-infection, therefore, it is incumbent that HIV patients on anti-retroviral therapy be carefully surveilled for the development of potential Hodgkin's lymphoma.

As noted previously, HIV/AIDS patients are at extremely high risk for lymphadenopathy; when these patients present with symptoms of fever, chills, night sweats and weight loss, furthermore, a long differential must be considered—with lymphomas high on the list. Most HIV-associated Hodgkin's cases will present with lymphadenopathy, typically in a cervical distribution (Sissolak, et al., 2010). Perhaps due to the unique pathobiology of HIV-associated Hodgkin's lymphomas, many HIV-associated Hodgkin patients present at a relatively young age (in addition to possibly presenting earlier on in the course of infection). Many of these patients will also present with advanced stage disease relative to the HIV-negative population (Sissolak, et al., 2010). High clinical suspicion warrants lymph node biopsy, which is required for accurate diagnosis. Most authorities also recommend an initial staging bone marrow biopsy given that 40-60% of cases present with bone marrow involvement (Sissolak, et al., 2010).

While a complete discussion of the possible histological subtypes of Hodgkin's lymphoma is beyond the scope of this chapter, it is warranted to discuss the histopathologic features of the most common form, namely the mixed cellularity subtype of classical Hodgkin's lymphoma. As in all the classical Hodgkin lymphoma subtypes, mixed cellularity subtype is characterized by the presence of scattered Reed-Sternberg cells (see Figure 12). These have a characteristic morphology: the cells are large (~15-40 μm) with abundant lightly basophilic cytoplasm and they have a central bilobed nucleus, each lobe having a central large inclusion-like eosinophilic nucleolus. More importantly relative to the other forms of Hodgkin's lymphoma, the mixed cellularity subtype demonstrates a diffuse effacement of normal lymph node architecture by a mixed population of inflammatory cells consisting of variable number of eosinophils, small lymphocytes, histiocytes, plasma cells and neutrophils. Also, this subtype lacks the characteristic fibrous bands of sclerosis that typify the nodular sclerosing subtype.

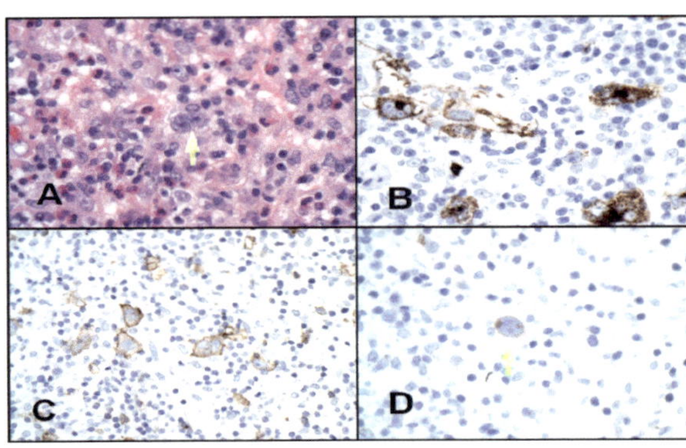

Fig. 12. Hodgkin's lymphoma: A: High-power view demonstrating Reed-Sternberg cell (arrow); B & C: CD15 and CD30 immunostains, respectively; D: EBV stain positive in Reed-Sternberg cell (arrow)

The immunophenotype is also characteristic of mixed cellularity Hodgkin's lymphoma. In particular, the Reed-Sternberg cell is characteristically positive for CD15 (a membrane protein involved in cell adhesion present on a number of hematolymphoid lineage cells) and CD30 (a marker of cell activation). Reed-Sternberg cells seen in Classical Hodgkin's lymphoma are also characteristically negative for the standard B-cell markers CD19 and CD20. Proof of the B-cell nature of Reed-Sternberg cells, however, may be derived from their frequent positive staining for PAX5, a B-cell transcription factor. Most cases of HIV-associated Hodgkin's lymphoma are also positive for EBV co-infection, often identifiable using the immunostain for the EBV-latent membrane protein antigen. This is in contrast to notably fewer cases of EBV positivity outside of HIV-infection (Carbone, et al., 2009).

Treatment approaches for HIV-associated Hodgkin's lymphomas are often similar to those used in non-HIV patients. Limited disease may be treated by a combination of adriamycin, bleomycin, vinblastine and dacarbazine chemotherapy, often with adjuvant radiation therapy to the involved area (if restricted to an amenable nodal region). Advanced cases are not typically amenable to radiation therapy (Sissolak, et al., 2010). Advanced cases may also be considered for bone marrow transplant. The use of rituximab as an adjuvant biological agent may also be considered; those cases demonstrating a large complement of CD20 cells (whether Reed-Sternberg or not) may respond (Sissolak, et al., 2010). Notably, studies looking at the appropriateness of traditional treatments for Hodgkin's disease in the context of HIV-positivity remain ongoing and optimal regimens may yet be discovered. Despite the potential etiologic impact of antiretroviral therapy in cases of HIV-associated Hodgkin's lymphoma, its use is still warranted given the reduction in risk of opportunistic infection (and other HIV-associated malignancies) in order that optimal chemotherapeutic regimens be instituted (Carbone, et al., 2009).

3.4 Plasmablastic lymphoma

Plasmablastic lymphoma is a highly aggressive B-cell lymphoma characterized histologically by a diffuse proliferation of large cells with plasmacytoid features. This entity was only recently recognized and has been shown to occur not only in HIV/AIDS patients but in other immunodeficient individuals, in particular in patients chronically immunosuppressed from solid organ transplants (Rafaniello Raviele, et al., 2009). In its most recent editions, probably owing to its unique clinicopathologic features, plasmablastic lymphoma was classified as an entity unto itself (Raphaël, et al., 2008). Many authors (and other previous classifications) consider plasmablastic lymphoma to be a variant of diffuse large B-cell lymphoma; Chang and colleagues, for example, demonstrated that plasmablastic lymphoma shows a number of overlapping genomic lesions with diffuse large B-cell lymphoma by comparative genomic hybridization techniques (Chang, et al., 2009). Nonetheless, from a treatment and prognostic perspective, plasmablastic lymphoma appears to differ from diffuse large B-cell lymphoma and its classification as a distinct entity is reasonable (Montes-Moreno, et al., 2010).

A number of reports have noted plasmablastic lymphoma arising from transformation from various low-grade lymphomas. Ouansafi and colleagues demonstrated evolution of a follicular lymphoma to plasmablastic lymphoma by means of sequence comparison of the immunoglobulin heavy chain gene rearrangements in both tumours (Ouansafi, et al., 2010). Another report of a plasmablastic lymphoma was described arising in concert with a monoclonal population of plasma cells suggesting potential transformation of the former from the latter (Qing, et al., 2011). Even more intriguing is the case report of concurrent plasmablastic lymphoma and classical Hodgkin's lymphoma arising in a patient with relative immunosuppression from history of chronic lymphocytic leukemia/lymphoma; this case was notably EBV positive (Foo, et al., 2010). The grand majority of cases, however, appear not to represent transformation from a lower grade lesion.

Estimates of the incidence of plasmablastic lymphoma are based on the few reported cases and small series; a recent review of the literature reported approximately 180 cases of plasmablastic lymphoma (Rafaniello Raviele, et al., 2009). While this number is undoubtedly an underestimate (since at least one other unreported case from our own institution in the previous 5 years was encountered), it speaks to the rarity of this entity. The majority of cases are encountered in the HIV/AIDS setting and many, though not all, of the remaining cases are associated with transplant related immunosuppression (Rafaniello Raviele, et al., 2009). The majority of cases, furthermore, were found to be EBV positive (Rafaniello Raviele, et al., 2009). While most cases of plasmablastic lymphoma have demonstrated an odd predilection for the oral cavity, many reports have noted a number of broad ranging almost invariably extranodal sites. A number of reported cases have demonstrated involvement of the central nervous system (Ustun, et al., 2009); involvement of the gastrointestinal tract has also been reported (Rafaniello Raviele, et al., 2009); there are even unique reports of plasmablastic lymphoma involving the penis and vulva (Sun, et al., 2011; Chabay, et al., 2009). Studies have furthermore demonstrated some intriguing clinicopathological factors pertaining to the primary site of plasmablastic lymphomas. Hanra and colleagues for instance, in comparing oral and extraoral cases of plasmablastic lymphoma, demonstrated a distinct survival difference favouring the oral forms (Hansra, et al., 2010).

Plasmablastic lymphoma has also demonstrated different clinicopathologic features in the HIV/AIDS population relative to other immunosuppressed populations. Castillo et al. demonstrated that HIV positive cases of plasmablastic lymphoma tend to occur in younger, typically male patients with a notable preponderance for the oral cavity (Castillo, et al., 2010). Castillo et al. also demonstrated a distinct survival difference between the HIV positive and negative cases of plasmablastic lymphoma, favouring those from HIV positive patients (Castillo, et al., 2010).

Regardless of the primary site or of HIV status, plasmablastic lymphoma demonstrates consistent histological characteristics (see Figure 13). Plasmablastic lymphoma shows a monomorphic morphology comprised of large cells with abundant often-eosinophilic cytoplasm and eccentrically located hyperchromatic nucleus often containing one or more nucleoli. The tumoural cells demonstrate a uniformly diffuse architecture, often with a number of interspersed apoptotic bodies and mitotic figures. Intermingled macrophages or smaller plasma cells may be noted; in some cases in which the latter are particularly abundant, the plasmablastic lymphoma with "plasmacytic differentiation" may be applied.

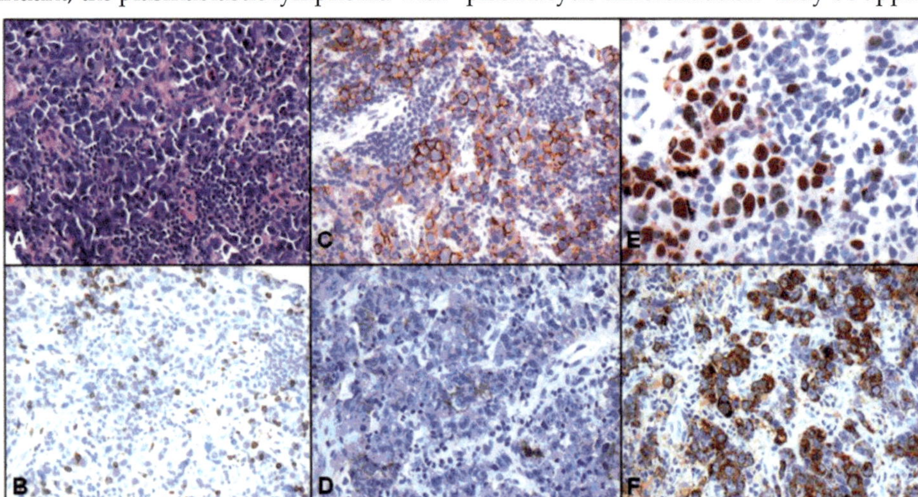

Fig. 13. A: Plasmablastic Lymphoma. B: LCA positive in reactive small T lymphocytes and negative in large neoplastic cells. C: CD138 positive in large neoplastic cells. D: EMA positive in large neoplastic cells. E: MUM-1 positive in large neoplastic cells. F: Lambda light chain positive in large neoplastic cells

In order to distinguish plasmablastic lymphoma for other diffuse lymphomas (and to rule out a simple but more common diffuse large B-cell lymphoma), immunophenotyping is crucial. In plasmablastic lymphoma, in addition to demonstrating minimal positivity for leukocyte common antigen (CD45), CD20 and CD79a, the tumoural cells are invariably positive for CD138; these features are of striking resemblance to the normal immunophenotype of plasma cells. Other post germinal centre markers such as MUM-1 and CD38 are also often positive. Some additional pathologic features that may potentially confuse the diagnosis include positivity for CD3, CD4 and CD56, all of which have been reported to be positive in some cases of plasmablastic lymphoma (Rafaniello Raviele, et al., 2009). Given the primary immunophenotypic differential diagnosis of a plasma cell malignancy (i.e. based on the combination of CD38, CD138, MUM-1 positivity with CD45, CD20 and CD79a negativity), the plasmablastic moniker is assigned given the histomorphology in combination with the absence of clinical features in support of a plasma cell dyscrasia. Plasma cell neoplasms also do not demonstrate positivity for EBV. Other possible differential diagnoses include carcinomas and melanomas, which can be ruled out by the way of an immunohistochemical panel of cytokeratins and melanoma markers. Goedhals et al. explored the electron microscopic features of ten plasmablastic lymphomas and found that 90% of cases demonstrated the consistent plasma cell features of eccentric nuclei with concentric perinuclear endoplasmic reticulum (Goedhals, et al., 2006)

The outcomes in cases of plasmablastic lymphoma are usually poor. In their in depth review, Raviele and colleagues noted disease related deaths in 59.6% of cases of oral-type plasmablastic lymphoma at an average of 10.4 months post-diagnosis as compared to 58.6%at an average of 6.2 months for the extra-oral type (Rafaniello Raviele, et al., 2009). Raviele and colleagues also noted a survival advantage to the use of highly active anti-retrovirals (Rafaniello Raviele, et al., 2009). Given the rarity of plasmablastic lymphoma, there are few studies addressing optimal chemotherapeutics; one large series of published cases noted that the most common chemotherapeutic regimen in plasmablastic lymphoma cases is CHOP (Castillo, et al., 2010). Other more intensive regimens have also been used (e.g. the CODOX-M, often used for HIV-associated Burkitt's lymphoma cases). Two case reports have noted responses to chemotherapy with bortezomib (Bibas, et al., 2010; Bose, et al., 2009); trials looking at optimal treatment regimens are lacking, however.

3.5 Primary effusion/body cavity lymphoma

Primary effusion/body cavity lymphoma is a rare aggressive lymphoma with a peculiar propensity for the serous cavities of the body, namely the peritoneum, pleura and pericardium. These lymphomas are also not primarily associated with a solid component though they may later develop nearby solid tumours and may extend to involve of lymph nodes. Primary effusion lymphoma is characteristically a disease of HIV/AIDS patients, though rare cases have been reported in HIV negative patients. Primary effusion lymphomas are also almost invariably positive for HHV-8 and may show co-infection with EBV.

Knowles and colleagues diagnosed the first cases of primary effusion lymphoma in 1989. Three cases were originally reported, all occurring in homosexual HIV-positive males with clinical features of AIDS. Each case presented with a body cavity effusion containing cytologically malignant cells and quickly died. The effusions were all noted to contain populations of large cells with generous eosinophilic to amphophilic cytoplasm, anisonucleosis and clumped chromatin. Several multinucleated giant cells and abnormal mitotic figures were also noted. The malignant effusion cells were positive for CD45, indicating a hematolymphoid origin, but were negative for B- and T-cell markers as well as a variety of myelomonocytic markers. Subsequent restriction fragment analysis of the DNA obtained from the neoplastic cells revealed immunoglobulin gene rearrangements, suggesting a B-cell origin. The three original cases were also found to be EBV positive; these cases were not tested for HHV-8 positivity in the original publication

Since the first reported cases, several more have been reported; this entity is nonetheless very rare relative to the other HIV/AIDS-associated lymphomas and accounts for approximately 3% (Boulanger, et al., 2005). The WHO notes that this lymphoma is most commonly encountered in HIV patients, but that some cases have been encountered in HIV-seronegative patients and even within the context of immunocompetence (Raphaël, et al., 2008). Primary effusion/body cavity lymphoma cells are almost invariably HHV-8 positive. This is of particular interest in those cases encountered in immunocompetent patients since, as a result of the high prevalence of HHV-8 infection, there is a notably increased risk in peoples (especially males) of the Mediteranean (Said & Cesarman, 2008).

In one of the largest and more recent series of primary effusion/body cavity lymphomas, Boulanger and colleagues reported a wide age range (33-78 years) with only one female of 28 cases (Boulanger, et al., 2005). While the majority of cases were noted to originate in patients from populations with low HHV-8 seroprevalence, Boulanger et al. did note that a substantial number (38%) of patients originated from geographic areas with seroprevalence higher than 5% (Boulanger, et al., 2005). Most cases were noted to present with effusions, predominantly pleural (Boulanger, et al., 2005). Primary effusion/body cavity lymphoma typically remains restricted to the original presenting body cavity (Carbone, et al., 2010). Involved serosal surfaces are often diffusely thickened (Carbone, et al., 2010). Interestingly, 42% of Boulanger et al.'s cases presented with additional extra-cavitary lesions. It has also been documented that many primary effusion/body cavity lymphoma patients have preceding or complicating Kaposi's sarcoma (Boulanger, et al., 2005). Most patients are also profoundly immunosuppressed; in the HIV-positive cohort of Boulanger et al. for example, the average CD4 count was below 200 cells/μL (Boulanger, et al., 2005).

Diagnosis of primary effusion/body cavity lymphoma is typically made on cytologic examination of effusion contents (see Figure 14). As Carbone and colleagues note, the malignant cells of primary effusion/body cavity lymphoma have an appearance resembling a combination of immunoblastic and anaplastic features (Carbone, et al., 2010). A variable degree of plasma cell differentiation may also be noted; a background of pronounced cellular debris and numerous mitoses often accompanies these features. A mixture of reactive inflammatory cells as well as admixed mesothelial cells will also be noted. These morphological features result in a differential diagnosis that may include Burkitt's lymphoma (which may also involve body cavities); as with most lymphomas, however, the immunophenotype will typically indicate the diagnosis. The effusive nature of this lymphoma is highly conducive to flow cytometry. Primary effusion/body cavity lymphoma, as noted previously, demonstrates CD45, CD138 and MUM-1 positivity in the context of dim or negative immunostaining for B-cell markers. This immunohistochemical pattern reflects the plasmablastic phenotype of primary effusion/body cavity lymphoma. Interestingly, a few cases have noted aberrant T-cell antigen expression (Carbone, et al., 2010). The diagnostic clincher, however, is the demonstration of HHV-8 positivity in the tumour cells; this can usually be accomplished reliably with immunohistochemical staining for the HHV-8 latency-associated nuclear antigen.

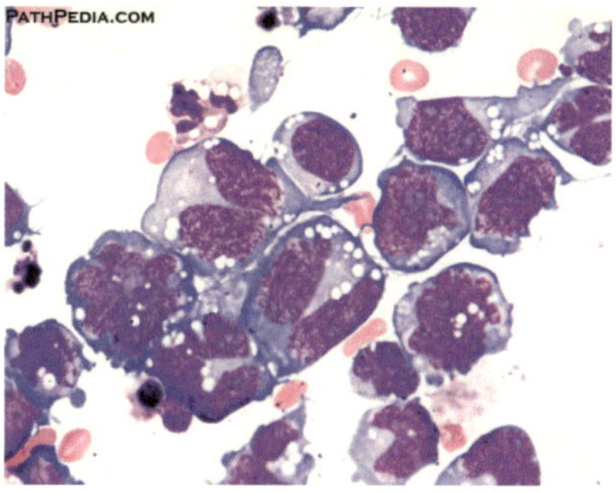

Fig. 14. Primary Effusion Lymphoma: Large cells with clear-coloured cytoplasmic bodies (vescicles containing immunoglobulin); note the eccentrically placed nuclei in a number of the cells, others with large atypical lobated nuclei and prominent nucleoli. Compare the size. difference of the neoplastic cells with the small normally sized (dark stained) round lymphocyte nucleus at the bottom left.

Despite its rarity, a number of studies have explored the molecular pathogenesis of primary effusion/body cavity lymphoma. Gene expression profile studies in primary effusion/body cavity lymphoma have demonstrated a unique profile relative to other aggressive lymphomas; these results tend to substantiate the distinct clinicopathologic distinction of primary effusion/body cavity lymphomas from other lymphomas (Ueda, et al., 2010). Other studies have demonstrated a number of complex cytogenetic abnormalities as well as a reduction in tumour-suppressor gene expression in primary effusion/body cavity lymphoma (Luan, et al., 2010; O'Hara, et al., 2009); these features may further contribute to the aggressiveness of this lesion.

Most published cases appear to be treated with CHOP or derivations thereof. Fewer cases have been treated with a more "aggressive" approach in line with regimens such as doxorubicin, cyclophosphamide, vindesine, bleomycin, prednisone. Some reported cases were also tried on an antiviral regimen (e.g. interferon alpha and cidofovir); the efficacy of these drugs in this context is uncertain, however. Unfortunately, regardless of the chemotherapy regimen, outcomes are poor. In Boulanger and colleagues' cohort, for example, only 14 of 28 patients received clinical remission and only 32% were alive after a median follow-up of 3.2 years (Boulanger, et al., 2005). Most patients who relapse, furthermore, will die of disease (Boulanger, et al., 2005). As in other HIV-associated lymphomas, prognosis appears to be improved with the early incorporation of anti-retroviral medications (Boulanger, et al., 2005; Carbone, et al., 2010).

3.6 T-cell lymphomas

T-cell lymphomas occurring in HIV/AIDS are substantially rarer that B-cell lymphomas. In their large cohort study of 302,834 AIDS patients, Biggar and colleagues noted that only 1.4%of non-hodgkin's lymphomas were of T-cell phenotype (Biggar, et al., 2001). Nonetheless, considering the extreme rarity of T-cell lymphomas in general, Biggar and colleagues estimated a relative risk of 15 of a T-cell lymphoma in the HIV positive population relative to the HIV negative population (Biggar, et al., 2001).

The first documented HIV positive T-cell lymphoma was noted in 1988 by Nasr and colleagues (Nasr, et al., 1988). This case consisted of a large cell lymphoma demonstrating loss of CD3 but with preservation of CD2 and CD4 immunoreactivity. Although CD30 and ALK-1 immunoreactivity were not reported in this case, the reported morphologic features seem most in keeping with anaplastic large cell lymphoma. The earliest reported T-cell lymphoma in a patient with suspected AIDS, however, predated Nasr and colleagues' case by four years; this case was reported in Japan in a patient with AIDS-defining clinical characteristics but co-infected by human t-cell lymphoma/leukemia virus-1 (Kobayashi, et al., 1984).

The most common T-cell lymphoma encountered in HIV-positive patients appears to be peripheral T-cell lymphoma, unspecified (Biggar, et al., 2001; Arzoo, et al., 2004). Several cases of anaplastic large cell lymphoma, NK/T-cell lymphoma and angioimmunoblastic T-cell lymphoma have also been reported, however (Biggar, et al., 2001; Arzoo, et al., 2004; Perez, et al., 2010; Castillo, et al., 2011). A few cases of enteropathy-associated T-cell lymphoma as well as adult T-cell leukemia/lymphoma have also been reported, though little specific information pertaining to the role of HIV in these cases could be gleaned (Arzoo, et al., 2004; Castillo, et al., 2011).

In the largest case series to date, Castilo and colleagues noted that the bulk of HIV-associated T-cell lymphomas occurred in males, typically presenting at high stage (stage III-IV), and often accompanied by B-symptoms (fever, night sweats and weight loss) (Castillo, et al., 2011). Similar clinical characteristics were noted in other smaller cohorts (Arzoo, et al., 2004; Perez, et al., 2010). Many T-cell lymphomas in HIV patients will also present with skin findings, apparently in greater proportions than HIV-associated B-cell lymphomas (Arzoo, et al., 2004).

Peripheral T-cell lymphoma, unspecified, typically occurs in lymph nodes and consists of medium to large-sized lymphocytes with irregular nuclei. The neoplastic T-cells usually show a diffuse pattern of involvement, preferentially involving the paracortical zones, often sparing the lymphoid follicles (see Figure 16). HIV-associated anaplastic large cell lymphoma also demonstrates a range of histological features. A range of cell size may be noted from the typical large anaplastic cell to the so-called small cell variant (see Figure 17). These cells may form loosely cohesive clusters, diffuse sheets and, as is often seen in lymph nodes, may present as subtle subcapsular aggregates. Angioimmunoblastic lymphoma, in contrast, is most common described as a diffuse process often completely obliterating the lymph node architecture; most commonly the lymph node will be replaced by an arborizing network of proliferating endothelial cells interspersed by an infiltrate of atypical lymphocytes, often accompanied by various non-neoplastic inflammatory cells. Mycosis fungoides is characterized by band like superficial dermal infiltrates of atypical lymphocytes (often described as "cerebriform") (see Figure 18). When these atypical cerebriform lymphocytes are noted in the peripheral blood or in lymph nodes, the Sezary syndrome is suspected (sezary syndrome does not always demonstrate the same epidermotropism as mycosis fungoides, however, and the skin changes in this context may be non-specific). NK/T-cell lymphomas occur most often in the aerodigestive tract where they often manifest as mucosal ulceration by atypical lymphocytes. These atypical lymphocytes may have ample cytoplasm and irregular convoluted nuclear membranes. An angioinvasive pattern is also common to NK/T-cell lymphoma, typically with associated areas of necrosis.

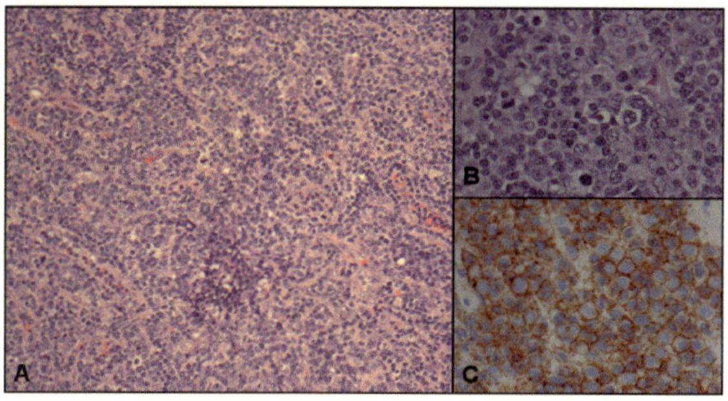

Fig. 15. Peripheral T-cell Lymphoma: A: Atypical cells expanding paracortical interfollicular regions; B: High-power demonstrating atypical cells (larger than normal interfollicular cells) with mitotic figures present; C: Diffuse CD3 positivity confirming T-cell lineage

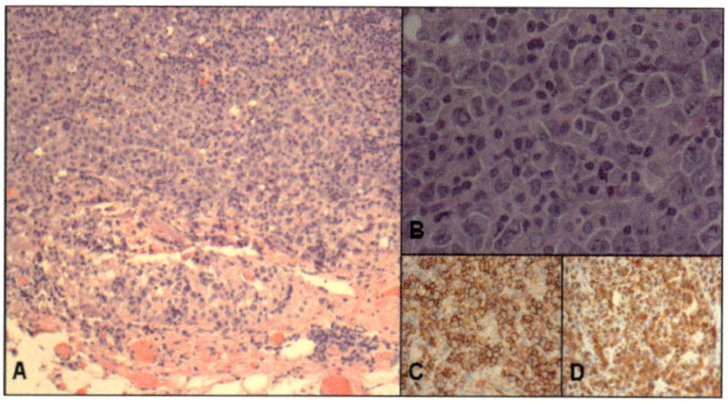

Fig. 16. Anaplastic Large Cell Lymphoma: A: Low-power view of lymph node involved by anaplastic large cell lymphoma showing subcapsular sinus involvement by tumour cells; B: High-power view of tumour cells demonstrating the characteristic hallmark cells (large nuclei with convoluted semi-lunar shapes); C: CD30 immunostain (diffuse positivity in tumour cells); D: ALK-1 immunostain (diffuse positivity in tumour cells)

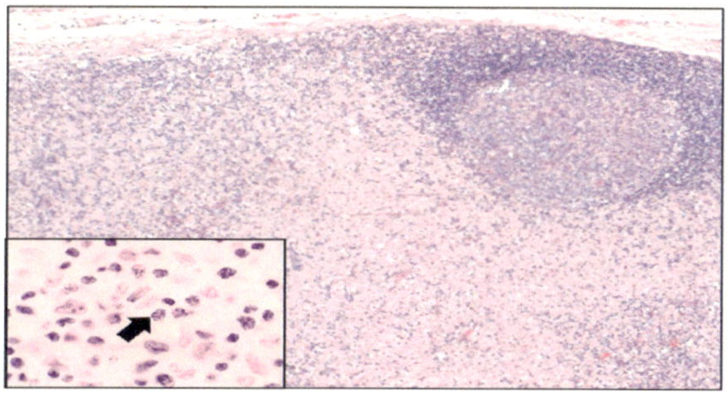

Fig. 17. Mycosis Fungoides: Lymph node demonstrating paracortical expansion by atypical lymphoid infiltrate; inset: large (cerebriform) sezary cells of mycosis fungoides

The typical T-cell lineage markers CD2, CD3, CD5, CD7, CD4, CD8 and CD43 are variably positive in T-cell lymphomas; these markers are useful at demonstrating aberrant phenotype (such as an aberrant CD4:CD8 ratio) or to hint at T-cell lineage neoplasm when the other T-cell markers are negative. The normal progression of T-cell marker ontogenesis proceeds from CD7 to CD2, CD3 and CD5 (in immature T-cells) and then onto CD4 and CD8 (in mature T-cells); the loss of one of the so-called pan-T-Cell markers CD2, CD3, CD5 or CD7 is helpful in the identification of an aberrant (plausibly neoplastic) phenotype. In one of the largest series of HIV-associated anaplastic large cell lymphomas, Perez and colleagues noted that the majority of cases were positive for one or more of CD45, CD2, CD3, CD5, CD4 and CD43 (Perez, et al., 2010); the uniting feature in all cases of ALCL, however, is diffuse strong CD30 positivity. Although the CD30 stain is not entirely specific to anaplastic large cell lymphoma (since this stain is a marker of activated cells), its presence in a diffuse pattern in cells with typically anaplastic morphology is characteristic. Also commonly positive in anaplastic large cell lymphoma is CD45 (also known as leukocyte common antigen, a marker indicating hematolymphoid origin). Interestingly, ALK-1 was noted to be positive in only two of their cases; this is in stark contrast to the non HIV-associated anaplastic large cell lymphomas, which are typically ALK-1 positive (Perez, et al., 2010; Nava, et al., 2008). Although this lack of ALK-1 positivity may represent a distinct molecular feature of HIV-associated anaplastic large cell lymphoma, to our knowledge, no studies have explored this as yet. The neoplastic T-cells in angioimmunoblastic T-cell lymphoma, in addition to staining positive for a number of pan-T-cell markers, are typically positive for CD4 but negative for CD3. These cells also stain positive for a number of markers of follicular centre origin including CD10 and BCL-6. The lymphocytic infiltrates in mycosis fungoides syndrome will often demonstrate a lack of CD3 and CD8 staining often with pronounced CD4 positivity. NK/T-cell lymphoma also demonstrates positivity for one or more pan-T-cell markers, in addition to positivity for CD56 and (unlike most T-cell lymphomas) EBV. These features can easily be demonstrated efficiently, and with only minimal tissue, using flow cytometry.

Most patients with HIV-associated peripheral T-cell lymphomas are treated with a CHOP-based chemotherapy regimen, though a variety of other regimens have also been employed (Castillo, et al., 2011). While most patients seem to demonstrate a complete or partial response to initial therapy, the majority die of progressive disease (Castillo, et al., 2011). A statistically significant improvement in the survival curve of HIV-associated peripheral T-cell lymphomas was also noted in patients treated with anti-retrovirals (Castillo, et al., 2011).

3.7 Lymph node findings in HIV/AIDS related Kaposi's sarcoma

We will limit the discussion of Kaposi's sarcoma in HIV/AIDS to those aspects pertaining to lymph node disease. Whether due to its underlying viral etiology or to the endothelial differentiation of the malignant cell of interest, Kaposi sarcoma often manifests itself in lymph nodes. The disease was first described in 1872 by Moritz Kaposi as a pigmented sarcoma of skin (Mesri, et al., 2010), this form probably represented the modern sporadic subtype seen predominantly in the Mediterranean. In the 1950s, Kaposi's sarcoma was encountered in Africa (Mesri, et al., 2010); this may have represented the first discovery of Kaposi's sarcoma in association with the as yet unknown HIV. When the HIV outbreak was identified, Kaposi's sarcoma was observed to be the most frequent (and AIDS defining) malignancy in this immunocompromised population. It was not until 1996 that a viral pathogen was discovered in association with Kaposi's sarcoma, later named the Kaposi sarcoma herpes virus, or HHV-8 (Mesri, et al., 2010).

Ioachim and colleagues undertook an intriguing study of extra-cutaneous Kaposi's sarcoma in AIDS patients; they noted that lymph nodes were the third most common extra-cutaneous sites of involvement by Kaposi's sarcoma in AIDS cases, next to the gastrointestinal tract and the lungs (Ioachim, et al., 1995). Cases demonstrating primarily nodal involvement may be entirely asymptomatic, with the exception of lymphadenopathy. In these cases the clinical differential diagnosis can be lengthy and histological diagnosis is required.

Lymph nodes involved by Kaposi's sarcoma are typically enlarged and demonstrate preserved architecture in areas not invaded by the tumour, often with follicular hyperplasia (see Figure 18). Involvement of lymph nodes by Kaposi's sarcoma typically begins in the form of triangular nodules with later encroachment into the cortex and medulla; these initial nodules may form wedges with bases parallel to the node capsule. Circular whorled-patterned nodules are also common and can be found throughout the nodal parenchyma. The cells within Kaposi's nodules are spindled with intervening slit-like vascular spaces. The neoplastic cells are usually fairly uniform with plump nuclei; mitoses may be present but are usually not numerous. Characteristic hyaline globules may be seen within Kaposi cells and in nearby histiocytes. Infiltration of tumour foci by lymphocytes, plasma cells and hemosiderin-laden macrophages is also frequent.

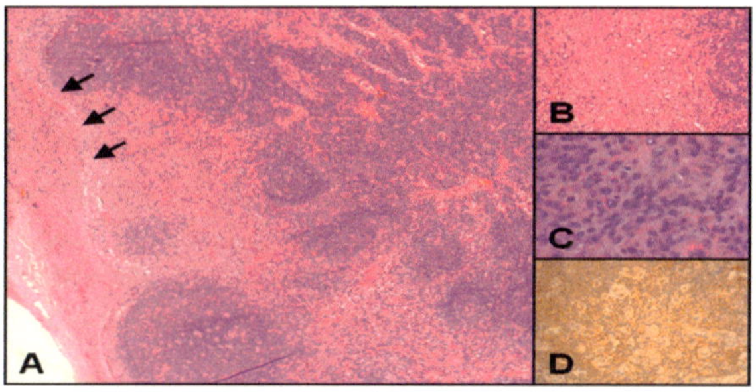

Fig. 18. Kaposi's Sarcoma: A: Low-power view of a lymph node involved by subcapsular nodules of Kaposi's sarcoma; B: Focus of neoplastic endothelial cells encroaching upon a follicle; C: High-power view of neoplastic endothelial cells with notable tumour cell cytoplasmic hyaline globules; D: HHV-8 immunostain demonstrating diffuse positivity

The morphologic differential diagnosis includes many vascular lesions, though the morphologic features are usually characteristic in Kaposi's sarcoma. Bacillary angiomatosis may show nodule formation but typically does not contain the uniformly plump monotonous spindle cells with intervening slit-like spaces seen in Kaposi's sarcoma. The vascular proliferation and hyalinization that may be seen in HIV-associated lymphadenopathy or Castleman's disease may be confused with Kaposi's sarcoma. Angiosarcomas should also be included in the differential diagnosis, though this typically demonstrates are much more sarcomatoid appearance with more marked atypia, necrosis and numerous mitoses. Confusion is avoided by using an immunohistochemical panel including markers for endothelial cells (such as CD31, CD34 or Factor VIII) in combination with a stain for HHV-8.

Antiretroviral therapy is used both to prevent Kaposi's sarcoma but also to treat it. Nonetheless, HIV patients with Kaposi's sarcoma may not respond curatively to antiretroviral optimization and some cases treated with antiretrovirals de novo have been known to develop more severe disease due to the so-called immune reconstitution inflammatory syndrome (in which the presumed increased in inflammatory mediators results in unintentional cytokinetic stimulation of the sarcoma) (Mesri, et al., 2010; Di Lorenzo, et al., 2007). Localized disease may respond to surgery or radiation therapy (though lymph node disease is frequently not localized) and more widespread disease is treated with chemotherapeutic regimens, typically including liposomal anthracyclines and taxanes (Di Lorenzo, et al., 2007). Newer biological therapies including the vascular endothelial growth factor receptor and tyrosine kinase inhibitors are currently being investigated (Di Lorenzo, et al., 2007). Some early studies exploring the use of antivirals (such as gancyclovir and foscarnet) have noted encouraging results though more definitive studies are ongoing (Di Lorenzo, et al., 2007).

4. Conclusion

In the three decades since the beginning of the modern HIV/AIDS epidemic, a great deal of advancement has been made in the understanding of retrovirology, immunology and hematolymphoid pathology. In these 30 years, the recognition of a unique and fastidious retrovirus causing AIDS has occurred, its biologic interaction with human cells has been detailed, and the variety of possible resulting illnesses following infection have been documented. In particular, the range of malignant disease that may occur in HIV/AIDS has been widely enumerated and, thankfully, has shown a distinct reduction in incidence and prevalence since the introduction of antiretroviral therapy, truly a modern medical elixir able to prolong life in a medical context once tantamount to a death sentence.

The above discussion should not only serve to highlight the unique clinical features of HIV-associated hematolymphoid disorders but also demonstrate the unique pathologic work-up necessary to ensure accurate classification and clinical follow-up. In particular, we emphasized the need to obtain tissue biopsies in any scenario in which a potential malignancy is considered. Furthermore, for the pathologist readership, it is imperative to properly handle and work-up a lymph node biopsy from any case in which there is a suspicion of lymphoma; we especially encourage the use of flow cytometry which is an invaluable tool in the diagnosis of lymphoid neoplasms and is extremely helpful in proper classification. Also, in addition to the standard H&E evaluation, a panel of immunohistochemical stains is usually needed to properly identify the lineage, malignant potential and classification of a lymphoid lesion. Many hematolymphoid malignancies require further molecular or cytogenetic work-up as well, the latter requiring fresh tissue.

5. References

Agarwal, P. A., Menon, S., Smruti, B. K. & Singhal, B. S.(2009).Primary central nervous system lymphoma: a profile of 26 cases from Western India.*Neurol.India,*Vol.57, No.6,(Nov-Dec),pp.756-763,0028-3886

Anderson, C. D. & Barrie, H. J.(1960).Fatal pneumocystis pneumonia in an adult. Report of a case. *Am.J.Clin.Pathol.,* Vol.34, (Oct), pp.365-370, 0002-9173

Arzoo, K. K., Bu, X., Espina, B. M., Seneviratne, L., Nathwani, B. & Levine, A. M.(2004).T-cell lymphoma in HIV-infected patients.*J.Acquir.Immune Defic.Syndr.,*Vol.36,No.5,(Aug 15),pp.1020-1027,1525-4135

Bakaki, P., Kayita, J., Moura Machado, J. E., et al.(2001).Epidemiologic and clinical features of HIV-infected and HIV-uninfected Ugandan children younger than 18 months.*J.Acquir.Immune Defic.Syndr.,*Vol.28,No.1,(Sep 1),pp.35-42,1525-4135

Besson, C., Goubar, A., Gabarre, J., et al.(2001).Changes in AIDS-related lymphoma since the era of highly active antiretroviral therapy.*Blood,*Vol.98,No.8,(Oct 15),pp.2339-2344,0006-4971

Bibas, M., Grisetti, S., Alba, L., Picchi, G., Del Nonno, F. & Antinori, A.(2010).Patient with HIV-associated plasmablastic lymphoma responding to bortezomib alone and in combination with dexamethasone, gemcitabine, oxaliplatin, cytarabine, and pegfilgrastim chemotherapy and lenalidomide alone.*J.Clin.Oncol.,*Vol.28,No.34,(Dec 1),pp.e704-8,1527-7755; 0732-183X

Biggar, R. J., Engels, E. A., Frisch, M., Goedert, J. J. & AIDS Cancer Match Registry Study Group(2001).Risk of T-cell lymphomas in persons with AIDS.*J.Acquir.Immune Defic.Syndr.,*Vol.26,No.4,(Apr 1),pp.371-376,1525-4135

Biggar, R. J., Engels, E. A., Ly, S., et al.(2005).Survival after cancer diagnosis in persons with AIDS.*J.Acquir.Immune Defic.Syndr.,*Vol.39,No.3,(Jul 1),pp.293-299,1525-4135

Biggar, R. J., Jaffe, E. S., Goedert, J. J., Chaturvedi, A., Pfeiffer, R. & Engels, E. A.(2006).Hodgkin lymphoma and immunodeficiency in persons with HIV/AIDS.*Blood,*Vol.108,No.12,(Dec 1),pp.3786-3791,0006-4971

Bose, P., Thompson, C., Gandhi, D., Ghabach, B. & Ozer, H.(2009).AIDS-related plasmablastic lymphoma with dramatic, early response to bortezomib.*Eur.J.Haematol.,*Vol.82,No.6,(Jun),pp.490-492,1600-0609; 0902-4441

Boulanger, E., Gerard, L., Gabarre, J., et al.(2005).Prognostic factors and outcome of human herpesvirus 8-associated primary effusion lymphoma in patients with AIDS.*J.Clin.Oncol.,*Vol.23,No.19,(Jul 1),pp.4372-4380,0732-183X

Boyko, W. J., Schechter, M. T., Craib, K. J., et al.(1987).The Vancouver Lymphadenopathy-AIDS Study: 7. Clinical and laboratory features of 87 cases of primary HIV infection.*CMAJ,*Vol.137,No.2,(Jul 15),pp.109-113,0820-3946

BURKITT, D.(1958).A sarcoma involving the jaws in African children.*Br.J.Surg.,*Vol.46,No.197,(Nov),pp.218-223,0007-1323; 0007-1323

Caldwell, R. G., Wilson, J. B., Anderson, S. J. & Longnecker, R.(1998).Epstein-Barr virus LMP2A drives B cell development and survival in the absence of normal B cell receptor signals.*Immunity,*Vol.9,No.3,(Sep),pp.405-411,1074-7613

Caponetti, G. C., Pantanowitz, L., Marconi, S., Havens, J. M., Lamps, L. W. & Otis, C. N.(2009).Evaluation of immunohistochemistry in identifying Bartonella henselae in cat-scratch disease.*Am.J.Clin.Pathol.,*Vol.131,No.2,(Feb), pp.250-256,1943-7722; 0002-9173

Carbone, A., Cesarman, E., Gloghini, A. & Drexler, H. G.(2010).Understanding pathogenetic aspects and clinical presentation of primary effusion lymphoma through its derived cell lines.*AIDS,*Vol.24,No.4,(Feb 20),pp.479-490,1473-5571; 0269-9370

Carbone, A., Gloghini, A., Serraino, D. & Spina, M.(2009).HIV-associated Hodgkin lymphoma.*Curr.Opin.HIV.AIDS.,*Vol.4,No.1,(Jan),pp.3-10,1746-6318; 1746-630X

Carpenter, C. C., Flanigan, T. P. & Lederman, M. M.(2004).Chapter 107: HIV Infection and the Acquired Immunodeficiency Syndrome, In:*Cecil essentials of medicine,*Andreoli, T. E. and Cecil, R. L., pp.917-935,W.B. Saunders,0721601472,Philadelphia, Pa.

Casper, C., Nichols, W. G., Huang, M. L., Corey, L. & Wald, A.(2004).Remission of HHV-8 and HIV-associated multicentric Castleman disease with ganciclovir treatment.*Blood,*Vol.103,No.5,(Mar 1),pp.1632-1634,0006-4971; 0006-4971

Castillo, J. J., Beltran, B. E., Bibas, M., et al.(2011).Prognostic factors in patients with HIV-associated peripheral T-cell lymphoma: a multicenter study.*Am.J.Hematol.,*Vol.86,No.3,(Mar),pp.256-261,1096-8652; 0361-8609

Castillo, J. J., Winer, E. S., Stachurski, D., et al.(2010).Clinical and pathological differences between human immunodeficiency virus-positive and human immunodeficiency virus-negative patients with plasmablastic lymphoma.*Leuk.Lymphoma,*Vol.51,No.11,(Nov),pp.2047-2053,1029-2403; 1026-8022

Chabay, P., De Matteo, E., Lorenzetti, M., et al.(2009).Vulvar plasmablastic lymphoma in a HIV-positive child: a novel extraoral localisation.*J.Clin.Pathol.,*Vol.62,No.7,(Jul),pp.644-646,1472-4146; 0021-9746

Chang, C. C., Chomel, B. B., Kasten, R. W., Tappero, J. W., Sanchez, M. A. & Koehler, J. E.(2002).Molecular epidemiology of Bartonella henselae infection in human immunodeficiency virus-infected patients and their cat contacts, using pulsed-field gel electrophoresis and genotyping.*J.Infect.Dis.,*Vol.186,No.12,(Dec 15),pp.1733-1739,0022-1899

Chang, C. C., McClintock, S., Cleveland, R. P., et al.(2004).Immunohistochemical expression patterns of germinal center and activation B-cell markers correlate with prognosis in diffuse large B-cell lymphoma.*Am.J.Surg.Pathol.,*Vol.28,No.4,(Apr),pp.464-470,0147-5185

Chang, C. C., Zhou, X., Taylor, J. J., et al.(2009).Genomic profiling of plasmablastic lymphoma using array comparative genomic hybridization (aCGH): revealing significant overlapping genomic lesions with diffuse large B-cell lymphoma.*J.Hematol.Oncol.,*Vol.2,(Nov 12),pp.47,1756-8722

Cotell, S. L. & Noskin, G. A.(1994).Bacillary angiomatosis. Clinical and histologic features, diagnosis, and treatment.*Arch.Intern.Med.,*Vol.154,No.5,(Mar 14),pp.524-528,0003-9926

Di Lorenzo, G., Konstantinopoulos, P. A., Pantanowitz, L., Di Trolio, R., De Placido, S. & Dezube, B. J.(2007).Management of AIDS-related Kaposi's sarcoma.*Lancet Oncol.,*Vol.8,No.2,(Feb),pp.167-176,1470-2045

Dispenzieri, A.(2007).POEMS syndrome.*Blood Rev.,*Vol.21,No.6,(Nov),pp.285-299,0268-960X

Doll, D. C. & List, A. F.(1982).Burkitt's lymphoma in a homosexual. *Lancet,* Vol.1, No.8279, (May 1), pp.1026-1027,0140-6736

Dunleavy, K., Little, R. F., Pittaluga, S., et al.(2010).The role of tumor histogenesis, FDG-PET, and short-course EPOCH with dose-dense rituximab (SC-EPOCH-RR) in HIV-associated diffuse large B-cell lymphoma.*Blood,*Vol.115,No.15,(Apr 15),pp.3017-3024,1528-0020; 0006-4971

Eliopoulos, A. G., Gallagher, N. J., Blake, S. M., Dawson, C. W. & Young, L. S.(1999).Activation of the p38 mitogen-activated protein kinase pathway by Epstein-Barr virus-encoded latent membrane protein 1 coregulates interleukin-6 and interleukin-8 production.*J.Biol.Chem.,*Vol.274,No.23,(Jun 4), pp.16085-16096, 0021-9258

EPSTEIN, M. A., ACHONG, B. G. & BARR, Y. M.(1964).Virus Particles in Cultured Lymphoblasts from Burkitt's Lymphoma.*Lancet,*Vol.1,No.7335,(Mar 28),pp.702-703,0140-6736

Ezzat, H., Filipenko, D., Vickars, L., et al.(2007).Improved survival in HIV-associated diffuse large B-cell lymphoma with the addition of rituximab to chemotherapy in patients receiving highly active antiretroviral therapy.*HIV.Clin.Trials,*Vol.8,No.3,(May-Jun),pp.132-144,1528-4336

Foo, W. C., Huang, Q., Sebastian, S., Hutchinson, C. B., Burchette, J. & Wang, E.(2010).Concurrent classical Hodgkin lymphoma and plasmablastic lymphoma in a patient with chronic lymphocytic leukemia/small lymphocytic lymphoma treated with fludarabine: a dimorphic presentation of iatrogenic immunodeficiency-associated lymphoproliferative disorder with evidence suggestive of multiclonal transformability of B cells by Epstein-Barr virus. *Hum.Pathol.*, Vol.41, No.12, (Dec), pp.1802-1808,1532-8392; 0046-8177

Fromont, E. G., Riche, B. & Rabilloud, M.(2009).Toxoplasma seroprevalence in a rural population in France: detection of a household effect.*BMC Infect.Dis.*,Vol.9,(May 28),pp.76,1471-2334

Gaidano, G., Carbone, A. & Dalla-Favera, R.(1998).Pathogenesis of AIDS-related lymphomas: molecular and histogenetic heterogeneity .*Am. J. Pathol.*, Vol.152, No.3, (Mar), pp.623-630, 0002-9440

Gasquet, S., Maurin, M., Brouqui, P., Lepidi, H. & Raoult, D.(1998).Bacillary angiomatosis in immunocompromised patients.*AIDS*,Vol.12,No.14,(Oct 1),pp.1793-1803,0269-9370

Goedhals, J., Beukes, C. A. & Cooper, S.(2006).The ultrastructural features of plasmablastic lymphoma.*Ultrastruct.Pathol.*,Vol.30,No.6,(Nov-Dec),pp.427-433,1521-0758; 0191-3123

Grimes, M. M., LaPook, J. D., Bar, M. H., Wasserman, H. S. & Dwork, A.(1987).Disseminated Pneumocystis carinii infection in a patient with acquired immunodeficiency syndrome.*Hum.Pathol.*,Vol.18,No.3,(Mar),pp.307-308,0046-8177

Gucalp, A. & Noy, A.(2010).Spectrum of HIV lymphoma 2009. *Curr. Opin. Hematol.*, Vol.17,No.4,(Jul),pp.362-367,1531-7048; 1065-6251

Guech-Ongey, M., Simard, E. P., Anderson, W. F., et al.(2010).AIDS-related Burkitt lymphoma in the United States: what do age and CD4 lymphocyte patterns tell us about etiology and/or biology?*Blood*,Vol.116,No.25,(Dec 16),pp.5600-5604,1528-0020; 0006-4971

Hansra, D., Montague, N., Stefanovic, A., et al.(2010).Oral and extraoral plasmablastic lymphoma: similarities and differences in clinicopathologic characteristics. *Am. J. Clin. Pathol.*, Vol.134,No.5,(Nov),pp.710-719,1943-7722; 0002-9173

Hazenberg, M. D., Hamann, D., Schuitemaker, H. & Miedema, F.(2000).T cell depletion in HIV-1 infection: how CD4+ T cells go out of stock. *Nat. Immunol.*, Vol.1, No.4,(Oct), pp.285-289,1529-2908

Ioachim, H. L., Adsay, V., Giancotti, F. R., Dorsett, B. & Melamed, J.(1995).Kaposi's sarcoma of internal organs. A multiparameter study of 86 cases.*Cancer*,Vol.75,No.6,(Mar 15),pp.1376-1385,0008-543X

Ioachim, H. L., Cooper, M. C. & Hellman, G. C.(1985).Lymphomas in men at high risk for acquired immune deficiency syndrome (AIDS). A study of 21 cases.*Cancer*,Vol.56,No.12,(Dec 15),pp.2831-2842,0008-543X

Ioachim, H. L., Cronin, W., Roy, M. & Maya, M.(1990).Persistent lymphadenopathies in people at high risk for HIV infection. Clinicopathologic correlations and long-term follow-up in 79 cases.*Am.J.Clin.Pathol.*,Vol.93,No.2,(Feb),pp.208-218,0002-9173

Ioachim, H., L. & Medeiros, J., L.(2009a).Chapter 18: Bacillary Angiomatosis of Lymph Nodes, In:*Ioachim's Lymph Node Pathology*,Ioachim, H., L. and Medeiros, J., L., pp.115-118,Wolters Kluwer, Lippincott Williams & Wilkins,0-7817-7596-5,Philadelphia, PA

Ioachim, H., L. & Medeiros, J., L.(2009b).Chapter 1: The Normal Lymph Node, In:*Ioachim's Lymph Node Pathology*,Ioachim, H., L. and Medeiros, J., L., pp.2-14,Wolters Kluwer, Lippincott Williams & Wilkins,0-7817-7596-5,Philadelphia, PA

Ioachim, H., L. & Medeiros, J., L.(2009c).Chapter 15: Human Immunodeficiency Virus Lymphadenitis, In:*Ioachim's Lymph Node Pathology*,Ioachim, H., L. and Medeiros, J., L., pp.99-105,Wolters Kluwer, Lippincott Williams & Wilkins,0-7817-7596-5,Philadelphia, PA

Ioachim, H., L. & Medeiros, J., L.(2009d).Chapter 28: Pneumocystis Lymphadenitis, In:*Ioachim's Lymph Node Pathology*,Ioachim, H., L. and Medeiros, J., L., pp.156-158,Wolters Kluwer, Lippincott Williams & Wilkins,0-7817-7596-5,Philadelphia, PA

Ioachim, H., L. & Medeiros, J., L.(2009e).Chapter 29: Toxoplasma Lymphadenitis, In:*Ioachim's Lymph Node Pathology*,Ioachim, H., L. and Medeiros, J., L., pp.159-164,Wolters Kluwer, Lippincott Williams & Wilkins,0-7817-7596-5,Philadelphia, PA

Ioachim, H., L. & Medeiros, J., L.(2009f).Chapter 42: Castleman Lymphadenopathy, In:*Ioachim's Lymph Node Pathology*,Ioachim, H., L. and Medeiros, J., L., pp.227-237,Wolters Kluwer, Lippincott Williams & Wilkins,0-7817-7596-5,Philadelphia, PA

Ioachim, H., L. & Medeiros, J., L.(2009g).Chapter 57: Hodgkin Lymphoma: Classical, In:*Ioachim's Lymph Node Pathology*,Ioachim, H., L. and Medeiros, J., L., pp.306-324,Wolters Kluwer, Lippincott Williams & Wilkins,0-7817-7596-5,Philadelphia, PA

Jacobson, C. A. & LaCasce, A. S.(2010).Lymphoma: risk and response after solid organ transplant.*Oncology (Williston Park)*,Vol.24,No.10,(Sep),pp.936-944,0890-9091; 0890-9091

Jasmer, R. M., Gotway, M. B., Creasman, J. M., Webb, W. R., Edinburgh, K. J. & Huang, L.(2002).Clinical and radiographic predictors of the etiology of computed tomography-diagnosed intrathoracic lymphadenopathy in HIV-infected patients.*J.Acquir.Immune Defic.Syndr.*,Vol.31,No.3,(Nov 1),pp.291-298,1525-4135

Jones, S. A., Horiuchi, S., Topley, N., Yamamoto, N. & Fuller, G. M.(2001).The soluble interleukin 6 receptor: mechanisms of production and implications in disease.*FASEB J.*,Vol.15,No.1,(Jan),pp.43-58,0892-6638

Kamani, J., Mani, A. U., Egwu, G. O. & Kumshe, H. A.(2009).Seroprevalence of human infection with Toxoplasma gondii and the associated risk factors, in Maiduguri, Borno state, Nigeria.*Ann.Trop.Med.Parasitol.*,Vol.103,No.4,(Jun),pp.317-321,0003-4983

Kaplan, J. E., Benson, C., Holmes, K. H., et al.(2009).Guidelines for prevention and treatment of opportunistic infections in HIV-infected adults and adolescents: recommendations from CDC, the National Institutes of Health, and the HIV Medicine Association of the Infectious Diseases Society of America.*MMWR Recomm Rep.*,Vol.58,No.RR-4,(Apr 10),pp.1-207; quiz CE1-4,1545-8601; 1057-5987

Kobayashi, M., Yoshimoto, S., Fujishita, M., et al.(1984).HTLV-positive T-cell lymphoma/leukaemia in an AIDS patient.*Lancet*,Vol.1,No.8390,(Jun 16),pp.1361-1362,0140-6736

Kostianovsky, M. & Greco, M. A.(1994).Angiogenic process in bacillary angiomatosis.*Ultrastruct.Pathol.*,Vol.18,No.3,(May-Jun),pp.349-355,0191-3123

Lamas, C. C., Mares-Guia, M. A., Rozental, T., et al.(2010).Bartonella spp. infection in HIV positive individuals, their pets and ectoparasites in Rio de Janeiro, Brazil: serological and molecular study.*Acta Trop.*,Vol.115,No.1-2,(Jul-Aug),pp.137-141,1873-6254; 0001-706X

Latif, A. S., Katzenstein, D. A., Bassett, M. T., Houston, S., Emmanuel, J. C. & Marowa, E.(1989).Genital ulcers and transmission of HIV among couples in Zimbabwe.*AIDS*,Vol.3,No.8,(Aug),pp.519-523,0269-9370

Leoncini, L., Raphaël, M., Stein, H., Harris, N., L., Jaffe, E., S. & Kluin, P. M.(2008).Burkitt Lymphoma, In:*WHO Classification of Tumours of Haematopoietic and Lymphoid Tissues*,Swerdlow, S., H., Campo, E., Harris, N., L., et al, pp.262-264,IARC,9283224310,Lyon, France

Levine, A. M., Seneviratne, L., Espina, B. M., et al.(2000).Evolving characteristics of AIDS-related lymphoma.*Blood*,Vol.96,No.13,(Dec 15),pp.4084-4090,0006-4971

Lewden, C., Salmon, D., Morlat, P., et al.(2005).Causes of death among human immunodeficiency virus (HIV)-infected adults in the era of potent antiretroviral therapy: emerging role of hepatitis and cancers, persistent role of AIDS.*Int.J.Epidemiol.*,Vol.34,No.1,(Feb),pp.121-130,0300-5771

Lindstrom, I., Kaddu-Mulindwa, D. H., Kironde, F. & Lindh, J.(2006).Prevalence of latent and reactivated Toxoplasma gondii parasites in HIV-patients from Uganda.*Acta Trop.*,Vol.100,No.3,(Dec),pp.218-222,0001-706X

Luan, S. L., Boulanger, E., Ye, H., et al.(2010).Primary effusion lymphoma: genomic profiling revealed amplification of SELPLG and CORO1C encoding for proteins important for cell migration.*J.Pathol.*,Vol.222,No.2,(Oct),pp.166-179,1096-9896; 0022-3417

Maguina, C., Guerra, H. & Ventosilla, P.(2009). Bartonellosis. *Clin.Dermatol.*, Vol.27, No.3, (May-Jun), pp.271-280,1879-1131; 0738-081X

Mantina, H., Wiggill, T. M., Carmona, S., Perner, Y. & Stevens, W. S.(2010).Characterization of Lymphomas in a high prevalence HIV setting.*J.Acquir.Immune Defic.Syndr.*,Vol.53,No.5,(Apr),pp.656-660,1944-7884; 1525-4135

Mbulaiteye, S. M., Anderson, W. F., Bhatia, K., Rosenberg, P. S., Linet, M. S. & Devesa, S. S.(2010).Trimodal age-specific incidence patterns for Burkitt lymphoma in the United States, 1973-2005.*Int.J.Cancer*,Vol.126,No.7,(Apr 1),pp.1732-1739,1097-0215; 0020-7136

McCune, J. M.(2001).The dynamics of CD4+ T-cell depletion in HIV disease. *Nature*, Vol.410, No.6831,(Apr 19),pp.974-979,0028-0836; 0028-0836

Mesri, E. A., Cesarman, E. & Boshoff, C.(2010).Kaposi's sarcoma and its associated herpesvirus.*Nat.Rev.Cancer.*,Vol.10,No.10,(Oct),pp.707-719,1474-1768; 1474-175X

Minnick, M. F., Smitherman, L. S. & Samuels, D. S.(2003).Mitogenic effect of Bartonella bacilliformis on human vascular endothelial cells and involvement of GroEL.*Infect.Immun.*,Vol.71,No.12,(Dec),pp.6933-6942,0019-9567

Mitchell, R. S., Beitzel, B. F., Schroder, A. R., et al.(2004).Retroviral DNA integration: ASLV, HIV, and MLV show distinct target site preferences. *PLoS Biol.*, Vol.2, No.8, (Aug), pp.E234,1545-7885; 1544-9173

Montes-Moreno, S., Gonzalez-Medina, A. R., Rodriguez-Pinilla, S. M., et al.(2010).Aggressive large B-cell lymphoma with plasma cell differentiation: immunohistochemical characterization of plasmablastic lymphoma and diffuse large B-cell lymphoma with partial plasmablastic phenotype. *Haematologica*, Vol.95, No.8, (Aug), pp.1342-1349,1592-8721; 0390-6078

Mosialos, G., Birkenbach, M., Yalamanchili, R., VanArsdale, T., Ware, C. & Kieff, E.(1995).The Epstein-Barr virus transforming protein LMP1 engages signaling proteins for the tumor necrosis factor receptor family.*Cell*,Vol.80,No.3,(Feb 10),pp.389-399,0092-8674

Mukherhee, S.(2010).Part 2: An Impatient War An Anatomist's Tumor, In:Anonymous pp.151-161,Scribner, A division of Simon & Schuster, Inc.,978-1-4391-0795-9,New York, NY

Mylona, E. E., Baraboutis, I. G., Lekakis, L. J., Georgiou, O., Papastamopoulos, V. & Skoutelis, A.(2008).Multicentric Castleman's disease in HIV infection: a systematic review of the literature.*AIDS.Rev.*,Vol.10,No.1,(Jan-Mar),pp.25-35,1139-6121

Nador, R. G., Chadburn, A., Gundappa, G., Cesarman, E., Said, J. W. & Knowles, D. M.(2003).Human immunodeficiency virus (HIV)-associated polymorphic lymphoproliferative disorders.*Am.J.Surg.Pathol.*,Vol.27,No.3,(Mar),pp.293-302,0147-5185

Nasr, S. A., Brynes, R. K., Garrison, C. P. & Chan, W. C.(1988).Peripheral T-cell lymphoma in a patient with acquired immune deficiency syndrome.*Cancer,*Vol.61,No.5,(Mar 1),pp.947-951,0008-543X

Nava, V. E., Cohen, P., Kalan, M. & Ozdemirli, M.(2008).HIV-associated anaplastic large cell lymphoma: a report of three cases.*AIDS,*Vol.22,No.14,(Sep 12),pp.1892-1894,1473-5571; 0269-9370

Navarro, J. T., Lloveras, N., Ribera, J. M., Oriol, A., Mate, J. L. & Feliu, E.(2005).The prognosis of HIV-infected patients with diffuse large B-cell lymphoma treated with chemotherapy and highly active antiretroviral therapy is similar to that of HIV-negative patients receiving chemotherapy.*Haematologica,*Vol.90,No.5,(May),pp.704-706,1592-8721; 0390-6078

Nielsen, K., McSherry, G., Petru, A., et al.(1997).A descriptive survey of pediatric human immunodeficiency virus-infected long-term survivors.*Pediatrics,*Vol.99,No.4,(Apr),pp.E4,1098-4275; 0031-4005

Norkin, L.(2010).The Retroviruses: Lentiviruses, Human Immunodeficiency Virus, and AIDS, In:*Virology Molecular Biology and Pathogenesis,*Norkin, L., pp.597-671,ASM Press,9781555814533,Washington, DC

Noy, A.(2010).Controversies in the treatment of Burkitt lymphoma in AIDS.*Curr.Opin.Oncol.,*Vol.22,No.5,(Sep),pp.443-448,1531-703X; 1040-8746

O'CONOR, G. T. & DAVIES, J. N.(1960).Malignant tumors in African children. With special reference to malignant lymphoma.*J.Pediatr.,*Vol.56,(Apr),pp.526-535,0022-3476

O'Hara, A. J., Wang, L., Dezube, B. J., Harrington, W. J.,Jr, Damania, B. & Dittmer, D. P.(2009).Tumor suppressor microRNAs are underrepresented in primary effusion lymphoma and Kaposi sarcoma.*Blood,*Vol.113,No.23,(Jun 4),pp.5938-5941,1528-0020; 0006-4971

Oksenhendler, E., Boulanger, E., Galicier, L., et al.(2002).High incidence of Kaposi sarcoma-associated herpesvirus-related non-Hodgkin lymphoma in patients with HIV infection and multicentric Castleman disease.*Blood,*Vol.99,No.7,(Apr 1),pp.2331-2336,0006-4971

Orem, J., Maganda, A., Mbidde, E. K. & Weiderpass, E.(2009).Clinical characteristics and outcome of children with Burkitt lymphoma in Uganda according to HIV infection.*Pediatr.Blood Cancer.,*Vol.52,No.4,(Apr),pp.455-458,1545-5017; 1545-5009

Osborne, J., Moore, P. S. & Chang, Y.(1999).KSHV-encoded viral IL-6 activates multiple human IL-6 signaling pathways.*Hum.Immunol.,*Vol.60,No.10,(Oct),pp.921-927,0198-8859

Ouansafi, I., He, B., Fraser, C., et al.(2010).Transformation of follicular lymphoma to plasmablastic lymphoma with c-myc gene rearrangement. *Am. J. Clin. Pathol.,*Vol.134,No.6,(Dec), pp.972-981,1943-7722; 0002-9173

Pantaleo, G., Graziosi, C., Demarest, J. F., et al.(1993).HIV infection is active and progressive in lymphoid tissue during the clinically latent stage of disease.*Nature,*Vol.362,No.6418,(Mar 25),pp.355-358,0028-0836; 0028-0836

Pape, M., Kollaras, P., Mandraveli, K., et al.(2005).Occurrence of Bartonella henselae and Bartonella quintana among human immunodeficiency virus-infected patients.*Ann.N.Y.Acad.Sci.,*Vol.1063,(Dec),pp.299-301,0077-8923

Park, S., Lee, J., Ko, Y. H., et al.(2007).The impact of Epstein-Barr virus status on clinical outcome in diffuse large B-cell lymphoma.*Blood,*Vol.110,No.3,(Aug 1),pp.972-978,0006-4971

Perez, K., Castillo, J., Dezube, B. J. & Pantanowitz, L.(2010).Human Immunodeficiency Virus-associated anaplastic large cell lymphoma.*Leuk.Lymphoma,*Vol.51,No.3,(Mar), pp.430-438,1029-2403; 1026-8022

Prasad, H. K., Bhojwani, K. M., Shenoy, V. & Prasad, S. C.(2006).HIV manifestations in otolaryngology.*Am.J.Otolaryngol.,*Vol.27,No.3,(May-Jun),pp.179-185,0196-0709

Qing, X., Sun, N., Chang, E., French, S., Ji, P. & Yue, C.(2011).Plasmablastic lymphoma may occur as a high-grade transformation from plasmacytoma. *Exp. Mol. Pathol.,* Vol.90, No.1, (Feb),pp.85-90,1096-0945; 0014-4800

Rafaniello Raviele, P., Pruneri, G. & Maiorano, E.(2009).Plasmablastic lymphoma: a review.*Oral Dis.,*Vol.15,No.1,(Jan),pp.38-45,1601-0825; 1354-523X

Raphaël, M., Said, J., Borisch, B., Cesarman, E. & Harris, N., L.(2008).Lymphomas associated with HIV infection, In:*WHO Classification of Tumours of Haematopoietic and Lymphoid Tissues,*Swerdlow, S., H., Campo, E., Harris, N., L., et al, pp.340-342, IARC, 9283224310, Lyon, France

Relman, D. A., Loutit, J. S., Schmidt, T. M., Falkow, S. & Tompkins, L. S.(1990).The agent of bacillary angiomatosis. An approach to the identification of uncultured pathogens.*N.Engl.J.Med.,*Vol.323,No.23,(Dec 6),pp.1573-1580,0028-4793

Robbins, S. L., Kumar, V. & Cotran, R. S.(2010).Chapter 6: Disease of the Immune System, In:*Robbins and Cotran Pathologic Basis of Disease,*Robbins, S. L., Kumar, V. and Cotran, R. S., Saunders/Elsevier,9781416031215,Philadelphia, PA

Roca, B.(2009).Castleman's Disease. A Review.*AIDS.Rev.,*Vol.11,No.1,(Jan-Mar),pp.3-7,1139-6121

Sacktor, N., Lyles, R. H., Skolasky, R., et al.(2001).HIV-associated neurologic disease incidence changes:: Multicenter AIDS Cohort Study, 1990-1998.*Neurology,*Vol.56,No.2,(Jan 23),pp.257-260,0028-3878

Said, J. & Cesarman, E.(2008).Primary effusion lymphoma, In:*WHO Classification of Tumours of Haematopoietic and Lymphoid Tissues,*Swerdlow, S., H., Campo, E., Harris, N., L., et al, pp.260-261,IARC,9283224310,Lyon, France

Shin, D. W., Cha, D. Y., Hua, Q. J., Cha, G. H. & Lee, Y. H.(2009).Seroprevalence of Toxoplasma gondii infection and characteristics of seropositive patients in general hospitals in Daejeon, Korea.*Korean J.Parasitol.,*Vol.47,No.2,(Jun),pp.125-130,1738-0006; 0023-4001

Sierra, S., Kupfer, B. & Kaiser, R.(2005).Basics of the virology of HIV-1 and its replication.*J.Clin. Virol.,*Vol.34,No.4,(Dec),pp.233-244,1386-6532

Sissolak, G., Sissolak, D. & Jacobs, P.(2010).Human immunodeficiency and Hodgkin lymphoma.*Transfus.Apher.Sci.,*Vol.42,No.2,(Apr),pp.131-139,1473-0502

Soulier, J., Grollet, L., Oksenhendler, E., et al.(1995).Kaposi's sarcoma-associated herpesvirus-like DNA sequences in multicentric Castleman's disease.*Blood,*Vol.86,No.4,(Aug 15),pp.1276-1280,0006-4971

Spina, M., Tirelli, U., Zagonel, V., et al.(1998).Burkitt's lymphoma in adults with and without human immunodeficiency virus infection: a single-institution clinicopathologic study of 75 patients.*Cancer,*Vol.82,No.4,(Feb 15),pp.766-774,0008-543X

Stoler, M. H., Bonfiglio, T. A., Steigbigel, R. T. & Pereira, M.(1983).An atypical subcutaneous infection associated with acquired immune deficiency syndrome.*Am.J.Clin.Pathol.,*Vol.80,No.5,(Nov),pp.714-718,0002-9173

Stone, M. J.(2010).Samuel Wilks: the "grand old man" of British medicine.*Proc.(Bayl Univ.Med.Cent),*Vol.23,No.3,(Jul),pp.263-265,0899-8280; 0899-8280

Sun, J., Medeiros, L. J., Lin, P., Lu, G., Bueso-Ramos, C. E. & You, M. J.(2011).Plasmablastic lymphoma involving the penis: a previously unreported location of a case with aberrant CD3 expression.*Pathology,*Vol.43,No.1,(Jan),pp.54-57,1465-3931; 0031-3025

Thirlwell, C., Sarker, D., Stebbing, J. & Bower, M.(2003).Acquired immunodeficiency syndrome-related lymphoma in the era of highly active antiretroviral therapy.*Clin.Lymphoma,*Vol.4,No.2,(Sep),pp.86-92,1526-9655

Ueda, K., Ito, E., Karayama, M., Ohsaki, E., Nakano, K. & Watanabe, S.(2010).KSHV-infected PEL cell lines exhibit a distinct gene expression profile.*Biochem.Biophys.Res.Commun.,*Vol.394,No.3,(Apr 9),pp.482-487,1090-2104; 0006-291X

Ustun, C., Reid-Nicholson, M., Nayak-Kapoor, A., et al.(2009).Plasmablastic lymphoma: CNS involvement, coexistence of other malignancies, possible viral etiology, and dismal outcome.*Ann.Hematol.,*Vol.88,No.4,(Apr),pp.351-358,1432-0584; 0939-5555

Vaccher, E., Tirelli, U., Spina, M., et al.(1996).Age and serum lactate dehydrogenase level are independent prognostic factors in human immunodeficiency virus-related non-Hodgkin's lymphomas: a single-institute study of 96 patients. *J.Clin.Oncol.,*Vol.14,No.8,(Aug), pp.2217-2223,0732-183X

Verani, A., Gras, G. & Pancino, G.(2005).Macrophages and HIV-1: dangerous liaisons.*Mol.Immunol.,*Vol.42,No.2,(Feb),pp.195-212,0161-5890; 0161-5890

Vockerodt, M., Morgan, S. L., Kuo, M., et al.(2008).The Epstein-Barr virus oncoprotein, latent membrane protein-1, reprograms germinal centre B cells towards a Hodgkin's Reed-Sternberg-like phenotype.*J.Pathol.,*Vol.216,No.1,(Sep),pp.83-92,0022-3417

Wain-Hobson, S.(1996).HIV. One on one meets two.*Nature,*Vol.384,No.6605,(Nov 14),pp.117-118,0028-0836

Wang, D., Liebowitz, D. & Kieff, E.(1985).An EBV membrane protein expressed in immortalized lymphocytes transforms established rodent cells.*Cell,*Vol.43,No.3 Pt 2,(Dec),pp.831-840,0092-8674

Wen, K. W. & Damania, B.(2010).Kaposi sarcoma-associated herpesvirus (KSHV): molecular biology and oncogenesis.*Cancer Lett.,*Vol.289,No.2,(Mar 28),pp.140-150,1872-7980; 0304-3835

Whelan, P. & Scadden, D. T.(2006).Cancer in the Immunosuppressed Patient, In:*Oncology,*Anonymous pp.1689-1716,Springer,978-0-387-31056-5,New York, NY

WHO Department of HIV/AIDS Stop TB Department(2010).Guidelines for intensified tuberculosis case-finding and isoniazid preventive therapy for people living with HIV in resource-constrained settings.Vol.1,No.1,(December 2010),pp.1-50,978 92 4 150070 8

Wolf, T., Brodt, H. R., Fichtlscherer, S., et al.(2005).Changing incidence and prognostic factors of survival in AIDS-related non-Hodgkin's lymphoma in the era of highly active antiretroviral therapy (HAART).*Leuk.Lymphoma,*Vol.46,No.2,(Feb),pp.207-215,1042-8194; 1026-8022

Wolff, K., Johnson, R. & Suurmond, D.(2005).Bacillary Angiomatosis, In:*Fitzpatrick's Color Atlas & Synopsis of Clinical Dermatology,*Wolff, K., Johnson, R. and Suurmond, D., pp.648-650,McGraw-Hill,0071440194,New York, NY

WRIGHT, D. H.(1963).Cytology and histochemistry of the Burkitt lymphoma. *Br. J. Cancer,* Vol.17,(Mar),pp.50-55,0007-0920

Yousif, A., Farid, I., Baig, B., Creek, J., Olson, P. & Wallace, M.(1996).Prevalence of Bartonella henselae antibodies among human immunodeficiency virus-infected patients from Bahrain.*Clin.Infect.Dis.,*Vol.23,No.2,(Aug),pp.398-399,1058-4838

Ziegler, J. L., Drew, W. L., Miner, R. C., et al.(1982).Outbreak of Burkitt's-like lymphoma in homosexual men.*Lancet,*Vol.2,No.8299,(Sep 18),pp.631-633,0140-6736

21

Sexual Dysfunctions

Marco de Tubino Scanavino
Institute of Psychiatry, University of São Paulo
Brazil

1. Introduction

Although HIV-positive individuals kept a central role in the maintenance of the epidemic, only from the 12th World AIDS Conference, held in Geneva in 1998, the sexuality of people living with HIV/AIDS received more systematic attention (Schiltz and Sandfort 2000). After receiving the diagnosis of HIV infection is common for people to become involved in a state of negative mood and decrease the frequency of sexual activity and those who remain with sexual practices most likely do so without adequate protection (Rosser, Gobby and Carr 1999). The adhesion to safe sex practices after diagnosis of HIV infection may have a negative impact on sexual functioning of most subjects (Newshan, Taylor and Gold 1998). The individuals that have partnership are significantly more likely to maintain sexual activity than those without (Stein et al. 2005). On the professionals, the sexual functioning is often overlooked among the care of HIV positive patients. Generally, information about the relationship between hormonal factors, psychological factors, drug effects, disease stage, and sexual functioning are not spoken by health professionals (Newshan et al. 1998). In addition, one must consider that individuals who acquire HIV through sexual or parenteral (excluding blood transfusions) are already part of a population at higher risk for sexual dysfunction, as many risk factors for HIV are also to the occurrence of sexual dysfunction, such as conflicts with the orientation or sexual identity, depression, and psychological problems related to self-image (Hijazi, Nandwani and Kell 2002).

Several factors may modify the sexual response. Beginning in youth, sexual dysfunctions are highly prevalent in all age groups. Symptoms of sexual dysfunction include erectile dysfunction, loss of libido, premature or delayed ejaculation, orgasmic disturbances, arousal difficulties, and dyspareunia, among others (Lewis et al. 2004).

For the Diagnostic and Statistical Manual of Mental Disorders, Fourth Edition, Text Revision (DSM-IV-TR) ((APA) 2000), the fundamental concepts of the principals sexual dysfunctions are: *Dyspareunia* is recurrent or persistent genital pain associated with sexual intercourse in men or women. *Female orgasmic disorder* is the delay of orgasm following normal excitement and sexual activity. Due to the widely varied sexual response in women, it must be judged by a clinician to be significant taking into account the person's age and situation. *Female sexual arousal disorder* is inability to attain or maintain until completion of sexual activity adequate lubrication in response to sexual excitement. *Hypoactive sexual desire disorder* is deficient or absent sexual fantasies and desire for sexual activity. This judgment must be made by a clinician taking into account the individual's age and life circumstances. *Male erectile disorder (impotence)* is recurring inability to achieve or maintain an erection until completion of the sexual activity. *Male orgasmic disorder* is delay or absence of orgasm following normal excitement and sexual activity. Due to the widely varied sexual response in men, it must be judged by a clinician to be significant, taking into account the person's age and situation. *Premature ejaculation* is the ejaculation with minimal sexual stimulation before or shortly after penetration and before the person wishes it. The condition is persistent or occurs frequently and causes significant distress (APA, 2000).

Factors such as lack of ability, poor sex education, and psychological conflicts play an important role in the development of sexual dysfunction at the start of sexual activity (Lewis et al. 2004). Life habits and morbid conditions become important risk factors for sexual dysfunction during aging; these factors include hypertension, diabetes, depression, heart disease, sex hormone deficiency, smoking, sedentary life style, and drug addiction (Moreira et al. 2001). Socioeconomic factors, such as education, employment and marital status, have also been related to sexual difficulties (Nicolosi et al. 2003).

Highly active antiretroviral therapy (HAART) has previously been shown to provide the best clinical management for HIV-infected patients, as it decreases the prevalence of hypogonadism and advanced HIV disease, which are principal causes of sexual dysfunction in people infected with HIV (Danoff 1996, Collazos 2007). However the prevalence on sexual dysfunctions in the HAART years show high rates (Collazos 2007). In this chapter we analyze the etiologic factors involved on sexual dysfunctions of HIV/AIDS people. We also describe the most prevalent sexual dysfunctions in males, and females. We propose steps for assessment, and diagnosis of the sexual dysfunction in HIV/AIDS people. We talk about the principal therapeutic strategies for recover healthy sexual function of this people. Finally, we comment on the prognostic factors.

2. Epidemiology

The prevalence rates of sexual dysfunctions in HIV/AIDS patients were reviewed: 46% presented with erectile dysfunction (range 9-74%), 39% with ejaculatory disturbances (range 36-42%), 44% with decreased libido (range 24-73%), and 27% with orgasmic disorders (range 7-49%). The high interval of range is because so much different designs and methods used in the HIV sexual dysfunctions studies (Collazos 2007). There are differences on the most prevalent sexual dysfunctions among men, and women.

The most prevalent female sexual dysfunctions are low sexual desire, orgasmic dysfunction, and dyspareunia (Hijazi et al. 2002, Luzi et al. 2009). A higher frequency (36%) of sexual inactivity during the last 12 months in female with AIDS has been reported by a Brazilian study (de Tubino Scanavino and Abdo 2010), which is in according with another study of females with HIV/AIDS, of which 28% reported having no sexual partners for an average of 69 months (Lambert, Keegan and Petrak 2005). We already know that HIV/AIDS females that has partners keep more the sexual activity than who does not have. But in the Brazilian study the female also does not maintain sexual arousal until the end of the sex, and probably this may partly explain the sexual inactivity because these women seem to find sex unsatisfactory (de Tubino Scanavino and Abdo 2010).

On men infected by HIV the most prevalent sexual dysfunctions are erectile dysfunction and premature ejaculation. In Brazil, a case-control study nested in a cross-sectional population study with people who reported AIDS found that almost 50% of the male reported ejaculatory symptoms, and 33% of the men living with AIDS reported erectile dysfunction (de Tubino Scanavino and Abdo 2010). In this study 12% of men with AIDS also reported dyspareunia, while no men without AIDS reported it (de Tubino Scanavino and Abdo 2010). Male dyspareunia is not commonly reported in the literature, possibly because it is not regularly investigated in studies of male sexual function.

3. Etiology

There are four important factors associated with sexual dysfunctions in HIV/AIDS patients: mental, hormonal, pharmachological, and other morbid conditions.

3.1 Mental factors

At the first moment, the condition of being HIV seropositive may cause feelings of loss of sexual attractiveness, reduction of sexual desire and sexual satisfaction. Moreover, they may be confronted with the absence of sexual partners, particularly when revealing their serological status. In addition, the sexual response may be undermined by fear or guilt in coming to contaminate partnerships (Newshan et al. 1998, Schiltz and Sandfort 2000).

A representative French study with HIV outpatients showed association among sexual difficulties and the discrimination by friends and partners, suffering by lipodystrophy, very disturbing HIV related symptoms. The authors recommend psychological support for HIV experience for improves the sexual life (Bouhnik et al. 2008). Feelings of guilt by have acquiring the HIV on sexual transmission may become a psychogenic factor and influence negatively the sexual response. Maybe because of this point, sexual dysfunctions are more prevalent on homosexual men than intravenous drug users (Sollima et al. 2001). In fact, gay and bisexual men have higher rates of sexual dysfunctions (Catalan and Meadows 2000) or just complaint more to the physicians on the disorder due to valorize more the sexual function than others.

Depression is one of the most important mental factors associated with sexual dysfunctions (Ciesla and Roberts 2001). A study on 300 HIV infected men found the older age and depression were associated with erectile dysfunction, and current higher CD4 account was protective (Crum-Cianflone et al. 2007).

The most common factors associated with female sexual dysfunction are the psychosocial aspects of HIV infection and the negative body image associated with use of medications that cause lipodystrophy (Bell et al. 2006, Hijazi et al. 2002, Luzi et al. 2009).

3.2 Hormonal factors

Hypogonadism was one of the most frequent causes of sexual dysfunction before HAART. Currently, HIV infected individuals may have testosterone levels higher than non infected individuals. Moreover, estradiol is often higher in men (50% of them) on HAART possibly because the augmentation of the peripheral conversion of the androgens to estrogens in lipid tissues (Bell et al. 2006, Goldmeier et al. 2002). But the role of estradiol in HIV sexual dysfunctions is not clear. The expected decrease in blood of the gonadotropin hormones was not confirmed (Collazos et al. 2002a), and one study observed improving on sexual function despite higher blood levels of estradiol (Collazos et al. 2002b). On the other side, an study on rabbits found estrogen receptors in cavernous body, and found pathophysiological changes in erectile function when rabbits are under continuous estrogen intake (Srilatha and Adaikan 2004). Another study with older men found that the balance between testosterone

(decreased) and oestradiol (higher) are associated with erectile dysfunction (Srilatha, Adaikan and Chong 2007).
Hyperprolactinemia may be associated with sexual dysfunction as it decreases the gonadotropin releases and have been found in part of the HIV individuals, but one study does not found difference in prolactin levels between patients with and without sexual difficulties (Collazos et al. 2002b).

3.3 Pharmacological factors

HAART era shows high rates of sexual dysfunction despite the improvement of health conditions. Anedotical report from studies suggest association among protease inhibitors and sexual dysfunctions, but just a few studies found a kind of evidence on it. These studies have found a possible effect on testosterone receptor by protease inhibitors (Yang et al. 2005, Baker, Vaughn and Fanestil 1978). Other evidences to explain sexual dysfunction by an effect of HAART are scarce. Future studies on pharmacological issues may specify the etiologic role of antiretrovirals to sexual dysfunction.
It has been reported ejaculatory dysfunction associated by use of didanosine (Hijazi et al. 2002). The neuropathy is a possible complication by use of some antiretrovirals and may be a sexual dysfunction factor for some patients (Rogstad et al. 1999).
However, HIV infected individuals use a lot of other medications that are associated with decrease on sexual response. Medications such as ketoconazole, fluconazole, ganciclovir, megestrol, methadone and cimetidine may decrease the level of testosterone and cause sexual dysfunction (Newshan et al. 1998, Daniell 2002). Antihypertensives, diuretics, hypolipemics, benzodiazepines, antidepressants, and antipsychotics are also associated with sexual dysfuncitons (Asboe et al. 2007, Lue 2000, Daniell 2002, Bruckert et al. 1996).

3.4 Comorbid conditions

Some morbid conditions are common in HIV people and some of them are often associated with sexual dysfunction as hepathopathy, diabetes, hyperlipidemia, hypertension, vascular disease, alcohol dependence (Moreira et al. 2001).

4. Diagnosis

When a patient comes for receiving care on sexual function, he needs time and more than one meeting with the health professional, to bind and reveal your intimate life problems.
But if a patient seeks medical care for other reasons but also has sexual problems, difficultly he will talk about spontaneously. Moreover, sexual life is poored investigated by practitioners, indeed in mental health settings. It also occurs on HIV/AIDS clinical context. In a research in the United Kingdom on HIV clinics, 60% of the physicians do not ask on sexual functioning of female HIV infected (Bell et al. 2006) despite the sexual difficulties are very prevalent on HIV women.
For this reason, in order to investigate sexual function of HIV people, the first point to consider is an appropriate doctor patient relationship (Lawlor and Braunack-Mayer 2004), which is basic to investigate clinical and sexual symptoms of the patients. It is important an attitude of open minded and free of judgments by the professional.

The diagnosis of sexual dysfunctions follows some steps for diagnosis: consistent doctor-patient relationship, investigation of clinical history and physical examination, investigation of the sexual life history, assessment on sexual response, and check the hormonal serum levels.

4.1 Clinical history and physical examination

The clinical history compreends the assessment on the immunological conditions, comorbidities, and medications. Severe immunological damage may indicates AIDS diagnosis. The poor health condition undermine physical and sexual response. Nevertheless the hypogonadism should be investigated. On the physical examination the gynecomaestia and testicular atrophy may indicates hypogonadism (Rosen et al. 2006). Hypogonadism is defined as low levels of testosterone (< 300 nh/dL) in early morning, with associated clinical manifestations, including sexual dysfunction, weight and muscle mass loss, fatigue, depressed mood, and anemia (Crum et al. 2005).
We already spoke on the most frequent comorbidity and the use of some medications which also influence the sexual response.

4.2 Sexual history

The sexual history should starts investigating the concepts on sexuality of the family (father and mother), following to the patient's sexual history, finishing with focus about some specific gender issues.

4.2.1 Sexuality on origin family

When sexuality is very repressed, it could undermine to live a broad experience of sex and love in adolescence and young adult life (Basson 2008), which are fundamental to sexual maturing process. The non psychological and sexual maturing and possible internal conflicts influence the sexual response. When somebody lives in a dysfunctional family in childhood and has early contact with the erotic experience (sexual abuse or permissive family ambience), it could be traumatic and harm the personality development, as the children experience feelings of being unprotected, unsafety, shame or guilt. Then, this person could presents sexual problems (aversion, excessive drive, sexual difficulties) later in your life (Noll, Trickett and Putnam 2003).
On sexual violence suffered during childhood and adolescence many studies have reported serious psychological effects and sexual consequences (Gwandure 2007, Greenberg 2001, Whetten et al. 2006). Victims of violence often have a high frequency of the stress post-traumatic disorder, depression, suicidal ideation and low self-esteem (Gwandure 2007) (Greenberg 2001, Whetten et al. 2006). This psychopathological issues are risk factors for HIV / AIDS in adult life, as negative moods promote sexual practices without the use of condoms and, therefore, exposure to virus (Gwandure 2007). Thus, research has documented the association between childhood sexual abuse and higher frequency of sexual risk behavior in adult life (Gwandure 2007, Greenberg 2001, Whetten et al. 2006, Sikkema et al. 2008). At the same time, in several studies of HIV-positive individuals is described childhood sexual abuse, which frequency varies between 24% and 76% (Whetten et al. 2006, Bedimo, Kissinger and Bessinger 1997, Kalichman et al. 2002, Liebschutz et al. 2000, Segurado et al. 2008).

4.2.2 Own sexual history

The own sexual history is very important. The first sexual experiences with boys or girls, the first complete sexual relationship, the exercise of masturbation are all significant steps in sexual maturing process, which compreend gaining knowledge on your body (erogenous zones) and of the others. When somebody has sexual difficulties in early sexual experiences and are not prepared to deal with, it could promote negative attitude regarding sex, and new experiences will be avoided, undermining the sexual maturing (Lewis et al. 2004). A person with sexual inexperiece is under higher risk for sexual dysfunction (Lewis et al. 2004), and, in turn, a person with sexual dysfunction is under higher risk for unsafe sex behavior (Rosen et al. 2006), even if become infected by HIV.

4.2.3 Gender issues

Some specific gender issues are also important to be investigated. For men, homosexual orientation presents a special vulnerability for sexual dysfunction, maybe because the process to accept the sexual orientation, the difficulties to deal with low acceptance by family and society, and the problems with gender identity (Coleman, Rosser and Strapko 1992). Some studies have reported higher rates of sexual dysfunction in HIV infected men who have sex with men (Cove and Petrak 2004).

For women, the mental health is a strong point to be investigated. Depression is a strong risk factor for sexual dysfunction (Cyranowski et al. 2004) and when treated can improve substancially the sexual dysfunction symptoms (Clayton et al. 2007).

Less investigated but so important is self-image and body image. Self-image compreends the perception from herself of the female issue, and the erotic issue. They are steps of sexual developing and are determinant to woman fells secure to engage in sexual experiences in adult life. The prejudice on body image by lipodystrophy has been considered the most important factor for sexual dysfunction in HIV infected women (Luzi et al. 2009) and could also influence to women do not engage in sex with partners.

Another important point on female sexual function is the presence of positive feelings for the partner (Basson 2008) and the sexual partner hability, as we know a lot of women just have positive sexual experiences when they are estimulated by a partner in an appropriate context, which involve affect and foreplay (Basson 2008).

4.2.4 Difference between organic and psychogenic sexual dysfunction

It is also relevant in sexual history to distinguish between characteristcs of organic or psychogenic sexual dysfunction (Table 1) (Speckens et al. 1993, Hatch, de la Peña and Fisher 1987). The psychogenic occurs more often in younger individuals, the onset is rapid, it could be related with adverse life events (when it appears soon after HIV diagnosis, e.g.) or problematic onset sex lives, the presentation is not constant and it changes depending on the partners, or the situations, and could not be presented in masturbation. Moreover, the organic occurs more often in older men, the onset is insidious, it does not have relation with life adverse events, the presentation is constant, and it also occurs in masturbation. For men, when the nocturnal penile erection is present it is suggestive of psychogenic etiology. Considering HIV infection we could think that individuals just seropositive with good health conditions probably presents sexual dysfunction by psychogenic etiology, and individuals with poor imunological conditions or AIDS diagnosis probably presents sexual dysfunction by organic factors.

Characteristics	Organic	Psychogenic
Age of onset	Older	Younger
Onset	Insidious	Quick
Pattern	Constant	Variable
Masturbation	Yes	No
Adverse life events and/or problems on the onset of sex life	No	Yes
Men: penile nocturnal Erection	No	Yes

Table 1. Clinical difference between organic and psychogenic sexual dysfunction

4.3 Assessment on sexual response

Some standardized instruments for quick assessment of sexual response can be used, as the health practitioners often find it difficult to investigate the sex lives of patients. For female we can use The Female Sexual Function Index (FSFI) to assess female sexual function. The FSFI is a self-responsive questionnaire with 19 multiple choice questions divided into six main domains. The questionnaire evaluates phases of the sexual cycle (desire, excitement and orgasm), sexual satisfaction and dyspareunia in the last four weeks (Rosen et al. 2000). For male there is The International Index of Erectile Function (IIEF) which addresses the relevant domains of male sexual function (erectile function, orgasmic function, sexual desire, intercourse satisfaction, and overall satisfaction), is psychometrically tested, readily self-administered in research or clinical settings (Rosen et al. 1997).

The Figure 1 shows generally items for investigating sexual function (de Tubino Scanavino and Abdo 2010).

In general items evaluating sexual function involves the follows (de Tubino Scanavino and Abdo 2010): "Did you have sexual intercourse during the last 12 months?", "Do you need to be stimulated by your partner to begin sexual intercourse?", "Is stimulation (foreplay) necessary for you for a long time before sexual intercourse?", "If there is no previous reciprocal stimulation (foreplay), do you and your partner proceed to genital sexual intercourse?", "Do you masturbate regularly?", "Do you usually have sexual desire?", "Do you feel pain during sexual intercourse?". Items evaluating female sexual function involves the follows: "When you kiss and hug during sexual intercourse, do you feel sexual arousal and does the vagina become wet?", "Do you maintain sexual arousal and a wet vagina until the end of sexual intercourse?", "Do you reach orgasm during sexual activity (inside the vagina or outside on the clitoris)?". Items evaluating male sexual function involves the follows: "Do you feel the pleasure of getting an erection and keeping it until the end of sexual intercourse?", "Do you always manage to maintain an erection (hard penis) until the end of sexual intercourse?", "Do you ejaculate (expel white liquid through the penis) quicker than you want?", "Do you ejaculate (expel white liquid through the penis) later than you want?", "Do you ejaculate (expel white liquid through the penis) at the desired time for you?".

Items for men and women	"Did you have sexual intercourse during the last 12 months?", "Do you need to be stimulated by your partner to begin sexual intercourse?", "Is stimulation (foreplay) necessary for you for a long time before sexual intercourse?", "If there is no previous reciprocal stimulation (foreplay), do you and your partner proceed to genital sexual intercourse?", "Do you masturbate regularly?", "Do you usually have sexual desire?", "Do you feel pain during sexual intercourse?".
Items specifically for women	"When you kiss and hug during sexual intercourse, do you feel sexual arousal and does the vagina become wet?", "Do you maintain sexual arousal and a wet vagina until the end of sexual intercourse?", "Do you reach orgasm during sexual activity (inside the vagina or outside on the clitoris)?".
Items specifically for men	"Do you feel the pleasure of getting an erection and keeping it until the end of sexual intercourse?", "Do you always manage to maintain an erection (hard penis) until the end of sexual intercourse?", "Do you ejaculate (expel white liquid through the penis) quicker than you want?", "Do you ejaculate (expel white liquid through the penis) later than you want?", "Do you ejaculate (expel white liquid through the penis) at the desired time for you?".

Fig. 1. Items for assessment the sexual function (de Tubino Scanavino and Abdo 2010).

4.4 Laboratory assessment

Laboratory assessment may involve a sexual hormones screening including testosterone, estrogen, estradiol, prolactin, gonadotropin. It is important check the serum free testosterone or the levels of sex hormone-binding globulin because it usually is increased in HIV infected individuals (Hofbauer and Heufelder 1996). When organic etiology is suspected, more profound evaluations can take place, such as Doppler ultrasonography (arterial obstruction) or nerve conduction study (neuropathy).

The Figure 2 summarizes the steps for the diagnosis.

5. Treatment

The treatment of sexual dysfunctions on HIV/AIDS patients involves pharmacotherapy, psychotherapy interventions, and psychoeducational approaches on safer sex.

5.1 Pharmacotherapy

For pharmacologycal management may be considered the changing of the antiretroviral used, the association of phosphodiesterase-5 inhibitors, testosterone replacement when hypogonadism was diagnosed, and letrozole if estradiol is increased.

1. Consistent doctor-patient relationship			
2. Clinical history and physical examination	Immunological Co-morbidities Hypogonadism		
3. Sexual history	Family	Repression Sexual abuse	
	Own sexual history	The onset Masturbation exercise First complete intercourse	
	Gender issues	Men who have sex with men	Sexual orientation Gender issues
		Women	Mental health Self-image Body image Feelings for the partner Hability of the partner
	Characteristics of the dysfunction	Organic Psychogenic	
4. Assessment on sexual response	Desire Arousal Orgasm Resolution Satisfaction		
5. Laboratory assessment	Hormonal	Testosterone Estradiol Gonadotropin Prolactin Estrogen Sex hormone-binding globulin	
	Metabolic	Carbohydrate Lipid profile	

Fig. 2. Steps for the diagnosis

5.1.1 Antiretrovirals

If medication is the principal factor you can try another drug that has poor influence on sexual response, such as nevirapine (Collazos 2007, Collazos et al. 2002c) or atazanavir (Bernal et al. 2005).

5.1.2 Phosphodiesterase-5 inhibitors

The use of phosphodiesterase-5 inhibitors is highly recommended in male sexual dysfunction, but one should be careful about drug interactions with antiretrovirals, particularly with protease inhibitors (especially ritonovir) because both are metabolized by the cytochrome P-450 system. Because the increases of serum concentration of phosphodiesterase-5 inhibitors when associated with protease inhibitors and cetoconazol, the dosage should be reduced (Merry et al. 1999, Rosen et al. 2006). The phosphodiesterase-5 inhibitors most often used are sildenafil, tadalafil and vardenafil.

Poppers (amyl nitrate) are contraindicated by men user of phosphodiesterase-5 inhibitors because lowers blood pressure especially in combination with phosphodiesterase-5 inhibitors.

5.1.3 Testosterone replacement

If the patient reaches the diagnostic criteria for hypogonadism there is some options for testosterone replacement.

On the other side, testosterone replacement is not prescribed for HIV patients without decreases on free testosterone blood levels because does not improve sexual dysfunctions have been reported in this condition, and they will be exposed to the adverse effects (Collazos 2007). Sometimes testosterone replacement could be problematic even to hypogonadal male, as in the report of three HIV infected patients with erectile dysfunction whose present low testosterone and SHBG despite are receiving long-term oxandrolone in addition to testosterone replacement therapy, beyond HAART. Discontinuation of oxandrolone led to the normalization or improvement of testosterone levels in all three patients with symptomatic improvement in one patient. The authors hypothesized the first pass metabolism of orally administered oxandrolone may decrease hepatic synthesis of SHBG, allowing exogenously supplied testosterone to be excreted (Wasserman, Segal-Maurer and Rubin 2008).

By the way, the testosterone replacement shows good results in sexual dysfunction of most of hypogonadal HIV infected individuals (Cofrancesco, Whalen and Dobs 1997, Rabkin, Rabkin and Wagner 1997, Rabkin, Wagner and Rabkin 1999, Rabkin, Wagner and Rabkin 2000, Seftel et al. 2004) and the replacement by testosterone gel topic shows good benefits (Schrader et al. 2005).

5.1.4 Letrozole

Finally, some improvement in sexual desire has been reported in a few patients on HAART who were treated with letrozole, an aromatase inhibitor that inhibits the conversion of testosterone to estradiol. Thirteen men who have sex with men on HAART with low sexual desire as well as raised estradiol levels were randomly allocated to receive either parenteral testosterone or letrozole for six weeks. Standardized instruments pointed out improvement in desire, and frequency of sexual acts in both treatment arms (Richardson et al. 2007).

5.2 Psychotherapy

The psychotherapic approaches on sexual dysfunction of HIV infected people involve supportive, processual, psychosexual, and psychoeducational therapies.

5.2.1 Supportive
If the most important factor is the psychogenic can use supportive therapy in early period after HIV diagnosis. It should foccuses in demystify the stigmas from HIV/AIDS as mortal disease and as associated to non conventional sex behavior. The supportive approach would diminish the fear and guilt.
A structured supportive approach could be necessary for the women who suffered sexual violence could overcoming and retake sexual life.

5.2.2 Processual
People who have severe sexual conflicts because grown in a family with high sexual repression or suffered childhood sexual abuse, a processual approach could be recomended as psychoanalysis.

5.2.3 Psychosexual
Psychosexual therapy such as sensitive focus or masturbation training are indicated when the acceptance of HIV seropositivity is solved and the sexual dysfunctions remains.

5.2.4 Psychoeducational
As most of the population did not receive sexual education, the psychoeducational approach is always useful involving anatomy concepts, the differences between male and female sexual response, e.g.

5.3 Psychoeducational approach on safer sex
Psychoeducational approach on safer sex is offered concomitant with the treatment of the sexual dysfunction. Always the approach involves the patient and his or her partner. Safer sex counseling is fundamental for explaining the risk for contact with different strains of HIV, and favouring the development of the resistence to antiretrovirals.
Finally, psychoeducational approach should stimulate lifestyle modification including safer sex, exercise, recreational drugs information, modifications of cardiovascular risk factors (Rosen et al. 2006).
The Figure 3 summarizes the treatment.

6. Prognosis

The sexual function before HIV diagnosis, the current physical and mental health, and the psychosocial support are important factors to improve sexual response. A medical team updated with knowledge on human sexuality is essential for diagnosis, and treatment of the sexual dysfunctions. When these conditions are preserved the results on therapeutics are good (Wasserman et al. 2008, Richardson et al. 2007, Schrader et al. 2005).
The problem is that in many times the sexual issues are not investigated by health professionals, and just a few of patients will talk about sexual problems spontaneously. As sexual dysfunction is so prevalent in general population and in people living with HIV, a lot of them, keep without caring on sexual difficulties. On addiction, sexual dysfunction has impact on quality of life, very often influencing negative attitudes by the individual, including bad adherence to antiretroviral regimens, and to safer sex strategies (Trotta et al. 2007, Trotta et al. 2008). Moreover, HIV infected people with sexual dysfuntion have

Intervention	Problem	Management strategy
1. Pharmacotherapy	Antiretrovirals	Change medication
	Association with Phosphodiesterase-5 inhibitors	Reduce the dosage Does not use with poppers
	Hypogonadism	Testosterone replacement
	Estradiol increased (low sex desire)	Letrozole
2. Psychotherapy	Early period after HIV diagnosis	Supportive therapy
	Women who suffered sexual violence	Supportive therapy
	Severe sexual repression Childhood sexual abuse Dysfunctional family	Psychoanalysis
	Poor sexual education Poor knowledge on human sexuality	Psychoeducational therapy
3. Psychoeducational on safer sex	Poor knowledge on sexual health	Strategies for safer sex to the patient and to the partner

Fig. 3. Interventions

increased risk of transmission of drug-resistant strains because the higher sexual risk behavior, and inadvertent use of phosphodiesterase-5 inhibitors without medical recommendations with higher likelihood of negative interaction with antiretrovirals (Trotta et al. 2007, Trotta et al. 2008).

Another important point is on the scarcity of health professional team with expertise in human sexuality. A so private issue needs professionals with hability to approach on these intimate issues of the patients. Otherwise the patients do not open your sexual problems to them.

When the patient receives attention on your sexual life, he feels valuable, and will be more open to engage in positive ways as on adherence to medications as on safer sex strategies.

7. Conclusion

Sexuality is a very important point to quality of life. A person who becomes infected by HIV particularly by sexual contact could be extremely confused about continuing engaging in sexual intercourses. The consequences mostly are negative attitudes toward life, harm on quality of life, sexual risk behaviors, and bad adherence to antiretrovirals. People who are living with HIV/AIDS are extremely important to epidemia control. Take care of your sexual life may improve your self steam and your protective behaviors.

By the way, the approach on sexual dysfunction in HIV infected people involves multiple variables and includes the assessment on clinical history (morbid conditions, medications), sexual history (family and own), sexual function (male and female), and laboratory studies (hormonal, metabolic). The management strategies by health professionals with expertise in human sexuality involves pharmacology and psychotherapy interventions. Always the psychoeducational approach on safer sex will be developed in parallel with others interventions. The recovery of the sexual function, associated with a good adherence to safe sex practices, will improve the quality of life of the people living with HIV/AIDS and help controlling the epidemia.

8. References

American Psychiatric Association (APA) (2000): Diagnostic and Statistical Manual of Mental Disorders, Fourth Edition, Text Revision. Washington, DC: American Psychiatric Association.

Asboe, D., J. Catalan, S. Mandalia, N. Dedes, E. Florence, W. Schrooten, C. Noestlinger & R. Colebunders (2007) Sexual dysfunction in HIV-positive men is multi-factorial: a study of prevalence and associated factors. *AIDS Care,* 19, 955-65.

Baker, M. E., D. A. Vaughn & D. D. Fanestil (1978) Inhibition by protease inhibitors of binding of adrenal and sex steroid hormones. *J Supramol Struct,* 9, 421-6.

Basson, R. (2008) Women's sexual function and dysfunction: current uncertainties, future directions. *Int J Impot Res,* 20, 466-78.

Bedimo, A. L., P. Kissinger & R. Bessinger (1997) History of sexual abuse among HIV-infected women. *Int J STD AIDS,* 8, 332-5.

Bell, C., D. Richardson, M. Wall & D. Goldmeier (2006) HIV-associated female sexual dysfunction - clinical experience and literature review. *Int J STD AIDS,* 17, 706-9.

Bernal, E., M. Masiá, S. Padilla & F. Gutiérrez (2005) Unexpected improvement of sexual dysfunction during atazanavir therapy. *AIDS,* 19, 1440-1.

Bouhnik, A. D., M. Préau, M. A. Schiltz, Y. Obadia, B. Spire & V. s. group (2008) Sexual difficulties in people living with HIV in France--results from a large representative sample of outpatients attending French hospitals (ANRS-EN12-VESPA). *AIDS Behav,* 12, 670-6.

Bruckert, E., P. Giral, H. M. Heshmati & G. Turpin (1996) Men treated with hypolipidaemic drugs complain more frequently of erectile dysfunction. *J Clin Pharm Ther,* 21, 89-94.

Catalan, J. & J. Meadows (2000) Sexual dysfunction in gay and bisexual men with HIV infection: evaluation, treatment and implications. *AIDS Care,* 12, 279-86.

Ciesla, J. A. & J. E. Roberts (2001) Meta-analysis of the relationship between HIV infection and risk for depressive disorders. *Am J Psychiatry,* 158, 725-30.

Clayton, A., S. Kornstein, A. Prakash, C. Mallinckrodt & M. Wohlreich (2007) Changes in sexual functioning associated with duloxetine, escitalopram, and placebo in the treatment of patients with major depressive disorder. *J Sex Med,* 4, 917-29.

Cofrancesco, J., J. J. Whalen & A. S. Dobs (1997) Testosterone replacement treatment options for HIV-infected men. *J Acquir Immune Defic Syndr Hum Retrovirol,* 16, 254-65.

Coleman, E., B. R. Rosser & N. Strapko (1992) Sexual and intimacy dysfunction among homosexual men and women. *Psychiatr Med,* 10, 257-71.

Collazos, J. (2007) Sexual dysfunction in the highly active antiretroviral therapy era. *AIDS Rev,* 9, 237-45.

Collazos, J., E. Martinez, J. Mayo & S. Ibarra (2002a) Sexual hormones in HIV-infected patients: the influence of antiretroviral therapy. *AIDS,* 16, 934-7.

Collazos, J., E. Martínez, J. Mayo & S. Ibarra (2002b) Sexual dysfunction in HIV-infected patients treated with highly active antiretroviral therapy. *J Acquir Immune Defic Syndr,* 31, 322-6.
Collazos, J., J. Mayo, E. Martínez & S. Ibarra (2002c) Association between sexual disturbances and sexual hormones with specific antiretroviral drugs. *AIDS,* 16, 1294-5.
Cove, J. & J. Petrak (2004) Factors associated with sexual problems in HIV-positive gay men. *Int J STD AIDS,* 15, 732-6.
Crum, N. F., K. J. Furtek, P. E. Olson, C. L. Amling & M. R. Wallace (2005) A review of hypogonadism and erectile dysfunction among HIV-infected men during the pre- and post-HAART eras: diagnosis, pathogenesis, and management. *AIDS Patient Care STDS,* 19, 655-71.
Crum-Cianflone, N. F., M. Bavaro, B. Hale, C. Amling, A. Truett, C. Brandt, B. Pope, K. Furtek, S. Medina & M. R. Wallace (2007) Erectile dysfunction and hypogonadism among men with HIV. *AIDS Patient Care STDS,* 21, 9-19.
Cyranowski, J. M., J. Bromberger, A. Youk, K. Matthews, H. M. Kravitz & L. H. Powell (2004) Lifetime depression history and sexual function in women at midlife. *Arch Sex Behav,* 33, 539-48.
Daniell, H. W. (2002) Hypogonadism in men consuming sustained-action oral opioids. *J Pain,* 3, 377-84.
Danoff, A. (1996) Endocrinologic complications of HIV infection. *Med Clin North Am,* 80, 1453-69.
de Tubino Scanavino, M. & C. H. Abdo (2010) Sexual dysfunctions among people living with AIDS in Brazil. *Clinics (Sao Paulo),* 65, 511-9.
Goldmeier, D., G. Scullard, M. Kapembwa, H. Lamba & G. Frize (2002) Does increased aromatase activity in adipose fibroblasts cause low sexual desire in patients with HIV lipodystrophy? *Sex Transm Infect,* 78, 64-6.
Greenberg, J. B. (2001) Childhood sexual abuse and sexually transmitted diseases in adults: a review of and implications for STD/HIV programmes. *Int J STD AIDS,* 12, 777-83.
Gwandure, C. (2007) Sexual assault in childhood: risk HIV and AIDS behaviours in adulthood. *AIDS Care,* 19, 1313-5.
Hatch, J. P., A. M. de la Peña & J. G. Fisher (1987) Psychometric differentiation of psychogenic and organic erectile disorders. *J Urol,* 138, 781-3.
Hijazi, L., R. Nandwani & P. Kell (2002) Medical management of sexual difficulties in HIV-positive individuals. *Int J STD AIDS,* 13, 587-92.
Hofbauer, L. C. & A. E. Heufelder (1996) Endocrine implications of human immunodeficiency virus infection. *Medicine (Baltimore),* 75, 262-78.
Kalichman, S. C., K. J. Sikkema, K. DiFonzo, W. Luke & J. Austin (2002) Emotional adjustment in survivors of sexual assault living with HIV-AIDS. *J Trauma Stress,* 15, 289-96.
Lambert, S., A. Keegan & J. Petrak (2005) Sex and relationships for HIV positive women since HAART: a quantitative study. *Sex Transm Infect,* 81, 333-7.
Lawlor, A. & A. Braunack-Mayer (2004) Doctors' views about the importance of shared values in HIV positive patient care: a qualitative study. *J Med Ethics,* 30, 539-43.
Lewis, R. W., K. S. Fugl-Meyer, R. Bosch, A. R. Fugl-Meyer, E. O. Laumann, E. Lizza & A. Martin-Morales (2004) Epidemiology/risk factors of sexual dysfunction. *J Sex Med,* 1, 35-9.

Liebschutz, J. M., G. Feinman, L. Sullivan, M. Stein & J. Samet (2000) Physical and sexual abuse in women infected with the human immunodeficiency virus: increased illness and health care utilization. *Arch Intern Med,* 160, 1659-64.

Lue, T. F. (2000) Erectile dysfunction. *N Engl J Med,* 342, 1802-13.

Luzi, K., G. Guaraldi, R. Murri, M. De Paola, G. Orlando, N. Squillace, R. Esposito, V. Rochira, R. Vincenzo, L. Zirilli & E. Martinez (2009) Body image is a major determinant of sexual dysfunction in stable HIV-infected women. *Antivir Ther,* 14, 85-92.

Merry, C., M. G. Barry, M. Ryan, J. F. Tjia, M. Hennessy, V. A. Eagling, F. Mulcahy & D. J. Back (1999) Interaction of sildenafil and indinavir when co-administered to HIV-positive patients. *AIDS,* 13, F101-7.

Moreira, E. D., C. H. Abdo, E. B. Torres, C. F. Lôbo & J. A. Fittipaldi (2001) Prevalence and correlates of erectile dysfunction: results of the Brazilian study of sexual behavior. *Urology,* 58, 583-8.

Newshan, G., B. Taylor & R. Gold (1998) Sexual functioning in ambulatory men with HIV/AIDS. *Int J STD AIDS,* 9, 672-6.

Nicolosi, A., E. D. Moreira, M. Shirai, M. I. Bin Mohd Tambi & D. B. Glasser (2003) Epidemiology of erectile dysfunction in four countries: cross-national study of the prevalence and correlates of erectile dysfunction. *Urology,* 61, 201-6.

Rabkin, J. G., R. Rabkin & G. J. Wagner (1997) Testosterone treatment of clinical hypogonadism in patients with HIV/AIDS. *Int J STD AIDS,* 8, 537-45.

Rabkin, J. G., G. J. Wagner & R. Rabkin (1999) Testosterone therapy for human immunodeficiency virus-positive men with and without hypogonadism. *J Clin Psychopharmacol,* 19, 19-27.

--- (2000) A double-blind, placebo-controlled trial of testosterone therapy for HIV-positive men with hypogonadal symptoms. *Arch Gen Psychiatry,* 57, 141-7; discussion 155-6.

Richardson, D., D. Goldmeier, G. Frize, H. Lamba, C. De Souza, A. Kocsis & G. Scullard (2007) Letrozole versus testosterone. a single-center pilot study of HIV-infected men who have sex with men on highly active anti-retroviral therapy (HAART) with hypoactive sexual desire disorder and raised estradiol levels. *J Sex Med,* 4, 502-8.

Rogstad, K. E., R. Shah, G. Tesfaladet, M. Abdullah & I. Ahmed-Jushuf (1999) Cardiovascular autonomic neuropathy in HIV infected patients. *Sex Transm Infect,* 75, 264-7.

Rosen, R., C. Brown, J. Heiman, S. Leiblum, C. Meston, R. Shabsigh, D. Ferguson & R. D'Agostino (2000) The Female Sexual Function Index (FSFI): a multidimensional self-report instrument for the assessment of female sexual function. *J Sex Marital Ther,* 26, 191-208.

Rosen, R. C., J. A. Catania, A. A. Ehrhardt, A. L. Burnett, T. F. Lue, K. McKenna, J. R. Heiman, S. Schwarcz, D. G. Ostrow, S. Hirshfield, D. W. Purcell, W. A. Fisher, R. Stall, P. N. Halkitis, D. M. Latini, J. Elford, E. O. Laumann, F. L. Sonenstein, D. J. Greenblatt, R. A. Kloner, J. Lee, D. Malebranche, E. Janssen, R. Diaz, J. D. Klausner, A. L. Caplan, G. Jackson, R. Shabsigh, J. H. Khalsa, D. M. Stoff, D. Goldmeier, H. Lamba, D. Richardson & H. Sadeghi-Nejad (2006) The Bolger conference on PDE-5 inhibition and HIV risk: implications for health policy and prevention. *J Sex Med,* 3, 960-75; discussion 973-5.

Rosen, R. C., A. Riley, G. Wagner, I. H. Osterloh, J. Kirkpatrick & A. Mishra (1997) The international index of erectile function (IIEF): a multidimensional scale for assessment of erectile dysfunction. *Urology,* 49, 822-30.

Rosser, B. R. S., J. M. Gobby & W. P. Carr. 1999. The unsafe sexual behavior of persons. 18-28.

Schiltz, M. A. & T. G. Sandfort (2000) HIV-positive people, risk and sexual behaviour. *Soc Sci Med,* 50, 1571-88.

Schrader, S., A. Mills, M. Scheperle & J. E. Block (2005) Improvement in sexual functioning and satisfaction in nonresponders to testosterone gel: clinical effectiveness in hypogonadal, HIV-positive males. *Clin Cornerstone,* 7 Suppl 4, S26-31.

Seftel, A. D., R. J. Mack, A. R. Secrest & T. M. Smith (2004) Restorative increases in serum testosterone levels are significantly correlated to improvements in sexual functioning. *J Androl,* 25, 963-72.

Segurado, A. C., E. Batistella, V. Nascimento, P. E. Braga, E. Filipe, N. Santos & V. Paiva (2008) Sexual abuse victimisation and perpetration in a cohort of men living with HIV/AIDS who have sex with women from São Paulo, Brazil. *AIDS Care,* 20, 15-20.

Sikkema, K. J., P. A. Wilson, N. B. Hansen, A. Kochman, S. Neufeld, M. S. Ghebremichael & T. Kershaw (2008) Effects of a coping intervention on transmission risk behavior among people living with HIV/AIDS and a history of childhood sexual abuse. *J Acquir Immune Defic Syndr,* 47, 506-13.

Sollima, S., M. Osio, F. Muscia, P. Gambaro, A. Alciati, M. Zucconi, T. Maga, F. Adorni, T. Bini & A. d'Arminio Monforte (2001) Protease inhibitors and erectile dysfunction. *AIDS,* 15, 2331-3.

Speckens, A. E., M. W. Hengeveld, G. A. Lycklama à Nijeholt, A. M. van Hemert & K. E. Hawton (1993) Discrimination between psychogenic and organic erectile dysfunction. *J Psychosom Res,* 37, 135-45.

Srilatha, B. & P. G. Adaikan (2004) Estrogen and phytoestrogen predispose to erectile dysfunction: do ER-alpha and ER-beta in the cavernosum play a role? *Urology,* 63, 382-6.

Srilatha, B., P. G. Adaikan & Y. S. Chong (2007) Relevance of oestradiol-testosterone balance in erectile dysfunction patients' prognosis. *Singapore Med J,* 48, 114-8.

Stein, M., D. S. Herman, E. Trisvan, P. Pirraglia, P. Engler & B. J. Anderson (2005) Alcohol use and sexual risk behavior among human immunodeficiency virus-positive persons. *Alcohol Clin Exp Res,* 29, 837-43.

Trotta, M. P., A. Ammassari, R. Murri, P. Marconi, M. Zaccarelli, A. Cozzi-Lepri, R. Acinapura, N. Abrescia, P. De Longis, V. Tozzi, A. Scalzini, V. Vullo, E. Boumis, P. Nasta, A. Monforte, A. Antinori & A. a. A. S. Group (2008) Self-reported sexual dysfunction is frequent among HIV-infected persons and is associated with suboptimal adherence to antiretrovirals. *AIDS Patient Care STDS,* 22, 291-9.

Trotta, M. P., A. Ammassari, R. Murri, A. Monforte & A. Antinori (2007) Sexual dysfunction in HIV infection. *Lancet,* 369, 905-6.

Wasserman, P., S. Segal-Maurer & D. Rubin (2008) Low sex hormone-binding globulin and testosterone levels in association with erectile dysfunction among human immunodeficiency virus-infected men receiving testosterone and oxandrolone. *J Sex Med,* 5, 241-7.

Whetten, K., J. Leserman, K. Lowe, D. Stangl, N. Thielman, M. Swartz, L. Hanisch & L. Van Scoyoc (2006) Prevalence of childhood sexual abuse and physical trauma in an HIV-positive sample from the deep south. *Am J Public Health,* 96, 1028-30.

Yang, Y., T. Ikezoe, T. Takeuchi, Y. Adachi, Y. Ohtsuki, S. Takeuchi, H. P. Koeffler & H. Taguchi (2005) HIV-1 protease inhibitor induces growth arrest and apoptosis of human prostate cancer LNCaP cells in vitro and in vivo in conjunction with blockade of androgen receptor STAT3 and AKT signaling. *Cancer Sci,* 96, 425-33.

22

AIDS Changed America with the Twin Breast Cancer Epidemic: Exploring the Consequences of Condomization

Arne N. Gjorgov
Retired Lecturer Epidemiologist, Skopje, Republic of Macedonia

1. Introduction

Breast cancer as an epidemic disease which suddenly emerged along with the AIDS in the United States at the beginning of the 1980s, continued its unabated rise ever since and steadily continued its unprecedented epidemic advance worldwide. Initially affecting mainly the advanced, developed and 'rich' countries of the West, the breast cancer epidemic is now increasingly affecting the developing, less-advanced and 'poor' countries of all parts of the world. The 'latent period' of transition from the 'West" to the East and South, took less than a decade to extend. The epidemic of breast cancer along with the other accompanying, widespread diseases in women of all ages became better apparent now and is increasingly attracting more attention and concern

More than 34 years ago, a case-control study was initiated and completed in the U.S. in order to test an *a priori* hypothesis that a reduced or eliminated exposure to human seminal factors during the reproductive life-spans of women is an etiologic risk factor of developing breast cancer in American married women (Gjorgov, 1978a,b; Gjorgov, 1979; 1980, 1990, 1991, 1994a,b,c, 1996, 1998b). The hypothesis-testing study was jointly carried out at the University of North Carolina, School of Public Health (Epidemiology), at Chapel Hill, NC, and at the University of Pennsylvania School of Medicine and Hospital, in Philadelphia, PA, between 1974 and 1978, more than eight years before mutual epidemics of AIDS and breast cancer ever emerged. The results of the study corroborated the evidence of a significant association between exposure to barrier contraception (condom use and withdrawal practice) and the development of breast cancer in American and other women. In addition, the results provided evidence of a potential for primary (non-chemical) prevention/protection against breast cancer at individual, familial and community levels. Quantifying the risk, the results of the study indicated that women who used condoms and/or practiced withdrawal had a risk of developing breast cancer of 5.2 times greater (95%CI 3.1 - 8.7) than women who used non-barrier methods for fertility-control and family-planning purposes (diaphragm, IUDs, rhythm, oral-contraceptive pills, cream-jellies, and tubal ligation). By using Bayes' conditional theorem, it was estimated that 17% of women in the mainstream population using condoms / withdrawal were likely to develop breast cancer, versus 3.9% of women using non-barrier contraceptive methods. The evidence challenged head on the widespread misperception that all women are at an 'equal risk of breast cancer' and that the disease is a 'random' event in the lives of women (Gjorgov, 1980; 2009b). The newly revealed carcinogenic and other devastating effects and consequences of condomization of female sexuality showed to be operative even at a frequency of use of 50% of condom use. The quantification in the study of the latent period of development of breast cancer was shown to be between 2½ and 5 years, rather than the prevailing arbitrary assumptions of 15-20 years. Almost 80 percent of the etiologic fraction of the putative risk factor, which could indicate a potential preventive gain, was attributed in the study to the condomized and coitus interruptus birth control. One of the most favored inferences of the study was that the marriage is a profoundly biological woman-man union, with physiologic impact on spouses/couples, particularly on woman, along with the customary definition of marriage is a social, economic, psychological, traditional, and legal man-woman unit. Anticipation turned postulate has been that condomization could adversely affect this oldest human institution, the marriage.

The major unforeseen development in the epidemiology of breast cancer, lingering during the past three decades, beginning from the early 1980s, and continuing through the 1990s and 2000s, is the introduced policy of condomization of women's sexuality, as a supposed 'safe' prophylaxis against the HIV/AIDS transmission in the populations. As postulated, the newly introduced mechanical device, the condom, in the intimate (sexual) reproductive ecosystem, has substantially changed (corrupted) the primordial inter-human microenvironment, by eliminating the postulated putative protective factors (the prostaglandins?), that is, by introducing on an unprecedented scale technical effects of absolute male sterility in intimate (sexual) woman-man communication and other marital relations. The new development seem almost for certain to have had substantially supported / confirmed both an indirect causality of the tested evidence of the condom to breast cancer link, and the potential of primary (non-chemical, natural) prevention of the current, excess and unabated breast cancer epidemic.

There is a variety of gender- (sex-) specific diseases or dysfunction in women of all ages, related or not to the perpetual changes of the physiology of the reproductive system and changes of functions and events during the women's the child-bearing life-span. The definition of female-specific diseases is a pragmatic one and consists of specific female organs and systems (the internal and external reproductive organs), and mutual organs in both genders (breast, thyroid, bones) which are preponderantly and 'specifically' present in female. The central postulate is that the condomization is deleterious to all of the normal life functions of women and their reproductive events.

By entering the New Millennium, the beginning of the 21st Century in particular, the twin epidemics and burden of the HIV/AIDS transmission and breast cancer epidemic are likely to remain a major medical problem and great public health burden. The objective of this study was to try to explore the magnitude of the unknown impact and "unintended consequences" of a social action (Fox, 2004), such as the mass condomization, upon the health and lives of women. Accordingly, the study will attempt to provide answer(s) to what is the problem and what has to be done about the worsening morbidity and mortality of women in the changing world, what has been done--or not done--in the past, and especially what seems to be needed to investigate and to be done in the future, in terms of prevention and protection of reproductive health, life processes, truthful birth control, and (un)happiness of women in today's contemporary societies. The methods of the study are assessments of the trends, postulated etiology (root causes), epidemiology and the potential of primary prevention of the most frequent diseases of women of all ages, the cancer of the breast as an epidemic diseases, especially in the industrialized and affluent world of the West, in the last three decades, since the early 1980s, and ever since.

Cancer of the breast is the truly a major marker of the condomization impact upon the health and lives of women in urgent need for solution. Other manifestations of the ill-effect of condomization of women's sexuality are also taken into considerations. All-inclusive data of female specific diseases and phenomena were collected from epidemiologic and clinical studies as well as from psychological and social investigations of female predominance, higher incidence, prevalence and mortality rates, and female to male ration (F:M) of various conditions and diseases **(Table 1).** Because of data limitations, only some of the most frequent afflictions of women and girls were subject to review in the study.

Exclusively female diseases and dysfunctions:
Ovarian cancer, (incidence and death rates), cysts, polycystic syndrome (PCOS), and dysfunctions, Endometrial cancer (incidence and death rates), other pelvic tumors-fibroids Cervical cancer (incidence and death rates), and lesions Vulvodynia, Pain during sex Endometriosis, Female sexual dysfunctions (FSD), Dysmerrhea, menstrual irregularities, cessation, breast pain, hot flashes, craps Abortion: Spontaneous, habitual, artificial, and 'missed abortion'; Pseudocyesis Chronic pelvic pain, Pelvic congestion syndrome, Bloating
Specific, predominantly female diseases: Ratio female : male
Breast cancer, incidence cases and rates is 100 : 1 in males; Thyroid cancer, incidence cases and rates is 3.5 - 7 : 1 in females to males; Osteoporosis, fractures, prevalence, more than 80 : 20 in female to males; Anorexia-bulimia ('eating') disorders, prevalence, in 90 : 10 girls / young women to boys / young men.
Other female predominant diseases: Ratio female : male (referred)
Thyroid disease (Hashimoto), prevalence 10 : 1 Graves disease, prevalence 7 : 1 Sjogren's syndrome, prevalence 9 : 1 Lupus erythematosus, prevalence 8 : 1 Rheumatoid arthritis, prevalence 2.5 : 1 Scleroderma, prevalence 3 : 1 Multiple sclerosis, prevalence 3 : 1 (National Academy of Sciences,.2011)

Table 1. Comprehensive woman's health: specific sex- (gender-) diseases in women, and female-to-male ratios

It should be mentioned here that some of the gender specific morbidly is also observed in domestic female animals, such as the **BSE**, *bovine spongiform encephalopathy,* and created in laboratory animals' mammary carcinomas and other tumors as well. It has been assumed, perhaps with some justification, that the persistent disproportion of higher female prevalence rates and aggregates of the specific gender diseases in females is also related to their specific, reproductive and natural functions. (Gjorgov, 1996b)

2. Evidence-based and theoretical etiology of the breast cancer epidemic

The provided evidence and inferences of the initial, hypothesis-testing study of etiology and prevention of breast cancer showed to be new and different from the widely and routinely accepted conceptions about the women's ill-health. The etiological link between the use of condom and breast cancer development in American and other married women, corroborated in a field study, was subsequently confirmed in a dramatic way by the explicitly predicted, natural experiment of the breast cancer outbreak/epidemic and the perplexing, rapid rise (Dinse et al. 1999), related to condomization campaigns and rumors for prophylaxis against the emergent mysterious infections.

The biological plausibility off the purported causal link of the carcinogenic effects between the of use of barrier methods of contraception, that is, use of condoms and/or withdrawal (*coitus interruptus*) and breast cancer in American and other women has been also corroborated elsewhere (Lê et al., 1989 in France, and Pikhut et al, 1991 in the former USSR). The indirect causality of breast cancer exposure to condom use was defined as an inverse ecological risk factor due to the absence, elimination or reduction of certain protective biological factors in the seminal fluid (the prostaglandins?), thus inducing technical effects of absolute male sterility in the prime biological woman-man communications. It has also been observed that the dichotomy of sexuality and procreative functions of female is much more complex, moving through incrementally deteriorating phases, than it has been presumed. Although intertwined, the distinct sexuality and reproduction capacities in women might offer a 'window of opportunity' to act coherently in achieving the imperatives of both control of the individual fertility and control of the global population growth.

Population-growth control could hardly proceed successfully by applying incorrect, deadly, and deceptive values of the technological method. The carcinogenic effects and life-threatening consequences of the barrier contraceptive methods, such as the new/old, high-tech condom device, along with the ancient technique of withdrawal, are cases in point: they cannot be assumed to be appropriate methods upon which a mass application of a proper population-growth control policy could be maintained. The contemporary social life and norms are practically incompatible with the bygone tradition of large families and multi-parity households. It has been calculated and observed that a woman has to have at least eight or more full term normal pregnancies (FTNPs), i.e., children, in order to be virtually protected against breast cancer. The Nature has not changed and made no adjustments to facilitate the modern human tendency for reduced reproduction. The modern medical history, not yet written, has already shown that any misconception and even inadvertent error in the sphere of human reproduction is bound to inflict tremendous harm on women and society, such as the mass condomization of female sexuality in the mainstream population. It is the purpose of this study to try to clarify the damage of the condom-related "reproductive freedom" fallacy and the scientific and individual ignorance and errors in condomized control of fertility, without passing judgment.

Although the main attention and concern has been focused on the 'hormonal,' oral contraceptive pills, the condom use and the uncritical campaigns for its use in any situation resulted in grave consequences on health and lives of women and girls, in terms of the on-going breast cancer epidemic and rampant 'eating' disorders. Even though the use of condoms dates for more than one century (in England at least), the condoms have been overlooked as the possible cause of the widespread ill-effects and grave consequences in women. The introduction of mass condomization of female sexuality has completely corrupted and destroyed the micro-environment of intimate (sexual) human ecosystem, by creating technical effects of sterile mating and un-physiological primordial woman-man communication and other relations. The unspoken ideas and intuitive popular knowledge of sex as a necessary part of life, health and survival of woman in marriage, and perhaps her beauty, was replaced by a conceptual vacuum in research, attitude and mindsets of sex and sexuality as a trivial, only 'recreational' gender activity.

3. Sources, population and methods

3.1 Sources

Global breast cancer data are updated in five-year reports published by the World Health Organization International Agency on Cancer Research (IARC), in Lyon, France, titled: "Cancer Incidence in Five Continents" (CI5s), volumes III-IX. (Waterhouse et al, 1977, 1982; Muir et al., 1987; Parkin et al, 1992; Parkin et al., 1997, 2002; Cirado et al., 2007). For achieving the objectives volumes III to IX, 1968 to 2002, inclusive, in duration of 35 years for most centers.

3.2 Population

Population under study consists of contingencies of women affected by breast cancer and other malignant diseases, collected by the national or regional Cancer Registries in 180 to 300 countries and population situations globally, with data quantified in average incidence rates (crude and age-standardized), collected in five-year periods, and reported by the regular editions of the WHO-IARC CI5 volumes.

3.3 Methods

For appraisal of existing, reliable and controlled data, collected internationally by the World Health Organization throughout several decades. Common statistical procedures [means, standard deviations, 95% CI (confidence intervals) of the risks, correlation coefficients, two-way statistical significances at $P<.01$ and $P<.05$ levels] were used for testing the differences, the temporal and spacial changes of the epidemic disease. Correlation and regression analyses, in order to test the statistical significance of the trends and rates of the diseases, and possible extrapolations. The necessary graphical figures and tables of the results and trends are also presented. The analysis of the multitude of data was done by using the SPSS (Statistical Package for Social Sciences), Version 16, 2008.

4. Epidemiological and clinical results and consequences

4.1 Perplexing breast cancer incidence rise worldwide

The rapid rise of breast cancer in the U.S. was first noted by the media, perplexed over the "highest breast cancer incidence rate (of 92.1) ever seen" in the U.S., in 1984. The type of tidal wave ('tsunami') onslaught of breast cancer heralded an emerging, unprecedented epidemic of a malignant (not contagious) disease in the medical history. Thus reaching for a first time in human medical history an unprecedented epidemic of malignant disease. Starting by 1987, the crude incidence rate (based on the number of new cases) was almost entirely replaced by age-adjusted incidence rates (computed on out of sight number of new cases). Correlation between the breast cancer incidence rates and prevalence rates of condom use were invariably positive at statistically significant levels, as presented in **Table 2** (Gjorgov, 1998; Gjorgov, 2000; UN Secretariat, 1994):

Region and number of countries/centres	Breast cancer age-adjusted incidence rates,+ 1983-1987 (Lowest and highest rates)	Condom-use prevalence, estimates, in %++ 1987	Correlation coefficient (Spearman r)
• **WORLDWIDE (166)**	6.4 - 104.2	1 - 15	.860**
• **NORTH AMERICA (46)** (USA and Canada)	52.2 - 104.2	10 - 15	.748**
• **SOUTH AMERICA (12)** (Columbia, Costa Rica, Cuba, Equador, Paraguay, Puerto Rico, Martinique, Brazil and other)	26.2 - 40.5	2 - 3	.548*
• **WEST EUROPE (42)** (Portugal, Spain, Italy, France, Norway, Finland, Denmark, Sweden, Holland, Iceland, West Germany, Switzerland and other)	35.7 - 73.5	5 – 13	.777**
• **EAST EUROPE (17)** (Czechoslovakia, GDR, Poland, Estonia, Latvia, Slovenia, Romania, Russia, and other)	31.1 - 43.7	3 - 5	.438
• **UK, AUSTRALIA, NEW ZEALAND (22)**	56.1 - 64.3	10 – 14	.564**
• **AFRICA** and **ASIA (27)** (Algeria, Gambia, Mali; China, India, Japan & other)	6.4 - 24.6	1 - 3	.558**
• **DEVELOPMENTAL STAGE**			
Developed regions (140)	35.7 - 104.2	5 - 15	.834**
Developing countries/regions (25)	6.4 - 43.7	1 - 3	.594**
• **RACE**			
White women (131)	31.1 - 104.2	2 - 15	.855**
Africans & Afro-Americans (12)	10.2 - 71.6	1 – 12	.541*
Orientals (23)	16.9 - 64.0	2 - 3	.821**
• **URBANIZATION**			
Urban populations (21)	31.1 - 104.2	3 - 15	.907**
Rural populations (26)	6.4 - 58.8	1 - 10	.932**

SOURCES: Parkin DM et al. 1992; United Nations Secretariat,.1994; Gjorgov AN., 1998, 2000 *p < .05 (significance level); **p < .01 and/or **p < .0001 (significance levels)

Table 2. Breast Cancer: Age-adjusted Rates (per 100,000) and Condom-Use Prevalence (percentages), 1983-1987, and Correlation coefficients, by Global Regions, Developmental Stage, Race, and Rural-Urban Places,

Quantifying the impact of condomization on breast cancer epidemic, it was estimated that an increase of condom use by 1 (one) percentage point, the gradient of increase of the breast cancer incidence will correspond to rate of 3.85 per 100,000 female population, globally. For North America, the increase of breast cancer incidence would correspond to a rate of 4.4/100,000 per one percent condom-use prevalence increase, and increase between 2.1 and 3.6 breast cancer incidence rates for various European countries. (Gjorgov, 1998a).

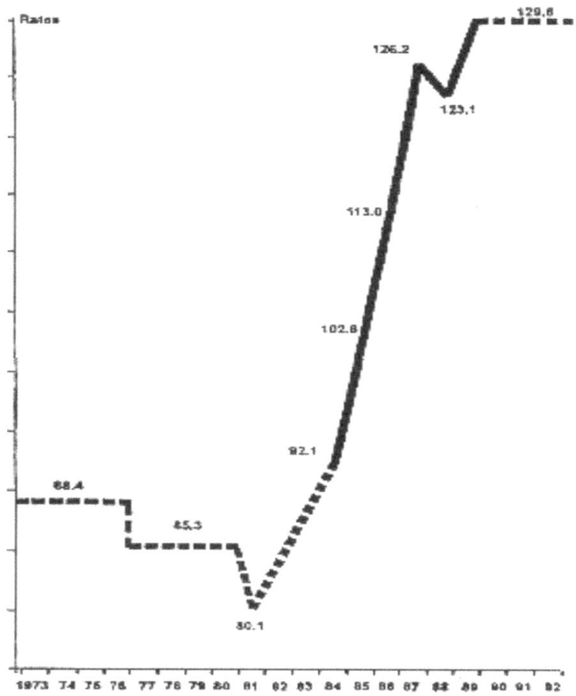

Fig. 1. Breast cancer rise in the United States, 1973-1987. Crude incidence rates, per 100,000 (female) population

Whether the condomization was intended for the feminist's allure only and latter adjusted for prophylaxis of the newly discovered HIV virus, is hard to come by. In one of available sources, the assertion about 'political decision' for condom-use promotion remained ambivalent: Ehrchardt "For the male condom, no controlled trials were demanded before it gained approval as an HIV prophylactic" (Ehrchardt, 1992).

Globally, the average number of breast cancer cases rose by 22% in the last two periods, between 1993-1997 and 1998-2002 (between CI2 VIII and IX Editions), showing difference in the medians of cases 1893.0 and 2735.5, and mode between 595 and 1840, respectively. The upsurge of breast cancer as an epidemic disease emerged rapidly in the United States after 1981, the first and 'the highest ever recorded' reported by the mass media incidence rates, foreboding the trends during the time period 1981 and 1986 and later. The escalation of breast cancer of 57.7 percent increase was recorded in a short period of six years between 1981 and 1986, with 80.1 incidence rate (per 100.000 female population) and 126.2 incidence rate, respectively (**Figure 1**).

4.2 Breast cancer epidemic changes in time, places and populations

The force of the rising incidence of breast cancer has been seen all over the world, the attempts of denigrating its surprise emergence and astonishing effect and magnitude notwithstanding. The new development of breast cancer as an epidemic disease could be best seen in **Figure 2**, as recorded for **Connecticut**, in the last 35 years.

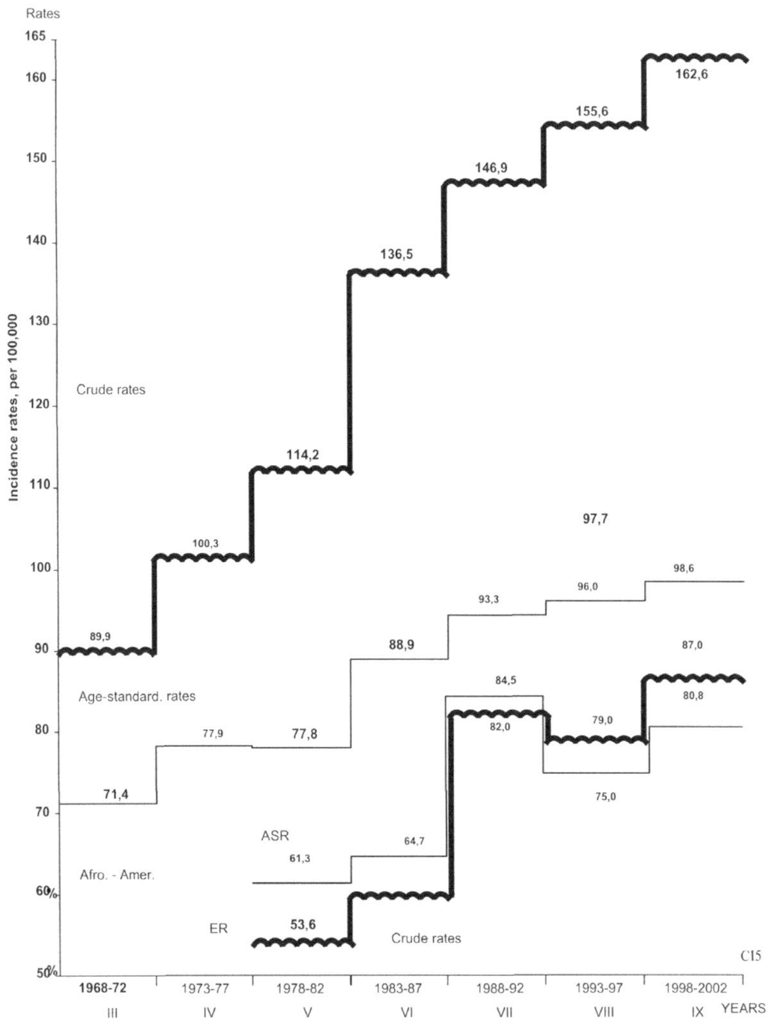

Fig. 2. Breast cancer trends in Connecticut, 1968-2002. Crude and age-adjusted incidence rates, per 100,000

The **Figure 2** reliably confirms the fact of a steep and steady increase of the breast cancer epidemic, for both races, since the Cancer Registry of Connecticut in New Haven, was first cancer registry in the world, established in 1936. (It may be of interest to note that there was a fluctuation of the breast cancer incidence rates for the Afro-Americans, an event rarely observed before.)

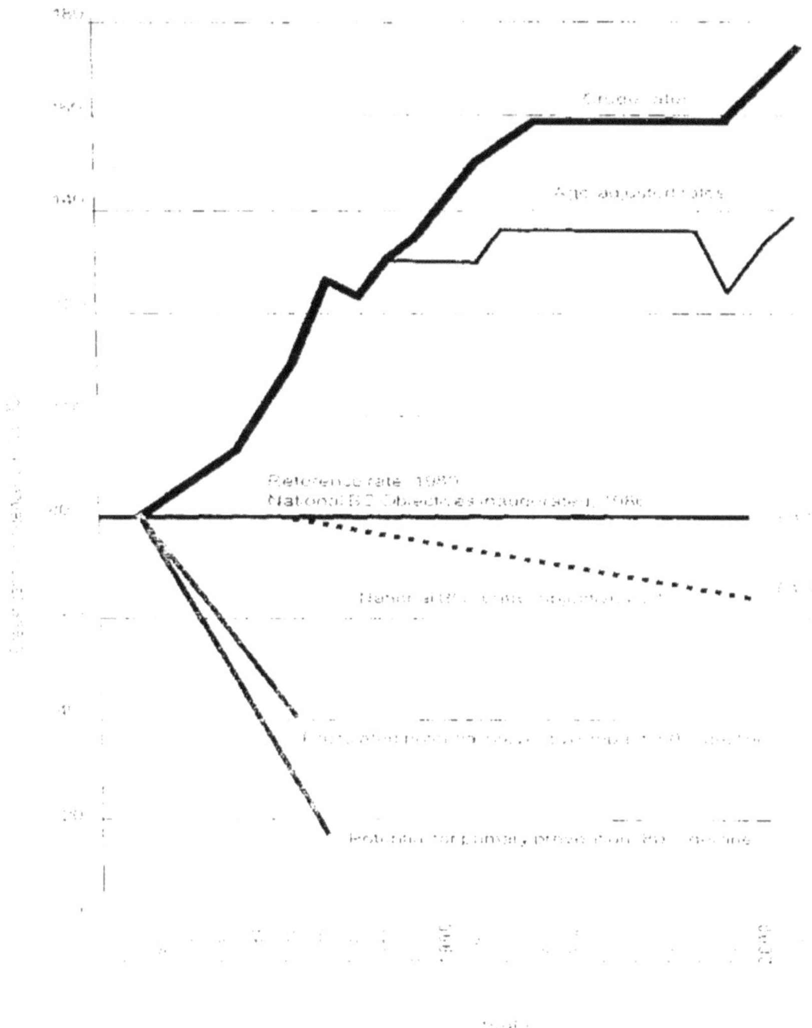

Fig. 3. Breast cancer trends in the U.S., 1980-2002. Observed crude and age-adjusted incidence rates: Projected 21% decline 1986-2000, and Postulated preventive impact, in percentages tested.

The overall epidemiology of the breast cancer epidemic in the **United States** is presented in the **Figure 3**. There is a dual presentation of the trends of the breast cancer progression in the past two-and-a-half decades, from 1980 to 2002. The breast cancer rising trends are presented in crude and age-adjusted incidence rates. The two incidence rates differ considerably, mainly because the age-adjusted rates, showing lower rates, were derived according to moving U.S. census populations, instead to the conventional World Standard Population 1960 (WSP). In the same **Figure 3** is presented the official, wrong prediction (in 1986) of 'declining' breast cancer trend until 2000, and also are presented two personal predictions of the future, postulated downward trends of 50 to 80 percent of breast cancer in the U.S.

Additional data support the analogous development of breast cancer rise in other parts of the country, such as the **San Francisco Bay Area (Figure 4)**, which was subsequently and perhaps justifiably called "the Breast Cancer Capital of the World," for the highest incidence in America in the 1983-1987 period, reaching the excess incidence rate.
The first, the NCI confident forecast of decline of breast cancer incidence rates between 1986 until 2000, by 21 percent, was patently wrong from the outset. The predicted decline of breast cancer, published in 1986 proved to be quite off center: the incidence rates of the disease almost doubled by the end of the 20th Century. The wrongly computed forecast of decline probably reflected the same percentage of decline of the disease during the 1970s, and was computed maybe before the statistical data were in following the 1981unexpected breast cancer jump; The second prediction of decline of the breast cancer incidence rates between 50 to 80 percent, as related to the 1980 situation, remained theoretical estimates, based on etiological fraction percent, contingent on implementation of primary prevention and elimination of the corroborated etiological risk factor of semi-official policy of condomization of the mainstream population(s) against the HIV/AIDS transmissions, along with the application of Bayes' probability theorem computation, and yet to be

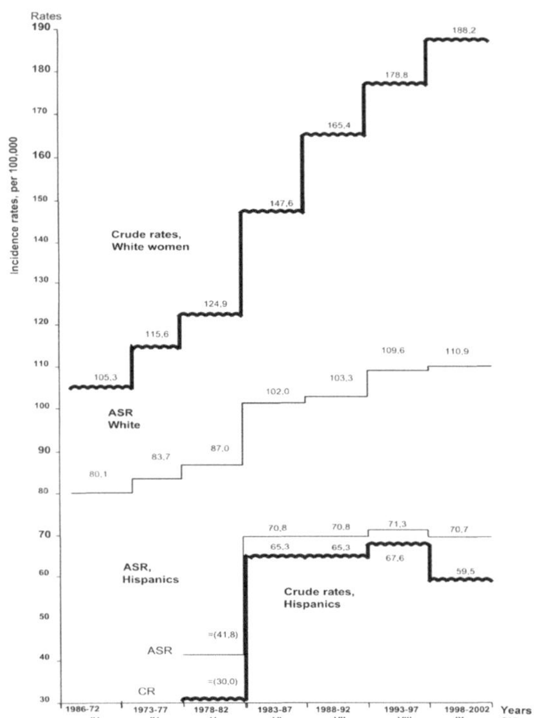

Fig. 4. Breast cancer in San Francisco Bay Area, CA, 1986-2002, by race. Crude and age-adjusted incidence rates, per 100,000

The same pattern of rapid rise of breast cancer was recorded in **Seattle, WA**, with an extraordinary jump of 27.8 percent of crude incidence rate (from 95.8 to 121.8) within one period of 1978-82 (before AIDS epidemic) to 1983-87 (the initial tide of the AIDS outbreak in the U.S.). (Figure not presented.) According to the data in the latest (IX) volume of the CI5, it seems that the infamous title of "Breast cancer capital of the world" has shifted from the San Francisco Bay Area to the Ferrara Region, Italy, with a crude incidence rate of 201.8 in the 1998-2002 period, and an increase of 263 percent in the number of breast cancer cases (from 527 to 1833) since 1998-1992.

In other parts of the Western world, the **Oxford** Region, the UK experienced immediate high increase of breast cancer and without apparent delay after the U.S. (**Figure 5**). The steady rise of the breast cancer incidence has been happening continuously and all 5-year time periods after 1980. In the mid-1990s, the Cancer Research UK organized, in cooperation with other European countries and North-American regions, so-called population-based, chemo-preventive community trials against epidemic breast cancer, by giving the drug *tamoxifen* to great number healthy women, in duration of five years, The enthusiastic chemo-preventive trials ended prematurely, with impractical results for breast prevention. No other idea or projects were envisioned or proposed for testing a potential primary (non-chemical) prevention of breast cancer. Circumstantial and fragmentary evidence seems to suggest that the idea of global condomization has originated at the 'R. Doll' Institute of Epidemiology in Oxford, probably thought of during the decade 1960s.

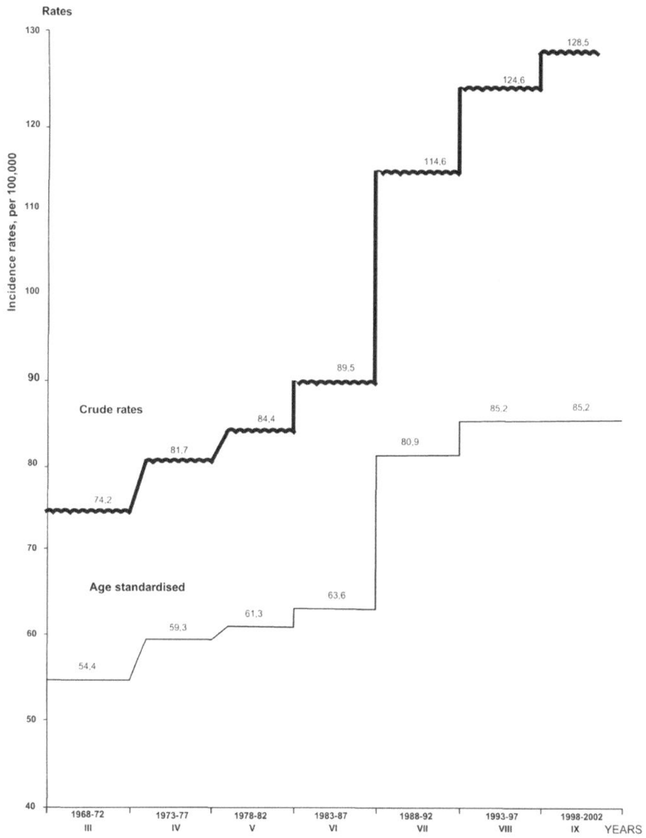

Fig. 5. Breast cancer in Oxford, UK, 1968-2002. Crude and age-adjusted incidence rates, per 100,000

At least two more high-risk regions of breast cancer epidemic in Europe deserve mention, in France and Sweden. The breast cancer epidemic in **France** (**Figure 6**) may prove of interest because of the fact that the North-Rhine Region is both one of the best developed regions, and one with the highest incidence rates in EU. The City of Strasbourg, where the multinational European Parliament is located, is also an important place where much of the debates and policies about breast cancer control, mainly for rectifying the early-detection screening policy, has been and is expected to continue to eventually consider primary prevention of the breast cancer epidemic soon.

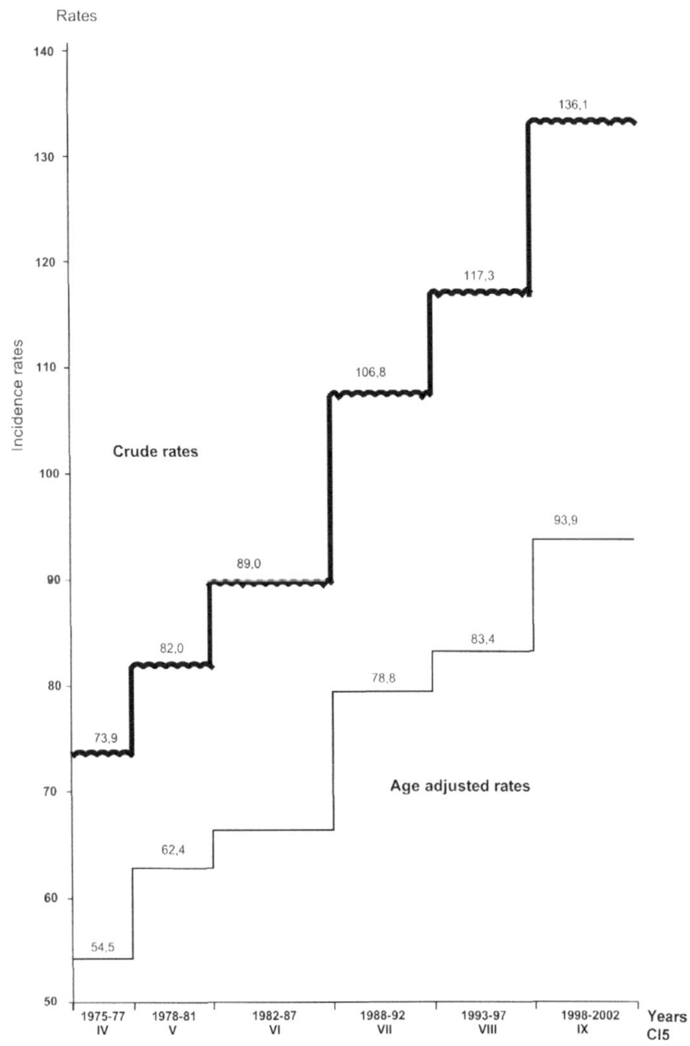

Fig. 6. Breast cancer in Bas-Rhin, France, 1975-2002. Crude and age-adjusted incidence rates, per 100,000

Sweden has always been a lead-country of high breast cancer incidence (**Figure 7**). The country has an interesting epidemiology of the disease, since the current, global breast cancer epidemic seems to have started much earlier there, during the decade of the 1970s, ten years before the epidemic was first recorded in the U.S. in the 1980s. Part of the puzzle lies in the information that condomization ("for non-contraceptive use") was first introduced in Sweden (Hinman, 1978; Valdiserri, 1988), in the 1970s decade, before campaigns of condomization were carried out in the rest of the world.

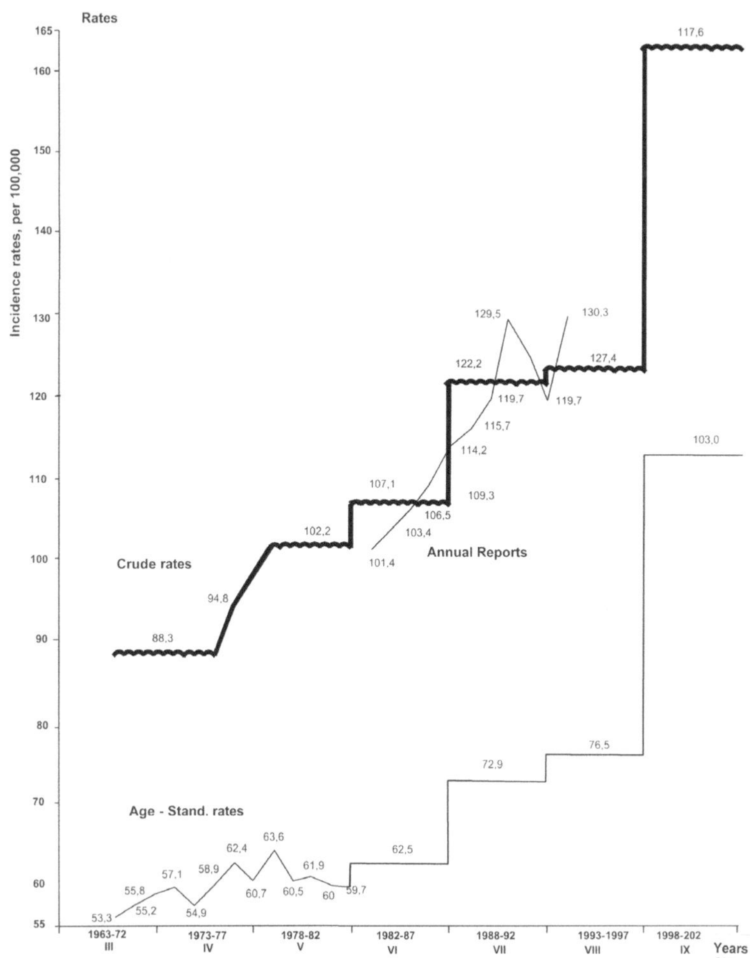

Fig. 7. Breast cancer in Sweden, 1971-2002. Crude and age-adjusted incidence rates, per 100,000

On the other side of the globe, in Australia, the rise of the breast cancer epidemic in the **New South Wales** showed the familiar European model of advent (**Figure 8**). According to the separate Annual Reports of the Cancer Registry of the Province NSW, the rise of breast cancer was apparently steeper than presented by the presentation in 5-year periods of the WHO-IARC CI5 reports.

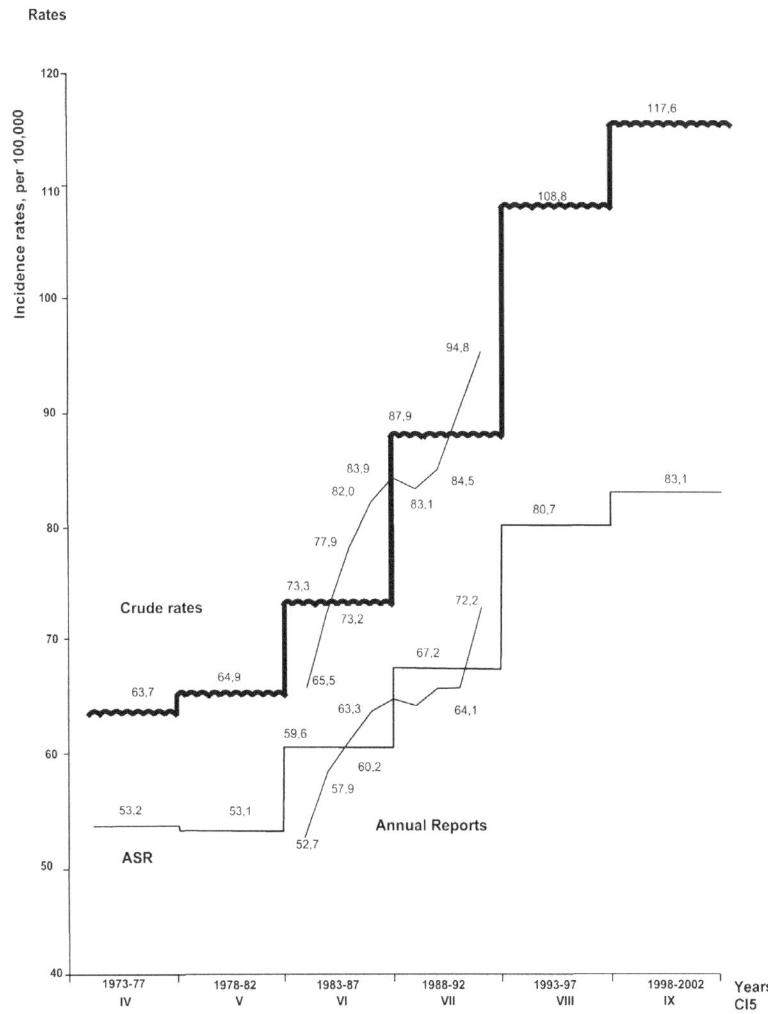

Fig. 8. Breast cancer in New South Wales, Australia, 1973-2002. Crude and age-adjusted incidence rates, per 100,000

In Asia, the experience of **Kuwait (Figure 9**) of the breast cancer epidemic rise was somewhat peculiar. First, Kuwait long enjoyed the distinction to be listed as a country with the lowest rate of breast cancer in the world. I worked and as Director of the National Cancer Registry at the Kuwait Cancer Control Centre for a long while, was able to observe the situation and the ensuing profound changes with regard breast cancer. (Gjorgov, 1986). Second, the breast cancer onslaught happened fast and affected very young, married multipara-women (not less than 4 pregnancies), between 23 to 35 years of age. The surgeons from Europe, worked in the local hospitals, were the first to voice alarm of the unusual in their practice pattern of performing mastectomies to such a young-age group of patients. Third, contrary to the American and European experience, the Non-Kuwaiti, immigrant women, had persistently had a higher incidence rate of breast cancer than the Kuwaiti women. During the past three decades, the increase of breast cancer in Kuwaiti women did not reach the higher incidence of the immigrant, Non-Kuwaiti women in the country.

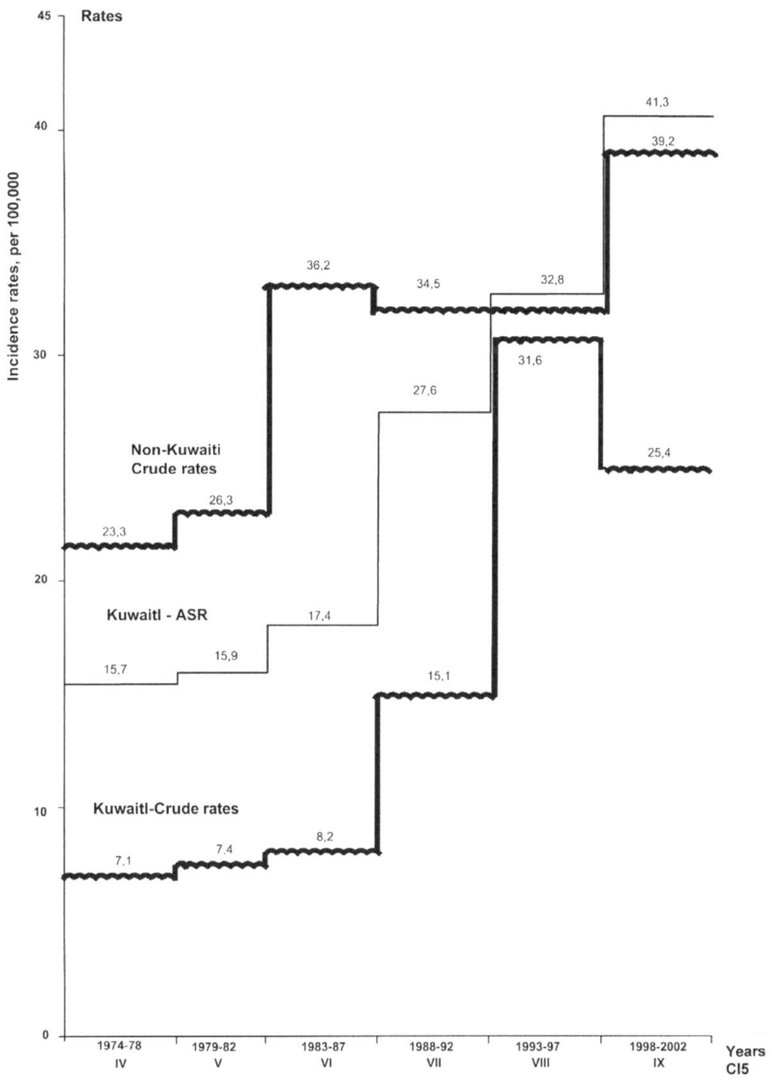

Fig. 9. Breast cancer in Kuwait, 1974-2002, by Kuwaiti and Non-Kuwaiti women. Crude and age-adjusted incidence rates, per 100,000

The other regions and countries of the world followed suit. In **Miyagi, Japan**, the **Figure 10** shows a steadily but moderately increasing breast cancer incidence rates. Nevertheless, the slow-moving breast cancer epidemic revealed an extraordinary evidence / proof of the peculiar characteristics of the breast cancer epidemic, the increase of the incidence in the younger women, most notably in the reproductive age-span of women (**Figure 11**).

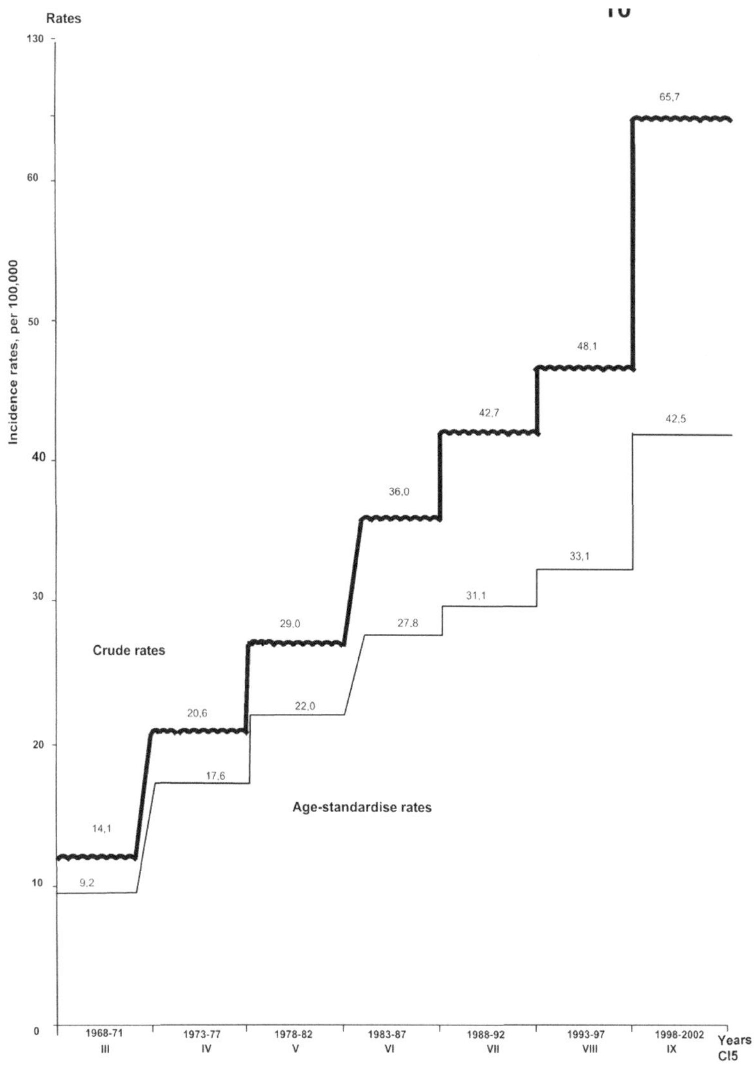

Fig. 10. Breast cancer in Miyagi, Japan, 1968-2002. Crude and age-adjusted incidence rates, per 100,000

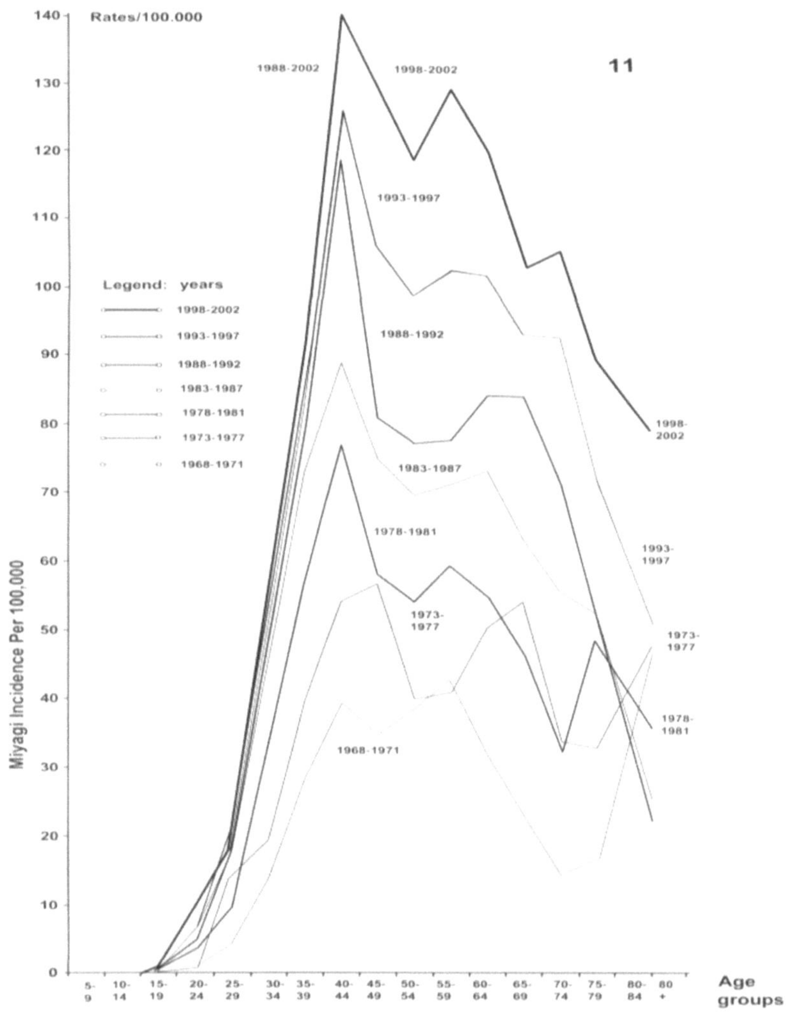

Fig. 11. Breast cancer Age-specific incidence rates in Miyagi, Japan, 1968-2002, by five-year periods, per 100,000

The conventional view that breast cancer is a "disease of affluence" had to be changed in the meantime by the epidemiology and empirical research of the disease in Afro-American women in the U.S., as well as in less industrialized (Krieger, 2002) and other "poor" countries. Three more situations could demonstrate the sudden changes in the trends of breast cancer developments (in %) in a number of centers in the **United States (Figure 12)** and in **Europe (Figure 13)**, from negative-decreasing to positive-increasing breast cancer trends.

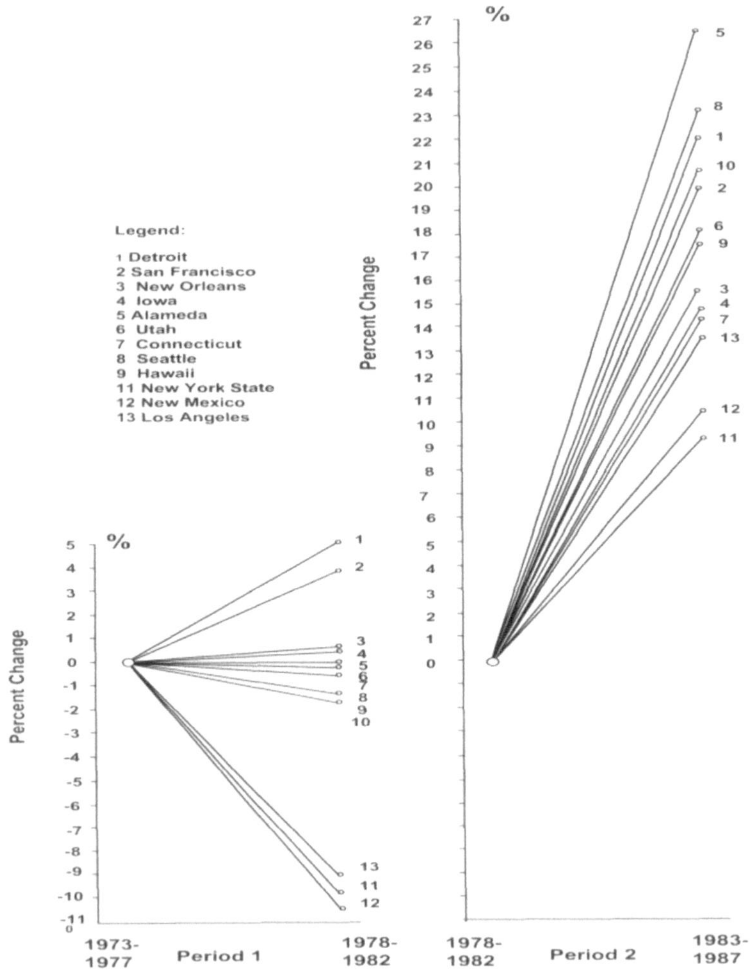

Fig. 12. Shift of breast cancer trends in the United States, 1983-1987, by time periods and regions. Changes of age-adjusted incidence rates, in percentages.

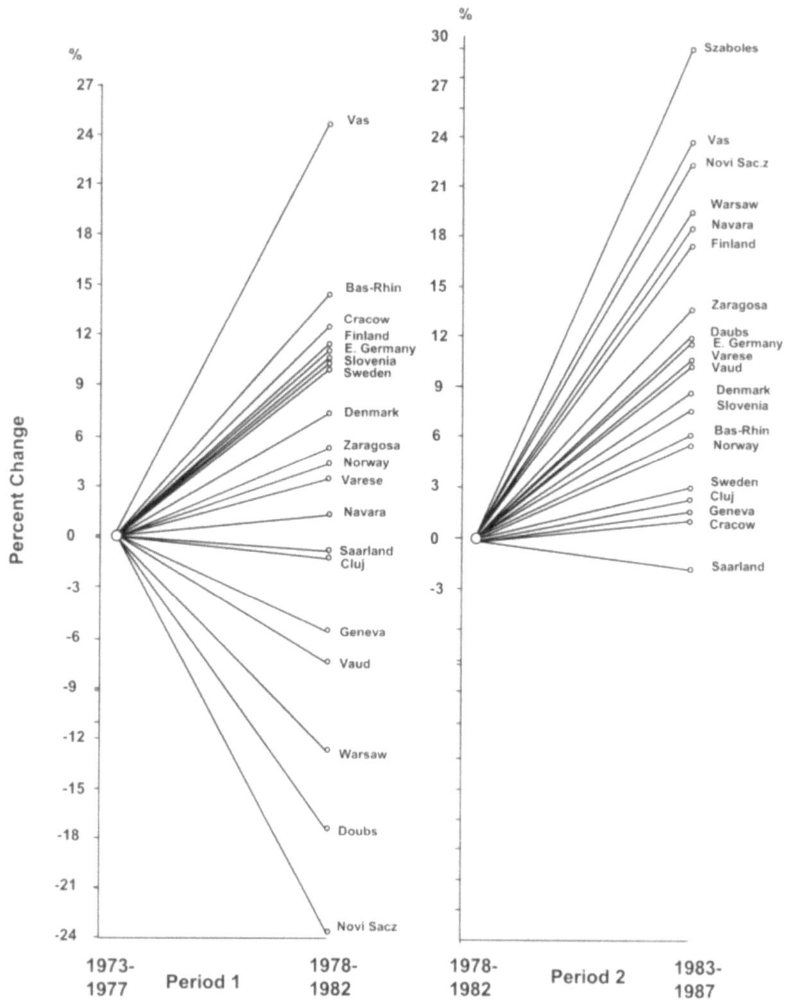

Fig. 13. Shift of breast cancer trends in Europe, 1983-1987, by time periods and countries. Changes of age-adjusted incidence rates, in percentages.

4.3 Inner developments of the breast cancer epidemic

The distribution of the age-specific incidence rates among young women, bellow 45 years of age, during the seven period of five-year intervals (35 years duration), between 1968 and 2002, clearly demonstrates the shift of the breast cancer epidemic towards younger, reproductive-age groups, ostensibly most frequently exposed to the purported risk factor of condomization. In addition to the situation in **Miyagi** (**Figure 11**), an extraordinary evidence of breast cancer descending in young women is evident in **Shanghai,** China (**Figure 14**). Perhaps a foreboding development of the disease in the country, the extraordinary shift of breast cancer incidence towards younger women was recorded in Shanghai in just a single five-year period, 1973-1978. In 2008, an alarming among many other studies appeared that rightly claimed that "China is on the point end of a breast cancer epidemic" (Linos et al. 2008). However, the solution in averting the predicted, impending breast cancer epidemic was seen and recommended in reductions of "modifiable risk factors," such as, alcohol intake, parity, hormone use, and adult weight gain... Condomization as a means for the restrictive reproductive policy was neither investigated nor mentioned in the study.

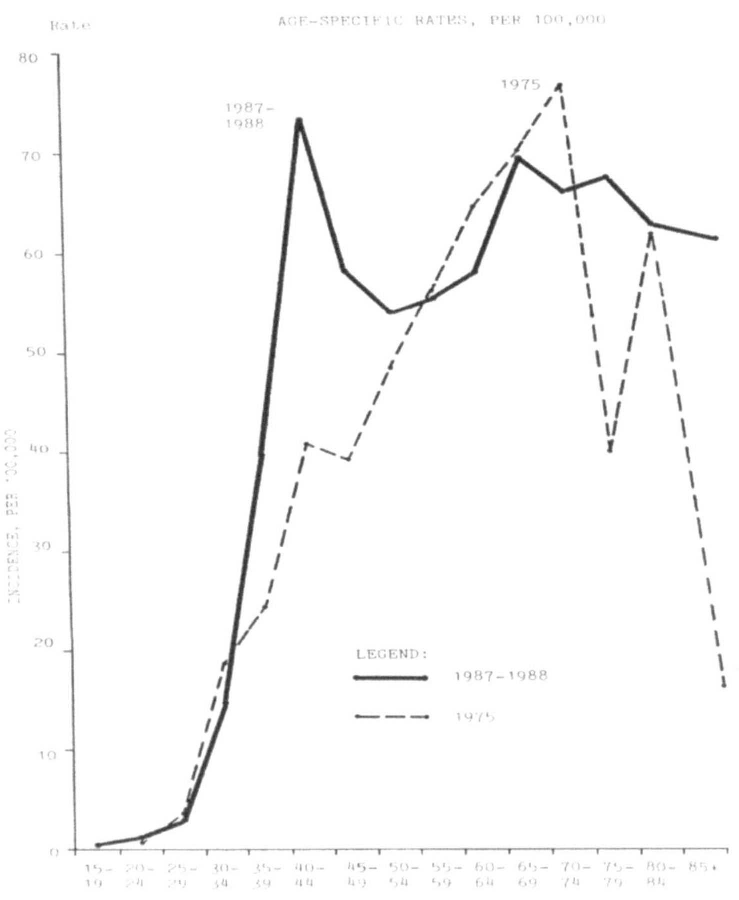

Fig. 14. Breast Cancer in Shanghai, China, 1975 and 1987-1988: "Debut" peak. Age-specific incidence rates, per 100,000

The unexpected shift towards young women was manifested in a remarkable peak of the disease in the of 35-39 year age-group, as a "debut" phenomenon, assuming that condomization was the first and perhaps the main mode of fertility control and family planning. Almost exactly the same situation was observed in Warsaw City (Poland), with the "debut" peak in 1987, compared with the age-specific distribution before the condom-use campaigns, in the period 1968-1972. (Figure not shown.) In the Volume VII of the CI5 (Parkin et al., 1997), and to a lesser degree in the Volumes VIII (Parkin, 2002) and IX (Cirado, 2007), there were more than 60 cases of age-specific distribution in which the first highest incidence of breast cancer was located in younger age groups, bellow 50, and even below 40 years of age. The "debut" phenomenon was mainly seen in countries with low baseline breast cancer incidence and where the breast cancer epidemic has been developing at a faster pace afterwards, such as, for instance, Italy.
The debut peaks showed that they are not static phenomena and not a rare situation. Data from the Malta National Cancer Registry (2010) showed that "debut" peaks popped up in the past decades in almost every year in a ten-year decade, and continued to be still present in subsequent cohorts of women **(Table 3).** Not less than 50-60 breast cancer age-specific distributions in the 1988-1992 period (CI5-VII) showed the highest peaks in younger women. The pattern of "debut" peaks is reminiscent to the epidemiological pattern of breast cancer age-specific incidence in Europe before and immediately after the WWII, with the so-called 'Clemmesen's hook' (Storm, 2011), similar but not equal with the "debut" phenomenon, because it happens to young women, in the prime of their reproductive sexuality, rather than at the end of the reproduction life time of menopause.

Age groups	**1998**	**1999**	**2000**	**2001**	**2002**	**2003**	**2004**	**2005**	**2006**	**2007**
15-19	0	0	0.07	0	0	0	0	0	0	0
20-24	0	0	0.07	0	0	0	0	0	0	0
25-29	0	0.08	0	0	0	0	0	0	0	0
30-34	0.17	0.18	0.09	0.60	0.33	0.24	0.08	0.07	0.15	0.35
35-39	0.36	0.29	0.37	030	0.79	0.40	0.41	0.58	0.33	0.41
40-44	1.13	1.68	0.75	0.60	0.87	1.09	1.39	1.44	1.27	1.48
45-49	1.76	1.43	1.57	1.68	0.97	1.02	0.80	2.05	1.32	1.40
50-54	2.47	1.60	1.91	2.22	2.19	1.77	2.14	1.53	1.80	1.92
55-59	2.29	2.26	2.29	2.18	2.07	2.68	2.33	2.00	2.52	2.04
60-64	1.50	2.56	2.62	1.59	2.89	3.59	2.61	3.76	3.20	3.00
65-69	3.23	3.27	3.09	2.34	1.64	2.28	2.13	3.50	3.30	3.65
70-74	4.12	2.28	3.21	2.56	3.15	1.27	3.58	2.19	3.62	3.44
75-79	2.09	4.71	3.83	3.07	2.50	4.26	2.95	4.53	4.41	3.82
80-84	4.12	3.75	6.34	3.43	2.36	3.48	2.86	4.39	2.87	3.85
85+	3.60	3.95	1.55	4.10	3.02	3.72	4.63	3.65	2.90	4.22
Crude rates	**106.75**	**110.34**	**110.44**	**100.75**	**99.57**	**108.40**	**109.67**	**128.81**	**127.50**	**131.74**
Age-adj. rates	**72.61**	**72.30**	**70.55**	**64.35**	**64.99**	**67.70**	**66.84**	**79.56**	**75.82**	**77.78**

Table 3. Cancer of the breast: Maltese Islands-Trends in Incidence 1998-2007. Incidence rates, by age and year of cancer registration (February 2010)

Most likely, the "debut" phenomenon is closely related with another puzzling issue of the breast cancer epidemic, the growing cases of ductal carcinoma in-situ (DCIS), or simply in-situ breast cancer, whose incidence, has gone up exponentially, up to 30 percent of the annual number of registered breast cancer cases, since the 1980s (National Cancer Institute, 2001). The in-situ (DCIS) cases in fact, testify of the evolving nature and lack of understanding of the global breast cancer epidemic. The in-situ breast cancer epitomizes also the conceptual vacuum in professional dealing with the breast cancer epidemic, because of misconception of DCIS as a random event in lives of women; not reporting of DCIS in the annual reports of incidence rate of breast cancer; exaggerated and not true claims of excellent ("nearly 100%") survival rate; unduly and unreasonably defined in-situ cases as non-breast cancer (0-zero stage); the systemic background of the in-situ cases is ignored and treatment is as a local disease. The early-detection screening, for finding most and more of the DCIS cases, has always been mired with uncertainty of further course of the in-situ finding into aggressive and metastatic breast cancer, the extent of treatment, and the dilemma about the usefulness of the early detection as the basic tenet of the breast cancer strategy.

4.4 Reproductive age and breast cancer

Age of women as such has almost invariably been defined among the strongest risk factor of breast cancer. The assertion of randomness has frequently accompanied the age factor. The international experience, however, points out to the long held observation that this assessment is not universally correct and that is in principle wrong. **Figure 15** shows that breast cancer in **Korea** is confined to middle-aged women, to the reproductive-age span women, with declining incidence after the peri-menopausal age of 50. In most of Asian populations (Japan, Malaysia, India), the breast cancer profiles exhibit the same pattern.

The pattern of breast cancer age distribution in Korea was similar to those in many European countries, which could still be seen in Porto, Portugal, evocative to the old rather than new European models. (Figure not presented)

Hidden behind the common reference of "cancer incidence increase" lies the fact that the increase is created to a high extent by the rise of breast cancer, while the category of "the rest of cancers" is actually decreasing. [The categories of breast cancer and "all cancers without skin cancer (C44)" are given as such and, for the purposes of this study, is computed a new category of "rest of cancers," meaning 'all cancers' minus breast cancer)]. The data of the **SEER** (Surveillance, Epidemiology, and End Results) program, containing nine registration centers in the U.S. and, since it stands for about 10 percent of the U.S. population, considered representative sample of the country, showed that the number of breast cancer rose by 11.6 percent, while the "rest" of cancers increased by 8.7 percent, between the two consecutive periods of 1993-97 and 1998-2002. The **Figure 16** presents data of increasing breast cancer age-adjusted incidence rates (16.8%) compared to the decreasing "rest" of cancer (-7.5%) in Afro-American women during the aforementioned two 5-year periods. There was exactly the same reciprocal increase of breast cancer (7.7%) and decrease (-4.3%) of the 'rest of cancers' in Afro-American women in Connecticut, and unexpected decrease (of -4.9%) of the 'rest' of cancers (age-adjusted incidence rates), and increase (1.2%) in white women in the San Francisco Bay Area, CA.

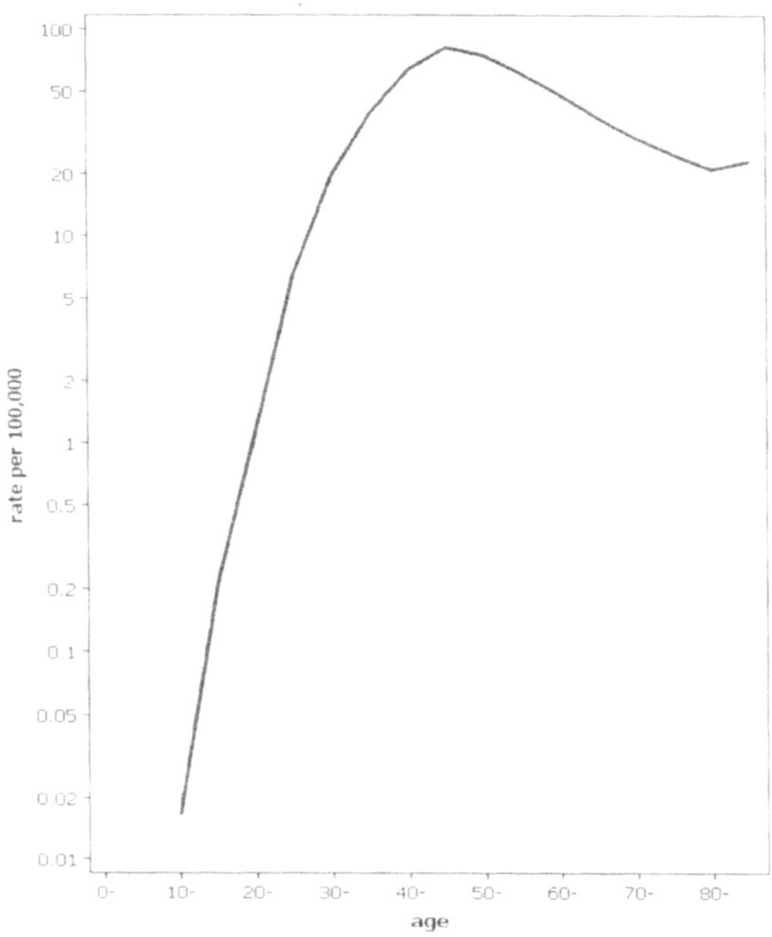

Fig. 15. Breast Cancer in Korea, 1988-2002. Age-specific incidence rates, per 100,000

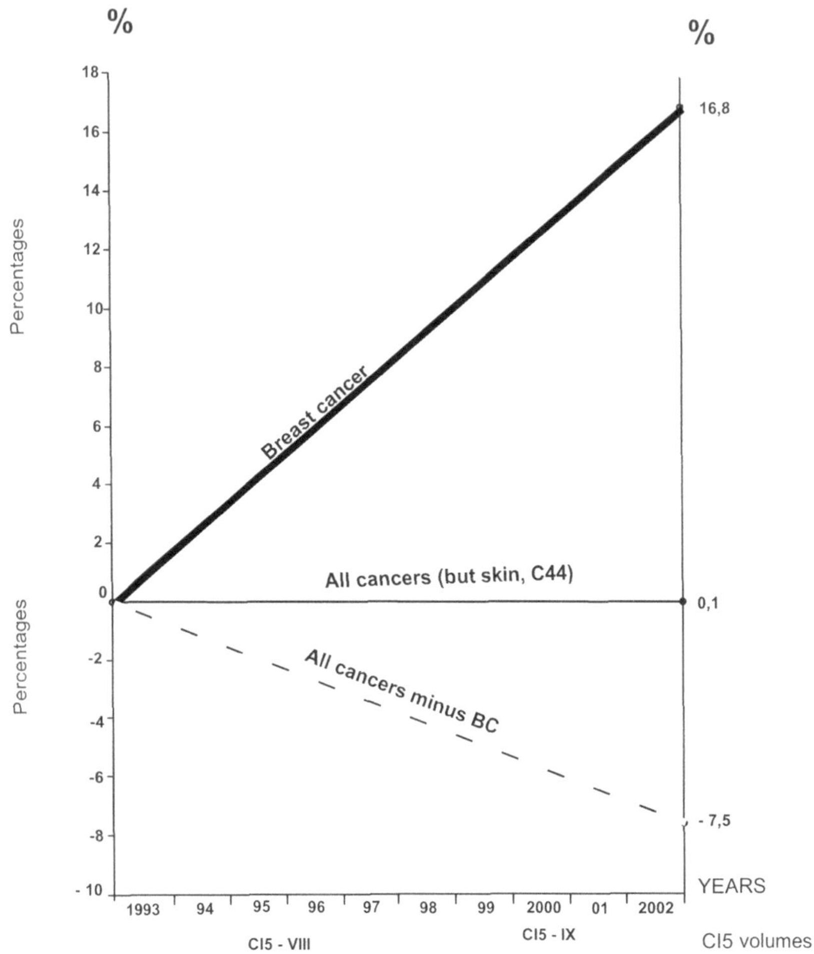

Fig. 16. Diverging trends of increase of breast cancer, and decrease of the 'rest' of all cancers in Afro-American women, 1993-2002, SEER - 9 regions. Age-standardized incidence rates, per 100,000

The differences in incidence rates and the diverging, comparative trends of increase and decrease of breast cancer and the 'rest' of cancers in women of both races (white and Afro-American), living in a reasonably same environment, gives credence to the evidence that the environmental chemicals/toxins, and of the women's nature culprit estrogen theory, are not the likely risk factors of the disease. The root cause of the modern-time women's suffering (breast cancer), is in certain other areas, such as, the "inverse" etiological risk factor at play at personal, intimate (sexual) and familial levels, as postulated.

Exactly the same pattern of diverging trends of rising breast cancer incidence rates as contrasted to decreasing incidence all other forms of cancer ('rest" of cancers) has been determined in Sweden in the past, Poland (Warsaw City) at the recent past and other centers in the world, according to the latest CI5 data (1998-2002). The same source shows that breast cancer incidence rates increased for 14.1% in Hong Kong, while the "rest" of cancer declined for minus 6.7% between decades 1993-97 and 1998-2002. The Shanghai City, a fast developing urban conglomerate, and similar to Hong Kong in population and number of breast cancer cases, showed the same trends of increase, of 29.8%, of breast cancer (age-adjusted incidence rates), and increase of 9.7% of the "rest" of cancers. Once again, the differing end-results of breast cancer between the two Chinese metropolises may corroborate the evidence that increase of the disease in Hong Kong, along with the decrease of the "rest" of cancers, is more related to other than poisonous risk factors in the environment, than the (fast) increase of breast cancer in Shanghai (together with the "rest" of cancers), which might be related to ecological pollution of presumed exposures to noxious workplace environments. The notion of better controlled environment-related cancers, defined as "rest" of cancers and excluding breast cancer, might be seen in the following examples for the two periods between 1993-97 and 1998-2002: Higher breast cancer rise and trailing rise of the "rest" of cancers is observed in Sweden, at country level again, with 3.3% breast cancer rise and -1.6% decline of the "rest" of cancers), Geneva (Switzerland, with a 6.2% breast cancer rise and -3.0% decline of the "rest" of cancers), Tyrol (Austria, with 4.9% breast cancer rise, and a practically stalled rise of "rest" of cancers, of 0.3%). Virtually, almost all centers of cancer registration in the world, for the two aforementioned periods, showed much higher percentages of breast cancer rises as compared with the increase of the "rest" of cancers.

The intermediate figures and other tabulated data which are to be presented, will try to corroborate once again the underlying tested theory (hypothesis) of the exposure forces of the misconceived barrier contraception as the main risk factor, attributed as the root cause of the epidemic of the gender-specific diseases. Almost no other known alteration in the inter-human environment or corruption of the intimate (sexual) woman-man ecosystem has taken place in the population(s), but the misconceived ubiquitous mass condomization, making this overlooked fallacy an exceedingly hazardous "minefield" to the health, lives and happiness of women and girls in the modern world. In contemporary dictionary of profit-driven healthcare system, the biological risk factors and exposure to ever-rising breast cancer and other epidemic diseases in women are considered as "keeping the healthy people in the risk pool" and "death spiral." From the deliberately maintaining the "risk pool" leading to scare, anxiety and "death spiral" of cost and uncertainties, new health-care dynamics are created, by which the insurance companies recruit eternal number of cases of breast-cancer affected women for "downstream" clinical activities, deceptively defined and disguised as "preventive health care for women," and which include "preventive screening," "preventive mammography programs" for "early detection," and clinical treatments (surgery and chemotherapy). (The failed, previously carried out community "chemo-prevention" trials on healthy women with *tamoxifen* against breast cancer, in a number of European and North American regions, in the 1990s, is not an active option anymore.)

Most of the results and data evaluated in the study would stay open-ended, to monitor the further developments of the increasing trends of the breast cancer epidemic, until after the decision and public option for intervention is implemented for practical elimination of the breast cancer epidemic and the accompanied diseases-tumors of female reproductive system. (Practical elimination of the excess breast cancer epidemic worldwide might be defined as is a virtual 'eradication' of the disease(s) to low incidence rates of sporadic cases the disease(s) at individual, familial and community levels.)

4.5 Ovarian cancer

Besides breast cancer, an integral part of the comprehensive research of the reproductive health of women is the ovarian and endometrial cancers. In this regard, observations and results in joint breast-ovarian cancer research experience are presented. The following commentary to highly publicized results in prevention of ovarian cancer by oral contraceptive pills is presented: Adjacent to cancer of the ovary are considered the polycystic syndrome, menstrual irregularities, endometriosis, female sexual dysfunction, low pelvic pain, craps, bloating.

The following critical comment was communicated to Prof. Valerie Beral, the Director of the **Cancer Research UK** and the lead author of the "Study: the Pill Protects against Ovarian Cancer," as reported by Washington Post Online, January 25, 2008 (Fragments):

> "The Oxford study reported only a partial truth about the prevention / protection against ovarian cancer in the United Kingdom and elsewhere. Yet, the research of the root cause of the epidemic extent of ovarian cancer has NOT been done.
>
> Despite the brief, but interrupted, heated exchange with the author and other presiding colleagues 14 years ago, at the 'Lancet International Breast Cancer Challenge Conference' (Brugge, Belgium, April 1994), about the tested evidence… that the CONDOMIZATION of women's sexuality, as the main root cause of the rising epidemics of epidemic breast cancer and other malignancies (ovarian and endometrial cancers), has been ignored and circumvented time and again, and not investigated to date…
>
> It is a real wonder that there were such women who used oral contraceptive pills during the long era of indiscriminate promotion of 'condom culture;' a minority of 'non-politically correct' women and couples who rejected, even periodically the use of condoms, perhaps by listening to their inner sense of impaired sexuality and health consequences. For, many millions of women suffered and died mainly in the Western world, including the UK, during the twin breast and ovarian epidemics. The deadly, false belief of the exposure to (use of) condoms as a "safe" device for fertility-control and family-planning purposes has apparently taken a heavy human toll, and puts many more lives in jeopardy.
>
> Despite the controversial assertion (that OC pills 'increase' breast cancer while decreasing ovarian cancer), the fact remains that the OC pills (with prevalent use during the 1970s), did not create the breast cancer epidemic, but the condomization of female sexuality (since the beginning of the 1980s), has predictably precipitated the unprecedented natural experiment of rapid breast cancer rise as an epidemic disease, or has 'coincided' with the emergence of the current, unabated breast / ovarian / gynecological cancer epidemics. According to previous evidence, the preventive effect is recognized not because of the OC-pill chemical content, i.e., "the first medication…(which) cuts ovarian cancer," as claimed by the authors of the aforementioned statistical study, but rather because of the non-use or abandoned barriers contraceptive methods (mainly condoms), associated with the observed protection of ovarian / breast cancer.
>
> The OC-pill claim as protective factor also contradicted the added statement by the authors of 'other protective measures' against ovarian cancer which included 'advice' for "having children or getting tubes tied." Those two human conditions (pregnancies or tubal ligation) oppose the presumed OC-pill preventive effects, for they contain neither exogenous, OC pill's estrogens nor any other medication. Consequently, the role of the

OC pills as a presumed preventive measure against cancer in women should be questioned and rejected as an interpretation of its effects, as highlighted previously in a discussion about 'Tubal ligation and risk of ovarian cancer" in the same journal, Lancet 2001; 358: 1467-70 (pp. 843-44).
Women may change the contraceptive methods during their reproductive lifetimes, and may frequently, even sporadically still use condoms, because of planned ignorance of its carcinogenic effects. It is anticipated that the termination of the main and perhaps the sole risk factor of breast / ovarian cancers, the universal condomization of women's sexuality, will bring about immediate health gain in the community. A practical 'eradication' of the diseases to levels of sporadic cases, is expected to reached in a speedy decline of the current, excess epidemics of breast and ovarian cancers, in a mirror image of the rapid rise of the sex- (gender-) specific malignant epidemics as they entered the human race more than two-and-a-half decades ago. What might help in defining and providing primary prevention of ovarian and breast cancer epidemics in the advanced courtiers of the West, including the UK, is the empowerment of the British and other women with the "Right to Know" legislation about life and death matters."

4.6 Thyroid cancer

An initial hypothesis-testing study, in the mid-1970s, showed evidence of a significant association between the exposure to condom use and the breast cancer development in American and other married women. During the mid-1980s, another field study corroborated the evidence of a postulated association between condom use and thyroid cancer in women as well. The study also confirmed the close relationship between these two female "sex- (gender-) specific" diseases of the breast and thyroid glands along with other accompanying diseases, tumors and cancers of female reproductive tract (Gjorgov, 1999).
A feedback was communicated to the New York Times, entitled: "Pseudo Answers to the Thyroid Cancer Contingency: Times Essentials" - "The Rising Incidence of Thyroid cancer," by **Carolyn Sayre** (NY Times, Oct. 15, 2010), as follows:

"The thyroid disorders and tumors, along with the other epidemic diseases that afflict women, such as breast cancer, showed to have the same etiologic root cause: the CONDOMIZATION of women's sexuality. I have investigated in the field of thyroid cancer and I strongly believe that the aforementioned Times essentials of thyroid cancer are incomplete and out of reality.
Firstly, the information in the article should have provided separate data of women (i.e., for the so-named in the article "certain groups"?) and should not referred to "people" rather than women throughout the article. The existing evidence suggests that the female thyroid cancer may etiologically differ from that in males. Besides the assumed environmental causes, the reproductive causes apparently play a major, additional causative role in the development of thyroid cancer in women. The female-male difference of the root causes of thyroid cancer in the past three decades (since the beginning of 1980s) may confirm or provide further evidence of the potential of primary (non-chemical) prevention of the disease in women to a great extent. The existing epidemiological evidence points out to a situation that thyroid cancer falls into the same category of the female sex- (gender-) specific diseases, along with breast cancer. While the ratio of breast cancer is about 100 in women to 1 in men, the ratio of thyroid cancer in

women is unanimously around or greater than three times of that of men.
Perhaps no one should be so mystified about the emerging, epidemic thyroid diseases nowadays, including the erratic thyroid cancer. Along with the other epidemic diseases which afflict women, such as breast cancer and the thyroid disorders have, almost certainly, the same etiologic root cause: the condomization of women's sexuality.
Inferring from the NYT article, it could be assumed that out the 45,000 thyroid cancer cases in the U.S. there were at least 1,125,000 thyroid-nodule biopsies, out of which about 843,750 thyroid-nodule biopsies were performed to about 33,750 women a year. It may confirm the assessment that the magnitude of the number of biopsies and other diagnostic procedures equal the scale of clinical diagnostic activities conducted to the epidemic of breast cancer.
It is anticipated that both widespread, epidemic diseases in women, breast cancer and thyroid disorders / nodules, could practically be eliminated ('eradicated' to sporadic cases), by a still pending, primary (non-chemical) prevention of the current breast cancer epidemic.."

(The comment was first communicated to the 'mystifying emergence' of Oprah's Thyroid Club almost three years earlier, on October 25, 2007),

The idea of similarity of risk factors of breast and thyroid cancers along with other female specific cancers, diseases and other phenomena was not widely known. The availability of the exceptionally rich cancer data in the WHO-IARC editions of the 'Cancer Incidence in Five Continents' (in last six editions) offered an opportunity to test the association, on global as well as regional scale (North America, South America, Europe, Asia, Australia, Africa), in addition to race (white, Afro-American), and developmental stage (developed and developing countries). The following **Table 4** presents the correlation coefficients and significance levels, of world data.

Country / Population	Vol. III: 1968-1972	Vol. IV: 1973-1977	Vol. V: 1878-1982	Vol. VI: 1983-1987	Vol. VII: 1988-1992	Vol. VIII: 1993-1997	Vol. IX: 1998-2002
# of places	**80**	**104**	**159**	**166**	**183**	**211**	**300**
Breast Ca.	.212*	.265*	.205*	.323*	.166*	.284**	.225**
Cervix Ca.	-.027	-.142	.041	-.060	-.118	-.208**	-.084
Uterus Ca.	.400**	.232**	.274**	.205**	,230**	..322**	.271**
Ovary Ca.	.078*	.080	.294**	.158*	.029	.224**	.538**

Legend:
+Age-adjusted according to World Standard Population (WSP), *Statistical significance $p<.05$
**Statistical significance $p<.01$ or $p<.001$

Table 4. Thyroid Cancer: Correlation coefficients with Breast cancer and other Cancers of reproductive system in women, World data: 1968-2002. Age-adjusted incidence rates, per 100,000.female population.

The results showed positive associations for breast, ovarian and endometrial cancer on global scale, and negative association with the cancer of the cervix uteri. The results are in accord with the postulated condomization exposure of women. The correlations coefficients

controlling for regional, especially on American and European variables and other developmental and racial variables reiterated the conclusion of a common root cause of breast and thyroid cancers. A series of dietary factors investigated in the study showed no significant results. The study was published in the journal
"Libri Oncologici" in Zagreb, Croatia. A brief summary of the "(Gjorgov, 1998a), is presented below:

Risk Factors Of Female Thyroid Cancer In Kuwait: A Retrospective Study (Summary)
Background. A case-control study was conducted in Kuwait during 1984-1985, in order to ascertain the reproductive characteristics, contraceptive practice, and dietary habits of 101 women with primary thyroid cancer (TC), aged 19-65 years, and a comparative group of 98 control women, free of the disease, and matched by age and nationality status. Information was obtained by personal interview with a questionnaire. **Objectives.** The study investigated the relationship between the risk factors in the domain of fertility control, known or postulated to be related to breast cancer, and the risk of TC in women. **Results.** The study showed that both groups of cases and controls were homogeneous and comparable in almost all studied factors. Differences at statistically significant levels were observed, however, in two contraceptive exposures: the TC patients reported more frequent and more extended use of condoms than the controls ($P<.05$), whereas the controls reported more extended exposure to oral contraceptives than the TC cases ($P<.01$). The highest relative risk (odds ratio) to the disease, OR = 4.3 (95%CI: 0.5--39.2), and adjusted OR = 7.1 (95%CI: 0.6--78.9), was observed for women with condom use of more than two years. In regard to the dietary factors, no appreciative differences were found for most of the investigated food items, except a difference of borderline significance of higher consumption of sugared products among the TC cases, and a significant difference of a higher consumption of sugared drinks among the controls. **Conclusions.** The findings of barrier contraceptive risk factors (condoms) in this study may help explain the similarity and analogy of the epidemiology of these predominantly female sex-specific neoplasms, cancer of the thyroid and cancer of the breast.
Key words: Reproduction, Contraception, Barrier methods, Condom, Non-barrier methods, Oral contraceptive, Diet

4.7 Other reproductive-health adverse effects

4.7.1 Adverse effects of condomization on female sexual dysfunction

Besides the new investigations into some new phenomena falling under a diagnosis of "FSDs" (female sexual dysfunctions), as further collateral, potential side effects of changed inter-human (woman-man) micro-environment could also come under consideration for investigation both the increased frequencies of divorce, and the more frequent reports of women's unhappiness. The assumption of condomization being associated with allegedly newly defined condition 'FSD' - Female sexual dysfunction - and the ensuing discussion in the **British Medical Journal**-Online, 2003, is presented in the following rapid response (Gjorgov, 2003):

Condomization of female sexuality - the cause of the FSD (Female Sexual Dysfunction) (Gjorgov, 2003)
"In the recent article about the female sexual dysfunction (FSD) (Moynihan, 2003) and in the ensuing rapid reactions and debate about the subject matter, the keystone factor of the

female sexuality is amazingly missing across the board: the factor MAN. This background of culturally conditioned deficit convinced me that the research on FSD is being taken out of context. In addition, it seems that the FSD is not a static condition, developing by random choice and aimless. As emphasized in the article and the comments, the FSD has certainly a poorly understood etiology, but it might be evolving into some realms of unknown end-result(s).

More than 25 years ago, a hypothesis-testing study[2] on primary breast cancer prevention and etiology was completed jointly at the University of North Carolina School of Public Health, at Chapel Hill, NC, and at the University of Pennsylvania School of Medicine and Hospital, in Philadelphia, PA, USA, during the mid-1970s. The study has tested and corroborated an a priori hypothesis on "semen factors" (deficiency) that an extended exposure to (use of) barrier contraception, specifically, the long-term condom use, and/or withdrawal practice, is significantly associated with the development of breast cancer in married American and other women, including the British women. Besides defining a new approach to the etiology of and the potential for a primary (non-chemical) prevention of breast cancer, another main contribution, I believe, of my cancer research has been the evidence-based inference that SEX along with marriage and love is a fundamental PHYSIOLOGICAL unit, above and beyond the psychological, social, economic, reproductive and legal linkage. The final report of the study, entitled, "BARRIER CONTRACEPTION AND BREAST CANCER" (Gjorgov, 1980) was published as a monograph by S. Karger Med. Publ., Basel-New York, in the distant 1980. (Since the book has been effectively banned from the public view and professional information, the breast cancer research was first published in the dissertation format, in 1979, by the University of Michigan Dissertation International, Ann Arbor, MI 48106; UMI publication # 79-14352.)

It was further indicated in the study that breast cancer is a systemic disease and not a random event, and that the breast carcinogenesis is most likely passing through nonspecific and unrecognized phases, manifesting itself in a number of trivial or undistinguishable symptoms in women's lives (Gjorgov, 1995), presumably such as the FSD, and eventually reaching a definite stage of overt breast cancer and other accompanying disease end-results, as predicted (Gjorgov, 1993, 1994a; Gjorgov, 1994b). An experimental trial (Gjorgov, 1999) of sterile mating on a colony of small laboratory animals corroborated the preventive efficacy of the semen factors (the prostaglandins) on mammary neoplastic tumors, and on the general impact on animal-female lives and health. The condom use introduces technical effects of absolute male sterility in marriages, placing an impregnable wall between the protective biology of man and woman, and converting their marriages into infertile male partners. It is quite conceivable that many a woman may feel the ill- effects ("female sex problems") because of the persistent and un-physiological condom use, and that the woman is reflexively trying to protect herself by escape, distancing, separation or reluctance against the unwittingly afflicting insults (!) upon her done by her technically sterile husband. It seems quite evident and certain that during the long evolution, Nature has not adjusted the species to sterile mating, including the humans.

Within the framework of the tested "semen-factor" (condom) hypothesis in breast cancer, partial comments, opinion and paraphrases on the FSD debate: - Perhaps "Body-mind" rather than "Mind-body" relationships is a better model than the psychiatric and social understanding of the FSD; - Contrary to what was mentioned, sex is NOT "Like Dancing": Sex is a physiological impact; - There is evidence that the continuing promotion of condoms use as a "normal sexual behavior" and/or (PC) contraceptive practice is lethal (breast cancer); - "Sexual functioning is an integral part of our lives" and perhaps of (gender) physical survival; - The feminist nonsense as a recipe for producing FSD: "masturbation" in females; - The "Conspiracy of Silence" for FSD is even more so for the unabated breast cancer epidemic; - The FSD, "as potentially epidemic condition" could and should be better handled in the services and domain of the Gynecologists-Obstetricians rather than the Urologists. - The "environmental intervention" in FSD, like in the breast cancer epidemic: Eradication of the "INVERSE" environmental factor, the barrier of the condom use that is eliminating, reducing or making absence the protective biological mechanisms in the intimate and subtle, inter-human (sexual) environment and ecosystem.

No wonder that the FSD is so prevalent in British and American women (reportedly, about 43%), for both are "high-risk" populations of breast cancer and are among the leading breast-cancer epidemic countries, with the highest breast cancer incidence and death rates in the world. Since the CONDOMIZATION of human sexuality seems to be the singular most important factor in the women's sexual dysfunction, my humble and evidence-based suggestion is simple and brief:

ABOLISH THE USE OF CONDOMS FOR CONTRACEPTIVE, FERTILITY-CONTROL AND FAMILY-PLANNING PURPOSES in the British marriages and couples, and make an urgent shift to the "non-barrier" methods of contraception (Gjorgov & Narod, 2001a). It is long overdue to make the British and other women happy."

4.7.2 Condomization, abortions, 'missed abortions,' and pseudopregnancy

The following letter to the **Editor of the New York Times**, referring to the editorial "Abortion, Condoms and Bush," by **Nicholas D. Kristof,** NYT November 5, 2006, tackles the issue of condoms, "missed abortion," and breast cancer:

Condoms, Condoms, Condoms...and Abortions. A critical reply

"Mr. Kristof seems biased and medically ill-informed by discussing a biological issue like abortions and condoms. What kind of abortion "rise" and "fall" throughout the past (three) decades and during (six) presidential periods? Discussion of temporal changes of all (i) the artificial, (ii) spontaneous, and (iii) so-called "missed" abortions? And, on top of this professional mix-up and mystery of abortions, a cause-and-effect link is added to the (predominant) use of condoms?

The (i) artificial abortions are carried out by demands, and reflect a fertility capacity of at least the woman. The artificial abortions burden the soul of the women in tremendous psychological pain, are reluctantly performed, and socially have always been quite controversial.

The (ii) spontaneous abortions reflect an infertility / sub-fertility status of both partners, usually married, and may indicate a hidden plight in building the family. The infertility condition is an acknowledged risk factor of development of breast cancer and other women's ill health.

The (iii) "missed abortion" is an utterance of professional, clinical perplexity. As a pastime term it could only be found in older editions of gynecology textbooks. The contemporary professionals try hard to avoid diagnosis of "missed abortion," for its occurrence is not understood, and indicates a situation of false pregnancy. The condition is connected with the use of condoms. The 'failure-rate' of the use of condoms as contraceptive device is (uncritically) estimated to be around 9 percent. In fact, the use of condoms is induction of technical effects of absolute male sterility in the intimate (sexual) relations. (The prolonged or repetitious condition of false pregnancy is presumed as the initial, still reversible stage of breast cancer and other sex- (gender-) specific diseases in women of all ages.)

In my informed view, the reported, intermittent phrasing of "sharp rise," "tiny increase" and/or "tiny fall" of abortions throughout time are misleading, inaccurate and incomplete. Actually, who knows whether the reports of abortions could ever be better exact?

On the other hand, the sharp rise and spiraling advent of the breast cancer epidemic in the country, in the last two-and-a-half decades (since the beginning of 1980s), the unending epidemic of malignant disease associated with the persistent condom use, is strangely overlooked in the column assessment.

The professional misjudgment and incompetence seem to be manifested in the confusion and equation of the use of condoms as a general category of family planning. The euphemism of "comprehensive sex education" practically means condom promotion / distribution in the schools, with condomization of the nascent sexuality of the schoolgirls, the youngest generation(s) of the American population, with unknown grave consequences / sequels.

As a young congressman, George H.W. Bush may have sponsored the 1970 public health program of family planning services which, almost certainly, may have included condoms, but, as President, he is recorded at a series on ABC television stations, in 1990, as rejecting distribution of condoms: "Not for me and not for the federal government... I don't think that just passing out condoms, giving up on lifestyle, giving up on family and fundamental values is correct... In terms of just national passing out of condoms to people, I am not in favor of that." So, President George W. Bush seems to be actually continuing the family roots. His energetic condom-paradigm shift and the potential of curbing the current breast cancer epidemic with the new anti-condom reproductive policy are anticipated to achieve an impending 'eradication' of the dreaded epidemic disease to the levels of sporadic cases in the country and far beyond."

NOTE: In less than a month, on Dec. 5, 2006, the New York Times run an article entitled; "All the signs of pregnancy except one: A baby," by Elizabeth Svoboda (Svoboda, 2006). Apparently, the NYT editors have investigated the above critique, confirming the information of false pregnancy which was repeatedly termed by its ancient Greek name, *pseudocyesis*. By quoting certain medical authorities, a skepticism was underlined that "human pseudocyesis will never be completely scientifically understood," and another assertion that it is "one of the classic examples how the mind affects the rest of the body." In fact, the condomization of female sexuality (pseudocyesis) may prove to be one of the classic examples of how the injured body affects the mind, rather than the way around. The issue of false pregnancy is associated with the condom-related "reproductive freedom" fallacy (Gjorgov, 1980, 1996a).

4.8 Anorexia-bulimia ('eating') disorders

The literature of Anorexia-Bulimia (conveniently called "eating") disorders match only that of breast cancer. The number of new cases of anorexia and bulimia disorders rose rapidly worldwide in the past three decades, 1980s, 1990s, and 2000s, the rampant condition is rising ever since, continuing its rise in the 2000s, especially in the developed West, such as, the U.S. and the E.U.

A descriptive study was conducted in young female patients in mid-200s, at the Psychiatric outpatient clinic at the Faculty of Medicine of the University Sts. Cyril and Methodius, in Skopje, Macedonia, in order to assess the sub-hypothesis that (illicit) barrier contraception (condom use and withdrawal practice) is a risk factor of anorexia-bulimia disorders in schoolgirls, college female students, and other young women and brides (Gjorgov, 2009a). The main results indicated of the study indicated that the anorexia-bulimia patients [with mean age of 23.3 years (sd= 3.1)] used overwhelmingly condom device and equally practiced withdrawal technique for contraceptive purposes, during most of their young sexual experience and initial reproductive lives, as opposed to negligible use of OC pills.

On the basis of the prior observation (the sub-hypothesis), a confident communication along with a suggestion was forwarded almost 14 years ago to the **Swedish Royal Family**, concerning the announcement of the worrisome 'eating' disorder condition in the future Queen of the country, as follows:

> M-me Elisabeth Tarras-Wahlberg, Spokeswoman, Skopje, December 10, 1997
> The Royal Palace, Stockholm, Sweden
>
> Dear Madam,
>
> This is a humble attempt to try to address, as a physician and researcher, the reported news in the media of a heavy body-weight loss of Her Royal Highness Princess Victoria and to try to suggest a new possible approach in the efforts for solving this worrisome situation.
>
> In my opinion, the heavy body-weight loss, so called *Anorexia nervosa,* is secondarily related to the problems of nutrition and diet. Rather, there is circumstantial evidence, that the life-threatening condition of *Anorexia nervosa* is perhaps causally related to the demands of reproductive and intimate life and to its applied technical barriers. The alternative hypothesis about the nature of *Anorexia nervosa* was deducted from a "byproduct" observation in my long research of the developmental processes in the field of breast cancer. Furthermore, the frequent condition of a prior excess body loss (and gain) in the affected, young, reproductive-aged women with breast cancer was controlled for and partially tested as a sub-hypothesis in my hypothesis-testing study of barrier contraception (the condom use and withdrawal practice) as an etiological risk factor associated to breast cancer in married American women.
>
> During my field and ecological studies of breast cancer, it became obvious that the condom use in your country has been quite prevalent, with all the postulated subsequent consequences of the widespread misconception that "the use of condom has no side effects." On the other hand, breast cancer in Sweden has been reported and registered as one of the highest in the world, and still raising, mainly because of

the widespread and long-term condom use in the general population, as postulated. In my separate study of the epidemiology and rising trends of breast cancer in Sweden, in 1992, the potential for prevention and control of the current breast cancer epidemic in the country was elaborated and suggested. Because the study could not be publish, copies of it were sent from Kuwait University to a number of health and political authorities and institutions in Sweden, as a personal communication.

Based on my research experience, I do believe that the exposure to the condom use (i.e., to technically induced sterile stimulation) induces some devastating effects to a normal, young, vivacious, healthy woman, among which the life-threatening response of *Anorexia nervosa* seems to be one of the most frequent condition in the advanced countries, such as Sweden. The assessment of H.H. the Princess' condition is done on incomplete information and on certain assumptions, which might not be correct. Nevertheless, the possible way out of the anorectic danger for such a lady, in my opinion, would be the absolute elimination of the condom as a fertility-control device, by reverting to any of the non-barrier contraceptive methods (the pills, diaphragm, rhythm, IUDs, creams-jellies), in order to be able to preserve the healthy reproductive and inter-human life, and to prevent neoplastic phenomena.

Enclosure: Clipping from the daily newspaper. Respectfully submitted, ...

(The letter was acknowledged with thanks for the 'wish to help.')

A similar communication was submitted recently to the Chairwoman of the **White House Council on Women and Girls** and Special Advisor the President, on December 10, 2010, concerning the rampant "eating' disorders cases in the U.S. and other developed countries of the West, as follows:

Dear Madam Special Advisor: Re: Eating Disorders Prevention

"Along with the Best wishes to Rep. Alcee L. Hastings and Patrick J. Kennedy and 34 Members of the Congress for their initiative to incorporate the global eating-disorders issue into the First Lady Michelle Obama "Let's Move Campaign" and the "Federal Response to Elimination of Eating Disorders (FREED) Act 2010."

Just to reiterate that there are no greater "strong environmental, cultural, and social factors" associated to or causing eating disorders, as mentioned in the letter to the First Lady (July 21, 2010), but the condomization of the nascent sexuality of schoolgirls, college and other women in the population. An all-inclusive approach to women's health and the new research of both the breast cancer epidemic and the rampant anorexia-bulimia disorders has identified as the main root cause of the specific sex- (gender-) diseases in women the misconceived and deadly, false belief of condom as a "safe" device for fertility-control and family-planning use.

My concern is, yet, that the blackout history of the past three decades may repeat itself, to continue stocking the unabated breast cancer epidemic in middle-age women (mothers), and extending the ill effects to the helpless anorexia-bulimia bewildered young women (daughters). The strongly reinforced, misleading, renewed condom-use offensive, oblivious of the greatest ill-health consequences to the half of the population, is poised to persist with the discrimination against women, girls and couples, by withholding the potentially life-saving information of a primary (non-chemical, non-profit) prevention / protection against the grave female-specific diseases at personal, familial and community levels. "

4.9 Osteoporosis

Osteoporosis far exceeds in frequency (incidence and prevalence) all other conditions in the female populations. During the past decades, since the early 1980s, osteoporosis and its sequels rapidly rose and continued its unabated rise, reaching excess epidemic proportions. As a "silent epidemic," osteoporosis has become highly prevalent as a great clinical and societal burden, and a heavy public health problem of highest priority, especially in the affluent North American, European and other communities. A systemic disease, affecting 7.8 million women in the U.S. and worldwide, osteoporosis is diagnosed by low bone mass than average and steadily deteriorating bone tissues, leading to bone fragility and increased fracture risk. In the U.S. and Europe, 1 in 3 or even 2 women over 50 years of age will develop the disease, and more and more affecting premenopausal women. Presently, there is a gap in the efforts to control, treat and prevent the osteoporosis. The predominant theories of diet, calcium and vitamin D deficiency, and other macro-environmental factors have advanced no progress in the etiology, treatment and prevention of the osteoporosis in women. The traditional and doctrinaire approaches have neither identified the etiological causes of the osteoporosis epidemic nor defined the ways of preventing the disease in the community and at individual and family levels. Within the framework of the Bone and Joint Decade 2000-2010, an attempt was made by submitting a project proposal to test a new hypothesis of an etiological relationship between the barrier contraception and the risk of osteoporosis development in women. The proposed hypothesis of the etiology of osteoporosis (and osteopenia) and of the potential of primary prevention of the condition in women postulates that the osteoporosis is a late, delayed and/or a prolonged consequence of the marital exposure to (use of) barrier forms of contraception (specifically, condoms and/or withdrawal, and male/family infertility) during the reproductive, pre-menopausal age span of women (Gjorgov, 2006).

Once again, various manifestations of affected bone health, such as the low back pain, showed distinct increase in prevalence the U.S., after the 1980s, the same alleged time period during all other ill-health developments occurred in women (**Figure 17**).

Osteoporosis, and its initial stage, osteopenia, are perplexed with misinformation and misconceptions. First, the proportion of women with osteoporosis over men with osteoporosis is almost nine times greater in women than in men, which fact is not always underlined for further considerations; Second, the condition fall into the setting of so called sex- (gender-) specific diseases in women (like breast cancer, in proportion 100:1 females to males; Third, the grave condition do not 'naturally' come with age (look at the Sybille figures of the Michelangelo frescoes); Fourth, not all women carry the same risk of osteoporosis; Fifth, the (mystified) "FRAX" osteoporosis / osteopenia risk assessment tool from the osteoporosis associations, consists of majority of the same spurious and secondary risk factors of breast cancer; Sixth, a primary (natural) prevention of the conditions has neither been mentioned nor considered. Since the idea of potential breast cancer prevention is that it should start long before the malignant tumors are diagnosed, it could be safe to suppose that the "natural" (non-chemical) prevention of the crippling conditions of osteoporosis/osteopenia should be attempted at the same time along with the prevention of the other gynecological lesions, or even earlier, during the peak of the reproductive lives of women. Information for prevention seems far superior to pharmaceutical marketing concerning the chemical control and 'treatment' of osteoporosis and osteopenia in women.

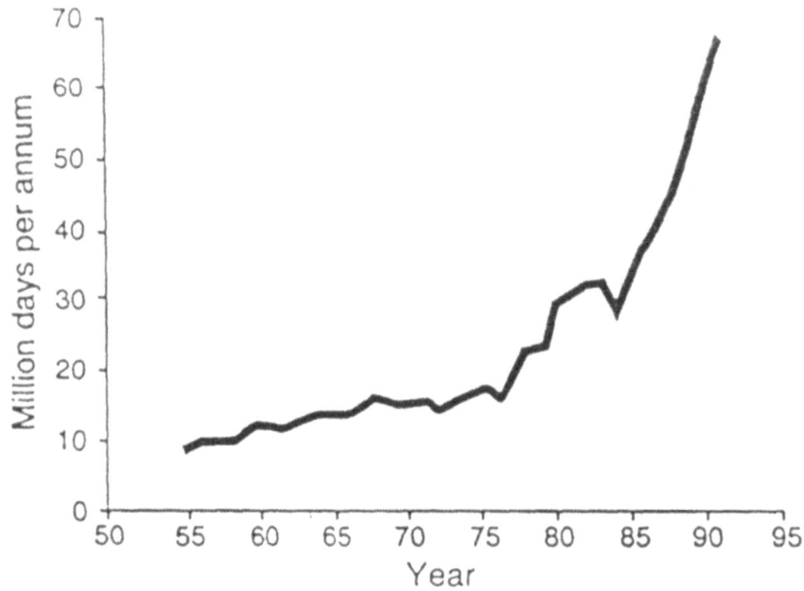

Fig. 17. Low back pain increasing trend in the U.S., 1955-1995.

5. Social and demographic consequences

5.1 Condomization adverse effects in marriage and divorce

The issues of contraception, marriage and divorces have been speculated upon frequently, mainly in the denominational quarters, in the U.S and elsewhere, under the sign of "controversial" issues and in some instance under feministic tendencies of interpretation. In the numerous judicial and social literature of the causes of divorce, some findings seem novel, such as he information that more women seek divorce than men nowadays (Ambekar, 2009) that divorces take husbands by surprise (Peatlng, 2005), that sex is a reason for divorce and that "dissatisfied women are less likely to have sex" (Kimbal, 2010). Some older sources of religious discussion were practically out of reach (Peters, 1998). It was early warning that the divorce rates have much risen recently. Hardly any of the recent studies in marriage, divorce and sexuality ever considered condoms as an impediment to marital relations.

Other recent reports confirmed the rapidly increasing divorce rates in the U.S., with a distinct jump at the end of the 1970s and the beginning of the 1980s, greatly surpassing any divorce rates in the U.S. over the recorded past 150 years (Stevenson & Wolfers, 2007a, 2007b; Wolfers, 2010). The surprising rise of the divorce rate, greater than that recorded after WWII, and subsequently fluctuating and slowly declining trend was presented in the first figure in the text. The explanation of the truly distinct changes of the divorce rates, with the mass and still high jump in divorce rates was not fully explained in the report. (**Figure 18**). The presumed 'driving forces' of divorce talked about a variety of conventional causes, such as, importance of marriage has changed, rising age at first marriage, high remarriage rates, rise of cohabitation, rise of out-of-wedlock fertility, and other social and economic reasons.

In a response to the authors, Betsey Stevenson and Justin Wolfers, a critical commentary of the missing biological dimension in their scholarly analysis of national data of divorce and marriage, underlying the following points:

"It seems we could not really know about the break-up of marriages, "long" or "new," if only the "broader economic and social consequences" are being considered, by forgetting the simple biological causes of the events.

By looking into the primary source of the news (*"Marriage and Divorce: Changes and their Driving Forces,"* by B. Stevenson & J. Wolfers, 2007 & 2009; Brining & Allen, 2000), besides the scholarly done review and presentation of official registry, raw data, the way of thinking, heavily influenced by the old-time feminism, seems very one-sided and insufficiently interpreted. The woman is analyzed manly as a technological, social, economy- and business- oriented personality, with no reference whatsoever to her (their) biological individuality.

It was rightly emphasized in the study that marriage and divorce laws and regulations along with technical changes in the family do not explain the rise of divorces over the past few decades. And yet, the women "who suffer" are those who in majority file for divorce. The figure 1 in the aforementioned study, presenting the rates of marriages and divorces (per 1000 American people), stretching for 145 years (1860-2005) is truly revealing. It seems to explain to a great extent the missing references to the most critical period of rapidly rising and still on-going period of exceptionally high-divorce rates in the country in the decades of 1980s, 1990s, and first part of the 2000s: the mass CONDOMIZATION of female sexuality. While the contraceptive pills and their impact upon the society have been studiously explained, the destructive impact of the promoted use of condoms over the past three decades has been strangely overlooked, with an utter oblivion to the current, excess breast cancer epidemic, the greatest scare, dread and real risk of women, along with the widespread gynecological tumors and other afflictions.

Given the corroborated evidence that the condom use is significantly associated with the breast cancer development in American and other married women, it is not a wonder that many a woman is filing for divorce and, supposedly looking for a "new partner." Intimate condomized relations induce technical effects of absolute sterile husband in the marriage, perhaps worse stressor than other ones mentioned in the debate blog, such as "poor health, poverty, and unemployment." If in the biological struggle the wife is not supported (by a fertile husband), it is a general belief / observation, and she is turning against him. (The racial differences in rates of divorce are also consistent with the differences in breast cancer incidence and prevalence rates, the levels of condom-use acculturation.)

The figure 1 in the study seems circumvented in the analysis of the causes of the sudden bulge of skyrocketed rates of divorces ever since the end of 1970s and still on-going (in 2005). (The condomization started with rumors at the end of the 1970s.) It may be safe to assume that it is the most likely a response of women "who suffer" and try to escape (mainly by divorce) from the unknown but felt devastating and carcinogenic effects of sterile mating, and the incremental bodily and breast-cancer changes. Since the figure 1 with unusual trends of divorce trends is rarely seen in the literature, it may be worth following up the trend data, to witness the probable rapid fall of the divorce rates along with the information of the root cause(s) for and elimination (fall) of the epidemic breast cancer incidence rates and the main risk factor, the condom-control of women, perhaps at the earliest anticipated date, after the year 2010."

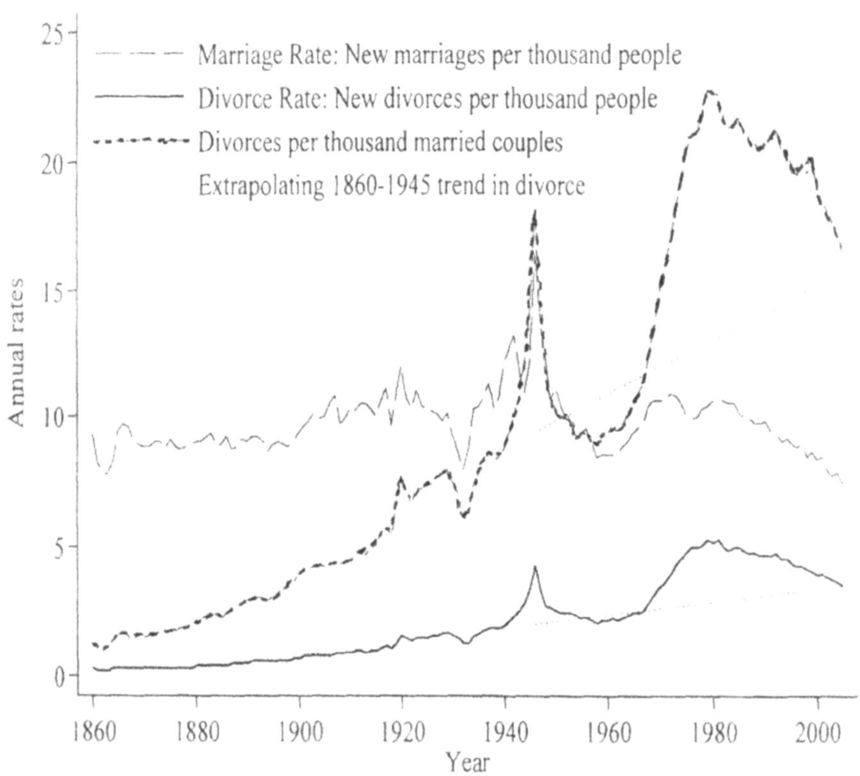

Fig. 18. Marriage and divorce rates in the United States, 1860-2000.

The unexplained changes in divorce rates reflected in other parts of the developed and affluent world. In **Australia**, a highly dramatic upsurge of divorce rates was recorded around 1978-1979, with a subsequent sharp decline and fluctuating changes afterwards (**Figure 19**) (Australian Historical Statistics, 2001). In the **UK**, the sudden almost threefold rise of the number of divorces was recoded somewhat earlier, in the mid-1978, and did not show appreciable decline for the next several years, until 2000 (**Figure 20**) (Office on National Statistics UK, 2004)...

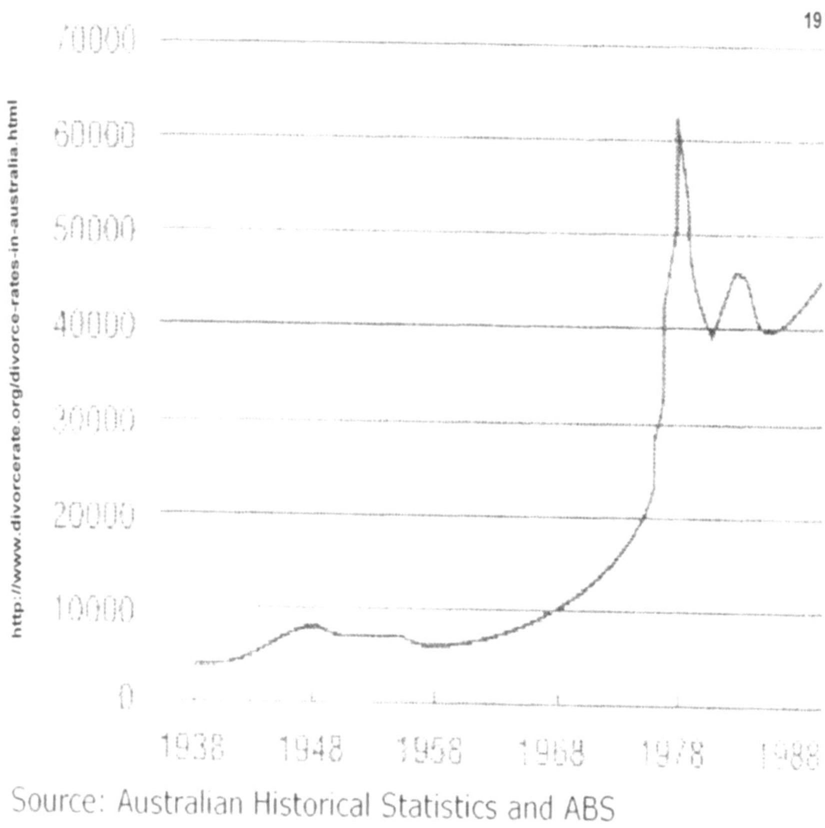

Fig. 19. Number of divorces in Australia, 1938-1991.

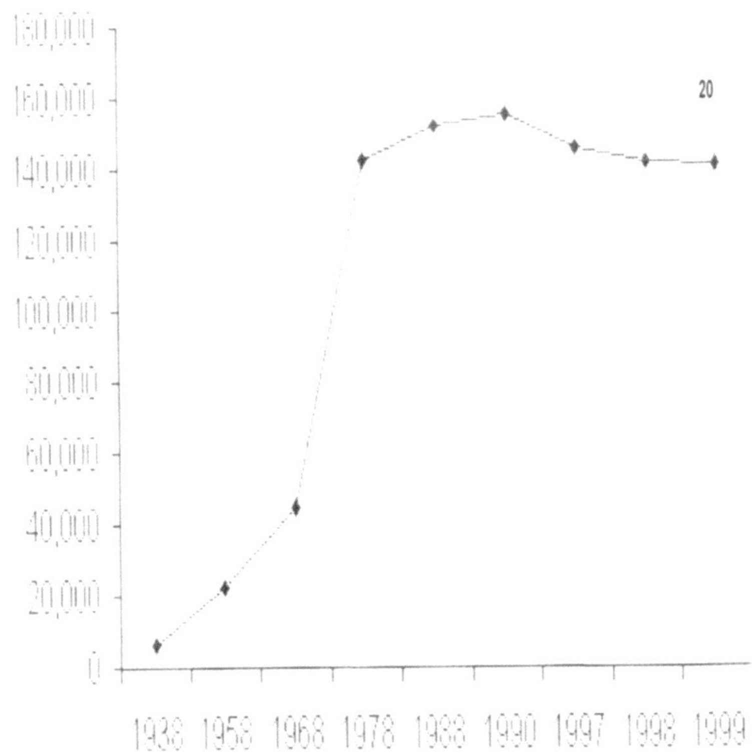

Fig. 20. Divorce rates in the UK, from 1938 to 1999.

In **Japan** there was also a wave of increased divorces as well (**Figure 21**) (Japanese Ministry of Health, 2002). However, the increase of the divorce rate in Japan showed at least three different demographic features: the increase was incremental and relatively lower, less than two rates (per 1000 population), against the increase in the U.S. (reaching more than 5.5 rate); and the peak of the divorce rates occurred about five years later than in the U.S. It is assumed that the changes in the divorce incidence rates may have the same driving force, stretching within a time period of several years, at the beginning of the 1980s.

The attempt for explanation of the observed social phenomena of high divorce outbreak did not reach considerations of condomization as a possible root cause of the observable fact. An attempt was made to address the issue of condoms as newly introduced environmental pollution in the inter-human intimate relations, in a comment to the article "Contraception and Divorce: Insight from American Annulment Cases," of 1998, by Dr. Edwards N. Peters, Edmund Card. Szoka Chair in Faculty Development, Canon of the Law Blog, Christmas 2010

"What prompted me to (belatedly) comment your article of 12 years ago is the ongoing routine of addressing condom as "contraception." In the mid-1970s, I conducted a hypothesis-testing study (jointly at two American universities) of the barrier contraception (condom use and withdrawal practice) and the development of breast cancer in American (and other) married women. The results corroborated the hypothesis and showed evidence of a significant condom and breast cancer association, together with the defined potential of primary (non-chemical) prevention of breast cancer as an epidemic disease. One of the main inferences was that marriage along with sexuality, love and family is a profound biological union between woman and man, along with the conventional definition of marriage as a social, economic, psychological, and legal unit.

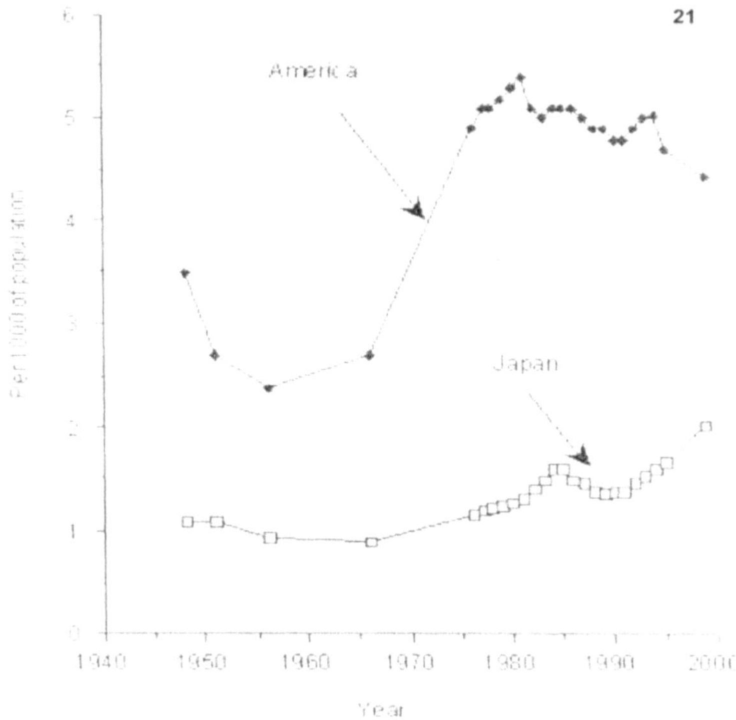

Fig. 21. American and Japanese divorce rates, from 1940 to 2000.

In a nutshell, condom is not a contraceptive method. This old/new (high-tech) barrier-device is literally a marriage-killer (divorce and a variety of psychosomatic phenomena and unhappiness) and woman-killer (breast cancer in mothers, and anorexia-bulimia disorders in young daughters). Condomization of female sexuality has been defined as the main and perhaps sole root cause of the unabated, excess breast cancer epidemic and other accompanying disorders of women and girls in the modern world. No other method of 'contraception' has been linked with the apparent natural experiment of the current breast cancer epidemic, or has shown the distinction to induce carcinogenic consequences on women on unprecedented scale in the country and societies globally. It seems that the study provided a basis of new understanding of contraception, and an attempt to use some of the (non-barrier) methods in preventive/therapeutical ways. In my view, the condomized control of women, rather the 'contraception' is the main causal factor for divorce, by which women supposedly try to escape from the deeply felt cancer-initiation process.

A real concern may present, time and again, the newly reinitiated, so-called "Rubber Revolution," the renewed, forceful and reckless condom promotion, entirely oblivious to the unabated, excess breast cancer epidemic, worldwide, and insensitive to the plight of the half of population, exposed to the highest risk of developing and suffering of the malignant epidemic disease(s) and other morbid phenomena."

The so-called Marriage calculator- divorce360 (Stevenson, 2010) could hardly fulfill its intended predictive purpose, since the analysis was based mainly on the educational levels and other social profiles of the spouses, and the failure (bias?) to consider the biological (sexual) dimension of marriage. Besides the calculator seems incomplete, because it lacks the necessary putative external risk factor quantified exposure, in order to serve as a Bayes' probability theorem requirements (Gjorgov, 2009b, 2010).

The dilemma of the official, but mistaken emphasis on strict promotion of use of condoms (in all sexual relations) in the U.S. House of Representatives (Lincoln, 1979) is given in the following personal communication to the **Honorable James H. Scheuer**, Chairman of the House Select Committee on Population, on May 29, 1979, in Philadelphia, PA:

"In reference to the conclusions of your Committee on Population concerning family planning policy, as reported by Richard Lincoln in *Family Planning Perspectives*, March/April 1979, the promotion of the "barrier" methods of contraception become an objective of first priority in the contraceptive research "of methods that are not known to be associated with hazardous side effects." No definition of "barrier" methods was presented in the journal's report (Lincoln, 1979) of the conclusions of your Committee. This is to inform you and your Committee that there are indications that some forms of barrier contraceptive methods are perhaps the most inadequate and hazardous methods for fertility regulation. This is also to present to you the available evidence of a recently completed study, indicating an association between the use of barrier contraceptive techniques and long-term health hazards in women. A barrier contraceptive, as defined in the study, is one which obstructs the passage and resorption of seminal content during sexual contact, such as the condom and withdrawal. The results of the tested hypothesis of the study corroborated the evidence that there is a significant relationship between barrier contraceptive practice and the development of breast cancer in women. The final findings corroborated the research hypothesis and the preliminary results of the study that women who used barrier contraceptive methods for extended periods of time in their marriages have a risk of developing breast cancer that is 4.6 - 5.2 times the risk of women who used other forms of fertility control. The results of the research also indicate that there is a potential for preventive action against the disease for a sizeable proportion of women in the population. It is estimated that by eliminating barrier contraceptive techniques, specifically the condom, and the incidence of breast cancer among married women in the United States could be reduced by as much as 50 percent. The results of the study consistently showed that the effects of a number of other reproductive and biological factors, such as age at first birth, parity, menarche, and others, had non-causal associations with the disease; The carcinogenic effect of the barrier contraceptive use was operative within a five-year exposure to condom use in marriage, with a cumulative effect; The study helps explain the increasing incidence of breast cancer, the international variation of the disease, and most of the reproduction-related risk indicators.

The final report, which is my dissertation, along with some other documents and material of the study would be gladly submitted to you and your Select Committee, if necessary. It is my belief that until further work in this field is done and confirmatory studies are conducted that this information of the devastating effects of condom use on woman's health should be made available to the users in community without unnecessary delay."

The recent report of the "Use of Contraception in the United States: 1982-2008" (Mosher and Jones, 2010) provided an abundance of data offering the opportunity to interpret the contraception figures, rates and trends in another way. There are a number of important findings which may shed a different light on the current discussion of the adverse impact of condomization upon society, and could be underlined, as such.

- It was stated in the Report that "in 2006-2008, 93 percent had ever had 'a partner' who used the male condom; 82 percent had ever used the oral contraceptive pill; and 59 percent had ever had 'a partner' who used withdrawal."
- The greatest increase of contraceptive methods recorded between 1982 and 1995 was for condoms, 79.5 percent of those who ever used the device, in comparison to OC pill, of only 7.9 percent increase. The increase of the condom 'ever used' prevalence in 1982 was 51.8 percent, and in 1995 82.0 percent, while the OC pill use remained virtually at a plateau, from ever-used prevalence of 94.5 percent in 1982 to 96.2 percent in 1995. For the next 13 years, until 2008, the increase of partners who have ever used condom was 93.0 percent (with 79.5 percent increase from 1982), while the OC pills ever used 82.3 percent (with 7.9 percent increase). The data may indicate that a combined (dual) use of condoms and OC pills might have been practiced, or an intermittent, non-consistent condom use.
- Changes in use of condom, pill and other contraceptive methods between 1982 and the subsequent years until 2008 clearly showed higher increases of all methods in certain ethnic groups in the U.S., corroborating the notion of condom acculturation as well. Thus, condom use by Hispanics at first sexual intercourse rose for 70.9 percent, for Afro-Americans 65.2 percent, and for whites 26.9 percent. OC pill dropped by -44.5 % for the Afro-American women, and withdrawal technique dropped by –17.3% for whites and -52.3% for Afro-Americans, but not for the Hispanics (which was low). The condom-use campaigns were not mentioned in taking place during the intervening years.
- Condom use by women aged 15-44 showed a declining trend after 1995, when the number of users (in thousands) declined from 13.1 to 11.1 in 2002, and to 10.0 in 2006-2008. The qualification of "persistent" condom use, which is considered practically impossible, because of the early adverse effects, use was not mentioned in the report.
- Prevalence of contraception use, both condoms and OC pills, was higher in younger groups up to age 30-34 than in the older groups 35-44, what is to be expected. The data of use of condom has obviously shifted to women of younger age which helps explain the "debut" breast cancer age-specific incidence peaks. The pill was used almost twice as much than condoms by women aged 20-24 (26.2 versus 13.4 by age, respectively); the condom was used in average of 10.0% by young women, and between 8.4 and 6.8 percent in older age groups 35-39 and 40-44. It looks like the ancient Roman "decimation" penal code is still powerful enough to make a strong impact on the community.
- Female sterilization was assessed at 27.1% in the 2006-2008 periods. There was age gradient of increase, showing a prevalence rate of 50.3% in the 40-44 age group. However, the unexpected high rate of "female sterilization" was not specified, in terms of proportion of elective tubal ligation and non-elective sterilizing surgical procedures. Tubal ligation is an established contraceptive method, but the hysterectomies and/or oophorectomies (one- or double-sided), are salvage surgical procedures carried out for

survival in many cases of breast, ovarian and other gynecological cancers. The blurred category of "female sterilization" showed a gradual increase of rates by parity, to highest proportion, of 58.7%, in women with three or more children. Once again, the purpose of the "sterilization" has not been specified, but helps explain the increasing survival rates of breast cancer in younger patients. (The male sterilization, vasectomy, assessed at 9.9% in the studied population sample, in 2006-2008, is still considered too controversial a method of contraception for pertinent comments.)

- Reasons for discontinuation of ever used contraceptive method, included prominent concern for the OC pill. To the question of "You had side effects," the pill users responded positively in 63.7 percent, while only 12.0 percent of condom users responded positively; to the question "Did not like changes to menstrual cycle," positive answer provided 10.6 percent of the pill-users, and none (zero percent) of the condom users. There was no side effect either recorded for condom use, even after more than 30 years of the condom - breast cancer link evidence first published.

The Scriptures and other classic literature throughout history seem to give ground for validity of the debates on the perennial issues of sexual relations, marriage, woman, love, conception, human seed, the "sin against nature" of sterile acts (coitus interruptus), prostitution, adultery and other human matters. A consensus in the polemic seems to be the belief that "husbands are the chief persons responsible for dissipation of their wives" (Flandrin, 1975; Gjorgov, 1977/1998). Many writers (Leo Tolstoy, Honoré de Balsac, Stefan Zweig, and many others), and other artists seem to have been ahead of the contemporary medical experts in assessing the natural forces of human intimate (sexual) relations. The Gustav Klimt's artistic vision of "Medicine" was unfairly discarded by the professors of the famous Faculty of Medicine of Vienna at the beginning of the 20th Century. The apotheosis of "Medicine" was angrily discarded by the professors, most likely because the artist portrayed superiority of nature (physical love) over medicine, and depicted his idea of the role of man as a biological complement and the key to functioning of (impact on) the captured woman's life, health, reproductive processes, fate, and exquisite beauty (Gjorgov, 2003b). (Remember the strange slay of Biblical Onan because of his 'mortal sin' of spilling the seed on the ground in sexual relations with his "dissatisfied" second wife?). No wonder that there were confounding 'clusters" of breast cancer in various public institutions around the world (Australia, the U.S.), given the multitude of fashionable, politically correct, condom-promoting zealots.

One of the major conclusions from the studies on marriage and divorce could be inferred that condomization has been implemented long before the AIDS epidemic emerged, during the second half of the decade of 1970s. That was the time of ascendance of feminism, with its primary anti-marriage mission. The promotion of condoms seemed as an "ideal" technical device for the "Our Bodies Ourselves" health-promotion movement. Although condom-promotion started with whispers and rumors, it was quite fervent, distributing condoms at the entries / exits of some of the hospitals, in a somewhat confidential way. The semi-secretive distribution extended for several year until he the solemnization of the mass condomization in the summer of 1986 (Koop, 1986).

The popular belief of the sexual relations exerting biological impact and health gain between woman and man, and for the woman in particular, is strongly imbedded in the minds of the people in the Mediterranean and Balkan regions, especially among the isolated Macedonian rural, mountainous, population (Gjorgov, 2001). It seems that the popular belief of physiological marital inter-dependence on woman reflects possibly the remnants of the classical Hippocratic teaching on seed. The dramatic developments of the contemporary, ever-rising breast cancer epidemic and reproductive health and nature of women and girls may incite a renewed philosophical debate for better understanding as to what is in having sex for a woman, whether women need (drive for) sex for a different biological 'purpose' than men do, and to eventually reconsider the unanswered persistent question "What the women want?" which Freud failed to answer.

It should be mentioned here that in the meantime a fleeting attempt was made by the Israel Health Minister in the 1990s to ban AIDS campaign promoting condom as a prophylactic against the HIV infection, recommending divorce instead for the healthy wife, rather than use of condoms (Siegel-Itzkovich, 1999). More importantly, on December 19, 2002, the U.S. agency CDC (Centers for Diseases control and Prevention) in Atlanta, GA, proclaimed official news, entitled: **"CDC Fact Sheet Not Promoting Condom Use Anymore"** (Meckler, 2002), which was enforced by the American President, who acted on extra information about the ill-effects of condom use. The CDC declaration seems to have had an immediate but short-lived impact on decline of the breast cancer epidemic in the U.S. in the 2003-2004 time period.

5.2 The hidden impact of condomization on life expectancy of women

A few years ago a series of reports appeared simultaneously indicating an unexpected decline in the life expectancy of American people (Ezzati et al., 2008; Brown, 2008; Danaei et al., 2010). The main point in these and other reports was that after a long while a shift in the in U.S. demography has happen, from the customary decrease to sudden increase of mortality The 'reversal of fortunes' as the shift was termed of the increasing mortality has happened in the last three decades, exactly after 1983. The fall of women's life expectancy was more pronounced than in men - of "one in five women" now experiencing lesser longevity and dying younger than before the beginning of 1980s. Although admitting that that the root causes for the downward trend is "impossible to know exactly," the search for causes was directed primarily on "modifiable behaviors and exposures," such as smoking, diet, and lack of exercise, along with the mortality of certain conditions of both sexes. "This is a story about smoking, blood pressure and obesity," was one of the over-confident statement of one of the Harvard researchers (Ezzati, 2008). Besides, the investigation included also diabetes, obesity and AIDS as possible causes of the fall in the life expectancy. The AIDS mortality, while insignificantly linked with the male life expectancy decline, did not relate to that of women.

A more recent background source, 'Explaining Divergent Levels of Longevity in High-Income Countries' review (Crimmins et al, 2011), offers more detailed information on the subject matter of declining life expectancy in the country, and in other comparative countries as well. The evidence in the review, indicated that: (1) the life expectancy is falling in the U.S., (2) the observable fact of falling life expectancy is particularly pronounced among women, (3) the new phenomenon of falling longevity occurred in the last 25 years (during the period 1980-2005), and (4) no risk factors, disease, or any other reason for the falling life expectancy in the U.S. and elsewhere has been determined for the evident, unexpected decline in life expectancy, especially in women (**Figure 22**).

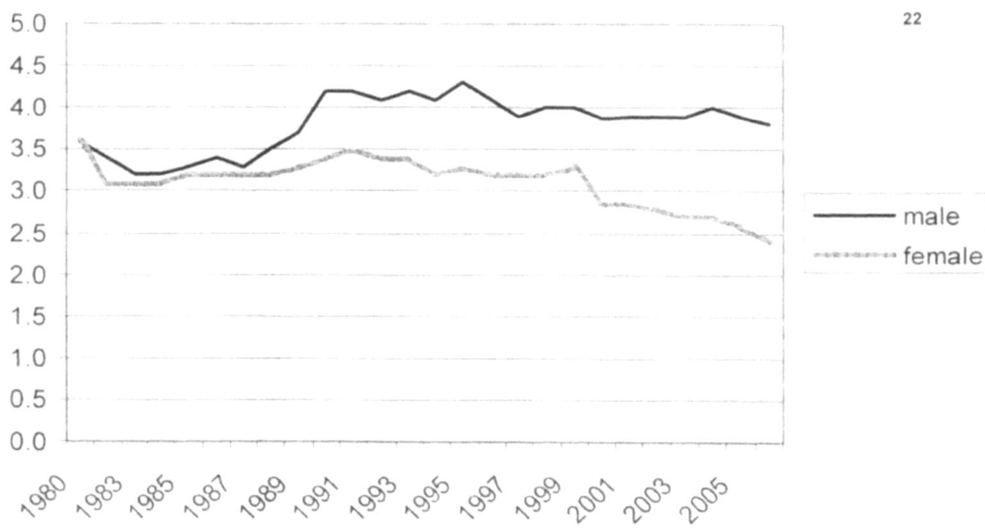

Fig. 22. Gender differences in declining life expectancy at age 50 for U.S. men and women, 1980-2006.

There must be some better way than unconvincing explanation of the confounding smoking and obesity factors, imparting them as the main culprit factors for the slashed longevity of American (and other) women. Missing factors in the review seem to be the unspoken breast cancer epidemic and the mass condomization of female sexuality. Breast cancer is generally treated in the analysis as a passing reference throughout the review. Conspicuously, the unabated and excess epidemic disease of breast cancer is hardly mentioned in the analysis. In the Chapter 8 of the review, entitled Hormone Therapy (in women), the main point of considerations was given on Coronary heart disease and Stroke, and Lung cancer, rather than on Breast cancer. Instead, Lung cancer was sited uncritically as a mortality factor for the decline of longevity even of men and women, because of neglected information that metastases of breast cancer to lungs account for more than 21 to 25 percent. The transmission of HIV/AIDS virus has not been found in the review as a risk factor for the enduring, 25-year decline of women's life expectancy.

The condomization of women's sexuality has been defined as a root cause of the current breast cancer epidemic along with the widespread, accompanying gynecological diseases, tumors and lesions of the organs of reproductive system and other phenomena in American women. The consequences, however, of the general condomization of women's and girls' sexuality in the mainstream population, in a misconceived attempt to stem the emergent AIDS epidemic by barrier birth-control device, has changed the demography of the American society, perhaps the most in the world. The never before experienced change of decline in longevity in of the people has been achieved by a profound corruption of the nature of the intimate (sexual) ecosystem of people, due to elimination of the biologically protective, primordial physiological impact of mutual woman-man relations. That is the change has been achieved by inducing technical effects of absolute male sterility in the marital and inter-gender micro-environment. Namely, the evidence of a significant association between condom use and breast cancer development in the population at large, rather than the transmission of HIV/AIDS virus in any high-risk group, or hormone therapy (for breast cancer) for that matter, may better explain the decline of longevity of American women. It is almost certain that the extent of condom promotion / distribution in the U.S. has been more persistent and more indiscriminate than in the other high-income, comparable countries.

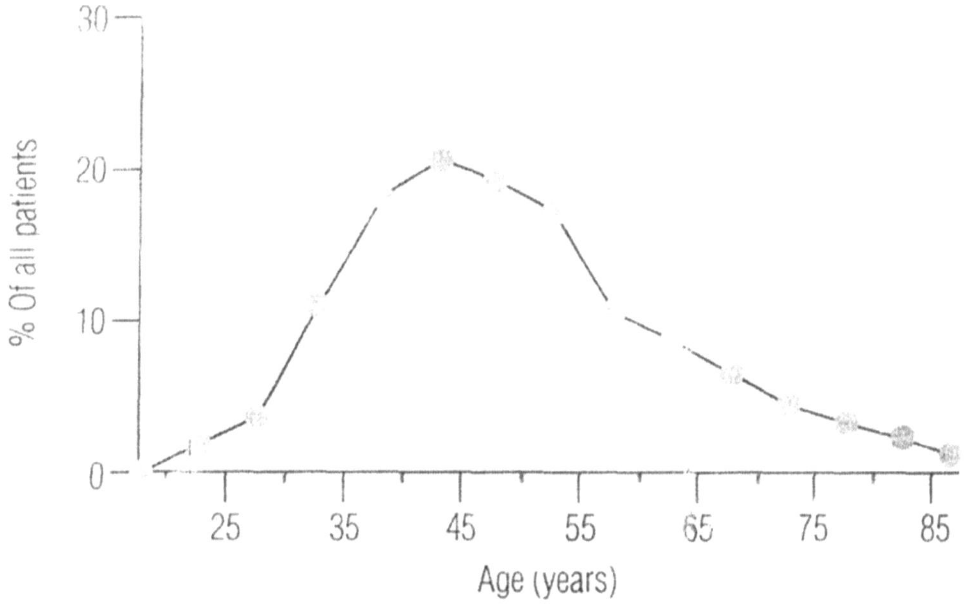

Fig. 23. Percentage of all deaths in women attributable to breast cancer (in 1990s).

The breast cancer epidemiology in the **U.K.**, in the mid-1990s (McPherson et al, 2000), included mortality figures of percentage of all deaths in women attributable to breast cancer (**Figure 23**). The proportion of breast cancer deaths was more than 20 percent in young women aged 40-45, and around 20% in the adjacent age groups 35-39 and 45-49.

In fact, the remarkable, long-term decline of life expectancy in American women may become a unique proof and testimony for both the medical, and perhaps political, misconception of social benefit of the indiscriminate, mass condomization, associated with the breast cancer epidemic, and the wrong-for-long misleading, deadly false belief of condom use as a "safe" hi-tech device for fertility-control and family-planning purposes. [The data of parallel decline on a lesser scale of male longevity might indicate that the devastating and carcinogenic effects of condomization on women's health and lives, resulting in epidemics of breast-ovarian-gynecological cancers, might exert some reciprocal, unknown social or any other biological effect on men as well.] The hope remains, however, that the elimination (practical 'eradication' to levels of rare, sporadic cases) of epidemic breast cancer, by elimination of the sole breast-cancer risk of condomized control of women's sexuality, to reflect rapidly on both decline of the breast cancer epidemic, and restoration of rising women's life expectancy, in a fast manner as the disease entered human race, after the point of departure of all events at the beginning of the 1980s.

6. The future: Prevention of the breast cancer epidemic

In the perspective of breast cancer, the future is present. The answer is the primary, non-chemical prevention of the breast cancer epidemic, although the idea about prevention seems lost and no-existent in the West (Ferlay et al, 2010; EuropaDonna, 2010). Based on 2002 to 2006 trend of increase, the projected future trend of breast cancer increase was estimated at 53% by 2030. Similar disturbing forecast of breast cancer increase of 66.3% in the England and Wales by 2025 has been computed by using a mathematical model based on abortion prevalence rates and several other secondary reproductive factors; the predicted increase being from 39,229 in 2004 to 65,252 in 2025 (Carroll, 2007). Other projected/predicted increase of breast cancer of 32.9% in the U.K., from 2005 till 2024, the present number of 41,900 new cases annually to 55,700 new breast cancer cases in 2024 was assessed by Cancer Research UK (2007). The basic assumption being that the present, sad situation of the breast cancer epidemic in the country will stretch helplessly in the next 20 years, and beyond, into infinity.

To the contrary, the breast cancer epidemic could change by a dramatic decline in the UK, by not less than -80%, from both the forecasted by Carrol excess number of 65,252 cases to eventually 13,050 in 2024, and the forecasted by the Cancer Research UK organization (2007) also excess number of 55,700 cases to 11,140 or less, by 2024, provided primary prevention is implemented in the meantime. The mentioned number of in-situ (DCIS) cases, defined as non-breast cancer (0-zero stage), is expected to decline to a level of one-third (1276 in-situ cases) or less, of the 3,827 cases in England & Wales in 2004 (Carroll, 2007), provided, again, primary prevention is initiated. This is just for laying the groundwork for testing *in vivo* the two opposite theories of breast cancer preventability in the near future.

The following comment was conveyed to **Nicholas D. Kristof**, the New York Columnist as a reply to his article "The secret war on condoms," NYT, Jan. 12, 2003:

> "**The War On Condoms Is The War Against Breast Cancer**
> With reference to your article, "The Secret War on Condoms" (NYT, January 10, 2003), your bitter denigration of the efforts and the politics of the U.S. President, George W. Bush, for dismissal of the condom use as a device for contraceptive, fertility-control and family-planning purposes is misplaced, one-sided and seemingly rational. Apparently, Mr. Bush is in command of extra information of the devastating, adverse and carcinogenic effects of the consistent condom use in married American and other women.
> It is not your fault, of course, that you might have been ignorant of a hypothesis-testing study, which defined and corroborated the true etiology of breast cancer in the country, determined a potential of a primary (non-chemical) prevention of the breast cancer epidemic in the community, predicted the imminent epidemic rise of the malignant disease and, I believe, provided ANSWER for solution and creation of a public health policy in the field of breast cancer and other accompanying diseases. The study was initiated, supported and completed during the mid-1970s, at the University of North Carolina School of Public Health, at Chapel Hill, NC, and at the University of Pennsylvania School of Medicine and Hospital, in Philadelphia, PA. The final report of the aforementioned study was published in the distant 1980, as well as in 1979 by the Michigan University Dissertation International, Ann Arbor, MI.
> However, there are strong indications that the research study has been concealed and secretly suppressed by the previous ("liberal") administrations, dealing with researchers

discovering other approaches with unemployment, academic and professional uprooting and deportation; very soon afterwards, the breast cancer epidemic suddenly and sharply rose and unabated continued its ever-rising increase. The estimate of the U.S. Senate has been that about 2,000,000 women became breast cancer victims during the decade of the 1990s, with 500,000 deaths of the disease. Nowadays, it has been reported that one million of new American breast cancer cases (most of them affluent victims) are registered in four years (rather than in five years, like in the 1990s). The incidence of breast cancer in the United States (as well as in Europe) has been at least seven times higher than the spread of AIDS, the deadly twin epidemic disease. Based on the available WHO data, during the two-decade period, 1981 till 2000, in the U.S have been registered 500,000 (accumulated) cases of AIDS, with about 150,000 deaths (and not less than four million women afflicted with breast cancer, including in-situ cases, with mote than a quarter of the affected women perished).

Apparently, by this backdrop of massacre of women, shattered families, widespread fear, real threat and tragedy in the Country and worldwide, the promotion of the indiscriminate, absolutistic and persistent exposure to (use of) condom in the mainstream population had to be reassessed and amended. The previous administration (at the highest possible levels), regretfully, missed the opportunity to properly address and entirely eliminate the breast cancer epidemic in the country and beyond, and to make the American women happy. With the resolute campaign of President George W. Bush against condom education among the teenagers in the schools, the ultimate objective of condomization of the society has been terminated and the cornerstone of a condom culture has been removed, I hope. In addition, I wonder as to whether a solution of the present gloomy breast cancer emergency or a sustainable prevention of breast cancer could be reached in the Country or elsewhere as long as an American study in primary breast cancer prevention and etiology, such as my monograph "*Barrier Contraception and Breast Cancer*" (1980), is effectively banned from public view, professional scrutiny and clinical assessment for a possible basis of a new breast cancer policy and efficient public health action in the field.

cc: Dr. Andrew C. von Achenbach, Director of the National Cancer Institute, January 12, 2003

cc: The Editors of the New York Times, February 12, 2003

The breast cancer epidemic has remained a perplexing epidemic, and is the case in point of a gender-specific, malignant disease, replacing the routine models of traditional epidemics of contagious, infectious diseases in the general population of both genders and all age groups. The traditionally known in the human history epidemics of infectious diseases have had defined source(s) of the contagious agent, are known to take a course of three main phases (slow or explosive beginning, reaching acme (the peak), and a protracted self-decline ('tail') of the natural end of the epidemics. It seems that the incidence, new HIV/AIDS cases, globally, have reached the peak at the beginning of the 1990s, and are presently showing sings of gradual, protracted, steady decline ever since (McNeil, 2010; USAIDS, 2010). Contrary to the medical experience, the breast cancer epidemic emerged fast, continued its unabated rise, never reached its culmination (acme), and never subsided in expected, tailed decline in the last three decades, since the beginning of 1980s. To the contrary, the new epidemic of breast cancer and other malignant disease(s) in women is not expected to vanish 'naturally,' by its own. Almost certainly, the current breast cancer epidemic is to be terminated by deliberate and conscious human intervention only. The data indicate that the increase of the 'cancer' epidemic in the West, and in other parts of the world, is fueled up mainly by the cancer of the breast and its steady epidemic increase. Apparently, to try to eliminate the current, unabated and excess breast cancer epidemic, a new way of thinking may be needed. The misconception about the breast cancer etiology and community burden hinders the efforts to understand, prevent and control the epidemic malignant breast disease. "What is of concern…is the way the medical-industrial complex uses the research. They would have us believe that because of various findings, such as cancer genes, the cure lies just around the corner. The truth is, however, it doesn't make much difference if a cure ever emerges. The search is a splendid money generator," by quoting other authors, declared the unheeded UK Working Group on the Primary Prevention of Breast Cancer (2007) and, in addition stated, that "there is no sign of leadership from government regarding... (prioritizing).. primary prevention" of breast cancer.

In the last three decades, breast cancer epidemic has spread to other, developing countries of Africa, South Asia, Latin America and elsewhere, as expected. The emerging breast cancer epidemic in the "poor" countries is attracting increasing attention in western countries, with projects and programs relied on old science, and the failing strategy of "palliative care" and "no cure" attitude to continue to be applied against the epidemic disease(s) everywhere. Practically, the inner nature and hormonal balance of woman is still considered to be at fault, which should and could be 'corrected' by chemical agents and human interventions.

The basic strategy of a breast cancer prevention is chemoprevention, particularly with the obsolete *tamoxifen* and other 'selective estrogen modulators,' conducting "downstream" clinical activities of early detection with mammographic screening, so-called 'preventive' mastectomies and oophorectomies, and ineffective counsels for "lessening" spurious risk factors of breast cancer, among which the condom use as a contraceptive method is never considered and maybe still suppressed (Mills, 1987; Bray et al., 2004; National Cancer Policy Board, 2005; Anderson, 2008; WHO-PAHO, 2008; Frenk, 2009; Lancet Editorial, 2009; Meriman, 2010; .Miller, 2010; European Breast Cancer Network, 2010).

Several years earlier, a communication was directed to **Dr. Mitra Roses Periago,** Director of the Pan-American Health Organization-PAHO, Washington, DC, February 14, 2006, regarding the "*Guidelines for International Breast Health and Cancer Control," Breast Journal* Suppl., January-February 2006, conveying the following critical comments (fragments):

"First and foremost, NO PREVENTION of breast cancer was ever mentioned in the PAHO Guidelines. The long-standing, tested evidence (Barrier Contraception and Breast Cancer," 1980), strongly indicating a potential of primary (non-chemical) prevention of breast cancer in American married women, was not taken under consideration in the Guidelines. The evidence, neither disputed nor rejected, showed that breast cancer is a preventable epidemic disease.

The PAHO Guidelines documented the fact that the expected epidemic wave of breast cancer, expanding from the affluent and prosperous Western World (North America and Europe, and others), has already reached the shores and lands of the developing world of Latin America, Africa, and Asia. The Guidelines displayed the growing rates of breast cancer in 'low-resource countries' as an equally serious, rapidly emerging political crisis and a grave public health issue and burden in both developed and developing world. The PAHO Guidelines for breast cancer control in developing countries, however, have relied

heavily on the efforts and experience of the inefficient and fruitless breast cancer control measures in stopping breast cancer before it starts in the developed countries of the West and the WHO. The added rhetoric and new terminology in the Guidelines about the new approaches, innovative research, stratification of the levels of needs, community-based programs, social support, and other envisioned activities against the epidemic of the cancer of the breast, may only replicate the conceptual vacuum and futility in understanding of the etiology and prevention of breast cancer (along with other tumors of the reproductive organs and ill-health phenomena in women) in new settings around the world…
The recent, dramatic "condom paradigm shift" entailed by the U.S. Government (2002) in favor of an "anti-condom" reproductive policy was, most probably, imposed by no accident… Informed observations seem to indicate that race might play a more lethal outcome to married 'non-white' women (Afro-American, Hispanics, Asian-American), exposed to absolute-sterile mating (condom use), than to 'white' women, in terms of breast cancer development, earlier death, shorter survival and physical devastation. If anything, empowerment of women and their husbands / partners with information of the real breast cancer risk would prove to be more useful in preventing the disease at individual, familial and community levels, than the planned regulations and guidelines..."

The following **Table 5** is an attempt to define and elaborate the proposal of the hypothesis 1978 (Gjorgov, 1978a,b, 1979, 1980) of the etiology of breast cancer, and a likely shift of the conceptual framework of the epidemic disease:

Old Paradigm	New Paradigm
1. No Prevention of Breast Cancer (BC)	1. Yes, Primary (non-chemical) Prevention of Breast Cancer
2. Public-health emphasis on mammography screening and early BC detection; Epidemiologically: (unreported) *in-situ* cases	2. Public-health emphasis on primary prevention; Instead of exposure to the BC risks; the *in-situ* cases counted as BC cases;
3. The risk factors of BC are not amenable	3. The main risk factor readily amenable; BC is preventable
4. Treatment and chemical prevention of the BC epidemic	4. Primary (non-chemical) prevention of BC as epidemic disease
5. Nutritional presumed causes (fat, alcohol, smoking, diet, environmental chemicals, toxins, etc), and Reproductive causes: Early menarche, Late births (>30 yrs), Family history, Low parity, No breast-feeding, OC pill use, Late menopause, Lack of exercise, 'Marital' Infertility issue, and other risk factors; Genes and mutations	5. Semen-factor deficiency tested hypothesis: The main etiological cause: the widespread use of Barrier methods: of contraception: Condom devices, Withdrawal practice and male sterility/infertility in marriages. Condom-use technical effects of absolute male sterility: condomization of female sexuality due to Sterile mating
6. Environmental toxic substances & Industrial waste as BC causes, Polluted living settings (home, food, water, working place, streets); Radiation; Gene mutations	6. Inverse environmental factor of BC: absence or elimination of putative protective factors in the intimate (sexual) ecosystem and inter-human micro-environment

Old Paradigm	New Paradigm
7. Toxic environmental waste as direct cause of BC	7. Toxic waste: Indirect cause of BC *via* male infertility
8. Estrogen-Progestin model; 'Toxic-loaded' bodies, HRT, Ignored carcinogenic effects of external steroids, 'Endocrine disrupters' as causes of the current BC epidemic	8. 'Deficiency' of Prostaglandins, seminal fluid; Inner endocrine imbalance in women-related to causes of BC; Foretold BC carcinogenicity of "exogenous hormones"(HRT)
9. Marriage as a social, psychological, economic & legal unit only. Biological independence of spouses-genders	9. Marriage (along sex & love): a biological union w/ profound physiological impact; Sex (gender) inter-dependence
10. BC: poorly known, 'random' disease; local treatment	10. BC a systemic disease, No known cure
11. Hopes & trials in BC chemoprevention (*Tamoxifen*)	11. High-tech devices (condoms, HRTs) gone wrong
12. BC: poorly understood disease, treated as a local one	12. BC: Systemic disease with no known cure
13. Focus on selected BC figures & emphasis to find cure	13. Research-based, hypothesis-tested evidence & data
14. 'Heroic' treatment procedures, endurance of women, learned helplessness and ignorance for self-protection against BC; Decisions of BC 'reduction' at the top, governmental levels	14. Empowerment of women and couples with information of the root cause & BC prevention; Cause-effectiveness assessment for protection made 'at the bottom,' personal and family levels
15. BC as a political crisis, because of progressively rising epidemic spread of the malignant disease in the society	15. Solution/answer to the current, excess BC epidemic, subject to the will and commitment of highest political level
16. The risk of BC unknown; Early detection & treatments as secondary prevention of early death, longer survival	16. Evidence-based definition of the main BC risk: Marital and persistent (long-term) exposure to (use of) condoms
17. Focus on selected BC figures and prejudiced data	17. Evidence-based and hypothesis-tested results / data
18. Long latent period of BC: between 10-20 years or, starting even "in the womb" (both unsubstantiated)	18. Short BC latent period: between 2½ to five years; Evidence confirmed / verified by forecasted BC natural experiment
19. No comprehensive theory (conceptual vacuum) of BC & women's ill health and associated BC equivalents of tumors of the reproductive system; BC linked to ovarian cancer mainly	19. Comprehensive approach to women's health: BC, Ovarian cancer / cysts, uterine cancer/lesions, thyroid cancer / nodules. Anorexia disorders; female osteoporosis; Body-mind phenomena
20. BC prevalent in older, postmenopausal women (>50)	20. Shift to young women (<50); debut peak condom users
21. Current BC epidemic-rapid rise: Denial / artifact claims	21. Rise of the BC epidemic predicted; Verified by events
22. Officially, not recognized & nonexistent BC epidemic	22. Evidence of rapid, unabated & ever-rising BC epidemic

Old Paradigm	New Paradigm
23. 'Second' most common malignant disease in women	23. BC - the commonest malignant disease in women
24. Competing high rates of Lung Cancer in women	24. Fueled by >20% BC metastases to the lungs
25. Higher BC incidence rates in white women	25. Higher BC rates in women of higher living standards
26. Ostensibly, BC mortality decline due to early detection and BC screening programs; (Consensus: *in-situ* cases not to be included in the total annual number of BC figure)	26. If there is a BC mortality decline, then probably due to therapy and surgical modalities, particularly hysterectomy, (with or without one-sided or two-sided oophorectomy)
27. Promotion of condoms as "safe" device for fertility-control and family-planning method	27. Elimination of condoms for contraceptive purposes in population as the main etiological risk of the BC epidemic
28. Priority: 'downstream' activities: screening for more cases & clinical salvage of BC affected women;	28. Priority: Prevention of the risks & cause(s) of current BC epidemic: shift to non-barrier birth-control methods
29. No definition of female response to sterile mating	29. Inner imbalance (Pseudopregnancy), Missed abortion
30. Primary (non-chemical) prevention of the BC epidemic not considered, despite the failed chemoprevention trials	30. Primary prevention ('eradication'), w/ estimated >80% reduction at individual, family and community levels
31. Chemo-prevention of BC: assuming "wrong" female nature to be corrected by Tamoxifen / Raloxifene & drugs	31. Nothing wrong with women's nature subject to chemical correction: Misconceived toxic-substance prevention of BC
32. Ovarian, endometrial and thyroid cancers and other gynecological diseases as unrelated to BC entities	32. Ovarian, endometrial, thyroid & gynecological cancers, lesions of same etiology, condomization of women all ages
33. Silence and suppression of the information of the potential for prevention of the current BC epidemic	33. Decision (pending?) for non-mutually exclusive primary prevention against the twin epidemics of BC and AIDS
34. Plan for action: Search for cure, better therapy, and new drugs and 'better armamentarium' for BC screening	34. Needed plan for action for BC prevention: Elimination of condom use for contraceptive purposes.
35. Overlooked impact of condomization upon issues of marriage, divorce, and women's mortality and life expectancy	35. Considerable protective impact upon social issues of marriage, divorce, and women's mortality and life expectancy

Table 5. Breast cancer hypothesis 1978 and shift of the conceptual framework. (Updated: March 2011)

In the strategy for the global Millennium Development Goals 2015 (MDGs) decisions, a similar situation presented itself regarding condomization of women in less-developed regions. In a letter to the United Nations Secretary-General, the **Hon. Ban Ki-moon**, on September 25, 2010, the following message about the harmful effects of condom-use programs was conveyed:

"As a former United Nations Fellow, Fulbright Scholar, physician and researcher, I like to take the liberty of trying to draw your attention to the grave consequences on women's and girls' reproductive health and lives of continuation of the fallacious condom policy in pursuing the future global Millennium Development Goals 2015 (MDGs).

The condomization of female sexuality, defined long ago as the root cause of the current breast cancer epidemic worldwide, is going o be perpetuated by the UN global MDG Plan for Action. The Plan is apparently oblivious to the global twin epidemic of breast cancer along with AIDS, and is projecting the mass condomization as the main critical plan for action for the Goal 5 and Goal 6 in particular. The breast cancer epidemic has been superseding manifold the HIV/AIDS epidemic in the developed, affluent world of the West, including the U.S., UK, and other EU countries, from the outset, in the early 1980s.

From the affluent, rich western world, the breast cancer epidemic is rapidly spreading to the so-called developing, 'poor' world of Africa and Asia, as anticipated. The typically affected by the disease young / younger women (the main condom users), testify in favor of the defined etiology of the raising breast cancer crisis in the developing regions of the world... Besides breast cancer, there is a myriad of accompanying gynecological tumors and diseases increasingly afflicting women of all races and age-cohorts during their reproductive life-span. It is anticipated that another, more fatal category of female suffering may soon appear, of women affected by both HIV/AIDS and breast cancer diseases combined.

The main culprit of the on-going global breast cancer crisis is the deadly false belief of the use of condom is a "safe" device for fertility-control and family-planning purposes. (By this token, let me mention some official data of the Korean women in the U.S. who have been and still are with the lowest recorded breast cancer incidence rates, which, in my experience, could be attributed to a traditionally low prevalence of condom use and, accordingly, to the assumed lowest condom acculturation in the new/old country.) Almost certainly, it was not by accident that the former President, George W. Bush, acting most likely on extra information, imposed a bold 'condom-paradigm shift,' in favor of an anti-condom reproductive policy, followed by a global ban on condom promotion and distribution, and termination of the unlimited condom funds to global agencies at home and abroad (including WHO, UNFPA, UNAIDS, World Bank and others)… At the present, I believe, the signs may seem encouraging that President Barack Obama would proceed with the same policy of non-condomization of the mainstream population, which policy is expected to prove to be extremely beneficial for elimination, i.e., for primary prevention (non-chemical, non-profit) of the current breast cancer epidemic, and for a better control of the other gender- (sex-) specific diseases in women of all ages. What seem to be happening now, instead, is that the United Nations and its agencies continue to sponsor / promote the relentless push of condoms, disguised as family planning methods, with lingering ill-effects and inevitably up-dating and transferring the current, breast cancer epidemic and other harmful experience of the West into poor world regions…

Ii is my belief that your post of UN Secretary-General embodies a unique opportunity to be able to try to help reassess the new scientific evidence about the epidemiological and social consequences of the never openly debated, arbitrary silenced issue of condomized control of women's and girls' sexuality, a deceptive protection of their reproductive health in the UN sponsored MDGs 5 & 6."

E-mailed and AIRMAILED

7. Conclusion

The perplexing worldwide breast cancer epidemic, defined as unintended consequence of widespread condomization of women's sexuality, carried out in fervent campaigns for both contraceptive and prophylactic (anti-HIV/AIDS) purposes continue to reign supreme, globally. It is the quintessence of a deadly female sex- (gender-) specific, malignant disease. The data indicate that the increase of the 'cancer' epidemic in the West, and in other parts of the world, is fueled up almost entirely by the breast cancer epidemic and its steady increase. The breast cancer epidemic is thriving mainly because of lack of commitment to eliminate the disease(s) to rare, sporadic cases, at personal, familial and community levels. The condomization of women's and girls' sexuality is directly related to multitude aspects of female ill health, disturbed functions, specific and accompanying diseases, life, death, marital malfunctions, and reduced longevity.

Most of the researchers in the field of cancer research and birth control seem to refer to a "recreational" value of sex, by searching only for technical aspects ("frequency") of intimate encounters and utterly ignoring the biological aspects and barriers to the primordial 'gender' communication, sexual relations. It is amazing that the authors have consistently missed the opportunity to consider barriers to sex as a part of life, particularly of women. The new epidemic of breast cancer and other malignant disease(s) in women is not expected to vanish 'naturally,' by its own. The data indicate that the increase of the breast cancer epidemic in the West, and in other parts of the world, is fueled up mainly by the deceptive condomization of female sexuality in mainstream populations. Almost certainly, the current breast cancer epidemic is to be terminated by deliberate and conscious human intervention only. To try to eliminate the current, unabated and excess breast cancer epidemic, a new way of thinking may be needed.

The answer to the current breast cancer contingency is to undertake a primary, non-chemical, no-profit, prevention of the epidemic. Since information in public health actions is superior to legislation, it seems better to take the first steps with subtle, nonjudgmental attitude. Perhaps the true information of the devastating and carcinogenic effects of condom use should be communicated to the consumers and displayed on the commercial product.

The information (warning) of the breast cancers risk being included in condom labeling. No doubt that women and couples, empowered with preventative, potentially life-saving information, will be able to make correct assessment of the risks and benefits values on matters of life and death, at a bottom, personal and familial, rather than at the detached at the top decision-making level.

8. Acknowledgments

Thanks to Ing, Emil Gjorgov, from the University American College Skopje, and Ing. Dr. Kosta Mangaroski, from the University St. Cyril and Methodius, Skopje, for the technical support.

9. References

Ambekar A. (2009). Causes and Effects of Divorce. Article. January 12. Internet web: www.articleswave.com/divorce-articles/causes-and-effects-ofdivorce.html

Anderson, BO., Yip, CH., Smith. RA. et al. (2008). Guideline implementation for breast healthcare in low-income and middle-income countries: overview of the Breast Health Global Initiative Global Summit 2007. Cancer 2008 Oct 15;113(8 Suppl):2221-43. Web: http://www.guideline.gov/content.aspx?id=13344#Section420

Australian Historical Statistics (2001). Divorce rates in Australia. Web: http://www.divorcerate.org/divorce-rates-in-australia.html

Bray, F; McCarron, P. & Parkin, DM. (2004). The changing global patterns of female breast cancer incidence and mortality. *Breast Cancer Research* 6: 229-239. Web. http://breast-cancer-research.com/content/6/6/229

Brining MF, Allen DW (2000). 'These boots are made for walking': Why most divorce filers are women. *American Law and Economics Review*, Vol. 2, pp. 126-169. Web: http://papers.ssrn.com/so13/papers.cfm?abstract_id=713110

Brown D (2008). Life Expectancy Drops for Some U.S. Women. Historic Reversal, Found in 1,000 Counties May Be Result of Smoking and Obesity. *Washington Post*, April 22. Internet web: http://www.washingtonpost.com/wp-dyn/content/article/2008/04/21/AR2008042102406_pf.html

Carroll, PS. (2007) 'The breast cancer epidemic: modeling and forecasts based on abortion and other risk factors', Journal of American Physicians and Surgeons, 12(3): 72-78. Web: http://www.jpands.org/vol12no3/carroll.pdf

Cirado MP, Edwards B, Shin HR, Storm H, Ferlay J, Heanue M, Boyle P. Eds. (2007). *Cancer Incidence in Five Continents*, Volume IX, WHO-IARC, Sci. Publ. 160, Lyon, France. (Digital data edition on Internet)

Cancer Research UK. (2007). Breast cancer - UK incidence statistics. Web: http://info.cancerresearchuk.org/cancerstats/types/breast/incidence/

Crieger, N. (2002). Is breast cancer a disease of affluence, Poverty or both? The case of African American women. *American Journal of Public Health* 92:611-612.

Crimmins EM, Preston SH, Cohen B (2011). Explaining Divergent Levels of Longevity In High-Income Countries. National Research Council of the National Academies. January 25. *National Academies Press*. Web: http://www.nap.edu/catalog/13089.html

Dinse, GE.; Umbach, DM.; Sasco, AJ. et al. (1999). Unexplained increases in cancer incidence in the United States from 1975 to 1994: Possible Sentinel Health Indicators. *Annual Review of Public Health* 20:173-209.

Danaei. G., Rimm, ER., Oza, S., et al. (2010). The promise of prevention: The effect of four preventable risk factors on national life expectancy and life expectancy disparities and county in the United States. PLoS Medicine, March, 7(3); e1000248. Web: http://www.ncbi.nlm.nih.gov/pmc/articles/PMC2843596/?tool=pmcentrez

Ehrchardt AA (1992). Trends in sexual behavior and the HIV pandemic. Editorial. *American Journal of Public Health* 82(11):1459-1461, November.

EuropaDonna. (2010). More women get breast cancer than any other cancer. (See Ferlay, J. et al., 2010) Web: http://europadonnaireland.ie/content/more

European Commission. (2006). *European Guidelines for quality assurance in breast cancer screening and diagnosis.* Fourth Edition. Perry, N. et al Editors. Health and Consumer Protection G.D., pp. 416.

Ezzati M, Friedman AB, Kulkarni SC, Murray CGL (2008). The reversal of fortunes: Trends in county mortality and cross-County mortality disparities in the United States. *PLoS Medicine*, April 22;5(4):e66, Web: http://www.plosmedicine.org/article/info%3Adoi%2F10.1371%2Fjournal.pmed.0050066

Ferlay, J.; Parkin, DM. and Steliarova-Foucher, E. (2010). Estimates of cancer incidence and mortality in Europe in 2008. Eur J Cancer, 46(4): 756-81. Web: http://www.ejcancer.info/article/S0959-8049(09)00926-5/pdf

Flandrin, J-L. (1975). Contraception, Marriage, and Sexual Relations in the Christian West. In: R. Foster & O. Ranum, Eds. Biology of Man in History, Chapter 1. Selection from the Annales Economies Societes, Civilisations. The John Hopkins University Press, Baltimore & London, 23-47.

Fox, MF. (2004). Robert King Merton. Life time of influence. Scientometrics, Vol. 60, No. 1, 47-50. Web: http://www.spingerlink.com/content/m0822078639422vu/bodyRef/PDF/11192_2004_Article_5149145.pdf

Frenk, J. (2009). Cancer is on the rise in developing countries. The shadow epidemic. Harvard School of Public Health. November 25. Web: http://www.hsph.harvard.edu/news/hphr/fall-2009/shadow-epidemic.html

Gjorgov, AN. (1978a). Barrier contraceptive practice and male infertility as related factors to breast cancer in married women. *Medical Hypotheses* (Montreal, Canada) 4(2): 79-88. Medline - Abstract # 03590510/78224510. Web: http://www.sementherapy.com/mirror/sciencedirect.com_002.htm

Gjorgov, AN. (1978b). Barrier contraceptive practice and male infertility as related factors to breast cancer in married women. Preliminary results. *Oncology* (Munich, Germany) 35: 97-100, Medlars II - Popline PIP/783908.

Gjorgov, AN. (1979). Barrier Contraceptive Practice and Male Infertility as Related Factors to Breast Cancer in Married Women. A Retrospective Study, pp 325. University of Michigan Dissertation International, Ann Arbor, MI 48106; UMI publication # 79-14352. Dissertation Abstract: Vol. XV, No. 1. Abstract: Web: http://www.hsc.edu.kw/vpo/library/theses/Author.asp?view=Gjorgov,%20Arne%20N#

Gjorgov, AN. (1980). *Barrier Contraception and Breast Cancer*. S.Karger Publ., Basel-Munchen-Paris-New York-Sydney: x+164.

Gjorgov, AN. (1986). Breast cancer in Kuwait, 1974-1983. An epidemiological study. *Journal of the Kuwaiti Medical Asso*ciation 20: 75-88.

Gjorgov, AN. (1989). Risk factors of female thyroid cancer in Kuwait. Retrospective study. (Leading article.) *Libri Oncologici* (Zagreb) 18(1-2):5-22. (Received for publication September 12th, 1988)

Gjorgov, AN. (1990). Breast cancer risk from use of condom: Interim evidence of an unplanned natural experiment. *Child and Family* (Oak Park, Illinois) 21: 97-101.

Gjorgov, AN. (1991). Breast cancer death rates in Yugoslavia, 1979-1987: An attempt to explain the new rising trends. *The Journal of the Medical Association of Macedonia.* 45(3-4): 67-73. (Summary in English).

Gjorgov, AN. (1993). Emerging worldwide trends of breast cancer incidence in the 1970s and 1980s: Data from 23 cancer registration centres. *European Journal of Cancer Prevention* (London) 2: 423-440.

Gjorgov, AN. (1994a). History of the condom: the overlooked adverse effects. *J Royal Society of Medicine* (London) 87: 570, September 1 (Opening of the Int'l Conf. on Population and Development, Cairo, Egypt, Sept. 2-14 (ICPD-1994). Web: http://www.ncbi.nlm.nih.gov/pmc/articles/PMC1294789/pdf/jrsocmed00081-0090c.pdf

Gjorgov, AN. (1994b). Worldwide BC Incidence: An Attempt at Interpretation of the Ecological Rising Trends and of the Potential for Prevention. Kuwait University. Poster at the *Lancet Breast Cancer Challenge Conference 1994*, Brugge, Belgium, April 21-23.

Gjorgov, AN. (1994c). Rising breast cancer incidence worldwide, 1980-1990. A potential for prevention. *J Med Assoc Macedon* 48(1-2): 118-123. (Summary in English).

Gjorgov, AN. (1996a). *Breast Cancer: Rationale for an Etiologic Hypothesis.* A Reappraisal of the Clinical, Experimental, and Theoretical Aspects of Neoplastic Processes, Pseudopregnancy Complex, and the Possible Role of the Seminal Prostaglandins. University of Pennsylvania School of Medicine, Philadelphia, PA, 1980, and Matica Mak. Publ., Skopje, 1996.

Gjorgov, AN. (1996b). Prevention and eradication of the *bovine spongiform encephalopathy* (*BSE*): A solicited response and proposal. *Macedonian Veterinary Review* (Skopje) 1996; 25(1-2): 97-101.

Gjorgov, AN. (1997/1998). Breast cancer death of Empress Theodora, wife of Justinian I of Byzantine, in the Sixth Century. *ASKLEPIOS, International Journal of History and General Theory of Medicine*, Vol. XI, pp. 117-121. Web: http://prodavnicanatajni.blog.mk/2006/11/30/seks-da-no-priroden/

Gjorgov, AN. (1998a). Ecological breast cancer incidence differentials and condom use prevalence worldwide, 1983-87: Corroboration of the potential for primary prevention. *Archive Balkan Medical Union* (Bucharest) 33; 111-123.

Gjorgov, AN. (1998b). Breast cancer and barrier contraception: Postulated and corroborated potential for prevention. Invited lecture. *Folia Medica* (Plovdiv) 1998; 30: 17-23. (PMID: 10205987 - MEDLINE.)

Gjorgov, AN.; Junaid, TA.; Burns, GR. & Temmim, L. (1999). Efficacy of preventive prostaglandin treatment of malignant mammary lesions in rats. An experimental trial. *Journal of* the *Balkan Union of Oncology* (*J-BUON*) - (Athens) 4:295-306. Ditto: (1996) *European Journal of Cancer Prevention* (London) 5(Suppl 2):104 (Abstract). Web: http://journals.lww.com/eurjcancerprev/citation/1996/12002/efficacy_of_preventive_prostaglandin_treatment_of.21.aspx and/or http://www.unet.com.mk/medics/mammary.htm

Gjorgov, AN. (2000). Continuing rise of the breast cancer epidemic worldwide, in the 1990s: Further evidence and corroboration of the potential for primary prevention. *Contributions of the Section of Biological & Medical Sciences of the Macedonian Academy of Sciences and Arts (MASA)*, Skopje, Vol. XXI, No. 1-2, pp 41-63.

Gjorgov, AN., Narod, S. et al. (2001a) Tubal ligation and risk of ovarian cancer. (Correspondence) Lancet, Sep. 8, 358:843-4. Web:

http://www.thelancet.com/journals/lancet/article/PIIS0140-6736(01)05991-8/fulltext

Gjorgov, AN. (2001b). Biological Foundations of Human Sexuality: Personal Notes on the Discordant Popular and Modern Attitudes. (Medical History Congress presentation, October 2001); *Asklepios, International Annual of History and Philosophy of Medicine* (Sofia) Vol. XIV: 160-164.

Gjorgov, AN. (2003a). Condomization of Female Sexuality - The Cause of FSD. *British Medical Journal*-Online, 26 January, Web: http://www.bmj.com/cgi/eletters/326/7379/45#29155

Gjorgov, AN. (2003b). Klimt's man-woman relation in his 'Medicine.' *British Medical Journal*-Online. Rapid response to 'Doctors versus artists: Gustav Klimt's Medicine'. 11 March. Web: http://www.bmj.com/cgi/eletters/325/7378/1506#30361

Gjorgov, AN. (2003c). Primary prevention of breast cancer versus the current policy of salvage treatment: Update of evidence and the proposition. *Macedonian Journal of Medicine* 49(1-2): 15-26.

Gjorgov, AN. (2006). A review of the osteoporosis in women and a new hypothesis for testing. *Macedonian Journal of Medicine* 52(1-2): 5-21.

Gjorgov, AN. (2008). Incomplete Study of 'Birth Control Pills Prevent Ovarian Cancer.' *The Washington Post* Blog, Comment, posted January 25. Web: http://digg.com/health/Birth_Control_Pills_Prevent_Ovarian_Cancer

Gjorgov, AN. (2009a). Anorexia and Bulimia Nervosa in Young Female Patients and Barrier Contraception Practice. *Asklepios, International Annual of History and Philosophy of Medicine* (Sofia) Vol. III New Series (XXII)::97-108.

Gjorgov, AN (2009b). Breast cancer risk assessment to barrier contraception exposure. New Approach. *Contributions Soc Biol Med Sci* MASA, XXX, 1, 217-233. (Macedonian Academy of Sciences and Arts), Web: http://e20.manu.edu.mk/prilozi/16ag.pdf

Gjorgov, AN. (2010). Reproductive Health of Women: An Attempt to Define Breast Cancer Prevention. *Macedonian Journal of Medical Sciences*, 3(2): 169-179, Jun. 15, Web: http://www.mjms.ukim.edu.mk/Online/MJMS_2010_3_2/MJMS.1857-5773.2010-0104v.pdf

Hinman, AR. (1978). The condom as prophylactic. Bull. N.Y. Acad. Med. 52(8):1004-1011. Web: http://www.ncbi.nim.nih.gov/pmc/articles/PMC1807317/?log$=activity

Japanese Ministry of Health (2002). Major causes of divorce – Japan gaining on USA and Canada. (Update 2007.) Web: http://hubpages.com/hub/Major_Causes_Of_Divorce

Kimball, M. (2010). Why Americans divorce. Women cite abuse, men site sex as top reasons for divorce. Internet web: www.divorce360.com/divorce-articles/causes-of-divorce/information/why-americans-divorce.aspx?artid=169

Koop, CE. (1986). Surgeon General's Report on AIDS. U.S. Public Health Service. *JAMA* 256:2783-2789.

Lancet Editorial. (2009). Breast cancer in developing countries. The Lancet 374:1567. November 7. Web: www.thelancet.com Vol 374 November 7, 2009 1567

Lincoln, R. (1979). The Select Committee Reports. *Family Planning Perspectives* 11(2):101-4, Mar-Apr. PMID: 456481 (Mesh Terms: Adolescent, Contraception, Emigration and Immigration, Family Planning Services, Fertility, Financing, Government, Humans, Cooperation, Population, Population Control, Research, Social Sciences)

Lê, Monique, G.; Bachelot, Annie & Hill, Catherine. (1989). Characteristics of reproductive life and risk of breast cancer in a case-control study of young nulliparous women. *Journal of Clinical Epidemiology* 42: 1227-1235.

Linos. E.; Spanos, D.; Rosner, BA. et al. (2008). Effects of reproductive and demographic changes on breast cancer incidence in China: A modeling analysis. *Journal of the National Cancer Institute* 100(19): 1352-1360.

Meckler, L. (2002). CDC Fact Sheet Not Promoting Condom Use Anymore. CDC Center for HIV, STD and TB Prevention, December 19. Web: http://www.aegis.com/news/ads/2002/AD022455.html

McNeil, DDG. (2010). UN reports decrease in new HIV infections. *The New York Times*, November 23-24. Web: http://www.nytimes.com/2010/11/24/world/africa/24infect.html and http://www.blueridgenow.com/article/20101124/ZNYT04/11243009

McPherson, K.; Steel, CN. & Dixon, JM. (2000). Breast cancer epidemiology, risk factor, and genetics. *BMJ* 321:1198-1206. 9 September. Web: http://www.bmj.com/content/321/7261/624.full

Malta National Cancer Registry (2010). Incidence of breast cancer in Females (1998-2007). *Dep't of Health Info. & Research.*

Meckler, L. (2002). CDC Fact Sheet Not Promoting Condom Use Anymore. Prevention News Update. December 19. Internet web: http://aegis.com/news/ads/2002/AD022455.html

Merriman, A. (2010). Emerging breast cancer epidemics: impact on palliative care. Breast Cancer Research 12(Suppl 4):S11. Web: http://breast-cancer-research.com/content/12/S4/S11

Miller, WR. (2010). Controversies in breast cancer 2010. Breast Cancer Research 12(Suppl 4): S1. Web: http://breast-cancer-research.com/content/12/S4/S1

Mills, JL. (1987). Reporting provocative results. Can we publish 'hot' papers without getting burned? Commentary. JAMA 258(23): 3428, December 18.

Moynihan R (2003). The making of a disease: Female sexual dysfunction. *BMJ*, 4 326:45-47, January.

National Academy of Sciences. (2011) Women's Health Research. Progress, Pitfalls, and Promise. Ch. 3. Research on Conditions with Particular Relevance to Women. (pp. 95-170) Table 3-1.

National Cancer Institute-NCI. (2002). SEER Cancer Statistics Review 1975-2000. Female breast cancer (In Situ) - Table IV-6.

Mosher WD, Jones J. (2010).Use of contraception in the United States: 1982–2008. *National Center for Health Statistics. Vital & Health Statistics* 23(29). Web: http://www.cdc.gov/nchs/data/series/sr_23/sr23_029.pdf

Muir, C., Waterhouse, J., Mack, T., Powell, J., Whelan, S., Eds. (1987). *Cancer Incidence in Five Continents*, Volume V, WHO-IARC, Publ. 120, Lyon, France.

National Cancer Policy Board-NCPB. (2005). Saving Women's Lives: Strategies for Improving Breast Cancer Detection and Diagnosis. Web: http://books.nap.edu/openbook.php?record_id=11916&page=269

Office of National Statistics (2004). Divorce rate in UK. Web: http://www.divorcerate.org/divorce-rates-in-uk.html

Parkin, DM.; Muir, CS.; Whelan, SL.; Gao, YT; Ferlay J. & Powell J. Eds. (1992). *Cancer Incidence in Five Continents*, Volume VI, WHO-IARC Sci. Publ. 120, Lyon, France.

Parkin DM, Whelan SL, Ferlay J, Raymond L, Young J. Eds. (1997). *Cancer Incidence in Five Continents*, Volume VII, WHO-IARC Sci. Publ. 143, Lyon, France.

Parkin DM, Whelan S, Ferlay J, Teppo L, Thomas DB. Eds. (2002). *Cancer Incidence in Five Continents*, Volume VIII, WHO-IARC, Sci. Publ. 155, Lyon, France. (Digital data edition on Internet).

Peatling, S. (2005). Divorce takes husbands by surprise. Article, March 17. Internet web: www.smh.com.au/news/National/Divorce-takes-husbands-by-surprise/2005/03/16/1110913668722.html

Peters, EN. (1998). Contraception and Divorce: Insights from American Annulment Cases. *Family Foundations (Nov.-Dec.).* CanonLaw.info. Web: http://www.canonlaw.info/a_contraceptionanddivorce.htm

Pikhut PM, Levshin VF, and Moskaleva LI. (1991). Methods of contraception and the risk of breast cancer development. *Sovyetskaya Medicina*, issue 12, pp. 70-72.

Siegel-Itzkovich, j. (1999). Israel health minister bans AIDS campaign promoting condoms. BMJ 319 (7223):1455 (December 4). Web: http://www.bmj.com/cgi/content/full/319/7223/1455/b?maxtoshow=&HITS=10718/05/01

Stevenson, B. & Wolfers, J. (2007a). Marriage and Divorce: Changes in their driving forces. *Journal of Economic Perspectives* Vol. 21, No. 2, pp. 27-52. Web: www.hartonupenn.edu/betseys/papers/JEP_Marriage_and_Divorce.pdf

Stevenson, B. & Wolfers, J. (2007b). Marriage and Divorce: Changes in their driving forces. NBER Working Paper Series, No 12944. National Bureau of Economic Research, Cambridge, MA. March. Web: http://www.nber.org/papers/w12944.pdf

Stevenson, B. & Wolfers, J. (2009). The paradox of declining female happiness. *American Economic Journal: Economic Policy* 1:2, 190-225. Web: http://www.aeaweb.org/articles.php?doi=10.1257/pol.1.2.190

Stevenson, B. (2010). Marriage calculator. Web: http://www.divorce360.com/content/getthedivorcecalculatorwidget.aspx

Storm, HH. (2011). Johannes Clemmesen - a pioneer and founder of Danish cancer epidemiology, has passed away on December 20, 2010, at the age of 102. Web: http://www.iarc.fr/media-centre/iarcnews/pdf/JohannesClemmesenEng.pdf

Svoboda, E. (2006). All signs of pregnancy except one: a baby. Article. *The New York Times*, December 5.

UK Working Group on the Primary Prevention of Breast Cancer. (2007). No More Breast Cancer. December. Web: http://www.nomorebreastcancer.org.uk/assets/main_v.1.pdf

UNAIDS (2010). Report on the global AIDS epidemic 2010. Web: http://www.unaids.org/globalreport/Global_report.htm

United Nations Secretariat. (1994). *Key issues in family planning, health and family well-being in the 190s and beyond.* International Conference on Population and Development, Cairo, 5-14 September. (ICPD, Cairo, 1994).

Valdiserri, RO. (1988). Cum Mastis Sic Clypeatis: The turbulent history of the condom. Bulletin of the N.Y. Academy of Medicine 64(3): 237-245.

Waterhouse, J.; Muir, C.; Correa, P. & Powell, J. Eds. (1977). *Cancer Incidence in Five Continents*, Volume III, WHO-IARC Publ. No. 15, Lyon, France.

Waterhouse. J.; Muir, C.; Shanmugaratnam, K. & Powell, J. Eds. (1982). *Cancer Incidence in Five Continents*, Volume IV, WHO-IARC Publ. No. 42, Lyon, France.

WHO-PAHO. (2008). Guidelines for International Breast Health and Cancer Control. Cancer - Volume 113, Issue Supplement 8 - 15 October (World Health Organization and Pan American Health Organization). Web: http://www.paho.org/English/AD/DPC/NC/pcc-breast-cancer-guidelines.htm and

Wolfers, J. (2010). How marriage survives. Op-Ed. New York Times, October 12. Web: http://www.nytimes.com/2010/10/13/opinion/13wolfers.html

Part 4

From the Clinic to the Patients: Transmission, Diagnosis and Therapies

Transmission of HIV Through Blood – How To Bridge the Knowledge Gap

Smit Sibinga, Cees Th and John P. Pitman
ID Consulting for International Development of Transfusion Medicine/ University of Groningen The Netherlands

1. Introduction

1.1 HIV and blood transfusion – The current state of the art

Of all blood donations 65% are made in developed (very high human development index or VH-HDI) countries, home to just 25% of the world's population. In 73 countries, donation rates are still less than 1% of the population (the minimum needed to meet basic needs in a country). Of these, 71 are either developing (low HDI) or transitional (medium to high HDI) countries; 42 countries collect less than 25% of their blood supplies from the safest source: voluntary non-remunerated blood donors. However, less than 50% of these donors donates regularly, the other half just one time only. In 2007, 31 countries (19%) still reported collecting paid donations, which is more than 1 million donations in total, where 41 countries (25%) were not able to screen all blood donations for one or more of the following transfusion-transmissible infections (TTIs) - HIV, hepatitis B, hepatitis C and syphilis (WHO 2010a).

Blood transfusion as a supportive haemotherapy contributes to saving lives and improving health, but millions of patients needing transfusion do not have timely access to or can afford safe blood. In 2007, 162 countries provided data to WHO on 85.4 million blood donations (World Health Organization [WHO] 2010a). These data come from countries that account for a total of 5.9 billion people, representing 92% of the global population. The report covers around 8,000 blood centres. In developed countries, the average annual collection per blood centre was 13,600 (range 49–289,075), in transitional countries 6,000 (range 20–499,212) and in developing countries 2,800 (range 114–23,251).

1.1.1 Blood supply

While the need for blood is universal, there is still a major imbalance between developing and advanced countries in the level of access to safe blood. It is estimated that blood donation by 1% of the total population (10 per 1,000 population) is generally the minimum needed to meet a nation's most basic requirements for blood; the requirements are higher in countries with more advanced health care systems and medical interventions.

Of the 85.4 milion donations in 2007, about 65 % were collected in developed countries. Blood donations per 1,000 population, which also reflect the general availability of blood in a country, vary widely and the lowest levels of availability are found in developing and transitional countries (WHO 2010a). The average donation rate in developed (VH-HDI) countries is 38.1 donations/1,000 population (range 4.92–68.01); in transitional (H and M-HDI) countries this rate is 7.5 (range 1.07–35.18) and in developing (L-HDI) countries an average of 2.3 (range 0.40–7.46) donations per 1,000 population were collected. In 2007, 73 countries (45%) reported collecting fewer than 10 donations per 1,000 population. Among them, 71 (97%) are either developing or transitional countries. Due to relatively high TTI marker prevalence the drop out of collected blood varies between 11 and over 20%, reducing the clinical availability substantially.

1.1.2 Blood donation

There are three major types of blood donation: voluntary unpaid donations (non-remunerated/altruistic), family/replacement donations (coerced), and paid donations. Donors who give blood voluntarily, regularly and for altruistic reasons have the lowest prevalence of HIV, hepatitis viruses and other blood-borne infections, as compared to people who donate for friends and family members or because of payment. Family and replacement donations are often hidden paid and seriously coerced. Sufficient supplies of safe blood can only be assured by regular donations from voluntary unpaid and anonymous donors. The 2007 WHO data reveal some improvements in such donations worldwide, but many developing and transitional countries still rely heavily on relatively unsafe one time only family/replacement donors and paid donors (fig 1).
This means a considerable gap in public awareness and knowledge about the essentials of blood donation as an act of social solidarity and blood transfusion as an integral element of the health care system.

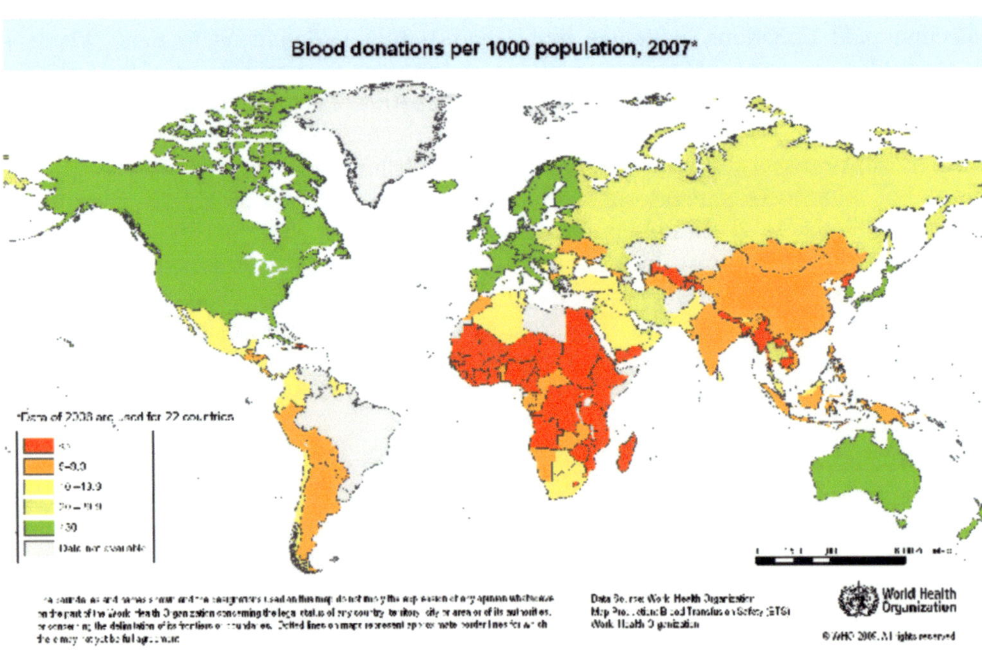

Fig. 1. Annual blood donations per 1,000 population, 2007. Source: Global Database on Blood Safety (GDBS), 2007 survey (WHO2010a)

1.1.2.1 Voluntary, unpaid donations

Of the 162 responding countries 57 (35%) report collecting 100% of their blood supplies from voluntary unpaid donors (fig. 2). Since World Blood Donor Day (14th June, birthday of Karl Landsteiner) celebration began in 2004, 111 countries (68.5%) reported an increase of the number of voluntary donations; 32 of these 111 (29%) have more than doubled the number of voluntary donations as compared to 2004 figures. All these 32 countries are developing or transitional countries. Additionally, 11 countries (Bosnia and Herzegovina, Burkina Faso, Cook Islands, Cape Verde, Kuwait, Guinea Bissau, Mauritania, Myanmar, Niue, Vanuatu and Vietnam) reported more than a 10% increase in voluntary unpaid donations in 2007, as compared to 2006 figures. However, a major problem remains the retention of voluntary non-remunerated blood donors.

1.1.2.2 Family/replacement donors and paid donors

Forty-two countries (26%) collect less than 25% of their blood supplies from voluntary unpaid blood donors. A significant amount of the blood supply in these countries is still dependent on family/replacement and paid blood donors. Thirty-one countries (18%) still report collecting paid donations in 2007, which represents more than 1 million donations in total.

The average donation rate in high-income countries is 45,400 donations per million people. This compares with 10,100 donations per million people in middle-income countries and 3,600 donations in low-income countries. If 1% to 3% of a country's population would donate blood, it would be sufficient to meet the country's needs. But in 77 countries, donation rates are still less than 1%.

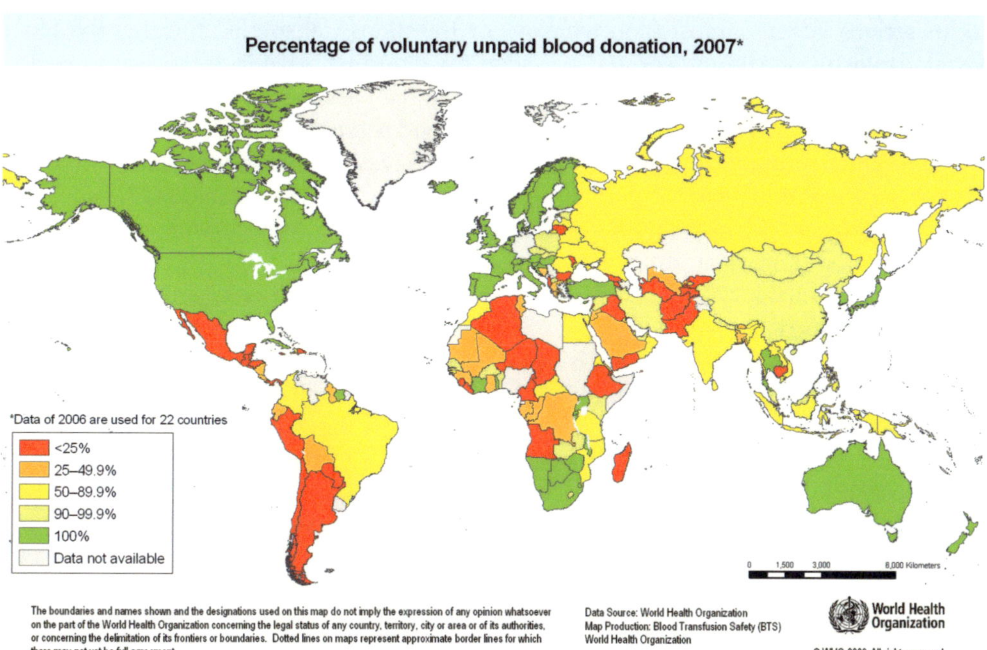

Fig. 2. Percentage voluntary non-remunerated blood donors, 2007. Source: Global Database on Blood Safety (GDBS), 2007 survey (WHO2010a)

1.1.3 Blood screening for transmissible infections

WHO recommends that all donated blood to be used for transfusion should be screened at minimum for HIV, hepatitis B, hepatitis C and syphilis (WHO 2010). Complete and accurate data on the screening of donated blood are not available from many developing countries, particularly those where blood services are not coordinated. Many countries do not have reliable testing systems because of staff shortages, lack of basic laboratory services, poor quality test kits or their irregular supply. Of the 162 countries that provided data on screening for transfusion-transmissible infections including HIV, hepatitis B, hepatitis C and syphilis, 41 (25%) are not able to screen all donated blood for one or more of these infections (fig. 3). The other 121 countries provided data on whether blood donations were screened in a quality-assured manner (use of standard operating procedures and participation in an external quality assessment scheme or EQAS). Overall, 88% of the blood collected are screened following these basic quality procedures: 89% in developed countries, 87% in transitional countries and 48% in developing countries. For the blood donations collected in the remaining 41 countries, which account for 22% of the global donations reported to WHO, the use of these basic quality assurance procedures for laboratory screening is still unknown. Additionally there is still a widespread mix of test kits used within countries, both ELISA and rapid test depending on availability and supply. Quality of performance and reliability of test results remain a problem of considerable concern.

1.1.4 Clinical use of blood

Data on the clinical use of donated blood is limited, but studies suggest that transfusions are often given unnecessarily when simpler, less expensive treatments can provide equal or greater benefit. Not only is this a waste of a scarce resource but it also exposes patients to the risk of serious adverse transfusion reactions or infections transmitted through the blood. Hospital transfusion committees and a system for reporting adverse transfusion reactions should be established in each hospital to implement the national policy and guidelines and to monitor the safe and rational use of blood and blood products at the local level. However, in a substantial proportion of the transition and developing countries there is still no national policy and no current guidelines or standards. In many situations haemoglobin transfusion triggers are high and surgical blood order equations and minimal blood order lists are not used (Kajja et al. 2010a, 2010b) .

In 2007, 120 countries (74%, including 46 developed, 48 transitional and 26 developing countries) identified and reported a total of 51,400 hospitals that perform blood transfusions, serving a population of around 3.6 billion. Not all countries were able to provide information on clinical practice (WHO 2010a). Data on hospitals performing transfusion provided by 96 countries (80%, including 38 developed countries, 40 transitional countries and 18 developing countries) illustrate the presence of a transfusion committee in 88% of these hospitals in developed countries, 33% in transitional and 25 % in developing countries. Mechanisms to monitor clinical transfusion practice (documentation) is present in 90% of the hospitals performing transfusion in developed countries, 52 % in transitional and 23 % in developing countries. However, a system for reporting adverse transfusion events (haemovigilance) in hospitals performing transfusion is found in 91% in developed countries, but only 46% in transitional and 23% in developing countries.

These 2007 WHO survey data illustrate a major gap in awareness and knowledge among policy makers and blood transfusion professionals, both in the procurement and the prescribing parts of the vein-to-vein blood transfusion chain in transitional (M-HDI) and even more prominent in developing (L-HDI) countries.

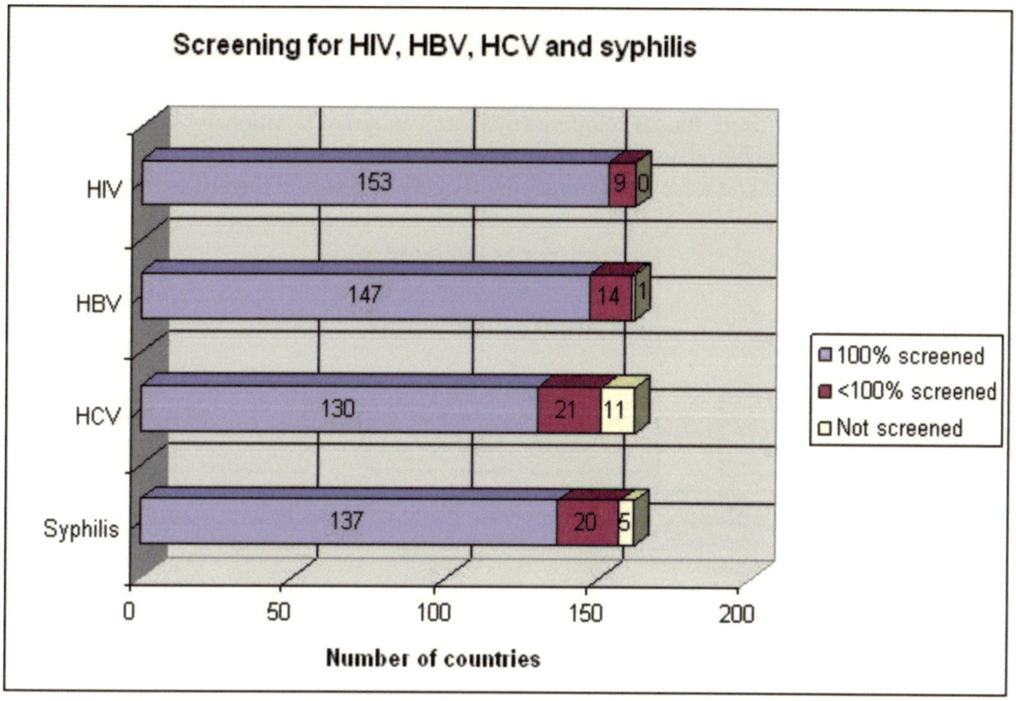

Fig. 3. Numbers of countries screening for HIV, HBV, HCV and syphilis Source: Global Database on Blood Safety (GDBS), 2007 survey (WHO 2010a)

1.2 Basics of the blood supply

Since UN together with its health organization WHO became operational in 1948, universal principles have been laid down in the UN Declaration of Universal Human Rights (UN 1948). For the health care and blood transfusion chain art. 25.1 - Right of Health through securing food, clothing, shelter and health care, and art. 26 - Right of Education, elementary and access to vocational education, are paramount.

In1975 the WHA passed a Resolution 28.72 (Utilization and Supply of Human Blood and Blood Products), indicating that blood is a national resource, to be 'shared' voluntarily and altruistically and to be given as a social act of solidarity, and that human blood and tissue should never be subject to commerce (WHO 1978)

These principles have been worked out by e.g. the International Society of Blood Transfusion (ISBT) in the Code of Ethics (ISBT 2000), but also by the EU in the Directives related to blood transfusion (EU 2003, Directive 2002/98/EC).

Blood transfusion in its vein-to-vein structure should be seen as a part of a larger project to develop a safe, sustainable, high quality and efficacious blood supply and transfusion system that is fully integrated into the health care system. Ensuring the safety and availability of blood and blood products is an essential public health responsibility. Measures to ensure blood safety also play a major role in preventing the transmission of HIV, hepatitis viruses and other blood born pathogens in health care settings. The Ministry

of Health (MoH) should provide effective leadership and governance in developing a national blood system that is fully integrated into the health care system. First the foundation, then the construction of the organization and the necessary infrastructure (Quality System and Quality Management System, facilities, etc), will need to be developed. These will be followed by the development of the human capacity needed at all levels, including in the hospitals (medical and paramedical staff).
In principle, the approach for developing such an integrated nationally supported and organized country wide blood supply and transfusion system for the future, and in line with internationally accepted and advocated principles of operation, would then be as follows (fig. 4)

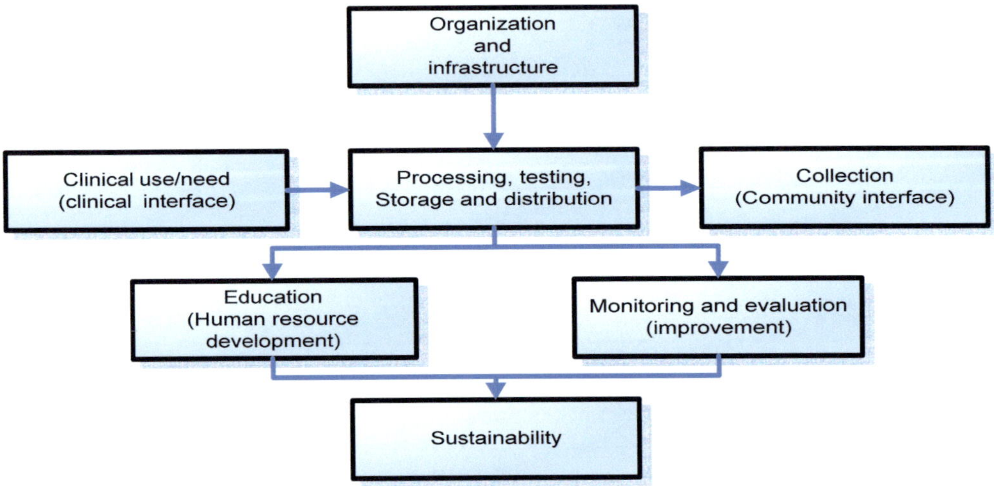

Fig. 4. Development scheme blood supply organization.

The set up should be based on a solid country specific legislative and regulatory system with sufficient authority to license operations according to international quality principles (cGMP, cGLP and cGCP)[1] supported by appropriate and standardized management principles based on ISO9001:2008. It starts with a clinical needs assessment to be followed by the logistics of the procurement and supply chain that has its roots in the community (public awareness) (Smit Sibinga 2006, WHO 2008c, Smit Sibinga et al 2009a,).
The implementation is not limited to public or private blood centres or establishments. The limitation is in the fragmentation with insufficient critical mass and economy of scale to guarantee quality and cost-effectiveness, nation wide access and affordability. National coordination and consistent and sustained governmental responsibility and support to protect citizens from unjustified and maleficent practices are the more important (Smit Sibinga 2000).
A nationally coordinated and integrated blood supply system needs competent and committed leadership and an appropriate budget to allow accessibility and affordability of haemotherapy, based on a proper and documented needs assessment. The financing system should be an integral part of a national health financing system based on cost recovery and a healthy insurance policy accessible and affordable for all citizens (WHO 2008, van Hulst et al. 2006).

[1] GMP = Good Manufacturing Practice, GLP = Good Laboratory Practice, GCP = Good Clinical Practice

The framework of such an integrated blood supply system could be based on the seven key elements (figure 4) as follows:

1. Organization and structure, including the necessary infrastructure to be strengthened and further developed. This element includes the development of an appropriate and implementable formal regulatory structure, development of a system of regional blood banks based on a sufficient economy of scale to become cost-effective. These institutions preferably should be part of a nationally coordinated blood transfusion service responsible for policy making, design of the necessary strategies, annual planning, the development of a national quality and quality management system based on internationally accepted standards and product specifications. Such quality and quality management system will have a uniform documentation system, which allows for the possibility of instituting a nation-wide ICT system for data management. The organization should have sufficient autonomy to operate its services. As the organization produces products (collection, processing and testing, storage and distribution) for clinical use, it is automatically product liable and should therefore operate independently from hospitals. Hospitals use the products for specific haemotherapy in patients and therefore have the legal obligation to protect consumer rights, which cannot be combined with product liability under the same final responsibility (conflict of interest). Another aspect of this first element is the need to develop appropriate and cGMP compliant working facilities, that guarantee a working environment that allows high quality operations to be performed by staff.
2. Clinical use needs full attention to develop evidence based transfusion practices all over the country. That means assessment of the current clinical practices and development of an in-hospital transfusion quality and quality management system. Hospitals will be supplied by regional procurement centers (blood centres) with a working stock that will be based on an inventory of actual needs per discipline - paediatrics, obstetrics, surgery and traumatology and haemato-oncology. The development of a well functioning clinical interface will lead to the change from the currently prevalent supply driven system to a demand driven system, based on mutual respect and understanding and key to the supplier-customer principle of quality operations (Kajja 2010).
3. Processing and testing of all units of blood collected will allow an efficient use of the blood collected and contribute to rational use of blood through component therapy. Testing for the key TTI markers (HIV, HBV, HCV and Syphilis) needs to be instituted with appropriate and standardized technology and methodology. Here, economies of scale are paramount to guarantee consistency of performance and cost containment. Where epidemiology indicates, additional tests can be considered such as brucellosis, Chagas or malaria. As screening tests focus on sensitivity, a system for confirmation needs to be developed at the national level - a reference laboratory that also could perform test kit and reagent validation before implementation is needed. Along with the development of component production, in-process quality control of the produced half and finished products (testing for standardized and uniform product specifications) will be part of the program.
4. Collection of source material - human blood or plasma - from voluntary non-remunerated and preferably regular blood donors, motivated and mobilized from identified low-risk groups in the community. This requires development of public awareness based on social marketing. The currently prevalent supply driven system of

the blood supply needs to be developed into a demand driven system, which means the availability of motivated potential donors willing to be mobilized to allow a balanced blood stock that is managed and the development of a contingency plan. Donor selection needs to be standardized and adjusted to internationally recommended minimum requirements for donor suitability.

5. Education (teaching and training) is the cornerstone of capacity building. A national assessment and inventory of available education (institutions, curricula) needs to be carried out to allow the development of an effective approach towards capacity building and human resource development at all levels involved. The in-country approach will focus on leadership development (senior and middle management) and development of operational competencies (professional knowledge and skills) through various education methodologies to allow larger groups of staff to benefit.
6. Monitoring and evaluation follows the implementation of a national quality and quality management system based on uniform documentation of what is being done, both at the management level (management information system) as well as at the operational level through an automated data processing system (ICT) with communication between all centres and the national Head Quarter and Ministry of Health. Use of simple statistical evaluation technology such as statistical process control (SPC) and application of Six Sigma (Gygi et al., 2005) will allow proper benchmarking focused on improvement through trend analysis. A nationwide compatible ICT system would allow proper quality management through coordinated monitoring and evaluation of uniform data collected through regional centres and hospitals (vein-to-vein).
7. Sustainability is not only dependent on financial resources, but comprehensively relates to all six elements as described above - organizational structure and infrastructure, competent and adequate human resources, a reliable and regular voluntary blood donor panel, a standardized procurement process, evidence based rational use of blood components and alternatives, and quality assurance through proper monitoring of set indicators and their evaluation through benchmarking focused on improvement. This follows the principle of the Deming cycle of improvement - **plan** (policy and strategies), **do** (implementation of managerial and operational processes), **check** (monitoring of the indicators/specifications and accurate data collection through documentation), **act** (evaluation of the collected data and the benchmarking).

1.3 Basics of the clinical use of blood

The clinical use of blood represents both the starting and the closing end of the demand and supply loop. Therefore, it does not make much sense to develop only the clinical interface if the basics of proper procurement (collection, processing and testing, storage and distribution), based on international principles (1948 UN Declaration of Universal Human Rights, 1975 WHA28/72 Utilization and Supply of Human Blood and Blood Products, International Red Cross and ISBT Code of Ethics) are not in place.

The in-hospital transfusion chain should include process analysis, process descriptions, related SOPs and operational documents such as a standard (national) blood request form, a standard compatibility test form, a transfusion outcome form, clinical guidelines and a haemovigilance report form (Kajja 2010).

The in-hospital transfusion chain consists of three distinctive processes, each containing a number of procedures, critical control points (CCPs/decisions) and documentation. (figure 5)

Each of these processes has a series of procedures and related documentation that needs to be developed:

1. The *blood ordering process* (ward/bedside) starts at the bedside with indication setting and decision making resulting in a standardized request and accompanying blood sample for compatibility testing. Traceability (documentation) is paramount to prevent adverse transfusion reactions due to clerical errors of identification (wrong blood in tube). It consists of six steps or procedures (diagnosis, indication, decision to transfuse or use alternatives, ordering, sample taking and transportation) and two operational documents (blood request form and sample label);
2. The *blood selection process* (laboratory) of blood components as requested and compatibility testing. It should be noted that compatibility testing is a laboratory diagnostic procedure. The blood selection process consists of four steps or procedures (reception and registration of request and sample, selection of blood, compatibility testing and transportation) and two operational documents (logbook and cross match form);
3. The *bedside transfusion process* (ward/bedside) of the selected units at the bedside, which needs careful identification of units and recipient (match), and the technical handling and observation of the transfusion, carried out by nursing staff and based on proper and uniform standard operating procedures with appropriate documentation to allow evaluation necessary to develop evidence based practice. It consists of two sub-processes:
   a. The preparation of the patient and the unit of blood before the transfusion - three steps or procedures (reception at the ward, patient and unit identification, vital signs);
   b. Transfusion and observation of the patient - four steps or procedures (connection to the patient, immediate observation, transfusion or discontinuation, observation of outcome).

These processes are closely interrelated, though distinctly different. The following steps are involved in the process:

1. Ward - Ordering (indication/decision/alternatives)

↓

2. Laboratory - Selection/compatibility

↓

3. Ward - a. Preparation: ID & vital signs

↓

b. Transfusion/observation

Fig. 5. In-hospital transfusion flow of steps.

Clinicians and nursing staff need to be trained in these steps and the related quality assurance and documentation to develop a proper and standardized monitoring and evaluation evidence based transfusion practice. To create ownership among the prescribing clinicians and nursing staff education should focus on consensus on items such as a uniform blood request form, terms of reference of a Hospital Transfusion Committee (HTC) and the outline of clinical guidelines (general and per prescribing discipline).

1.4 Gaps in the blood supply and clinical use

In many developing countries blood transfusion in the vein-to-vein concept is still in its first or second generation stage. This means that blood is most often collected and transfused in the absence of a formal policy environment and without adequate regulatory controls or standards. In such systems, blood collection and utilization are fragmented, often dependent on independent factors limited to specific hospitals, such as the availability of trained and competent staff, funds for procurement, and a population of blood donors willing to come on a voluntary and regular basis.

Following the vein-to-vein transfusion chain, major gaps exist in the following areas:

1. Organization and infrastructure -
   a. Legal and regulatory frameworks are often outdated or do not exist.
   b. Commitment of health authorities is lacking or isolated in fragmented centres.
   c. Management capacity to sustain blood collection, storage, testing and transfusion services differs from routine hospital or laboratory management.
   d. Organization and infrastructure for blood services requires national and facility-specific assessments and inputs.
   e. Chain of command and clear job descriptions contribute to quality control, stock management, and career development.
   f. Quality culture and professional discipline are dependent on successful pre-service and on-going in-service training opportunities.
   g. Poor hygiene and waste management may contribute to broader infection control problems within a facility and the local community.
2. Clinical use –
   a. Clinical awareness and accountability among clinicians is essential to avoid unnecessary transfusions and preserve limited blood stocks.
   b. Improper indication setting and decision making may increase transfusion recipients' risk.
   c. Informed consent of patients can create additional ethical and legal challenges for a facility when not obtained properly (Kajja et al. 2011)
   d. Poor documentation and traceability contribute to wastage; may facilitate fraud, and; create barriers to appropriate epidemiological follow-up and tracing in the event of an adverse transfusion event.
   e. Communication and understanding between suppliers and users is essential to ensure that suppliers (i.e., blood donors) contribute based on a humanitarian impulse, not one based on personal gain, and that users (patients and clinicians) recognize and consent to the risks related to transfusion.
3. Processing and testing –
   a. Standards of processing and quality control are a crucial line of defense in patient safety and preventing unnecessary wastage.
   b. Inconsistent supply logistics can interrupt quality-associated work routines, contribute to unnecessary wastage (out-dating and cold chain spoilage) and promote unequal service between regions or facilities (Kajja et al. 2010a, 2010b)

4. Collection of source material (community interface) –
   a. Community awareness about the need for blood and the risks of disease transmission via transfusion are essential to mobilize a safe donor pool.
   b. Types of blood donors must be actively motivated, selected and screened for safety.
5. Education –
   a. Education and staff competency: The basis for a quality assured and sustained system. (Smit Sibinga, 2009a)
6. Monitoring and evaluation –
   a. Applied research in the field of transfusion medicine through proper monitoring and evaluation (M&E) and continued statistical process control (SPC) can contribute to improved operations as well as global understanding of risks, barriers and best practices (Smit Sibinga, 2009b).

2. Principles and ethical aspects of blood donation and transfusion - How do these elements promote blood safety?

Like other medical specializations, the practice of transfusion medicine is bound by the ancient Greek Hippocratic mandate *Primum est non nocere* (first, do no harm). However, for transfusion specialists, this principle is not limited to the transfusion itself or to the recipient of the transfusion. Rather, it applies to a long chain of ethical decisions that stretches from the motivation of potential donors whose blood is used for transfusions to post-transfusion follow-up. This section will describe and explain how each link in this chain contributes to a safe blood supply and to safe transfusion practice.

2.1 Ethical aspects of blood donation

A brief history of blood donation and transfusion ethics

The ethical principles that govern the modern vein-to-vein transfusion system were developed relatively recently, that is to say, largely within the second half of the 20th century, when the science of transfusion medicine became an accepted and routine part of medical practice. (American College of Physicians [ACP], 1984) Indeed, from the 17th century, when physicians began experimenting with transfusing animal blood into humans, through the late 19th and early 20th century when blood groups were discovered and coagulation factors described, the field of transfusion medicine was marked by experimentation, trial and error, and few human subjects protections. (Feldschuh, 1990; McCullough, 1998; Kendrick, n.d.) The 1948 Nuremburg Code established a global framework for medical ethics following the atrocities committed by Nazi doctors during the Second World War. In Europe and North America, laws covering ethical concepts such as the requirement that patients give informed consent prior to medical procedures began to emerge in the 1950s and 1960s. (ACP, 1984) In the mid-1930s, the founding of the International Society of Blood Transfusion (ISBT), created a global forum for the development of specific ethical guidelines for the practice of blood transfusion. Two decades later, in 1955, the International Federation of Blood Donor Organizations (FIODS) was established to focus attention on ethical guidelines for the donation of blood and plasma. Both entities, as well as authors such as Richard Titmuss (The Gift Relationship: From Human Blood to Social Policy, 1971) (Titmuss, 1971), contributed to a body of ethical work that lead to the 1975 World Health Assembly resolution containing global recommendations for ethical blood donations and transfusions (WHA 28.72). Those recommendations included the following key elements of transfusion ethics:

1. Blood donations should be voluntary and unpaid.
2. Countries should collect an adequate supply of blood to be self-sufficient.
3. Countries should develop legislation and supporting regulations to monitor and control the quality of blood collections, blood service laboratory operations (infectious disease screening, compatibility testing, production of blood products), and transfusion practice.

These recommendations seem especially prescient following the emergence of the HIV/AIDS epidemic in the 1980s, and the identification of blood transfusion as a significant route of HIV infection (US CDC, 1982). Between 1980 and 2000, the ISBT and WHO refined and adapted these original principles into a global code of ethics whose purpose was "*to define the ethical principles and rules to be observed in the field of Transfusion Medicine.*" The ISBT code of ethics is discussed in detail below. Most countries worldwide have blood policies based on these fundamental principles (WHO, 2011a). Since 2000, these principles have guided numerous global resolutions related to HIV prevention and the emerging donor-supported field of 'blood safety'. (PEPFAR, 2005-2010; WHO, 2011b)

'*Safe blood starts with me*'. This commonly used blood donor motivation slogan captures one of the principal ethical issues in blood donation, namely that donors share an equal burden of responsibility with blood services to ensure the safety of the blood supply (Grainger et al., 1997). As the sole source of blood for transfusion, donors are indispensible. Yet, donors also have rights that must be respected and are, more critically, the principal vector for transfusion-transmissible infections. Ensuring the safety of donated blood, therefore, requires a balanced, combination approach, including active, education-based and non-coercive social mobilization practices by transfusion services and donation centres, and the *active and honest* participation of donors in the pre-donation screening process.

The ISBT Code of Ethics (2000, 2006 revision) contains 11 principles that expand on these concepts, especially as they relate to donor health and safety, donors' right to anonymity or confidentiality during and after donation, and donors' *ethical responsibility* not to donate if they believe their blood may be infected with HIV or another blood-borne pathogen.

The ISBT code can be collapsed into a chain with four basic links. This pre-donation chain describes the individual links that protect donors and the recipients of donated blood. As noted above, each of these links contributes to blood safety in a different way.

Link 1: Mobilizing blood donors without coercion

Identifying, mobilizing, educating, motivating and retaining an adequate pool of eligible and willing blood donors is the primary challenge faced by blood transfusion services worldwide. The problem is especially serious in the developing world, where public awareness of blood transfusion is low (Elhence, 2006), traditional or cultural beliefs about blood may serve as powerful disincentives to blood donation (Umeora et al., 2005), and high population prevalence rates for HIV and other TTIs may be a barrier to blood donor appeals to the general public (McFarland et al., 1998). In countries with serious blood shortages, the impulse to pay or coerce blood donors can be powerful (Parry, 1984). But since the 1980s, prompted largely by concerns about transfusion-transmitted hepatitis and HIV, blood services in the developed world have largely adopted policies promoting voluntary and anonymous blood donation and prohibiting or limiting the payment of donors (ISBT,

2006b).[2] In the developing world, national blood policies developed since 2000 increasingly reflect World Health Organization recommendations that call for blood donors to act on an altruistic impulse, not in exchange for money or other kinds of compensation, and for blood services to mobilize *voluntary, non-remunerated* donors. The WHO Aide-Mémoire on establishing national blood transfusion services considers this practice '*the foundation of a safe and adequate blood supply.*' (WHO, 2011c)

The ISBT Code of Ethics (2006 revision)

Blood Centers: Donors and Donation

(International Society for Blood Transfusion [ISBT], 2006a)

1. Blood donation including haematopoietic tissues for transplantation shall, in all circumstances, be voluntary and non-remunerated; no coercion should be brought to bear upon the donor. A donation is considered voluntary and non-remunerated if the person gives blood, plasma or cellular components of his/her own free will and receives no payment for it, either in the form of cash, or in kind which could be considered a substitute for money. This would include time off work other than that reasonable needed for the donation and travel. Small tokens, refreshments and reimbursements of direct travel costs are compatible with voluntary, non-remunerated donation. The donor should provide informed consent to the donation of blood or blood components and to the subsequent (legitimate) use of the blood by the transfusion service.
2. A profit motive should not be the basis for the establishment and running of a blood service.
3. The donor should be advised of the risks connected with the procedure; the donor's health and safety must be protected. Any procedures relating to the administration to a donor of any substance for increasing the concentration of specific blood components should be in compliance with internationally accepted standards.
4. Anonymity between donor and recipient must be ensured except in special situations and the confidentiality of donor information assured.
5. The donor should understand the risks to others of donating infected blood and his or her ethical responsibility to the recipient.

---

[2] Exceptions exist to this general trend, most notably in paid plasma donations in the United States. Other developed countries provide financial or material compensation to donors, or have laws granting blood donors time off from work in exchange for donations. (European Commission, 2003, as cited in Farrugia et al., 2010; U.S. Food and Drug Administration, 2002) While the push for 100% voluntary, non-remunerated blood donations in developing countries has been shown to effectively screen out donors at high risk of infection with HIV or other transfusion-transmissible infections (Sarkodie et al., 2001), an emerging body of evidence suggests that some donors who act for reasons other than personal altruism - for instance, family members or others who donate in emergencies or to replace blood units - may present no greater risk to the blood supply than first-time volunteer donors (Allain et al., 2009; Diarra et al., 2009). Indeed, WHO and others stress the importance of motivating and retaining repeat donors '*who give blood regularly*', as the best way to screen out potential donors with a high behavioural risk profile. Yet, despite regular reinforcement of this global guidance, many services continue to provide or experiment with some forms of remuneration for blood donors, e.g., cholesterol screening (Glynn et al., 2003), distribution of lottery ticket (Stutzer & Goette, 2010), or transportation to and from the donation clinic (ISBT, 2006). These divergent findings pose a substantial ethical challenge for blood service managers faced with a limited pool of willing blood donors and unmet demand for blood.

6. Blood donation must be based on regularly reviewed medical selection criteria and not entail discrimination of any kind, including gender, race, nationality or religion. Neither donor nor potential recipient has the right to require that any such discrimination be practiced.
7. Blood must be collected under the overall responsibility of a suitably qualified, registered medical practitioner.
8. All matters related to whole blood donation and haemapheresis should be in compliance with appropriately defined and internationally accepted standards.
9. Donors and recipients should be informed if they have been harmed.
10. Blood is a public resource and access should not be restricted.
11. Wastage should be avoided in order to safeguard the interests of all potential recipients and the donor.

Link 2: Education is key

Worldwide, the public must be educated to understand that blood donation supports the collective good - that a unit donated today could save the life of a neighbour, a friend, a loved one, a stranger, or even the donor himself, tomorrow (*'today me, tomorrow you'*). But donors must also be educated about the risks associated with donation, both for the donor and for the recipient of donated blood. Education materials and programs should emphasize two main areas of risk and consent.

Risks to the donor and consent required prior to donation:

- The potential for syncope (fainting), hyperventilation, bruising or damage to veins during the veinipuncture process.
- Since most countries test or strive to test 100% of donated blood for pathogens such as HIV, hepatitis B and C, and syphilis, donors must be informed of these tests and given an opportunity to receive their results with appropriate counselling. In South Africa, the South African National Blood Service (SANBS) includes a clear statement about testing and the potential emotional impact on donors: *'Every blood donation is tested for HIV/AIDS. Persons testing positive must be aware that this may have a psychological impact and profoundly influence their lifestyle.'* (South African National Blood Service [SANBS], 2006)

Risks to recipients of donated blood:

- Transmission of infectious pathogens, including HIV.
- Other adverse transfusion events, e.g. circulatory overload, TRALI, mis-matched blood group, allogenic reactions.

Social mobilization and donor education campaigns will differ depending on the target audience. In many developing countries, youth, especially high-school students, contribute a substantial proportion of the national blood supply (Jacobs et al., 1994). However, it should be noted that donation camps at schools usually are based on coercion through the school authorities. (Los et al., 2009) In addition to confirming the voluntary nature of school-based donations, blood services must also study the epidemiology of HIV and other transfusion-transmissible infections among school-aged donors to ensure that this group actually carries a lower risk of infection compared to the general population. Over the last 10 years, several successful models to promote blood donation among youth have been established worldwide. These include the Club 25 model created by the International Federation of Red Cross and Red Crescent Societies (See: http://www.ifrc.org/en/what-we-do/health/blood-services/international-club-25-new-blood-for-the-world/) and the annual WHO-sponsored World Blood Donor Day on June 14, the birthday of Karl Landsteiner.

Link 3: Pre-donation counselling and behavioural risk screening

Pre-donation screening occurs after a donor has decided to make a donation, but before the blood is collected. The use of behavioural screening - also often referred to as self-exclusion screening - allows donors a confidential space in which to reflect on their behavioural risk profile and to weigh the consequences of a contaminated donation, especially donations that carry a high risk of infection with HIV. Behavioural questionnaires provide the blood service with information about lifestyle practices that could increase the donor's risk of carrying a TTI, and work-related information (e.g. do you operate heavy equipment?) that could create a safety hazard for the donor immediately after a donation. Questionnaires also provide information on medicines the donor is taking or other health conditions that could cause adverse reactions in the transfusion recipient or an adverse reaction for the donor (e.g. dizziness or fainting).

In most countries, pre-donation screening includes a written questionnaire and a face-to-face interview with a trained nurse or a donor counsellor. Questionnaires should ask donors simple, yet direct, questions about their general health and lifestyle, especially risky sexual practices. The following questions, drawn from the South African National Blood Service (SANBS) pre-donation questionnaire, are representative of the kinds of behavioural questions donors should be asked in confidence prior to a donation:

- Have you ever been refused as a blood donor, or told not to donate?
- In the past six months have you had sexual activity with or without a condom: With more than one sex partner? With a regular sex partner excluding your spouse? With someone whose sexual background you do not know?
- In the past six months have you: Had sexual activity with a prostitute or anyone else who takes money or drugs or other favours for sex? Received money, drugs or other payment for sex? Been a victim of a sexual assault?
- Male donors: In the past 6 months have you had oral or anal sex with another man with or without a condom?
- In the past 12 months: Have you had a sexually transmitted disease (STD) e.g. syphilis, gonorrhoea, genital ulcers, VD or 'drop'?
- Have you ever used needles to take drugs, steroids, or anything not prescribed by your doctor or a nurse?
- Do you think your blood is safe for transfusion to a patient?
- To your knowledge does your sex partner have other sex partners?

While the safety rationale justifies this kind of intrusive personal questioning, some automatic exclusion criteria, notably YES answers to questions about homosexual sex, have sparked ethical debates about the fairness of excluding donors on the basis of sexual orientation (Martucci, 2010).

Link 4: Laboratory screening

The WHO Aide Mémoire for National Blood Programmes encourages '*testing of all donated blood, including screening for transfusion-transmissible infections, blood grouping and compatibility testing.*' However, this WHO recommendation must not be viewed in isolation. Indeed, the Aide Mémoire and other WHO guidance stresses that laboratory screening must be part of an 'integrated strategy' that includes the mobilization of low behavioural risk voluntary, non-remunerated donors, a quality assurance system within the laboratory, and the reduction of unnecessary transfusions (WHO, 2011a). Research from high HIV prevalence countries in

Africa has shown this integrated approach can have a positive impact on reducing the number of donations with incident or 'window period' HIV infections that the antigen/antibody assays used in most developing countries might not detect (Basavaraju, 2010).

The 2010 WHO Guidelines on Screening Donated Blood for Transfusion-Transmissible Infections recognize that operational limitations (*'lack of coordination ... inadequate infrastructure ... shortages of trained staff ... poor quality systems'*) may prohibit some blood services from screening all donated units, or create barriers to the implementation of a coordinated, integrated laboratory screening program. The guidelines identify the following negative outcomes that may occur when laboratory screening systems do not exist or fail:

- Inefficient screening systems and wastage of resources owing to differing levels of operation at multiple sites
- Lack of quality assurance and quality management systems
- Use of poor quality test kits and reagents
- Unreliable, inconsistent supplies and transport conditions of test kits and reagents due to poor logistics
- Equipment failure
- Variations in laboratory procedures and practices
- Double standards due to a mix of technologies and methodologies
- Incorrect storage or inappropriate use of test kits and reagents
- Inadequate procedures for identification, leading to the misidentification of patient or donor blood samples, donations or processed units of blood and blood components
- Technical failure in testing
- Misinterpretation of test results
- Inaccuracies in the recording or transcription of test results.
- Higher error rates in test results
- Increased risk of failure to detect TTIs
- Unnecessary hold time due to poor access to confirmatory tests
- Unnecessary discard of non-reactive blood
- Blood shortages and use of unscreened blood in urgent situations
- Incorrect donor notification and stigmatization. (WHO, 2009)

2.2 Ethical aspects of blood transfusion

As noted in section 1.2, Article 25 of the 1948 UN Declaration of Universal Human Rights (DUHR) makes reference to individuals' '*right to security in the event of ... sickness, disability ... or other lack of livelihood in circumstances beyond his control.*' The principle of obtaining patient consent prior to performing a blood transfusion or other medical procedure is derived from the broad concepts of *health* and *security ... in the event of sickness* described in the DUHR. Subsequent codes of medical ethics, including the Council of Europe's 2007 revision of its Guide to the Preparation, Use and Quality Assurance of Blood Components; these codes expanded on this basic definition of 'security' to cover all of the decisions preceding, during, and following a transfusion: From confirming the appropriate diagnosis and prescription order, to correct patient identification and adverse event monitoring during the transfusion itself. (Council of Europe, 2007) Occasionally, prescribers of blood will encounter patients who refuse a recommended transfusion on religious grounds. Clinicians may also face difficult decisions with patients who are minors and patients for whom a transfusion may extend life but not necessarily improve the quality of the patient's life; the creation of institutional ethics committees within hospitals and transfusion centres is recommended to educate staff about ethical issues; support ethical decision-making; develop ethics codes and policies, and; counsel staff and conduct ethical reviews (Perlin, 2001; Kajja et al. 2011).

Ethical considerations continue even after a successful transfusion, most notably in cases where recipients become infected with a transfusion-transmissible infection, or are deemed at risk of infection because new information about the donor of the transfused unit comes to light (e.g. HIV sero-conversion in the donor).

The ISBT code of ethics for hospitals and patients contains seven key principles related to the transfusion of blood and blood products.

ISBT Code of Ethics for Hospitals and Patients

(International Society for Blood Transfusion [ISBT], 2006a)

1. Patients should be informed of the known risks and benefits of blood transfusion and/or alternative therapies and have the right to accept or refuse the procedure. Any valid advance directive should be respected.
2. In the event that the patient is unable to give prior informed consent, the basis for treatment by transfusion must be in the best interests of the patient.
3. Transfusion therapy must be given under the overall responsibility of a registered medical practitioner.
4. Genuine clinical need should be the only basis for transfusion therapy.
5. There should be no financial incentive to prescribe a blood transfusion.
6. As far as possible the patient should receive only those particular components (cells, plasma, or plasma derivatives) that are clinically appropriate and afford optimal safety.
7. Blood transfusion practices established by national or international health bodies and other agencies competent and authorised to do so should be in compliance with this code of ethics.

It should be noted that these seven principles are predicated on an assumption that the ethical principles related to blood donors and the screening of blood for transfusion-transmissible infections have been respected. As with the ethical framework for blood donations, these principles can contribute to reduced risks of transfusion-transmissible infections by reducing or minimizing the number of inappropriate transfusions.

3. Assessment techniques and methodologies: Identifying and addressing gaps and needs in blood safety programs and blood transfusion services

Understanding the roles and responsibilities associated with the various departments and job descriptions within a blood transfusion service is a complex task, involving layers of policy, science, human behaviour, risk, ethics, finances, and, ultimately, medical practice. Further identifying gaps, risks and needs within each (or all) of these layers, is an additional step that blood transfusion services must take in order to address weaknesses, strengthen services, recruit and/or retain staff, improve quality and evaluate the impact of services and products provided to transfusion centres or hospitals and patients. The ultimate goal of these objectives is to improve the safety of blood and blood products used for transfusion. The U.S. Food and Drug Administration cites the '*safety, purity, and potency*' of blood products as the main rationale for conducting blood service quality audits and assessments (Food and Drug Administration, 2010).

To accomplish assessment and evaluation objectives, blood services may use a number of assessment and evaluation tools, many of which are drawn from business practices (e.g. Six Sigma, Total Quality Management, SWOT analyses) or the field of risk analysis. International organizations (WHO, ISBT, the IFRCRCS), national blood transfusion services, regulatory agencies, and Red Cross/Red Crescent Societies, as well as multilateral and bilateral donors (e.g. the European Union, the U.S. President's Emergency Plan for AIDS Relief, the Japan International Cooperation Agency) have also developed assessment tools and indicators to assist with the development, implementation and monitoring of blood safety projects and programs.

The field of evaluation has evolved and expanded substantially in the last 20 years. A recent PubMed literature search found nearly 250,000 papers dedicated to public health evaluations or assessments within the last decade. Beyond the scientific literature, thousands of programme reports, guides and other documents in the 'gray literature' are published each year. This massive diversity of material includes many different methodologies, some of which have been used by blood transfusion services to monitor, evaluate, assess or audit (Chevrolle et al., 2000) human resource needs (Ferrera et al., 2001), blood banking, stock management, laboratory and transfusion practices (Fretz, 2003; Dosunmu & Dada, 2005), training curricula (Wehrli, 2011), epidemiological surveillance (Roussel et al; Linden & Bianco, 2001), and quality systems (Berte, 1997; Mintz, 1995; Smit Sibinga, 2001).

This chapter will review the basic elements these tools are designed off to assess, monitor and evaluate. Examples derived from specific tools and indicators, such as the WHO Global Database on Blood Safety, will be presented to highlight the utility of assessment and evaluation in the development of strong blood transfusion services, especially in areas with high burdens of HIV and other transfusion-transmissible infections.

As mentioned above in section 1.2, blood services worldwide are built around a framework with seven basic components, each of which can be evaluated through techniques such as SWOT analyses (Strengths-Weaknesses-Opportunities-Threats), and addressed with the principles of the Deming cycle of improvement (Plan-Do-Check-Act):

1. Structure and organization
2. Clinical use of blood
3. Processing and testing
4. Blood collections
5. Education and Training
6. Monitoring and Evaluation
7. Sustainability

Within each of these elements, WHO and other blood safety technical assistance programs have developed assessment indicators to help blood services identify needs, gaps and risks.

3.1 The WHO global database on blood safety

A good place to begin to make sense of the diversity of available materials is the WHO Global Database on Blood Safety (GDBS). The GDBS was developed by WHO with expert input through the Global Collaboration on Blood Safety (GCBS) and launched in 1998. WHO member countries are asked to submit data to the GDBS every two years. The indicators collected by the GDBS are periodically revised and increasingly reflect collaborative work between WHO and development partners supporting blood safety programmes in countries.

The GDBS questionnaire contains 253 process, outcome and output indicators clustered around eight operational and technical areas (WHO, 2011d) :

1. Administrative Information
2. Organization and Management
3. Blood Donors and Blood Collection
4. Screening for Transfusion-Transmissible Infections
5. Blood Group Serology Testing of Blood Donations
6. Blood Component Preparation, Storage and Transportation
7. Hospital Transfusion Process and Clinical Use of Blood & Blood Components
8. Fractionated Plasma Products

Since its launch, WHO has received and compiled three reports (1998-1999; 2001-2002; 2004-2005); data collection for a fourth report was begun in 2008.

3.1.1 Mind the gaps – Recent GDBS findings

The identification of blood transfusion as a significant vector for HIV transmission in Africa in the 1990s (Colbunders, 1991) led to increasing attention and financing for blood safety programmes via global health programmes focused on HIV prevention.[3] As noted above, the epidemiology of transfusion-transmitted HIV also drove the passage of World Health Assembly (WHA) resolutions on the blood safety, and the development, over the last decade, of WHO's catalogue of blood safety guidelines and recommendations. In many countries this increased attention to blood safety as part of a comprehensive HIV prevention strategy has strengthened the whole national blood service - from vein-to-vein - in addition to reducing the transmission of HIV through transfusion. Still, despite progress, transfusion systems remain weak in many countries, especially those in the lower income strata. The most recent GDBS report (2004-2005) highlighted a number of these weaknesses, including:

- Less than 50% of countries report collecting blood exclusively from voluntary, non-remunerated blood donors.
- 40% of the 172 countries surveyed, reported having national haemovigilance systems.
- 53% reported having national regulatory bodies for blood transfusion.
- 80% of the world's population live in countries that collect only 45% of the global blood supply.

3.1.2 Addressing gaps – Achieving change

Experience and evidence from the field over the last decade has shown that blood services in countries with high prevalence HIV have been able to systematically reduce the prevalence of HIV in donated blood units by identifying and addressing gaps and weaknesses in their operations and structures. In 2008, the U.S. Centers for Disease Control and Prevention (CDC) presented data from the PEPFAR blood safety program that showed substantial gaps in the legislative and policy frameworks in 14 countries in sub-Saharan Africa and the Caribbean (US CDC, 2008).

Using indicators adapted from the WHO GDBS, CDC asked countries if a national blood policy was in place or if the national blood transfusion service (NBTS) was supported by a 'legislative framework' (e.g. laws and regulations). In 2003, only six of the 14 countries

[3] Half of the 101 countries that responded to a GDBS question about external support for their blood services indicated that they were receiving some kind of international assistance in 2004-2005.

reported having a national blood policy; the same year only four of the 14 countries reported having a 'legislative framework' to support NBTS activities. By 2007, all 14 countries had national blood policies in place or in development, and 10 of 14 countries had established or were developing 'legislative frameworks' based on WHO blood safety guidelines. (Table 1)

	Established national policy		Enacted legislative framework		No. of whole blood units collected					No. of whole blood units collected per 1,000 population[†]				
Country	2003	2007	2003	2007	2003	2004	2005	2006	2007	2003	2004	2005	2006	2007
Botswana	Yes	Yes	No	No	11,583	13,210	20,643	21,061	22,230	6.4	7.3	11.2	11.2	11.6
Côte d'Ivoire	Yes	Yes	Yes	Yes	67,780	77,972	86,321	86,082	92,009	3.8	4.3	4.6	4.5	4.8
Ethiopia[§]	No	Yes	No	No	17,208	17,941	19,203	21,019	22,220	0.2	0.2	0.2	0.3	0.3
Guyana	Yes	Yes	No	In development	4,008	4,896	4,531	5,192	5,475	5.4	6.6	6.1	7.1	7.5
Haiti	No	Yes	No	In development	8,711	9,513	10,823	13,622	17,094	1.0	1.0	1.2	1.4	1.8
Kenya	Yes	Yes	Yes	Yes	40,857	47,661	80,762	113,080	123,787	1.2	1.4	2.3	3.1	3.3
Mozambique	No	In development	No	In development	67,105	69,648	76,667	72,170	79,925	3.4	3.5	3.8	3.5	3.8
Namibia	No	Yes	No	In development	17,860	19,154	19,133	18,422	18,309	9.1	9.6	9.5	9.0	8.9
Nigeria[¶]	No	Yes	No	Yes	—	—	1,266	5,519	16,987	—	—	<0.1	<0.1	0.1
Rwanda	No	Yes	No	No	30,786	28,777	37,893	38,539	32,543	3.5	3.2	4.1	4.1	3.3
South Africa**	Yes	Yes	Yes	Yes	809,322	813,239	805,923	822,950	821,258	17.3	17.2	16.9	17.2	17.0
Tanzania[¶]	No	Yes	No	In development	—	—	12,597	63,411	109,471	—	—	0.3	1.6	2.7
Uganda	Yes	Yes	Yes	Yes	102,703	106,996	115,988	122,442	133,585	3.8	3.8	4.0	4.1	4.3
Zambia	No	In development	No	In development	40,616	38,477	61,982	54,308	68,056	3.7	3.4	5.4	4.6	5.7

* As described in: World Health Organization. Aide-memoire for national blood programmes. Geneva, Switzerland: World Health Organization; 2002. Available at http://www.who.int/bloodsafety/transfusion_services/en/Blood_Safety_Eng.pdf.
† Based on United Nations Population Division census estimates for 2003–2007.
§ Ethiopia Red Cross Society is the designated national blood transfusion service.
¶ Nigeria and Tanzania established their national blood transfusion services in 2004. The first year with 12 complete months of data available was 2005.
** Includes data from South Africa National Blood Service and Western Province Blood Service.

Table 1. Standards of national blood transfusion policies and legislative frameworks, number of whole blood units collected, and number collected per 1,000 population - U.S. President's Emergency Plan for AIDS Relief, 14 countries, 2003-2007

	% of persons with HIV infection*		% of blood collections reactive for HIV					% of blood collections received from voluntary, non-remunerated donors				
Country	2001	2007	2003	2004	2005	2006	2007	2003	2004	2005	2006	2007
Botswana	26.5	23.9	7.5	5.7	4.0	2.7	2.1	100	100	100	100	100
Côte d'Ivoire	6.0	3.9	1.6	1.4	1.5	1.4	1.2	100	100	100	100	100
Ethiopia[†]	2.4	2.1	—	3.6	3.4	2.5	3.0	38.8	27.5	23.2	28.1	28.4
Guyana	2.5	2.5	0.8	0.6	1.0	0.6	0.3	21.7	18.9	26.1	31.2	61.1
Haiti	2.2	2.2	1.7	1.8	1.6	1.9	1.4	5.2	5.4	14.9	27.4	51.9
Kenya	8.1	7.8[§]	1.5	1.7	1.9	2.5	1.2	99.0	95.3	97.6	98.9	99.5
Mozambique	10.3	12.5	8.6	6.9	6.4	8.3	7.2	58.0	58.3	59.6	52.0	72.3
Namibia	14.6	15.3	0.7	0.6	0.6	0.5	0.6	100	100	100	100	100
Nigeria[¶]	3.2	3.1	—	—	3.8	3.5	2.5	—	—	100	100	92.3
Rwanda	4.3	2.8	1.1	0.1	1.2	0.9	0.5	100	100	100	100	100
South Africa**	16.9	18.1	<0.1	<0.1	<0.1	<0.1	0.1	100	100	100	100	100
Tanzania[¶]	7.0	6.2	—	—	4.8	3.2	2.8	—	—	66.5	80.0	89.2
Uganda	7.9	5.4	2.0	1.9	1.6	1.5	1.3	95.5	96.3	99.0	99.9	100
Zambia	15.4	15.2	6.9	6.4	9.0	6.4	3.8	72.7	71.2	90.6	97.9	99.6

* Estimates from the Joint United Nations Programme on HIV/AIDS (UNAIDS), available at http://data.unaids.org/pub/globalreport/2008/jc1510_2008_global_report_pp211_234_en.pdf. Because UNAIDS methodology used to estimate 2003 prevalence was different from the methodology used for 2007, data are presented for 2001, the most recent pre-program year for which the same methodology was used as for 2007.
† Ethiopia Red Cross Society is the designated national blood transfusion service.
§ Preliminary estimate.
¶ Nigeria and Tanzania established their national blood transfusion services in 2004. The first year with 12 complete months of data available was 2005.
** Includes data from South Africa National Blood Service and Western Province Blood Service. Autologous donations and collections from designated donors are reported as donations from voluntary, non-remunerated donors.

Table 2. Estimated percentage of persons aged 15-49 years with human immunodeficiency virus (HIV) infection, percentage of blood collections reactive for HIV, and percentage of collections from voluntary, non-remunerated donors - U.S. President's Emergency Plan for AIDS Relief, 14 countries, 2003-2007

During the same four year period, all 14 countries reported lower or stable rates of HIV prevalence in donated units (Table 2).

Although a strict causal association cannot be derived (Noumsi et al., 2008) from these data, this report suggests a positive relationship between progress toward addressing policy and other operational gaps and improvements in the safety of donated blood for supportive haemotherapy.

4. Evidence based strategies to move from a supply-driven to a demand-driven blood transfusion system

4.1 Community specifics for tailor made solutions

In the majority of economically restricted countries the transfusion chain from vein-to-vein is determined by what happens to be available. The supply drives the system. When a clinical need occurs, either the scarce hospital or blood bank stock is being used and exhausted or family is urged to search for blood donors, whether family related, friends or what the market offers. Often that results in under-treatment of patients, unjustified use or no treatment at all. The data available for mother and infant death due to shortages illustrate this situation (WHO et al. 2010).

Most of these donors are seriously coerced, time pressure stimulates poor handling and the serious and realistic effect of transmission of infections such as HIV, HBV and HCV. Besides, it has been observed and documented that hidden stocks are being kept or just grow due to shortage in organization and poor logistics of the supply (Kajja I et al., 2010a). The chain quite often is interrupted at the clinical interface side, with a serious paucity of communication between producer/supplier and prescriber/consumer of blood and blood components. The root cause of this paucity is in limited and focused knowledge and related practices on either side of the chain. When regular need assessments are being done a better idea would grow about the epidemiology of blood transfusion in the hospitals, which then could lead to balanced and evidence based logistics of supply of human blood in anticipation of the needs.

As a consequence the blood supply and clinical use should be firmly embedded in the health care system with major involvement of the community to allow such anticipatory strategies. Community involvement means community education to understand why a continuous and not an incidental and *ad hoc* support is needed (Los & Smit Sibinga, 2001). It is the principle of '*today me, tomorrow you*' as a social act of solidarity. When the blood supply becomes a community issue, awareness and responsibility to support with healthy blood on a sharing principle, rather than being dragged into blood donation because of urgent needs of family and relatives who might die if you would not donate immediately (Los & Smit Sibinga, 2001). Questionnaires and testing, whether rapid or ELISA then move towards the edge of becoming a farce, seriously jeopardizing the safety of blood transfusion.

To find out what the knowledge, attitudes and practices of a community are in relation to blood donation and transfusion, a KAP (knowledge, attitudes, practices) study could certainly be beneficial. KAP studies can be done broad, focused on the community by and large or target specific groups, such as presumed low risk categories, known or registered blood donors, and non-donors. Each such KAP study will need a careful analysis to unravel the underlying anthropological and psychological information needed to understand how the mind is set of those who participated and how that relates to community feelings and behaviour as a whole. KAP studies should not be incidental, but be part of a mechanism to follow up and study the changes in mind set and behaviour of the community. Only then will it provide a useful tool for benchmarking progress in attitude and related practices (Los & Smit Sibinga, 2009; Los et al. 2009).

4.2 Prerequisites – Leadership, awareness, willingness, environment/climate, access

Unsafe blood transfusions have contributed to the enormous burden of HIV infections in various developing parts of the world, in particular in sub-Saharan Africa and the Central Asian region (World Bank et al., 2008), and still continue to add to this burden. The risk of HIV, HCV and HBV infection through unsafe blood and blood products is exceptionally high (95-100%) compared to other common routes of exposure: For example, 11-32% for mother-to-child transmission of HIV and HBV and 0.1%-10% for sexual contact. Sub-Saharan Africa has a particularly high level of transfusion-associated HIV compared with other developing regions due to a higher risk of infected blood being transfused. This results from a combination of factors: High rates of transfusion in some groups of patients (particularly women during labour, and children in the malaria Season), a higher incidence and prevalence of HIV infection, dependence on unsafe blood donors and inadequate or even absence of testing of blood for HIV in some countries (WHO 2008a, 2010a, 2010b). However, also the poor education level and poverty among larger groups in the community play an important role. Women and children account for a disproportionate number of HIV, HBV and HCV infections through unsafe blood because they are the main groups of patients receiving blood transfusion. In developing countries around 50% of the blood is transfused to women and 25% to children, largely under the age of 5 years. Up to 20% of maternal mortality and 15% of child deaths have been attributed to severe anaemia due to malaria. Timely access to safe blood transfusion is a life-saving measure in many of these clinical conditions and can also prevent serious illness in these patients.

Besides the need for identified, competent and designated leadership (Smit Sibinga 2009a, 2009b), there is the holistic need for awareness - politicians and policy makers, community in all its diversity, health professionals and related stakeholders such as hospital managers, religious leaders and educators. The government is final responsible for the well being of the community and should create the environment and climate for education and professional infrastructure to allow awareness and willingness to grow and sustain. The organization of the health care should guarantee access and affordability to all in need, and the blood supply and clinical prescribers should use and optimize the professional and social climate and environment to allow proper, safe and justified practices of procurement and clinical use of blood and blood components to be developed and implemented.

It has been demonstrated that a well organized and structured nationally supported blood supply and transfusion system yields a better and safer transfusion practice with a minimum residual risk for transmission of blood born infections, in particular HIV/AIDS, as compared to a non-cohesive and fragmented blood supply. Any structure should find its anchor in an appropriate legal framework - documented principles of blood donation and transfusion, adequate regulations and an operational system for audit and inspection of compliance with the principles and related operational standards and technical requirements (Hollan et al., 1990)

4.3 Role of education and vocational institutes

As mentioned in section 2.1 the key factor is competent human capacity at all levels, which means education of the community to create public awareness, the professionals to create professional awareness and politicians to create political awareness. The awareness to be raised relates to the risks for contracting infectious diseases such as HIV/AIDS, hepatitis, malaria and tuberculosis. Additionally these infectious diseases may be spread through a variety of contacts, e.g. the blood supply. Education provides knowledge through information, which is stored in the brains. A major question and related process is how to convert the acquired knowledge into appropriate action. The process depends highly on how the information is presented and how the knowledge is perceived. The perception ultimately triggers the action needed (WI Thomas & Thomas DS, 1928).

Education and vocational institutes do play a paramount role in the presentation of information and the way the acquired knowledge is perceived individually and collectively, leading to individual behaviour and collective or group behaviour - the moral and ethics of a community. To bridge the existing knowledge gap, analysis is needed of both the way, the environment and the contents of the information offered, and the intellectual mechanisms of the perception of the knowledge necessary for the triggering of appropriate action (Los & Smit Sibinga, 2009; Kajja, 2010).

Potential teachers and parents therefore need to be educated on how to pack and present the information and how to monitor and evaluate the perception of the knowledge. This continuum should have a high rank on the priority list of any nation, filling in one of the key universal human rights - the right of education. Competence is the intimate twinning through matching of acquiring knowledge and developing skills to act appropriately, whatever is concerned. When the community or public understands the need for a healthy life style, for sharing regularly a bit of healthy blood with those in need, by donating blood on an altruistic and regular basis, when the professionals in the health care understand the need to appropriately deal with the collection, processing, testing, storage and distribution of human blood as a transplant and at the clinical side with the in-hospital processes of prescription and ordering, selection and compatibility testing, and the ultimate transfusion and its monitoring and evaluation, the gap will be substantially narrowed and shallowed. However, without a proper understanding of the policy makers, the gap will not be bridged completely.

Evidence-based strategies for blood safety and availability have been successfully implemented in most developed countries and some transitional and developing nations. However, despite the proven effectiveness of these strategies, many countries are making slow progress towards their implementation. There is ample evidence that a nationally supported blood supply and clinical use of human blood, well regulated and professionally implemented on an adequate economy of scale, leads to a significant reduction in risk of transmission of infectious diseases.

Such nationally supported approach covers the entire nation and is based on education of all parties involved, understanding the importance and relevance of the necessary and ongoing provision of information and related actions.

Such systems recognize and address the potential weaknesses and gaps as listed above in the 6 major areas of transfusion medicine - 1. Organization and structure; 2. Clinical use (clinical interface); 3. Processing and testing; 4. Collection of source material (community interface); 5. Education; 6. Monitoring and evaluation (research and development).

Such systems are based on the needs of the community to be met by the supply through anticipation, proper planning and adequate logistics (Smit Sibinga, 2000). The demand then will drive the supply and no longer the other way around.

5. Directions for improvement – Values and realities

Over the past few decades, since the outbreak of the HIV/AIDS epidemic, much work has been done to provide a better understanding of the routing of transmission of the virus. There are prominent differences in the various cultures in the perception of the risks related to behaviour, personal and collective. That relates to different standards of moral and ethics, of values of life and realities of human attitudes and behaviour. Education remains a key factor in the provision of knowledge and related perception needed for action to prevent transmission, both vertical and horizontal. Blood transfusion in the vein-to-vein concept lacks behind in its development despite the continuum of initiatives developed by organizations such as the World Health Organization (WHO), the International Federation of Red Cross and Red Crescent Societies (IRC), the International Society of Blood Transfusion (ISBT) and the World Federation of Hemophilia (WFH) (Smit Sibinga, 2002). The WHO Blood Transfusion Safety Programme at WHO-HQ, Geneva, evolved from the WHO Global Programme on AIDS and the Global Blood Safety Initiative (GBSI) of the late 1980s. The leadership role of WHO has become visible through the development of a number of tools for education, collecting data, and providing guiding documents such as the series of *Aide Mémoires* to support and advise Governments in their attempts to structure national blood supply systems on a cost-effective, safe and sustainable basis. The Global Blood Safety Initiative started to map the situation of the blood supply and clinical use in the world and provide a series of expert advises, including two documents on education in transfusion medicine (WHO 1992a, 1992b).

5.1 WHA resolutions

With the goal of ensuring universal access to safe blood, WHO has been at the forefront of the movement to improve blood safety as mandated by successive World Health Assembly resolutions. In 2007 an important global meeting took place in Ottawa, Canada, addressing in a global consultation crucial aspects of a universal access to safe blood all part of the identified gaps (WHO, 2008a). More than 30 years after the first World Health Assembly resolution (WHA28.72) addressed the issue of blood safety, equitable access to safe blood and blood products and their safe and rational use still remain major challenges throughout the world. While the demand for blood is growing in the advanced world with longevity of life and increasingly sophisticated clinical procedures, national blood supplies are rarely sufficient to meet existing requirements in the restricted economy part of the world with some 80% of the global population.

Since that first World Health Assembly Resolution, a series of Resolutions has been created, endorsed and signed by the Member State representatives in an attempt to stimulate implementation at national level (Table 3). A recent one, WHA63.12 on Availability, Safety and Quality of Blood Products, was endorsed in May 2010 and urges Member States –

1. to take all the necessary steps to establish, implement and support nationally-coordinated, efficiently-managed and sustainable blood and plasma programmes according to the availability of resources, with the aim of achieving self-sufficiency, unless special circumstances preclude it;
2. to take all the necessary steps to update their national regulations on donor assessment and deferral, the collection, testing, processing, storage, transportation and use of blood products, and operation of regulatory authorities in order to ensure that regulatory control in the area of quality and safety of blood products across the entire transfusion chain meets internationally recognized standards;
3. to establish quality systems, for the processing of whole blood and blood components, good manufacturing practices for the production of plasma-derived medicinal products and appropriate regulatory control, including the use of diagnostic devices to prevent transfusion transmissible diseases with highest sensitivity and specificity;

4. to build human resource capacity through the provision of initial and continuing education (teaching and training) of staff to ensure quality of blood services and blood products;
5. to enhance the quality of evaluation and regulatory actions in the area of blood products and associated medical devices, including in vitro diagnostic devices;
6. to establish or strengthen systems for the safe and rational use of blood products and to provide education (teaching and training) for all staff involved in clinical transfusion, to implement potential solutions in order to minimize transfusion errors and promote patient safety, to promote the availability of transfusion alternatives including, where appropriate, autologous transfusion and patient blood management;
7. to ensure the reliability of mechanisms for reporting serious or unexpected adverse reactions to blood and plasma donation and to the receipt of blood components and plasma derived medicinal products, including transmissions of pathogens (haemovigilance);

The red thread through all these resolutions is the prevention of further spread of HIV/AIDS through contaminated blood transfusions and improving patient care, addressing the major knowledge gaps.

<table>
<tr><td colspan="2">The global need for blood safety and availability has been highlighted in the following WHA and Executive Board (EB) resolutions and regional resolutions (PAHO and AFRO) that provide specific direction on strategies and activities within individual regions:</td></tr>
<tr><td>1975:</td><td>WHA Resolution WHA28.72: Utilization and Supply of Human Blood and Blood Products</td></tr>
<tr><td>1987:</td><td>EB Resolution EB79.R1: Blood and Blood Products</td></tr>
<tr><td>1995:</td><td>WHA Resolution WHA48.27: Paris AIDS Summit</td></tr>
<tr><td>1999:</td><td>DC-PAHO/AMRO Resolution CD41.R15: Strengthening Blood Banks in the Region of the Americas</td></tr>
<tr><td>2000:</td><td>WHA Resolution WHA53.14: HIV/AIDS: Confronting the Epidemic</td></tr>
<tr><td>2001:</td><td>RC-AFRO Resolution AFR/RC51/R2: Blood Safety Strategy for the African Region</td></tr>
<tr><td>2002:</td><td>WHA Resolution WHA55.18: Quality of Care: Patient Safety</td></tr>
<tr><td>2003:</td><td>WHA Resolution WHA56.30: Global Health Sector Strategy for HIV/AIDS</td></tr>
<tr><td>2005:</td><td>WHA Resolution WHA58.13: Blood Safety: Proposal to Establish World Blood Donor Day</td></tr>
<tr><td rowspan="2">2007:</td><td>WHA Resolution WHA60.24: Health Promotion in a Globalized World</td></tr>
<tr><td>WHA Resolution WHA60.29: Health Technologies</td></tr>
<tr><td rowspan="5">2010:</td><td>WHA Resolution WHA63.10: Partnerships</td></tr>
<tr><td>WHA Resolution WHA63.12: Availability, Safety and Quality of Blood Products</td></tr>
<tr><td>WHA Resolution WHA63:18: Viral Hepatitis</td></tr>
<tr><td>WHA Resolution WHA63:19: WHO HIV/AIDS strategy for 2011-2015</td></tr>
<tr><td>WHA Resolution WHA63:20: Chagas Disease: Control and Elimination</td></tr>
</table>

Table 3. WHA Resolutions related to blood safety.

5.2 Millennium development goals

The United Nations Millennium Development Goals (MDG) are eight goals that in 2000 all 191 UN Member States have agreed to try to achieve by the year 2015 (UN, 2000). The United Nations Millennium Declaration, signed in September 2000 commits world leaders to combat poverty, hunger, disease, illiteracy, environmental degradation, and discrimination against women, all essential parts of the original 1948 UN Declaration of Universal Human Rights.

The eight MDGs are derived from this UN Millennium Declaration.

1. to eradicate extreme poverty and hunger;
2. to achieve universal primary education;
3. to promote gender equality and empower women;
4. to reduce child mortality;
5. to improve maternal health;
6. to combat HIV/AIDS, malaria, and other diseases;
7. to ensure environmental sustainability;
8. to develop a global partnership for development.

All eight goals have specific targets and indicators. Of these eight goals, the numbers 4, 5 and 6, and eight of the 18 targets relate directly to health and safe blood transfusion. The number 2 relates to education and the number 8 to the role of partnership for development, equally important to the development of safe and efficacious blood transfusion practices.

Some developing countries have made impressive progress in achieving the health-related Millennium Development Goals, targets and indicators. However, many more are still falling behind. Progress is particularly slow in sub-Saharan Africa but also in other developing and transition countries such as a number of the Newly Independent States (NIS), where knowledge gaps remain a major issue to address.

5.3 Success stories

There is a steadily growing number of success stories on bridging the knowledge gap and improving on the safety of the blood supply. We present just a few recent examples, largely from the African continent.

Eritrea (Baraki et al., 2010) - In 2006, despite the production of blood components in the National Blood Transfusion Centre (NBTC), about 90% of blood requests were for whole blood, an evidence of inappropriate use of blood and blood components in Eritrea. This could be the result of absence of proper and up to date guidelines and lack of training in appropriate use of blood and blood components, and alternatives. To change, the NBTC adapted clinical guidelines from the WHO document on appropriate use of blood (WHO, 2001). Copies of this document were distributed to all hospital staff in the country followed by training to the guidelines.

Objective of this Swiss Red Cross and Academic Institute IDTM (Groningen, NL) supported project was to assess the impact of distributing clinical guidelines and training (interventions) on knowledge, attitude and practice (KAP) of clinical prescribers in blood transfusion before and after the interventions. Correctly responded knowledge, attitude and practice (KAP) questions were collectively considered. Baseline: 3.8 percent of respondents correctly answered all KAP questions, which increased to 6.1 percent after the intervention. Of the total KAP questions, the average correct responses were 15.86 in the baseline and 17.45 in the follow-up assessment. The difference was positive and statistically significant ($p<0.000$) demonstrating the intervention had a major impact in changing the overall knowledge, attitude and practice of these health workers. When certain tools were audited, the compliance was found to be 38.1 percent among the assessed hospitals, though the auditing was limited to seven (7) major hospitals. This shows the intervention has made an impact when compared with the pre-intervention status.

When blood and blood components utilization comparison was made before (2006) and after the intervention (2008), demand for whole blood had decreased whereas the demands for all blood components had increased significantly (except FFP which remained unchanged).

This shows the progress made in Eritrea through focused education in addressing safe transfusion practice, and the measurable improvements in that practice.

Malawi (courtesy Dr. Jean C. Emmanuel) - Malawi (population of ± 11 million) is a Low Human Development Index (L-HDI) country. The European Union EC EDF VIII Project document set out to develop an independent and sustainable National Malawi Blood Transfusion Service (MBTS) following the recommendations and guidelines of the World Health Organisation (WHO), International Federation of Red Cross and Red Crescent Societies (IFRCRCS) and the International Society of Blood Transfusion (ISBT). The MBTS project plan was based on sustainable and effectively managed and organised independent National Blood Services. The platform for development was the establishment of a Finance and Administration department, with an experienced chartered cost accountant (CPA) as Director; with facilities and trained staff. Effective collaborative networks have been established with Ministry of Health (MoH) and Ministry of Finance (MoF), ensuring incorporation of a sustainable budget into the national annual fiscal budget, negotiated 'fee for service' from the private health insurance schemes for the private sector, and an equitable career structure for all staff with social benefits to ensure continuous capacity building and retention of staff. MBTS Trust Board appointed an experienced CEO; Finance & Administration Director and Medical Director.

In February 2000 a financing agreement, MAI/7001/002, was signed between the Republic of Malawi and the European Commission (EC) for € 7.8m in order to support the Malawi MoH to establish an independent National MBTS under a formally constituted and independent Malawi Blood Transfusion Service Trust. Project funding was increased with a further € 1.3m following a successful mid-term review (MTR). The Project Manager was appointed in March 2003 and development commenced. The Board of Trustees is responsible for the effective operation of MBTS and drafted appropriate legal frameworks, comprising the Constitution for the Board of Trustees and Legislation of the Service. MBTS is an officially registered Non Government Organisation (NGO) with a legal seal. MBTS is managed and organised by a competent Chief Executive Officer (CEO) who has internationally recognised qualifications, a Finance and Administrative Director and Medical Director with a Deputy; together form the Senior Management Team reporting directly to the Board. Developing collaborative working partnerships with the relevant NGOs, stakeholders and bodies in the private and public sector in Malawi is an important and ongoing strategy.

The overall objective of MBTS is to provide safe blood and blood products, reduce the incidence of HIV, and other diseases transmissible by blood, ensuring equitable access and availability of blood and promoting appropriate clinical use of blood. The goal was achieved within the planned project timeframe a sustainable, national blood transfusion service providing a safe, adequate and accessible supply for all those in need in recognised health care establishments from 100% voluntary non-remunerated safe blood donors, which meets the needs of all hospitals in Malawi through the three centres specifically designed and built within the project framework.

The five-year project ended 2007. An independent Mid Term Review (MTR) Team contracted by European Commission (EC), concluded that the project had been successfully implemented. As a result EC agreed to an extension to the funding of € 1.3m through EDF IX, for the construction of 3 Blood Centres.

Key achievements of the project:

- Establishment of an approved and effective Board of Trustees, CEO and Executive Team, with effective leadership, organisation and management, personnel (110 staff) all trained to international standards in all areas of work, with job descriptions, SOPs and implementing quality systems;
- MBTS policy, plan and legal framework approved as official legal instruments;
- Construction of 3 blood transfusion centres (completed 2008);
- Equipment and vehicles for 8 mobile collection teams including a blood donor bus;
- Recurrent expenditure secured in fiscal budget by 'subvention' from fiscal year beginning July 2006 to present;
- Project Manager/Technical Assistance funded by EC responsible for development and training ended 31 March 2007;
- All objectives, and planned outputs, were achieved on time;
- All donated blood is tested for HIV I/ II, p24 antigen; Hepatitis B & C; Syphilis and malaria with the introduction of a quality management system, and good laboratory practices. Trained senior staff have become trainers of district hospital blood bank staff and future MBTS staff;
- Blood Cold Chain (BCC) system in place for the transport of blood specimens for centralized testing and distribution of blood and blood products to all hospitals; provision of targeted hospitals with appropriate resources for the storage of blood and blood products for blood transfusion;
- District Hospital laboratory staff have been trained using WHO Distance Learning Materials (every technician has a personal copy);
- Training workshops, seminars and lectures on appropriate clinical use of blood facilitated by respective senior staff;
- Research ongoing on knowledge, attitudes and practices (KAP) on blood donation issues; evaluating prevalence of Hepatitis C (HCV); on evidence based rationale for individual patient identification arm bands; research paper co-authored on Clinical Paediatric Transfusion Guidelines;
- MBTS provides blood and products from 100% voluntary non-remunerated donors to all public and private hospitals;
- MBTS is a sustainable and effective Service with an approved fiscal budget and a "fee for service" through private medical insurance.

Sudan (Hassan Ali et al., 2010) - In Sudan blood transfusion services were fragmented - hospital based with 85% of blood collected from family and replacement donors. More than 300 hospital blood banks practice blood collection and transfusion; 40% are rural hospitals with transfusion rate of 5-100 units of blood per month besides large central and specialized urban hospitals with transfusion rate of 100-300 units of blood per month. About 300,000 units of blood are collected annually; 56% is screened using rapid tests and 44% by ELISA technique, with a TTI marker prevalence of HIV - 2%, HBV - 6%, HCV - 2% and syphilis - 5%. Apart from a few solitary guidelines and SOP-like instructions no quality system was in place. Almost exclusively whole blood is being transfused and adverse events are poorly observed. In 2009, in close collaboration with World Health Organization and the Academic Institute IDTM (Groningen, NL), a project to improve quality in blood transfusion through an appropriate quality management system was established, focused on the creation of a solid national blood supply and transfusion framework. Objectives were to review existing quality management programme and identify gaps, assist in the development of a draft national quality policy and develop a plan for quality improvement including capacity building. Through a series of field visits to main blood transfusion centres in three main States, the establishment of a National Steering Committee to create full ownership, capacity building through basic education in quality management and clinical transfusion medicine (quality culture) and enhancement of a voluntary blood donation programme strategy, the following goals were reached –

1. Endorsed National Blood Transfusion Policy (Ministry of Health);
2. Voluntary Blood Donor Association established and registered;
3. 50 senior blood bank quality managers from 10 States educated in the basics of quality management. Committees from these trainers have worked on developing a draft national quality manual;
4. 6 seminars for prescribers conducted in 3 States, to improve clinical blood transfusion knowledge and practice (in-hospital transfusion chain).

This demonstrates that international collaboration (WHO/IDTM) can generate major achievements in establishing a national framework and improving quality blood transfusion services in developing countries to achieve the goals of safe and adequate blood supplies and clinical awareness and knowledge at national level.

Uganda (Kyeyune et al., 2010) - In 1957, a centralized transfusion service - the Uganda Blood Transfusion Service (UBTS), was started at Nakasero. This supplied blood to the entire country for the following 20 years. The period from 1977 to 1987 saw political unrest disrupt national infrastructures and aggravated the human resource crisis in the health sector. This resulted into reversion to the original unregulated hospital based transfusion service nationwide. Like any other low HDI country, Uganda is still challenged by a low availability of voluntary non-remunerated blood donors (VNRBD); insufficient transport and storage facilities; low capacities in testing of donated blood and quality assurance in testing laboratories. Through a step-by-step approach these problems are being reversed using locally and internationally sourced technical and financial support. In May 1987, Uganda with the assistance of the Global Programme on AIDS (GPA) of the World Health Organization (WHO) held a financial donor conference in Kampala. As a result, the Uganda AIDS Control Programme (UACP) was formed. The European Commission (EC) through its AIDS Task Force (ATF) made a pledge of 1.5 million Euros to rehabilitate the central blood bank at Nakasero and the collection, processing and distribution of 10,000 units of whole blood to be supplied to hospitals within 100 kms from Nakasero Blood Bank. In the period 1989-2004, further funding from EC together with adequate technical advice and support enabled the UBTS to improve its infrastructure by opening four regional blood banks in Mbarara, Fort-Portal, Gulu, Mbale and two satellites in Arua and Kitovu. This was accompanied by development and adoption of a National Blood Transfusion Policy, and organization and coordination of a national safe blood transfusion service based on voluntary non-remunerated blood donors. This period saw significant reduction of HIV and hepatitis B sero-prevalence among donors. A quality assurance programme was instituted in the UBTS establishment, and opportunities for human resource development in-service training were initiated. The EC fund was phased out in 2004 amidst increasing demands for safe blood for an increasing population. From 2004 to date UBTS has enjoyed technical (TA provision) and financial support from the US PEPFAR project, focused on strengthening of the national blood transfusion service. This has been followed by renovation of existing and establishment of new facilities, increased blood collection from 107,000 units in 2004 to 165,500 units in 2009. Blood testing for hepatitis C was started in 2005 in addition to HIV, Hepatitis B and syphilis testing. Hospital transfusion committees to oversee clinical use of blood are being created, and a major emphasis is on quality system essentials and capacity building in the regional blood banks.

Uzbekistan (Makhmudova & Smit Sibinga, 2008) - Project focus: development of a Republican Blood Supply and Transfusion System based on international standards - safe, efficacious, sustainable and affordable.

The Government of Uzbekistan initiated measures to reform the Health Care System. Government and Asian Development Bank (ADB) signed a Loan Agreement (2004) for a major project: Woman and Child Health Development (WCHD); part is used to improve blood services. The blood services situation requires radical improvement: Donated blood is not safe, majority is collected from paid donors with serious risk of HIV, HCV and HBV transmission. The country lacks a national blood safety policy, strategic plan, appropriate legislative and regulatory framework. The Blood Safety Program (component 3) of WCHD comprises a nationwide blood supply system, initiated in 2004 and substantiated in 2006, based on WHO and Red Cross principles. The programme is public health oriented, addressing the need for a nationally supported system, cost-effective, motivation and mobilization of the community to convert the current paid and replacement system into a truly voluntary and regular blood donor system, upgrading procurement operations (regional and economy-of-scale). It addresses the need for equitable access of safe blood to all citizens, appropriate clinical practices, and a national budget system to allow sustained and continuous operations. Using public education and social marketing campaigns with the support of NGOs, a voluntary and regular donor programme will be implemented stepwise. Another major point is in establishing appropriate clinical transfusion practices. With support of international expertise, MoH has created a Republican reform plan to reduce the number of inadequate hospital based blood transfusion units. The plan focuses on consolidation of core activities - blood collection, processing and testing, storage and distribution in 6 regional centres, strategically spread over the country to be able to handle logistics of demand and supply, and provide cost-effective operations. Implementation is in phases to allow proper adaptation and guarantee of continued supply of blood over the transition period. The WCHD conducts training needs assessments, develops training modules based on WHO guidelines and provides education for clinicians and transfusion medicine specialists (capacity building). Another example of how to bridge the knowledge gap.

This demonstrates that donor funding when appropriately utilized and supported by adequate provision of guidance and technical advice can improve blood transfusion programmes in the low human development index countries.

5.4 Lessons learned

To reduce the burden of morbidity and mortality through HIV infected blood transfusions of particularly the poor and marginalized populations, the focus should be on an increasing access to clinical and diagnostic technology, safe blood, blood components and medical devices. This could be achieved through reducing the leading risk factors to human health

in which lack of education (knowledge) plays a major role. When a safe and professional environment for the vein-to-vein use of blood and blood components is created, the risk for transmissible and transfusion related diseases will be reduced. At the same time there should be developed a sustainable and integrated health care system by building competent leadership, management and operational capacity in the methodologies and technologies involved in the procurement and clinical use of blood and blood components as fundamental elements of a sustainable health care system.
That could only be achieved sustainably when enabling policies and an institutional environment are developed through appropriate national drug and blood policies (legal and regulatory framework), with all partners involved in the health technologies and within the framework of national health policies (integrated), which generate a common vision and a realistic and feasible plan for action.

6. Acknowledgement

The authors would like to acknowledge Dr. Yifdeamlak E. Baraki from Eritrea, Dr. Jean C. Emmanuel from Malawi, Dr. Abdul Hassan Ali from Sudan, Dr. Dorothy Kyeyune from Uganda and Dr. Mayya Makhmudova from Uzbekistan for their invaluable contribution to the success stories.

7. References

Adriani WPA, Smit Sibinga CTh. *How to develop a practical Quality Management System in resource limited countries,* Vox Sanguinis, Vol. 95, Issue 241 (Suppl), pp. 501

Allain JP, Sarkodie F, Asenso-Mensah K, Owusu-Ofori S. (2009). *Relative safety of first-time volunteer and replacement donors in west Africa,* Transfusion, Vol. 50, pp. 340-3

American College of Physicians Ad Hoc Committee on Medical Ethics (Eds.). (1984). *American College of Physicians Ethics Manual Part I: History of Medical Ethics, The Physician and the Patient, The Physician's Relationship to Other Physicians, The Physician and Society, Annals of Internal Medicine,* Vol. 101, Issue 1 (July 1984), pp. 129-137

Baraki Y, Swiss Red Cross, Smit Sibinga CTh. (2010). *The Impact of Introduction of Clinical Guidelines and Training in Appropriate Use of Blood and Blood Products (AUB) on Knowledge, Attitude and Practice of Blood Prescribers in Eritrea.* Transfusion, 2010;50 (2S):187A

Basavaraju S et al. (2010). *Reduced risk of transfusion-transmitted HIV in Kenya through centrally co-ordinated blood centres, stringent donor selection and effective p24 antigen-HIV antibody screening,* Vox Sanguinis, Vol. 99, Issue 3 (October 2010), pp. 212–219

Berte LM. (1997). *Tools for improving quality in the transfusion service,* American Journal of Clinical Pathology, Vol. 107, Issue 4 Suppl 1 (April 1997), pp. S36-42

Chevrolle F et al. (2000). *Blood transfusion audit methodology: the auditors, reference systems and audit guidelines,* Transfus Clin Biol, Vol. 7, Issue 6, (December 2000), pp. 559-62

Colebunders R et al. (1991). *Seroconversion rate, mortality, and clinical manifestations associated with the receipt of a human immunodeficiency virus-infected blood transfusion in Kinshasa, Zaire,* Journal of Infectious Diseases, Vol. 164, pp. 450–6

Council of Europe (2007). Chapter 30: Pre-transfusion Measures, In: Guide to the Preparation, Use and Quality Assurance of Blood Components, Accessed March 25, 2011, Available from: http://books.google.com.na/books?id=huNgp2KJ-wQC&pg=PA47&lpg=PA47&dq=council+of+europe+2005+Preparation,+Use+and+Quality+Assurance+of+Blood+Components&source=bl&ots=l6T4a7MmBy&sig=gljoQKBPlhZXCZIUCh6yNeoFBMc&hl=en&ei=vtKMTZ-DNM33gAfJh9mfDQ&sa=X&oi=book_result&ct=result&resnum=5&ved=0CDQQ6AEwBA#v=onepage&q=council%20of%20europe%202005%20Preparation%2C%20Use%20and%20Quality%20Assurance%20of%20Blood%20Components&f=false

Diarra A, Kouriba B, Baby M, Murphy E, Lefrere JJ. (2009). *HIV, HCV, HBV and syphilis rate of positive donations among blood donations in Mali: lower rates among volunteer blood donors,* Transfusion Clin Biol, Vol. 16, pp. 444-7

Dosunmu AO, Dada MO. (2005). *Principles of blood transfusion service audit, African Journal of Medical Science,* Vol. 34, Issue 4 (December 2005), pp. 349-53

European Union. (2003). Directive 2002/98/EC of the European Parliament and the Council of 27 January 2003 Setting standards of quality and safety for the collection, testing, processing, storage and distribution of human blood and blood components and amending Directive 2001/83/EC Official Journal of the European Union 2003 I.33/30-39

Farrugia A, et al. (2010). *Payment, compensation and replacement – the ethics and motivation of blood and plasma donation,*Vox Sanguinis, Vol. 99 (June 2010), pp. 202-211

Feldschuh J, with Weber D. (1990). *Safe Blood: Purifying the Nation's Blood Supply in the Age of AIDS,* The Free Press, 0-02-910065-8, New York

Ferrera V et al. (2001). *Methodology for the development of a program for following and maintaining the competency of human resources,* Transfusion Clin Biol, Vol. 8, Issue 1 (February 2001), pp. 30-43

Fretz C. (2003). *Self-Assessment Tools,* Transfusion Clin Biol, Vol. 10, Issue 2 (April 2003), pp. 94-8

Glynn SA, Williams AE, Nass CC, Bethel J, Kessler D, Scott EP, Fridey J, Kleinman SH & Schreiber GB. (2003). *Attitudes toward blood donation incentives in the United States: implications for donor recruitment,* Transfusion, Vol. 43, Issue 1 (January 2003), pp. 7-16

Grainger B, Margolese E, Partington E. *Legal and ethical considerations in blood transfusion,* Canadian Medical Association Journal 1997; 156 (11 suppl)

Gygi C, DeCarlo N, Williams B. (2005) *Six Sigma for Dummies.* Wiley Publishing Inc. ISBN: 0-7645-6798-5, Hoboken, NJ, USA

Hassan Ali A, Abdellah YE, Smit Sibinga CTh. (2010) *International Collaboration: an Approach to Establishing Blood Transfusion Quality System in Sudan,* Vox Sanguinis 2010;99 (suppl 1):92

Hollán SR, Wagstaff W, Leikola J, Lothe F. (eds.). (1990) *Management of blood transfusion services.* WHO Press, Geneva, CH

International Federation of Red Cross/Red Crescent Societies (IFRC).

International Society of Blood Transfusion [ISBT]. (2006) *International Forum: Paid vs. unpaid donors,* Vox Sanguinis, Vol. 90, No. 1, pp. 63-70.

International Society of Blood Transfusion [ISBT]. (2006) ISBT Code of Ethics for Blood Donation and Transfusion, In: Documentation, Accessed March 23, 2011, Available from: http://www.isbt-web.org/documentation/default.asp

Jacobs B et al. (1994). *Secondary school students: a safer blood donor population in an urban with high HIV prevalence in east Africa*, East Africa Medical Journal, Vol. 71, Issue 11 (November 1994), pp. 720-3

Kajja I, Bimenya G, Smit Sibinga C. (2010b) *The interface between blood preparation and use in Uganda,* Vox Sanguinis 2010;98:e257-e262

Kajja I, Bimenya GS, Eindhoven GB, ten Duis HJ, Smit Sibinga CTh. (2010b) *Surgical blood order equation in femoral fracture surgery,* Transfusion Medicine; 2010: doi: 10.1111/j.1365-3148.2010.01033.x

Kajja I, Bimenya GS, Eindhoven GB, ten Duis HJ, Smit Sibinga CTh. (2010a) *Blood loss and contributing factors in femoral fracture surger,* African Health Sciences 2010;10:18-25

Kajja I, Bimenya GS, Smit Sibinga CTh. (2011) *Informed consent in blood transfusion: Knowledge and administrative issues in Uganda hospitals,* Transfusion and Apheresis Science 2011; 44:33-39

Kajja I, Kyeyune S, Bimenya GS, Smit Sibinga CTh. (2010a) *Bottlenecks of blood processing in Uganda,* Transfusion Medicine, 2010;20:329-336

Kajja, I (2010). *The Current Hospital TransfusionPractices and Procedures in Uganda,* PhD Thesis, GrafiMedia RUG, ISBN 978-90-367-4619-9

Kendrick DB. (n.d.). Blood Program in World War II, In: *Medical Department United States Army in World War II,* Accessed March 25, 2011, Available from: http://history.amedd.army.mil/booksdocs/wwii/blood/default.htm

Kyeyune D, Kataaha P, Kajja I, Smit Sibinga CTh. (2010) *The Success Story of Donor Funding to Uganda Blood Transfusion Service,* Vox Sanguinis 2010;99 (suppl 1):513

Linden JV, Bianco C (Eds.) (2001). *Blood Safety and Surveillance,* Marcel Dekker, 0-8247-0263-8, New York

Los APM, Mutegombwa SM, Gabra GA, Smit Sibinga CTh. (2009) *Liaison role of school teachers to support blood collection, donor motivation and retention at schools in Africa: Could the Uganda experience serve as an example for other African countries?* Africa Sanguine 2009;12:5-10

Los APM, Smit Sibinga CTh. (2001) Community involvement: The Development – the Past, the Present and the Future of Blood Donation as a Form of Community Involvement. In: Transfusion Medicine: Quo Vadis? What has been achieved, what is to be expected. Smit Sibinga CTh & Cash JD. (Eds.). pp21-29.

Los APM, Smit Sibinga CTh. (2009) *Social marketing tools to improve blood collection and donor retention,* Vox Sanguinis 2009;96 (suppl. 1):124 (abstract P-147)

Makhmudova MR, Smit Sibinga CTh. (2008) *Creation of a National blood program in Uzbekistan,* Vox Sanguinis, 2008;95 (Suppl 1):218 (P440)

Martucci J. (2010). *Negotiating exclusion: MSM, identity, and blood policy in the age of AIDS,* Soc Stud Sci, Vol. 40, Issue 2 (April 2010), pp. 215-41

McCullough J. (1998). Transfusion Medicine, McGraw-Hill, 0-07-045113-3, New York

McFarland W et al. (1998). *Risk factors for HIV seropositivity among first-time blood donors in Zimbabwe,* Transfusion, Vol. 38, Issue 3 (March 1998), pp. 279-84

Mintz PD. (1995). *Quality assessment and improvement of transfusion practices,* Hematol Oncol Clin North Am., Vol. 9, Issue 1 (February 1995), pp. 219-32

Noumsi GT, Schneider WH, Lachenal G, Smit Sibinga CTh. *Use of blood donor screening data to access HIV dynamics in Cameroun,* Vox Sang 2008;95 (Suppl 1):261 (P559)

Parry E.H.O. (Ed.). (1984) Principles of Medicine in Africa, 2d Edition, Oxford Medical Publications, 0192613375, Nairobi

Perlin T. (2001). TKTK, In: Ethical issues in transfusion medicine, Macpherson CR, Domen RE, Perlin T, Editors, pp. TK-TK, AABB Press, 978-1563951381, Bethesda

Roussel P et al. (2001). *Methodologic contribution to blood transfusion materials surveillance,* Transfus Clin Biol, Vol. 8, Issue 4 (August 2001), pp. 359-73

Sarkodie F, Adarkwa M, Adu-Sarkodie Y, Candotti D, Acheampong JW & Allain JP. (2001). *Screening for viral markers in volunteer and replacement blood donors in West Africa,* Vox Sanguinis, Vol. 80, pp. 142–7

Smit Sibinga CT, Los APM, van der Tuuk Adriani WPA. *Project management as a recommendable approach to improve donor management in restricted economy countries (preliminary results),* Vox Sanguinis, 2006;91 (Suppl 3):191 (P-405)

Smit Sibinga CT. *Needs and essentials for Nationally supported structure and organisation of the blood supply: the Sanquin model,* Transfusion 2006;46(Supplement):192A

Smit Sibinga CTh, Kajja I. (2009). *How to determine the needs for safe blood in Africa – expectations and realities.* Programme and Abstracts book 5th International Congress AfSBT, Nairobi, KY 2009: F56 p.97

Smit Sibinga CTh, van der Does JA, Los APM, Molijn HM, van der Tuuk Adriani WPA. (2009) *Opzet en ontwikkeling van de bloedvoorziening in ontwikkelingslanden. Hoe doe je dat?* Tijdschrift voor Bloedtransfusie 2009;2:87-92.

Smit Sibinga CTh. (2000). *Transfusion medicine in developing countries,* Transfusion Medicine Reviews 2000;14:269-274.

Smit Sibinga CTh. (2001) *Risk management: an important tool for improving quality.* Transfusion and Clinical Biology 2001;8:214-17.

Smit Sibinga CTh. (2002). *GCBS, ICBS and other initiatives; Will there be a 'toto pro partum'?* In: Transmissible Diseases and Blood Transfusion. Smit Sibinga CTh, Dodd RY (eds.). pp 195-202. Kluwer Academic Publishers ISBN 1-4020-0986-0. Dordrecht/ Boston/London

Smit Sibinga CTh. (2006). *Needs and essentials for Nationally supported structure and organisation of the blood supply: the Sanquin model,* Transfusion, 2006;46(Supplement):192A

Smit Sibinga, CTh. (2007). *Detecting and Monitoring Reactions in the Developing World,* In: Transfusion Reactions. Popovsky, MA, ed. 3rd edition AABB Press, Bethesda, MD, USA, 449-65

Smit Sibinga CTh. (2008). *The need for post-academic leadership development and transfusion medicine related health sciences research.* The Academic Institute for International Development of Transfusion Medicine. Transfusion Today 2008;77:9

Smit Sibinga CTh. (2009). *Is the need for safety of the blood supply in Africa different from other resource limited parts of the world?* Programme and Abstracts book 5th International Congress AfSBT, Nairobi, KY June 2009: T29 p.72

Smit Sibinga CTh. (2009a). *Filling a gap in transfusion medicine education and research,* Transfusion Medicine Reviews 2009;23;284-291

Smit Sibinga CTh. (2009b). *Pioneers and pathfinders – C.Th. Smit Sibinga: an autobiography,* Transfusion Medicine Reviews 2009;23:160-165.

South African National Blood Service [SANBS]. (2006) Donor Form, Accessed March 23, 2011, Available from: http://www.sanbs.org.za/new_donors/Eng_SEQ.pdf

Stutzer A & Goette L. (2010). *Blood donor motivation: what is ethical? What works?* ISBT Science Series, Vol. 5 (2010), pp. 244–248

Thomas WI & Thomas DS (eds,). (1928). The child in America. Alfred Knopf, New York USA

Titmuss R. (1971). The Gift Relationship: From Human Blood to Social Policy, New Press, 1565844033, New York

Umeora OU at al. (2005). *Socio-cultural barriers to voluntary blood donation for obstetric use in a rural Nigerian village,* African Journal of Reproductive Health, Vol. 9, Issue 3 (December 2005), pp. 72-76

United Nations. (1948) Universal Declaration of Human Rights. 22 March 2011 Avalailable from: www.un.org/en/documents/udhr/index.shtml

United Nations. (2000). Millennium Development Goals. 22 March 2011 Availble from: www.un.org/millenniumgoals/

United States Centers for Disease Control and Prevention [CDC]. (1982). *Possible transfusion-associated acquired immune deficiency syndrome (AIDS) – California,* MMWR Morbidity and Mortality Weekly Report, Vol. 31, pp. 652-654

United States Centers for Disease Control and Prevention [CDC]. (2008. *Progress Towards Strengthening Blood Transfusion Srvices – 14 Countries, 2003-2007,* MMWR Morbidity and Mortality Weekly Report, Vol. 57, pp. 1273-1277

United States Food and Drug Administration [FDA]. (2010). CPG Sec. 230.150 Blood Donor Classification Statement, Paid or Volunteer Donor (05/07/2002 new), In: Compliance Policy Guides, Accessed March 27, 2011, Available from: http://www.fda.gov/ICECI/ComplianceManuals/CompliancePolicyGuidanceManual/ucm122798

United States Food and Drug Administration [FDA]. (2010). Compliance Manual, Part I: Background, In: Inspection of Licensed and Unlicensed Blood Banks, Brokers, Reference Laboratories, and Contractors, Accessed March 25, 2011, Available from: http://www.fda.gov/BiologicsBloodVaccines/GuidanceComplianceRegulatoryInformation/ComplianceActivities/Enforcement/CompliancePrograms/ucm095226.htm

United States President's Emergency Plan for AIDS Relief. (2011) 2005-2010 PEPFAR Annual Reports, In: Annual Report to Congress on the President's Emergency Plan for AIDS Relief, Accessed March 23, 2011, Available from: http://www.pepfar.gov/press/c19573.htm

van Hulst M, Sagoe KW, Vermande JE, van de Schaaf IP, van der Tuuk Adriani WP, Torpey K, Ansah J, Mingle JA, Smit Sibinga CT, Postma MJ. (2008). *Cost-effectiveness of HIV screening of blood donations in Accra (Ghana),* Value Health 2008;11:809-19.

van Hulst M, Smit Sibinga CTh, Postma MJ. (2009). *Health economics of blood transfusion safety – focus on sub-Saharan Africa,* Biologicals 2009;doi:10.1016/j.biologicals.2009:1-6

van Hulst R, Dhingra N, Smit Sibinga CT, Postma MJ. (2006). *Cost-effectiveness of interventions ensuring blood transfusion safety in Africa,* Transfusion 2006;46 (Supplement):169A

Wehrli J. (2011). *The nuts and bolts of curriculum and assessment,* Journal of Clinical Apheresis, Vol. 26, Issue 1 (ePub December 2010), pp. 29-46

World Bank in collaboration with U.S. CDC/CAR, USAID and WHO-EURO. (2008). *Blood Services in Central Asian Health Systems: A clear and present danger of spreading HIV/AIDS and other infectious diseases*. The International Bank for Reconstruction and Development/The World Bank, Washington DC, USA

World Health Organization. (1978). *WHA28.72 Utilization and supply of human blood and blood products*. WHO 1978, Geneva CH

World Health Organization. (1992a). *Report of the GCBS informal consultation on 'Assessment of Training Needs in Transfusion Medicine'*. WHO_LBS_92.6, 1992, Geneva, CH

World Health Organization. (1992b). *Report of the GCBS informal consultation on 'Collaboration in Training in Transfusion Medicine'*. WHO_LBS_92.71, 1992, Geneva, CH

World Health Organization (2001) *The Clinical Use of Blood. Handbook.* WHO/BTS/99.3, 2001, Geneva, CH

World Health Organization. (2008b). *Global Database on Blood Safety. Report 2004-2005*, WHO 2008 Geneva, CH

World Health Organization. (2008c). *Aide Mémoire for National Policy Makers. Good Policy Process for Blood Safety and Availability*. WHO/EHT/08.02. January 2008, Geneva, CH

World Health Organization. (2010a). *Global Blood Safety and Availability. Facts and figures from the 2007 survey*. WHO 2010, Geneva, CH

World Health Organization. (2010b). *Screening donated blood for transfusion-transmissible infections: recommendations*. World Health Organization. ISBN 978-92-4-154788-8

World Health Organization. (2008a). *Universal access to safe Blood Transfusion* WHO/EHT/08.03, Geneva, CH

World Health Organization. (2009). *Screening donated blood for transfusion-transmissible infections: recommendations*, In: Research Policy, Accessed March 26, 2011, Available from: http://www.who.int/rpc/guidelines/9789241547888/en/index.html

World Health Organization. (2011a). Blood Transfusion Safety, In: *National Blood Policies*, Accessed March 23, 2011, Available from: http://www.who.int/bloodsafety/transfusion_services/nat_blood_pol/en/

World Health Organization. (2011b). World Health Assembly/Executive Board Resolutions on Blood Safety, In: Blood transfusion safety documentation centre, Accessed March 23, 2011, Available from: http://www.who.int/bloodsafety/publications/en/index.html

World Health Organization. (2011c). Aide-Memoire on Blood Safety for National Blood Programmes, In: *Documentation*, Accessed March 23, 2011, Available from: http://www.who.int/bloodsafety/publications/en/index.html

World Health Organization. (2011d). *Global Database on Blood Safety, In: Blood transfusion safety*, Accessed March 25, 2011, Available from: http://www.who.int/bloodsafety/global_database/en/

24

Molecular Epidemiology of HIV-1 Infection in the Amazon Region

Antonio Carlos Rosário Vallinoto, Luiz Fernando Almeida Machado,
Marluísa de Oliveira Guimarães Ishak and Ricardo Ishak
Federal University of Para, Institute of Biological Sciences, Virus Laboratory, Brazil

1. Introduction

No other group of infectious agents has received increased attention from scientists in recent years than that of retroviruses. This reflects not only their importance as pathogens of humans and animals, but also its great value in studying the interactions between pathogens and host.

The family *Retroviridae* comprises a large number of viruses that have the ability to insert its genome into the host cell and infect primarily vertebrates, despite having been described infections in other animals such as snails and insects.

Viruses pathogenic to humans which cause infections worldwide can be divided into two main groups: the transformants and the cytopathic. The first, induce changes in the control of cell division and can lead to tumors, such as Human T-lymphotropic virus (HTLV), belonging to the genus *Deltaretrovirus* and is linked to neurological and hematological. Cytopathic retroviruses are members of the *Lentivirus* genus, such as the Human immunodeficiency virus (HIV), and are related to severe immunodeficiency condictions.

The ubiquotous conditions, now known by the name of acquired immunodeficiency syndrome (AIDS) is caused by HIV and was first recognized in the summer of 1981. The spread of an emerging virus in all regions of the world, caused great losses both in terms of human lives as well as in the economic point of view.

HIV infection results in a profound disorder in the host immune system, which is characterized by a decrease in the number of lymphocytes with the CD4 glycoprotein on their surface, especially helper T lymphocytes (ATL), with subsequent reversal of the ratio of CD4+ or CD8+ T lymphocytes.

In Brazil, the HIV-1 dissemination reflects the grandeur and diversity sociogeographic of the country and its regional heterogeneity. The first cases of HIV/AIDS in Brazil, dates from 1982 and were originated the Southeast individual, which today still has the highest number of reported cases of the disease. Subtypes B, F, C and D, in addition to samples of virus recombinants and dual infections in different geographical areas. In the present chapter, we describe the molecular epidemiology of HIV-1 infection in the Brazilian Amazon region, emphasizing its impact in the city of Belem, Capital of the Para State, which is the main port of entry into the Amazon, highlighting the occurrence of the circulating subtypes and the genetic profile of the host which is associated with the infection.

Currently HIV-1 genetic heterogeneity is classified into four phylogenetic groups: M, N, O and P, which may reflect four interspecific transmission events from chimpanzees (Plantier et al., 2009). Group M (major) is the most frequently involves with human infectious worldwide and is composed of nine genetically distinct subtypes, named A, B, C, D, F, G, H, J and K, whose gene sequences differ approximately 20% (Taylor et al., 2008).

In Brazil, HIV-1 is characterized by the occurrence of several subtypes of the M group, and includes subtype B, the most prevalent in the majority of the regions, followed by subtypes F, C, and D, (Monteiro et al., 2009) although some cities present a distinct pattern of distribution of these subtypes (Vicente et al., 2000; Soares et al., 2003). This diversity of subtypes could represent more than one port of entry of HIV-1 in the country, with the emergence of the epidemic occurring, probably in the late 1970's or early 1980's (Morgado et al., 1998).

The circulating recombinant forms of HIV (CRFs) have an important role in regional and global epidemics of the virus, particularly in regions where multiple subtypes circulate simultaneously. Currently over 40 CRFs are recognized worldwide (http://www.hiv.lanl.gov), and five have been described in Brazil, designated as CRF28_BF, CRF29_BF, CRF39_BF, CRF40_BF e CRF31_BC (Sanabani et al., 2006; De Sá Filho et al., 2006, http://www.hiv.lanl.gov/content/sequence/HIV/CRFs/CRFs.html), where CRF_BC represents 11% of the HIV-1 viruses circulating in the Southern region of the country (Santos et al., 2006).

In addition to the CRF, a large number of unique recombinant forms (URFs) have been characterized worldwide (McCutchan, 2006). Notoriously, a recombination is a potentially important mechanism that significantly contributes to HIV genetic variability with serious implications for diagnosis, drug treatment and optimal vaccine development (Sanabani et al., 2010).

2. HIV-1 infection in the Brazilian Amazon region

The molecular epidemiology of HIV-1 strains circulating in the Northern region of Brazil is poorly known (Table 1). The State of Para has 43.3% of the cases. Until June 2006, there were 5919 infected individuals, in which 80.4% were men and 19.6% were women (Brasil, 2008). The prevalence of the infection in the State of Amapa is still low, although the region borders French Guiana and a great number of indigenous populations move freely between the two countries. The cities of Belem (State of Para), Manaus (State of Amazonas) and Macapa (State of Amapa) can be considered as the main entry of HIV-1 in northern Brazil. The city of Belem has one of the largest ports in the Brazilian Amazon and receives a great input of tourists throughout the year, while the city of Macapa is located next to several Indian tribes and borders countries such as Guyana, which generates a large population movement between two locations. The city of Belem shows the highest diversity of subtypes of HIV-1 in Brazil, having been identified the subtypes B, F, D, C and recombinant CRF02_AG subtype reflecting in this way, the same epidemiological profile found in almost all regions of Brazil (Sabino et al., 1996; Morgado et al., 1998; Ramos et al., 1999, Tanuri et al., 1999; Vicente et al., 2000) and from South America (Marquina et al., 1996; Navas et al., 1999; Avila et al., 2002; Castro et al., 2003).

The population group studied presented epidemiological characteristics which indicated that the heterosexual transmission of HIV-1 associated with sexual promiscuity, was the main way of virus dissemination. HIV-1 occurred mostly in the group of individuals who reported having only primary and secondary education, as well as those with a heterosexual behavior. There was no statistically correlation between sex, educational level, sexual orientation and risk behavior for HIV-1, with subtypes B and F infection.

Subtype C was identified in Belem and phylogenetic analysis supports the hypothesis that the virus was imported from the Southeast and Southern Brazil. Additionally, the recombinant CRF02_AG subtype, circulating in Belém-PA probably was reported for the first time in the Amazon region and reinforces the importance of epidemiological surveillance for the virus in the country.

In Belem four subtypes were described in relation to *env*: B (88.3%), F (8.3%), D (1.7%), and C (1.7%); subtype B was the only one found in Macapa. In relation to the *pro* segment, there were four distinct subtypes in Belem: B (88.3%), F (9.3%), D (1.2%), and CRF02_AG (1.2%). In Macapa, subtypes B (97.1%) and F (2.9%) were detected. Six strains were characterized as mosaics: two were B^{env}/F^{pro} (1.6%), two F^{env}/B^{pro} (1.6%), one C^{env}/B^{pro} (0.85%), and one B^{env}/D^{pro} (0.8%) (Machado et al., 2009).

When compared to the State of Amazonas, there is a higher concentration of cases of disease in Manaus (capital), which holds approximately 90% of cases (Fundação de Medicina Tropical do Amazonas, 2006). Manaus has greater human genetic diversity because of their indigenous origin and sociocultural strong influence of migration from the Northeast region of Brazil since the 1800's when colonization occurred more intensely because of the business cycles of the rubber extractive exploratory projects, settlement of forest areas its transformation into an industrial area (Carneiro Filho, 1998).

There is evidence that the HIV / AIDS in the city of Manaus evolved with different patterns of distribution and expansion, whose characteristics define its consolidation in the initially affected districts still in the emergency epidemic, spreading later to other spaces receptive City (Silva et al., 2009).

In Manaus, it was found almost equal proportions of HIV-1 strains belonging to subtype B (51.6%) and F (48.4%), a finding that differs from previous results from studies conducted in urban areas of southeastern Brazil (Vicente et al., 2000).

Region	State	Subtypes	Gene(s)	References
North	Pará	B, F, D e C	*env*	Machado *et al.*, 2009
	Pará	B, F, D, CRF02_AG	*pro*	Machado *et al.*, 2009
	Pará	B^{env}/F^{pro}, F^{env}/B^{pro}, C^{env}/B^{pro}, B^{env}/D^{pro}		Machado *et al.*, 2009
	Amapá	B	*env*	Machado *et al.*, 2009
	Amapá	B e F	*pro*	Machado *et al.*, 2009
	Amazonas	B, F e B/F	*env*	Vicente *et al.*, 2000

Table 1. Geographic distribution of subtypes of HIV-1 in northern Brazil.

3. Genetic background of HIV-1 infected subjects

The pathogenesis of human immunodeficiency virus 1 infection is very complex and of course influenced by both viral and host factors (Cohen et al., 1997). Studies have focused the attention about the role of *MBL* gene variants and its serum concentration on the progression of AIDS in HIV-1-infected subjects (Garred et al., 1997; Prohászka et al., 1997).

Mannose-binding lectin (MBL) is a liver-derived pluripotent serum lectin that has a role in the host's innate immune system (Turner, 2003) by binding with high affinity to mannose or other carbohydrate components existent in viruses, bacteria and yeast (Kuipers et al., 2003). However, MBL function is directly associated with its serum concentrations which are determined by the interplay between promoter and structural gene mutations (Madsen et al., 1995; Jüliger et al., 2000).

Three mutations have been described in the structural region of the molecule (codons 52, 54 and 57) from which are derived three allelic variants named *MBL*D*, *MBL*B* and *MBL*C*, respectively. On the other hand, the wild allele is called *MBL*A* (Madsen et al., 1994). The occurrence of these variants have been associated with MBL serum deficiency and consequently to susceptibility/resistance to infection by various pathogens, including HIV-1 (Drogari-Apiranthitou et al., 1997; Garred et al., 1997; Prohászka et al., 1997; Luty et al., 1998; Hibberd et al., 1999; Peterslund et al., 2001; Klabunde et al., 2002; Roy et al., 2002; Song et al., 2003).

It was investigated the association between *MBL* gene polymorphism and the susceptibility to HIV-1 infection (Vallinoto et al., 2006). The study of 145 HIV-1-infected subjects and 99 healthy controls showed the presence of alleles *MBL*A*, *MBL*B* and *MBL*D*, whose frequencies were 69%, 22% and 09% among patients and 71%, 13% and 16% among healthy controls, respectively. The presence of the variant *MBL*B* was associated with higher plasma viral load levels, suggesting the importance of the *MBL* gene polymorphism in the clinical evolution of HIV-1-infected patients.

The prevalence of mutations in the -550 (H/L) and -221 (X/Y) mannose-binding lectin (MBL) gene promoter regions and their impact on infection by human immunodeficiency virus 1 (HIV-1) was investigated in a population of 128 HIV-1 seropositive and 97 seronegative patients (Vallinoto et al, 2008). The allele identification was performed through the sequence-specific primer polymerase chain reaction method, using primer sequences specific to each polymorphism. The evolution of the infection was evaluated through CD4+ T-lymphocyte counts and plasma viral load. The allele and haplotype frequencies among HIV-1-infected patients and seronegative healthy control patients did not show significant differences. CD4+ T-lymphocyte counts showed lower levels among seropositive patients carrying haplotypes LY, LX and HX, as compared to those carrying the HY haplotype. Mean plasma viral load was higher among seropositive patients with haplotypes LY, LX and HX than among those carrying the HY haplotype. When promoter and exon 1 mutations were matched, it was possible to identify a significantly higher viral load among HIV-1 infected individuals carrying haplotypes correlated to low serum levels of MBL. The current study shows that haplotypes related to medium and low MBL serum levels might directly influence the evolution of viral progression in patients. Therefore, it is suggested that the identification of haplotypes within the promoter region of the MBL gene among HIV-1 infected persons should be further evaluated as a prognostic tool for AIDS progression.

4. References

Avila, M.M., Pando, M.A., Carrion, G., Peralta, L.M., Salomon, H., Carrillo, M.G., Sanchez, J., Maulen, S., Hierholzer, J., Marinello, M., Negrete, M., Russell, K.L. & Carr, J.K. (2002). Two HIV-1 epidemics in Argentina: different genetic subtypes associated with different risk groups. *Journal of Acquired Immune Deficiency Syndrome. Apr* 1, 29(4):422-426, ISSN:1525-4135

Brasil. Ministério da Saúde. *Boletim Epidemiológico* (2008). AIDS, 12: 1-57, http://portal.saude.gov.br/portal/svs/visualizar_texto.cfm?idtxt=21168.

Carneiro Filho, A (1998). Manaus: fortaleza extrativismo-cidade, uma história da dinâmica urbana. *In*: Espaço e Doença Um Olhar Sobre o Amazonas. Rojas, L.B.I., Toledo, L.M. I.6.1-I.6.5, Fundação Oswaldo Cruz, Rio de Janeiro,.

Castro, E., Echeverría, G., Deibis, L., González de Salmen, B., Dos Santos Moreira, A., Guimarães, M.L., Bastos, F.I. & Morgado, M.G. (2003). Molecular epidemiology of HIV-1 in Venezuela: high prevalence of HIV-1 subtype B and identification of a B/F recombinant infection. *Journal of Acquired Immune Deficiency Syndrome*. Mar 1, 32(3): 338-344, ISSN:1525-4135

Cohen, O.J., Kinter, A. & Fauci, A.S. (1997). Host factors in the pathogenesis of HIV disease. *Immunology Reviews*, 159: 31-48, ISSN:0105-2896.

De Sa Filho, D.J., Sucupira, M.C., Caseiro, M.M., Sabino, E.C., Diaz, R.S. & Janini, L.M. (2006). Identification of two HIV type 1 circulating recombinant forms in Brazil. *AIDS Research and Human Retroviruses*, 22:1-13, ISSN: 0889-2229

Drogari-Apiranthitou, M., Fijen, C.A.P., Thiel, S., Platonov, A., Jensen, L., Dankert, J. & Kuijper, E.J. (1997). The effect of mannan-binding lectin on opsonophagocytosis of *Neisseria meningitides*. *Immunopharmacology*, 38: 93-99, ISSN:0162-3109.

Fundação de Medicina Tropical do Amazonas (2006). Coordenação Estadual do Programa de DST/Aids do Amazonas. Boletim Epidemiológico 1: 1-20.

Garred, P., Richter, C., Andersen, A.B., Madsen, H.O., Mtoni, I., Svejgaard, A. & Shao, J. (1997). Mannan-binding lectin in the sub-Saharan HIV and tuberculosis epidemics. *Scandinavian Journal of Immunology*., 46: 204–208, ISSN:0300-9475

Hibberd, M.L., Sumiya, M., Summerfield, J.A., Booy, R. & Levin, M. (1999). Association of variants of the gene for mannose-binding lectin with susceptibility to meningococcal disease. *Lancet*, 353: 1049-1053, ISSN:0099-5355

Jüliger, S., Luckner, D., Mordmüller, B., May, J., Weierich, A., Lell, B., Luty, A., Kremsner & Kun, F.J., 2000. Promoter variants of the human mannose-binding lectin gene show different binding. *Biochemical and biophysical research communications*, 275: 617-622, ISSN:0006-291X

Klabunde, J., Berger, J., Jensenius, J.C., Klinkert, M.Q., Zelck, U.E., Kremsner, P.G. & Kun, J.F. (2000). Schistosoma mansoni: adhesion of mannan-binding lectin to surface glycoproteins of cercariae and adult worms. *Experimental Parasitology*, 95: 231–239, ISSN:0014-4894

Kuipers, S., Aerts, P.C. & Van Dijk, H. (2003). Differential microorganism-induced mannose-binding lectin activation. *FEMS Immunology and Medical Microbiology*, 36: 33-39, ISSN:0928-8244

Luty, A.J., Kun, J.F. & Kremsner, P.G. (1998). Mannose-binding lectin plasma levels and gene polymorphisms in *Plasmodium falciparum* malaria. *Journal of Infectious Diseases*, 178: 1221-1224, ISSN:0022-1899

Machado, L.F., Ishak, M.O., Vallinoto, A.C., Lemos, J.A., Azevedo, V.N., Moreira, M.R., Souza, M.I., Fernandes, L.M., Souza, L.L. & Ishak, R (2009). Molecular epidemiology of HIV type 1 in northern Brazil: identification of subtypes C and D and the introduction of CRF02_AG in the Amazon region of Brazil. *AIDS Research and Human Retroviruses*, 25(10): 961-966, ISSN: 0889-2229

Madsen, H.O., Garred, P., Kurtzhals, J.A., Lamm, L.U., Ryder, L.P., Thiel, S. & Svejgaard, A. (1994). A new frequent allele is the missing link in the structural polymorphism of the human mannan-binding protein. *Immunogenetics*, 40: 37–44, ISSN:0093-7711

Madsen, H.O., Garred, P., Thiel, S., Kurtzhals, J.A.L.,Lamm, L.U., Ryder, L.P. & Svejgaard, A. (1995). Interplay between promoter and structural gene variants control basal serum level of Mannan-Binding Protein. *Journal of Immunology*, 155: 3013-3020, ISSN:0022-1767

Marquina, S., Leitner, T., Rabinovich, R.D., Benetucci, J., Libonatti, O. & Albert, J. (1996). Coexistence of subtypes B, F, and as B/F env recombinant of HIV type 1 in Buenos Aires Argentina. *AIDS Research and Human Retroviruses*. Nov 20, 12(17):1651-1654, ISSN: 0889-2229.

McCutchan, F.E. (2006). Global epidemiology of HIV. *Journal of Medical Virology.*, 78(Suppl 1): S7-S12, ISSN:0146-6615

Monteiro, J.P., Alcantara, L.C., de Oliveira, T., Oliveira, A.M., Melo, M.A., Brites, C. & Galvão-Castro, B. (2009). Genetic variability of human immunodeficiency virus-1 in Bahia state, Northeast, Brazil: High diversity of HIV genotypes. *Journal of Medical Virology*, 81(3): 391–399, ISSN:0146-6615

Morgado, M.G., Guimarães, M.L., Gripp, C.B., Costa, C.I., Neves Jr, I., Veloso, V.G., Linhares-Carvalho, M.I., Castello-Branco, L.R., Bastos, F.I., Kuiken, C., Castilho, E.A., Galvão-Castro, B. & Bongertz, V (1998). Molecular epidemiology of HIV-1 in Brazil: high prevalence of HIV-1 subtype B and identification of an HIV-1 subtype D infection in the city of Rio de Janeiro, Brazil. Evandro Chagas Hospital AIDS Clinical Research Group. *Journal of Acquired Immune Deficiency Syndrome*, Aug 15, 18(5): 488-494, ISSN:1525-4135

Navas, M.C., Letourneur, F., Gomas, E., Boshell, J. & Saragosti, S (1999). Analysis of the V3 loop sequences from 12 HIV type 1-infected patients from Colombia, South America. *AIDS Research and Human Retroviruses*, Aug 10, 15(12): 1141-1144, ISSN: 0889-2229

Peterslund, N.A., Koch, C., Jensenius, J.C. & Thiel, S. (2001). Deficiency of mannan-binding lectin (MBL), association with severe infections after chemotherapy. *Lancet*, 358: 637-638, ISSN:0099-5355

Plantier, J.C., Leoz, M., Dickerson, J.E., De Oliveira, F., Cordonnier, F., Lemée, V., Damond, F., Robertson, D.L., Simon, F (2009). A new human immunodeficiency virus derived from gorillas. *Nature Medicine*, Aug, 15(8): 871-872, ISSN:1078-8956

Prohaszka, Z., Thiel, S., Ujhelyi, E., Szlavik, J., Banhegyi, D., Fust, G. (1997). Mannan-binding lectin serum concentrations in HIV-infected patients are influenced by the stage of disease. *Immunology Letters*, 58: 171-175, ISSN:0165-2478

Ramos, A., Tanuri, A., Schechter, M., Rayfield, M.A., Hu, D.J., Cabral, M.C., Bandea, C.I., Baggs, J. & Pieniazek, D (1999). Dual and recombinant infections: an integral part of the HIV-1 epidemic in Brazil. *Emerging Infectious Diseases*, 5(1): 65-74, ISSN:1080-6040

Roy, S., Knox, K., Segal, S., Griffiths, D., Moore, C.E., Welsh, K.I., Smarason, A., Day, N.P., Mcpheat, W.L., Crook, D.W. & Hill, A.V.S. (2002). MBL genotype and risk of invasive pneumococcal disease: a case-control study. *Lancet*, 359: 1569-1573, ISSN:0165-2478.

Sabino, E.C., Diaz, R.S., Brigido, L.F., Learn, G.H., Mullins, J.I., Reingold, A.L., Duarte, A.J., Mayer, A. & Busch, M.P. (1996). Distribution of HIV-1 subtypes seen in an AIDS clinic in Sao Paulo City, Brazil. *AIDS*, 10(13): 1579-84, ISSN:0953-0096

Sanabani, S., Kleine Neto, W., Kalmar, E.M., Diaz, R.S., Janini, L.M. & Sabino, E.C. (2006). Analysis of the near full length genomes of HIV-1 subtypes B, F and BF recombinant from a cohort of 14 patients in Sao Paulo, Brazil. *Infection, Genetics and Evolution*, 6:368-377, ISSN:1567-1348

Sanabani, S.S., Pastena, E.R., Neto, W.K., Martinez, V.P. & Sabino, E.C. (2010). Characterization and frequency of a newly identified HIV-1 BF1 intersubtype circulating recombinant form in São Paulo, Brazil. *Virology Journal*, 16, 7:74, ISSN:1743-422X

Santos, A.F., Sousa, T.M., Soares, E.A., Sanabani, S., Martinez, A.M., Sprinz, E., Silveira, J., Sabino, E.C., Tanuri, A. & Soares, M.A (2006). Characterization of a new circulating recombinant form comprising HIV-1 subtypes C and B in southern Brazil. *AIDS*, 20: 2011-2019, ISSN:0953-0096

Silva, L.C., Santos, E.M., Silva, Neto, A.L., Miranda, A.E., Talhari, S. & Toledo, L.M. (2009). Pattern of HIV/AIDS infection in Manaus, State of Amazonas, between 1986 and 2000. *Revista da Sociedade Brasileria de Medicina Tropical*, Sep-Oct,42(5): 543-50, ISSN:0037-8682

Soares, E.A., Santos, R.P., Pellegrini, J.A., Sprinz, E., Tanuri, A. & Soares, M.A. (2003). Epidemiologic and molecular characterization of human immunodeficiency virus type 1 in southern Brazil. *Journal of Acquired Immune Deficiency Syndrome*, 34: 520–526, ISSN:1525-4135

Song, L.H., Binh, V.Q., Duy, D.N., Jüliger, S., Bock, T.C., Luty, A.J.F., Kremsner, P.G. & Kun, J.F.J. (2003). Mannose-binding lectin gene polymorphisms and hepatitis B virus infection in Vietnamese patients. *Mutation Research*, 522: 119-125, ISSN:0027-5107

Tanuri A, Vicente AC, Otsuki K, Ramos CA, Ferreira OC Jr, Schechter M, Janini LM, Pieniazek D & Rayfield M.A. (1999). Genetic variation and susceptibilities to protease inhibitors among subtype B and F isolates in Brazil. *Antimicrobial Agents Chemotherapy*, 43(2): 253-258, ISSN:0066-4804

Taylor, B.S., Sobieszczyk, M.E., McCutchan, F.E., Hammer, S.M. (2008). The challenge of HIV-1 subtype diversity. *The New England Journal of Medicine*, Apr 10, 358(15): 1590-1602, ISSN:0028-4793

Turner, M.W. (2003). The role of mannose-binding lectin in health and disease. *Molecular Immunology*, 40: 423-429, ISSN:0161-5890

Vallinoto, A.C., Menezes-Costa, M.R., Alves, A.E., Machado, L.F., Azevedo, V.N., Souza, L.L., Ishak, M.O.G. & Ishak, R. (2006). Mannose-binding lectin gene polymorphism and its impact on human immunodeficiency virus 1 infection. *Molecular Immunology*, *43*: 1358-1362, ISSN:0161-5890

Vallinoto, A.C.R., Muto, N.A., Alves, A.E.M., Machado, L.F.A., Azevedo, V.N., Souza, L.L.B., Ishak, M.O.G. & Ishak, R. (2008). Characterization of the polymorphisms in the mannose-binding lectin gene promoter among human immunodeficiency virus 1 infected subjects. *Mem Inst Oswaldo Cruz*, 103: 645–649, ISSN:1678-8060

Vicente, A.C., Otsuki, K., Silva, N.B., Castilho, M.C., Barros, F.S., Pieniazek, D., et al. (2000). The HIV epidemic in the Amazon Basin is driven by prototypic and recombinant HIV-1 subtypes B and F. *Journal of Acquired Immune Deficiency Syndrome*, 23: 327–331, ISSN:1525-4135.

Saliva Testing as a Practical Tool for Rapid HIV Screening

H. Blake[1], P. Leighton[2] and S. Sharma[3]
[1]*Division of Nursing, University of Nottingham, B Floor (South Block Link), Queen's Medical Centre, NG7 2HA, Nottingham,*
[2]*Division of Primary Care, University of Nottingham, Room 2104, C Floor South 3Block, Queen's Medical Centre, NG7 2UH, Nottingham*
[3]*Department of Psychology, University of Strathclyde, G1 1XQ, Glasgow,*
[1,2]*United Kingdom*
[3]*Scotland*

1. Introduction

Whilst the annual number of new HIV infections is steadily declining, levels of new infections overall are high and the number of people living with HIV has increased worldwide. An estimated 73,000 people in the UK are living with HIV, of which it is estimated that 24,000 are undiagnosed or unaware of their HIV status (Health Protection Agency, 2007). The prevalence of undiagnosed HIV infection would therefore seem a key driver for increased and routine HIV testing, both to lessen the potential for unwitting transmission of HIV and to support early detection and timely access to medical care in those infected. It has been shown that late diagnosis of HIV infection, resulting in delayed patient management, is associated with poorer survival (Losina et al., 2009). In the UK, the National Strategy for Sexual Health and HIV (Department of Health, 2001) aims to reduce the prevalence of undiagnosed HIV by increasing screening.

This is a rapidly advancing field and whilst it is beyond the scope of this chapter to encapsulate all the current evidence in this field, a brief overview is presented of saliva testing as a diagnostic tool, the benefits and the caveats. The contexts in which saliva testing for HIV are currently conducted is considered both in the UK and internationally. The evidence for the sensitivity and specificity of this method will be considered. Attitudes of recipients towards rapid HIV screening, in particular saliva testing, are considered together with attitudes towards the contexts in which testing is undertaken.

2. Diagnosis of HIV/AIDs

HIV screening is undertaken for a number of purposes, the UNAIDS/WHO summarise these as i) testing for screening blood, ii) testing for epidemiological surveillance and iii) testing for diagnosing infected individuals (UNAIDS, 1997). A variety of specific tests might be used to these ends. The British HIV Association (BHIVA) states that, "a potentially important mechanism for limiting the HIV epidemic is the widespread use of HIV testing in a variety of clinical settings," but provides no specific guidance on how the testing should be done (BHVA, 2005). The selection of the most appropriate test, and testing protocol, should not only be informed by test sensitivity and specificity, but also by a number of economic and logistic factors (Branson, 2003). The following sections outline some key information relating to procedures for HIV testing, categories of HIV testing, and HIV testing guidelines, and consider technical and process issues relating to HIV testing.

2.1 Testing for HIV

HIV testing has evolved from initial concerns, in the mid/early 1980s, for screening the supply of donated blood, to now reflect a broader range of concerns which include clinical diagnosis and strategic public health intervention (Branson, 2000a, 2000b). UNAIDS/WHO have identified four distinct categories of HIV testing: Diagnostic testing, Voluntary counselling and testing (VCT), Routinised testing in specific setting, and Mandatory testing.

Diagnostic HIV testing is testing undertaken where signs and symptoms related to an HIV infection are observed in any individual. Testing is carried out to ensure timely clinical diagnosis, and to ensure the provision of adequate clinical support and services. People with certain diseases, such as tuberculosis and any other sexually transmitted disease, are also tested for HIV infection on a regular basis to this end.

Voluntary counselling and testing, also referred to as 'client focused testing', categorises those programmes of HIV testing which are designed to promote HIV awareness and to broaden access to HIV testing. Such testing is carried out in the absence of individual symptoms and is combined with group and individual counselling around HIV issues to raise awareness and educate in relevant health, and health behaviour, areas. This kind of testing programme is often undertaken with those who are perceived to be at high-risk of exposure to the HIV virus, or those who are concerned that they have been recently exposed to HIV. Testing is provided in local health and community settings, and pre and post-test counselling is offered to all those being testing. Pre-test counselling is often delivered in group settings, with post-test and follow-up counselling delivered on a one-to-one basis. UNAIDS/WHO identify VCT as the most effective approach to testing for achieving behaviour change to prevent HIV transmission in public settings.

Routine HIV testing of those accessing clinical or medical services is often carried out in those settings where high risk client groups are prevalent. Such testing is carried out with the purpose of early (asymptomatic) identification, with associated benefits for reduced risk of unwitting transmission of the virus. Carried out in community health centres, specialist clinics or hospitals settings such testing includes that undertaken in sexual health clinics with people who are undergoing diagnostic testing for other sexually transmitted diseases. It also incorporates the testing of intravenous drug users in primary and secondary care settings. Routine testing of this kind often utilises rapid HIV tests, which are described in more detail in section 3.

Mandatory HIV testing may be carried out for all donors prior to procedures involving transfusion of blood, bodily fluids or any organ transplant. In some countries, HIV testing is compulsorily carried out at the time of immigration, pregnancy and during routine medical check-ups of military personnel.

The individual, and health service cost, benefits associated with early detection and early medical intervention in cases of HIV infection offer a strong argument for routine testing, even amongst those populations where the incidence of HIV is low (Paltiel, 2006). Whilst evidence for screening programmes reducing the transmission of HIV is unclear (Paltiel, 2006), a range of studies indicate that those who are aware of their HIV status amend their behaviour so as to limit the risk of HIV transmission to others (Marks et al., 2005; Crepaz et al., 2006; Chou et al., 2005).

In the United States (U.S.) in 2006, in an effort to improve the identification of HIV-positive individuals, the Center for Diseases Control and Prevention (CDC) released their current HIV testing guidelines. These recommended routine testing for those age 13 to 64 years regardless of risk factors, unless testing is specifically declined by the individual (opt-out testing) (Branson et al., 2006). In the U.S. the following criteria apply: opt-out HIV screening is recommended for patients in all healthcare settings, with people at high risk for HIV infection screened for HIV at least annually. Here, separate written consent for HIV testing is not required; general consent for medical care should be considered sufficient to encompass consent for HIV testing. Finally, prevention counselling should not be required with HIV diagnostic testing or as part of HIV screening programmes in healthcare settings (Branson et al., 2006). Although one-third of people with HIV infection in the UK remain undiagnosed, current UK guidelines recommend opt-out testing only for pregnant women and people attending genitourinary clinics (Hamill et al., 2007).

2.2 HIV tests

HIV testing involves the detection of antibodies produced by the body in an unsuccessful attempt to fight HIV infection, such antibodies being more easily detected than the virus itself. Testing can be carried out on whole blood, plasma, serum, urine, dried blood spots and saliva samples, but might only be carried out after a 3-8 week period following infection (Schopper & Vercauteren, 1996). During this 3-8 week window the HIV antigen is rarely identified - bar in exceptional circumstances at the peak of high circulation of virus particles (Carne, 1988; Chin, et al., 2007).

Initial developments in HIV screening centred upon the need to ensure that donated blood remained free of the HIV virus. A *testing paradigm* thus emerged to protect the supply of donated blood, a paradigm marked by "tests with high sensitivity, suitable for batch processing of high volumes of specimens in centralised laboratories with specialised equipment." (Branson, 2000a). The enzyme-linked immunosorbent assay (ELISA) was indicative of this; a screening test for blood, efficient in large-scale hospital settings and reliant upon specialist laboratory equipment. The ELISA is the most appropriate, and most commonly used, screening test for samples greater than 100 per day; the ELISA is most appropriate for population level surveillance of HIV infection (UNAIDS, 1997). Performed by trained medical staff the ELISA test is reliable, but incurs substantial costs and might only offer results a few days after testing. Whilst this cost and delay are less important in screening donated blood, for other forms of testing they might act as a barrier.

During the late 1980s and early 1990s the benefits of *voluntary counselling and testing* were increasingly recognised and other testing algorithms were developed to meet this end (Branson, 2000a). Concerns about false positives from the ELISA test led the U.S. Public Health Service recommending secondary testing with the Western Blot (WB) to ensure accuracy. Although once again, the significant time delay associated with this combination of tests, of up to 2 weeks before test results are returned to patients, was a significant barrier. Also ELISA both in isolation and in combination with the WB test has limited suitability for remote or smaller clinical settings where resources are limited and access to adequate facilities is restricted (McCarthy et al., 1993; Owens et al., 1996). With particular concern for testing in the developing world, and to reflect a growing number of simple and rapid assays, the UN/WHO offers an informative typology of testing combinations (UNAIDS, 1997; Branson, 2000a, 2003).

For blood screening, population surveillance (of high risk groups) and diagnosis of individuals from high risk populations (who are displaying signs/symptoms of HIV infection) a single screening assay is adequate; and, a reactive test should be considered sufficient for a HIV positive diagnosis. For population surveillance (low and mid-risk groups), asymptomatic individual diagnosis (high risk group) and symptomatic diagnosis (low and mid-risk social group) a second screening assay should follow an initial reactive test; if both initial and second assays are reactive then the specimen is considered positive. For asymptomatic diagnosis (low and mid-risk social group) a third screening assay should be carried out following initial and second reactive tests; the specimen is considered positive if the third test is also reactive.

2.3 Technical and process issues

Above all, HIV testing should be carried in accordance with ethical principles designed to protect human rights. Testing should be carried out in a confidential manner and the person being tested should be fully informed about the nature and procedures of the test. Tests should be undertaken with caution since clinicians may be both civilly and criminally liable if they take a blood sample for HIV testing without disclosing to the patient (i) the nature of the test, (ii) the possible consequences of a positive result, and (iii) without obtaining informed consent (Sherrad & Gatt, 1987).

Further, where a positive HIV test manifests, appropriate psychological counselling should be provided to the diagnosed individual (WHO, 2004). Other technical and process issues include consideration of the cost-effectiveness of testing, of the quality of tests and testing procedures, and of the potential for home testing and the associated benefits and caveats.

Cost-effectiveness

Evidence from the U.S. suggests that routine, voluntary HIV testing is not only of crucial public health importance but is also economically justified (Walensky et al., 2007). The cost of HIV testing kits is variable, although this expenditure accounts for a substantial portion of the budget in national AIDS programmes. Selecting the most appropriate and cost-effective products for each particular setting therefore includes careful consideration of a range of factors including cost of test kit, storage, equipment maintenance and training of personnel.

Quality of testing procedures

Ensuring that quality is maintained and standard operating procedures are followed is critical to the generation of reliable results. The majority of HIV diagnostic products perform very well when used according to specific instructions. However, there is a risk that kits may be produced that do not meet exacting standards for quality, or make fraudulent claims for endorsement by WHO or the U.S. Food and Drink Administration (Kurtzweil, 1999). This remains an ongoing challenge.

Home testing

Home testing has positive implications for offering an alternative to people who might otherwise not seek testing in traditional health care facilities. For example, in some countries, a high uptake has been achieved by delivering both HIV counselling and testing at home, in the highest uptake in rural areas, in young people and groups with low educational attainment; this has resulted in substantial reductions in existing inequalities in accessing such services (Mutale et al., 2010). However, there are serious caveats associated with home testing which must be considered and balanced against any perceived benefits. Firstly, there is a potential that such kits may be fraudulent (e.g. Kurtzweil, 1999) or less accurate than those administered by trained staff. Secondly, there may be a risk of abuse if individuals are forced to take tests against their will. Finally, there a need for immediate confirmation of results and also access to counselling for those with a positive test result. In the UK little HIV testing is currently performed outside GUM and antenatal settings (Tweed et al., 2010).

3. Rapid testing and saliva testing

The introduction of rapid and 'point of care' testing in HIV was primarily to increase identification of HIV infected individuals, to enable inexpensive and convenient methods of testing amongst rural, outreach and at-risk populations, and to improve consumer experience of the testing procedure (Holt, 2009). Such rapid tests use finger-stick capillary whole blood (FSB) or oral fluid (OF), thus avoiding the need for venous blood sampling and centrifugation (Pavie et al., 2010). Specific benefits associated with rapid testing include immediate communication of test results (in standard tests between 25% and 33% of those tested do not return to receive their results), and advantages in immediate medical staff awareness of HIV status so as to limit the potential for HIV transmission during medical procedures (Kane, 1999; Branson, 2000a).

Rapid tests modified to use oral fluid samples obviate the need for either venepuncture or finger prick blood analysis (Hamill et al., 2007). Oral fluid HIV tests offer additional advantages due to their non-invasive nature, can be performed anywhere, do not require specialist phlebotomy training or equipment, and reduce biohazardous risk (Delaney et al., 2006). Rapid, reliable and affordable tests, requiring no equipment and minimal training, are now also available for HIV infection in developing countries (Peeling & Mabey, 2010).

3.1 Nature of rapid testing and saliva testing

In recent decades, a number of rapid test assays have been developed that enable HIV antibody status to be determined quickly, efficiently and less invasively than traditional forms of testing. Most rapid tests can be conveniently carried out 'on site' by someone with basic training and for this reason these are often referred to as 'point-of-care testing' (Kendrick et al., 2005). These tests are designed to detect antibodies in several different body fluids including whole blood from finger-prick blood, plasma, urine, or saliva. Rapid tests are simple to perform, can be conducted in rural settings without laboratory equipment, and remove the need to process and store specimens and transport them from the field (Pascoe et al., 2009).

Rapid tests rely on samples of blood taken from fingertip or saliva sample obtained by rubbing an absorbent pad across the lower and upper gums in the mouth. Obtained blood or saliva sample is then transferred into a plastic device already containing a developer solution, followed by the insertion of an assay test strip into the device. After a brief waiting period of approximately 15-20 minutes the appearance of two lines on the test strip is interpreted as a positive test result, indicating the presence of HIV-1 antibodies; however, a single line indicates a negative test result, and no visible lines imply an invalid test.

The speed with which test results can be produced make rapid HIV tests very popular and extremely useful particularly in public outreach settings (Spielberg et al., 2005). In such settings there may be limited access to a HIV test centre and furthermore, there may be a reluctance to be assessed for HIV infection amongst certain groups (e.g. sex-workers, drug-injectors). Moreover, it is not uncommon that individuals who have agreed to take a HIV test, do not return for their conventional laboratory blood test results and thus remain unaware of their HIV virus carrier status, presenting a danger to society as potential HIV transmitters (Galvan et al., 2004). Use of rapid saliva tests also have the potential to prevent HIV infections occurring in health workers due to handling of blood during standard ELISA, WB or rapid blood tests.

The unique features manifested by all rapid tests are their non-invasive testing procedure and the immediacy of producing results. Another advanced characteristic of rapid tests is the level of anonymity offered since the saliva, blood or urine specimen can be collected at home, sent to the laboratory for testing and results declared via the telephone, without a need to visit the clinic in person.

3.2 Diagnostic accuracy of HIV rapid tests

All diagnostic tests have limitations and sometimes their use may produce erroneous or questionable results. The accuracy of tests is often described in terms of 'sensitivity' (the percentage of results that will be positive when HIV is not present) and 'specificity' (the percentage of results that will be negative when HIV is not present). False positives occur when the test incorrectly indicates that HIV is present in a non-infected person. Conversely, false negatives occur when the test incorrectly indicates that HIV is absent in an infected person.

In a review of the risks and benefits of HIV screening, the U.S. Preventive Services Task Force concluded in 2005 that, "...the use of repeatedly reactive enzyme immunoassay followed by confirmatory Western blot or immunoflourescent assay remains the standard method for diagnosing HIV-1 infection. A large study of HIV testing in 725 U.S. laboratories reported a sensitivity of 99.7% and a specificity of 98.5% for enzyme immunoassay, and studies in U.S. blood donors reported specificities of 99.8% and greater than 99.99%. With confirmatory Western blot, the chance of a false-positive identification in a low-prevalence setting is about 1 in 250,000 (95% CI, 1 in 173,000 to 1 in 379,000)" (Chou et al., 2005).

The specificity rate outlined above for enzyme immunoassay screening tests indicates that, in every 1,000 positive HIV test results, there will be around 15 false positive results. However, confirming the test result (e.g. repeating the test, if this option is available) may reduce the likelihood of a false positive to just 1 result in every 250,000 tests. The sensitivity rating outlined above indicates that, in every 1,000 negative HIV test results, there will be 3 false negative results. Nevertheless, the high negative predictive value of these tests is extremely high, meaning that a negative test result will be correct more than 9,997 times in 10,000 (99.97% of the time). Due to the high negative predictive value of HIV screening tests, the CDC recommends that a negative test results be considered conclusive evidence that an individual does not have HIV.

Non-specific reactions, hypergammaglobulinemia, or the presence of antibodies directed to other infectious agents that may be antigenically similar to HIV can produce false positive results. Auto-immune diseases, such as systemic lupus erythematosus, have also rarely caused false positive results. Most false negative results are due to the window period; other factors, such as post-exposure prophylaxis, can rarely produce false negatives (Hare et al., 2004).

Rapid tests have been used for more than two decades to test serum and plasma, particularly in developing countries and for emergency diagnosis. They are simple to use and have high specificity, however, false positives do occur and they have been criticised in previous years for lacking in sensitivity relative to reference enzyme immunoassays (EIA/ELISA), particularly during primary HIV infection and infection by variant strains (Makuwa et al., 2002). There is, however, research evidence to indicate that rapid HIV tests produce results of comparable sensitivity and specificity to the ELISA test (Franco-Paredes et al., 2006; Greenwald et al., 2006; Branson, 2000a). Laboratory testing of 1266 specimens at rural peripheral laboratories of varied combinations of seven rapid HIV tests even showed a specificity of 100% (Stetler et al., 1997). Empirical studies have shown promising findings in a range of settings and populations including HIV positive individuals (DeBattista et al., 2007), HIV negative individuals (Makasso, 2005), sexual health clinic attenders (DeBattista et al., 2007), pregnant adult women in Namibia (Hamers et al., 2008), acute care (Lee et al, 2011) and adults presenting for voluntary testing elsewhere in the developing world (Pascoe et al., 2009).

Furthermore, whilst some early work has suggested that salivary testing should be recommended only for epidemiological studies (Mortimer & Parry, 1992), more recent studies have continued to demonstrate that rapid oral fluid tests show a high standard of sensitivity and specificity (e.g. Debattista et al., 2007; Hamers et al., 2008; Delaney et al., 2006). Independent performance data for 4 FDA approved rapid HIV tests (Franco-Paredes et al., 2006) and a wider range of rapid tests (Branson, 2000a) highlight product testing with both sensitivity and specificity outcomes of 100% (Oraquick and Retrocell HIV-1/2) (Branson, 2000a). Data from 2006 showed that in testing, sensitivity and specificity exceeded 99% in 4 FDA approved tests (with the exception of Reveal G2 Plasma test where specificity is 98.6%) (Franco-Paredes et al., 2006). Comparisons between rapid HIV tests are inconsistent. It has been suggested that there may be differences in diagnostic accuracy, with tests being less sensitive on oral fluid than on finger-stick whole blood and less sensitive on finger-stick whole blood than on serum (Pavie et al., 2010). More recently, in a direct comparison of the performance of all 6 tests currently approved by the FDA for use in the U.S. (using whole blood, oral fluid, serum, and plasma specimens), it has been shown that *all* rapid tests have statistically equivalent performance characteristics, based on overlapping confidence intervals for sensitivity and specificity, compared with conventional ELISA (Delaney et al., 2011).

It should be noted that although rapid tests using saliva have been shown to have high sensitivity and specificity parameters (Delaney et al., 2011), these are essentially brief screening tests and it has long been recognised that in cases where the first screening test utilised saliva, the diagnosis should be reconfirmed through a rapid test that involves blood testing (Andersson et al., 1997). In fact, it is now generally accepted that a second confirmatory test which detects the presence of a specific type of antibody to HIV 1/2 *must* follow (Franco-Paredes, et al., 2006). WHO recommends that for diagnostic purposes, two assays be used with a third test for discrepant results (Strategy II and III); the first test must have the highest sensitivity and the second test a similar or higher specificity (UNAIDS/WHO, 2004). Accuracy may be altered in pregnancy, and to improve diagnostic accuracy and to reduce false-positive results it may be necessary to use two rapid tests during labour and delivery (Pai et al., 2007). Some further limitations have been identified with oral fluid assays (e.g. unlikely to detect those in early stages of HIV infection or with reduced viral load) these limitations also apply to other rapid assays (Pascoe et al., 2009).

A large number of studies have been published to date on various aspects of test performance specifically for oral mucosal transudate (OMT) and saliva tests. A number of brief narrative reviews published between 1994-2006 have focused predominantly on the description of oral rapid test technologies, although this early work has not evaluated diagnostic accuracy. Two more recent systematic reviews on diagnostic accuracy have been conducted (Wesolowski, 2006; Pai, 2007). These include a review undertaken by the CDC as part of a post-marketing surveillance of one rapid test (Wesolowski, 2006) and a systematic review focused exclusively on performance of all rapid tests in pregnant women (Pai, 2007). A recent meta-analysis has evaluated OMT, saliva based rapid and point of care tests in at-risk populations worldwide from 1986-2011 (Balram & Pai, 2010). This data provided evidence of good overall performance of oral fluid-based HIV tests in global settings. The authors recommended these oral rapid tests as first line screening alternatives to blood-based rapid test and suggest their enhanced use in global expanded HIV testing initiatives (Balram & Pai, 2010). Furthermore, rapid testing is deemed to be suitable for use in community-based clinical research settings, to assess eligibility both for trial participation and for the provision of on-site voluntary counselling and testing services (Everett et al., 2009).

3.3 Acceptability of HIV rapid tests

Non-invasive rapid HIV tests have been consistently shown to be a preferred method of testing amongst varied population groups in both youth (Peralta et al., 2001; Pugatch et al., 2001) and adults, including men who have sex with men (MSM) (Sy et al., 1998; Chen et al., 2010) and injecting drug users (Colfax et al., 2002; Greensides et al., 2003; Spielberg et al., 2000). Recent research has also considered the acceptability of testing amongst healthcare professionals.

Youth populations

Although universal testing of adolescents is currently recommended in the U.S., previous studies have demonstrated that only 41% to 61% of adolescents offered a non-rapid HIV test agree to testing (Mehta et al., 2007; Goodman et al., 1994). Furthermore, only between one and two-thirds of adolescents who are tested return to receive their results and post-test counselling (Goodman et al., 1994; Ilegbodu et al., 1994; Lazebnik et al., 2001; Tsu et al., 2002). A recent study by Mullins et al. (2010) showed that 70% of adolescents preferred rapid to traditional HIV testing, and that rapid testers were more likely to receive their results within the follow-up period. This study suggested that for adolescents non-invasive testing may have a greater impact on their choice of a rapid method than the availability of same day test results. A high preference for rapid oral tests in comparison to invasive blood tests has also been demonstrated elsewhere (Pugatch et al., 2001; Peralta et al., 2001). Studies of rapid testing in specific settings have shown that paediatric emergency departments have been highly rated by adolescents aged 14-21 years, as a preferred location for rapid HIV testing. This supports the need for increased development of prevention and testing programs in this setting (Haines et al., 2011). It has been acknowledged that rapid testing should be followed by HIV prevention opportunities and rapid linkage to care (Peralta et al., 2001).

Adult populations

A high level of acceptance for rapid testing and a preference for rapid oral tests in comparison to invasive blood tests has been demonstrated in adult 'at risk' populations

including MSM, high-risk heterosexual populations and injecting drug users (Speilberg et al., 2000; Greensides et al., 2003; Colfax et al., 2002; Sy et al., 1998, Chen et al., 2010).
Research has shown that the majority of adults tested (95%) preferred results to be disclosed by telephone, again highlighting the importance of privacy issues in testing procedures (Speilberg et al., 2000). Positive implications of, rapid testing also include potential for, and increased monitoring and awareness of HIV related risk-behaviour (Speilberg et al., 2000). In MSM, injecting drug users and high risk heterosexuals attending a sexual health clinic (Greensides et al., 2003; Colfax et al., 2002), concerns have been raised about rapid testing in relation to associated costs, privacy issues, accuracy and reliability of results, access to post-test counselling and information, lack of access to testing, and lack of knowledge about testing centres and procedures (Greensides et al., 2003). It has been suggested that concerns regarding the accuracy of the rapid test might limit test acceptance and should be addressed during pre-test information procedures (Merchant et al., 2009).
Nevertheless, despite these concerns, a strong preference has been identified for non-invasive quick testing procedures, in particular, rapid oral testing methods (Chen et al., 2010). Although rapid testing procedures appear to be preferred in these populations, a large proportion of these individuals (almost half) remain unaware of the availability of home collection kits for HIV testing in areas where these are accessible (Greensides et al., 2003; Colfax et al., 2002). Many individuals 'at risk' have reported that they would test more frequently if testing was available for clinic or home use (Chen et al., 2010). In certain populations, such as MSM, those who prefer rapid testing may be significantly more likely to have some formal education, to have discussed testing with a sexual partner, to be aware of rapid testing, and to have had a previous test (Cohall et al., 2010).
Research has investigated the potential for offering rapid testing in commercial and community venues, although a significant number of barriers have been raised. Again, concerns have been raised about the lack of confidentiality and privacy for testing in social venues, and about the potential lack of post-test support for those who test positive (Prost et al., 2007).

Healthcare populations

Studies of HIV testing have mainly considered *patient* preferences, although recent work has investigated the attitudes of *healthcare* staff towards testing (Arbelaez et al., 2009; Sahoni et al., 2010). For example, it has been shown that hospital staff satisfaction and overall attitudes towards HIV testing program in an emergency department is high, and that healthcare staff attitudes do not represent a barrier to program implementation (Sahoni et al., 2010). Rapid advances in technology have also led to widening of training opportunities for rapid testing across geographically remote healthcare facilities (Knapp et al., 2011). Further, research is emerging which considers the role of various healthcare professionals rapid diagnostic testing for HIV in various regions of the world (e.g. oral health care workers; Patton et al., 2011). Whilst conducting rapid screening in the dental clinic setting has been identified as a viable option (Dietz et al., 2008; Patton et al., 2011), oral healthcare professionals have expressed a lack of confidence that graduating dentists have the skills and willingness to conduct HIV counselling and testing in dental practice; in fact lack of training in prevention counselling has been identified as a primary barrier (Patton et al., 2002). Additional challenges to rapid testing have been identified in a range of medical settings including insufficient staffing, inadequate privacy or space, associated administration, time limitations and competing priorities.

4. Conclusions

This is a rapidly advancing field and as such this chapter presents an overview of the key issues with selected evidence. In conclusion, it seems that rapid screening tests and/or alternative biological samples (such as oral fluid) are now thought to be effective in HIV prevention strategies by reaching a larger population through improved accessibility and general consent in approaches to screening, immediate referral of HIV positives for medical treatment and partner notification. Oral fluid testing has been implemented in a range of settings. The test appears to perform well in field settings, and can be considered a good alternative to blood samples, suitable for use in epidemiologic surveys aiming to estimate HIV prevalence in general populations and in high risk groups. There are several limitations in that oral fluid assays may be unlikely to detect those in early stages of HIV infection or with reduced viral load, and have shown altered accuracy in pregnancy; however, such limitations also apply to other rapid assays.

Research has suggested that in adults the most important factors in HIV testing are test accuracy, time to results and privacy of results. Studies have also suggested that patients express a preference for oral testing over venepuncture sampling since it is rapid and less invasive, although preferences may vary in different settings. Less invasive methods are preferred also in youth. Indeed, offering less invasive rapid testing to at-risk youth may assist clinicians in increasing the proportion of teens who agree to undergo testing and receive their test result. In general rapid testing is better accepted by patients in both developed and resource-limited settings. Point of care tests specifically assist in making testing accessible in areas with limited laboratory facilities. These tests have the potential for reducing the number of people who do not return to clinics to learn of their test result, and thus reduce the proportion of infected individuals who remain unaware of their diagnosis.

Overall, the majority of studies have demonstrated high sensitivity and specificity of oral fluid-based rapid HIV test in comparison with routinely utilized methods. With recent research showing comparable accuracy for a range of currently approved tests and specimen types, it may be characteristics such as convenience, time to result, shelf life, and cost that will be likely determining factors for selection of a rapid screening test for a specific application (Delaney et al., 2011). This suggests that rapid tests with well documented performance characteristics should be made available in public health and clinical settings.

Specifically, it seems that saliva specimens can be easily collected under difficult field conditions with minimal training and provide a valuable alternative to testing blood for HIV-seroprevalence studies. Salivary testing for HIV may therefore be a convenient and potentially accurate epidemiological tool, although should be used with caution since single test systems may be less appropriate to diagnose HIV infection in an individual without follow-up testing. There is a drive for continual improvement of test performance, such that is has been suggested that all initial positive findings should be repeated by second test method with a second confirmatory specimen found positive prior to informing the patient. This may serve to mitigate the emotional distress and unnecessary treatments associated with false positive HIV testing.

5. References

Andersson, S., da Silva, Z., Norrgren, H., Dias, F. & Biberfeld, G. (1997). Field evaluation of alternative testing strategies for diagnosis and differentiation of HIV-1 and HIV-2 infections in an HIV-1 and HIV-2-prevalent area, *AIDS,* 11 (15), 1815-1822.

Arbelaez, C., Wright, E., Losina, E. & et al. (2009). Emergency provider attitudes and barriers to universal HIV testing in the emergency department. *J Emerg Med.* Oct 13 [Epub ahead of print].

Balram, B. & Pai, N. (2011). Salivary and oral fluid based HIV antibody assays for rapid diagnosis of HIV infection. The 9th Annual Cochrane Canada Symposium, Early Exposure to Cochrane: accessible, credible & practical, 16-17 Feb 2011, Vancouver, BC.

Branson, B. (2000a). Rapid Tests for HIV Anti-body, *AIDS Reviews,* 2, 76-83.

Branson, B. (2000b). Assessing Diagnostic Technologies Marketed to Less Industiralised Countries, *Journal of International Physicians in AIDS Care,* Feb 2000, 28-30.

Branson, B. (2003). Point of Care Rapid Tests for HIV Antibodies, *Journal of Laborqtory Medicine,* 27 (7/8), 288-295.

Branson, B., Handsfield, H., Lampe, M. & et al. (2006). Revised recommendations for HIV testing of adults, adolescents, and pregnant women in health-care settings. *MMWR Recomm Rep,* 55(RR-14), 1–17.

British HIV Association (2005). *Guidelines for the treatment of HIV-infected adults with antiretroviral therapy.* www.bhiva.org/cms1191541.asp.

Carne, C. (1988). *Testing and screening for HIV infection.* Health Education Authority: London.

Chen Y., Bilardi, J., Lee, D., Cummings, R., Bush, M. & Fairley, C. (2010). Australian men who have sex with men prefer rapid oral HIV testing over conventional blood testing for HIV. *Int J STD AIDS* 21(6):428-30.

Chin, B., Lee, S., Kim, G., Kee, M., Suh, S., & Kim, S. (2007). Early Identification of Seronegative Human Immunodeficiency Virus Type 1 Infection with Severe Presentation. *Journal of Clinical Microbiology,* 45, 1659-1662.

Chou, R., Huffman, L., Fu, R., Smits, A. & Korthuis, P. (2005). Screening for HIV: a review of the evidence for the U.S. Preventive Services Task Force, *Annals of Internal Medicine,* 143, 55-73.

Cohall, A., Dini, S., Nye, A., Dye, B., Neu, N. & Hyden, C. (2010). HIV testing preferences among young men of color who have sex with men. *Am J Public Health.* 100(10), 961-6. Epub 2010 Jan 14.

Colfax, G., Lehman, J., Bindman, A., Vittinghoff, E., Vranizan, K., & Fleming, P., et al. (2002). What happened to home HIV test collection kits? Intent to use kits, actual use, and barriers to use among persons at risk for HIV infection. *AIDS Care* 2 (14), 675-82.

Crepaz, N., Lyles, C., Wolitski, R., Passin, W., Rama, S., Herbst, J. & et al. (2006). Do prevention interventions reduce HIV risk behaviours among people living with HIV? A meta-analytic review of controlled trials [Editorial], *AIDS,* 20 (1), 143-157.

Debattista, J., Bryson, G., Roudenko, N., Dwyer, J., Kelly, M., Hogan, P., & Patten, J. (2007). Pilot of non-invasive (oral fluid) testing for HIV within a clinical setting. Sexual Health, 4 (2), 105-109.

Delaney, K., Branson, B., Uniyal, A., Kerndt, P., Keenan, P., Jafa, K., Gardner, A., Jamieson, D. & Bulterys, M. (2006). Performance of Oral Fluid HIV- 1/2 test: experience from four CDC studies, *AIDS,* 20, 1655-1660.

Department of Health (2001). *National Strategy for Sexual Health and HIV,* DoH, London.

Dietz, C., Ablah, E., Reznik, D. & Robbins, D. (2008). Patients' attitudes about rapid oral HIV screening in an urban, free dental clinic. *AIDS Patient Care STDS* 22(3):205-12.

Everett, D., Baisley, K., Changalucha, J., Vallely, A., Watson-Jones, D., Cook, C., Knight, L., Ross, D., Mugeye, K., McCormack, S., Lacey, C., Jentsch, U. & Hayes, R. (2009). Suitability of simple human immunodeficiency virus rapid tests in clinical trials in community-based clinic settings. *J Clin Microbiol* 47 (4), 1058-62. Epub 2009 Feb 25.

Franco-Paredes, C., Tellez, I., & del-Rio, C. (2006). Rapid HIV testing: A review of the literature and implications for the clinician. *Current HIV/AIDS Reports*, 3, 159-165.

Galvan, F., Brooks, R. & Leibowitz, A. (2004), Rapid HIV Testing: Issues in Implementation, *Aids Patient Care and STDS*, 18 (1), 15-18.

Goodman, E., Tipton, A., Hecht, L. & et al. (1994). Perseverance pays off: health care providers' impact on HIV testing decisions by adolescent females. *Pediatrics* 94 (6 Pt 1), 878–82.

Greensides, D., Berkelman, R., Lansky, A., & Sullivan, P. (2003). Alternative HIV Testing Methods Among Populations at High Risk for HIV Infection. *Public Health Reports*, 118, 531-539.

Greenwald, J., Burstein, G., Pincus, J. & Branson, B. (2006). A Review of Rapid HIV Antibody Tests, *Current Infectious Disease* Reports, 8, 125-131.

Haines, C., Uwazuoke, K., Zussman, B., Parrino, T., Laguerre, R. & Foster, J. (2011). Pediatric emergency department-based rapid HIV testing: adolescent attitudes and preferences. *Pediatr Emerg Care* 27 (1), 13-16.

Hamers, R., de Beer, I., Kaura, H., van Vugt, M., Caparos, L., & Rinke, de Wit T. (2008). Diagnostic accuracy of 2 oral fluid-based tests for HIV surveillance in Namibia. *Journal of Acquired Immune Deficiency Syndromes*, 48(1):116-8.

Hamill, M., Burgoine, M., Farrell, F., Hamelaar, J., Patel, G., Welchew, D. & Jaffe HW (2007). Time to move towards opt-out testing for HIV in the UK. *BMJ*, 334: 1352-4.

Hare, C., Pappalardo, B., Busch, M., Phelps, B., Alexander, S., Ramstead, C., Levy, J. & Hecht, F. (2004). Negative HIV antibody test results among individuals treated with antiretroviral therapy (ART) during acute/early infection. The XV International AIDS conference. pp. abstract No MoPeB3107.

Health Protection Agency (2007). Testing Times. HIV and other Sexually Transmitted Infections in the United Kingdom. London: Health Protection Agency,

Centre for Infections. November 2007. Holt, M. (2009). *Rapid HIV testing: A literature review*. Australian Federation of AIDS Organisation Inc.

Ilegbodu, A., Frank, M., Poindexter, A., & et al. (1994). Characteristics of teens tested for HIV in a metropolitan area. *J Adolesc Health* 15 (6), 479–84.

Kane, B. (1999). Rapid testing for HIV: Why so fast. *Annals of Internal Medicine*, 133 (6), 481-483.

Kendrick, S., Kroc, K., Withum, D., Rydman, R., Branson, B. & Weinstein, R. (2005). Outcomes of Offering Rapid Point-of-Care HIV Testing in A Sexually Transmitted Disease Clinic, *J Acquir Immune Defic Syndr*, 38 (2), 142-146.

Knapp, H., Chan, K., Anaya, H., Goetz, M. (2011). Interactive Internet-Based Clinical Education: An Efficient and Cost-Savings Approach to Point-of-Care Test Training. *Telemed J E Health*. Apr 14. [Epub ahead of print]

Kurtzweil, P. (1999). Internet sales of bogus HIV test kits result in first-of-kind wire fraud conviction. *FDA Consum*, 33 (4), 34-5.

Lazebnik, R., Hermida, T., Szubski, R. & et al. (2001). The proportion and characteristics of adolescents who return for anonymous HIV test results. *Sex Transm Dis* 28 (7), 401–4.

Lee, B.E., Plitt, S., Fenton, J., Preiksaitis, J.K., Singh, A.E. Rapid HIV tests in acute care settings in an area of low HIV prevalence in Canada. *J Virol Methods* 172 (1-2), 66-71. Epub 2010 Dec 28.

Losina, E., Schackman, B., Sadownik, S., Gebo, K., Walensky, R. & et al. (2009). Racial and Sex Disparities in Life Expectancy Losses among HIV-Infected Persons in the

United States: Impact of Risk Behavior, Late Initiation, and Early Discontinuation of Antiretroviral Therapy. *Clin Infect Dis* 49, 1570–1578.

McCarthy, B., Wong, J., Munoz, A., & Sonnenberg, F. (1993). Who should be screened for HIV infection? A cost-effectiveness analysis. *Archives of Internal Medicine*, 153, 1107-1116.

Makuwa, M., Souquie`re ,S., Niangui, M., Rouquet, P., Apetrei, C. & et al. (2002). Reliability of rapid diagnostic tests for HIV variant infection. *J Virol Methods,* 103, 183–190.

Marks, G., Crepaz, N., Senterfitt, J. & Janssen, R. (2005). Meta-analysis of high-risk sexual behavior in persons aware and unaware they are infected with HIV in the United States: implications for HIV prevention programs, *Jounral of Acquired Immune Deficiency Syndrome*, 39, 446-453.

Mehta, S., Hall, J., Lyss, S. & et al. (2007). Adult and pediatric emergency department sexually transmitted disease and HIV screening: programmatic overview and outcomes. *Acad Emerg Med,* 14 (3), 250–8.

Merchant, R., Clark, M., Seage, G. 3rd, Mayer, K., Degruttola, V. & Becker, B. (2009). Emergency department patient perceptions and preferences on opt-in rapid HIV screening program components. *AIDS Care,* 21 (4), 490-500.

Mortimer, P., Parry, J. (1992). Letter to the Editor: Salivary testing for HIV infection. *BMJ*, 305, 1093.

Mullins, T., Braverman, P., Dorn, L, Kollar, L., & Kahn, J. (2010). Adolescent Preferences for Human Immunodeficiency Virus Testing Methods and Impact of Rapid Tests on Receipt of Results. *Journal of Adolescent Health,* 46, 162–168.

Mutale, W., Michelo, C., Jürgensen, M.& Fylkesnes, K. (2010). Home-based voluntary HIV counselling and testing found highly acceptable and to reduce inequalities. *BMC Public Health,* 10, 347.

Owens, D., Nease, R. & Harris, R. (1996). Cost-effectiveness of HIV screening in acute care settings. *Archives of Internal Medicine*, 156, 394-404.

Paltiel, D., Walensky, R., Schackman, B., Seage, G., Mercincavage, L., Weinstein, M., & Freedberg, K. (2006). Expanded HIB Screening in the United States: Effects on Clinical Outcomes, HIV Transmission and Costs, *Annals of Internal Medicine,* 145 (11), 797-806.

Pai, N., Tulsky, J., Cohan, D., Colford, J. & Reingold, A. (2007). Rapid point-of-care HIV testing in pregnant women: a systematic review and meta-analysis. *Trop Med Int Health,* 12 (2), 162-73.

Pascoe, S., Langhaug, L., Mudzori, J., Burke, E., Hayes, R. & Cowan, F. (2009). Field Evaluation of Diagnostic Accuracy of an Oral Fluid Rapid Test for HIV, Tested at Point-of-Service Sites in Rural Zimbabwe, *Aids, Patient Care and STDs.*, 23 (7), 571-6.

Patton, L., Ranganathan, K., Naidoo, S., Bhayat, A., Balasundaram, S., Adeyemi, O., Taiwo, O., Speicher, D. & Chandra, L. (2011). Oral Lesions, HIV Phenotypes, and Management of HIV-Related Disease: Workshop 4A. *Adv Dent Res,* 23 (1), 112-116.

Patton, L., Santos, V., McKaig, R., Shugars, D. & Strauss, R. (2002). Education in HIV risk screening, counseling, testing, and referral: survey of U.S. dental schools. *J Dent Educ,* 66 (10), 1169-77.

Pavie, J., Rachline, A., Loze, B., Niedbalski, L., Delaugerre, C., Laforgerie, E., Plantier, J., Rozenbaum, W., Chevret, S., Molina, J. &, Simon, F. (2010). Sensitivity of Five Rapid HIV Tests on Oral Fluid or Finger-Stick Whole Blood: A Real-Time Comparison in a Healthcare Setting. PLoS ONE , 5(7): e11581. doi:10.1371/journal.pone.0011581

Peeling, R. & Mabey, D. (2010). Point-of-care tests for diagnosing infections in the developing world. *Clin Microbiol Infect,* 6 (8), 1062-1069.

Peralta, L., Constantine, N., Griffin D., Martin, L., & Ghalib, K. (2001). Evaluation of youth preferences for rapid and innovative human immunodeficiency virus antibody tests. *Archives of Pediatric and Adolescent Medicine*, 155 (7), 761-762.

Pugatch, D., Levesque, B., Lally, M., Reinert, S., Filippone, W., Combs, C., Flanigan, T. & Brown, L. (2001). HIV testing among young adults and older adolescents in the setting of acute substance abuse treatment. *Journal of Acquired Immune Deficiency Syndrome*, 27, 135-42.

Prost, A., Chopin, M., McOwan, A., Elam, G., Dodds, J., Macdonald, N. & Imrie, J. (2007). "There is such a thing as asking for trouble": taking rapid HIV testing to gay venues is fraught with challenges. *Sex Transm Infect*, 83, 185–188.

Sohoni, A., Gordon, D., Vahidnia, F. & White, D. (2010). Emergency Department Staff Satisfaction With Rapid Human Immunodeficiency Virus Testing. *Academic Emergency Medicine* 17, 561–565.

Schopper, D., & Vercauteren, G. (1996). Testing for HIV at home: what are the issues? *AIDS*, 10, 1455-1465.

Sherrard, M. & Gatt, I. (1987). Human immunodeficiency virus (HIV) antibody testing. Guidance from an opinion provided for the British Medical Association. *Br Med J (Clin Res Ed)*. 295 (6603), 911-912.

Smith, P., Buzi, R. & Weinman, M. (2005). HIV testing and counseling among adolescents attending family planning clinics. *AIDS Care,* 17 (4), 451–456.

Spielberg, F., Critchlow, C., Vittinghoff, E., Coletti, A.S., Sheppard, H., Mayer, K., Metzgerg, D., Judson, F., Buchbinder S., Chesney, M., & Gross, M. (2000). Home collection for frequent HIV testing: acceptability of oral fluids, dried blood spots and telephone results. HIV Early Detection Study Group. *AIDS*, 14 (12), 1819-1828.

Spielberg, F., Branson, B., & Goldbaum, G., et al. (2005). Choosing HIV counseling and testing strategies for outreach settings: a randomized trial. *Journal of Acquired Immune Deficiency Syndrome*, 38, 348–355.

Stetler, H., Granade, T., Nunez, C., Meza, R., Terrell, S., Amador, L. & George, R. (1997). Field evaluation of rapid HIV serologic tests for screening and confirming HIV-1 infection in Honduras, *AIDS*, 11, 369–375.

Sy, F., Rhodes, S., Choi, S., Drociuk, D., Laurent, A., Naccash, R., & Kettinger, L. (1998). The acceptability of oral fluid testing for HIV antibodies. A pilot study in gay bars in a predominantly rural state. *Sexually Transmitted Diseases*, 25 (4), 211-215.

Tsu, R., Burm, M., Gilhooly, J. & et al (2002). Telephone vs. face-to-face notification of HIV results in high-risk youth. *J Adolesc Health* 30 (3), 154–60.

Tweed, E., Hale, A., Hurrelle, M., Smith, R., Delpech, V., Ruf, M., Klapper, P., Ramsay, M. & Brant, L. (2010) Monitoring HIV testing in diverse healthcare settings: results from a sentinel surveillance pilot study. *Sex Transm Infect* 86 (5), 360-4. Epub 2010 Apr 28.

UNAIDS (1997). HIV Testing Methods - UNAIDS technical update, UNAIDS, Geneva.

UNAIDS/WHO (2004). HIV Assays: Operational Characteristics (Phase 1) Simple/Rapid tests (Report 14) 2004.

Walensky, R., Freedberg, K., Weinstein, M. & Paltiel, A. (2007). Cost-effectiveness of HIV testing and treatment in the United States. *Clin Infect Dis*, 45 (Suppl 4), S248-54.

Wesolowski, L., MacKellar, D., Facente, S., Dowling, T., Ethridge, S., Zhu, J., Sullivan, P. & Post-marketing Surveillance Team (2006). Post-marketing surveillance of OraQuick whole blood and oral fluid rapid HIV testing. *AIDS,* 20 (12), 1661-1666.

26

HAART and Causes of Death in Perinatally HIV-1-Infected Children

Claudia Palladino[1], Jose María Bellón[2], Francisco J. Climent[3], María del Palacio Tamarit[1], Isabel de José[4] and Mª Ángeles Muñoz-Fernández[1]

[1]*Laboratorio de Inmuno-Biología Molecular, Hospital General Universitario "Gregorio Marañón"*

[2]*Unidad de Investigación, Fundación de Investigación Biomédica Hospital "Gregorio Marañón"*

[3]*Servicio Infecciosas, Hospital "Ramón y Cajal"*

[4]*Servicio Infecciosas Infantil, Hospital Universitario "La Paz", Madrid, Spain*

1. Introduction

Children represent a population at higher risk of Human Immunodeficiency Virus type 1 (HIV-1) infection and AIDS-related death. Approximately 2.5 million (1.6–3.4) children are infected at present, accounting for 370,000 [230,000–510,000] new infections and 260,000 [150,000–360,000] deaths (Gray et al., 2001). About 90% of children living with HIV-1 are in sub-Saharan Africa. The paediatric HIV-1 epidemic is fuelled by HIV-1 infection in women of childbearing age. In fact, mother-to-child (perinatal) HIV-1 transmission during pregnancy, birth or breastfeeding accounts for the vast majority of HIV-1 cases in children. An estimated 2.4 million infected women give birth annually. This results in the birth of approximately 1,000 HIV-1–infected babies per day, of which 80% occur in resource-limited countries where there are no effective programs for prevention of mother-to-child transmission (MTCT) of HIV-1 . Almost two decades ago, the introduction of antiretroviral chemoprophylaxis to prevent MTCT of HIV-1 was an important milestone in paediatric HIV-1. The use of antiretroviral drugs and elective caesarean section have reduced the incidence of MTCT in industrialised countries to <2% since 1997 (The European Collaborative Study [ECS], 2005; Connor et al., 1994). However, such interventions to prevent MTCT of HIV-1 are still not widely accessible or available in most resource-limited countries where the rate of transmission is estimated at 12–40% (De Cock et al., 2000). Concerning the diagnosis and treatment of HIV-1, significant improvements have been made over the last few years, yet much more needs to be done. The first evidence of the efficacy of antiretroviral therapy (ART) in HIV-1–infected children was published 20 years ago (Pizzo et al., 1988). Since then, the introduction of highly active antiretroviral therapy (HAART) into medical care for HIV-1–infected children and adolescents has increased life expectancy and resulted in AIDS incidence decline in both industrialised countries and resource-limited settings (Judd et al., 2007; Patel et al., 2008; Puthanakit et al., 2007; Reddi et al., 2007). Some studies have also described the immunovirological impact of HAART (Fraaij et al., 2005; Scherpbier et al., 2006; Walker et al., 2004). Nevertheless, in developing countries early diagnosis is a major challenge and ART is often started late. The clinical impact of early treatment has been recognised (Faye et al., 2004; Violari et al., 2007); in fact, in the absence of treatment, 50% of infants die before their second birthday (Newell et al., 2004). Moreover, lack of resources restricts drug supply. Despite the number of children receiving ART increased from about 75,000 in 2005 to 360,000 in 2009, these represent en estimated ART coverage of 28% [21-43%] of all children less than 15 years who need ART in resource-limited settings (WHO, 2010). On the contrary, in industrialised countries antiretroviral drugs are widely available. In addition, new therapeutic options have been developed for the paediatric population in recent years, such as the protease inhibitor darunavir approved for children aged ≥ 6 years and adolescents (Blanche et al., 2009), or are under evaluation in ongoing clinical trials, including the second generation non-nucleoside reverse transcriptase inhibitor etravirine (ClinicalTrials.gov 2008b, 2009a), the new protease inhibitor tipranavir (Salazar et al., 2008), and the new families of antiretrovirals, such as the CCR5 antagonists and integrase inhibitors (ClinicalTrials.gov 2007, 2008a, 2009b).

2. Impact of antiretroviral therapy

Given that HIV-1 infection has turned into a chronic condition and that exposure to antiretrovirals is likely to be life-long, continuous assessment of the impact of HAART on progression of perinatal HIV-1 infection remains an important public health issue to improve health care strategies. Here, we report the evaluation of HAART effectiveness on the incidence of AIDS and death, and the trends in the underlying causes of death at population level over almost three decades in Madrid (Spain). In Western Europe, Spain continues to be one of the countries with the highest AIDS incidence rate and prevalence. Within Spain, the *Comunidad Autónoma de Madrid* is the area most affected by the infection, with a total of 18,866 AIDS cases up to 2010 (24% of the national cases) (Centro Nacional de Epidemiología [CNE], 2010). The high HIV-1 prevalence had a direct impact on the spread of the infection within the infant population and although the risk of perinatal transmission of HIV-1 has decreased below 2% in recent years, paediatric HIV-1 cases are still being diagnosed (Palladino et al., 2008). In the *Comunidad Autónoma de Madrid*, a total of 237 cumulative AIDS cases due to vertical transmission were reported to the National AIDS Registry from 1981 to 2010 (CNE, 2010). The introduction of HAART in late 1996 and its universal and free availability (Ministerio de sanidad y Consumo, 1998) offered the opportunity to control HIV-1 disease progression in the paediatric population (2005; Resino et al., 2006b). The aim of this study was to describe the mortality and AIDS rates and changes in underlying causes of death in HIV-1-infected paediatric patients. Moreover, risk factors associated with shorter first-line HAART duration among antiretroviral-naïve patients who began HAART after 1996 were examined.

2.1 Study population and methods

The HIV Paediatric Cohort of the *Comunidad Autónoma de Madrid* was established in 1995 as an open cohort of paediatric patients infected by HIV-1 through MTCT, for whom it was assumed that HIV-1 transmission occurred on the date of birth (de Martino et al., 2000). The cohort has included all HIV-1-infected patients identified in a multicenter network of nine referral paediatric hospitals from January 1982 (birth date of the first MTCT-infected child in Madrid). Children infected before 1995 were enrolled retrospectively, while those infected after 1995

were enrolled prospectively. Complete ascertainment of all records was carefully sought. Informed consent was obtained from mothers of all patients. The Institutional Ethics Committee approved the study. HIV-1 testing during pregnancy was offered to all women until 1998, when routine testing was introduced for all pregnant women. Patients were actively followed up every 3-6 months (Centers for Disease Control and Prevention [CDC] 1998). At the beginning of the study, the diagnosis of HIV-1 infection was based on the results of a serologic test for HIV-1 antibody, which was performed routinely for children born to seropositive women. When the result of the serologic test was positive, the infection was confirmed by paediatricians and/or through hospital summaries. Later, the diagnosis was done by positive results of HIV-1 PCR DNA and peripheral blood mononuclear cells viral culture assays on two separate samples (Resino et al., 2006a). The clinical classification and definition of AIDS-related events were based on international guidelines (CDC 1994). Children in the A or B clinical category who became older than 13 years were not categorised as having AIDS by $CD4^+$ cell count criteria when they had <200 cells/ml (CDC 1992).
Deaths were reported by paediatricians. The underlying cause of death (the disease/injury which initiated the morbid event leading to death) was confirmed by reviewing medical histories or autopsy certificates and interviewing paediatricians. Patients were cross-checked with the National Death Index to validate their causes of death classified as: "AIDS-defining" when attributable to a disease in the C clinical category (CDC 1992, 1994); "HIV-related" when attributable to a category A or B disease (CDC 1992, 1994) or to ARV adverse events; "non-HIV-related": all other causes. To report the underlying cause of death, when multiple concurrent causes contributed to death, patients were included as many times as the number of illnesses diagnosed. The study period comprised a pre-HAART era (1982-1996) and a post-HAART era (1997-2009), and was divided into six calendar periods (CP) on the basis of the changing HIV-1 therapy management. CP1 (1982-1989): it was chose as the reference period, when ART was not routinely available; CP2 (1990–1993): the standard of care was zidovudine monotherapy; CP3 (1994–1996): children were receiving dual-nucleoside regimen; CP4 (1997–1998): when HAART, a combination of three or more drugs, was introduced; CP5 (1999–2004): early-HAART period; CP6 (2005–2009): late-HAART period. Information on socio-demographic characteristics, mother's transmission category, clinical and immunovirological data and the antiretroviral therapy were recorded. Any change in two or more antiretroviral drugs that lasted ≥14 days, excluding dosage changes, in the presence of detectable HIV-1 RNA, was considered to indicate the start of a new regimen.

2.1.1 Statistical analysis

AIDS and mortality rates were calculated as the number of new AIDS and death cases per hundred person-years (p-y) of follow-up. Individuals were followed from the date of enrolment (i.e., date of HIV-1 diagnosis or first blood test) until the date of development of the event of interest (AIDS or death) or December 31, 2009 (administrative censoring date), whichever occurred first. The risk of progression to AIDS and death over time was estimated by survival analyses using Kaplan-Meier curves and Cox proportional hazards models. Time was calculated from the birth date so that comparisons across different calendar periods were based on individuals who were infected for the same length of time. All models were stratified by hospital and adjusted for potential confounders (gender, mother's transmission category and immunological category). Fisher exact test, χ^2 or Mann-Whitney U test were used to derive *P*-values. Poisson regression was used to compare mortality and infection rates between our cohort and the age-similar general population living in the *Comunidad Autónoma de Madrid*. The median duration of initial HAART regimen was determined by Kaplan-Meier analysis. Univariate proportional hazards regressions were used to identify factors associated with a shorter initial regimen. The variables examined included demographics, socio-economic characteristics, baseline laboratory values ($CD4^+$ cell count, HIV-1 RNA, haemoglobin), clinical status and adherence to initial HAART regimen. Then, multivariate regression analysis was performed including all factors for which the results of univariate analysis were statistically significant ($P<0.05$, 2-sided). Analyses were performed with SPSS 16 and Epidat 3.1.

3. Results

Overall, 484 children who acquired HIV-1 from their mothers between 1982 and 2009 were enrolled and followed for 5298.2 person-years (11.6 years; interquartile range (IQR): 5.2-16.7). HIV-1 infection occurred mainly in 1992 [IQR: 1988-1995]; 270 (56%) patients were girls and 299 (62%) had a mother who acquired the virus through injection drug use. Table 1 provides the characteristics of the children at the end of each calendar period (CP). The cohort had the highest number of enrolled children between 1994 and 1996; in the last period (2005-2009) there were 279 children included, of whom 13 were born in this period. The sex ratio remained stable over time (CP1: 1.0; CP6: 1.4), while the median age (CP1: 2.6 [1.0-4.4]; CP6: 14.8 [11.6-17.5]; $P<0.001$) and the proportion of immigrants (CP1: 3.1; CP6: 15.5; $P<0.0001$) increased. An increase of the median $CD4^+$ cell percentage at the end of each calendar period was observed (CP2: 22.5 [11.9-32.1]; CP4: 26.5 [18.2-33.7]; CP6: 33.4 [28.0-39.7]) and a concomitant decrease of HIV-1 RNA since 1997 (median $\log_{10}$ copies/ml CP4: 4.31 [3.80-4.91]; CP6: 2.60 [1.70-3.55]). The proportion of children with <400 copies/ml was 9% (13/151) in CP3, 20% (39/196) in CP4, 60% (150/248) in CP5, and 80% (160/199) in CP6. Two adolescents died in CP2 achieving undetectable HIV-1 RNA at death. The $CD8^+$ cell percentage remained stable (CP2: 42.0 [29.0-52.0]; CP4: 43.7 [35.6-52.5]; CP6: 38.9 [31.7-45.7]). The changes over time in antiretroviral therapy management are described in Fig. 1. Monotherapy was used in the early 1990s and dual-nucleoside therapy in mid-1990s. An increasing proportion of children receiving HAART from 1997 onward was observed; by 2005, up to 80% of the children were on HAART.

3.1 Time to AIDS or death

Information on 471 children, of whom 285 (61%) developed an AIDS-defining disease, was available for the progression to AIDS analyses. The AIDS incidence rate increased over time until 1989 (32.6 per 100 p-y), it arose again during the first half of the 1990s (13.2 in 1991; 18.8 in 1995) and waned off thereafter (3.2 in 1999; 0.0 in 2009) (Fig. 2). The cumulative incidence curves showed a reduction in the proportion of patients developing AIDS after 1997 compared to the period 1982-1989 (Fig. 3A). Multivariate Cox analysis showed a more pronounced decline in the last period (CP6) (AHR: 0.07; 95%CI: 0.04-0.16) than in the CP5 (AHR: 0.23; 95%CI: 0.15-0.37) (Table 2). A total of 159/484 (33%) deaths occurred. The death incidence rate was 7.4 per 100 p-y at risk in 1986, it peaked in 1995 (10.1 per 100 p-y) and declined thereafter (0.7 in 1999; 0.0 in 2009) (Fig. 2). The incidence of death decreased since 1997 compared to the period 1982-1989 (Fig. 3B, Table 2). Multivariate analysis showed more marked improvements in survival in the CP6 (AHR: 0.16; 95%CI: 0.05-0.50) than in the CP5 (AHR: 0.25; 95%CI: 0.11-0.56).

Characteristics	Period					
	CP1 *(80-89)*	*CP2* *(90-93)*	*CP3* *(94-96)*	*CP4* *(97-98)*	*CP5* *(99-04)*	*CP6* *(05-09)*
N. of HIV-1-infected patients	168	280	317	282	315	279
Age, years (median, IQR)	2.6 (1.0 - 4.4)	4.0 (1.8 - 6.6)	5.0 (2.6 - 8.0)	6.7 (3.8 - 9.6)	11.1 (7.8 - 14.0)	14.8 (11.6-17.5)
Date of birth, n. of patients						
1980-1989	168	144	115	85	79	47
1990-1993	-	136	115	93	90	85
1994-1996	-	-	87	73	68	63
1997-1998	-	-	-	31	29	27
1999-2004	-	-	-	-	49	44
2005-2009	-	-	-	-	-	13
Sex ratio, n. of girls	1.00	1.19	1.23	1.27	1.32	1.41
Geographic origin, n. (%)						
Spain	156 (92.9)	264 (94.3)	298 (94.0)	256 (90.8)	271 (86.0)	235 (84.0)
Central America	0 (0)	3 (1.1)	4 (1.3)	8 (2.8)	10 (3.2)	9 (3.2)
South America	3 (1.8)	4 (1.4)	6 (1.9)	6 (2.1)	8 (2.5)	8 (2.9)
North Africa	0 (0)	0 (0)	1 (0.3)	1 (0.4)	1 (0.3)	2 (0.7)
Sub-Sahara Africa	0 (0)	3 (1.1)	5 (1.6)	8 (2.8)	19 (6.0)	20 (7.2)
Other	2 (1.2)	2 (0.7)	2 (0.6)	3 (1.1)	5 (1.6)	4 (1.4)
Unknown/Unavailable	7 (4.2)	4 (1.4)	1 (0.3)	-	1 (0.3)	1 (0.4)
Maternal transmission, n. (%)						
Injecting drug use	119 (70.8)	189 (67.5)	196 (61.8)	168 (59.6)	185 (58.7)	154 (55.2)
Heterosexual	29 (17.3)	56 (20.0)	69 (21.8)	69 (24.5)	78 (24.8)	74 (26.5)
IDU / Heterosexual	13 (7.7)	23 (8.2)	29 (9.1)	24 (8.5)	23 (7.3)	19 (6.8)
Transfusion	3 (1.8)	3 (1.1)	7 (2.2)	6 (2.1)	6 (1.9)	6 (2.2)
Unknown/Unavailable	4 (2.4)	9 (3.2)	16 (5.0)	15 (5.3)	23 (7.3)	26 (9.3)
Clinical category C, n. (%)	69 (41.3)	106 (38.3)	137 (44.1)	102 (37.4)	124 (40.8)	102 (37.5)
Death, n. (%)	21 (12.5)	49 (17.5)	63 (19.9)	12 (4.3)	10 (3.2)	4 (1.4)

Table 1. Demographic and clinical characteristics of the HIV-1-infected patients enrolled in the HIV Paediatric Cohort of the *Comunidad Autónoma de Madrid* at the end of each calendar period (CP). IQR: interquartile range; clinical classification was based on the 1994 revised CDC guidelines. IDU: injecting drug use.

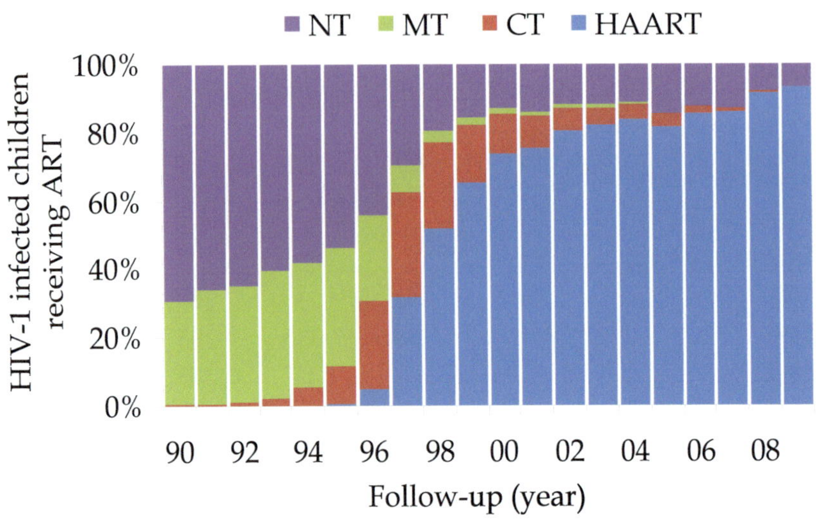

Fig. 1. Use of antiretroviral therapy among HIV-1 vertically infected children enrolled in the HIV Paediatric Cohort of the *Comunidad Autónoma de Madrid*. NT: not treated; MT: monotherapy; combined/dual-nucleoside therapy; HAART: highly active antiretroviral therapy.

		AIDS	
Calendar period	**N.**	**N. of cases**	**Adjusted HR (95% CI)**
1982 - 1989	167	69	1.00
1990 - 1993	232	61	0.49 (0.33 - 0.69)
1994 - 1996	255	81	0.64 (0.44 - 0.91)
1997 - 1998	199	28	0.39 (0.25 - 0.63)
1999 - 2004	216	37	0.23 (0.15 - 0.37)
2005 - 2009	178	9	0.07 (0.04 - 0.16)
		Death	
Calendar period	**N.**	**N. of cases**	**Adjusted HR (95% CI)**
1982 - 1989	168	21	1.00
1990 - 1993	280	49	1.33 (0.77 - 2.28)
1994 - 1996	317	63	1.71 (1.00 – 2.94)
1997 - 1998	282	12	0.54 (0.25 - 1.14)
1999 - 2004	315	10	0.25 (0.11 - 0.56)
2005 - 2009	279	4	0.16 (0.05 - 0.50)

Table 2. Effect of calendar period on the risk of AIDS and death. Note: Adjusted hazard ratios were derived from a standard Cox proportional hazard model that included calendar period (external time-dependent covariate), gender, mother's transmission category, immunological category and it is stratified by hospital.

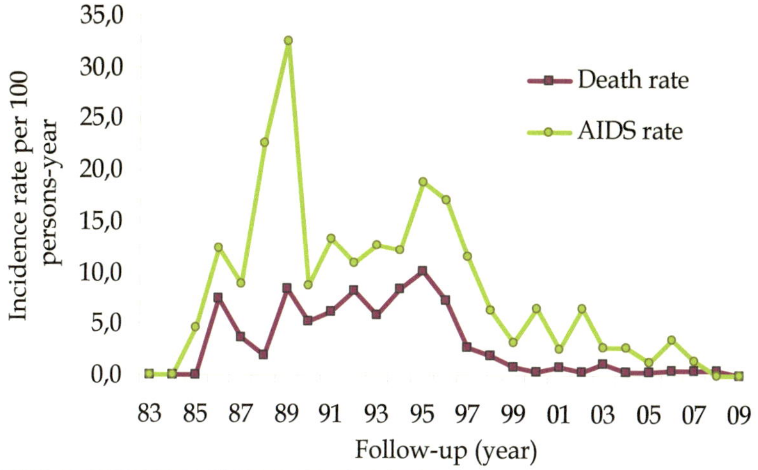

Years	AIDS			Death		
	p-y	N.	Rate	p-y	N.	Rate
1982	2	0	0,0	2	0	0,0
1983	10	0	0,0	10	0	0,0
1984	24	0	0,0	24	0	0,0
1985	44	2	4,6	45	0	0,0
1986	65	8	12,4	68	5	7,4
1987	79	7	8,9	84	3	3,6
1988	89	20	22,6	105	2	1,9
1989	98	32	32,6	133	11	8,3
1990	103	9	8,7	154	8	5,2
1991	121	16	13,2	177	11	6,2
1992	147	16	10,9	206	17	8,3
1993	158	20	12,7	221	13	5,9
1994	173	21	12,2	239	20	8,4
1995	170	32	18,8	248	25	10,1
1996	164	28	17,1	248	18	7,3
1997	156	18	11,5	256	7	2,7
1998	158	10	6,3	263	5	1,9
1999	155	5	3,2	269	2	0,7
2000	155	10	6,5	275	1	0,4
2001	155	4	2,6	278	2	0,7
2002	155	10	6,5	283	1	0,4
2003	152	4	2,6	276	3	1,1
2004	151	4	2,6	271	1	0,4
2005	150	2	1,3	263	1	0,4
2006	142	5	3,5	244	1	0,4
2007	136	2	1,5	233	1	0,4
2008	132	0	0,0	217	1	0,5
2009	128	0	0,0	209	0	0,0

Fig. 2. Annual AIDS and mortality incidence rates per 100 person-years (p-y) in the HIV Paediatric Cohort of the *Comunidad Autónoma de Madrid*.

In the population aged 0-19 years of the *Comunidad Autónoma de Madrid*, the mortality decreased from 4.2 deaths per 10,000 inhabitants in 1996 to 3.5 in 2007. In spite of the mortality decline in our cohort, it still was 10.4-fold (95%CI: 5.8-18.8; *P*<0.001) higher than in age-similar general population after 1999. Since 1999, the HIV-1–infected infants had a higher mortality rate than children/adolescents (IRR: 6.9; 95%CI: 2.3-20.3; *P*<0.001), as in the general population (IRR: 18.9; 95%CI: 17.9-19.9; *P*<0.001). A lower decrease of mortality among HIV-1–infected infants (IRR: 2.6; 95%CI: 0.9-7.4; *P*=0.069) between pre-HAART and post-HAART era than among older patients (IRR: 12.5; 95%CI: 7.6-20.4; *P*<0.001) was observed. On the contrary, mortality decreased equally in infants (IRR: 1.8; 95%CI: 1.8-1.9; *P*<0.001) and children/adolescents (IRR: 1.5; 95%CI: 1.5-1.6; *P*<0.001) in the general population.

3.2 Causes of death

Overall, 169 causes of death were documented for 151/159 (95%) patients (Table3). The 81% (137/169) were AIDS-defining, 12% (20/169) HIV-related and 7% (12/169) non-HIV-related. Multiple causes of death were reported in 16/151 (11%) patients, 3.2 (0.6–6.3) years old at death, of which 7 were infants: 13/129 (10%) died in pre-HAART era and 3/22 (14%) in post-HAART era. Concomitant pathologies were diagnosed in 101/151 (67%) patients (Table 4). The majority (83%) of the subjects died in the post-HAART era had a low/medium socio-economic status. From 1999 to 2007, the risk of death from infections was 115.9 times (95% CI: 42.0–265.8; *P*<0.001) higher in our cohort than in the *Comunidad Autónoma de Madrid*. It was not possible to evaluate the risk of death from other causes than infections due to the low number of events.

AIDS-defining causes were 82% (118/144) in pre-HAART and 76% (19/25) in post-HAART era. The most frequent contributing events were opportunistic infections (58%, 79/137) (Table 4), wasting syndrome (19%, 26/137) and lymphoid interstitial pneumonia (12%, 16/137). The largest components of opportunistic infections were bacterial (20%, 28/137), fungal (mainly *Pneumocystis jiroveci*; 15%, 20/137), and mycobacterial infections (mainly *Mycobacterium tuberculosis*; 10%, 14/137). These three etiologic pathogens were associated with the only cases of death occurred in 2005-2007. No statistically significant changes over time were observed in the proportions of the causes of death. HIV-related causes were 11% (16/144) in pre-HAART and 16% (4/25) in post-HAART era. Overall, the leading causes of death were infections (75%, 15/20), mainly bacterial (65%, 13/20), and bleeding (15%, 3/20). The causes of death reported in post-HAART era were: bacterial infection, pulmonary bleeding caused by thrombocytopenia, pulmonary arterial hypertension and lactic acidosis (1 case each). Non-HIV-related causes were 7% (10/144) in pre-HAART and 8% (2/25) in post-HAART era. Infections were the main cause of death (75%, 9/12), mainly viral infections (67%, 8/12), followed by cancer (17%, 2/12) and hepatic pathology (8%, 1/12). The only causes of death reported in post-HAART era were cancer and hepatic failure (1 case each).

3.3 Duration of HAART regimen

Of 484 patients included in the HIV Paediatric Cohort of the *Comunidad Autónoma de Madrid*, 105 (22%) were naïve to antiretrovirals when HAART began as of January 1997. It was possible to analyse the duration of the first HAART regimen in 82 of them. Half of the patients were girls (42; 51%) and had a median age at HAART initiation of 3.6 years (0.6-7.3).

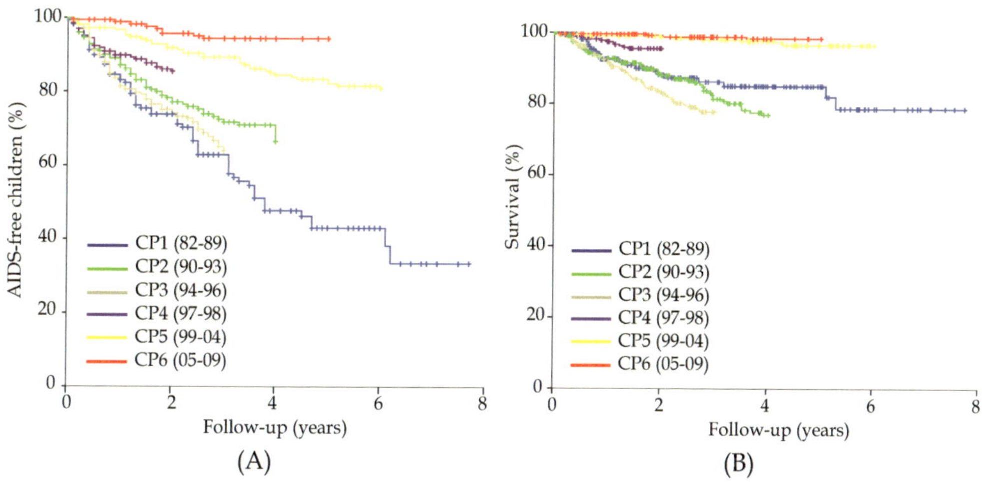

Fig. 3. Kaplan-Meier curves for HIV-1-infected children enrolled in the HIV Paediatric Cohort of the *Comunidad Autónoma de Madrid* without AIDS (A) and for survival (B) in different calendar periods.

Cause of death	Pre-HAART (1982-1996) N=144 (85.2%)	Post-HAART (1997-2009) N=25 (14.8%)
Cancer	6 (4.2)	3 (12.0)
NHL	5 (3.5)	2 (8.0)
HL	1 (0.7)	--
Others	--	1 (4.0)
Infections	90 (62.5)	13 (52.0)
Bacterial infections	34 (23.6)	7 (28.0)
Pneumonia	20 (13.9)	3 (12.0)
Sepsis	14 (9.7)	3 (12.0)
Meningitis	--	1 (4.0)
Fungal infections	17 (11.8)	3 (12.0)
Pneumonia	13 (9.0)	3 (12.0)
Esophageal	4 (2.8)	--
Mycobacterial infections	13 (9.0)	3 (12.0)
Nontuberculous	8 (5.6)	2 (8.0)
Tuberculosis	5 (3.5)	1 (4.0)
Viral infections	15 (10.4)	--
Pneumonia	5 (3.5)	
Sepsis	6 (4.2)	
AGE	3 (2.1)	
PML	1 (0.7)	
Parasitic infections	11 (7.6)	--
Cryptosporidiasis	9 (6.3)	
Toxoplasmosis	1 (0.7)	
Leishmaniasis	1 (0.7)	
Other causes	48 (33.3)	9 (36.0)
Wasting	22 (15.3)	4 (16.0)
Pulmonary	15 (10.4)	2 (8.0)
Encephalopathy	9 (6.3)	--
Hepatic	--	1 (4.0)
Bleeding	2 (1.4)	1 (4.0)
Lactic acidosis	--	1 (4.0)

Table 3. All causes of death for HIV-1–infected children enrolled in the HIV Paediatric Cohort of the *Comunidad Autónoma de Madrid* stratified by pre-HAART era and post-HAART era. Pulmonary cause of death includes lymphoid interstitial pneumonia cases and 1 case of pulmonary hypertension. AGE: acute gastroenteritis; HL: Hodgkin's lymphoma; NHL: non-Hodgkin's lymphoma; PML: progressive multifocal leukoencephalopathy (JC virus). Percentage may not total 100 because of rounding.

	Pre-HAART (1982-1996)	Post-HAART (1997-2009)
Opportunistic infection	**N=67/129 (51.9%)**	**N=12/22 (54.5%)**
Recurrent bacterial infection	22 (32.8)	6 (50.0)
Pneumocystis jiroveci	13 (19.4)	3 (25.0)
Cryptosporidiosis	9 (13.4)	0
Nontuberculous mycobacteria	6 (9.0)	2 (16.7)
Mycobacterium tuberculosis	5 (7.5)	1 (8.3)
Candidasis	4 (6.0)	0
Cytomegalovirus	6 (9.0)	0
Toxoplasmosis	1 (1.5)	0
JC virus	1 (1.5)	0
Comorbidity*	**N= 87/129 (64.9%)**	**N=14/22 (60.9%)**
Wasting	52 (38.8)	11 (47.8)
Encephalopathy	50 (37.3)	7 (30.4)
Hepatic	17 (12.7)	2 (8.7)
Miocardiophaty	20 (14.9)	2 (8.7)
Hematologic alterations	15 (11.2)	3 (13.0)
Candidiasis	10 (7.5)	--
Hypertension	3 (2.2)	--
Nephropathology	3 (2.2)	--
Giardiasis	1 (0.7)	--
HSV	1 (0.7)	--

Table 4. Prevalence of opportunistic infections and comorbidity in the deceased patients of the HIV Paediatric Cohort of the *Comunidad Autónoma de Madrid*, stratified by pre-HAART and post-HAART era. HSV: Herpes simplex virus. *Note: Patients can be counted more than once.

The majority originated from Spain (58; 71%) and 19 (23%) were adopted or lived in institutions. The socio-economic status was medium-high for 28 (56%) out of 50 patients and low for 22 (44%). At baseline, the median CD4$^+$ cell count was 707 (19%) cells/ml (212-1,443) and HIV-1 RNA was 100,000 (5.0 $\log_{10}$) copies/ml. The median duration of the first HAART regimen was 40.5 months (20.9-80.2). Fifty (61%) subjects were still on the same regimen at the end of the follow-up (Fig. 4, circle chart), being the median HAART duration in this group of 64.5 months (28.6-95.1). The rest of the study group (32/82; 39%) switched to a second regimen after 25.9 months (12.4-39.2) of first regimen. The median first-line HAART duration was significantly different between the two groups (P<0.0001). Among the 32 patients who experienced first-line HAART discontinuation, up to 6 switches to successive regimens were observed and had a median duration of 25.9 months (20.7-29.2) (Fig. 4, bar chart). The cumulative incidence curves for time to initial HAART regimen discontinuation showed a longer median HAART duration for the 65/82 (79%) children who started the therapy after 6 months of age compared with the 17 (21%) infants who started at or before 6 months (P=0.033) (Fig 5A). In addition, this analysis showed a longer median HAART duration for the 31 (60%) out of 52 subjects with good/perfect adherence compared with the 21 (40%) subjects with poor/intermediate adherence (P<0.0001) (Fig. 5B). Initial HAART regimen discontinuation remained associated to younger ages (AHR: 4.56; 95%CI: 1.76–11.86; P=0.002) and poor adherence (AHR: 5.02; 95%CI: 2.02–12.47; P=0.001) in the multivariate analysis performed for 52 patients (Table 5). The most frequently prescribed first-line regimen was based on protease inhibitors, while one-quarter of the patients received therapy based on non-nucleoside reverse-transcriptase inhibitors (Fig. 6). Two nucleosides backbone therapy remains the cornerstone for all patients but one who had 3 nucleosides. For patients who discontinued the first-regimen, there was a difference, approaching statistical significance, between the duration of the PI-based therapy (30.0 months [13.1-40.5]) and the NNRTI-based therapy (15.2 [5.5-23.2]; P=0.054).

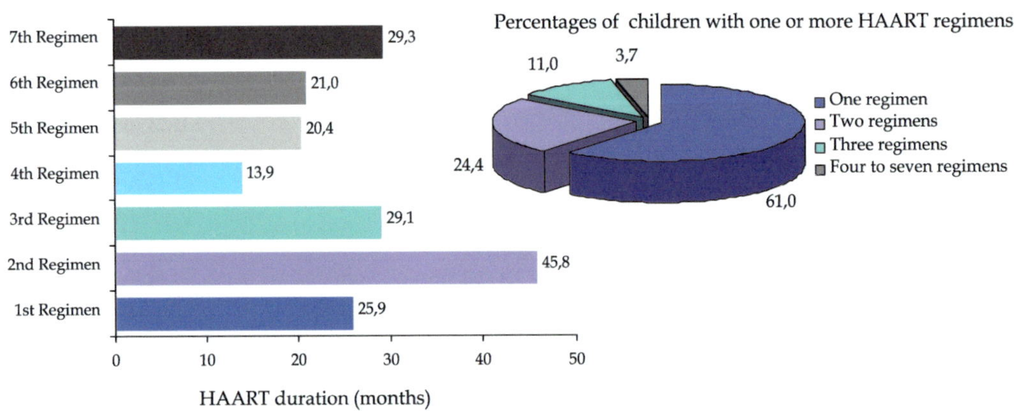

Fig. 4. Relative proportion of patients according to the number of HAART regimens among the 82 antiretroviral-naïve patients who start HAART since 1997 (circle chart); months of HAART regimen duration among the 32 patients with regimen switch (bat chart).

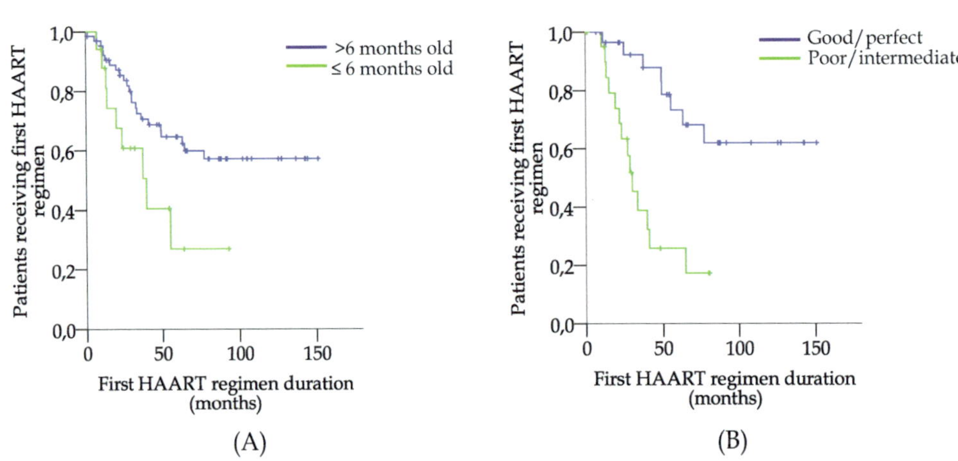

Fig. 5. Kaplan-Meier curves for time to discontinuation of first HAART regimen according to the age of HAART initiation (A) and to adherence to first HAART regimen (B).

	First HAART regimen discontinuation		
	N.	N. of cases (%)	Adjusted HR (95% CI)
Age at HAART initiation			
> 6 months	40	14 (35.0)	1.00
≤ 6 months	12	8 (66.7)	4.56 (1.76 - 11.86)
Adherence to first HAART regimen			
Good/perfect	31	8 (25.8)	1.00
Poor/intermediate	21	14 (66.7)	5.02 (2.02 - 12.47)

Table 5. Effect of age at HAART initiation and adherence on the risk of first HAART regimen discontinuation. Note: Adjusted hazard ratios were derived from a standard Cox proportional hazard model.

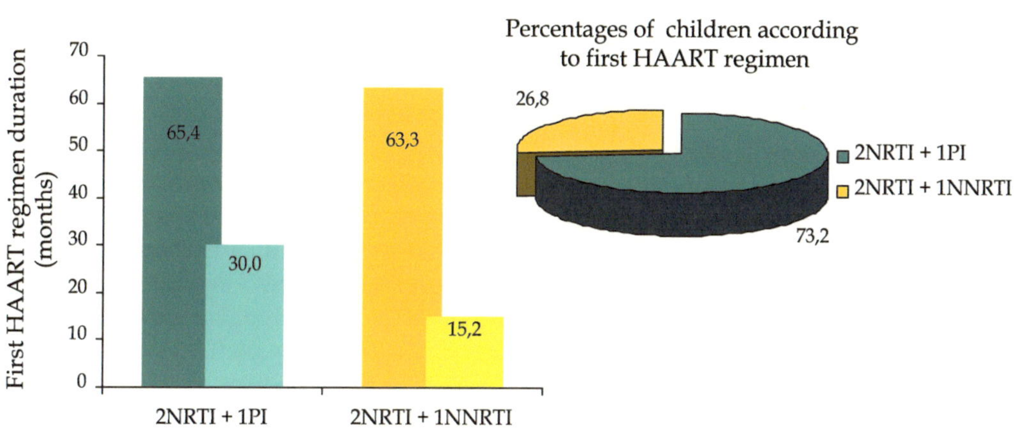

Fig. 6. Relative proportion of initial HAART regimen types among the 82 antiretroviral-naïve patients who started HAART since 1997 (circle chart); months of HAART regimen duration in patients who did not suspended the first HAART regimen (dark coloured bars) and who suspended the first regimen (light coloured bars). NRTI: nucleoside reverse-transcriptase inhibitor; NNRTI: non-nucleoside reverse-transcriptase inhibitor; PI: protease inhibitor.

4. Discussion

The results of this multicenter study on 484 patients infected by HIV-1 through perinatal transmission from the region of Madrid, show that the immunovirological response observed after the introduction of HAART has improved steadily since 1997. Also, an increase in clinical outcome with calendar period was observed. The marked reduction in progression to AIDS and death (by 93% and 84%, respectively) in recent years compared to 1982-1989 suggests a relationship between clinical outcome and HAART, which became widely available from 1997 onward. However, in the latter period, a low but stable mortality rate was recorded, in accordance with those recently reported by others (Brady et al., 2010; Judd et al., 2007).

Remarkably, mortality continued to be more than ten-fold higher in our cohort than in age-similar general population after 1996 and mainly affected patients of low/medium socio-economic status (Palladino et al., 2008). In addition, HIV-1–infected infants were still at higher risk for death compared with older paediatric patients, being this pattern mirrored in the general paediatric population and maybe attributable to the immature of the immune system (Gortmaker et al., 2001). Finally, the mortality trend had a strikingly lower decrease among infants than among children aged ≥ 1 year in our cohort, where it decreased equally in both groups in the general population. These findings highlight the HIV-1-infected infants as a major target for healthcare policy. We observed very high AIDS and mortality incidence rates during the first years of follow-up. These data on mortality are consistent with historical European series (ECS, (1994). and with data on HIV-1 progression in children living in setting where they do not receive medical care (Brahmbhatt et al., 2006; Marinda et al., 2007). In fact, zidovudine monotherapy administration to paediatric patients started only in 1988 (Pizzo et al., 1988) and in our cohort the majority of the children were still untreated in this year. Moreover, the high HIV-1 prevalence among the female population fuelled by the so called "epidemic of heroin" had a direct impact on the spread of the infection in infants.

Our study shows that monotherapy exerted some benefit in the management of symptomatic children (Butler et al., 1991; McKinney et al., 1991; Resino et al., 2006b). Nevertheless, it had a time-limited effect due to ongoing viral replication that inevitably leads to the emergence of resistant HIV-1 quasispecies, which was also promoted by the lack of drug dosage adjustments for children at that time. The dual-nucleoside therapy proved to be more effective than monotherapy (Englund et al., 1997; Resino et al., 2006b). However, in our setting its effect on mortality or AIDS prevention between 1994- 1996 was similar to that exerted by monotherapy. This finding might be partially attributable to the regimen switch to dual-drug therapy (mainly zidovudine plus didanosine) after several years of zidovudine treatment in many children, when zidovudine was not more completely active. Thus, even with perfect adherence, dual-drug therapy was only partially suppressive being administered as functional monotherapy and due to cross-resistance within the nucleoside analogue class. In addition, during this period more than 40% of the children were still untreated and more than 35% were on monotherapy. Previous studies reported the effectiveness of HAART on the risk of death in the setting of large paediatric cohorts, but these had limited follow-up and lacked assessment of the progression to AIDS (de Martino et al., 2000; Gortmaker et al., 2001). In 2000, the Italian Register for HIV Infection in Children (de Martino et al., 2000) observed a reduction in the mortality rate of 71% in individuals undergoing triple-combination therapy compared with untreated patients, while Gortmaker and colleagues found a 67% reduction comparing HAART with other therapy (Gortmaker et al., 2001). Important reductions of 76% have also been reported recently by a 10-year follow-up survey (Patel et al., 2008). Our analyses found a stronger reduction (84%), but it is not directly comparable with previous published data due to the longer follow-up and to the difference in the performed analyses. In fact, we dealt with the trend of the risk of death in different calendar periods considered as an external time-dependent covariate. The high prevalence of comorbidities, along with multiple causes of death, resulted in increasing complexity of the management of patients with HIV/AIDS.

In terms of specific causes of death, AIDS–defining events were the most represented, with proportions higher than that recently observed in adults (Martinez et al., 2007; Palella et al., 2006). This finding might be directly linked to a late HIV-1 diagnosis at the beginning of the epidemic and to the persistence of opportunistic infections, that were the leading AIDS-defining causes of death (Brady et al., 2010; Selik & Lindegren 2003), although less represented since HAART advent (Currier et al., 1998; Kaplan et al., 2001). As in previous studies, bacterial infections were the largest component of opportunistic infections (Gona et al., 2006; Langston et al., 2001). Although specific information for their aetiology was mainly unavailable, we supposed that pneumococcus (*Streptococcus pneumoniae*) might has been the prominent microbial on the basis of recent reports (Cotton et al., 2008; Gortmaker et al., 2001; Kapogiannis et al., 2008). In addition, the pneumococcal conjugate vaccine available since 2000 (Black et al., 2000) and recommended for all HIV-infected children, has a lower efficacy in these patients than in HIV-uninfected children (Bliss et al., 2008). Some bacterial infections occurred with normal $CD4^{+}$ cell percentage (≥25%), consistently with previous report (Gona et al., 2006), maybe because the HIV-1 infection does not allow the correct development of primary immune function leading to the production of polyclonal, non-specific immunoglobulin increasing the risk of infections with encapsulated bacteria (Brady et al., 2010; Cotton et al., 2008; Gortmaker et al., 2001; Kapogiannis et al., 2008). The population-based analysis yielded consistent results with studies of HIV–infected patients (Kapogiannis et al., 2008; Martinez et al., 2007), highlighting a higher incidence of infections in our cohort than in the general population of similar age from the same region. Along with host immune factors (Janoff et al., 1992), antimicrobial resistance (Cotton et al., 2008; Jaspan et al., 2008), comorbidity and co-infections might have contributed to the high risk of death from opportunistic infections. The introduction of both *Pneumocystis* pneumonia prophylaxis (CDC 1995; Simonds et al., 1995) and HAART in our cohort has been accompanied by substantial reductions in mortality caused by *Pneumocystis* pneumonia (Gona et al., 2006; Kaplan et al., 2000), which have continued to occur in post-HAART era only in infants born to women with late HIV-1 diagnosis or unmonitored pregnancy, causing failure to implement *Pneumocystis* pneumonia prophylaxis (Gibb et al., 2003; Simpson et al., 2000). The cases of *M. avium* complex infection in our cohort have decreased over time (Gona et al., 2006). The cases reported in CP2 were diagnosed in children 6-11 years old, probably as a complication of advanced immunologic deterioration and the difficulty to realize a complete adherence to HAART and *M. avium* complex chemoprophylaxis. On the other hand, our data have shown an increase in the median age at death over time that might reflect improved management and prolongation in the time to development of a first bacteremia (Kapogiannis et al., 2008). More prolonged survival might allow chronic underlying comorbid conditions to become more clinically relevant in the next future. The proportion of HIV–related causes of deaths (12%) increased over time even if not statistically significant. Interestingly, the case of lactic acidosis was related to HAART regimen (stavudine + didanosine + efavirenz) that caused mitochondrial toxicity, whose rate is known to be increased by stavudine + didanosine co-administration (Blanco et al., 2003; Cote et al., 2002). Among non-HIV–related causes of death, the 7% of all the underlying causes, the fulminant hepatic failure occurred in 2008 was HCV-associated. We did not observe the increase of conditions, including diabetes mellitus, cancer, cardiovascular, liver and renal diseases that have become frequent in HIV-1–infected adults (Crum et al., 2006;

Lewden et al., 2008; Novoa et al., 2008; Palella et al., 2006; Sackoff et al., 2006; Smit et al., 2006). The lack of increase of non-HIV-related causes of death might be due to the long duration pathogenesis of these diseases as well as to their rarity, which might have limited power to identify such evolution.

The duration of initial HAART regimens for antiretroviral-naïve children has not been reported. On the contrary, several studies have assessed this public health issue in HIV-1-infected adults (Chen et al., 2003; Miller et al., 1999; Palella Jr et al., 2002; Phillips et al., 2001). The median duration of the first regimen observed in our study population was more than 3 years, the double of the duration described by Cheng and colleagues (2003) in a group of 405 antiretroviral-naïve adults and longer than that observed by Palella et al. (2002) who enrolled patients with previous antiretroviral experience. Notably, our study had a longer follow-up which could in part explain this difference. Among the therapy-naïve paediatric patients enrolled in the HIV Paediatric Cohort of the *Comunidad Autónoma de Madrid*, poor adherence has been identified as primary risk factor for initial HAART regimens discontinuation and short duration. This result is in agreement with the association between adherence and response to antiretroviral therapy reported for paediatric patients, being incomplete adherence the primary cause of treatment failure (Chiappini et al., 2006; Gray et al., 2001; Hainaut et al., 2003; Resino et al., 2003). In addiction, the age at HAART initiation was found to be another independent risk factor for first HAART regimen discontinuation. The impact of HAART on the morbidity and mortality in Spanish HIV-1 vertically infected children has been discussed elsewhere (Resino et al., 2006b; Sanchez et al., 2003). However, an assessment of underlying causes of mortality and a population effectiveness analysis have never been performed in the context of an observational paediatric cohort in Spain. A number of limitations of this study should be noted. First, temporal changes in the spectrum of causes of deaths were not statistically significant; whether this result has been due to the limited number of deaths occurred after 1996 should be cautiously taken into account. Second, a survivor bias due to the partially retrospective enrolment might have caused mortality underestimation in infants at the beginning of the epidemic. Nevertheless our cohort remains more than representative of the HIV-1 epidemic in one of the Spanish regions most affected by the disease over almost three decades.

5. Conclusion

Despite the population effectiveness of HAART in reducing HIV-1-associated mortality, new challenges could arise for national surveillance systems as prolonged survival and long-term antiretroviral exposure might contribute to additional and different causes of death in perinatally infected patients in the future.

6. Acknowledgments

The authors thank patients for their participation and the HIV HGM BioBank belonging to the Spanish AIDS Research Network (RED RIS) and Red Nacional de BioBancos, and The cohort of the Spanish Paediatric HIV Research Network CoRISpe cohort node 1.

This study was partially supported by grants from Red Temática de Investigación Cooperativa Sanitaria ISCIII (RETIC RD06/0006/0035), Fundación para la Investigación y Prevención del SIDA en España (FIPSE 240800/09 and 380910/10), Paediatric European

Network for Treatment of AIDS (PENTA), Fundación Caja Navarra, Fondo de Investigación Sanitaria (FIS INTRASALUD PI09/02029). The Spanish MICINN through the Juan de la Cierva program (JCI-2009-05650) (to C.P.).

7. References

Black, S., Shinefield, H., Fireman, B., Lewis, E., Ray, P., Hansen, J. R., Elvin, L., Ensor, K. M., Hackell, J., Siber, G., Malinoski, F., Madore, D., Chang, I., Kohberger, R., Watson, W., Austrian, R., & Edwards, K. (2000). Efficacy, safety and immunogenicity of heptavalent pneumococcal conjugate vaccine in children. Northern California Kaiser Permanente Vaccine Study Center Group. *Pediatr Infect Dis J*, Vol. 19, No. 3, (Mar 2000), pp. 187-195, 0891-3668 (Print) 0891-3668 (Linking)

Blanche, S., Bologna, R., Cahn, P., Rugina, S., Flynn, P., Fortuny, C., Vis, P., Sekar, V., van Baelen, B., Dierynck, I., & Spinosa-Guzman, S. (2009). Pharmacokinetics, safety and efficacy of darunavir/ritonavir in treatment-experienced children and adolescents. *AIDS*, Vol. 23, No. 15, (Sep 2009), pp. 2005-13, 1473-5571 (Electronic) 0269-9370 (Linking)

Blanco, F., Garcia-Benayas, T., Jose de la Cruz, J., Gonzalez-Lahoz, J., & Soriano, V. (2003). First-line therapy and mitochondrial damage: different nucleosides, different findings. *HIV Clin Trials*, Vol. 4, No. 1, (Jan-Feb 2003), pp. 11-19, 1528-4336 (Print) 1528-4336 (Linking)

Bliss, S. J., O'Brien, K. L., Janoff, E. N., Cotton, M. F., Musoke, P., Coovadia, H., & Levine, O. S. (2008). The evidence for using conjugate vaccines to protect HIV-infected children against pneumococcal disease. *Lancet Infect Dis*, Vol. 8, No. 1, (Jan 2008), pp. 67-80, 1473-3099 (Print) 1473-3099 (Linking)

Brady, M. T., Oleske, J. M., Williams, P. L., Elgie, C., Mofenson, L. M., Dankner, W. M., & Van Dyke, R. B. (2010). Declines in mortality rates and changes in causes of death in HIV-1-infected children during the HAART era. *J Acquir Immune Defic Syndr*, Vol. 53, No. 1, (Jan 2010), pp. 86-94, 1944-7884 (Electronic) 1525-4135 (Linking)

Brahmbhatt, H., Kigozi, G., Wabwire-Mangen, F., Serwadda, D., Lutalo, T., Nalugoda, F., Sewankambo, N., Kiduggavu, M., Wawer, M., & Gray, R. (2006). Mortality in HIV-infected and uninfected children of HIV-infected and uninfected mothers in rural Uganda. *J Acquir Immune Defic Syndr*, Vol. 41, No. 4, (Apr 2006), pp. 504-508, 1525-4135 (Print) 1525-4135 (Linking)

Butler, K. M., Husson, R. N., Balis, F. M., Brouwers, P., Eddy, J., el-Amin, D., Gress, J., Hawkins, M., Jarosinski, P., Moss, H., & et al. (1991). Dideoxyinosine in children with symptomatic human immunodeficiency virus infection. *N Engl J Med*, Vol. 324, No. 3, (Jan 1991), pp. 137-44, 0028-4793 (Print)

Centers for Disease Control and Prevention. (Dec 1992). Revised classification system for HIV-1 infection and expanded surveillance case definition for AIDS among adolescents and adults. *Morbidity and Mortality Recomm Rep*, Vol. 41, No. RR-17, pp. 1-19, 17.02.2011, Available from: <http://www.cdc.gov/mmwr/preview/mmwrhtml/ 00018871.htm>

Centers for Disease Control and Prevention. (Sep 1994). Revised classification system for human immunodeficiency virus infection in children less than 13 years of age. *Morbidity and Mortality Weekly Report CDC Surveill Summ*, Vol. 43, No. RR-12, pp. 1-10, 17.02.2011, Available from:

<http://www.cdc.gov/mmwr/preview/mmwrhtml/ 00032890.htm>

Centers for Disease Control and Prevention. (Apr 1995). Revised guidelines for prophylaxis against Pneumocystis carinii pneumonia for children infected with or perinatally exposed to human immunodeficiency virus. *Morbidity and Mortality Weekly Report,* Vol. 44, No. RR-4, pp. 1-11, 17.02.2011, Available from: <http://www.cdc.gov/mmwr/PDF/rr/rr4404.pdf>

Centers for Disease Control and Prevention. (Apr 1998). Guidelines for use of antiretroviral agents in pediatric HIV infection. *Morbidity and Mortality Weekly Report,* Vol. 47, No. RR-4, pp. 1-31, 17.02.2011, Available from <http://www.cdc.gov/mmwr/preview/mmwrhtml/00053104.htm>

Centro Nacional de Epidemiología. Instituto de Salud Carlos III. (Jun 2010) Vigilancia epidemiológica del SIDA en España, 28.10.2010, Available from: <http://cne.isciii.es. Accessed January 15, 2011>

Chen, R. Y., Westfall, A. O., Mugavero, M. J., Cloud, G. A., Raper, J. L., Chatham, A. G., Acosta, E. P., Taylor, K. H., Carter, J., & Saag, M. S. (2003). Duration of highly active antiretroviral therapy regimens. *Clin Infect Dis,* Vol. 37, No. 5, (Sep 2003), pp. 714-722, 1537-6591 (Electronic) 1058-4838 (Linking)

Chiappini, E., Galli, L., Tovo, P. A., Gabiano, C., Gattinara, G. C., Guarino, A., Badolato, R., Giaquinto, C., Lisi, C., & de Martino, M. (2006). Virologic, immunologic, and clinical benefits from early combined antiretroviral therapy in infants with perinatal HIV-1 infection. *AIDS,* Vol. 20, No. 2, (Jan 2006), pp. 207-215, 0269-9370 (Print) 0269-9370 (Linking)

ClinicalTrials.gov. (2007). Safety and Effectiveness of Raltegravir (MK-0518) in Treatment-Experienced, HIV-Infected Children and Adolescents. NCT00485264. 25.01.2011, Available from: <http://clinicaltrials.gov/ct2/show/NCT00485264?term=NCT00485264&rank=1>

ClinicalTrials.gov. (2008a). An Open Label Pharmacokinetic, Safety And Efficacy Study Of Maraviroc In Combination With Background Therapy For The Treatment Of HIV-1 Infected, CCR5 -Tropic Children. NCT00791700. 28.02.2011, Available from: <http://clinicaltrials.gov/ct2/show/study/NCT00791700>

ClinicalTrials.gov. (2008b). Safety and Antiviral Activity of Etravirine (TMC125) in Treatment-Experienced, HIV Infected Children and Adolescents. NCT00665847. 25.01.2011, Available from: <http://clinicaltrials.gov/ct2/show/results/NCT00665847>

ClinicalTrials.gov. (2009a). Continued Access to Etravirine (ETR) in Treatment Experienced HIV-1 Infected Children and Adolescents. NCT00980538. Available from: <http://clinicaltrials.gov/ct2/show/NCT00980538>

ClinicalTrials.gov. (2009b). Pharmacokinetic Effects of New Antiretroviral Drugs on Children, Adolescents and Young Adults. NCT00977756. 25.01.2011, Available from: <http://clinicaltrials.gov/ct2/show/NCT00977756>

Connor, E. M., Sperling, R. S., Gelber, R., Kiselev, P., Scott, G., O'Sullivan, M. J., VanDyke, R., Bey, M., Shearer, W., Jacobson, R. L., & et al. (1994). Reduction of maternal-infant transmission of human immunodeficiency virus type 1 with zidovudine treatment. Pediatric AIDS Clinical Trials Group Protocol 076 Study Group. *N Engl J Med,* Vol. 331, No. 18, (Nov 1994), pp. 1173-80, 0028-4793 (Print) 0028-4793 (Linking)

Cote, H. C., Brumme, Z. L., Craib, K. J., Alexander, C. S., Wynhoven, B., Ting, L., Wong, H., Harris, M., Harrigan, P. R., O'Shaughnessy, M. V., & Montaner, J. S. (2002). Changes in mitochondrial DNA as a marker of nucleoside toxicity in HIV-infected patients. *N Engl J Med*, Vol. 346, No. 11, (Mar 2002), pp. 811-820, 1533-4406 (Electronic) 0028-4793 (Linking)

Cotton, M. F., Wasserman, E., Smit, J., Whitelaw, A., & Zar, H. J. (2008). High incidence of antimicrobial resistant organisms including extended spectrum beta-lactamase producing Enterobacteriaceae and methicillin-resistant Staphylococcus aureus in nasopharyngeal and blood isolates of HIV-infected children from Cape Town, South Africa. *BMC Infect Dis*, Vol. 8, (Apr 2008), pp. 40, 1471-2334 (Electronic) 1471-2334 (Linking)

Crum, N. F., Riffenburgh, R. H., Wegner, S., Agan, B. K., Tasker, S. A., Spooner, K. M., Armstrong, A. W., Fraser, S., & Wallace, M. R. (2006). Comparisons of causes of death and mortality rates among HIV-infected persons: analysis of the pre-, early, and late HAART (highly active antiretroviral therapy) eras. *J Acquir Immune Defic Syndr*, Vol. 41, No. 2, (Feb 2006), pp. 194-200, 1525-4135 (Print) 1525-4135 (Linking)

Currier, J. S., Williams, P. L., Grimes, J. M., Squires, K. S., Fischl, M. A., & Hammer, S. M. (1998). Incidence rates and risk factors for opportunistic infections in a phase III trial comparing indinavir + ZDV + 3TC to ZDV + 3TC. *Proceedings of the 5th Conference on Retroviruses and Opportunistic Infections*, Chicago, Illinois, USA, Feb 1-5, 1998

De Cock, K. M., Fowler, M. G., Mercier, E., de Vincenzi, I., Saba, J., Hoff, E., Alnwick, D. J., Rogers, M., & Shaffer, N. (2000). Prevention of mother-to-child HIV transmission in resource-poor countries: translating research into policy and practice. *JAMA*, Vol. 283, No. 9, (Mar 2000), pp. 1175-1182, 0098-7484 (Print) 0098-7484 (Linking)

de Martino, M., Tovo, P. A., Balducci, M., Galli, L., Gabiano, C., Rezza, G., & Pezzotti, P. (2000). Reduction in mortality with availability of antiretroviral therapy for children with perinatal HIV-1 infection. Italian Register for HIV Infection in Children and the Italian National AIDS Registry. *JAMA*, Vol. 284, No. 2, (Jul 2000), pp. 190-197, 0098-7484 (Print) 0098-7484 (Linking)

Englund, J. A., Baker, C. J., Raskino, C., McKinney, R. E., Petrie, B., Fowler, M. G., Pearson, D., Gershon, A., McSherry, G. D., Abrams, E. J., Schliozberg, J., & Sullivan, J. L. (1997). Zidovudine, didanosine, or both as the initial treatment for symptomatic HIV-infected children. AIDS Clinical Trials Group (ACTG) Study 152 Team. *N Engl J Med*, Vol. 336, No. 24, (Jun 1997), pp. 1704-1712,

Faye, A., Le Chenadec, J., Dollfus, C., Thuret, I., Douard, D., Firtion, G., Lachassinne, E., Levine, M., Nicolas, J., Monpoux, F., Tricoire, J., Rouzioux, C., Tardieu, M., Mayaux, M. J., & Blanche, S. (2004). Early versus deferred antiretroviral multidrug therapy in infants infected with HIV type 1. *Clin Infect Dis*, Vol. 39, No. 11, (Dec 2004), pp. 1692-1698, 1537-6591 (Electronic) 1058-4838 (Linking)

Fraaij, P. L., Verweel, G., van Rossum, A. M., van Lochem, E. G., Schutten, M., Weemaes, C. M., Hartwig, N. G., Burger, D. M., & de Groot, R. (2005). Sustained viral suppression and immune recovery in HIV type 1-infected children after 4 years of highly active antiretroviral therapy. *Clin Infect Dis*, Vol. 40, No. 4, (Feb 2005), pp. 604-608, 1058-4838 (Print)

Gibb, D. M., Duong, T., Tookey, P. A., Sharland, M., Tudor-Williams, G., Novelli, V., Butler, K., Riordan, A., Farrelly, L., Masters, J., Peckham, C. S., & Dunn, D. T. (2003). Decline in mortality, AIDS, and hospital admissions in perinatally HIV-1 infected children in the United Kingdom and Ireland. *BMJ*, Vol. 327, No. 7422, (Nov 2003), pp. 1019

Gona, P., Van Dyke, R. B., Williams, P. L., Dankner, W. M., Chernoff, M. C., Nachman, S. A., & Seage, G. R., 3rd. (2006). Incidence of opportunistic and other infections in HIV-infected children in the HAART era. *JAMA*, Vol. 296, No. 3, (Jul 2006), pp. 292-300, 1538-3598 (Electronic) 0098-7484 (Linking)

Gortmaker, S. L., Hughes, M., Cervia, J., Brady, M., Johnson, G. M., Seage, G. R., 3rd, Song, L. Y., Dankner, W. M., & Oleske, J. M. (2001). Effect of combination therapy including protease inhibitors on mortality among children and adolescents infected with HIV-1. *N Engl J Med*, Vol. 345, No. 21, (Nov 2001), pp. 1522-1528,

Gray, L., Newell, M. L., Thorne, C., Peckham, C., & Levy, J. (2001). Fluctuations in symptoms in human immunodeficiency virus-infected children: the first 10 years of life. *Pediatrics*, Vol. 108, No. 1, (Jul 2001), pp. 116-122, 1098-4275 (Electronic) 0031-4005 (Linking)

Hainaut, M., Ducarme, M., Schandene, L., Peltier, C. A., Marissens, D., Zissis, G., Mascart, F., & Levy, J. (2003). Age-related immune reconstitution during highly active antiretroviral therapy in human immunodeficiency virus type 1-infected children. *Pediatr Infect Dis J*, Vol. 22, No. 1, (Jan 2003), pp. 62-69, 0891-3668 (Print) 0891-3668 (Linking)

Janoff, E. N., Breiman, R. F., Daley, C. L., & Hopewell, P. C. (1992). Pneumococcal disease during HIV infection. Epidemiologic, clinical, and immunologic perspectives. *Ann Intern Med*, Vol. 117, No. 4, (Aug 1992), pp. 314-324, 0003-4819 (Print) 0003-4819 (Linking)

Jaspan, H. B., Huang, L. C., Cotton, M. F., Whitelaw, A., & Myer, L. (2008). Bacterial disease and antimicrobial susceptibility patterns in HIV-infected, hospitalized children: a retrospective cohort study. *PLoS One*, Vol. 3, No. 9, (Set 2008), pp. e3260, 1932-6203 (Electronic) 1932-6203 (Linking)

Joint United Nations Programme on HIV/AIDS. (July 2010). UNAIDS Outlook Report, Geneva, Switzerland: UNAIDS, p. 7, 20.01.2011, Available from: <http://data.unaids.org/pub/Outlook/2010/20100713_outlook_report_web_en.pdf >

Judd, A., Doerholt, K., Tookey, P. A., Sharland, M., Riordan, A., Menson, E., Novelli, V., Lyall, E. G., Masters, J., Tudor-Williams, G., Duong, T., & Gibb, D. M. (2007). Morbidity, mortality, and response to treatment by children in the United Kingdom and Ireland with perinatally acquired HIV infection during 1996-2006: planning for teenage and adult care. *Clin Infect Dis*, Vol. 45, No. 7, (Oct 2007), pp. 918-924

Kaplan, J. E., Hanson, D., Dworkin, M. S., Frederick, T., Bertolli, J., Lindegren, M. L., Holmberg, S., & Jones, J. L. (2000). Epidemiology of human immunodeficiency virus-associated opportunistic infections in the United States in the era of highly active antiretroviral therapy. *Clin Infect Dis*, Vol. 30 Suppl 1, No., (Apr 2000), pp. S5-14, 1058-4838 (Print) 1058-4838 (Linking)

Kaplan, J. E., Sepkowitz, K., Masur, H., Sirisanthana, T., Russo, M., & Chapman, L. (2001). Opportunistic infections in persons with HIV or other immunocompromising conditions. *Emerg Infect Dis*, Vol. 7, No. 3 Suppl, (Aug 2001), pp. 541, 1080-6040 (Print) 1080-6040 (Linking)

Kapogiannis, B. G., Soe, M. M., Nesheim, S. R., Sullivan, K. M., Abrams, E., Farley, J., Palumbo, P., Koenig, L. J., & Bulterys, M. (2008). Trends in bacteremia in the pre- and post-highly active antiretroviral therapy era among HIV-infected children in the US Perinatal AIDS Collaborative Transmission Study (1986-2004). *Pediatrics*, Vol. 121, No. 5, (May 2008), pp. e1229-1239, 1098-4275 (Electronic) 0031-4005 (Linking)

Langston, C., Cooper, E. R., Goldfarb, J., Easley, K. A., Husak, S., Sunkle, S., Starc, T. J., & Colin, A. A. (2001). Human immunodeficiency virus-related mortality in infants and children: data from the pediatric pulmonary and cardiovascular complications of vertically transmitted HIV (P(2)C(2)) Study. *Pediatrics*, Vol. 107, No. 2, (Feb 2001), pp. 328-338, 1098-4275 (Electronic) 0031-4005 (Linking)

Lewden, C., May, T., Rosenthal, E., Burty, C., Bonnet, F., Costagliola, D., Jougla, E., Semaille, C., Morlat, P., Salmon, D., Cacoub, P., & Chene, G. (2008). Changes in causes of death among adults infected by HIV between 2000 and 2005: The "Mortalite 2000 and 2005" surveys (ANRS EN19 and Mortavic). *J Acquir Immune Defic Syndr*, Vol. 48, No. 5, (Aug 2008), pp. 590-598, 1525-4135 (Print) 1525-4135 (Linking)

Marinda, E., Humphrey, J. H., Iliff, P. J., Mutasa, K., Nathoo, K. J., Piwoz, E. G., Moulton, L. H., Salama, P., & Ward, B. J. (2007). Child mortality according to maternal and infant HIV status in Zimbabwe. *Pediatr Infect Dis J*, Vol. 26, No. 6, (Jun 2007), pp. 519-526

Martinez, E., Milinkovic, A., Buira, E., de Lazzari, E., Leon, A., Larrousse, M., Lonca, M., Laguno, M., Blanco, J. L., Mallolas, J., Garcia, F., Miro, J. M., & Gatell, J. M. (2007). Incidence and causes of death in HIV-infected persons receiving highly active antiretroviral therapy compared with estimates for the general population of similar age and from the same geographical area. *HIV Med*, Vol. 8, No. 4, (May 2007), pp. 251-258, 1464-2662 (Print) 1464-2662 (Linking)

McKinney, R. E., Jr., Maha, M. A., Connor, E. M., Feinberg, J., Scott, G. B., Wulfsohn, M., McIntosh, K., Borkowsky, W., Modlin, J. F., Weintrub, P., & et al. (1991). A multicenter trial of oral zidovudine in children with advanced human immunodeficiency virus disease. The Protocol 043 Study Group. *N Engl J Med*, Vol. 324, No. 15, (Apr 11 1991), pp. 1018-1025

Miller, V., Staszewski, S., Sabin, C., Carlebach, A., Rottmann, C., Weidmann, E., Rabenau, H., Hill, A., Lepri, A. C., & Phillips, A. N. (1999). CD4 lymphocyte count as a predictor of the duration of highly active antiretroviral therapy-induced suppression of human immunodeficiency virus load. *J Infect Dis*, Vol. 180, No. 2, (Aug 1999), pp. 530-533, 0022-1899 (Print) 0022-1899 (Linking)

Ministerio de sanidad y Consumo. (Nov 1998). Encuesta hospitalaria sobre la utilización de recursos y características de los pacientes VIH/SIDA, 17.02.2011, Available from: <www.msc.es/sida/epidemiologia>

Newell, M. L., Coovadia, H., Cortina-Borja, M., Rollins, N., Gaillard, P., & Dabis, F. (2004). Mortality of infected and uninfected infants born to HIV-infected mothers in Africa: a pooled analysis. *Lancet*, Vol. 364, No. 9441, (Oct 2004), pp. 1236-1243, 1474-547X (Electronic) 0140-6736 (Linking)

Novoa, A. M., de Olalla, P. G., Clos, R., Orcau, A., Rodriguez-Sanz, M., & Cayla, J. A. (2008). Increase in the non-HIV-related deaths among AIDS cases in the HAART era. *Curr HIV Res*, Vol. 6, No. 1, (Jan 2008), pp. 77-81, 1873-4251 (Electronic) 1570-162X (Linking)

Palella, F. J., Jr., Baker, R. K., Moorman, A. C., Chmiel, J. S., Wood, K. C., Brooks, J. T., & Holmberg, S. D. (2006). Mortality in the highly active antiretroviral therapy era: changing causes of death and disease in the HIV outpatient study. *J Acquir Immune Defic Syndr*, Vol. 43, No. 1, (Sep 2006), pp. 27-34, 1525-4135 (Print) 1525-4135 (Linking)

Palella Jr, F. J., Chmiel, J. S., Moorman, A. C., & Holmberg, S. D. (2002). Durability and predictors of success of highly active antiretroviral therapy for ambulatory HIV-infected patients. *AIDS*, Vol. 16, No. 12, (Aug 2002), pp. 1617-1626, 0269-9370 (Print) 0269-9370 (Linking)

Palladino, C., Bellon, J. M., Perez-Hoyos, S., Resino, R., Guillen, S., Garcia, D., Gurbindo, M. D., Ramos, J. T., de Jose, M. I., Mellado, M. J., & Munoz-Fernandez, M. A. (2008). Spatial pattern of HIV-1 mother-to-child-transmission in Madrid (Spain) from 1980 till now: demographic and socioeconomic factors. *AIDS*, Vol. 22, No. 16, (Oct 2008), pp. 2199-2205, 1473-5571 (Electronic) 0269-9370 (Linking)

Patel, K., Hernan, M. A., Williams, P. L., Seeger, J. D., McIntosh, K., Van Dyke, R. B., & Seage, G. R., 3rd. (2008). Long-term effectiveness of highly active antiretroviral therapy on the survival of children and adolescents with HIV infection: a 10-year follow-up study. *Clin Infect Dis*, Vol. 46, No. 4, (Feb 2008), pp. 507-515

Phillips, A. N., Miller, V., Sabin, C., Cozzi Lepri, A., Klauke, S., Bickel, M., Doerr, H. W., Hill, A., & Staszewski, S. (2001). Durability of HIV-1 viral suppression over 3.3 years with multi-drug antiretroviral therapy in previously drug-naive individuals. *AIDS*, Vol. 15, No. 18, (Dec 2001), pp. 2379-2384, 0269-9370 (Print) 0269-9370 (Linking)

Pizzo, P. A., Eddy, J., Falloon, J., Balis, F. M., Murphy, R. F., Moss, H., Wolters, P., Brouwers, P., Jarosinski, P., Rubin, M., Broder, S., Yarchoan, R., Brunetti, A., Maha, M., Nusinoff-Lehrman, S., & Poplack, D. G. (1988). Effect of continuous intravenous infusion of zidovudine (AZT) in children with symptomatic HIV infection. *N Engl J Med*, Vol. 319, No. 14, (Oct 1988), pp. 889-896, 0028-4793 (Print) 0028-4793 (Linking)

Puthanakit, T., Aurpibul, L., Oberdorfer, P., Akarathum, N., Kanjananit, S., Wannarit, P., Sirisanthana, T., & Sirisanthana, V. (2007). Hospitalization and mortality among HIV-infected children after receiving highly active antiretroviral therapy. *Clin Infect Dis*, Vol. 44, No. 4, (Feb 2007), pp. 599-604, 1537-6591 (Electronic)

Reddi, A., Leeper, S. C., Grobler, A. C., Geddes, R., France, K. H., Dorse, G. L., Vlok, W. J., Mntambo, M., Thomas, M., Nixon, K., Holst, H. L., Karim, Q. A., Rollins, N. C., Coovadia, H. M., & Giddy, J. (2007). Preliminary outcomes of a paediatric highly active antiretroviral therapy cohort from KwaZulu-Natal, South Africa. *BMC Pediatr*, Vol. 7, (Mar 2007), pp. 13-25, 1471-2431 (Electronic)

Resino, S., Bellon, J. M., Gurbindo, D., Leon, J. A., & Munoz-Fernandez, M. A. (2003). Recovery of T-cell subsets after antiretroviral therapy in HIV-infected children. *Eur J Clin Invest*, Vol. 33, No. 7, (Jul 2003), pp. 619-627, 0014-2972 (Print) 0014-2972 (Linking)

Resino, S., Alvaro-Meca, A., de Jose, M. I., Martin-Fontelos, P., Gutierrez, M. D., Leon, J. A., Ramos, J. T., Ciria, L., & Munoz-Fernandez, M. A. (2006a). Low immunologic response to highly active antiretroviral therapy in naive vertically human immunodeficiency virus type 1-infected children with severe immunodeficiency. *Pediatr Infect Dis J*, Vol. 25, No. 4, (Apr 2006a), pp. 365-368, 0891-3668 (Print)

Resino, S., Resino, R., Bellon, J. M., Micheloud, D., Gutierrez, M. D., de Jose, M. I., Ramos, J. T., Fontelos, P. M., Ciria, L., & Munoz-Fernandez, M. A. (2006b). Clinical outcomes improve with highly active antiretroviral therapy in vertically HIV type-1-infected children. *Clin Infect Dis*, Vol. 43, No. 2, (Jul 2006b), pp. 243-252, 1058-4838 (Print)

Sackoff, J. E., Hanna, D. B., Pfeiffer, M. R., & Torian, L. V. (2006). Causes of death among persons with AIDS in the era of highly active antiretroviral therapy: New York City. *Ann Intern Med*, Vol. 145, No. 6, (Sep 2006), pp. 397-406, 1539-3704 (Electronic) 0003-4819 (Linking)

Salazar, J. C., Cahn, P., Yogev, R., Negra, M. D., Castelli-Gattinara, G., Fortuny, C., Flynn, P. M., Giaquinto, C., Ruan, P. K., Smith, M. E., Mikl, J., & Jelaska, A. (2008). Efficacy, safety and tolerability of tipranavir coadministered with ritonavir in HIV-1-infected children and adolescents. *AIDS*, Vol. 22, No. 14, (Sep 2008), pp. 1789-1798, 1473-5571 (Electronic) 0269-9370 (Linking)

Sanchez, J. M., Ramos Amador, J. T., Fernandez de Miguel, S., Gonzalez Tomee, M. I., Rojo Conejo, P., Ferrnado Vivas, P., Clemente Vivas, J., Ruiz Contreras, J., & Nogales Espert, A. (2003). Impact of highly active antiretroviral therapy on the morbidity and mortality in Spanish human immunodeficiency virus-infected children. *Pediatr Infect Dis J*, Vol. 22, No. 10, (Oct 2003), pp. 863-867, 0891-3668 (Print)

Scherpbier, H. J., Bekker, V., van Leth, F., Jurriaans, S., Lange, J. M., & Kuijpers, T. W. (2006). Long-term experience with combination antiretroviral therapy that contains nelfinavir for up to 7 years in a pediatric cohort. *Pediatrics*, Vol. 117, No. 3, (Mar 2006), pp. e528-536, 1098-4275 (Electronic) 0031-4005 (Linking)

Selik, R. M., & Lindegren, M. L. (2003). Changes in deaths reported with human immunodeficiency virus infection among United States children less than thirteen years old, 1987 through 1999. *Pediatr Infect Dis J*, Vol. 22, No. 7, (Jul 2003), pp. 635-641, 0891-3668 (Print) 0891-3668 (Linking)

Simonds, R. J., Lindegren, M. L., Thomas, P., Hanson, D., Caldwell, B., Scott, G., & Rogers, M. (1995). Prophylaxis against Pneumocystis carinii pneumonia among children with perinatally acquired human immunodeficiency virus infection in the United States. Pneumocystis carinii Pneumonia Prophylaxis Evaluation Working Group. *N Engl J Med*, Vol. 332, No. 12, (Mar 1995), pp. 786-790, 0028-4793 (Print) 0028-4793 (Linking)

Simpson, B. J., Shapiro, E. D., & Andiman, W. A. (2000). Prospective cohort study of children born to human immunodeficiency virus-infected mothers, 1985 through 1997: trends in the risk of vertical transmission, mortality and acquired immunodeficiency syndrome indicator diseases in the era before highly active antiretroviral therapy. *Pediatr Infect Dis J*, Vol. 19, No. 7, (Jul 2000), pp. 618-624, 0891-3668 (Print) 0891-3668 (Linking)

Smit, C., Geskus, R., Walker, S., Sabin, C., Coutinho, R., Porter, K., & Prins, M. (2006). Effective therapy has altered the spectrum of cause-specific mortality following HIV seroconversion. *AIDS*, Vol. 20, No. 5, (Mar 2006), pp. 741-749, 0269-9370 (Print) 0269-9370 (Linking)

The European Collaborative Study. Mother-to-child transmission of HIV infection in the era of highly active antiretroviral therapy. *Clin Infect Dis*, Vol. 40, No. 3, (Feb 2005), pp. 458-465, 1537-6591 (Electronic) 1058-4838 (Linking)

The European Collaborative Study (1994). Natural history of vertically acquired human immunodeficiency virus-1 infection. *Pediatrics*, Vol. 94, No. 6 Pt 1, (Dec 1994), pp. 815-819, 0031-4005 (Print) 0031-4005 (Linking)

Violari, A., Cotton, M., Gibb, D., Babiker, A., Steyn, J., Jean-Phillip, P., J., M., & Team., o. b. o. t. C. S. (2007). Antiretroviral therapy initiated before 12 weeks of age reduces early mortality in young HIV-infected infants: evidence from the Children with HIV Early Antiretroviral Therapy (CHER) Study. Fourth Internationa AIDS Society Conference, Sydney, Australia, July 22–25, 2007, 17.02.2011, Available from; <http://www.ias2007.org/pag/Abstracts.aspx?AID=5557>

Walker, A. S., Doerholt, K., Sharland, M., & Gibb, D. M. (2004). Response to highly active antiretroviral therapy varies with age: the UK and Ireland Collaborative HIV Paediatric Study. *AIDS*, Vol. 18, No. 14, (Sep 2004), pp. 1915-1924, 0269-9370 (Print) 0269-9370 (Linking)

WHO/UNAIDS/UNICEF. (Sep 2010). Towards Universal Access: Scaling up Priority HIV/AIDS Interventions in the Health Sector: Progress Report 2010. Geneva, Switzerland: World Health Organization, pp. 1-146, 20.01.2011, Available from: <http://www.who.int/hiv/pub/2010progressreport/en/>

Cannabinoids – Influence on the Immune System and Their Potencial Use in Supplementary Therapy of HIV/AIDS

Alicja Szulakowska and Halina Milnerowicz
Department of Biomedical and Environmental Analyses, Faculty of Pharmacy,
Silesian Piasts University of Medicine in Wroclaw
Poland

1. Introduction

Cannabis sativa (Fig. 1.) has been valued for its medicinal as well as its psychotropic properties dating back to ancient times. In nineteenth century W.B. O'Shaughnessy used marijuana for pain relief and Jean-Jacques Moreau de Tours - French psychiatrist, said, that cannabis is very helpful in therapy of psychiatric disorders (Booth, 2004). Main constituents of *Cannabis sativa* were discovered in 1960's and named after the plant - cannabinoids. The identification of the chemical structure of *cannabis* components and the possibility of obtaining its pure constituents were related to a significant increase in scientific interest in this plant. This interest was renewed in the 1990's with the description of cannabinoid receptors and the identification of an endogenous cannabinoid system in the brain (Zuardi, 2006).
The most notable of the cannabinoids are: tetrahydrocannabinol (THC) - the most psychoactive substance found in the cannabis plant and cannabidiol - constituent which has displayed sedative effects. Both constituents can be found in the brown resin secreted by the hair which covers female plants (Truta et al., 2002). Cannabinoids bind to the cannabinoid receptors (CB receptors), change metabolism of the cells, moderate neurotransmission and hormones extraction, what affect main functions of the human body (Demuth et al., 2006, ElSohly et al., 2005).
The cannabinoid receptor family currently includes two types: CB1, characterized mostly in neuronal cells and brain, and CB2, characterized in immune cells (lymphocytes and macrophages) and tissues (spleen and tonsils) (Demuth et al., 2006). Both receptors are proteins and consist of seven transmembrane–spanning domains (Fig. 2.)(Joy et al., 1999). The CB1 molecule is larger than CB2. However, both receptor molecules are alike in four of the seven regions embedded in the cell membrane (known as the transmembrane regions). The intracellular loops of the two receptor subtypes are quite different, which might affect the cellular response to the ligand (Szulakowska&Milnerowicz, 2007). Human body also produces substances that activate CB receptors, they are known as endocannabinoids. The studies have revealed a broad role of endocannabinoids and cannabinoid receptors in a variety of physiological processes as neuromodulation, pain and appetite sensation, motor learning (Saito et al., 2010).

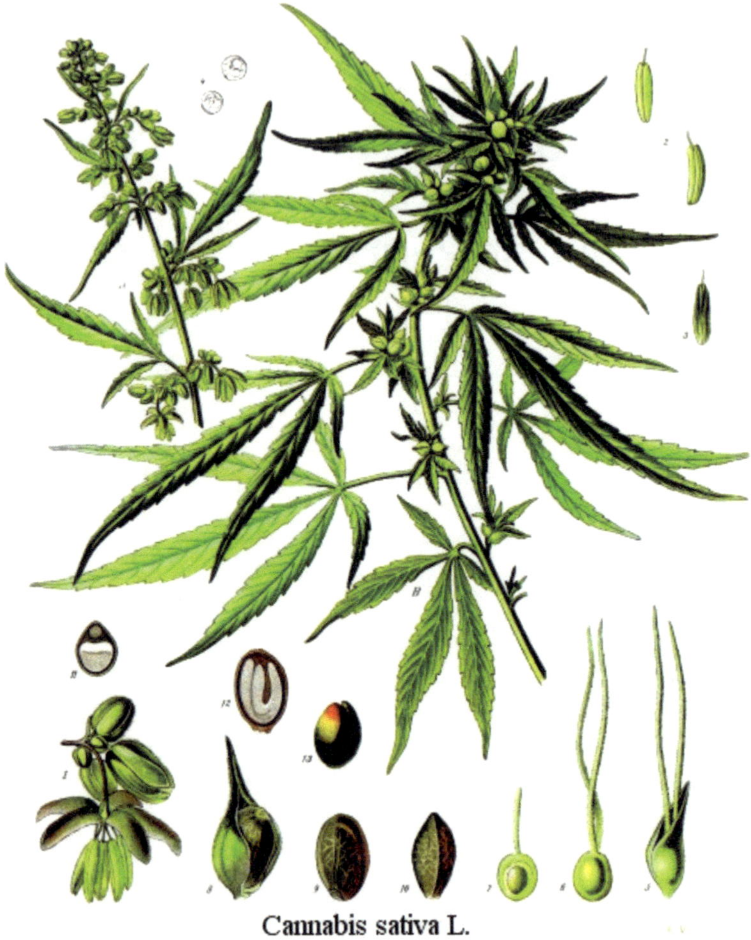

Fig. 1. *Cannabis sativa* (Kohler, 1887).

2. Cannabinoids and the immune system

The study of marijuana cannabinoid biology has led to many important discoveries in immunology; not only existence of a new physiological system - the endocannabinoid system, but also its role in the regulation of the immune system. Studies examining the effect of cannabinoids on immunity have shown that many cellular and cytokine mechanisms are suppressed by these agents (Klein&Cabral, 2006).

2.1 Cellular effects

Scientists have already suggested in 1970s that cannabinoids can change the number and function of T cells. Various functions from cytotoxic T cell killing to antibody production by B cells have been examined. Nong and Co. have studied the T-cell rosetting capacity of lymphocytes in CD4 and CD8 subsets – it was impaired in peripheral blood cells from marijuana users. Scientists examined also the effects on the number of lymphocytes in CD4 and CD8 subsets. The percentage of CD4 T cells was increased in peripheral blood cells from marijuana smokers, with a mean CD4/CD8 ratio of 1.95 as opposed to 1.27 in controls (Nong et al., 2002; Massi et al., 2006). Finally, Klein and Co. proved that cannabinoids affect cytotoxic T lymphocytes (CTL) - after incubation with THC, the cytolytic activity of CTL was depressed by about 60% (Klein et al., 1991). It also appeared that cannabinoids can disrupt proliferation and cytolytic activity in natural killer cells (NK), which plays very important role in host defences against tumors and microbes (Massi et al., 2006).

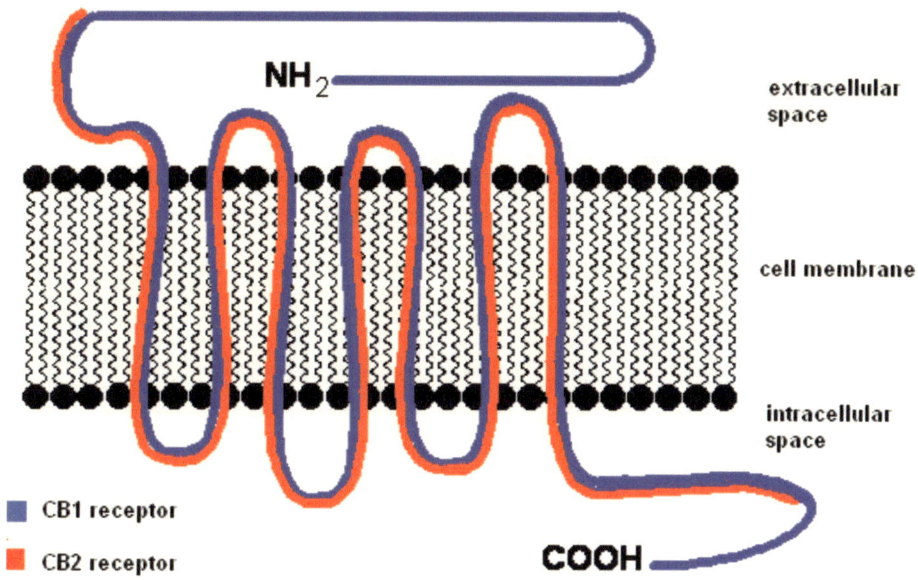

Fig. 2. Cannabinoid receptors CB1 and CB2 (Joy et al., 1999).

Functions of macrophages are also impaired by cannabinoids through either a receptor- or non-receptor-mediated mechanism. Studies with pulmonary alveolar macrophages showed that cannabinoids significantly lowered the level of tumor necrosis factor α (TNFα) in the bronchoalveolar lavage (Klein et al., 1991). Scientists proved that cannabinoids influenced the ability of macrophages to process antigens necessary for the activation of CD4+ T lymphocytes (McCoy et al., 1999), reduced chemotaxis (Sacerdote et al., 2000) and affect the production of arachidonic acid metabolites in macrophage cultures (Berdyshev et al., 2000). The influence of cannabinoids on NO production is still unclear (Massi et al., 2006).

2.2 Cytokines and hormones

Cannabinoids can modulate the action of cytokines mostly by affecting immune cells, for example macrophages or Th cells, their immunomodulatory properties are complex, what was shown in the Table 1.

Scientists proved that cannabinoids can modulate immune response also by affecting hormones release. For example administration of THC, may increase level of adrenocorticotropic hormone and corticosterone, what is causing downstream release of immunoregulatory molecules as cortizol and sex hormones and inhibition of immune response (Massi et al., 2006; Tanasescu&Constantinescu, 2010; Baker et al., 2007).

Name of the cytokine	Cannabinoid infulence	General result	References
IFNγ	Decreased level	Anti-inflammatory action	(Zheng et al., 1992, 1996)
TNFα	Decreased level	Anti-inflammatory action	(Zheng et al., 1992, 1996)
Il-1	Decreased level	Anti-inflammatory action	(Kozela et al., 2010)
Il-2	Decreased level	Anti-inflammatory action	(Zhu et al., 1993)
Il-4	Increased level	Action unclear	(Klein et al., 2000)
Il-6	Decreased level	Anti-inflammatory action	(Kozela et al., 2010)
Il-10	Decreased level	Action unclear	(Sacerdote et al., 2005)
Il-12	Decreased level (THC)/increased level (CBD)	Anti-inflammatory action (THC)/ Anti-inflammatory action	Massi et al., 2006; Klein et al., 2000; Sacerdote et al., 2005)

Table 1. Cannabinoid influence on cytokines profile

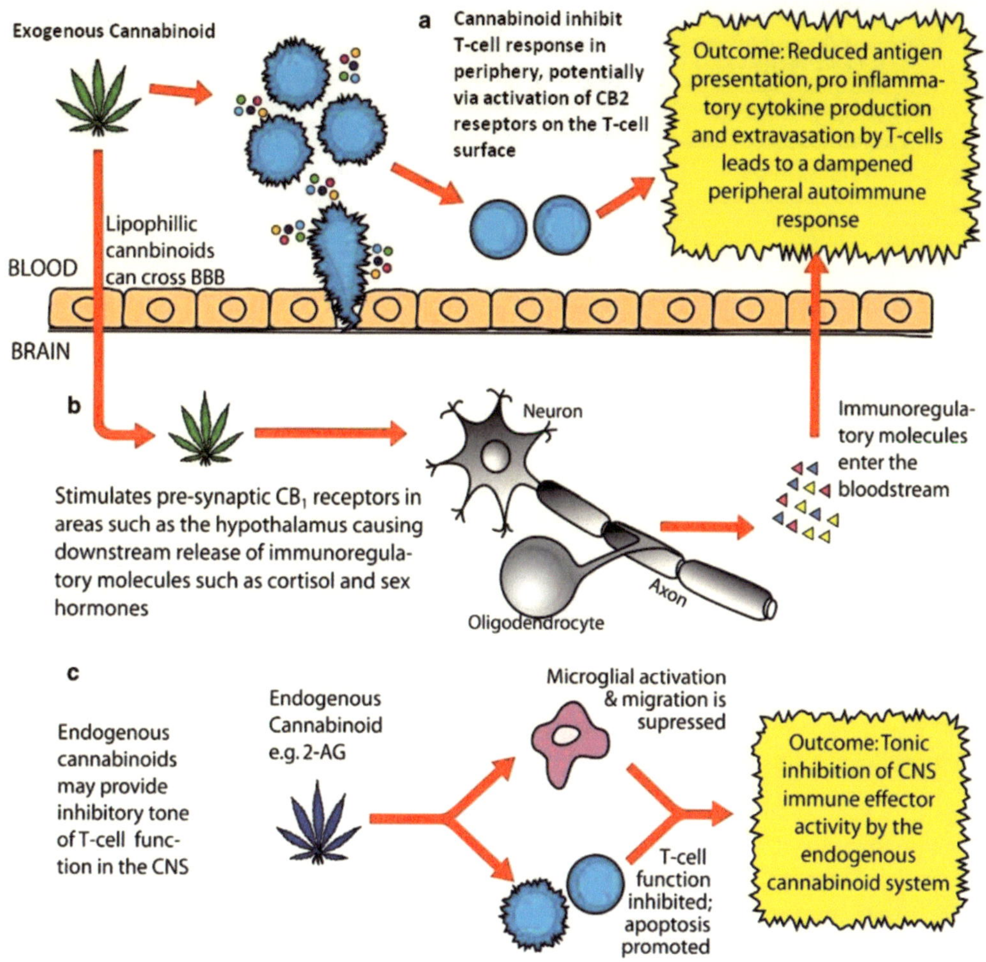

Fig. 3. Immune regulation by cannabinoids. Exogenously administered cannabinoids (a, b) or endocannabinoids (c) may inhibit the action of the immune response in either the periphery (a, b) or the central nervous system (CNS; c) via either a direct (a, c) or indirect (b) action on leukocytes (from Baker et al., 2007).

Cannabinoids can modulate immune reactions in the periphery but also in the brain, influence T cell subset balance and cytokine expression. Generally, they alter many functions of the immune response, what was shown in the Fig. 3. (Baker et al., 2007).

3. Immunological consequences of cannabinoids use by HIV/AIDS patients

Anti-inflammatory potential action of cannabinoids tends to be evident from the studies discussed in the previous paragraph. Cannabinoids do induce apoptosis in immune cells and alleviate inflammatory responses (Rieder et al., 2010). Even though the progressive failure of the immune system is a cause of AIDS disease, no conclusive data have been obtained as to potential risk associated with HIV infection and the use of cannabinoids. In 2003 Abrams and co. examined short-term effects of cannabinoids in patients with HIV-1 infection. Scientists measured HIV RNA level and CD4+ and CD8+ cell subsets, during 21 days of oral and smoked marijuana administration among 67 patients with HIV-1 infection. At days 0 and 21, HIV RNA was undetectable in 50% to 55% of patients in each group, the mean changes were decreases in both cannabinoid groups: marijuana group and dronabinol group. The unadjusted mean increases in CD4+ cell counts were greater for patients receiving cannabinoids than for patients receiving placebo. CD8+ cell counts were on average 20% greater for patients receiving marijuana than for patients receiving placebo and marginally greater (average 10%) for patients receiving dronabinol than for those receiving placebo. Authors concluded that smoked and oral cannabinoids did not seem to be unsafe in patients with HIV infection with respect to HIV RNA levels, CD4+ and CD8+ cell counts (Abrams et al., 2003).

Kosel and co. decided to examine effects of cannabinoids on the pharmacokinetics of indinavir and nelfinavir - protease inhibitors used as a component of highly active antiretroviral therapy to treat HIV infection and AIDS. Patients on stable regimens containing indinavir or nelfinavir were randomized to one of three treatments: 3.95% THC marijuana cigarettes, dronabinol 2.5 mg capsules or placebo capsules administered three times daily. The treatment lasted 14 days. Authors concluded that their results after marijuana treatment (statistically significant decrease in maximum concentration of nelfinavir - C(max)) by -17.4% (P=0.46) and the magnitude of changes in indinavir concentration - C(max) by -14.1% (P=0.039)), are likely to have no short-term clinical consequence. The use of cannabinoids is unlikely to impact antiretroviral efficacy (Kosel et al., 2002).

4. Therapeutic use of marijuana for people living with HIV/AIDS

Over 40 million people are affected by HIV/AIDS in the world. There is still no cure available for this disease, although remarkable improvements in the quality and life expectancy have been achieved. Most of the patients are on long-term treatment with combinations of antiretroviral therapies and cope with the side effects of these therapies (nausea, vomiting, pain, reduced appetite, weight loss, headaches, diarrhea, constipation, anxiety and depression) (Woolridge et al., 2005). Recently, therapeutic use of marijuana has emerged as an important issue for people living with HIV/AIDS. Fogarty et al. reported that people with HIV/AIDS who use marijuana indicate improved moods, sensory experiences, creativity, increased socialising, elation and changes in appetite (Fogarty et al., 2007; Woolridge et al., 2005). In 2005 Woolridge et al. surveyed 143 HIV positive people who reported using marijuana to manage side effects of long-term anti-retroviral treatment. Results were shown in the table below (Table 2.) (Woolridge et al., 2005).

The ability of cannabinoid to treat pain, nausea, appetite loss, muscle spasm and a wide variety of other symptoms causes that more and more HIV/AIDS patients reach for marijuana as an alternative remedy. The actual numbers of HIV/AIDS patients that use marijuana to treat HIV related symptoms is a difficult number to quantify, but some researchers report that this number is quite significant (Cannon, 2010).

In 1998/1999, in Canada approximately 15% of 977 responders were using marijuana for medical purposes (Braitstein et al., 2001). In California in 2001 – 33.3% of the 442 responders reported the use of marijuana (Cannon, 2010). Regarding this data, in 2007 scientists examined people living with HIV/AIDS in Australia. The results show that among 408 participants, 59.8% reported some use of marijuana in the past six months. 244 (55.7% of those) reported recreational use only of marijuana and 44.3% admitted mixed use of marijuana for therapeutic and recreational purposes (Fogarty et al., 2007). In 2007/2008 in South Africa only 3.7% of 618 admitted that was using marijuana in the past six month, mostly for stress relief (85.7%) and to a lesser extent for recreational purposes (relaxation) (23.5%) and pain relief (17.6%) (Peltzer et al., 2008). These results from different places in the world show that substantial proportion of people living with HIV/AIDS use marijuana for therapeutic purposes, despite considerable legal barriers, suggesting that cannabis represents another option in their health management (Fogarty et al., 2007). The small percentage of South Africans with HIV/AIDS using marijuana for therapeutic purposes may be caused by poverty (marijuana is more expensive than other alternative, supplementary methods like micronutrients, religious healing) and limited access to information about alternative therapy (Peltzer et al., 2008).

Symptom	Number of complaints	Much better [%]	Little better [%]	No change [%]	Little worse [%]	Much worse [%]
Lack of appetite	111	79	18	2	0	1
Pain in muscle	65	63	31	6	0	0
Nausea	62	56	37	3	2	2
Anxiety	98	64	49	3	2	2
Nerve pain	53	51	40	9	0	0
Depression	94	56	30	9	4	1
Tingling	46	37	48	9	7	0
Numbness	42	36	36	24	5	0
Weight loss	62	45	24	31	0	0
Headaches	46	35	30	33	2	0
Tremor	24	37	29	21	13	0
Constipation	24	21	29	46	4	0
Tiredness	60	17	33	33	15	2
Diarrhea	48	13	23	56	6	2
Vision dimness	22	9	27	55	9	0
Weakness	48	10	21	54	15	0
Memory loss	38	13	5	34	34	13
Slurred speech	9	11	0	78	11	0

Table 2. Effect of marijuana on Complaint of Symptoms in 143 HIV Patients (from Woolridge et al., 2005).

4.1 Pain management

Neuropathic pain and muscular pain is reported by people living with HIV/AIDS. Patients describe pain as "aching", "burning" and "painful numbness" of legs and hands mostly (Cannon, 2010). Despite management with opioids and other pain modifying therapies, neuropathic pain continues to reduce the quality of life among 30% or more of HIV-infected individuals. Scientists suppose that pain perception is modulated by cannabinoid receptors in the central and peripheral nervous system (Ellis et al., 2009) via endocannabinoids, an endogenous system of retrograde neuromodulatory messengers that work in tandem with endogenous opioids (McCarberg, 2007).

Cannabinoids have been shown to inhibit the experience of pain in both - animal and human studies. It was demonstrated in 2007 in a study conducted by Abrams et al. He decided to determine the effect of smoked cannabis on the neuropathic pain of HIV-associated sensory neuropathy and an experimental pain model. Scientists asked fifty patients to smoke either cannabis or identical placebo cigarettes with the cannabinoids extracted three times daily for 5 days. Reduction in pain intensity was measured. It occurred that smoked cannabis reduced daily pain by 34% with placebo. Greater than 30% reduction of pain was reported by 52% in the cannabis group and by 24% in the placebo group. The first cannabis cigarette reduced chronic pain by a median of 72% vs 15% with placebo (Abrams et al., 2007). Similar trial was conducted by American scientists in 2009. Ellis et al. examined 127 HIV-associated distal sensory predominant polyneuropathy and measured change in pain intensity by the Descriptor Differential Scale (DDS) from a pretreatment baseline to the end of each treatment week. Treatments were placebo and delta-9-tetrahydrocannabinol, smoked four times daily for 5 consecutive days during each of 2 treatment weeks, separated by a 2-week washout. Among all the patients, pain relief was greater with cannabis than placebo and the proportions of subjects achieving at least 30% pain relief with cannabis vs placebo were 0.46 and 0.18. Results were shown in Fig. 4. (Ellis et al., 2009). This study's findings are equivalent to those achieved by Abrams et al. in 2007 and consistent with other recent research supporting the short-term efficacy of cannabis for neuropathic pain (Ellis et al., 2009; Abrams et al., 2007).

Results of other studies show that cannabis can treat not only the neuropathic pain but also muscular and chronic pain. Woolridge study demonstrated that 94% of participants reported positive results for muscular pain management using marijuana (Cannon, 2010; Woolridge et al., 2005). Finally, as it was mentioned in the previous paragraph, 30% reduction in chronic pain was reported by 52% of the smoked cannabis group (Cannon, 2010; Abrams et al., 2007).

Scientists suppose that analgetic properties of cannabinoids are effect of additional receptor and non-receptor mechanisms of their activity. Synergy between opioids and cannabinoids may produce opioid-sparing effects, as well as extend the duration of analgesia and reduce opioid tolerance and dependence, what is very important in long-term palliative treatment (McCarberg, 2007; Karst&Wippermann, 2009).

4.2 Management of wasting syndrome

Wasting is big problem for people living with HIV/AIDS and is linked to disease progression and death. It is defined as the involuntary loss of more than 10% of normal body weight in addition to at least 30 days of diarrhea, fever and generalized weakness. It is caused by several factors:

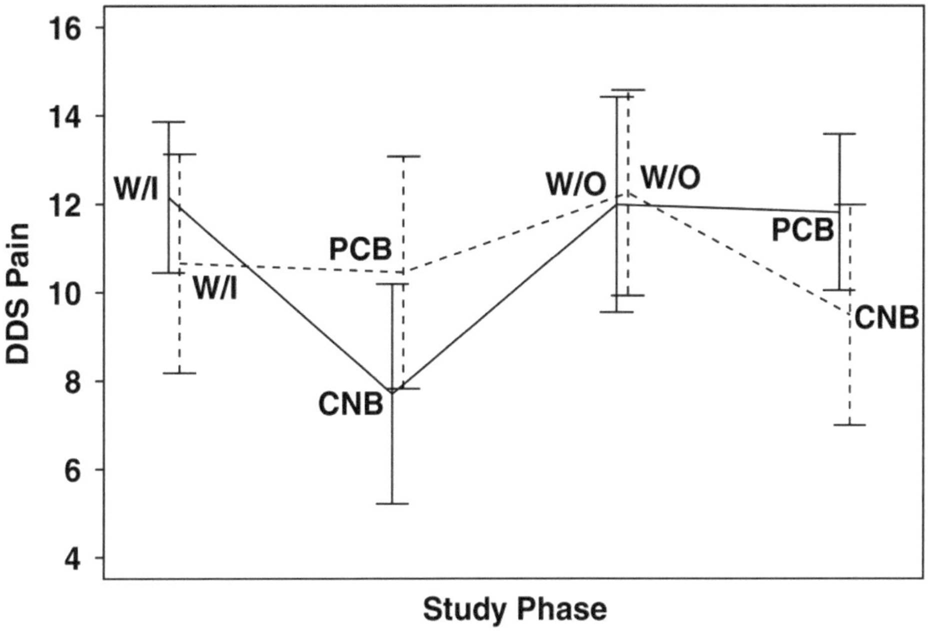

Fig. 4. DDS pain severity scores for participants in the cannabis (CNB) and placebo (PCB) arms before study treatment (W/I), during each of the 2 treatment weeks (1, 2) and during the Washout (W/O) between treatment weeks (from Ellis et al., 2009).

- Low food intake - low appetite is common among HIV/AIDS patients and is mostly caused by anti-retroviral drugs (their side effects such as nausea, changes in the sense of taste, or tingling around the mouth also decrease appetite). Moreover, opportunistic infections in the mouth, throat or stomach may also reduce food intake.
- Poor nutrient absorption - opportunistic infections of the gastrointestinal tract can interfere with the absorption of nutrients. Moreover, HIV may directly affect the intestinal lining and reduce nutrient absorption; diarrhea may affect nutrient absorption indirectly - it flushes the system of needed nutrients and calories.
- Altered metabolism - HIV/AIDS affects food processing and protein building. It is probably caused by the increased activity of the immune system. People need more calories just to maintain their body weight (Cannon, 2010; The Body, 2011).

5. Antiemetic action

Scientists suppose that emesis (the side effect of anti-retroviral therapy) is caused by the stimulation of receptors in the central nervous system or the gastrointestinal tract. This stimulation appears to be caused by the drug used in treatment itself or a metabolite of the drug. The high concentration of cannabinoid receptors in the nucleus of the solitary tract, suggest that exogenous cannabinoids bind to receptors and prevent them from binding with drugs and metabolites (Szulakowska&Milnerowicz, 2007). Recent findings suggest that the mechanism of anti-emetic action of cannabinoids is more complex - CB1 agonist suppresses vomiting, which is reversed by CB1 antagonism, and CB1 inverse agonism promotes vomiting. Parker et al. proved that cannabinoid agonists –THC suppress nausea. It occurred that cannabidiol (CBD) can also be used in the supplementary therapy of HIV/AIDS. The antiemetic effects of CBD may be mediated by indirect activation of somatodendritic 5-HT (1A) receptors in the dorsal raphe nucleus; activation of these autoreceptors reduces the release of 5-HT in terminal forebrain regions and inhibit nausea and emesis (Parker et al., 2010).

In 2001 Tramer et al. decided to search systematically for randomised controlled comparisons of the antiemetic efficacy of cannabinoids with any antiemetic or placebo (control) in chemotherapy, radiotherapy, surgery or HIV/AIDS. Scientist analyzed data from 30 randomised controlled trials published between 1975 and 1997 (1366 patients). Across all the trials, cannabinoids were more effective than active comparators and placebo. Results were shown in the Table 3. (Tramer et al., 2001).

	Cannabinoids % (number of patients)	Control % (number of patients)
Control of nausea and vomiting		
Complete control of nausea *vs* placebo	70 (81/116)	57 (66/115)
Complete control of vomiting *vs* placebo	66 (76/116)	36 (41/115)
Complete control of nausea *vs* active comparator	59 (122/207)	43 (93/215)
Complete control of vomiting *vs* active comparator	57 (111/194)	45 (90/201)
Patients' rating		
Cannabinoids *vs* placebo	76 (153/202)	13 (27/202)
Cannabinoids *vs* active comparator	61 (371/604)	26 (156/608)

Table 3. Control of nausea and vomiting and patients' preference for treatment in trials of cannabinoids against active antiemetic or control treatment (Tramer et al., 2001).

6. Appetite stimulation

Cannabinoids can also stimulate appetite and food intake. This property is connected with the presence of functional cannabinoid type 1 receptors in the digestive system, especially the liver. Hepatocytes express CB1 receptors, the activation of which increase the expression of lipogenic genes and *de novo* fatty acid synthesis, which contributes to the development of diet-induced obesity. Cannabinoids can also stimulate AMP-activated protein kinase in the hypothalamus, whereas they inhibit it in the liver and adipose tissues (Osei-Hyiaman, 2007). Moreover, scientists proved that CBs can activate fatty acid synthase (FAS), whereas the inhibition of FAS is a result of profound anorexia. These finding thus suggest that the same molecular pathway is involved in both central appetitive and the peripheral anabolic effects of cannabinoids (Szulakowska&Milnerowicz, 2007; Osei-Hyiaman et al., 2005).

In 2007 Haney et al. decided to check tolerability and efficacy of smoked marijuana and oral dronabinol in HIV-positive marijuana smokers. This placebo-controlled within-subjects study evaluated marijuana and dronabinol across a range of eating topography and mood. Scientists administered 4 times daily for 4 days each dronabinol and marijuana, but only one drug was active per day. Administration of drugs was separated by four days of placebo washout. Results were shown in the Fig. 5. In comparison to placebo, marijuana and dronabinol increased daily caloric intake and body weight. It is probably caused by the increased number of eating occasions - marijuana and dronabinol increased the number of eating occasions but didn't alter the number of calories intake. Moreover, marijuana and dronabinol produced significant shifts in the distribution of macronutrient administration by enhancing the proportion of calories derived from fat. The final effect of increased caloric intake and macronutrients administration was weight gain - 1.2 kg after 4 days of dronabinol and 1.1 kg after 4 days of marijuana (Haney et al., 2007).

6.1 Mood control

Scientists consider that prevalence of psychiatric disorders (mostly depression) is really high among the people living with HIV/AIDS. In 2001 in the USA nearly half of the population screened positive for a psychiatric disorder (36% major depression, 26.5% dysthymia, 15.8% generalized anxiety disorder, 10.5% panic attack)(Bing et al., 2001). Psychiatric disorders may be triggered by side effects of medications or the effects of HIV on the brain. Research show that depression can limit the energy needed to keep focused on staying health and may accelerate HIV's progression to AIDS (The Body, 2002).

Clinical data suggests that cannabinoids can strongly modulate mood of the people living with HIV/AIDS. Marijuana and dronabinol can help to overcome psychiatric disorders like anxiety, depression and sleeping disorders. In 2004 Prentiss et al. reported that 60.3% of 133 people living with HIV/AIDS and coping with psychological disorders recently used marijuana to alleviate the symptoms. Only few of them (9.1%) reported smoking marijuana/using dronabinol ineffective (Prentiss et al., 2004). Moreover, Haney et al. showed also that cannabinoids from marijuana or dronabinol can improve mood without producing disruptions in psychomotor functioning and add benefit of improving rating of sleep (Haney et al., 2007). In general, people living with HIV/AIDS reported that using marijuana cause reduction in stress, relief from anxiety and improve sleep (Cannon, 2010; Fogarty et al., 2007).

Scientists suppose that anti-depressive properties of THC and CBD are probably effect of involvement of these cannabinoids in the modulation of serotonergic signaling by their capacity to increase the availability of circulating tryptophan (precursor necessary for the biosynthesis of the 5-HT). The compensation of tryptophan degradation might be an important mechanism, by which THC and CBD may improve mood disturbances - mainly cause by alteration of serotonergic activity) (Jenny et al., 2010).

7. Medical marijuana use – Legal issues

Scientists from all over the world have explored the use of medical marijuana. Many of them have clearly reported that cannabinoids have therapeutic benefits (Cannon, 2010). According to this information, many countries, including Canada, Australia, The Netherlands and Switzerland, have legalized marijuana for medical purposes. The process of legislation of medical marijuana began in the United States in 2005. Today medical marijuana is legal at least in thirteen states (Active State Medical Marijuana Programs, 2011). Table 4. shows a summary of the main features of medical marijuana programs in different countries (Cannon, 2010).

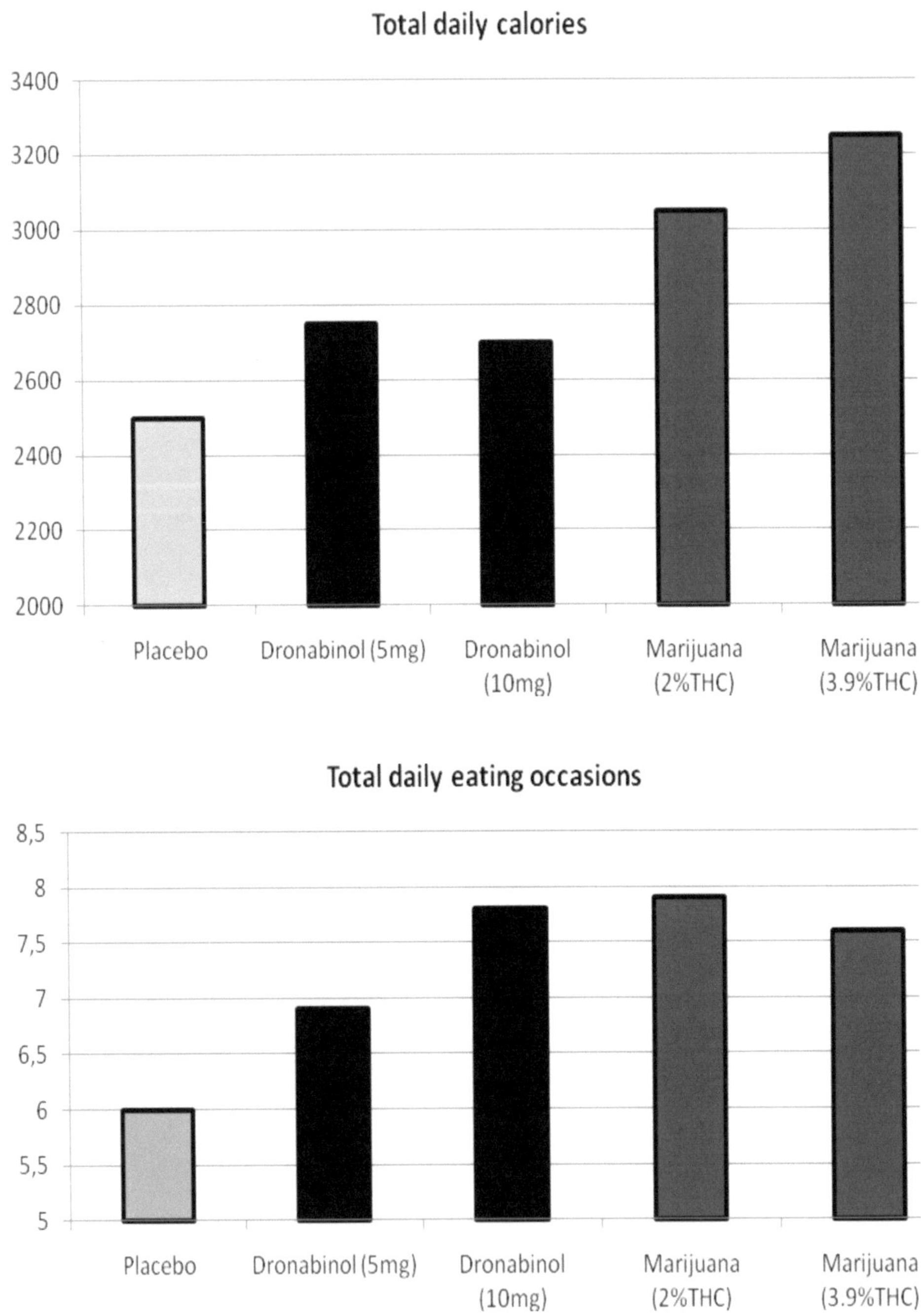

Fig. 5. Mean total daily caloric intake and total number of eating occasions as a function of marijuana (MJ) and dronabinol (Dronab) dose (Haney et al., 2007).

Country	Legal issues	Eligible health conditions	Access
United States of America	Legal for medical purposes in 13 states	HIV/AIDS Cancer Arthritis Anorexia Chronic pain Spasticity Glaucoma Migraine	Patients must receive a prescription from a physician
Canada	Legal for medical purposes	HIV/AIDS Cancer Multiple Sclerosis Spinal cord injury/disease Severe arthritis Epilepsy Part of a palliative care treatment program	Patients must become licensed by the Medical Marijuana Resource Centre to access marijuana
The Netherlands	Illegal - exception for personal use	HIV/AIDS Cancer Multiple Sclerosis Tourette's Syndrome Chronic pain Spasticity	Patients must voluntarily apply through the Department of Public Health to join the program and be issued with an identification car

Table 4. A summary of the main features of the medical marijuana programs in different countries (Cannon, 2010).

8. Conclusion

There is constant debate whether cannabis should be considered therapeutic for HIV/AIDS patients. According to the literature, management of HIV-associated symptoms is one of the most common applications ascribed to medical marijuana (Prentiss et al., 2004). More and more studies have characterized the extent of cannabis use for medical benefit to address HIV-related symptoms like nausea (Parker et al., 2010), lack of appetite (Tramer et al., 2001), emesis (Parker et al., 2010), pain (McCarberg, 2007), depression (Bing et al., 2001), anxiety Haney et al., 2007) and weight loss (Fogarty et al., 2007). However, it has to be mentioned, that use of cannabinoids can have side effects. Several scientists have warned about the negative effects of marijuana use on the cardiovascular, respiratory and nervous system (Cannon, 2010; Corless et al., 2009), and psychological dysfunction including loss of memory (Seamon et al., 2007) and pointed out the necessity for further investigation of the effects of cannabinoids. Moreover, recent legislative efforts to support legalization of medical marijuana suggest the need for more precise understanding of the typical patterns and determinants of marijuana use, and better characterization of the epidemiology of cannabis use for relief of symptoms commonly associated with HIV/AIDS (Cannon, 2010; Abrams et al., 2007).

9. References

Abrams, D.I.; Hilton, J.F.; Leiser, R.J.; et al. (2003). Short-Term Effects of Cannabinoids in Patients with HIV-1 Infection. A Randomized, Placebo-Controlled Clinical Trial, *Ann Intern Med,* 139, 258-266.

Abrams, D.I.; Jay, C.A.; Shade, S.B.;Vizoso, H.; Reda, H.; Press, S.; Kelly, M.E.; Rowbotham, M.C.; Petersen, K.L. (2007). Cannabis in painful HIV-associated sensory neuropathy. A randomized placebo-controlled trial, *Neurology,* 68, 7, 515-521.

Active State Medical Marijuana Programs, *NORML,* http://www.norml.org/index.cfm?Group_ID=3391#Maryland (downloaded April 20, 2011).

Baker, D.; Jackson, S.J.; Pryce, G. (2007). Cannabinoid control of neuroinflammation related to multiple sclerosis, *British Journal of Pharmacology,* 152, 649–654.

Berdyshev, E.V. (2000). Cannabinoid receptors and the regulation of im-mune response. *Chem Phys Lip,* 108, 169-190.

Bing, E.G.; Burnam, M.A.; Longshore D. et al. (2001). The estimated prevalence of psychiatric disorders, drug use and drug dependence among people with HIV disease in the United States: results from the HIV Cost and Services Utilization Study. *Archives of General Psychiatry,* 58, 721-728.

The Body: The Complete HIV/AIDS Resource, (2002). Depression and HIV: Fact Sheet 2-5005, *The Body: The Complete HIV/AIDS Resource,* viewed 10 March 2011, http://www.thebody.com/content/art6295.html#sup1

The Body: The Complete HIV/AIDS Resource, (2007). Wasting Syndrome: Fact Sheet 519, *The Body: The Complete HIV/AIDS Resource,* viewed 10 March 2011, http://www.thebody.com/content/art6127.html

Both, M. (2004). *Cannabis: A history,* Thomas Dunne Books

Braitstein, P.; Kendall, T.; Chan, K.; Wood, E.; Montaner, J.S.; O'Shaughnessy, M.V.; Hogg, R.S. (2001). Mary-Jane and her patients: sociodemographic and clinical characteristics of HIV-positive individuals using medical marijuana and antiretroviral agents, *AIDS,* 15, 4, 532-533.

Cannon, R. (2010). The medicinal use of marijuana for people living with HIV/AIDS in South Australia, *AIDS Council of South Australia information paper No. 2,* ISBN 978-0-9808084-3-8.

Corless, I.; Lindgren, T.; Holzemer, W.; Robinson, L.; Moezzi, S.; Kirksey, K.; Coleman, C.; Tsai, Y.F.; Sanzerro, L.; Hamilton, M.J.; Sefcik, E.F.; Canaval, G.E.; Rivero Mendez, M.; Kemppainen, J.K.; Bunch, E.H.; Nicholas, P.; Nokes, K.M.; Dole, P.; Reynolds, N. (2009). Marijuana Effectiveness as an HIV Self-Care Strategy, *Clinical Nursing Research,* 18, 2, 172-193.

Demuth, D.G.; Molleman, A. (2006). Cannabinoid signaling, *Life Sci,* 78, 549–563.

Ellis,R.J.; Toperoff,W.; Vaida,F.; van den Brande,G.; Gonzales,J.; Gouaux,B.; Bentley,H.; Atkinson, J.H. (2009). Smoked Medicinal Cannabis for Neuropathic Pain in HIV: A Randomized, Crossover Clinical Trial, *Neuropsychopharmacology,* 2009, 34, 3, 672-680.

ElSohly, M.A.; Slade, D. (2005). Chemical constituents of marijuana: The complex mixture of natural cannabinoids, *Life Sci,* 78, 539-548.

Fogarty, A.; Rawstorne, P.; Prestage, G.; Crawford, J.; Grierson J.; Kippax, S. (2007). Marijuana as therapy for people living with HIV/AIDS: social and health aspects, *AIDS Care*, 19, 2, 295-301.

Haney, M.; Gunderson, E.W.; Rabkin, J.; Hart, C.L.; Vosburg, S.K.; Comer, S.D.; Foltin, R.W. (2007). Dronabinol and Marijuana in HIV-positiive Marijuana Smokers. Caloric intakie, Mood, and Sleep, *J Acquir Immune Defic Syndr*, 45, 5, 545-554.

Jenny, M.; Schrocksnadel, S.; Uberall, F.; Fuchs, D. (2010). The Potential Role of Cannabinoids in Modulating Serotonergic Signaling by Their Influence on Tryptophan Metabolism, *Pharmaceuticals*, 3, 2647-2660.

Joy, J.E.; Watson S.J.Jr.; Benson J.A.Jr. (1999). *Marijuana and Medicine:Assessing the Science Base*, National Academy Press, Washington D. C., 1999

Karst, M.; Wippermann, S. (2009). Cannabinoids against pain. Efficacy and strategies to reduce psychoactivity: a clinical perspective, *Expert Opin Investig Drugs*, 18, 2, 125-133.

Klein, T.W; Kawakami, Y; Newton, C; Friedman, H. (1991). Marijuana com-ponents suppress induction and cytolytic function of murine cyto-toxic T cells in vitro and in vivo, *J Toxicol Environ Health* , 32, 465-477.

Klein, T.W; Newton A; Nakachi, N; Friedman, H. (2000). Delta 9-tetrahydrocannabinol treatment suppresses immunity and early IFN-gamma, IL-12, and IL-12 receptor beta 2 responses to Legionella pneumophila infection, *J Immunol*, 164, 12, 6461-6.

Klein, T.W.; Cabral, C.A. (2006). Cannabinoid-induced immune suppression and modulation of antigen-presenting cells, *J Neuroimmune Pharmacol*, 1,1, 50-64.

Kohler, F.E. (1887). Medizinal Pflantzen.
http://upload.wikimedia.org/wikipedia/commons/1/19/Koeh-026.jpg
(downloaded March 11, 2011)

Kosel, B.W.; Aweeka, F.T.; Benowitz, N.L.; Shade, S.B.; Hilton, J.F.; Lizak, P.S.; Abrams, D.I. (2002). The effects of cannabinoids on the pharmacokinetics of indinavir and nelfinavir, AIDS, 16, 4, 543-50.

Kozela, E; Pietr, M; Juknat, A; Rimmerman, N; Levy, R; Vogel, Z. (2010) Cannabinoids Δ^9-Tetrahydrocannabinol and Cannabidiol Differentially Inhibit the Lipopolysaccharide-activated NF-κB and Interferon-β/STAT Proinflammatory Pathways in BV-2 Microglial Cells, *J Biol Chem*, 285, 3, 1616–1626.

Massi, P; Vaccani, A; Parolaro, D. (2006). Cannabinoids, immune system and cytokine network, *Curr Pharm Des*, 12, 24, 3135-46.

McCarberg, B.H. (2007). Cannabinoids: their role in pain and palliation, *J Pain Palliat Care Pharmacother*, 21, 3, 19-28.

McCoy, K.L; Matveyeva, M; Carlisle, S.J; Cabral, G.A. (1999). Cannabinoidinhibition of the processing of intact lysozyme by macrophages:evidence for CB2 receptor participation, *J Pharmacol Exp Ther*, 289, 1620-1625.

Nong, L; Newton, C; Cheng, Q; Friedman, H; Roth, M.D; Klein, T.W. (2002). Altered cannabinoid receptor mRNA expression in peripheralblood mononuclear cells from marijuana smokers, *J Neuroimmunol*, 127, 169-176.

Osei−Hyiaman, D.; DePetrillo, M.; Pacher, P.; Liu, J.; Radaeva, S.; Bátkai, S.; Harvey−White, J.; Mackie, K.; Offertáler, L.; Wang, L.; Kunos, G. (2005). Endocannabinoid activation at hepatic CB1 receptors stimulates fatty acid synthesis and contributes to diet−induced obesity, *J Clin Invest*, 115, 5, 1298–1305.

Osei−Hyiaman, D. (2007). Endocannabinoid system in cancer cachexia. Nutrition in wasting disease, *Curr Opin Clin Nutr Metab Care*, 10, 4, 443–448.

Parker, L.A.; Rock, E.; Limebeer, C. (2010). Regulation of nausea and vomiting by cannabinoids, *Br J Pharmacol*, "Accepted article", doi: 10.1111/j.1476-5381.2010.01176.x

Peltzer, K.; Friend-du Preez, N.; Ramlagan,S.; Fomundam, H. (2008). Use of traditional complementary and alternative medicine for HIV patients in KwaZulu-Natal, South Africa, *BMC Public Health*, 8, 255.

Prentiss, D.; Power, R.; Balmas, G.; Tzuang, G.; Israelski, D.M. (2004). Patterns of marijuana use among patients with HIV/AIDS followed in the public health care setting, *J Acquir Immune Defic Syndr*, 35, 1, 38-45.

Rieder, S.A.; Chauhan, S.; Singh, U.; Nagarkatti, M.; Nagarkatti, P. (2010). Cannabinoid-induced apoptosis in immune cells as a pathway to immunosuppression, Immunobiology, 215, 8, 598–605.

Sacerdote, P; Massi, P; Panerai, A.E; Parolaro, D. (2000). In vivo and in vitro treatment with the synthetic cannabinoid CP-55,940 decreases the in vitro migration of macrophages in the rat: involvement of bothCB1 and CB2 receptors, *J Neuroimmunol*, 109, 155-163.

Sacerdote, P; Martucci, C; Vaccani, A; Bariselli, F; Panerai, A.E; Colombo, A; Parolaro, D; Massi, P. (2005). The nonpsychoactive component of marijuana cannabidiol modulates chemotaxis and IL-10 and IL-12 production of murine macrophages both in vivo and in vitro., J Neuroimmunol, 159, 1-2, 97-105.

Saito, V.M.; Wotjak, C.T.; Moreira, F.A. (2010). Pharmacological exploitation of the endocannabinoid system: new perspectives for the treatment of depression and anxiety disorders?, *Rev. Bras. Psiquiatr*, 32, 1, 7-14.

Seamon, M.; Fass, J.; Maniscalco-Feichtl, M.; Abu-Shraie, N.A. (2007). Medical Marijuana and the developing role of the pharmacist, *American Journal of Health-System Pharmacy*, 64, 1037-1044.

Szulakowska, A.; Milnerowicz H. (2007). Cannabis sativa in the light of scientific research, *Adv Clin Exp Med*, 16, 6, 807-815.

Tanasescu, R; Constantinescu, C.S. (2010). Cannabinoids and the immune system: an overview, Immunobiology, 215, 8, 588-97.

Tramèr, M.R.; Carroll, D.; Campbell, F.A.; Reynolds, D.J.M.; Moore, R.A.; McQuay, H.J. (2001). Cannabinoids for control of chemotherapy induced nausea and vomiting: quantitative systematic review, *BMJ*, 323, 7303, 16.

Truta, E.; Gille, E.; Toth, E.; Maniu, M. (2002). Biochemical differences in Cannabis sativa L. depending on sexual phenotype, *J Appl Genet*, 43, 4, 451–462.

Woolridge, E.; Barton, S.; Samuel, J.; Osorio, J.; Dougherty, A.; Holdcroft, A.; (2005). Cannabis use in HIV for pain and other symptoms,*Journal of Pain and Symptom Management*, 29, 4, 358-367.

Zheng, Z.M; Specter, S; Friedman, H. (1992). Inhibition by delta-9-tetra-hydrocannabinol of tumor necrosis factor alpha production bymouse and human macrophages, *Int J Immunopharmacol*, 14, 1445-1452.

Zheng, Z.M;Specter, S.C. (1996). Δ9-Tetrahydrocannabinol suppresses tumornecrosis factor alpha maturation and secretion but not its transcrip-tion in mouse macrophages, *Int J Immunopharmacol*, 18, 53-68.

Zhu, W; Igarashi, T; Qi, Z.T; Newton, C; Widen, R.E; Friedman, H.(1993) Delta-9-tetrahydrocannabinol (THC) decreases the number of high and intermediate affinity IL-2 receptors of the IL-2 dependentcell line NKB61A2, *Int J Immunopharm*, 15, 401-408.

Zuardi, A. (2006). History of cannabis as a medicine: a review, *Rev Bras Psiquiatr*, 28,2, 153-157.

28

Small Livestock, Food Security, Nutrition Security and HIV/AIDS Mitigation

John Cassius Moreki[1] and Richard Dikeme[2]
[1]*Department of Animal Science and Production, Botswana College of Agriculture*
[2]*Botswana Network of People Living with HIV and AIDS, Botswana*

1. Introduction

Livestock contribute to people's livelihoods in many ways, and their contributions tend to be particularly important for poorer people. These include source of cash income, liquid asset, inputs to crop production (draught power and manure), diversification of risk/ buffer to crop production, cultural value (livestock may be sacrificed at the time of a certain festival) and source of food (Conroy, 2005). Sale of livestock and their products can be a valuable source of income. For example, animals, especially small livestock (i.e., goats, sheep, poultry and rabbits) can be sold to meet immediate family needs such as food, clothing, medical expenses, school fees etc.

Livestock play an important role in supporting the social and economic safety nets of households and communities. They are central to people's livelihoods, food security and nutrition; they act as a "bank" to be called upon in times of stress or need (either sold, traded, or slaughtered). Also, livestock are central in many of the major events of life, i.e. birth ceremonies, weddings and funerals. However, it appears that little is known about how traditional community institutions, particularly around livestock production (e.g. women's poultry groups, grazing support and dairy cooperatives) are holding up under the stress induced by HIV and AIDS and related chronic illnesses (FAO, 2003). The study of Mutenje et al. (2008) in the Muzarabani and Bindura districts of Mashonaland Central Province in Zimbabwe found that livestock, particularly poultry and smallstock (sheep and goats), play a significant role in smoothing income fluctuations due to HIV and AIDS. The workers reported that about 90% of HIV and AIDS-afflicted households, headed mainly by women or children, used poultry and goats as consumption-smoothing strategies when faced with negative income shocks.

Africa is the hardest hit continent in the world in terms of HIV epidemic (Topouzis, 1999; FAO, 2005). The HIV and AIDS pandemic in sub-Saharan Africa is widely recognised as development disaster threatening poverty reduction, economic growth and not merely a health issue (Mohiddin & Johnson, 2006). HIV and AIDS affects households' nutrition by decreasing food consumption and impairing nutrient absorption (Hanze et al., 2005). According to FAO (2005), people that live with HIV and AIDS (PLWHA) have special nutritional needs to assist them to remain active and productive workers and to ward off the opportunistic infections that accompany the disease and in prolonging their lives. The PLWHA need good nutrition to stay as healthy as possible. However, good nutrition cannot cure AIDS or prevent HIV infection, but it can delay the progression from HIV to full-blown AIDS and related diseases, and improve the quality of life of PLWHA. Slater & Wiggins (2005) argued that households may sell off large livestock, such as cattle, and use smaller stock units, such as goats and chickens, that can be reared closer to the homestead, and that can be sold off in small quantities to release cash for purchase of medicines for the sick or basic needs where regular sources of income are lost. Small livestock, especially village chickens (also referred to as family chickens) are the most significant livestock species in terms of levels of ownership, supply of protein, and the potential for earning cash income. It has been demonstrated in Botswana, Lesotho and Zambia that livestock, especially village poultry can play an important role in mitigating the impacts of HIV and AIDS on household and community food security and nutrition, as well as, economic empowerment of the vulnerable groups.

As women are the main carers of sick people, chickens can play an important role in providing them with additional resources to perform the important task of caring for people living with HIV and AIDS (Alders et al., 2007a, 2007b). In Mozambique, Alders et al. (2009) reported that village chickens play an important role in households where there is lack of able-bodied workers, such as those affected by HIV and AIDS or those family members living with disabilities. In households headed by widows, children or grandparents, chickens represent the easiest species to raise for sale and home consumption, providing high quality protein and micronutrients, which play an important role in the nutrition of HIV and AIDS patients. Furthermore, village poultry production also provides women and children with experience in small-scale business management and improved knowledge about human nutrition (Alders et al., 2009).

Among the small livestock species reared by individuals and communities in the rural villages, village poultry predominates; hence the emphasis of this chapter is on village poultry. Livestock, especially poultry species, have shown to provide an effective first step in alleviating abject rural poverty (Mack et al., 2004). According to Rural Self-Help Development Association (RSDA) (2011), throughout Africa village poultry are a valuable asset to local populations as they contribute to food security, poverty alleviation and promote gender equality, especially in the disadvantaged groups (HIV and AIDS infected and affected people, women, poor farmers etc.) and less favoured areas of rural Africa where the majority of the poor people reside. The study of Moreki et al. (2010a) in Chobe district of Botswana reported the main reasons for rearing village chickens to be family consumption (75%), source of income (75%), prestige (36%), traditional healing ceremonies (6.82%) and barter (6.82%). These findings clearly show that village poultry have a bearing in the lives of rural populace. Pica-Ciamarra & Otte (2009) in India concluded that backyard poultry farming remains important for rural households, as it ensures a steady flow of high quality food and, through cash income, reduces vulnerability.

2. Advantages of small livestock over larger stock

Unlike larger stock such as cattle, small livestock require less space; they are less capital intensive and are easy to manage as they can be reared within or near homesteads. This makes it much easier for women who are mainly carers of sick people and children to look after both the sick and small livestock simultaneously; hence cutting on labour costs. The rearing of small livestock near or within homesteads ensures regular supply of food to the families in terms of eggs, meat and milk. Lengkeek et al. (2008) argued that PLHWA are less able to perform heavy work, to work for long periods or follow strict work schedules; hence the need to rear smallstock such as a poultry which are easy to keep as they require few inputs. According to Winrock International (1992), livestock contribute directly to the sustainability of the farming systems by providing manure, which is the principal soil amendment and fertilizer available to large numbers of African farmers. A recent study of Simainga et al. (2010) in Zambia reported that the majority of the respondents in Mongu and Kalabo districts used manure from village chickens to fertilize gardens in order to produce vegetables for the households. Figure 1 shows vegetables that were fertilized with chicken manure in Botswana.

According to Sitholimela (2000) in South Africa, the advantages of goats over cattle include: they are easily handled by women and children, e.g., they can be easily milked, dewormed and vaccinated; they require less feed; produce significant quantities of meat and milk for households' consumption; have a short generation interval and produce more progenies. In addition, they are easy to sell to meet immediate households' needs and can be bartered for household commodities such as grain and seeds. To the majority of rural communities in the developing countries, livestock is regarded as "a walking bank" or "a bank in the hoof" because they provide readily available petty cash in times of need.

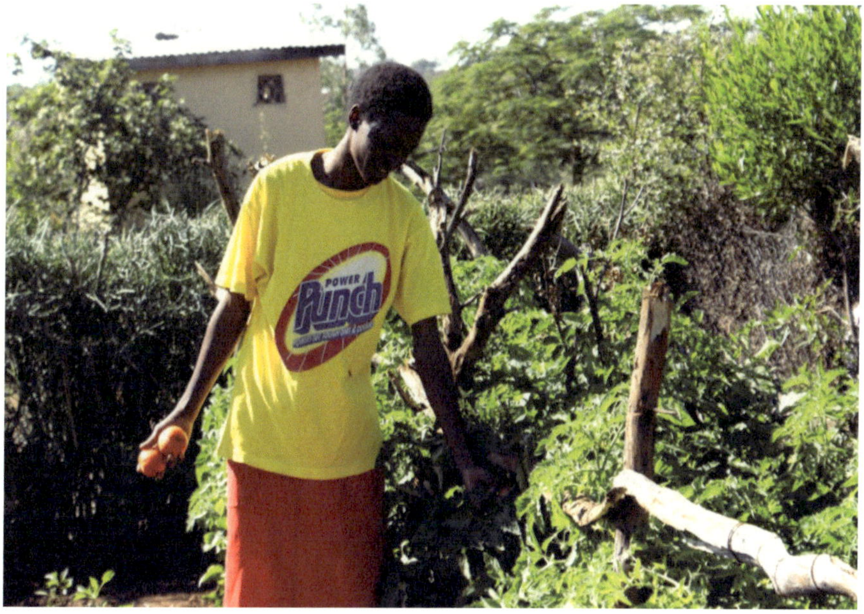

Fig. 1. Tomato plants fertilized with manure

3. The first rung on the livestock ladder

Small livestock, especially village poultry can provide the start of the owner climbing the "livestock ladder", leading to other livestock species such as goats and cattle (Dolberg, 2003). Botswana Network of People Living with HIV/AIDS (BONEPWA) (2010) reported that from October 2005 to October 2010, the beneficiaries of a chicken project supported by Swedish International Development Corporation Agency (SIDA) purchased 250 goats from the proceeds of chickens. Figure 2 shows chickens that were sold to buy goats while the purchased goats are shown in Figures 3 and 4. In a recent field day held in Bobonong in

Botswana, one beneficiary of SIDA supported project reported having bought a cow from the chicken proceeds. This clearly indicates that the rearing of small livestock enables rural families to start owning larger livestock such as cattle, which are considered status symbols in most African countries. BONEPWA (2010) concluded that the rearing of small livestock provides their owners the opportunity to climb the societal ladder by owning larger stock.

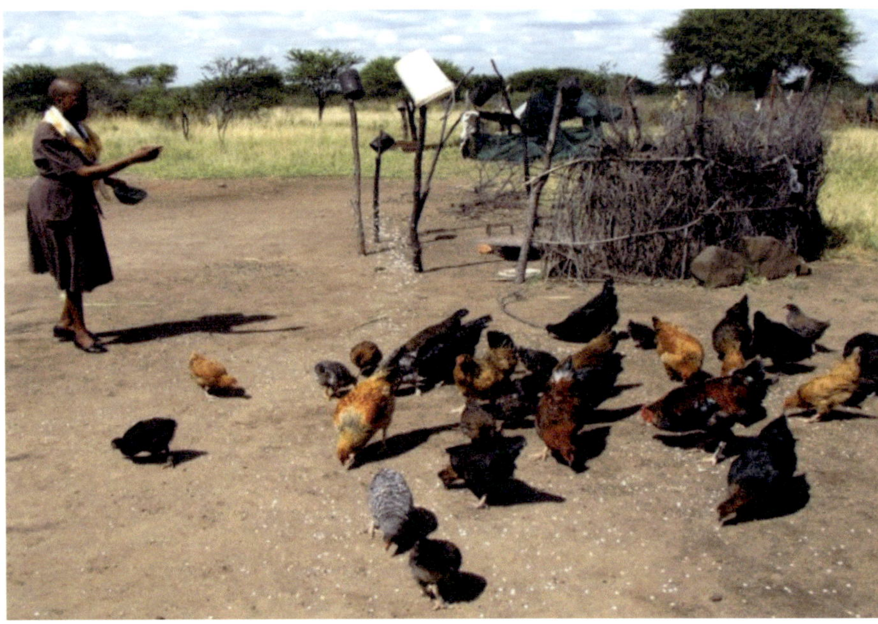

Fig. 2. Part of the chickens that were sold to buy goats

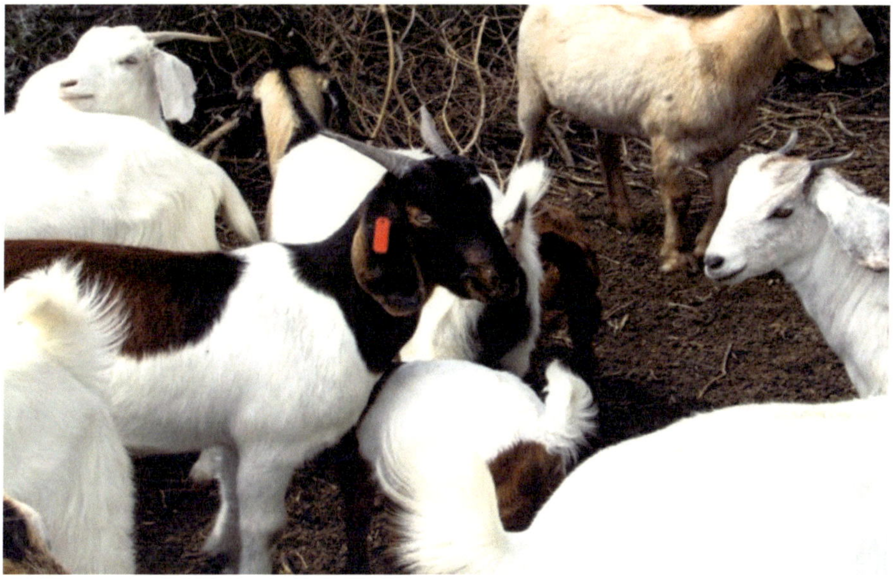

Fig. 3. Some of the goats bought with money from chicken sales

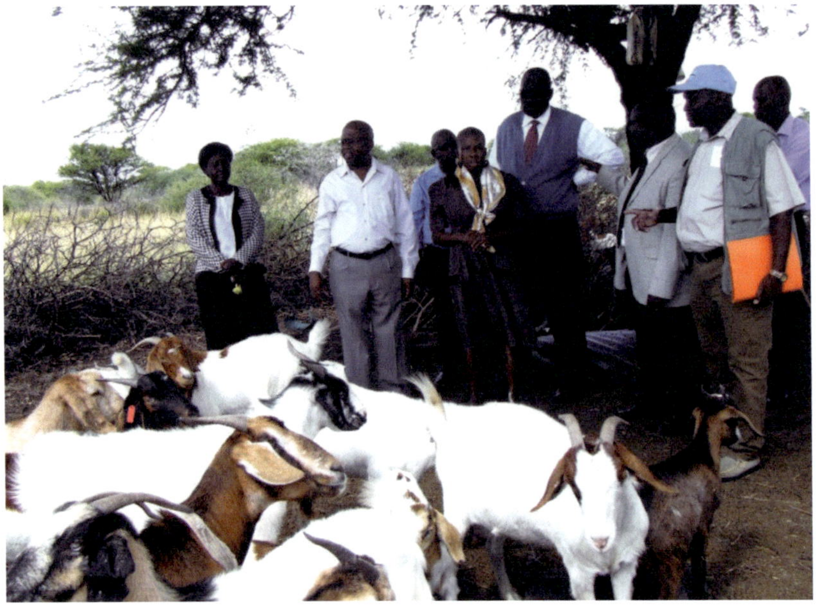

Fig. 4. Goats being appreciated by development workers in Botswana

4. Nutrition and household income generation

The roles played by small livestock in household nutrition and income generation are briefly discussed in the sections below.

4.1 Nutrition

Livestock products such as meat, egg and milk products supply proteins, vitamins and minerals and extra energy, and help to strengthen muscles and the immune system. People with weak health (immune system) are more vulnerable to infections, including diseases transmitted by animals or through contaminated food and water. Even people with access to anti-retrovirals need a balanced diet to fully benefit from such treatment (FAO, 2005).

As shown in Figure 5, goats provide milk which is a balanced diet. Milk is a rich source of nutritionally available minerals (Allen & Miller, 1981) and it contains more of calcium and phosphorus than cow and human milk (Jenness, 1978). From human nutrition's view point, milk and milk products are a source of selenium which plays an important role in the immune system. Goat milk increases the resistance of the body against AIDS. Selenium helps to protect the organism against oxidation stress, participates in the synthesis and metabolism of thyroid hormones, proteosynthesis, it is important for reproduction and its anti-carcinogenic effect plays an important role as well (Schrauzer, 2000). Melse-Boonstra et al. (2007) reported that observational studies on selenium and HIV and AIDS consistently show a positive association between selenium status and delayed disease progression or increased mortality. The study of Barrionuevo et al. (2003) showed that goat-milk has an important and beneficial effect on the bioavailability of copper, zinc and selenium. Belewu and Adewole (2009) concluded that goat milk is affordable, available and nutritious; hence a wide variation of knowledge on the nutrition and hypollergic characteristics of goat milk could promote the direct use of the milk in the nutrition of orphans and vulnerable children.

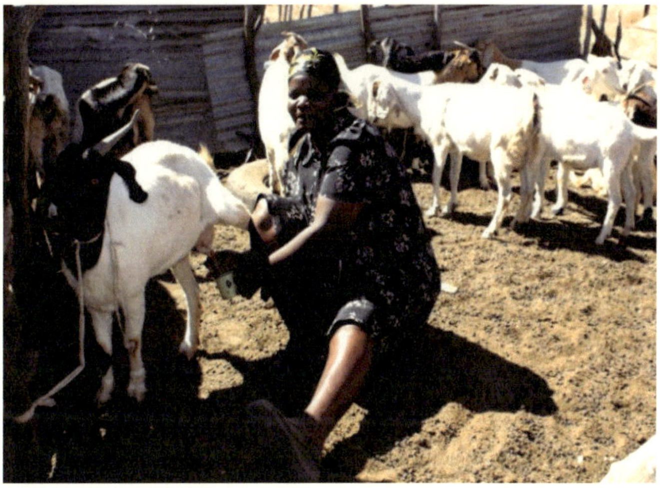

Fig. 5. A woman milking a goat in Bobonong, Botswana

Good nutrition is crucial for PLWHA who need more calories and protein than uninfected individuals. Malnourished HIV-infected people progress more quickly to AIDS and nutrition is critically important to people on retro-viral therapy. The ways of improving the nutrition component of mitigation strategies include promoting block farming, school gardening, community kitchens for orphans and vulnerable children, home-based care nutrition support and nutrition campaigns and training (Economic Commission for Africa, 2006). The rearing of village poultry in Botswana, Lesotho and Zambia has also demonstrated played by village chickens a crucial role in nutrition and food security among PLWHA. RSDA (2011) in Lesotho reported that some people consider village chickens as an option to mitigate HIV and AIDS after realizing that chickens can be the easiest way of obtaining daily nutritional requirements. Moreki et al. (2011) in their study in Botswana reported that all the respondents (46) acknowledged the contribution of chickens in human nutrition. In that study, the respondents said chickens provided relish and hence were the main supplier of good quality protein to the households. Furthermore, the sale of chickens contributed to improved habitable shelter. The proceeds from the sale of chickens contributed to the purchase of building materials for construction of houses. Figure 6 shows the house that was painted following sale of chickens in Nata in Botswana.

Eggs, in particular, offer a great nutritional bargain: they contain approximately 315 kilojoules and are one of the best quality food sources known. Eggs supply an array of vitamins such as A and B12, and they are one of the best food sources of vitamin K, a bone-boosting nutrient. In addition, eggs provide choline, a B vitamin that plays a role in brain development (Alders et al., 2003). Also, eggs are an ideal carrier for enriching human diets with important dietary minerals such as selenium and iodine. Jacques (2006) stated that selenium is involved in the proper functioning of the immune system or inhibiting the progression from HIV to AIDS. The disease is reported to be less prevalent in countries with high selenium soil content than those with low selenium content. Selenium is involved in the conversion of thyroxine (T4) to triodothyronine (T3), indicating its importance in the functioning of the thyroid gland. Seafoods are a rich source of selenium, as are some livestock products, including eggs and chicken meat.

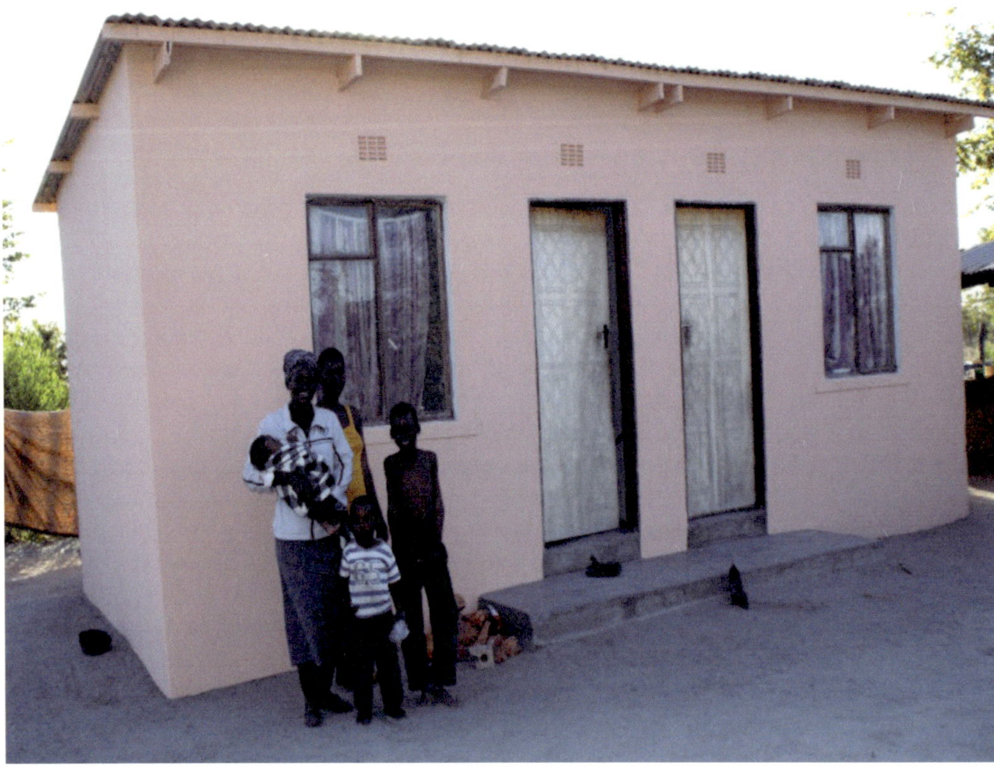

Fig. 6. House painted using money from chicken sales in Botswana

Some of the mitigation strategies mentioned previously attempted to provide some ideas for those working with livestock and communities to mitigate the impact of HIV/AIDS on livestock production and household food security. In addition to these potential interventions, it is important to consider the nutritional needs of the affected individuals and households, review existing support institutions (whether it be extended family, community-based organisations, etc.) and assess, with the community, and particularly those affected, the best way forward to ensure livestock production within, or for, those households. Labour and financial constraints of households must be considered before strategies are discussed or plans developed.

4.2 Income generation

Small livestock can provide income generation for family activities such as education, nutrition, health and clothing. Copland and Alders (2009) stated that village poultry have constantly commanded a price premium over commercial birds and there is a wide market demand for village poultry products. In Zambia, Simainga et al. (2011) reported that income from sale of chickens and eggs was used for groceries, school fees and uniforms, transport to hospitals or medical facilities, medication and talk time (air time).

5. Ownership of small livestock

Generally, small livestock are owned by women. In Botswana, Mrema & Rannobe (1996) reported that women own more goats than their male counterparts who have more resources and can afford to own cattle. Furthermore, village poultry are owned and managed by women and children and are often essential elements of female-headed households (Alders et al., 2003; Guéye, 2004; Bagnol, 2005). The study of Moreki et al. (2010b) showed that 83.2% of women owned chickens compared to 16.8% for men. A recent study (Moreki et al., 2010c) also showed that 73.5% of women own goats. The authors argued that, chickens are generally regarded as livestock that women raise mainly because they are perceived to be of less commercial value than other livestock such as cattle. In the opinion of Moreki et al. (2010b), in Botswana men tend to be responsible for cattle and larger animals and women for smaller animals such as sheep, goats and poultry. These results led Moreki et al. (2010c) to conclude that sheep and goats rearing plays an important role in food security, in addressing issues of gender imbalances, as well as, in poverty eradication in furtherance of the Millennium Development Goals (United Nations, 2010).

6. Marketing

Small livestock and products are sold on a one-on-one basis, which is referred to as direct marketing. Usually, small livestock are sold when there is immediate need for cash. Unlike in commercial livestock, no cold chain is required as stock is sold live and products raw. Recently, Simainga et al. (2011) in Zambia reported that women, especially mothers are involved in chicken sales than men, indicating that women owned chickens and decided on their sales, as well as, how money was used. However, it is likely that women consulted their spouses on how the money was used.

7. HIV and AIDS and small livestock production

Smallstock play a vital role in many rural livelihoods, providing food, income and security. The products of smallstock are rich in protein, minerals and vitamins. They are sources of income and manure for use as compost or fuel, and a store of wealth and insurance. Small livestock may enable women to have more economic independence if they control the income earned from the sale of livestock and their products. Tending to the ongoing every-day requirement of smallstock can normally be integrated into the time and labour constraints facing many HIV/AIDS affected households (Anon, 2006).

According to BONEPWA (2010), the majority of support group members infected and affected by HIV and AIDS in Botswana has attested that through ownership and sale of small livestock (i.e., chickens, guinea fowl and goats), they were able to reduce the number of patients that default from taking anti-retroviral drugs, as they are able to sell chickens to buy medication and food, and also pay for transport to the hospitals for treatment. The effects of HIV and AIDS scourge at household level has reduced since beneficiaries are now able to feed their households resulting in reduced dependency on government hand-outs, family members and relatives. Some of the patients who were bedridden due to AIDS have recovered and are caring for their livestock. This has led to one support group member to say *"we are finding ourselves to be useful members of the community since we are back into our productive lives after spending a long time in sick beds"*. This indicates that small livestock production plays a pivotal role in food and nutrition security, as well as, restoring self-esteem among the affected community members.

8. Conclusion

This review has demonstrated that small livestock have an important role to play in poverty alleviation, improving food and nutrition security, as well as, in economic empowerment of PLWHA and other vulnerable groups. Successful HIV and AIDS mitigation strategies involving goats and chickens in Botswana, Lesotho and Zambia indicate that small livestock play a vital role in the fight against the HIV and AIDS scourge, mainly through provision of nutrition and income generation. Therefore, support from government and non-governmental organizations is crucial if the benefits are to be extended to the rest of the rural communities, the majority of whom are poverty-stricken

9. Acknowledgements

The authors wish to acknowledge assistance they received from BONEPWA+, RSDA and Golden Valley Agricultural Research Trust in Botswana, Lesotho and Zambia, respectively

10. References

Alders, R.; Cambaza, A.B. & Harun, M. (2003). Village chickens, food security and HIV/AIDS mitigation. Retrieved from www.kyeemafoundation.org/content/.../HIV-AIDS%20paper%20Nov03.pdf

Alders, R.; Bagnol, B.; dos Anjos, F. & Young, M. (2007a). Promotion of HIV/AIDS mitigation and wildlife conservation through improved village poultry production in Southern Africa, Retrieved from http://www.fao.org/AG/againfo/home/events/bangkok2007/en/background_4.html

Alders, R.; Bagnol, B.; Harun, M. & Young, M. (2007b). Village poultry, food security and HIV/AIDS mitigation. LEISA Magazine 23.3 September 2007.

Alders, R.; Bagnol, B.; Chicamisse, M.; Serafim, J. & Langa, J. (2009) The role of village chickens in HIV/AIDS mitigation in Manica and Sofala provinces of Mozambique. In, Alders R.G., Spradbrow P.B. and Young M.P. (eds) 2009. Village chickens, poverty alleviation and the sustainable control of Newcastle disease. Proceedings of an international conference held in Dar es Salaam, Tanzania, 5-7 October 2005. ACIAR Proceedings No. 131, 235 pp.

Allen, J.C. & Miller, W.J. (1981). Transfer of selenium from blood to milk goats and non-interference of copper with selenium metabolism. Journal of Dairy Science 64: 814-821.

Anon (2006). HIV/AIDS and small livestock development. Retrieved from http://www.smallstock.info/issues/HIV.htm

Bagnol, B. (2005). Improving village chicken production by employing effective gender-sensitive methodologies. Retrieved from http://aciar.gov.au/files/node/11133/PR131%20part%201.pdf

Barrionuevo, M.; Lopez Aliaga, I.; Alférez, M.J.M.; Mesa, E; Nestáres, T. & Campos, M.S. (2003). Beneficial effect of goat milk on bioavailability of copper, zinc and selenium in rats. Journal of Physiology and Biochemistry 59: 111-118.

Belewu, M.A. & Adewole, A.M. (2009). Goat milk: A feasible dietary Based approach to improve the nutrition of orphan and vulnerable children. Pakistan Journal of Nutrition 8: 1711-1714.

Botswana Network of People Living with HIV and AIDS (2010). Annual Technical Report - October 2009 to September 2010: Village chicken component. Gaborone, Botswana.

Conroy, C. (2005). Participatory Livestock Research: A Guide. ITDG Publishing. The Netherlands. 3-4. ISBN 1-85339-577-3.

Copland, J.W. & Alders, R.G. (2009). The comparative advantages of village poultry or smallholder poultry in rural development. In, Alders R.G., Spradbrow P.B. and Young M.P. (eds) 2009. Village chickens, poverty alleviation and the sustainable control of Newcastle disease. Proceedings of an international conference held in Dar es Salaam, Tanzania, 5-7 October 2005. ACIAR Proceedings No. 131. 207-209.

Dolberg, F. (2003). Review of household poultry production as a tool in poverty reduction with focus on Bangladesh and India. FAO Pro-Poor Livestock Policy Initiative Working Paper No. 6. Food and Agriculture Organizations of the United Nations. Rome.

Economic Commission for Africa (2006). Mitigating the impact of HIV/AIDS on smallholder agriculture, food security and rural livelihoods in Southern Africa: Challenges and action plan., Retrieved from www.uneca.org/sros/sa/publications/HIV-AIDSandAgriculture.pdf

FAO (2003). Measuring impacts of HIV/AIDS on rural livelihoods, Retrieved from http://www.fao.org/sd/2003/PE0102_en.htm

FAO (2005). Ministerial Seminar on *Education for Rural People in Africa: Policy Lessons, Options and Priorities* hosted by the Government of Ethiopia 7-9 September 2005, Addis Ababa, Ethiopia. Retrieved from http://www.fao.org/hivaids/publications/Addis_ERP-AIDS.pdf

Guèye, E.F. (2004). Gender aspects in family poultry management systems in developing countries. http://www.fao.org/ag/AGAinfo/themes/en/infpd/documents/papers/2004/12gender318.pdf

Hlanze, Z.; Gama, T. & Mondlane, S. (2005). The Impact of HIV/AIDS and Drought on Local Knowledge Systems for Agrobiodiversity and Food Security. Retrieved from ftp://ftp.fao.org/docrep/fao/009/ag251e/ag251e00.pdf

Jenness, P.E. (1978). The nutritive value of dairy products. Dairy Industries International 43: 7-16.

Lengkeek, A.; Koster, M. & Salm, M. (2008). Mitigating the effects of HIV/AIDS in small-scale farming. Agromisa Foundation, Wageningen. ISBN Agromisa: 978-90-8573-090-3. Retrieved from http://www.anancy.net/documents/file_en/Agrodok-45-Mitigating_the_effects_of_HIV_AIDs_in_small-scale_farming.pdf

Jacques, K.A. (2006). Zoonotic disease: Not just from birds, not just in the flu. In, T.P. Lyons, K.A., Jacques and J.M. Hower (eds.) Nutritional biotechnology in the feed and food industries: Proceedings of Alltech's 22nd Annual Symposium, Lexington, Kentucky, USA. 23-26 April 2006. Nottingham University Press, UK. 149-159.

Mack, S.; Hoffmann, D. & Otte, J. (2004. The contribution of poultry to rural development, Retrieved from http://193.43.36.103/AG/AGAInfo/themes/en/infpd/documents/papers/2004/contribution1618.pdf

Melse-Boonstra, A.; Hogenkamp, P. & Lungu, O.I. (2007). Mitigating HIV/AIDS in Sub-Saharan Africa through selenium in food. Farmer Publication, Lusaka. Golden Valley Agricultural Research Tust (GART). 11.

Mohiddin, A. & Johnston, D. (2006). HIV/AIDS mitigation strategies and the State in sub-Saharan Africa – the missing link? Retrieved from http://www.globalizationandhealth.com/content/2/1/1

Moreki, J.C.; Dikeme, R. & Poroga, B. (2010a). The role of village poultry in food security and HIV/AIDS mitigation in Chobe District of Botswana. Retrieved from http://www.lrrd.org/lrrd22/3/more22055.htm

Moreki, J.C.; Mokokwe, J.; Keboneilwe, D. & Koloka O.A. (2010b). Evaluation of the Livestock Management and Infrastructure Development Support Scheme in seven districts of Botswana, Retrieved from http://www.lrrd.org/lrrd22/5/more22087.htm

Moreki, J.C.; Thutwa, M.; Koloka, O.; Ntesang, K. & Ipatleng, T. (2010c). Utilization of smallstock package of Livestock Management and Infrastructure Development Support Scheme, Botswana, Retrieved from http://www.lrrd.org/lrrd22/12/more22232.htm

Moreki, J.C.; Poroga, B. & Dikeme, R. (2011). Strengthening HIV/AIDS food security mitigation mechanisms through village poultry. Retrieved from http://www.lrrd.org/lrrd23/2/more22055.htm

Mrema, M. & Rannobe, S. (1996). Goat production in Botswana: Factors affecting production and marketing among small-scale farmers. In, Lebbie S H B and Kagwini E (Editors) Proceedings of the Third Biennial Conference of the African Small Ruminant Research Network UICC, Kampala, Uganda. 5-9 December 1994. Retrieved 12 February 2010, Retrieved from http://www.fao.org/wairdocs/ilri/x5473b/x5473b0v.htm

Mutenje, M.J.; Mapiye, C.; Mavunganidze, Z.; Mwale, M.; Muringai, V.; Katsinde, C.S. & Gavumende, I. (2008). Livestock as a buffer against HIV and AIDS income shocks in the rural households of Zimbabwe. Development Southern Africa 25. Abstract, Retrieved from http://www.informaworld.com/smpp/content~db=all~content=a790526994

Pica-Ciamarra, U & Otte, J. (2009). Poultry, food security and poverty alleviation in India: Looking beyond the farm-gate. Pro-poor Livestock Policy Initiative - A Living from Livestock Research Report. Retrieved from www.fao.org/ag/AGAInfo/.../en/pplpi/.../rep-0902_indiapoultry.pdf

Schrauzer, G.N. (2000). Anticarcinogenic effects of selenium. Cell Molecular Life Sciences 57: 1864-1873.

Simainga, S.; Banda, F. & Sakuya, N. & Moreki, J.C. (2010). Health management in village poultry in Kalabo and Mongu Districts in the Western Province of Zambia. Livestock Research for Rural Development 22(9), Retrieved from www.lrrd.org/lrrd22/9/sima22171.htm

Simainga, S.; Moreki, J.C.; Banda, F. & Sakuya, N. (2011). Socio-economic study of family poultry in Mongu and Kalabo Districts of Zambia. Livestock Research for Rural Development 23(02), Retrieved from http://www.lrrd.org/lrrd23/2/sima23031.htm

Rural Self-Help Development Agency. (2011). The study on socio-economic status of village chickens at Ha Molemane (Berea), Phamong (Mohales' Hoek), Tebang, Ha Notsi, and Ribaneng (Mafeteng) of Lesotho. Maseru, Lesotho. pp.111.

Sitholimela, I. (2000). The effect of land tenure system on goat production in Kwazulu-Natal. M. Inst. Agrar. (Animal Production) Thesis. University of Pretoria, Republic of South Africa.

Slater, R. & Wiggins, S. (2005). Responding to HIV/AIDS in agriculture and related activities. Natural Resource perspectives, Number 98, March 2005. www.odi.org.uk/resources/download/1237.pdf

Topouzis, D. (1999). The implications of HIV/AIDS for household food security in Africa. United Nations Commission for Africa, Food Security and Sustainable Development Division, October 1999. Retrieved from www.uneca.org/popia/gateways/Women_Back_doc_4.pdf

United Nations (2010). The Millennium Development Goals Report. The United Nations Department of Economics and Social Affairs (DESA) - June 2010. Retrieved from http://www.org/milleniumgoals/pdf/MDG%20Report%202010%20En%20r15%20-low%20res%2020100615%20-.pdf>

Winrock International (1992). Assessment of Animal Agriculture in Sub-Saharan Africa. Morrilton, Arkansas. Winrock International. 12. ISBN 0-933595-76-X. Retrieved from HIV/AIDS has severe short- as well as long-term impacts on food security.